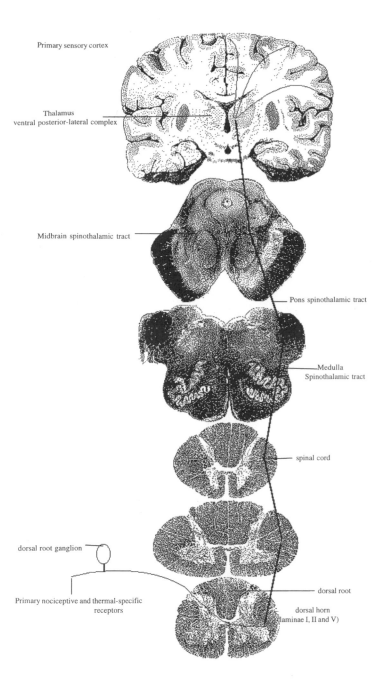

Primary sensory cortex

Thalamus
ventral posterior-lateral complex

Midbrain spinothalamic tract

Pons spinothalamic tract

Medulla
Spinothalamic tract

spinal cord

dorsal root ganglion

Primary nociceptive and thermal-specific
receptors

dorsal root

dorsal horn
(laminae I, II and V)

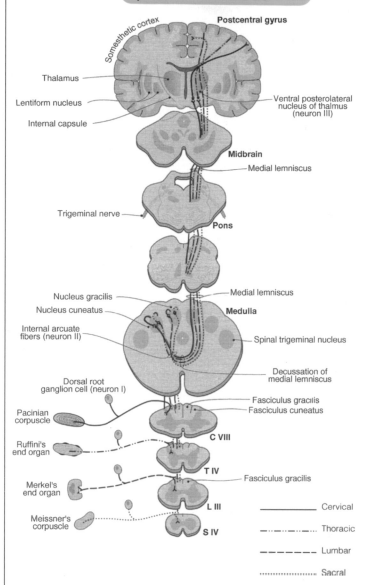

Somesthetic cortex

Postcentral gyrus

Thalamus

Lentiform nucleus

Internal capsule

Ventral posterolateral
nucleus of thalmus
(neuron III)

Midbrain

Medial lemniscus

Trigeminal nerve

Pons

Nucleus gracilis

Nucleus cuneatus

Internal arcuate
fibers (neuron II)

Medial lemniscus

Medulla

Spinal trigeminal nucleus

Decussation of
medial lemniscus

Dorsal root
ganglion cell (neuron I)

Pacinian
corpuscle

Ruffini's
end organ

Merkel's
end organ

Meissner's
corpuscle

Fasciculus gracilis
Fasciculus cuneatus

C VIII

T IV

L III

S IV

Fasciculus gracilis

————— Cervical

—·—·—·—·· Thoracic

— — — — Lumbar

················· Sacral

Pain and temperature pathway. Primary nociceptive
and thermospecific afferents with their cell body in the
dorsal root ganglia. These afferents send their central
projection to the superficial laminae of the dorsal horns
(laminae I to IV). Second-order neurons project mainly
into the contralateral spinothalamic tract ascending
through the lateral brainstem to the ventral posterior
lateral and to the anterior and intralaminar thalamic
nuclei. These third-order afferent neurons project into
the primary sensory cortex.

The formation and course of the posterior columns in
the spinal cord and the medial lemniscus in the
brainstem. The posterior columns are formed from
uncrossed ascending and descending branches of
spinal ganglion cells. Ascending fibers in the fasciculi
gracilis and cuneatus synapse on cells of the nucleus
gracilis and cuneatus. Fibers forming the medial
lemniscus arise from cells of the nuclei gracilis and
cuneatus, cross in the lower medulla, and ascend to the
thalamus. Impulses mediated by this pathway include
proprioceptive, vibratory, and discriminative touch.
Spinal ganglia and afferent fibers entering the spinal
cord at different levels are coded as in legend.
(Modified from Carpenter MB: Human Neuroanatomy.
Baltimore, MD. Williams & Wilkins, 1983.)

Saunders Manual of

Neurologic
Practice

Saunders Manual of
Neurologic Practice

Randolph W. Evans, MD
Chief of Neurology Section
Park Plaza Hospital
Clinical Associate Professor
Department of Neurology
University of Texas Medical School at Houston and
Department of Family and Community Medicine
Baylor College of Medicine
Houston, Texas

Saunders
An Imprint of Elsevier Science

SAUNDERS

An Imprint of Elsevier Science

The Curtis Center
Independence Square West
Philadelphia, Pennsylvania 19106

SAUNDERS MANUAL OF CRITICAL CARE   ISBN 0–7216–9761–5
Copyright © 2003 Elsevier Science (USA)

Notice

Neurology is an ever-changing field. Standard safety precautions must be followed, but as new research and clinical experience broaden our knowledge, changes in treatment and drug therapy may become necessary or appropriate. Readers are advised to check the product information currently provided by the manufacturer of each drug to be administered to verify the recommended dose, the method and duration of administration, and contraindications. It is the responsibility of the treating physician, relying on experience and knowledge of the patient, to determine dosages and the best treatment for each individual patients. Neither the Publisher nor the editors assume any liability for any injury and/or damage to persons or property arising from this publication.

THE PUBLISHER

Library of Congress Cataloging-in-Publication Data

Saunders manual of neurologic practice / [edited by] Randolph W. Evans.
       p. ; cm.
    ISBN 0–7216–9761–5
    1. Neurology—Handbooks, manuals, etc. I. Evans, Randolph W.
    [DNLM: 1. Nervous System Diseases. 2. Diagnostic Techniques, Neurological.   WL
140 S257 2003]
    RC343.4 .S386 2003
    616.8—dc21

                                                2002036647

GWI/CC

Printed in the United States of America

Last digit is the print number: 9 8 7 6 5 4 3 2 1

This book is dedicated with love to my wife, Marilyn,
our children, Elliott, Rochelle, and Jonathan, and to my parents,
Dr. Richard I. Evans and the late Zena A. Evans.

It is also dedicated with much appreciation to my teachers,
Professors Arnold Schwartz, K. Michael Welch,
and Stanley H. Appel.

Contributors

J. STEVEN ALEXANDER, Ph.D.
Associate Professor of Cellular and Molecular Physiology, Louisiana State University Health Sciences Center, Shreveport, Louisiana
Arnold-Chiari Malformation and Syringomyelia

MARIA E. ALEXIANU, M.D.
Chief Resident in Neurology, New York University School of Medicine; Chief Resident, Department of Neurology, New York University Medical Center, New York, New York
Muscle Cramps; Fasciculation

AHMAD AL-KHATIB, M.D.
Attending Neurologist, St. Rita's Medical Center, Lima, Ohio
Carpal Tunnel Syndrome and Other Median Neuropathies

EVAN ALLEN, M.D.
Director, The Sarasota Stroke Center, Healthsouth Rehabilitation Center of Sarasota, Sarasota, Florida
Organ Transplantation

AMER AL-SHEKHLEE, M.D.
Assistant Professor of Neurology, Case Western Reserve University School of Medicine; Attending Neurologist, University Hospitals Health System, Cleveland, Ohio
Other Upper Limb Mononeuropathies

TETSUO ASHIZAWA, M.D.
Professor and Chairman, Department of Neurology, University of Texas Medical Branch, Galveston, Texas
Molecular Genetic Testing

MISHA-MIROSLAV BACKONJA, M.D.
Associate Professor, University of Wisconsin; Attending Physician, University of Wisconsin Hospital and Clinics, Madison, Wisconsin
Neuropathic Pain

CHRISTOS BALLAS, M.D.
Instructor, Department of Psychiatry, University of Pennsylvania School of Medicine, Philadelphia, Pennsylvania
Auditory Hallucinations; Mood Disorders; Anxiety Disorders; Psychotic Disorders; Somatoform Disorders; Personality Disorders; Substance-Related Disorders; Attention Deficit Hyperactivity Disorders

GEORGE D. BAQUIS, M.D.
Director, Electromyography Laboratory, Baystate Medical Center, Springfield; Assistant Professor of Neurology, Tufts University Medical School, Boston, Massachusetts
Paresthesias; Sexual Dysfunction; Sphincter Dysfunction

RUSSELL BARTT, M.D.
Assistant Professor of Neurological Sciences, Rush Medical College, Rush University; Attending Physician, Cook County Hospital, Chicago, Illinois
Human Immunodeficiency Virus and Human T-lymphotropic Virus Type 1

DANIEL M. BLOOMFIELD, M.D.
Assistant Professor of Medicine, Columbia University College of Physicians and Surgeons; Assistant Attending, New York Presbyterian Hospital: Columbia Presbyterian Campus, New York, New York
Vasovagal Syncope

KAREN I. BOLLA, Ph.D.
Associate Professor of Neurology, Psychiatry and Behavioral Sciences, and Environmental Health Sciences, Department of Neurology, Johns Hopkins School of Medicine, Baltimore, Maryland
Metals, Organic Solvent, and Pesticide Intoxication

KANOKWAN BOONYAPISIT, M.D.
Attending Neurologist, Siriraj Hospital, Bangkok, Thailand
Clinical Electromyography

PAUL W. BRAZIS, M.D.
Professor of Neurology and Consultant in Neurology and Neuro-ophthalmology, Mayo Clinic—Jacksonville, Jacksonville, Florida
Approach to Visual Symptoms and Signs; Optic Neuritis; Optic Neuropathy; Pupillary Disorders; Ptosis, Lid Lag, and Lid Retraction; Ocular Motor Palsies; Nystagmus; Orbital Disorders; Papilledema and Pseudotumor Cerebri; Visual Illusions and Hallucinations

AMITABHA CHANDA, M.B.B.S., M.S., M.Ch.
Assistant Professor and Consultant Neurosurgeon, National Neurosciences Centre, Kolkata, India
Subdural and Epidural Hematomas

THOMAS C. CHELIMSKY, M.D.
Assistant Professor of Neurology, Case Western Reserve University; Director, Pain Center, and Autonomic Disorders, University Hospitals of Cleveland, Cleveland, Ohio
Reflex Sympathetic Dystrophy and Causalgia

STUART R. CHIPKIN, M.D.
Associate Professor of Medicine, Tufts University School of Medicine, Boston; Chief, Division of Endocrinology, Diabetes and Metabolism, Baystate Medical Center, Springfield, Massachusetts
Endocrine Disorders; Pituitary Tumors

ERIK A. COHEN, M.D.
Fellow in Endocrinology, Bayside Medical Center, Springfield, Massachusetts
Endocrine Disorders; Pituitary Tumors

HOWARD COLMAN, M.D., Ph.D.
Instructor, Department of Neuro-oncology, University of Texas M.D. Anderson Cancer Center, Houston, Texas
Meningiomas

EDWARD C. COVINGTON, M.D.
Director, Chronic Pain Rehabilitation, Cleveland Clinic Foundation, Cleveland, Ohio
Treatment of Chronic Neck and Back Pain

PATRICIA K. COYLE, M.D.
Professor of Neurology, School of Medicine, State University of New York at Stony Brook, Stony Brook, New York
Chronic Meningitis

JOSEP DALMAU, M.D., Ph.D.
Associate Professor of Neurology, Department of Neurology, University of Arkansas for Medical Sciences, Little Rock, Arkansas
Paraneoplastic Neurologic Syndromes

MICHAEL W. DEVEREAUX, M.D.
Professor of Neurology, Case Western Reserve University, University Hospitals of Cleveland, Cleveland; Vice President of Clinical Integration, University Hospitals Health System, Cleveland; Medical Director, University Hospitals Health System Richmond Heights Hospital, Richmond Heights, Ohio
Approach to Neck and Low Back Disorders

ACLAN DOGAN, M.D.
Resident, Department of Neurological Surgery, Oregon Health and Science University, Portland, Oregon
Spinal Cord Injury

EUGENE DULANEY, M.D.
Clinical Assistant Professor of Neurology, University of Vermont College of Medicine; Attending Neurologist, Fletcher-Allen Health Care, Burlington, Vermont
Radiculopathy and Cauda Equina Syndrome

KEVIN C. ESS, M.D., Ph.D.
Pediatric Epilepsy Fellow, and Director, Tuberculosis Sclerosis Clinic, Washington University; Pediatric Epilepsy Fellow, St. Louis Children's Hospital, St. Louis, Missouri
Neurofibromatoses; Tuberous Sclerosis Complex and Other Neurocutaneous Disorders

RANDOLPH W. EVANS, M.D.
Chief of Neurology Section, Park Plaza Hospital; Clinical Associate Professor, Department of Neurology, University of Texas Medical School at Houston and Department of Family and Community Medicine, Baylor College of Medicine, Houston, Texas
The Neurologic History and Examination; Headaches; Neurological Eponyms; Lumbar Puncture and Cerebrospinal Fluid Evaluation; Migraine; Tension-type, Chronic Daily Headache, and Drug-induced Headache; Cluster Headache; Brief Head and Facial Pains; First or Worst Headaches; Headaches During Childhood and Adolescence; Headaches in Women; Headaches in Patients Over the Age of 50; Other Headaches; Mild Head Injury and the Postconcussion Syndrome; Whiplash Injuries; Mountain Sickness; Decompression Sickness; Lightning and Electrical Injuries; Hyperventilation Syndrome

BRUCE J. FISCH, M.D.
Professor of Neurology and Director, Epilepsy Center of Excellence, Louisiana State University School of Medicine, New Orleans, Louisiana
Electroencephalography

MARC FISHER, M.D.
Professor of Neurology, University of Massachusetts Medical School; University of Massachusetts/Memorial Healthcare, Worcester, Massachusetts
Localization in Neurovascular Disease; Transient Ischemic Attacks; Acute Ischemic Stroke; Spontaneous Intracerebral Hemorrhage; Subarachnoid Hemorrhage and Saccular Aneurysm; Spinal Cord Stroke; Stroke in Younger Adults; Cerebral Venous Thrombosis; Stroke in Pregnancy and the Postpartum Period

HARALD GELDERBLOM, M.D.
Research Instructor of Neurosciences, University of Medicine and Dentistry of New Jersey—New Jersey Medical School, Newark, New Jersey
Spirochetal Infections (Neurosyphilis and Lyme Neuroborreliosis)

DAVID S. GELDMACHER, M.D.
Associate Professor, Department of Neurology, University of Virginia; Director, Memory Disorders Program, Department of Neurology, University of Virginia Health System, Charlottesville, Virginia
Memory and Praxis Complaints; Dementia Overview; Alzheimer's Disease

PIERRE GIGLIO, M.D.
Clinical Fellow, Department of Neuro-oncology, University of Texas M.D. Anderson Cancer Center, Houston, Texas
Embryonal and Pineal Region Tumors; Skull-Based and Sellar Region Tumors

KIMBERLY L. GOSLIN, M.D., Ph.D.
Clinical Assistant Professor of Neurology, Oregon Health Sciences University; Neurology Division, The Oregon Clinic, Portland, Oregon
Inflammatory Spondyloarthropathies; Systemic Lupus Erythematosus; Sjögren's Syndrome; Rheumatoid Arthritis; Progressive Systemic Sclerosis; Fibromyalgia; Behçet's Disease; Sarcoidosis; Temporal Arteritis and Polymyalgia Rheumatica; Neurologic Manifestations of the Vasculitides

JOHN E. GREENLEE, M.D.
Professor and Chair, University of Utah School of Medicine; Attending Neurologist, Veterans Affairs Medical Center, Salt Lake City, Utah
Brain and Spinal Abscess

MORRIS D. GROVES, M.D., J.D.
Assistant Professor, and Director of Inpatient Services, Department of Neuro-oncology, University of Texas M.D. Anderson Cancer Center, Houston, Texas
Epidemiology and Pathophysiology in Neuro-oncology; Clinical Presentations; Spinal Cord Tumors; Metastatic Brain Tumors; Meningeal and Spinal Metastases; Neurologic Complications of Chemotherapy and Radiotherapy

DAVID H. GUTMANN, M.D., Ph.D.
Professor, Donald O. Schnuck Family Professor, and Director, Neurofibromatosis Program, Washington University; Professor, St. Louis Children's Hospital, St. Louis, Missouri
Neurofibromatoses; Tuberous Sclerosis Complex and Other Neurocutaneous Disorders

SAMRINA HANIF, M.D.
Research Assistant, Department of Rehabilitation Medicine, New York University School of Medicine; Clinical Research Assistant, Tisch Hospital, New York University Medical Center, New York, New York
Amyotrophic Lateral Sclerosis

YADOLLAH HARATI, M.D., F.A.C.P.
Professor, Department of Neurology, and Director, Muscle and Nerve Pathology Laboratory, Baylor College of Medicine, Houston, Texas
Muscle and Nerve Biopsy; Guillain-Barré Syndrome; Other Acute Neuropathies; Diabetic Neuropathies; Chronic Inflammatory Demyelinating Polyradiculoneuropathy; Porphyrias; Genetically Determined Peripheral Neuropathies; Manifestations of Myopathies; Congenital Myopathies; Dermatomyositis and Polymyositis; Inclusion Body Myositis; Other Acquired Myopathies; Glycogen and Lipid Storage Myopathies

SIGMUND HSU, M.D.
Assistant Professor, Department of Neuro-oncology, University of Texas, M.D. Anderson Cancer Center, Houston, Texas
Glial Tumors

AJAY JAWAHAR, M.D.
Instructor, Gamma Knife, Department of Neurosurgery, Louisiana State University Health Sciences Center, Shreveport, Louisiana
Moderate and Severe Head Injury

BASHAR KATIRJI, M.D., F.A.C.P.
Professor of Neurology, Case Western Reserve University School of Medicine; Director, Neuromuscular Division, EMG Laboratory and Muscle Disease Center, University Hospitals of Cleveland, Cleveland, Ohio
Clinical Electromyography; Peripheral Nerve Injuries; Brachial Plexopathies; Neurogenic Thoracic Outlet Syndrome; Carpal Tunnel Syndrome and Other Median Neuropathies; Ulnar and Radial Neuropathies; Other Upper Limb Mononeuropathies; Peroneal, Sciatic and Tibial Neuropathies; Other Lower Limb Mononeuropathies; Mononeuropathies During Pregnancy and Labor

RICHARD P. KLUCZNIK, M.D.
Assistant Professor, Interventional Neuroradiology, The Methodist Hospital, Baylor College of Medicine, Houston, Texas
Magnetic Resonance Angiography and Cerebral Angiography

JENNIFER S. KRIEGLER, M.D.
Associate Professor of Neurology, Case Western Reserve University, Cleveland; Co-Director, American Migraine Center, Lyndhurst, Ohio
Myofascial Pain Syndrome and Sacroiliac Joint Dysfunction

DAVID S. KUSHNER, M.D.
Associate Professor of Neurology, University of Miami School of Medicine; Medical Director, Brain Injury Program, Healthsouth Rehabilitation Hospital, Miami, Florida
Neurorehabilitation; Neurorehabilitation of Brain Injuries

ANDREW G. LEE, M.D.
Associate Professor of Ophthalmology, Neurology, and Neurosurgery, University of Iowa Hospitals and Clinics, Iowa City, Iowa
Approach to Visual Symptoms and Signs; Optic Neuritis; Optic Neuropathy; Pupillary Disorders; Ptosis, Lid Lag, and Lid Retraction; Ocular Motor Palsies; Nystagmus; Orbital Disorders; Papilledema and Pseudotumor Cerebri; Visual Illusions and Hallucinations

JIN-MOO LEE, M.D., Ph.D.
Assistant Professor, Washington University School of Medicine; Attending Physician, Barnes-Jewish Hospital, St. Louis, Missouri
Organ Transplantation

KERRY H. LEVIN, M.D.
Clinical Associate Professor of Neurology, Pennsylvania State College of Medicine, Hershey, Pennsylvania; Staff Neurologist, Cleveland Clinic, Cleveland, Ohio
Diagnostic Testing for Neck and Back Disorders

JONATHAN N. LEVINE, M.D.
Assistant Professor, Baylor College of Medicine; Neuroradiologist, The Methodist Hospital, Houston, Texas
Magnetic Resonance Imaging: Basic Principles and Techniques; Computed Tomography: Basic Principles and Techniques

STEVEN LOVITT, M.D.
Assistant Professor of Medicine and Pathology, University of Texas Health Science Center; Faculty Physician, Audie Murphy Veterans Affairs Hospital; Co-Director, Muscular Dystrophy Association Clinic of South Texas, San Antonio, Texas
Muscle and Nerve Biopsy; Guillain-Barré Syndrome; Other Acute Neuropathies; Porphyrias; Manifestations of Myopathies; Congenital Myopathies

HAZEM MACHKHAS, M.D.
Assistant Professor, Department of Neurology, Baylor College of Medicine; Director, Outpatient Neurology Clinics Neuroly Care Line, Veterans Affairs Medical Center, Houston, Texas
Clinical Evaluation of Peripheral Neuropathies; Diabetic Neuropathies; Chronic Inflammatory Demyelinating Polyradiculoneuropathy; Genetically Determined Peripheral Neuropathies; Muscular Dystrophies; Dermatomyositis and Polymyositis; Inclusion Body Myositis; Other Acquired Myopathies; Glycogen and Lipid Storage Myopathies; Skeletal Muscle Channelopathies; Side Effects of Immunosuppressive Therapies

DANIEL W. MILLER, M.D.
EMG and Neuromuscular Fellow, University Hospitals of Cleveland, Cleveland, Ohio
Mononeuropathies During Pregnancy and Labor

ALIREZA MINAGAR, M.D.
Assistant Professor of Neurology, Department of Neurology, Louisiana State University Health Sciences Center, Shreveport, Louisiana
Parkinson's Disease; Progressive Supranuclear Palsy; Huntington's Disease; Dystonia; Tourette's Syndrome; Essential Tremor; Wilson's Disease; Multiple System Atrophy; Myoclonus; Multiple Sclerosis; Acute Disseminated Encephalomyelitis; Arnold-Chiari Malformation and Syringomyelia; Drug-Induced Movement Disorders

ANIL NANDA, M.D., F.A.C.S.
Professor and Chairman, Department of Neurosurgery, Louisiana State University Health Sciences Center in Shreveport School of Medicine, Shreveport, Louisiana
Moderate and Severe Head Injury; Subdural and Epidural Hematomas; Cranial Neuropathy; Spinal Cord Injury

WILLIAM G. ONDO, M.D.
Assistant Professor of Neurology, Department of Neurology, Baylor College of Medicine, Houston, Texas
Gait, Balance, and Falls; Transient Global Amnesia and Other Amnestic Disorders

ERDEM ORBERK, M.D.
Resident, Department of Neurology, University of Massachusetts Medical School; University of Massachusetts/Memorial Healthcare, Worcester, Massachusetts
Localization in Neurovascular Disease; Transient Ischemic Attacks; Acute Ischemic Stroke; Spontaneous Intracerebral Hemorrhage; Subarachnoid Hemorrhage and Saccular Aneurysm; Spinal Cord Stroke; Stroke in Younger Adults; Cerebral Venous Thrombosis; Stroke in Pregnancy and the Postpartum Period

ANDREW R. PACHNER, M.D.
Professor of Neurosciences, University of Medicine and Dentistry of New Jersey—New Jersey Medical School, Newark, New Jersey
Spirochetal Infections (Neurosyphilis and Lyme Neuroborreliosis)

RUSSELL C. PACKARD, M.D., F.A.C.P.
Professor of Neurology and Neuropsychiatry, and Director, Neuropsychiatry Residency, Texas Tech University School of Medicine, Lubbock, Texas
Fatigue; Vitamin Deficiency and Toxicity; Illicit Drugs

KATIE PLUNKETT, M.S.
Instructor, Department of Molecular and Human Genetics, Baylor College of Medicine, Houston, Texas
Molecular Genetic Testing

DAVID C. PRESTON, M.D.
Associate Professor of Neurology, Department of Neurology, Case Western Reserve University School of Medicine; Director, Neuromuscular Service, University Hospitals of Cleveland, Cleveland, Ohio
Spondylosis and Facet Syndrome

NATTE RAKSADAWAN, M.D.
Neuromuscular Fellow, New York University School of Medicine, and New York University Medical Center, New York, New York
Spinal Muscular Atrophy; Hereditary Spastic Paraplegia

MUHAMMAD RAMZAN, M.D.
Assistant Professor of Neurology, University of Massachusetts Medical School; University of Massachusetts/Memorial Healthcare, Worcester, Massachusetts
Localization in Neurovascular Disease; Transient Ischemic Attacks; Acute Ischemic Stroke; Spontaneous Intracerebral Hemorrhage; Subarachnoid Hemorrhage and Saccular Aneurysm; Spinal Cord Stroke; Stroke in Younger Adults; Cerebral Venous Thrombosis; Stroke in Pregnancy and the Postpartum Period

KAREN L. ROOS, M.D.
John and Nancy Nelson Professor of Neurology, Indiana University School of Medicine, Indianapolis, Indiana
Bacterial Meningitis; Encephalitis

RICHARD B. ROSENBAUM, M.D.
Clinical Professor of Neurology, Oregon Health and Sciences University; Neurology Division, The Oregon Clinic, Portland, Oregon
Inflammatory Spondyloarthropathies; Systemic Lupus Erythematosus; Sjögren's Syndrome; Rheumatoid Arthritis; Progressive Systemic Sclerosis; Fibromyalgia; Behçet's Disease; Sarcoidosis; Temporal Arteritis and Polymyalgia Rheumatica; Neurologic Manifestations of the Vasculitides

CARL E. ROSENBERG, M.D.
Adjunct Assistant Professor, Department of Neurology, Case Western Reserve University, Cleveland, Ohio
Sleep and Testing; Insomnia and Circadian Rhythm Disorders; Periodic Limb Movements and Restless Legs; Obstructive Sleep Apnea; Parasomnias; Narcolepsy and Hypersomnias

DAVID B. ROSENFIELD, M.D.
Professor, Department of Neurology, Director, Stuttering Center Speech Motor Control Laboratory, and Professor, Department of Otorhinolaryngology and Communicative Sciences, Baylor College of Medicine; Professor, The Methodist Hospital, Houston, Texas
Speech Disorders; Language Disorders

MICHAEL J. RUCKENSTEIN, M.D., M.Sc., F.A.C.S.
Associate Professor, Department of Otorhinolaryngology—Head and Neck Surgery, University of Pennsylvania; Hospital of the University of Pennsylvania, Philadelphia, Pennsylvania
Diagnostic Testing; Hearing Loss; Tinnitus; Vertigo

CONCEPCION E. SANTILLAN, M.D.
Assistant Professor, Department of Neurology, Case Western Reserve University School of Medicine; Neurologist, University Hospitals of Cleveland, Cleveland, Ohio
Spondylosis and Facet Syndrome

STEVEN C. SCHACHTER, M.D.
Associate Professor of Neurology, Harvard Medical School; Director of Research, Department of Neurology, Beth Israel Deaconess Medical Center, Boston, Massachusetts
Syncope vs Seizure; Etiology and Manifestations; Epilepsy Syndromes; Medical Treatment; Status Epilepticus; Surgical Treatment; Epilepsy and Pregnancy; Starting and Stopping Medications; Driving and Other Restrictions; Iatrogenic Seizures

MICHAEL E. SEIFF, M.D.
Private Practice, Nevada Neurosurgery, Las Vegas, Nevada
Hydrocephalus

OLA A. SELNES, Ph.D.
Associate Professor, Johns Hopkins University School of Medicine and Johns Hopkins Hospital, Baltimore, Maryland
Neuropsychological Testing

WILLIAM A. SHEREMATA, M.D.
Professor of Neurology and Director of Multiple Sclerosis Center, Department of Neurology, University of Miami, Miami, Florida
Multiple Sclerosis; Acute Disseminated Encephalomyelitis

LISA M. SHULMAN, M.D.
Associate Professor of Neurology, and Co-Director, Maryland Parkinson's Disease and Movement Disorders Center, University of Maryland School of Medicine, Baltimore, Maryland
Parkinson's Disease; Progressive Supranuclear Palsy; Huntington's Disease; Dystonia; Tourette's Syndrome; Essential Tremor; Wilson's Disease; Multiple System Atrophy; Myoclonus; Drug-Induced Movement Disorders

CATHY A. SILA, M.D.
Associate Medical Director, Cerebrovascular Center, Section of Stroke and Neurologic Intensive Care, Department of Neurology, Cleveland Clinic, Cleveland, Ohio
Vascular Surgery

BRIAN W. SMITH, M.D.
Assistant Professor of Neurology, Tufts University School of Medicine, Boston; Attending Neurologist, Baystate Medical Center, Springfield, Massachusetts
Endocrine Disorders; Venoms and Bacterial Toxins; Pituitary Tumors; Cognitive Side Effects of Medications

YUEN T. SO, M.D., Ph.D.
Associate Professor, Department of Neurology, Stanford University; Director, Neurology Clinic, Stanford University Medical Center, Stanford, California
Alcoholism

DAVID SOLOMON, M.D., Ph.D.
Assistant Professor of Neurology, University of Pennsylvania School of Medicine, Philadelphia, Pennsylvania
Dizziness; Benign Positional Vertigo; Bell's Palsy and Other VII Lesions; Disorders of Smell and Taste; Facial Numbness; Disorders of Cranial Nerves IX and X; Disorders of Cranial Nerves XI and XII and Multiple Cranial Neuropathies

JEFFREY P. STAAB, M.D., M.S.
Assistant Professor of Psychiatry, Departments of Psychiatry and Otorhinolaryngology – Head and Neck Surgery, University of Pennsylvania School of Medicine; Director of Adult Clinical Services, Department of Psychiatry, Hospital of the University of Pennsylvania, Philadelphia, Pennsylvania
Auditory Hallucinations; Mood Disorders; Anxiety Disorders; Psychotic Disorders; Somatoform Disorders; Personality Disorders; Substance-Related Disorders; Attention Deficit Hyperactivity Disorders

RON TINTNER, M.D.
Associate Professor, Department of Neurology, Baylor College of Medicine, Houston, Texas
Vascular Dementia; Subcortical Dementia

IVO W. TREMONT-LUKATS, M.D.
Clinical Fellow, Department of Neurology, University of Texas M.D. Anderson Cancer Center, Houston, Texas
Other Tumors

SUDHAKAR TUMMALA, M.D.
Fellow, University of Texas Medical School at Houston, and Memorial Hermann Hospital, Houston, Texas
Clinical Presentations; Neurologic Complications of Chemotherapy and Radiotherapy

PRASAD VANNEMREDDY, M.D.
Assistant Professor of Research, Department of Neurology, Louisiana State University Health Sciences Center, Shreveport, Louisiana and Professor of Neurosurgery, Nizam's Institute of Medical Sciences, Hyderabad, India
Cranial Neuropathy

LOUIS H. WEIMER, M.D.
Associate Clinical Professor of Neurology, Columbia University College of Physicians and Surgeons, New York, New York
Autonomic Testing; Postural Hypotension

WILLIAM J. WEINER, M.D.
Professor and Chairman, Neurology, and Director, Maryland Parkinson's Disease and Movement Disorders Center, University of Maryland School of Medicine, Baltimore, Maryland
Parkinson's Disease; Progressive Supranuclear Palsy; Huntington's Disease; Dystonia; Tourette's Syndrome; Essential Tremor; Wilson's Disease; Multiple System Atrophy; Myoclonus; Drug-Induced Movement Disorders

MICHAEL I. WEINTRAUB, M.D., F.A.C.P., F.A.A.N.
Clinical Professor of Neurology and Medicine, New York Medical College, Valhalla; Adjunct Clinical Professor of Neurology, Mount Sinai School of Medicine, New York; Formerly Chief of Neurology, Phelps Memorial Hospital, Sleepy Hollow, New York
Medical-Legal Issues and Neurology

G. BRYAN YOUNG, M.D., F.R.C.P.C.
Professor of Neurology, Departments of Medicine and Critical Care, University of Toronto; Director of EEG Laboratory and Consultant in Neurology, Sunnybrook and Women's College Health Sciences Center, Toronto, Ontario, Canada
Encephalopathies, Coma, Herniation, and Brain Death; Hypoventilation, Hypoxia, and Carbon Monoxide Poisoning; Liver and Kidney Failure; Electrolyte and Glucose Abnormalities; Hypothermia and Hyperthermia

DAVID S. YOUNGER, M.D.
Clinical Associate Professor of Neurology, New York University School of Medicine; Director, Neuromuscular Diseases, and Jerry Lewis Muscular Dystrophy Association (MDA) Clinic, New York University Medical Center, New York, New York
Muscle Weakness; Myasthenia Gravis and Myasthenic Syndromes; Amyotrophic Lateral Sclerosis; Spinal Muscular Atrophy; Hereditary Spastic Paraplegia; Muscle Cramps; Fasciculation

JOSEPH R. ZUNT, M.D., M.P.H.
Assistant Professor, University of Washington Harborview Medical Center, Seattle, Washington
Creutzfeldt-Jakob Disease; Cerebral Malaria; Neurocysticercosis

Preface

Saunders Manual of Neurologic Practice is designed to help busy physicians evaluate and manage neurologic disorders. Information is presented in a standardized outline format with key points color highlighted and boxed for easy reference. Each chapter includes about five recent or classic references. This comprehensive although not encyclopedic volume covers most of the common and uncommon disorders (with an emphasis on common disorders) seen by neurologists as well as primary care physicians and other specialists who care for patients with neurologic disorders. This **Manual** follows others in this very successful series including **Medical Practice, Pediatrics, and Critical Care.**

There are 25 parts and 205 chapters. The first part, "Approach to Symptoms and Signs," explores the neurologic exam, common symptoms and signs, and the persons behind common eponyms (including Thomas Willis who coined the word "neurology" in 1664). The second part, "Diagnostic Testing," examines the basic principles and techniques, indications, contraindications, normal and abnormal findings, and complications of testing. The first two parts provide an introduction to neurology for the medical student, resident, and non-neurologist. The next 22 parts cover specific neurologic disorders. The final part reviews common psychiatric disorders. The figures in the front and back endsheets provide a brief summary of essential neuroanatomy. I hope this book fills the need for a quick and authoritative reference source in the office or hospital with practical information for the neurologist, non-neurologist, student, and resident to better serve our patients with neurologic disorders.

I thank our 87 outstanding contributors for their excellent chapters. I appreciate the encouragement, advice, and hard work of our acquisition editors, Allan Ross and Susan Pioli, the developmental editor, David Orzechowski, and the director of production, Berta Steiner.

Randolph W. Evans, MD
Houston, Texas
October, 2002

Contents

Detailed table of contents begins on following right hand page

Contents

Part IV
Dementia and Amnestic Disorders

Part V
Movement Disorders

Part VI
Multiple Sclerosis and Other Demyelinating Diseases

Part VII
Epilepsy

1 The Neurologic History and Examination

Randolph W. Evans

Introduction

1. The neurologic history and examination are the cornerstone of clinical neurology.
2. The information obtained is the basis for formulating the differential diagnosis and the clinicoanatomic approach. Where is the lesion (cortical, subcortical, brainstem, cerebellum, spinal cord, nerve root, peripheral nerve, neuromuscular junctions, muscle)? What is the pathology? Is diagnostic testing indicated to answer the questions?
3. An incomplete history or examination can easily result in misdiagnosis, inappropriate diagnostic tests, or the wrong treatment. Contrary to the opinion of some nonneurologists, a magnetic resonance imaging (MRI) scan is not a substitute for the history and physical examination.
4. The specifics of a neurologic history and physical examination vary from patient from patient.
   a. An otherwise healthy 20-year-old with back pain does not require formal mental status testing.
   b. Family history is unlikely to be relevant in a 90-year-old with a stroke.
   c. A screening neurologic examination is performed on everyone. A more detailed, focused examination may be performed depending on the history and any abnormal examination findings.
5. As the physician's knowledge of neurologic disorders expands, he or she becomes more efficient, spending less time by becoming more selective in the use of diagnostic testing.
6. This chapter reviews the essentials of the history and examination. Other chapters in this section and throughout the book expand on the topics as specific disorders are discussed.

Neurologic History

1. Overview
   a. The history is incredibly important. Many diseases are diagnosed from the history alone. As you go through the history, you can also perform a verbal physical examination. As you begin, you may already have an idea of what you are going to find, and you can see if you were right.
      (1) Mental status is assessed with the history, including speech and language, vocabulary, memory, affect, personality, and other factors.
      (2) Proximal muscle strength can be assessed by asking if patients have trouble brushing their hair or getting up from a chair.
      (3) In cases of diplopia, is the separation of images increased in a particular direction of gaze?
   b. Osler said, "Listen to the patient. He is telling you the diagnosis." I concur. But if you listen to the patient passively (especially a circumferential historian), you may spend all day and not get any closer to the diagnosis. Effective history-taking is an active process.
      (1) Give the patient a few minutes to discuss the reason for the encounter.
      (2) Persistently try to get answers to relevant questions (while being polite and respectful) and then listen closely to the patient's responses. Use both open and close-ended questions.
      (3) Actively generate hypotheses about the problem from the beginning to the end of the clinical encounter and then sequentially try to prove or disprove them.
      (4) You may need to obtain more history during the examination, after discussions with the patient, after the visit, or as diagnostic test results are available.
      (5) In many cases you may wish to ask patients what they think is wrong with them.
         (a) In some cases they are accurate, but in many others they are not even close.
         (b) They may be extremely worried inappropriately, so it is often helpful to explain why their diagnosis is incorrect. Examples include the patient with essential tremor who thinks he has Parkinson's or the patient with migraines who believes that he has a brain tumor or aneurysm.

(c) Patients often research their symptoms on the Internet before they see the physician. For some reason, many neurologic patients incorrectly conclude that they have multiple sclerosis or amyotrophic lateral sclerosis (ALS).

PEARLS

- "Listen to the patient. He is telling you the diagnosis."

- Effectively taking the patient's history is an active process.

  —Give the patient a few minutes to discuss the reason for the visit.

  —Be persistent in getting answers to relevant questions and listen closely to the responses.

  —Actively generate hypotheses about the problem—which must be sequentially proved or disproved—from the beginning to the end of the examination.

  —Ask patients what they think is wrong.

---

c. Assess whether the patient is a reliable historian.
   (1) Additional information may be required from family members, coworkers, friends, or observers (e.g., if a patient has a seizure) and may be essential if the patient has altered mental status.
   (2) In some cases, reviewing the medical records is essential. Unfortunately, patients often do not bring their records or the referring physician does not provide them. In nonurgent cases, you may have to obtain the records before providing recommendations.
   (3) Do not accept second-hand information as clinically pertinent without confirming the information or test results yourself.

d. Do not neglect your relationship with the patient.
   (1) You may be brilliant and invariably make accurate diagnoses and recommend appropriate evaluations or treatment, but if patients get the idea that you do not care or are not friendly, or if you do not clearly explain things, they may be dissatisfied and seek another doctor or be more likely to sue you (see Appendix).
   (2) Remember the importance of nonverbal communication (e.g., smiling, making eye contact, or giving a pat on the shoulder) and verbal empathy during the encounter.

e. In some cases, you may wish to repeat the history to ensure that the patient has nothing to add or change.

2. The chief complaint
   a. Starting point: Why is the patient there?
   b. Sometimes they do not know, with the reason for the encounter being a problem noted by family members, friends, or the referring physician.

3. History of present illness: identifying information
   a. Age and gender: Diseases and susceptibility vary with age and gender.
   b. Traditionally, neurologic reports have identified handedness.
      (1) This is important only in selected cases. About 96% of those who are right-handed and 70% of those who are left-handed have a dominant left hemisphere.
      (2) Although the obvious circumstance for asking about handedness is hemispheric dysfunction, handedness may also be important in cases of entrapment neuropathy or radiculopathy.
   c. A description of ethnicity has been traditionally included, although this is an anachronism.
      (1) There are a few genetic neurologic diseases where ethnicity is a factor (e.g., sickle cell disease, Tay-Sachs disease).
      (2) Such a description is becoming more challenging in our melting pot country where persons from different groups have children. Ethnic labels are often medically useless because of the diverse origin of those to whom a label is given. However, where a person has lived or their culture may certainly be relevant for various acquired diseases.
   d. Include specifics about symptom onset (acute, subacute, chronic, insidious), duration, course (progressive, relapsing or remitting, static), and associated symptoms and signs.
   e. Include specifics about pain, including location, radiation, quality, severity, frequency, precipitating, and relieving factors.
   f. Obtain a list of the prior health care providers seen, diagnostic tests, and treatments.

4. Past medical history
   a. Obtain a history of past medical illnesses, operations, allergies, medications, and review of systems. Other disorders and treatments may cause or affect neurologic disorders or alter recommendations for treatment.

b. A social history is important as well, including habits, education, occupation, and travel history.

c. The family history is of course essential when you are evaluating one of the many genetically determined neurologic diseases. However, the patient may have incorrect or incomplete information. Examination and testing of relatives is necessary in some cases.

The Neurologic Examination

1. "Neuro grossly intact" typically means that a formal examination was not performed, and such a notation may not be helpful to subsequent physicians.

   a. Record your actual examination or state that no neurologic deficits were noted during the interview and observation of the patient. Even better, perform a screening examination.

2. A screening examination is usually adequate unless the history or examination suggests abnormalities requiring a more extensive work-up. It can be performed in just a few minutes.

3. Mental status: evaluate during the interview.

   a. Other chapters in this section review the elements of a detailed evaluation.

   b. Gradations of consciousness (the set of neural processes that allow a person to perceive, comprehend, and act on the internal and external environments)

      (1) Arousal: the degree to which the persons appears to be able to interact with the environment

      (2) Awareness: reflects the depth and content of the aroused state

      (3) Alert: requires intact cognitive functions of both cerebral hemispheres (provide awareness) and preservation of arousal mechanisms of the reticular activating system

      (4) Delirium: transient, usually reversible, cerebral dysfunction with a decreased attention span and a waxing and waning type of confusion. Disorientation, illusions, and hallucinations may be present.

      (5) Lethargic: less alert than usual but can be easily aroused

      (6) Stupor: decreased alertness but can be stimulated with effort into responding

      (7) Obtundation: appears to be asleep much of the time when not stimulated

      (8) Coma: eyes closed, no attempt to avoid noxious stimuli; unarousable and unconscious

      (9) Vegetative state: arousal without awareness

      (10) Locked-in state

         (a) Conscious of their environment but cannot move any extremities, cannot talk, or do not have horizontal eye movements (de-efferented state).

         (b) The only communication may be through vertical eye movements and blinking.

         (c) The lesion is in the brainstem and involves the motor pathway, the efferent abducent nerve fibers, and the corticobulbar fibers.

         (d) It can be due to a pontine infarct or hemorrhage and central pontine myelinolysis.

      (11) Rather than using jargon that may be interpreted differently by different physicians, describe the patient's specific level of consciousness and the response to stimuli (verbal, visual, painful).

   c. Table 1–1 provides the Mini-Mental State Examination, which is an extremely useful screening test.

4. Cranial nerves

   a. I (olfactory): not routinely tested

      (1) May wish to check in cases of head injury or with specific smell complaints

      (2) Use nonvolatile substance such as coffee. Volatile substances can stimulate trigeminal afferents in the nose.

   b. II (optic): may include visual acuity of each eye, visual fields, and funduscopy

   c. III (oculomotor), IV (trochlear), VI (abducens): lateral and vertical eye movement, and pupillary light response

      (1) Rules for evaluating diplopia

         (a) The distance between the true and false image increases with gaze in the direction of action of the paretic muscle (e.g., with a right sixth nerve palsy, the distance increases with horizontal gaze to the right).

         (b) Horizontal diplopia occurs with lesions of the medial or lateral rectus muscle. Vertical diplopia occurs with a superior or inferior rectus or oblique muscle lesion.

         (c) The most peripherally seen image is the false image. It comes from the eye with the paretic muscle.

TABLE 1–1. MINI-MENTAL STATE EXAMINATION (MMSE)

MAXIMUM SCORE	SCORE	CRITERIA
		Orientation
5	( )	What is the (year) (season) (date) (day) (month)
5	( )	Where are we? (state) (country) (town or city) (hospital or building) (floor)
		Registration
3	( )	Ask the patient if you may test his/her memory. Then say the names of three unrelated objects, clearly and slowly, about 1 second for each (e.g., apple, table, penny). After you have said all three, ask the patient to repeat them. This first repetition determines the score (0 to 3), but keep saying them until he/she can repeat all three (up to six trials).
		Attention and Calculation
5	( )	Ask the patient to begin with 100 and count backward by 7. Stop after five subtractions (93, 86, 79, 72, 65). Score the total number of correct answers. If the patient cannot or will not perform the serial 7s task, ask him/her to spell the word "World" backward. The score is the number of letters in the correct order (e.g., DLROW = 5; DLRW = 4; DLORW, DLW = 3; OW = 2; DRLWO = 1).
		Recall
3	( )	Ask the patient to recall the three items repeated above (e.g., apple, table, penny).
		Language
2	( )	*Naming:* Show the patient a wristwatch and ask him/her what it is. Repeat for a pen.
1	( )	*Repetition:* Ask the patient to repeat the phrase, "No ifs, ands, or buts," after you.
3	( )	*Three-Stage Command:* Give the patient a piece of blank paper and ask him/her to take a piece of paper in the right hand, fold it in half, put it on the floor." Score 1 point for each part correctly executed.
1	( )	*Reading:* Ask the patient to read the following sentence and do what it says. Score 1 point only if the patient actually closes his/her eyes.

Close Your Eyes

1	( )	*Writing:* Give the patient a blank piece of paper and ask him/her to write a sentence spontaneously. It must contain a subject and verb and be sensible. Correct grammar and punctuation are not necessary.
1	( )	*Copying:* Ask the patient to copy the figure of intersecting pentagons exactly as it is. All ten angles must be present and two must intersect to form a four-sided figure to score 1 point. Tremor and rotation are ignored.

Maximum Total Score 30	Total Score ( )	MMSE score of less than 24 of a possible 30 has a diagnostic sensitivity of 80% to 90% and a specificity of 80% for impaired cognitive performance. The MMSE is sensitive to the effects of age and education.

Adapted from Folstein MF, Folstein SE, McHugh PR: "Mini-Mental State": a practical method for grading the cognitive state of patients for the clinician. J Psychiatr Res 12:189–198, 1975.

(2) The swinging flashlight test (to check for a Marcus Gunn pupil or relative afferent pupillary defect)

    (a) The patient fixates on an object in the distance in a darkened room. Shining the light on one pupil and then quickly on the other elicits equal pupillary constriction followed by escape to an intermediate pupil size.

    (b) Immediate dilation of the pupil or no initial change in pupil size followed by dilation of the pupils is abnormal and consistent with a relative afferent pupillary defect due to disease of the retina, optic nerve, optic chiasm, or optic tract and amblyopia.

  d. V (trigeminal): light touch and pinprick sensation of the face.

    (1) Also supplies muscles of mastication. Attempted jaw opening results in deviation of the jaw to the paretic side.

  e. VII (facial): smile, close eyes

  f. VIII (vestibulocochlear): Whisper, have the patient listen to a ticking watch, or lightly rub your fingers together. Test each ear

    (1) Weber test: Vibrating 256 Hz tuning fork is placed on the middle of the head.

Lateralization occurs on the same side as the middle ear involvement and the opposite side of the cochlear disease.

(2) The Rinne test: Vibrating tuning fork is placed against the mastoid. When it is no longer heard, it is held in front of the ear. The tuning fork should be heard longer with air than bone conduction unless there is disease of the middle ear or blocking of the external auditory canal.

(3) Vestibular testing includes the Dix-Hallpike maneuver and caloric testing discussed in Section IX.

g. IX (glossopharyngeal), X (vagus): elevation of soft palate in midline when saying "aah"; gag reflex

h. XI (spinal accessory): Shrug the shoulder and turn the head against resistance.

i. XII (hypoglossal): Stick out the tongue and move it from side to side. The tongue deviates to the weak side.

5. Motor examination

a. Tone (resistance to passive movement): abnormalities

(1) Spasticity due to corticospinal tract lesions. The flexors of the arms and the extensors and adductors of the leg have a greater increase in tone—hence the hemiplegic posture and gait. Clasp-knife phenomenon (resistance to rapid passive movement with sudden giving way near the completion of joint flexion or extension) may be present due to heightened stretch reflexes.

(2) Rigidity due to extrapyramidal lesions that may result in cogwheeling (catches and releases) or lead-pipe (uniform) resistance

(3) Gegenhalten phenomenon (paratonia): pseudovoluntary resistance by the patient against any passive movement of the limb. Each attempt by the examiner to move the limb is met with an equal opposing force, which gives rise to the appearance of increased tone. Gegenhalten is usually associated with diffuse cerebral disease and dementia.

(4) Hypotonia due to cerebellar dysfunction, a lower motor neuron lesion, or an acute upper motor neuron lesion

b. Inspect muscle. Check for atrophy, hypertrophy, fasciculations.

c. Strength. Most often used is the Medical Research Council 0-5/5 scale (see Part I, Table 7–2).

(1) When testing, give the patient the mechanical advantage (the muscle should be partially contracted).

(2) Decreased rapid alternating movements of hands and feet and pronator drift (pronation and downward drift of the outstretched supinated arm) with normal strength testing can be subtle signs of corticospinal tract disease.

(3) Look for a pattern of weakness such as hemiparesis (Table 1–2), paraparesis (Table 1–3), symmetrical proximal paresis (typical for myopathy although there are exceptions), and symmetrical distal paresis (e.g., due to polyneuropathy).

d. Observe for the presence for involuntary movements, such as tremor, dystonia, and chorea.

6. Coordination testing with finger–nose–finger and heel-to-shin

a. Other tests for cerebellar function include

TABLE 1–2. PATTERNS OF WEAKNESS THAT AID IN LOCALIZATION

Distribution of Weakness: UMN or LMN Signs	Location of Lesion
Limbs and lower face on same side (spastic hemiparesis, UMN)	Contralateral cerebral hemisphere
All four limbs (spastic tetraparesis, UMN), speech (spastic dysarthria), swallowing with hyperactive jaw and facial jerks (pseudobulbar palsy, UMN)	Bilateral cerebral hemispheres
Hemiparesis (UMN) plus cranial nerve signs (LMN)	Brain stem
Tetraparesis (UMN) plus cranial nerve signs (LMN)	Brain stem
All four limbs (spastic tetraparesis, UMN)	Mid or upper cervical cord
Lower limbs (UMN) and hands (LMN)	Low cervical cord
Lower limbs (spastic paraparesis, UMN)	Thoracic spinal cord
	Bilateral, medial motor cortex
All limbs: proximal > distal (LMN)	Muscle (myopathy or dystrophy)
Legs: distal > proximal (LMN)	Nerve (polyneuropathy)
Ocular muscles, eyelids, jaw, face, pharynx, tongue (LMN)	Neuromuscular junction (NMJ)
Jaw, face, pharynx, tongue; sparing ocular muscles, eyelids (UMN and LMN)	Motor neuron disease
Specific muscle groups in one limb (LMN)	Nerve root, plexus, or peripheral nerve

Abbreviations: LMN, lower motor neuron; UMN, upper motor neuron.
From Hammerstad JP: Strength and reflexes. In Goetz CG, Pappert EJ (eds), Textbook of Clinical Neurology. Philadelphia, W.B. Saunders, 1998, p. 245.

TABLE 1–3. ANATOMIC LOCALIZATION OF PARAPARESIS

LOCATION OF LESION	PATTERN OF WEAKNESS, REFLEXES, AND ASSOCIATED SIGNS
Bilateral medial hemispheres (leg area motor cortex)	Spastic paraparesis with no sensory level
Thoracic	Paraparesis with hyperreflexia of legs, normal reflexes in arms; thoracic sensory level
Lumbar	Paraparesis, loss of reflexes, double incontinence with flaccid bladder and sphincters

From Hammerstad JP: Strength and reflexes. In Goetz CG, Pappert EJ (eds), Textbook of Clinical Neurology. Philadelphia, W.B. Saunders, 1998, p. 256.

rebound, check reflex, and arrhythmic rapid alternating movements.

7. Deep tendon reflexes
   a. Grading
      (1) 0: absent
      (2) 1+: decreased
      (3) 2+: normal
      (4) 3+: increased
      (5) 4+: increased with clonus (note how many beats, sustained or not)
   b. If you can count, you can remember the roots for each reflex. Additional roots are in parentheses. S1,2 (ankle), L(2)3,4 (knee), C5,6 (biceps and brachioradialis), C(6)7,8 (triceps).
   c. If a reflex is absent or depressed, try reinforcement (Jendrassik maneuver), which can be done by isometrically flexing the fingers of the hands, making a fist with one or both hands, or mentally focusing on the extremity being tested.
8. Plantar response (Babinski)
   a. Stimulating the skin on the lateral edge of the sole of the foot, starting at the heel, advancing to the ball of the foot, and then continuing medially to the base of the great toe normally results in flexion of the toes.
   b. An abnormal response is extension of the great toe with or without fanning of the other toes and withdrawal of the leg. Look for the first movement of the great toe. Do not mistake withdrawal for an abnormal finding. An extensor response is normal during the first year of life but later is due to pathology of the corticospinal tract.
9. Primitive reflexes: Glabellar, snout, grasp, suck, root, and palmomental reflexes may be present due to bilateral frontal lobe disease (also callled "frontal release reflexes").

10. Sensory examination
    a. Light touch (mediated by spinothalamic tract and dorsal columns) can be used for general screening.
    b. Pinprick and cold sensation (e.g., from a tuning fork) are mediated by the spinothalamic tract and vibration sense (128 Hz tuning fork). Proprioception is mediated by the dorsal columns.
       (1) Some patients become upset when they see you pull out a sharp safety pin (a new one for each patient). Try cold sensation. If results are inconsistent, compare pinprick to cold sensation.
       (2) Compare the least vibration the patient can detect versus your own ability to continue to feel the vibration.
       (3) Proprioception is tested by holding the distal portion of the toe or finger by its sides. The patient should be able to detect 1 degree of movement of a finger and 2 to 3 degrees of movement of a toe.
    c. Romberg test
       (1) Test of proprioception
       (2) Performed by asking the patient to stand, feet together with eyes open and then with eyes closed. Patients with significant proprioceptive loss can stand still with their eyes open because vision compensates for the loss of position sense, but they sway or fall with their eyes closed because they are unable to keep their balance.
    d. When primary sensory modalities are intact, contralateral parietal lobe sensory integration function can be assessed.
       (1) Graphesthesia (identifying numbers written on the palm using a dull pointed object)
       (2) Stereognosis (identifying common objects such as a quarter or dime when placed in the palm and then felt with the fingers).
       (3) Double simultaneous stimulation (touching homologous parts of the body on one side, the other side, or both sides at once with the patient identifying which side or if both sides are touched while their eyes are closed). Extinction of one side is the abnormal finding.
    e. Look for patterns seen with disorders of different levels of the neuraxis.
       (1) Neuropathy. Compare proximal to distal sensation.
       (2) Dermatomal and single peripheral nerves.

(See figures inside the back cover of this book.)

    (3) Compare left to right sides.

    (4) Check for a sensory level over the trunk. (Remember that a sensory level indicates the lowest level of compromise, but the lesion can be higher in the thoracic or cervical spinal cord.)

11. Gait: Assess while watching the patient walk in or out of the examination room.

    a. Tandem to assess balance

    b. Walking on heels and toes to assess balance as well as L5 roots (walking on heels) and S1 roots (walking on toes) in patients with low back pain

    c. Squatting or getting up from a chair to assess proximal lower extremity strength

Key Elements: Screening Neurologic Examination

- Mental status: evaluate during the interview
- Cranial nerves
  - —II: gross visual acuity of each eye, funduscopy, confrontation visual fields
  - —III, IV, VI: horizontal and vertical eye movements, response of pupils to light
  - —V: pinprick and touch sensation of the face
  - —VII: smile, close eyes
  - —VIII: ticking watch, rubbing fingers together, or whispering in each ear
  - —IX, X: palate elevates in midline; gag reflex
  - —XI: turning the head against resistance to each side; shrugging the shoulders
  - —XII: sticking out the tongue, moving it from side to side
- Motor
  - —Tone, bulk, and strength
  - —Check proximal and distal muscles
- Cerebellar
  - —Finger–nose–finger, heel-to-shin
- Reflexes
  - —Deep tendon reflexes (mnemonic: 1,2 . . . 3, 4 . . . 5,6 . . . 5,6 . . . 7,8)
  - —Plantar response

- Sensory
  - —Pinprick or cold sensation and light touch
  - —Proprioception, vibratory sense
- Gait

Coma Examination

See also Part I, Chapter 14, Encephalopathies, Coma, Herniation, and Brain Death.

1. The Glasgow Coma Scale (see Section XIII, Chapter 2, Moderate and Severe Head Injury) is often used to follow traumatic and nontraumatic cases.

2. Abnormal respiratory patterns

    a. Cheyne-Stokes (periodic)

        (1) Escalating hyperventilation followed by decremental hypoventilation and finally apnea with recurring cycle lengths of 40 to 100 seconds

        (2) Due to bilateral hemispheric dysfunction, structural lesions, and metabolic encephalopathy

    b. Posthyperventilation apnea

        (1) Apnea for more than 12 seconds following five deep breaths

        (2) Indicator of depressed central nervous system (CNS) function

    c. Central neurogenic hyperventilation

        (1) Continuous deep breathing with 40 to 70 respirations per minute

        (2) Due to bilateral hemispheric, lower midbrain, or upper pons dysfunction

    d. Apneustic respiration

        (1) Prominent prolonged end-inspiratory pauses

        (2) Lesion in the lower half of the pons

    e. Cluster or Biot's breathing

        (1) Variably irregular rate and amplitude

        (2) Lesion in the lower pons or upper medulla

    f. Ataxic

        (1) Infrequent, irregular breaths

        (2) Lesions in lower pons or upper medulla

    g. Apnea

        (1) No respiration

        (2) Lesion possibly in the medulla down to C4, peripheral nerve, neuromuscular junction, or muscle

3. Pupils

    a. Lesions below the pons and above the thalamus usually do not cause pupillary abnormalities (except for Horner's syndrome associated with medullary or cervical spinal cord lesions).

b. Metabolic and diencephalic lesions: small reactive pupils

c. Tectal lesions: pupils large and fixed and may display hippus

d. Third nerve (uncal) lesion: pupils large and fixed

e. Pontine lesions or opioid overdose: pinpoint pupils

f. Midbrain lesion: pupils at midposition and fixed

4. Eye movements

a. Observation of the resting position of the eyes

(1) Horizontal conjugate gaze deviation may be due to an ipsilateral hemispheric lesion, contralateral pontine lesion, or contralateral hemispheric epileptic focus.

(2) Deviation of the visual axes can be due to skew, a decompensated phoria, paralysis of one or more of the ocular motor nerves, or restrictive ophthalmopathy (e.g., blowout orbital fracture).

(3) Skew deviation (vertical misalignment of the eyes) can be due to a brainstem lesion.

(4) Eyes deviated downward suggest a dorsal midbrain or thalamic lesion but can also be seen with subarachnoid hemorrhage or hypoxic encephalopathy.

(5) Tonic upgaze may be due to diffuse injury to the cortex and cerebellum during anoxia.

b. Observation of spontaneous eye movements

(1) Roving (slow conjugate or disconjugate) eye movements are usually seen with metabolic encephalopathies or bilateral lesions above the brainstem.

(2) Ocular bobbing consists of a rapid downward movement of both eyes, followed by slower return to the primary position. May be present with pontine lesions or metabolic encephalopathy.

(3) Inverse ocular bobbing or ocular dipping, which consists of a slow downward movement followed by a rapid return to midposition, is often associated with diffuse cerebral damage.

(4) Slow, horizontal, conjugate deviations of the eyes that alternate every few seconds ("ping-pong" gaze) is due to an intact pons disconnected from bilateral hemispheres.

(5) Periodic alternating gaze deviation (horizontal conjugate deviation of the eyes with alternation every 2 minutes) can be present with hepatic encephalopathy.

c. Reflex eye movement

(1) Oculocephalic reflex ("doll's eyes")

(a) When the head is rotated laterally in a patient with intact brainstem function, the eyes should move in a direction opposite to the movement of the head.

(b) It tests the function of pathways that start at the pontomedullary junction (eighth nerve and nucleus), synapse in the contralateral caudal pons (paramedian pontine reticular formation and sixth nerve and nucleus), ascend through the medial longitudinal fasciculus, and synapse in the ipsilateral midbrain (third nerve and nucleus).

(c) Absence of the response suggests brainstem dysfunction, which should be confirmed with caloric testing.

(d) In cases of trauma, do not check until the stability of the neck has been verified by radiographs.

(2) Caloric testing

(a) If the oculocephalic reflex is absent, ice water caloric testing is a stronger stimulus.

(b) Check to see that the tympanic membranes are intact.

(c) Angle the patient's head at 30 degrees to align the horizontal semicircular canals perpendicular to the floor.

(d) Ice water (30–60 mL) is used to irrigate the external auditory canal using a large syringe and a butterfly catheter with the needle removed. Wait a few minutes, and then irrigate the other ear.

(e) The cold water inhibits the ipsilateral vestibular system.

(f) If the brainstem is intact, the eyes deviate slowly and conjugately to the side of the cold water (slow phase of nystagmus).

(i) The fast corrective component of eye movement, which is away from the stimulated ear, is mediated by the frontal lobe eye fields and is absent in a comatose patient.

(ii) The mnemonic COWS ("cold—opposite, warm—same") should more correctly be "fast COWS" as the direction of the nystagmus is reported by the fast phase. Because there is no fast phase, the only response is the slow phase, which is toward the cold irrigated ear.

(iii) Absence of response to caloric testing is due to a structural lesion of the pons or a metabolic disorder such as sedative drug intoxication.

(iv) Downward deviation of one or both eyes following unilateral cold water irrigation suggests sedative drug intoxication.

5. Motor responses

a. Observe for the presence of spontaneous movement. If not present, apply a noxious stimulus such as sternal rubbing, twisting a nipple, or nail bed or supraorbital compression.

b. Decorticate posturing (flexion at the elbow and wrist bilaterally, with shoulder adduction and extension of the legs) is seen with lesions above the brainstem, specifically above the red nucleus.

c. Decerebrate posturing (internal rotation and adduction of the shoulder with extension at elbows, wrists, and legs) is usually associated with a bilateral midbrain or pontine lesion.

d. Unilateral or asymmetrical posturing is suggestive of structural disease in the contralateral cerebral hemisphere or brainstem.

Key Clinical Features: Coma Examination

- Respiratory pattern
- Pupils
- Eye movements
  - Resting position
  - Spontaneous
  - Reflex
- Motor responses

Anatomic Localization

1. Attempt first to explain the symptoms and signs with one focal lesion. (Recall Occam's razor or the law of parsimony. William of Occam (1284-1347) wrote, "Plurality should not be posited without necessity"). Of course, some diseases can be multifocal.

2. In problem cases, review the pertinent neuroanatomy.

3. Patterns of weakness aid in localization (Table 1–2).

4. Look for paraparesis (Table 1–3) and hemiparesis (Table 1–4).

5. The upper motor neuron syndrome consists of

TABLE 1–4. ANATOMIC LOCALIZATION OF HEMIPARESIS

Location of Lesion	Characteristics of Hemiparesis and Associated Signs
Cerebral cortex	Contralateral arm is affected more than leg or face; sometimes tongue (deviates to weak side) Left hemisphere: aphasia, apraxia Right hemisphere: inattention to left half of body, visual space; constructional apraxia Homonymous hemianopia on weak side Decreased graphesthesia, extinction of sensory stimuli
Internal capsule	Contralateral arm equal to leg; face may be spared No sensory loss or aphasia
Brainstem	Contralateral arm equal to leg plus ipsilateral cranial nerve palsy
Midbrain	Third nerve palsy (Weber syndrome)
Pons	Sixth and seventh nerve palsies (peripheral); ipsilateral conjugate gaze palsy possible (Foville's syndrome)
Medulla	Twelfth nerve palsy
Cervical spinal cord (hemicord)	Ipsilateral weakness of arm and leg, sparing face; ipsilateral loss of proprioception and vibration Contralateral loss of pain and temperature (Brown-Séquard syndrome)

From Hammerstad JP: Strength and reflexes. In Goetz CG, Pappert EJ (eds), Textbook of Clinical Neurology. Philadelphia, WB Saunders, 1998, p. 256.

weakness, spasticity, hyperactivity of the tendon reflexes, and an extensor plantar response (Babinski sign).

6. Lower motor neuron syndrome includes muscular weakness, atrophy, fasciculations, and loss of deep tendon reflexes.

Differential Diagnosis

1. It follows anatomic localization.

2. Try to explain the clinical picture with a single disease, although more than one disease could be present.

3. Unusual presentations of common diseases are more frequent than rare diseases (when you hear hoofbeats think of horses, not zebras).

4. When the diagnosis is not certain, arrange the possibilities in a hierarchy from most to least likely. (As bank robber Willie Sutton said, "That's where the money is.")

5. Try not to exclude any treatable diseases from the list of possibilities.

6. Attempt to be flexible in your reasoning. Do not make a diagnosis as if it were set in stone, never reconsidering other possibilities. Reevaluate as indicated based on the review of prior records, symptoms, signs, response to treatment, and results of diagnostic testing.

7. Intelligently order diagnostic testing. Consider pretest probabilities, sensitivity, and specificity.

8. If the case is a difficult one and you are just not sure, explore the avenues.

    a. Do some research by looking at pertinent books or journal articles or check with other colleagues.

    b. If you are still not sure, get a second or even a third opinion. The cognitive services of neurologists are much less expensive than ordering tests in a shotgun fashion.

    c. As is pertinent, review diagnostic studies with the physician who interpreted them (e.g., the radiologist) and make certain there was adequate clinical information.

    d. If you are still stumped, consider getting second opinions on the diagnostic test results, such as imaging studies or nerve and muscle biopsies.

9. Surprisingly often, despite the best efforts, a diagnosis is not forthcoming. Considerations here include rare presentations, a new disease, and functional disorders.

Functional Weakness and Sensory Disturbance

1. Functional weakness

    a. Observe the patient at all times during the history, examination, in the waiting room, or in the hospital. Look for inconsistency e.g., dragging a leg during gait testing but walking into the exam room normally.

    b. Look for other findings to go along with a hemiplegia such as facial weakness, and asymmetry of tone and reflexes.

    c. Hoover's sign: to evaluate functional hemiplegia

        (1) Everyone extends their hip when flexing their contralateral hip.

        (2) With the patient lying supine with legs extended, place your hands under the patient's heels and ask the patient to push down both heels. With an organic plegia, the pressure should only be felt from the good leg.

        (3) Then, keeping your hand under the "weak" heel, place your other hand on the top of the normal leg. Ask the patient to concentrate hard on the good leg and lift or extend the leg against your resistance. In hysterical plegia, the allegedly paralyzed heel will press down against your hand.

    d. "Give-way" weakness

        (1) When checking muscle function, there is variable or collapsing weakness.

        (2) Strength may improve with encouragement.

        (3) Strength may be difficult to assess if the patient has pain with use.

    e. With a functional gait disorder, the patient may drag the entire leg as a single unit. The hip may be rotated, the ankle may maintain an inverted or everted posture, and there is no hip circumduction. Other functional patterns include sudden knee buckling; walking with flexion of hips and knees; cautious, broad-based steps with decreased stride length and height ("walking on ice"); inconsistent patterns with fluctuation of impairment; and excessive slowness of movements or hesitation.

2. Functional sensory disturbance

    a. Typically affects all modes of sensation in a hemisensory distribution or affecting an entire extremity.

    b. Loss of pinprick sensation on one side with midline splitting or splitting of vibration sense over the sternum or frontal bone is often but not always functional. Midline splitting can occur in thalamic stroke.

3. The diagnosis of functional weakness and sensory loss can be very difficult.

    a. Even experienced physicians can be incorrect. Many medical malpractice suits are the result of incorrectly diagnosing an organic disease as functional.

    b. Patients may appear to have a functional exam because they do not understand what they are asked to do or are trying to please the doctor.

    c. Many patients with solely organic disease will have functional findings on exam.

    d. Patients can also have both functional and organic disorders.

Bibliography

Internet Text and Video Resources

Blumenfeld H. An interactive online guide to the neurological examination (with video demonstrations)—Yale University. *http://www.neuroexam.com.*

Larsen PD, Stensaas SD. NeuroLogic: an anatomical approach to the neurological exam. *http://medlib.med.utah.edu/neurologicexa_m/home_exam.html.*

Sodicoff M. The neurological examination. Temple University. *http://courses.temple.edu/neuroanatomy/lab/neuexam.htm.*

Internet Neurology Case Studies

Baylor College of Medicine. *http://www.bcm.tmc.edu/neurol/case.html.*

Books

Brazis PW, Masdeu JC, Biller J: Localization in Clinical Neurology, 4th ed. Philadelphia, Lippincott Williams & Wilkins, 2001.

Caplan LR, Hollander J: The Effective Clinical Neurologist, 2nd ed. Oxford, Butterworth Heinemann, 2001.

2 Dizziness

David Solomon

Definition

1. Dizziness is experienced when the psychophysical mechanism necessary for normal spatial orientation fails, which is often due to disorders of sensory, integrative, and motor mechanisms
2. In general usage, this symptom is too vague to be of any specific diagnostic value. It can have a broad range of etiologies, including presyncope and vestibular or anxiety disorders (see Part IX, Chapter 4, Vertigo).

Epidemiology and Risk Factors

1. A common "geriatric syndrome" with dizziness as a chief complaint has been described in a large series of elderly patients without prominent vestibular problems.
   a. The most common findings are
      (1) Anxiety
      (2) Depressive symptoms
      (3) Impaired hearing
      (4) Taking more than five medications daily
      (5) Postural hypotension
      (6) Impaired balance
      (7) History of myocardial infarction
2. Patients with sensory deficits involving a combination of somatosensory, visual, and vestibular modalities (e.g., macular degeneration, peripheral neuropathy)
3. Widespread white matter changes seen on brain magnetic resonance imaging (MRI)
4. Migraine
5. Uncompensated vestibular loss

Etiology and Pathophysiology

1. Causes of presyncopal dizziness, lightheadedness, or disorientation
   a. Hyperventilation: causes cerebral vasoconstriction and hypoperfusion
   b. Orthostatic hypotension: drop in systolic blood pressure of greater than 20 mm Hg, or elevation in pulse rate of more than 20 beats/minute, or both when going from supine to upright position
      (1) Antihypertensives

(2) Alpha-blockers used for prostatic hypertrophy
   c. Vasovagal attacks (only occasionally precipitated by vertigo)
   d. Decreased cardiac output (arrhythmia, myocardial infarction, congestive heart failure, aortic stenosis)
   e. Postconcussion syndrome
   f. Hypoglycemic dizziness
      (1) Catecholamine-related symptoms (palpitations, sweating, tremor, pallor)
      (2) Insulin
      (3) Less commonly: alcohol consumption with fasting or insulin-secreting tumors
   g. Intoxication should always be sought as a cause of dizziness owing to over-the-counter or prescription medications
      (1) Gaze-evoked nystagmus and gait ataxia commonly are associated with the use of alcohol, barbiturates, benzodiazepines, and anticonvulsants.

Clinical Features

1. Presyncopal
   a. Symptoms are global and described as "woozy," "about to black out," "tunnel vision," or "lightheaded." They are frequently experienced by healthy individuals who rise quickly from a chair and have a few seconds of disorientation because of inadequate orthostatic compensation.
   b. Usually due to insufficient central nervous system (CNS) perfusion.
   c. Symptoms are worse when standing and diminish with lying down.
   d. They may be associated with tachycardia or bradycardia, pallor, and diaphoresis.
   e. An exception is a cardiac arrhythmia, which could decrease cerebral blood flow in any position.
2. Hyperventilation
   a. May be insidious, with an increase in the frequency of sighs or depth of breathing
3. Imbalance and unsteadiness with standing and walking
   a. Often multifactorial

    b. Visual loss, new spectacle correction, bifocals

    c. White matter disease

    d. Cervical spinal stenosis

    e. Vitamin B_{12} deficiency

4. Labyrinthine

    a. Mainly horizontal nystagmus present in straight-ahead gaze

5. Brainstem or cerebellar etiology if the following are present.

    a. Five D's

      (1) Dysarthria

      (2) Dysphagia

      (3) Dysmetria (appendicular ataxia)

      (4) Diplopia

      (5) Down-beating or direction-changing nystagmus (or both)

    b. Hemifacial or hemibody sensory or motor deficit

    c. Horner's syndrome

    d. Hiccups, visual inversion, drop attacks, visual loss, confusion

Key Clinical Signs and Symptoms

- Patients describe being "woozy" or "about to black out," having "tunnel vision," or feeling "light-headed."

- Hyperventilation (may be insidious)

- Imbalance and unsteadiness with standing and walking

- Horizontal nystagmus in straight-ahead gaze

- Visual loss

Differential Diagnosis

1. Psychophysiologic or anxiogenic dizziness

    a. Anxiety

    b. Panic syndrome

    c. Agoraphobia

2. Postconcussion syndrome

3. Cardiovascular

4. Drug toxicity

5. Hypoglycemia

6. Exercise-induced dizziness

7. Labyrinthine vertigo (unilateral dysfunction)

    a. Etiology of episodic vertigo by duration

      (1) 1–2 Seconds

        (a) Head movement with uncompensated vestibular loss

        (b) Crisis of Tumarkin (a feature of Ménière's syndrome)

        (c) Drop attack (vertebrobasilar insufficiency)

      (2) Less than 60 seconds

        (a) Benign paroxysmal positional vertigo

      (3) Minutes

        (a) Transient ischemic attack (TIA)

      (4) Hours

        (a) Ménière's syndrome

        (b) Migraine

      (5) Days

        (a) Vestibular neuronitis

        (b) Cerebellar or brainstem stroke

8. Bilateral vestibular loss

    a. Not associated with vertigo

    b. Oscillopsia (apparent visual motion) with head movement and imbalance

    c. Worsening gait in darkness or on soft surfaces

    d. Most often due to aminoglycoside ototoxicity

      (1) Gentamicin is the usual drug that causes vestibular toxicity.

      (2) Hearing is usually unaffected.

      (3) It can occur even with normal peak and trough levels.

      (4) It can be associated with a family history of aminoglycoside ototoxicity susceptibility.

Laboratory Testing

1. Glucose

2. Thyroid-stimulating hormone (TSH)

3. Vitamin B_{12}

4. Cardiac evaluation: tilt table, electrocardiography (ECG), Holter monitoring

5. Electronystagmography and audiography

6. Emergently image the patient with acute dizziness with MRI of the brain if accompanied by

    a. Unilateral or asymmetrical hearing loss

    b. Brainstem or cerebellar symptoms other than vertigo

    c. Stroke risk factors (diabetes, hypertension, history of myocardial infarction)

    d. Acute onset associated with neck pain

    e. Direction-changing spontaneous nystagmus

    f. New-onset severe headache

    g. Inability to stand or walk

Key Tests

- Glucose
- TSH
- Vitamin B_{12}
- Cardiac evaluation: tilt table, ECG, Holter monitor
- Electronystagmography and audiogram
- MRI

Radiologic Features

1. Posterior fossa mass lesion
2. Vertebral or basilar artery disease
3. Cervical spinal stenosis or cord compression
4. Abnormal echocardiogram
   a. Aortic stenosis
   b. Poor cardiac ejection fraction

Treatment

1. Medications
   a. Avoid vestibular suppressants (anticholinergics and antihistamines) except during the acute phase of vertigo. There is no role for chronic treatment of dizziness with meclizine (Antivert)
   b. Migraine prophylaxis
   c. Specific serotonin reuptake inhibitors (e.g., sertraline)
2. Orthostatic hypotension
   a. Increased water and salt intake
   b. Midodrine
   c. Fludrocortisone
3. Hyperventilation symptoms are alleviated by breathing in and out of a paper bag.

Key Treatment

- Medications
  —Vestibular suppressants (anticholinergics and antihistamines) should be avoided except during the acute phase of vertigo.
  —Migraine prophylaxis
  —Specific serotonin reuptake inhibitors (e.g., sertraline)
- For orthostatic hypotension
  —Increased water and salt intake
  —Midodrine
  —Fludrocortisone
- For hyperventilation symptoms
  —Breathing in and out of a paper bag

Prevention

1. Avoid polypharmacy.
2. Initiate vestibular exercises promptly after labyrinthine loss.
3. Monitor patients receiving aminoglycoside therapy.
   a. Measure dynamic visual acuity by having the patient read from an eye chart while rotating the head horizontally once per second.
   b. A loss of more than two lines of visual acuity should prompt discontinuation of aminoglycoside therapy if possible.

Bibliography

Drachman DA: Occam's razor, geriatric syndromes, and the dizzy patient. Ann Intern Med 132:403–404, 2000.
Evans RW: Neurologic aspects of hyperventilation syndrome. Semin Neurol 15:115–125, 1995.
Staab JP, Ruckenstein MJ, Solomon D, Shepard NT: Serotonin reuptake inhibitors for dizziness with psychiatric symptoms. Arch Otolaryngol Head Neck Surg 128:554–560, 2002.
Tinetti ME, Williams CS, Gill TM: Dizziness among older adults: a possible geriatric syndrome. Ann Intern Med 132:337–344, 2000.

3 Approach to Visual Symptoms and Signs

Paul W. Brazis
Andrew G. Lee

Visual Symptoms

Past medical history emphasis with complaint of visual loss:

1. Past medical and surgical history
2. Past ocular history
3. What was the best previous vision?
4. When was the last eye exam?
5. History of patching eyes as child, surgery, or glasses?
6. History of amblyopia?
7. Cone down questioning to specific visual problem.
   a. Afferent visual system (e.g., visual loss—field or acuity).
      (1) Onset (e.g., upon waking, following a headache)
      (2) Course
         (a) Acute, subacute, chronic?
         (b) Stable, progressive?
         (c) Precipitating factors (e.g., trauma, illness)?
         (d) Transient or persistent?
      (3) Duration of visual loss—seconds, minutes, hours, days)
      (4) Monocular or binocular?
      (5) Associated pain or headache? Auras?
      (6) Associated "positive" phenomena (e.g., scintillations or other visual hallucinations)?
   b. Efferent visual system (e.g., diplopia, pupil abnormality, ptosis)
      (1) Monocular or binocular diplopia? Monocular diplopia usually indicates ocular disease (e.g., cataract) or less often cerebral cortical or nonorganic problem. Binocular diplopia usually means motility impairment.
      (2) Horizontal diplopia?
         (a) Horizontal diplopia usually means weakness of lateral rectus muscle or medial rectus muscle.
         (b) Worse at distance than near usually indicates lateral rectus paresis (e.g., abducens nerve palsy)
         (c) Worse on gaze to left means weakness of left lateral rectus or right medial rectus paresis.
      (3) Vertical diplopia?
         (a) Usually indicates paresis of one of the vertically acting muscles in either eye (right or left inferior rectus, superior rectus, inferior oblique, superior oblique).
         (b) Is vertical separation of images worse on left or right gaze? If worse on gaze to right, may be weakness of right superior rectus, right inferior rectus, left superior oblique, or left inferior oblique muscles.
         (c) Is separation worse on downgaze or upgaze? If separation is worse on gaze right and down, this indicates weakness of the right inferior rectus or left superior oblique muscle.
      (4) Is diplopia or ptosis worse as day progresses or with fatigue? Raises question of myasthenia gravis, but many other causes of motility impairment will also be more apparent with physical or mental fatigue.
   c. Pain and sensory symptoms (e.g., headache, eye pain, facial numbness, or paresthesias)
      (1) Palliative and precipitating factors
      (2) Associated symptoms (e.g., migraine aura)
      (3) Location, character, duration, periodicity, etc.

Diplopia History

- Monocular or binocular?

- Vertical or horizontal?

- Worse on left or right gaze?

- Worse on gaze up or down?

- Worse at distance or near?

Bibliography

Brazis PW, Masdeu JC, Biller J: Localization in Clinical Neurology, 4th ed. Philadelphia, Lippincott Williams & Wilkins, 2001, pp. 133–270.

Lee AG, Brazis PW: Clinical Pathways in Neuro-Ophthalmology. An Evidence-Based Approach. New York, Thieme, 1998.

4 Paresthesias

George D. Baquis

Definition

1. Paresthesias are abnormal spontaneous sensations described as tingling, pins and needles, or prickling. They are a common reason for patients to seek medical attention, can occur at multiple anatomic sites, and can be transient benign symptoms or harbingers of serious neurologic disease.

2. They may be accompanied by pain, other sensory symptoms including analgesia or hypesthesia (loss of sensation), dysesthesia (evocation of unpleasant discomfort by painless stimuli), or hyperpathia (exaggerated heightened response to painful stimuli).

3. Symptoms can arise from multiple anatomic sites within the central and peripheral nervous system. Their significance is determined by mode of onset, location, temporal course, accompanying symptoms, neurologic examination, and diagnostic test findings.

Etiology

1. Somatic sensation originates from specialized skin receptors including pacinian corpuscles, Meissner's corpuscles, and Merkel discs (mechanical skin deformation); hair receptors (hair movement); Ruffini nerve endings (stretch); and Golgi tendon organs (muscle stretch).

2. Information is transmitted through peripheral nerves of differing diameters to the central nervous system. More heavily myelinated type A alpha fibers conduct touch and pressure. Thinly myelinated type A delta or unmyelinated type C fibers conduct pain and temperature.

3. The sensory nerve cell bodies (dorsal root ganglia) are positioned at the spinal neural foramina located external to the spinal cord. These cells project axons through the posterior nerve roots and synapse with other neurons at multiple levels within the spinal cord and brainstem.

4. Discrete nerve pathways within the spinal cord that can be selectively affected by neurologic disease include the posteriorly located gracilis and cuneatus fasciculi (touch, pressure, joint position sense, and vibration), lateral spinothalamic tracts (pain and temperature), and anterior spinothalamic tracts (touch pressure). Neurons within the brainstem and spinal cord secondarily synapse

within the thalamus, which projects to the somatosensory cortex.

Clinical Examination

1. A 128 Hz tuning fork, cotton, and a disposable safety pin are used to test modalities of pinprick and temperature, vibration, light touch, and joint position. Patterns of altered sensation should be described or diagrammed. Variations in threshold occur over different body surfaces, and thresholds change with age.

2. Testing should proceed from affected abnormal areas to those of normal sensation.

3. Comparison of the abnormal side to the homologous normal side can be helpful.

4. Discriminative modalities such as two-point discrimination, localization of cutaneous stimulation, recognition of objects by palpation, and identification of numbers written on the palm or fingertips can be impaired by diseases affecting the somatosensory cortex or thalamocortical projections.

5. Assessment of the observed behavioral response to painful stimulation supplements the verbal descriptions of those patients who do not understand instructions or cannot participate fully for formal sensory testing.

PEARLS

- Testing should proceed from affected abnormal areas to those of normal sensation.
- Comparison of the abnormal side to the homologous normal side can be helpful.

Clinical Features

1. Anatomic patterns
   a. Mononeuropathies: Paresthesias can be the most prominent symptom of a focal mononeuropathy. Objective sensory loss may be less than anatomically expected because of overlap between adjacent nerve territories. A positive Tinel's sign may be elicited over the affected nerve at sites of focal injury or nerve regeneration.

b. Radiculopathies: Radiating pain can accompany paresthesias and may be aggravated by movement or coughing. Altered cutaneous sensation follows a dermatomal pattern and can be accompanied by muscular weakness and depression of the tendon reflex corresponding to the affected nerve root. The area of objective sensory loss may be less than expected from the anatomic distribution because of dermatomal overlap. Because movement aggravates pain, guarding is a common response. Thoracic radiculopathies can mimic visceral pain syndromes. The distribution of paresthesias and sensory loss may be difficult to distinguish from a peripheral nerve injury.

c. Polyneuropathies: Distal foot and leg tingling may be associated with loss of sensation that progressively spreads in a symmetrical "stocking" pattern affecting lower limbs before upper limbs in a length-dependent fashion. Distal weakness and depressed tendon reflexes may accompany altered sensation. Sensory ganglionopathies can be painful, and profound ataxia may result from large fiber involvement. Multifocal symptoms may result from a mononeuropathy multiplex.

d. Myelopathies: A transverse truncal sensory level may accompany an uncomfortable squeezing thoracic or abdominal girdling tightness, which is usually several levels below the structural spinal cord lesion. Paresthesias, loss of sensation, ataxia, and pain can result from diseases that affect large proprioceptive sensory fibers traveling in the gracilis and cuneatus fasciculi. With cervical spine posterior column disease, neck flexion may evoke brief abrupt electrical sensations that spread to the arms, back, or legs—the sign of Lhermitte. Distal paresthesias can be difficult to distinguish from those of distal polyneuropathies.

e. Brainstem diseases: Crossed sensory symptoms and signs are characteristic of diseases affecting the lateral medulla and lower pons. Cranial nerve palsies may accompany the sensory abnormalities.

f. Thalamic lesions: Pure hemisensory impairment of all sensory modalities can result from disease of the contralateral ventral posterolateral and ventral posteromedial thalamic nuclei. Symptoms may be more severe than clinical examination findings, which may be patchy.

g. Somatosensory cortex: Contralateral paresthesias and pain can result from small parietal hemispherical lesions, but larger lesions usually also affect other cortical functions such as language (left hemisphere) or behavior and spatial attention (right hemisphere).

2. Diseases

a. Intermittent paresthesias

(1) Transient ischemic attacks (TIAs): The sudden onset of tingling or prickling that may last minutes to hours with complete resolution

(2) Migraine: Paresthesias originate in a localized region of a limb and gradually migrate over several minutes, spreading to contiguous limb. Resolution can be followed by a severe headache.

(3) Somatosensory seizures: Isolated hemifacial or limb paresthesias are rarely an ictal symptom, and motor features may accompany sensory symptoms. Unilateral somatosensory symptoms of benign rolandic epilepsy may shift from side to side.

(4) Hyperventilation: Paresthesias of the face, hands, and feet can be associated with lightheadedness, dry mouth, blurred vision, and tetany. Symptoms resolve within several minutes of cessation of overbreathing. Anxiety is a common cause and symptoms may lead to panic attacks. Hyperventilation can cause a seizure in predisposed individuals, and this may complicate the diagnosis.

(5) Metabolic: Hypophosphatemia can cause paresthesias that affect perioral, periorbital, and facial regions.

(6) Limb positioning, transient nerve compression, and entrapment neuropathies: Paresthesias occur in the distribution of affected nerves and resolve over minutes after a change in limb position. Focal entrapment neuropathies of the median nerve at the wrist, ulnar nerve at the wrist or elbow, and peroneal nerve at the fibula evoke characteristic symptoms that can be recurrent or persistent. The nocturnal paresthesias of carpal tunnel syndrome typically awaken patients at night and affect the first three fingers. Ulnar nerve entrapment at the cubital tunnel or tardy ulnar palsy at the elbow cause hand weakness accompanied by small finger tingling. Altered skin sensation which splits the fourth finger is suggestive of a peripheral nerve etiology. Hand shaking or other movement is a common response to peripheral nerve entrapment. Prolonged symptoms from recurrent or multiple compression mononeuropathies should raise

consideration of hereditary polyneuropathy with predisposition to pressure palsies.

b. Subacute or chronic paresthesias

(1) Multiple sclerosis: Paresthesias are localized and result from demyelinating plaques which can affect any central nervous system myelinated region. Symptoms last from days to months, and resolution can be incomplete.

(2) Stroke: The abrupt onset of hemisensory paresthesias may be the only symptom of a posterior thalamic lacunar stroke, and sensory loss on neurologic examination is often mild. Symptoms resolve over weeks to months and may be accompanied by the difficult-to-treat pain syndrome of Dejerine-Roussy.

(3) Polyneuropathy: Distal paresthesias are frequently the initial manifestation of distal polyneuropathies. Pure sensory polyneuropathies or ganglionopathies are uncommon and can cause facial, truncal, and limb paresthesias. Severe pain can be difficult to treat. Limb and truncal ataxia can occur if large fiber proprioceptive function is lost and can be difficult to distinguish from cerebellar dysfunction. Excessive pyridoxine intake, Sjögren's syndrome, and remote affect of cancer are among many described causes of purely sensory polyneuropathies, but often no diagnosis can be established.

(4) Focal structural disease (neoplasia, syrinx): Intracerebral tumors, vascular malformations, and cysts need to be considered when paresthesias are persistent, localized, and accompanied by abnormal focal neurologic examination findings. Syringomyelia and other central spinal cord diseases can cause a shoulder cape distribution of temperature sensory loss with spared proprioception that accompanies limb and facial paresthesias.

(5) Psychiatric origin: Paresthesias may not conform to known neuroanatomic patterns, may have abrupt sharply defined margins, and may be discordant with other neurologic findings (for example, absence of lower limb joint position and vibration sensation with normal coordination and balance). However, elaboration of psychiatric symptoms upon those of nonpsychiatric origin is common and can be diagnostically challenging.

(6) Other: The numb chin syndrome can represent a mental neuropathy and is an ominous symptom associated with metastatic cancer. Lambert-Eaton myasthenic syndrome, a paraneoplastic disorder associated with small cell lung cancer, can cause parestheisias through an effect on cholinergic sensory fibers, but other symptoms usually predominate. Paresthesias may be present with complex regional pain syndromes in the absence of a peripheral nerve injury.

Key Signs

- Numb chin

- Truncal sensory level

- Sensory loss with ataxia

- Coexistent muscular weakness or tendon reflex abnormalities

- Recurrent or persistent localized paresthesias

Prognosis and Treatment

1. The severity of paresthesias does not predict underlying disease or course of illness.

2. Several patterns should raise clinical concern and prompt consideration of further diagnostic testing (see Key Signs).

3. The anatomic origin and underlying disorder causing paresthesias are often not clear from a clinical office evaluation. Additional diagnostic testing may be needed to exclude serious disease and alleviate patient concerns (see Key Tests).

4. Prognosis and treatment are determined by the underlying clinical disorder.

Key Tests

Polyneuropathy, Radiculopathy, and Mononeuropathy

- Electromyography and nerve conduction testing

Structural and Inflammatory Brain and Spinal Cord Disease

- Magnetic resonance imaging (MRI)

Epilepsy

- Electroencephalography (EEG)

- Ambulatory EEG monitoring

Demyelinating Diseases
• Somatosensory evoked potentials

Small Fiber Sensory Polyneuropathy
• Quantitative computerized sensory examination (CASE IV)

Bibliography

Fisher CM: Concerning paresthesias. Trans Am Neurol Assoc 87:196–198, 1962.

Gardner EP, Martin JP, Jessell TM: The bodily senses. In Kandel ER, Schwartz JH, Jessell TM (eds): Principles of Neural Science, 4th ed. New York, McGraw-Hill, 2000, pp. 430–450.

Haerer AF: The exteroceptive sensations. In DeJong's The Neurologic Examination, 5th ed. Philadelphia, J.B. Lippincott, 1994, pp. 47–66.

Mitsumoto H, Wilbourn AJ: Causes and diagnosis of sensory neuropathies: a review. J Clin Neurophysiol 11:553–567, 1994.

Stewart JD: The diagnosis of focal neuropathies. Focal Peripheral Neuropathies, 3rd ed. Philadelphia, Lippincott Williams & Wilkins, 2000, pp. 45–69.

Woolsey RM, Young RR: The clinical diagnosis of disorders of the spinal cord. In Young RR, Woolsey RM (eds): Diagnosis and Management of Disorders of the Spinal Cord. Philadelphia, W.B. Saunders, 1995, pp. 135–144.

5 Neuropathic Pain

Misha-Miroslav Backonja

Introduction

1. After respiratory symptoms, pain is the most common reason for visits to primary care physicians and among the most common reasons for visits to neurologists.

2. Advances in neurobiology of pain, from basic science to clinical investigations, are now clearly demonstrating that chronic pain is a neurologic disorder, and that it refers in particular to neuropathic pain disorders such as diabetic painful neuropathy, postherpetic neuralgia, radiculopathies, and post-traumatic neuralgias, among many others.

3. The practical diagnostic implication regarding neuropathic pain is that the neurologic exam is abnormal; the therapeutic implication is that neuropathic pain disorders respond best to neuromodulating agents such as anticonvulsants, and when opioids are used large doses are required.

4. Evaluation of the chronic neuropathic pain patient requires something beyond the standard history and neurologic examination and should also include additional assessment tools, such as a neuropathic pain examination and a musculoskeletal examination.

5. The specific evaluations and assessments that should be performed for all chronic pain patients include

   a. Pain history

   b. Pain-specific sensory examination

   c. Musculoskeletal and myofascial evaluation

   d. Basic psychological assessment

   e. If there is a suspicion of Complex Regional Pain syndrome (CRPS), traditionally known as reflex sympathetic dystrophy (RSD), then a CRPS/RSD-specific examination should also be performed.

 Key Evaluations—Chronic Pain

- Pain history
- Pain-specific sensory examination
- Musculoskeletal and myofascial evaluation
- Basic psychological assessment

Evaluation of Patients with Chronic Pain

1. Pain assessment is the first and the crucial part of any diagnostic process that leads to pain diagnosis; it is performed during the initial evaluation and repeated regularly during the treatment follow-ups.

2. The essential first step in pain assessment is the clinician's acknowledgment that the patient is experiencing pain and that the pain is real.

3. Important elements of pain assessment include location, intensity, and specific descriptors. Other key elements of pain assessment include the temporal course of symptoms; associated symptoms; evaluation of mood; sleep and the functional level; past treatments; the use of tobacco, alcohol, and illegal drugs; and coping skills.

4. Follow-up assessments and monitoring of symptoms can be made using the Neuropathic Pain Scale.

5. The Brief Pain Inventory is a questionnaire that is useful for assessing the impact of pain on patient function and quality of life.

6. The pain and symptoms assessment should assist the clinician in deciding whether the patient requires further evaluation and treatment from other pain medicine specialists, such as a psychologist, psychiatrist, physiatrist, or vocational counselor.

THE PHYSICAL EXAMINATION IN GENERAL

General Medical Examination and Examination of the Musculoskeletal System

1. An important aspect of the general medical examination to be emphasized in this chapter includes the status of the skin, noting the following as either present or absent: skin color (red, pale, bluish, mottled), rashes, swelling, and temperature abnormalities.

2. The status of joints, muscles and ligaments, and any swelling, laxity, or tenderness must also be considered. If any abnormality is present it could suggest a systemic disorder, such as systemic lupus erythematosus or rheumatoid arthritis, many of which could have neurologic involvement as part of the syndrome complex.

3. Abnormalities of skin and joints also suggest and support the evidence for a possible diagnosis of CRPS/RSD.

NEUROLOGIC EXAMINATION

1. Pain that is unsupported by significant physical findings ought not to be dismissed as psychogenic pain or malingering.
2. An important consideration is traditional neurologic reliance on sharp-dull discrimination of pinprick testing as inadequate for pain diagnosis because traditional sharp-dull discrimination is not conducive for testing of allodynia, hyperalgesia, and all other positive sensory phenomena.

Sensory System Examination

1. The patient with neuropathic pain is the only and the best judge of the pain symptoms.
2. The examination itself is carefully described beforehand to the patient and the patient is reassured that the limits of the examination will be set by the patient.
   a. During the course of the sensory examination, the patient will have been instructed to answer questions regarding the perception of the stimulus in simple terms: yes, no, or do not know.
   b. The stimulus should be first applied to the normal body part, thus introducing the stimulus to the patient and establishing how the examination is to be conducted.
   c. The initial questions are simple, unambiguous, and should ask only if the perceived sensation is normal or abnormal.
   d. The next question is whether each stimulus is uncomfortable, unpleasant, or painful.
   e. Last of all, patients are encouraged to use their own terms to describe perception of each stimulus.
   f. The area affected by the abnormal sensation with application of stimuli is then mapped.

Sensory Signs: Negative Sensory and Positive Sensory Phenomena

1. Negative sensory symptoms and signs are perceived as decreased or less.
2. Positive sensory symptoms and signs are associated with additional sensory phenomena.

Positive Sensory Phenomena

1. Mechanical allodynia: Abnormal sensation of pain from usually nonpainful mechanical stimulation, such as pain from clothing or bed sheets, may be one of the most disabling physical symptoms.

   a. Examining the patient for allodynia entails lightly touching the painful region with a fingertip, cotton swab, or paintbrush.
   b. There is a distinction between static and dynamic mechanical allodynia, depending on how the stimulus is applied:
      (1) Static allodynia is obtained by applying a single stimulus, such as light pressure, to a defined area. This pain phenomenon is a result of sensitized C-nociceptors.
      (2) Dynamic allodynia is a result of activation of A-beta non-nociceptive afferents and it is obtained by moving the stimulus, such as a brush or a cotton swab, across the hypersensitive area.
2. Thermal allodynia: An abnormal sensation of pain from usually nonpainful thermal stimulation such as cold or warmth, including worsening of pain when the painful region is exposed to a cold or warm external environment.
   a. Examining the patient for thermal allodynia entails placing a cool stimulus, such as a cool tuning fork, and a warm stimulus, such as a warm (not hot) test tube of water or a warm tuning fork, directly on the painful region for a few seconds. The patient may report a delay in experiencing the thermal stimulus and then describe a strong or irritating sensory experience that continues longer than normal.
   b. The two types of thermal allodynia have very different underlying mechanisms.
      (1) Warm allodynia is a result of sensitized C-nociceptors.
      (2) Cold allodynia is the result of central sensitization and dysfunctional inhibitory mechanisms.
3. Summation: An abnormally increasing painful sensation to a repeated stimulus. Although the stimulus remains constant, the patient will describe the pain as growing and growing. Summation is frequently seen as a part of hyperalgesia and hyperpathia, although it may be seen in mechanical allodynia from light touch stimulation or from vibration.
4. After-sensation: The abnormal persistence of a sensory perception provoked by a stimulus even though the stimulus has ceased. Neuropathic pain patients may report that the pain, dysesthesia, or paresthesia lingers for seconds or minutes after mechanical, thermal, or painful stimuli.
5. Hyperalgesia: An exaggerated pain response from a usually painful stimulus. Hyperalgesia does not have a symptom analogue and can only be determined by physical examination.
   a. Examining the patient for hyperalgesia entails

stimulating the painful region with a sharp object, like a safety pin, using both a single pinprick stimulus (static hyperalgesia) and multiple pinprick stimuli (dynamic hyperalgesia).

(1) Repeated stimuli are applied to exactly the same area for a few seconds or as long as tolerated by the patient.

(2) At the bedside the simplest way to test for thermal hyperalgesia is by using a glass tube filled with ice-cold water.

(3) Hyperalgesia is present if an exaggerated pain response is observed and reported by the patient to either single or multiple pinprick stimuli, or both.

(4) Summation and after-sensation are frequently present.

(5) Often areas of hyperalgesia are adjacent to areas of sensory deficits within the region of neuropathic pain; i.e., sensory changes may be patchy within the affected region.

b. Underlying mechanisms range from sensitization of nociceptors, such as in mechanical static and heat hyperalgesia; to central sensitization due to activity low threshold innocuous receptors, such as in dynamic hyperalgesia; to central sensitization and inhibitory dysfunction, such as in cold hyperalgesia.

6. Hyperpathia: The most complex abnormal sensation, hyperpathia refers to an abnormally painful and exaggerated reaction to a stimulus, especially to repetitive stimuli, in a patient who at first perceives the stimulus as less intense due to an increased pain threshold.

a. The pain is typically described as "explosive" by the patient.

b. Summation and after-sensation are usually present; for example, during repetitive stimulation with a pin, the patient may at first perceive very little, but after a few seconds the patient reports a great deal of pain and responds with a pronounced reaction.

7. Paresthesia: An abnormal sensation that is not described as unpleasant or painful, paresthesia can be either a spontaneous sensation, such as the report of pins and needles perceived at rest, or can be evoked on physical examination by nonpainful or painful stimulation, such as light touch, thermal application, or pinprick.

8. Dysesthesia: An abnormal sensation described as unpleasant by the patient. As with paresthesia, dysesthesia may be spontaneous or provoked by maneuvers during the physical examination; once the patient reports the provoked sensations as painful, they should be considered to be allodynia.

Key Positive Sensory Phenomena

- Allodynia
- After-sensation
- Hyperalgesia
- Hyperpathia
- Paresthesia
- Dysesthesia

Motor System Examination

1. Patients with neuropathic pain experience motor symptoms and signs, which could also be viewed as negative and positive motor symptoms and signs.

a. On the level of the motor system, negative signs include hypotonia, decreased muscle strength, and decreased endurance.

b. Positive motor signs include increased muscle tone, tremor, dystonia, and dyskinesias.

c. Motor system evaluation of the patient with neuropathic pain syndromes frequently also reveals incoordination, ataxia, and apraxia as well. The type and the degree of motor abnormality varies from syndrome to syndrome, depending on how much the sensorimotor system is affected, and whether that effect is direct or indirect.

d. Motor symptoms and signs should not be overlooked during the pain evaluation because they are significant indicators that the nervous system beyond the pain-transmitting fiber is affected and dysfunctional.

Key Symptoms and Signs

Negative Signs

- Hypotonia
- Decreased muscle strength
- Decreased endurance

Positive Signs

- Increased muscle tone
- Tremor
- Dystonia
- Dyskinesia

MUSCULOSKELETAL AND MYOFASCIAL EVALUATION

1. Myofascial pain syndrome is a chronic pain disorder maintained by chronic tightness and spasm of muscles and soft tissues.

2. In patients with definite neuropathic pain syndromes, it is critical to assess whether a secondary myofascial component is present, because myofascial pain requires a distinct treatment strategy.

3. The musculoskeletal examination should include assessment of mechanical limitations in the range of motion of the spine (cervical, thoracic, and lumbosacral) and of the upper and lower limbs.

4. Myofascial examination entails palpating soft tissues for evidence of tightness and trigger points, focal areas of tightness and tenderness which when palpated reproduce the patient's original pain complaint and other symptoms.

5. Myofascial pain generally develops as a secondary phenomenon, evolving from disuse or overuse of musculature as a consequence of the primary neuropathic pain syndrome. In some patients, however, it is the primary cause of chronic pain.

SPECIFIC ASPECTS OF CPRS/RSD EXAMINATION

1. To make the clinical diagnosis of CRPS/RSD, specific symptoms and signs need to be investigated, beyond the symptoms and signs of neuropathic pain: does the patient experience abnormal swelling, skin temperature changes—cold, hot, or alternating—skin color changes, or sudomotor abnormalities—increased or decreased sweating—localized to the region of pain.

2. Temperature asymmetries could be documented using a skin-probe thermometer, an infrared thermometer and thermography, or contact thermography.

3. Patients may have motor abnormalities including negative and positive motor phenomena and, in some cases, neglect-like syndrome.

PSYCHOLOGICAL ASSESSMENT

1. Most patients with chronic pain, regardless of the cause and etiology, experience some psychological symptoms in the course of their illness.

2. For the vast majority of chronic pain patients, psychological disturbances are secondary, evolving from the unrelieved pain and its drastic effects on the quality of life, and are not the primary cause of the pain.

3. Regardless of whether psychological issues are primary or secondary for any given patient, they need to be properly assessed and treated specifically.

4. Common psychological diagnoses in chronic pain patients include depression, anxiety and panic disorders, and post-traumatic stress disorder.

5. If psychological conditions are thought to be even possibly a component of the clinical picture, then referral to a psychologist or psychiatrist, preferably one with chronic pain expertise, is necessary.

HOW TO SUMMARIZE FINDINGS ON HISTORY, PAIN ASSESSMENT, AND PHYSICAL EXAMINATION

1. The diagnosis of neuropathic pain is usually straightforward, based on a history of nerve injury, the patient's description of the pain, and the possible presence of allodynia, hyperalgesia, hyperpathia, summation, or after-sensation on physical examination: it is not only the number of symptoms and signs but also the severity of those that are present that contributes to the diagnosis of a neuropathic pain syndrome.

2. It is the rule rather than the exception that patients with chronic neuropathic pain have more than one type of pain; for example, an elderly man who suffers from postherpetic neuralgia who at midthorax may have constant pain that keeps him awake all night is also likely to have mechanical allodynia, which prevents him from wearing any clothing, and secondary myofascial pain in the shoulder. This combination leads to sleep deprivation, social isolation, and limited use of the man's arm.

3. Myofascial examination is important in all patients, even those with well-defined neuropathic pain, where myofascial dysfunction may be a prominent secondary pain.

4. The diagnostic process should also include evaluation of psychological diagnoses and psychosocial issues, which may be integral components of the patient's overall clinical situation.

5. Ancillary laboratory, electrophysiologic, and imaging studies may be used to confirm the clinical impression, but by no means are they necessary. Also, it should be remembered that the absence of abnormal laboratory findings does not exclude the diagnosis of neuropathic pain.

6. Therapeutic trials with pharmacological agents and nerve blocks may be used to corroborate the diagnosis, but the absence of pharmacological effect does not rule out neuropathic pain.

Bibliography

Backonja M-M, Galer BS: Pain assessment and evaluation of patients with neuropathic pain. Neurol Clin North Am 16:775–790, 1998.

Galer BS, Butler S, Jensen MP: Case reports and hypothesis: a neglect-like syndrome may be responsible for the motor disturbance in reflex sympathetic dystrophy (Complex Regional Pain Syndrome-1). J Pain Symptom Manage 10: 385–391, 1995.

Galer BS, Jensen MP: Development and preliminary validation of a pain measure specific to neuropathic pain: the Neuropathic Pain Scale. Neurology 48:332–338, 1997.

Travell JG, Simons DG: Myofascial pain and dysfunction: the trigger point manual. Baltimore, Williams & Wilkins, 1992.

Wasner G, Baron B, Backonja M-M: Post-traumatic painful neuralgias: complex regional pain syndromes (reflex sympathetic dystrophy and causalgia)—CRPS/RSD: clinical characteristics, pathophysiological mechanisms and therapy. Neurol Clin North Am 16:851–868, 1998.

6 Headaches

Randolph W. Evans

Introduction

1. Headaches are a near universal experience with a 1-year period prevalence of 90% and a lifetime prevalence of 99%.

2. Twenty-eight million Americans have migraines per year. Five percent of women and 2.8% of men have headaches 180 days or more per year.

3. Headaches are one of the most common complaints of patients seen by neurologists (20% of outpatient visits) and primary care physicians.

4. During a 1-year period in the United States, 9% of adults see physicians for headaches and 83% self-medicate.

5. The differential diagnosis of headaches is one of the longest in medicine, with over 300 different types and causes (Table 6–1). It is critical for the physician to diagnose headaches as precisely as possible.

6. Although most headaches are of benign and poorly understood origin, some secondary headaches can have serious and sometimes potentially life-threatening causes.

7. Since their introduction in 1988, the International Headache Society (IHS) criteria have become the worldwide standard for classification (an updated classification will be issued in 2003).

   a. Primary headaches, for which there is no other underlying cause, include migraine, tension type, cluster, and miscellaneous headaches (such as benign exertional headaches).

   b. There are many secondary headaches (Table 6–1), and these are classified according to cause.

8. A careful history, examination, and, in some cases, diagnostic testing will usually allow the accurate diagnosis of headaches.

9. In some cases, a precise diagnosis may not be possible. For example, some benign headaches have both migraine and tension type features. Patients with chronic daily headaches may be difficult to classify.

Pain-Sensitive Structures

1. Similar headaches can have different causes arising from various pain-sensitive structures.

2. Although all pain is felt in the brain, the brain

TABLE 6–1. MAJOR CATEGORIES OF HEADACHE DISORDERS

Migraine
Tension-type headache
Cluster headache and chronic paroxysmal hemicrania
Miscellaneous headaches unassociated with a structural lesion
   Idiopathic stabbing, external compression, cold stimulus, benign cough, benign exertional, associated with sexual activity
Headache associated with head trauma
Headache associated with vascular disorders
   Acute ischemic cerebrovascular disorder, intracranial hematoma, subarachnoid hemorrhage, unruptured vascular malformation, arteritis, carotid or vertebral artery pain, venous thrombosis, arterial hypertension, associated with other vascular disorder
Headache associated with nonvascular intracranial disorder
   High and low cerebrospinal fluid pressure, intracranial infection, intracranial sarcoidosis and other noninfectious inflammatory disease, related to intrathecal injections, intracranial neoplasm, associated with other intracranial disorder
Headache associated with substances or their withdrawal
   Acute and chronic substance use or exposure, withdrawal after acute and chronic use, associated with substances with uncertain mechanism
Headache associated with noncephalic infection
   Viral infection, bacterial infection, other infection
Headache associated with metabolic disorder
   Hypoxia, hypercapnia, mixed hypoxia and hypercapnia, hypoglycemia, dialysis, other metabolic abnormality
Headache or facial pain associated with disorder of cranium, neck, eyes, ears, nose, sinuses, teeth, mouth, or other facial or cranial structures
Cranial neuralgias, nerve trunk pain, and deafferentation pain
   Persistent pain of cranial nerve origin, trigeminal neuralgia, glossopharyngeal neuralgia, nervus intermedius neuralgia, superior laryngeal neuralgia, occipital neuralgia, central causes of head and facial pain other than tic douloureux

List excerpted from: Headache Classification Committee of the International Headache Society. Classification and diagnostic criteria for headache disorders, cranial neuralgia, and facial pain. Cephalalgia 8(suppl 7);1–96, 1988.

parenchyma, itself, is not pain sensitive. Likewise, the arachnoid, ependyma, and dura (except portions near blood vessels) are not sensitive to pain.

3. Cranial nerves V, VII, IX, and X, the circle of Willis and proximal continuations, meningeal arteries, large veins in the brain and dura, and structures external to the skull (including scalp and neck muscles, cutaneous nerves and skin, the mucosa of paranasal sinuses, teeth, cervical nerves and roots, and the external carotid arteries and branches) are sensitive to pain.

4. The location and source of the pain may be the same—e.g., cheek or forehead pain resulting from maxillary or frontal sinusitis.

5. Because of referral patterns, the location of the pain may not be the same as the source. For

example, supratentorial structures are innervated by the ophthalmic division of the trigeminal nerve, and the infratentorial or posterior fossa structures are supplied by C_2 and C_3. Thus, a cerebellar hemisphere lesion generally refers pain posteriorly and an occipital lobe lesion refers pain anteriorly.

6. The caudal nucleus of the trigeminal nerve, which is located between the mid pons and the third cervical segment, also receives painful messages from the upper cervical roots and from the trigeminal nerve. Thus, pain from the upper cervical spine or posterior fossa can be referred to the front of the head.

The Headache History

1. The headache history is usually essential to establishing the diagnosis.
2. Table 6–2 provides the key elements of the headache history.
3. Table 6–3 gives examples of questions to ask to gather the key elements.
4. Some patients have more than one type of

TABLE 6–2. KEY ELEMENTS OF THE HEADACHE HISTORY

Temporal profile
  Age of onset
  Time to maximum intensity
  Frequency
  Time of day
  Duration
  Recurrence
Headache features
  Location
  Quality of pain
  Severity of pain
Associated symptoms and signs
  Before headache
  During
  After
Aggravating or precipitating factors
  Trauma
  Medical conditions
  Triggers
  Trigger zones
  Activity
  Pharmacologic
Relieving factors
  Nonpharmacologic
  Pharmacological
Evaluation and treatment history
  Physicians and other health care providers
Psychosocial history
  Substance use
  Occupational and personal life
  Psychological history
  Sleep history
  Impact of headache
Patient's own diagnosis
Family history
Complete medical and surgical history

From Evans RW: Chapter 1. Diagnosis of headaches. In Evans RW, Mathew NT (eds), Handbook of Headache. Philadelphia, Lippincott Williams & Wilkins, 2000, p. 4, with permission.

TABLE 6–3. HELPFUL QUESTIONS TO ASK FOR THE HEADACHE HISTORY

Do you have different types of headaches or just one?
Where does the headache hurt?
When did you first start having these headaches?
What were you doing when the headache started?
How long before the headache is of maximal intensity?
How long does the headache last?
Does the headache recur?
How often do they occur?
What is the pain like? Is it a pressure, throbbing, pounding, aching, or stabbing?
Is the pain mild, moderate, or severe?
On a scale of 1 to 10, with 10 the worst and 1 the least, how would you rate the headache?
Do you have trouble with your vision before or during the headache?
Do you have other symptoms (e.g. nausea, vomiting, lightsensitivity, noise sensitivity, discomfort with eye movement, etc.) with the headache?
Are there signs present? (fever, ptosis, miosis, etc.)
Do you have triggers of your headaches? (e.g., menses, stress, foods, beverages, lack of sleep, oversleeping, strong odors, trigger zones, etc.)
What makes the headache worse? (e.g., coughing, bending over, physical activity, etc.)
What makes the headache better? (e.g., sleep, lying down in a quiet room, etc.)
Do your headaches have any impact on your life?
Do you take over-the-counter medications, vitamins, or herbs for your headaches? If so, how much and how often? Do you drink caffeinated beverages, and, if so, what types and how many?
What presciption drugs have you tried and with what effect?
What doctors have you seen in the past for your headaches?
What other treatments have your tried and with what success? (e.g., acupuncture, chiropractic, biofeedback, stress management, massage, etc.)
Have you been under much stress lately?
Have you been depressed?
Do you have any parents or siblings with a history of migraines or bad headaches?

From Evans RW: Chapter 1. Diagnosis of headaches. In Evans RW, Mathew NT (eds), Handbook of Headache. Philadelphia, Lippincott Williams & Wilkins, 2000, p. 5, with permission.

headache. Both open-ended questions ("What are your headaches like?") and close-ended inquiries ("Do you have nausea with the headache?") are necessary. Often, it is helpful to ask about a history of mild headaches versus bad headaches.

5. Some patients are not able to remember or articulate features of the headache ("It's just a headache."). When patients have chronic headaches, it may be necessary to ask them to keep a headache diary in which they record features of their headache(s) over time and then return for a later appointment.
6. Temporal profile
   a. Age of onset
      (1) Migraine headaches usually begin before the age of 40; they uncommonly develop after the age of 50.
      (2) Temporal arteritis typically begins after age 50, rarely earlier.
   b. Time to maximum intensity

(1) Thunderclap headache, a severe headache with maximum intensity within 1 minute, can be caused by subarachnoid hemorrhage, carotid artery dissection, and migraine.

(2) Severe headaches can also have a gradual onset such as migraine or viral meningitis.

c. Frequency: Primary headaches have widely variable frequencies ranging from a few migraines in a lifetime to cluster headaches occurring up to 8 times daily.

d. Time of day

   (1) Cluster headaches often occur during certain times of the day and may awaken the sufferer at about the same time nightly.

   (2) Headaches that awaken people are usually benign (such as migraine, cluster, and hypnic). Headaches from brain tumors, meningitis, and subarachnoid hemorrhage may also disrupt sleep.

   (3) Tension-type headaches often occur in the afternoon.

e. Duration

   (1) Migraine: 4 to 72 hours in adults and 2 to 48 hours in children

   (2) Cluster headache: 15 to 180 minutes

   (3) Tension-type headache: 30 minutes to days

   (4) Trigeminal neuralgia is characterized by volleys of pain lasting a few seconds to less than 2 minutes

f. Recurrence (the return of headache within 24 hours of an initial response after acute treatment): About 30% of the time after using a triptan for migraine, the headache recurs about 12 hours later.

7. Heachache features

a. Location

   (1) Cluster headaches are always unilateral, whereas about 60% of migraines are unilateral.

   (2) Trigeminal neuralgia is typically unilateral, occurring more often in the second or third trigeminal distributions than in the first.

   (3) Headaches from brain tumors or subdural hematomas can be bilateral or unilateral.

b. Quality of pain

   (1) In about 50% of cases, migraine pain is throbbing, pounding, or pulsatile.

   (2) Tension-type headaches cause a pressure, aching, tight, or squeezing sensation.

   (3) Cluster headaches are described as boring or burning.

   (4) Trigeminal neuralgia is often an electrical or stabbing pain.

   (5) Headaches caused by brain tumors can produce a variety of pains ranging from a dull steady ache to throbbing.

c. Severity of pain

   (1) When asking patients about severity, use of a pain scale—1 (minimal pain) to 10 (the worst pain)—is helpful, even though the ranking is, of course, subjective.

   (2) Migraine pain can vary from mild to severe in general, and also from attack to attack.

   (3) Severity of pain does not equate with the presence of life-threatening causes. The majority of severe headaches are migraine or cluster types.

   (4) The new onset of severe headache should be taken very seriously. Some patients with headaches due to brain tumors or subdural hematomas may report a mild headache similar to the tension-type headache and relieved by simple analgesics.

8. Associated symptoms and signs

a. Before the headache

   (1) About 60% of migraineurs will have a prodrome in the hours to days before the headache. Complaints may include changes in mental state (irritability, depression, euphoria, etc.), neurologic (trouble with concentration; light, noise, and smell hypersensitivity), and general (diarrhea or constipation, thirst, sluggish feeling, food cravings, or neck stiffness).

   (2) About 20% of migraines are those with an aura. They generally develop over 5 to 20 minutes and last less than 60 minutes. The headache can begin before, during, or after the aura. The most common auras in descending frequency are visual, sensory, motor symptoms, and speech and language abnormalities.

   (3) Complaints prior to onset of the headache are also very important in diagnosing causes of headache. Low-grade fever and upper respiratory symptoms or diarrhea followed by headache are frequently present in viral meningitis.

b. During

   (1) Migraine is accompanied by nausea in 90%, vomiting in 30%, and light and noise sensitivity in 80%. The same symp-

toms are often present in association with headaches from subarachnoid hemorrhage or meningitis.

(2) Ipsilateral conjunctival injection, tearing, and nasal congestion or drainage typically occur during cluster headaches. Ipsilateral ptosis and miosis occur in about 30% of cases.

c. After

(1) After the headache resolves, many migraineurs complain of feeling tired and drained with decreased mental acuity. Depression or euphoria is sometimes reported.

(2) In some systemic disorders, high fever and headache may be followed by other symptoms or signs.

9. Aggravating or precipitating factors

a. Trauma

(1) Head and neck trauma are frequently followed by headaches.

(2) Headaches beginning after mild head injury are usually benign but raise concerns of a subdural or epidural hematoma in up to 2% of cases.

b. Medical conditions

(1) Pregnancy: Pre-eclampsia and cortical venous thrombosis should be considered postpartum. During the second and third trimesters of pregnancy, migraines usually decrease in frequency.

(2) In 90% of cases, pseudotumor cerebri occurs in obese women.

(3) Paroxysmal hypertension with headache suggests pheochromocytoma.

(4) New onset headaches in someone who is positive for human immunodeficiency virus (HIV) could be due to a variety of causes, including cryptococcal meningitis.

(5) Headache in a person with a history of cancer (especially lung, breast, melanoma, colorectal, and hypernephroma) raises concerns about metastatic disease.

(6) Persons with polycystic kidney disease have a 10% risk of having an intracranial saccular aneurysm.

c. Triggers

(1) Some 85% of migraineurs have one or more triggers.

(2) During periods of cluster headaches, alcohol can be a trigger.

(3) Tension-type headaches can be triggered by stress.

d. Trigger zones

(1) Stimulation of certain areas of the face or mucous membranes of the mouth may trigger pain in trigeminal neuralgia.

(2) Glossopharyngeal neuralgia may similarly be triggered by swallowing, chewing, talking, coughing, or yawning.

e. Activity and posture

(1) Coughing, sneezing, weight lifting, bending, stooping, orgasm, or straining with a bowel movement may trigger benign exertional headaches, cough headaches, or benign orgasmic cephalgia.

(2) When any of the activities listed above trigger a first or worst severe headache lasting hours, subarachnoid hemorrhage should be considered.

(3) Exertional headache or jaw pain can occasionally signal angina pectoris.

(4) Physical activity and coughing may exacerbate migraine, post–lumbar puncture headaches, and headaches caused by brain tumors with mass effect.

(5) Low cerebrospinal pressure headaches can be brought on with sitting or standing and can be relieved by lying supine.

(6) Headaches caused by raised intracranial pressure may worsen in the supine position.

(7) The pain of acute frontal, ethmoid, and sphenoid sinusitis worsens when lying supine and improves with sitting upright. Pain from acute maxillary sinusitis is less when supine and worse in the upright position.

f. Pharmacologic

(1) Frequent use of many prescription or over-the counter drugs can cause rebound headaches in susceptible people and may cause preventive medications to be ineffective.

(2) Headaches can be triggered or their infrequency increased by the use of various medications including oral contraceptives

g. Relieving factors

(1) Non-pharmacologic

(a) Migraine headaches may resolve with sleep or improve with lying down in a dark, quiet room or by application of ice.

(b) Tension-type headaches may improve with relaxation for some people and with exercise in others.

(2) Pharmacologic

(a) Responses to prescription and over-the-counter treatments including dosages and side effects should be obtained in detail.

(b) Also ask about the use herbs such as feverfew and vitamins such as riboflavin.

10. Evaluation and treatment history of other physicians and health care providers

11. Psychosocial history

a. Substance use

(1) Ask about use and quantities of tobacco, alcohol, caffeine, and illicit drugs.

(2) Rebound headaches commonly occur from drinking as little as 2 to 3 cups of coffee daily.

b. Occupational and personal life and psychological history. Ask about stressors, depression, anxiety, occupational toxins, and a school history in students.

12. Sleep history

a. The obese patient who snores may have sleep apnea causing headaches in the morning.

b. Sleep deprivation due to restless legs syndrome may contribute to migraine and tension-type headaches.

c. Patients with sleep disturbance and frequent headaches may benefit from use of sedating tricyclic antidepressants.

d. Sleep difficulties may be due to depression or anxiety.

13. Impact of headache

a. What effect do the headaches have on occupational and personal life?

b. Is the patient missing a lot of work, school, leisure activities, or home activities?

14. Patient and family's own diagnosis

a. Headache may be incorrectly attributed to "sinus," aneurysm, or a brain tumor.

b. Explain how your diagnosis is probable and theirs is unlikely and that testing is usually not necessary for primary headaches.

15. Family history

a. A history of migraine is also present in perhaps 80% of first-degree relatives. Because over 50% of those with migraine are not aware of the diagnosis, you may need to ask about a history of bad or sick headaches or perimenstrual headaches in family members.

b. Perhaps 10% of persons with a history of first-degree relatives with intracranial saccular aneurysm(s) have the same disorder. A family history of neurofibromatosis should also raise concern.

16. Complete medical and surgical history

a. A complete medical and surgical history is crucial not only to consider systemic causes of headache but also to be aware of possible contraindications to medications such as bronchial asthma and nonsteroidal anti-inflammatory drugs or beta-blockers or coronary artery disease and triptans.

b. A history of medication allergies or sensitivities is mandatory.

c. A complete review of systems is also important. Galactorrhea and amenorrhea may occur in a woman with a pituitary macroadenoma causing headaches. Progressive weight loss and headaches may be present in cases of metastatic cancer or AIDS. Syncope and headaches could be due to a colloid cyst of the third ventricle.

Physical Examination

1. Abnormal vital signs such as fever or significantly elevated blood pressure may indicate the cause of the headache.

2. A focused general examination may be informative.

a. An erythematous oropharynx and posterior cervical adenopathy in a teenager with new-onset headaches may indicate infectious mononucleosis as the cause.

b. In cases of possible meningitis or subarachnoid hemorrhage, neck stiffness or meningeal signs should be checked for.

c. Findings of cervical region or suboccipital trigger points can suggest a myofascial cause of headaches. Temporomandibular joint tenderness, clicking, or limitation of movement may be associated with headaches.

d. In headaches caused by frontal or maxillary sinusitis, there is usually tenderness to palpation over the affected sinus and nasal drainage.

e. In patients over the age of 50 with new-onset headaches, the superficial temporal artery should be checked for induration or a reduced or absent pulse, which may be associated with temporal arteritis. Examining the carotid arteries for pulses and bruits is important in patients at risk for atherosclerotic disease. The carotid bulb may be tender in cases of carotidynia or carotid dissection.

f. The skin examination may be useful, e.g., in revealing rash due to viral exanthems and multiple café-au-lait spots due to neurofibromatosis.

3. Every patient seen for headaches should have, at the least, a screening neurological examination, which can be performed within a few minutes. Although the exam is usually normal, you do not want to diagnose a patient with tension-type headaches when you might have found evidence of papilledema, a mild lateral rectus paresis, unequal pupils, a mild hemiparesis, or the presence of a Babinski sign if you had only performed a brief exam.

A Summary of the Features of Headaches

The features of the three most common primary headaches are summarized in Table 6–4 and those of some secondary headaches in Table 6–5.

Diagnostic Testing

1. For most headaches, the diagnosis can be made on the basis of the detailed history and examination without any diagnostic testing at all.

2. A computed tomography (CT) scan of the head will detect most pathology causing headaches and is the preferred study for acute head trauma and subarachnoid hemorrhage.

3. A standard magnetic resonance imaging (MRI) scan of the brain is preferred for the evaluation of headaches. May demonstrate pathology not seen on standard CT (paranasal sinuses, pituitary, posterior fossa, cortical veins (such as superior sagittal sinus thrombosis), cervicomedullary junction (e.g., Chiari I malformation), intracranial aneurysms, carotid dissection, infarcts, white matter abnormalities, congenital abnormalities, and neoplasms.

4. The yield of CT scan or MRI scan in patients with any headache and a normal neurologic examination is about 2%.

5. Table 6–6 provides reasons to consider use of neuroimaging for headaches. Table 6–7 gives reasons to consider use of neuroimaging for children with headaches.

6. Patients who meet IHS criteria for migraine rarely have abnormal neuroimaging findings.

7. Electroencephalography (EEG) is not useful in the routine evaluation of patients with headache. EEG may be helpful if the patient has headaches and symptoms suggesting a seizure disorder or alteration of consciousness.

8. Blood tests are generally not helpful for the diagnosis of headaches, although there are numerous indications.

   a. Arteritis (erythrocyte sedimentation rate or C-reactive protein in temporal arteritis) and

TABLE 6–4.   FEATURES OF SOME PRIMARY HEADACHES

FEATURE	MIGRAINE	EPISODIC TENSION-TYPE	EPISODIC CLUSTER
Epidemiology	18% of women, 6% of men	90% of adults	0.4% for men
	4% of children before puberty	35% of children ages 3–11	0.08% for women
Female/male	3/1 after puberty, 1/1 before	5/4	1/5
Family history	80% of first-degree relatives	Frequent	Rare
Typical age at onset (years)	92% before age 40, 2% after age 50	20–40	20–40
Visual aura	In 20%	No	No
Location	Unilateral 60%, bilateral 40%	Bilateral>unilateral	Unilateral
			Especially orbital, periorbital, frontotemporal
Quality	Pulsatile or throbbing in 50%	Pressure, aching, tight, squeezing	Boring, burning, or stabbing
Severity	Mild to severe	Mild to moderate	Severe
Onset to peak pain	Minutes to hours	Hours	Minutes
Duration	4–72 hours	Hours to days	15–180 minutes
	May be <1 hour in children		
Frequency	Rare to frequent	Rare to frequent	1–8 per day during clusters
Periodicity	Menstrual migraine	No	Yes
			Average bouts 4–8 weeks
			Average 1 or 2 bouts yearly
Associated features	Nausea in 90%, vomiting in 30%, light and noise sensitivity in 80%	Occasional nausea	Ipsilateral conjunctival injection, tearing, and nasal congestion or drainage
			Ptosis and miosis in 30%
Triggers	Present in 85%	Stress, lack of sleep	Alcohol, nitrates
	Numerous		
Behavior during headache	Still, quiet, tries to sleep	No change	Often paces
Awakens from sleep	Can occur	Rare	Frequently

From Evans RW: Chapter 1. Diagnosis of headaches. In Evans RW, Mathew NT (eds), Handbook of Headache. Philadelphia, Lippincott Williams & Wilkins, 2000, pp. 12–13, with permission.

TABLE 6–5.   FEATURES OF SOME SECONDARY HEADACHES

Headache Type	Epidemiology	Age of Onset	Location	Quality and Severity	Frequency	Associated Features	Comments
Trigeminal neuralgia	4.3/100,000/ year ♀/♂ = 1.6/1	Usually over 40 If <40, consider multiple sclerosis	Unilateral 96% 2nd or 3rd >1st trigeminal division	Stabbing Electrical bursts Burning Last few seconds–<2 minutes	Few to many/ day	Trigger zone present >90%	Usuallly due to vascular compression of V. Scan needed to exclude occasional tumor
Brain tumor	Persons/yr in US 24,000 primaries 170,000 with metastases	Any age	Often bifrontal Unilateral or bilateral Any location	Variable–can be pressure or throbbing Mild–severe	Occasional to daily. Usually progressive	Papilledema in 40% At time of diagnosis, headache present in 30%–70%	Primaries in adults: lung 64%, breast 14%, unknown 8%, melanoma 4%, colorectal 3%, hypernephroma 2%
Pseudotumor cerebri	1/100,000/yr 90% are female 90% are obese	Mean of 30	Often bifronto-temporal but can occur in other locations or be unilateral	Pulsatile Moderate to severe	Daily	Papilledema in 95% Transient visual obscurations in 70% Intracranial noises in 60% VI nerve palsy in 20%	MRI scan preferred to better exclude cortical venous thrombosis and posterior fossa lesions
Subarachnoid hemorrhage	30,000/yr in USA due to saccular aneurysm	Mean of 50	Usally bilateral Any location	Usually severe but can be mild and gradually increasing	Paroxysmal	Often with nausea, vomiting, stiff neck, focal findings, syncope. Stiff neck absent in 36%	CT scan abnormal on first day 95%, third 74%, 1 week 50%. Lumbar puncture may be essential to diagnosis
Temporal arteritis	In age >50, annual incidence 18/ 100,000 ♀/♂ = 3/1	Rare before 50 Mean age of 70	Variable Unilateral or bilateral Often temporofrontal	Often throbbing May be sharp, dull, burning, or lancinating Mild–severe	Intermittent to continuous	50% have PMR Jaw claudication in 38% 50% have absent pulse or tender STA	ESR WNL in up to 36% CRP usually elevated STA biopsy false negative up to 44%
Acute paranasal sinusitis	More common in children (in whom frontal and sphenoid sinusitis are rare) than in adults	Any age	Frontal— forehead, maxillary— cheek, ethmoid— between eyes, sphenoid— variable	Dull, aching Can be severe	Acute defined as lasting from 1 day to 3 weeks	Fever in about 50%. Nasal congestion and purulent nasal drainage usually present (less often in sphenoid)	Well visualized on routine MRI but not on routine CT scan of head. CT scan of the sinuses is the best study.
Subdural hematoma	Occurs in 1% after mild head injury In chronic cases, up to 50% without history of head injury	Any age	Unilateral or bilateral	Mild–severe May be aching, dull, or throbbing	Paroxysmal to constant	50% with normal neuro exam Alteration in consciousness and focal findings may be present	MRI may detect the occasional isodense subdural hematoma which can be missed on CT scan

Abbreviations: CRP = C-reactive protein; ESR = erythrocyte sedimentation rate; PMR = polymyalgia rheumatica; STA = superficial temporal artery; WNR = within normal limits.
From Evans RW: Chapter 1. Diagnosis of headaches. In Evans RW, Mathew NT (eds), Handbook of Headache. Philadelphia, Lippincott Williams & Wilkins, 2000, pp. 14–16, with permission.

infection (infectious mononucleosis, Lyme disease, HIV)

b. Antiphospholipid antibodies (white matter lesions on MRI), complete blood counts and metabolic studies (anemia, renal failure, hypercalcemia), and endocrine studies (hypothyroidism, pituitary tumors)

c. Baseline for monitoring adverse effects of certain medications (e.g., valproic acid or carbamazepine)

9. Lumbar puncture: MRI or CT scan is always performed before a lumbar puncture for the evaluation of headaches, except where acute meningitis is suspected.

a. Lumbar puncture can be diagnostic for meningitis or encephalitis, meningeal carcinomatosis or lymphomatosis, subarachnoid hemorrhage, and high (e.g., pseudotumor cerebri) or low cerebrospinal fluid (CSF) pressure.

b. After neuroimaging, examples where lumbar

puncture is often indicated: first or worst headache; headache with fever or other symptoms or signs suggesting an infectious cause; a subacute or progressive headache (e.g., an HIV-positive patient or a person with carcinoma); and an atypical chronic headache (e.g., to rule out pseudotumor cerebri in an obese woman without papilledema).

TABLE 6–6.   REASONS TO CONSIDER NEUROIMAGING FOR HEADACHES

Temporal and headache features
1. The "first or worst" headache
2. Subacute headaches with increasing frequency or severity
3. A progressive or new daily persistent headache
4. Chronic daily headache
5. Headaches always on the same side
6. Headaches not responding to treatment

Demographics
7. New-onset headaches in patients who have cancer or who test positive for HIV infection
8. New-onset headaches after age 50
9. Patients with headaches and seizures

Associated symptoms and signs
10. Headaches associated with symptoms and signs such as fever, stiff neck, nausea, and vomiting
11. Headaches other than migraine with aura associated with focal neurologic symptoms or signs
12. Headaches associated with papilledema, cognitive impairment, or personality change

From Evans RW: Chapter 1. Diagnosis of headaches. In Evans RW, Mathew NT (eds), Handbook of Headache. Philadelphia, Lippincott Williams & Wilkins, 2000, p. 19, with permission.

TABLE 6–7.   REASONS TO CONSIDER NEUROIMAGING FOR CHILDREN WITH HEADACHES

1. Persistent headaches of less than 6 months duration that do not respond to medical treatment
2. Headache associated with abnormal neurologic findings, especially if accompanied by papilledema, nystagmus, or gait or motor abnormalities
3. Persistent headaches associated with an absent family history of migraine
4. Persistent headache associated with substantial episodes of confusion, disorientation, or emesis
5. Headaches that awaken a child repeatedly from sleep or occur immediately on awakening
6. Family history or medical history of disorders that may predispose one to central nervous system lesions and clinical or laboratory findings suggestive of central nervous system involvement

Data from Medina LS, Pinter JD, Zurakowski D, et al.: Children with headache: clinical predictors of surgical space-occupying lesions and the role of neuroimaging. Radiology 1997;202:819–824.

Bibliography

Evans RW: Headache case studies for the primary care physician. Med Clin North Am, March 2000, in press.

Evans RW, Mathew NT: Handbook of Headache. Philadelphia, Lippincott Williams & Wilkins, 2000.

Lance JW, Goadsby PJ: Mechanism and Management of Headache, 6th ed. Oxford, Butterworth Heinemann, 1998.

Olesen J. Tfelt-Hansen P, Welch KMA, (eds): The Headaches, 2nd ed. Philadelphia, Lippincott Williams & Wilkins, 2000.

Silberstein SD, Lipton RB, Dalessio SJ: Wolff's Headache and Other Head Pain, 7th ed. New York, Oxford University Press, 2001

7 Muscle Weakness

David S. Younger

The diagnosis of muscle weakness is an art that depends on both experience and logical clinical reasoning because it encompasses much of clinical neurology (Table 7–1).

History

1. The history and examination represent the starting point in the diagnosis of a motor disorder of the peripheral nervous system.
2. The goal of the history and examination is twofold: first, to establish the neurologic symptoms and signs, including temporal progression and associated findings, and then to formulate a categorical diagnosis and localize the disease process in a specific motor unit: the spinal cord anterior horn cell, root, peripheral nerve, neuromuscular junction (NMJ), or muscle.
3. It is useful to ask about fatigue, cramps, myalgia, fasciculation, stiffness, and spasms.
   a. Fatigue and myalgia in the absence of specific weakness suggest depression or systemic illness.
   b. Frequent cramping with myalgia is seen in myoadenylate deaminase deficiency. Muscle cramps, aching, and fasciculations can be present in benign cramp-fasciculation syndrome.
   c. Muscle contractures are separated diagnostically from true cramps and dystonic postures or spasms by electromyography (EMG).
   d. Stiffness is exquisitely painful in the stiff-man syndrome and painless when caused by rigidity or spasticity alone in lesions of the extrapyramidal pathways or corticospinal tracts (CST).
4. Patients should also be asked about specific sensory symptoms, and the response should be recorded in their own words. If there is sensory

TABLE 7–1. SCOPE OF THE EVALUATION OF WEAKNESS

1. History
2. Physical examination
3. Family pedigree
4. EMG-NCS
5. Blood studies
6. Lumbar CSF analysis
7. Nerve biopsy
8. Muscle biopsy
9. Neuroimaging studies

Abbreviations: EMG-NCS: electromyography-nerve conduction studies; CSF: cerebrospinal fluid.

involvement, there must be more than a myopathy, and the cause should be sought in a lesion in the peripheral nerves, dorsal root ganglia, or dorsal columns of the spinal cord.

5. The tempo of the disease may provide a clue to the exact cause of weakness.
   a. Fluctuation and variability of weakness over days, weeks, or months is likely to be due to myasthenia gravis (MG).
   b. Precipitous weakness transiently worsening over days is likely due to myoglobinuria and may be the first sign of heritable enzymatic myopathy. In contrast, recurrent attacks of slight to severe weakness lasing a few hours upon awakening, sparing oropharyngeal muscles is usually due to periodic paralysis.
   c. Limb weakness and sensory loss developing over several weeks while a patient is in the intensive care unit is virtually always due to critical illness neuropathy.
   d. Leg weakness beginning in the legs of a young boy and evolving over years is most likely due to Duchenne or Becker muscular dystrophy (DMD and BMD), characterized by deficiency of dystrophin in a muscle specimen; limb-girdle or distal muscular dystrophy characterized by deficiency in one of several sarcoglycans in adolescents and young adults; and inclusion body myositis (IBM) in an older adult of either gender.
6. The rule that proximal or girdle weakness equals myopathy and distal weakness implies neuropathy is useful when distal weakness is accompanied by sensory loss and early loss of tendon reflexes.
7. Clues to the cause of muscular weakness may be obtained in a family pedigree and should include the name, sex, age, and specific symptoms and physical characteristics of similarly affected family members and others with associated neurologic illnesses.
   a. Affected relatives should be examined and photographed, and the records of deceased family members should be reviewed closely.
   b. Although a pedigree may indicate the pattern of inheritance in an affected cohort, it may not be informative if the patient is an index case, or if failure of expressivity of the gene defect leads to a phenotypically normal heterozygote.
   c. The possible modes of single-gene inheritance

include autosomal dominant, autosomal recessive, and X-linked dominant transmission.

8. The distinctive biology of mitochondrial DNA (mtDNA) has added new concepts and terminology to classical mendelian genetics. Mitochondrial disorders are now classified according to whether the gene defect lies in nuclear DNA, mtDNA, or in faulty communication between the two genomes.

   a. The human mitochondrial genome is contained in a tiny molecule of 16,569 base pairs, of which 37 genes encode structural proteins, including subunits of complexes I, III, IV (cytochrome c oxidase), and subunits of complex V.

   b. Several biologic factors explain the heterogeneity of human mitochondrial disease, including the absolute dose of mitochondrial genomes present in specific organs such as brain, heart, and skeletal muscle, depending upon the requirement for oxidative energy; and whether a mutation affects some or all of the mtDNA, leading to varying proportions of mutant mtDNA among tissues over the lifetime of the patient. Such variations explain the appearance of particular syndromes at different ages.

Key Clinical Features

The following should be investigated concerning muscle weakness:

• Fatigue

• Cramps

• Myalgia

• Fasciculation

• Stiffness

• Spasms

• Specific sensory symptoms

• Tempo of the disease (e.g., fluctuation and variability of weakness over days, weeks, or months)

• History of similarly affected family members

Physical Examination

1. A detailed examination is the next step in the elucidation of weakness. It generally begins with an assessment of mental status for memory loss or frank dementia.

2. The examination of cranial motor function includes assessment of ocular motility, strength in facial and neck muscles, and tests for audition, vestibular function, and patterns of speech.

   a. Two useful signs for MG include the lid-twitch sign, elicited by asking the patient to gaze fully downward and then slowly bringing the eyes upward to a straight-ahead position; and Hering's sign, in which ptosis is accentuated by passive opening of the contralateral lid.

   b. Several unmistakable cranial signs of bulbar amyotrophic lateral sclerosis (ALS) usually seen in combination with dysarthria include mentalis muscle twitcing, scalloping and twitching of the tongue, and copious pharyngeal secretions.

3. Individual limb muscles should be examined and graded on a scale of 0 to 5 (Table 7–2).

4. Coordination is tested by rapid successive movements and finger-to-nose pointing.

5. Gait and station testing

   a. A young boy with suspected DMD is asked to rise from a low chair or deep squat, with arms folded on the chest, a maneuver described by Gower and named in his honor.

   b. Children with DMD are asked to stand upright from a seated position, characterized first by pushing with one arm in a bent-forward position while climbing up the legs with both arms.

   c. The patient should be observed erect with both eyes open and closed (Romberg sign), and gait should be assessed while on toes, heels, and walking tandem. Hopping on either foot may also be useful.

6. Sensory exam

   a. Proprioception, vibratory sensation, and light touch sensation subserved by large myelinated sensory nerve fibers should be tested appropriately in the hands and feet.

   b. Thermal and pinprick sensation, subserved by small unmyelinated fibers residing in dermal and epidermal skin tissues, should be tested and rated by the patient.

7. Tendon reflexes are best tested with the patient seated, hands folded in the lap and legs dangling; knee jerks are considered absent after reinforcement. Similarly, ankle reflexes should be tested with the patient kneeling.

   There are unmistakable patterns of neurologic signs that may be crucial to diagnosis and may

TABLE 7–2. GRADING OF LIMB MUSCLE STRENGTH

0: No contraction
1: Flicker or trace of contraction
2: Active movement with gravity eliminated
3: Active movement against gravity
4: Active movement against gravity and resistance
5: Normal power

then direct further evaluation toward the likeliest causes.

a. Focal weakness, wasting, and tendon areflexia, sparing sensation, are classic lower motor neuron (LMN) signs of a primary or secondary lesion of the anterior horn cells or their axons, respectively termed *neuronopathy* and *motor neuropathy*. These lesions further separable by EMG and nerve conduction studies (NCS).

b. Overly brisk reflexes in limbs with LMN signs, accompanied by Hoffmann's sign, Babinski's sign, and clonus, are an unequivocal upper motor neuron (UMN) sign of a lesion in CST.

c. The combination of LMN and UMN signs in a suspected patient makes the clinical diagnosis of ALS "inescapable".

d. UMN signs alone are the presenting feature of spastic paraparesis that most often proves to be due to multiple sclerosis (MS), compressive tumor of the foramen magnum or spinal cord, dural vascular malformation of the cord, cervical spondylotic myelopathy, herniated thoracic nucleus pulposus, hereditary spastic paraplegia (HSP), spinocerebellar ataxia, multisystem atrophy (MSA) syndrome, bilateral strokes, neurosyphilis, vacuolar myelopathy due to retroviral infection, or syringomyelia.

e. Primary lateral sclerosis (PLS), previously eschewed for its lack of proof in life, is an acceptable clinical diagnosis for idiopathic spastic paraparesis of late life when genetic and acquired causes are excluded.

Laboratory Evaluation

1. EMG-NCS studies

a. These studies are necessary in the investigation of suspected myopathy, disorders of the NMJ, peripheral neuropathy, entrapment neuropathies, plexopathy, radiculopathy, and amyotropic lateral sclerosis (ALS).

b. The electrical features of myopathy include normal NCS in association with short-duration low-amplitude motor unit potentials (MUP), with excessive polyphasia, and early rapid recruitment upon submaximal effort.

c. Detailed EMG-NCS studies can separate peripheral neuropathy into demyelinating and axonal forms.

(1) Demyelinating peripheral neuropathy is distinguished by significant slowing of segmental velocities; prolongation of distal and F-wave latencies; motor conduction block, defined as a drop of 50% or more of the proximal compound muscle action potential (CMAP); and absence of spontaneous activity on needle EMG. A reduction of 20% in the CMAP amplitude is strongly suggestive of a block in the absence of abnormal temporal dispersion.

(2) Axonal neuropathy is recognized by normal or mildly slow nerve conduction velocities, reduced CMAP and sensory nerve action potential (SNAP) amplitudes, normal distal latencies, and normal or mildly prolonged F-wave latencies, in association with active or chronic distal spontaneous activity, long-duration MUP, and reduced recruitment pattern in weak muscles.

d. The NMJ disorders are clinically, electrophysiologically, and pathologically heterogeneous.

(1) They have in common loss of the safety factor for NMJ transmission, with an abnormal response to repetitive nerve stimulation.

(2) An abnormal decremental response of 12% or more of successive CMAPs after 3 Hz motor nerve stimulation, with aggravation of the block for several minutes after brief exercise indicates a postsynaptice defect such as MG.

(3) Lambert-Eaton myasthenic syndrome (LEMS) is due to antibodies directed against presynaptic voltage-gated calcium channels, and demonstrates low-amplitude CMAP responses on conventional NCS, which increase by 100% to 200% after 20 Hz or more of repetitive nerve stimulation.

(4) Single-fiber electromyography supplements repetitive nerve stimulation by quantifying transmission at individual end plates while the patient voluntarily activates the muscle fiber under examination. It is a technique that requires strict patient cooperation and examiner proficiency.

(5) Electrodiagnostic studies can provide more accurate information than the clinical examination in the differentiation of a brachial plexus lesion from proximal mononeuritis multiplex or a nerve root lesion, such as in the differentiation of axillary, suprascapular, and musculocutaneous neuropathies, from the C5 root or an upper trunk brachial plexus lesion.

e. Radiculopathy, or root lesion, leads to peripheral motor deficits in a myotomal distribution.

(1) Nerve root impingement caused by intervertebral disc herniation may be accompanied by neuropraxic or axonopathic injury. Because these lesions are proximal to the

dorsal root ganglion, they can be identified when narrowing of the lateral recess or nerve root foramina is recognizable as active denervation, and when F-response latencies are prolonged without alteration of the SNAP.

(2) In practice, F-wave measurements are of limited usefulness because they can only be recorded from a limited number of muscles.

(3) H responses are more sensitive but are similarly restricted to abnormality of the S1 segment.

2. Transcranial magnetic stimulation (TCMS)

a. TCMS is potentially useful in motor disorders associated with primary degeneration of CST such as ALS and PLS.

b. Circular high-power coils are positioned on the scalp, centered over the vertex (Cz) to record CMAP and distal latencies in the arms and over frontal cortex (Fz) for the legs.

c. The motor roots are stimulated with a cathode positioned over C7 and L1.

d. The central motor conduction time (CMCT) is calculated by subtracting the distal motor latencies obtained after nerve root stimulation from those obtained by cortical stimulation.

e. CMAP amplitudes recorded after cortical stimulation are expressed as a percentage of those obtained from root stimulation.

f. An abnormally prolonged CMCT and reduced CMAP amplitudes correlate with the presence of CST involvement in patients with ALS, PLS, and possibly MS

3. Neuroimaging studies

a. Radiologic studies are also important in the laboratory evaluation of patients with weakness.

b. Magnetic resonance imaging (MRI) is the most widely used neuroimaging study for central nervous system (CNS) disorders. The intravenous contrast agent gadopentetate dimeglumine crosses the blood–brain barrier and is associated with few side effects. It shortens T_1 and T_2 relaxation times of spin echo images and accumulates in lesions as areas of increased signal intensity when compared with precontrast images.

c. MRI of the spine has supplanted myelography in the evaluation of patients with spinal cord disorders, and it can be used to image the cross-sectional planes of individual limbs at sites of focal muscle wasting due to myopathy,

and along selected nerves enlarged by lymphomatous infiltrates.

d. MR spectroscopy supplements exercycle ergometry and treadmill protocols in patients with defects of muscle oxidative metabolism.

e. Positron emission tomography complements MRI in the CNS evaluation of mitochondrial encephalomyopathy, Parkinson's disease, MSA, and vasculitis, among other degenerative disorders.

4. Blood tests and antibody assays

a. An elevated serum creatine kinase (CK) is usually the first laboratory abnormality in myopathy, and it is always accompanied by increased levels of serum glutamic-oxaloacetic acid, glutamic-pyruvic acid transaminases, lactate dehydrogenase, and aldolase.

b. The forearm ischemic test is a useful adjunct in the diagnosis of defects of glycogenolytic or glycolytic pathways that impair lactate production during ischemic exercise.

(1) Baseline specimens of CK, ammonia, and lactate are drawn and placed on ice.

(2) The patient vigorously squeezes a rolled-up sphingomanometer cuff, pushing the mercury column to mean arterial pressure, and after deflation of the cuff, sequential specimens are drawn 1, 3, 6, and 10 minutes after 1 minute of ischemic exercise.

(3) Many patients develop severe muscle cramping during exercise and should stop immediately by deflating the cuff to prevent muscle necrosis.

(4) In normal subjects there is a 3- to 5-fold increase in lactate in the first two samples, with a gradual decline to baseline, which does not occur in defects of the glycolytic pathway.

(5) Serum ammonia rises 3- to 5-fold in normal controls and in patients with glycogen metabolism defects.

(6) If the patient's lactate rises after exercise but the ammonia fails to rise significantly, the diagnosis of myoadenylate deaminase deficiency can be considered.

c. Autoimmune serology plays a pivotal role in the diagnosis of NMJ disorders.

(1) Acetylcholine receptor binding, blocking, and modulating antibodies, and striational antibodies and should be tested in patients with MG.

(2) Suspected patients with LEMS should be studied for antibodies to P/Q and N-type voltage-gated calcium channels.

(3) The specific blood studies that should be performed in patients with peripheral neuropathy should be guided by the clinical presentation and postulated etiologic diagnosis.

Tests for anemia, diabetes, renal and hepatic disease, vitamin B_{12} deficiency, thyroid function (thyroxine, triiodothyronine, thyrotropin), monoclonal and polyclonal paraproteinemia (serum protein electrophoresis, immunofixation, quantitative immunoglobulins—IgG, IgA, and IgM), antibodies to hepatitis B and C, antibodies to antinuclear antigen and neutrophilic cytoplasmic antigen, erythrocyte sedimentation rate, cryoglobulinemia, amyloid (Bence Jones proteinuria), and alterations in T and B cell subsets present in lymphoproliferative disorders and human deficiency virus infection (HIV) are all relatively inexpensive and may reveal information at the outset of the evaluation.

(4) The emergence of peripheral neuropathic disorders associated with monoclonal and polyclonal antibodies directed against peripheral nerve antigens has made it possible to consolidate panels of commercially available autoimmune serology according to the suspected diagnosis:

(a) Antibodies to myelin-associated glycoprotein (MAG) are useful in patients with demyelinating sensorimotor neuropathy; IgM, GM1, and GD1b antibodies, in patients with multifocal motor neuropathy (MMN) (which may simulate ALS but differs in the presence of conduction block and shows responsiveness to treatment with intravenous immunoglobulin IVIg and cyclophosphamide)

(b) Polyclonal IgM GM1 antibodies react with GD1a in the acute axonal neuropathy form of Guillain-Barré syndrome (GBS) with preceding *Campylobacter* enteritis

(c) Polyclonal IgG GM1 antibodies with specificity to GQ1b are useful in the Miller-Fisher form of GBS (characterized clinically by areflexia, ataxia, and ophthalmoplegia).

(d) Paraneoplastic serology is useful in the early diagnosis of occult malignancy, which when treated effectively can result in improvement in the associated paraneoplastic neurologic disorder. Anti-Hu or anti-neuronal nuclear antibody type 1–associated paraneoplastic encephalomyelitis and sensory neuropathy, is a primarily sensory disorder; however, up to 40% of affected patients demonstrate anterior horn cell involvement and can present clinically with frank LMN signs.

5. Lumbar puncture

a. Properly performed, lumbar puncture is safe and informative in a variety of disorders that can result in syndromes of weakness.

b. For example, acellular cerebrospinal fluid (CSF) with a raised protein content supports the diagnosis of Kearns-Sayre syndrome of mitochondrial encephalomyopathy, as well as GBS and chronic inflammatory demyelinating polyradiculoneuropathy (CIDP).

c. Pleocytosis and a mild protein elevation occur in poliomyelitis.

d. Patients with suspected active neuroborreliosis should undergo lumbar CSF analysis because virtually all patients with one or more aspects of Garcin's triad of meningitis, cranial neuritis, and radiculitis will likely demonstrate lymphocytosis, intrathecal production of *Borrelia burgdorferi*–specific antibody, and demonstrable organisms by polymerase chain reaction (PCR).

6. Genetic analysis

a. A decade of intensive research in the molecular genetics of motor disease has begun to unravel the nature of the clinical diversity of muscular dystrophy, mitochondrial encephalomyopathy, membrane motor disorders, congenital MG, Charcot-Marie-Tooth (CMT) disorders, and other hereditary neuropathies; HSP, SCA, childhood spinal muscular atrophy, and ALS.

b. These achievements have resulted in more precise diagnosis and genetic counseling through improved carrier detection and prenatal screening.

7. Muscle and nerve biopsy

a. Properly handled, muscle biopsy is especially useful in the routine evaluation of suspected inflammatory myopathy owing to possible polymyositis, dermatomyositis, and IBM; glycolytic and lipid-storage myopathy; muscular dystrophy, mitochondrial encephalomyopathy; myoglobinuria, systemic vasculitis, and sarcoidosis.

b. The muscle chosen for biopsy should be involved clinically and electrophysiologically but not end-stage. Most authorities agree that muscle biopsy should ideally be performed at centers with expertise in neuromuscular disease to assure thorough evaluation.

c. Nerve biopsy provides the necessary histologic proof of certain motor disorders such as peripheral nerve vasculitis, polyglucosan body disease, neurolymphomatosis, and amyloidosis; it also adds precision to the diagnosis and prognosis of CIDP, diabetic neuropathy, MMN; and metachromatic leukodystrophy, Krabbe disease, adrenomyeloneuropathy, and ceroid lipofuscinosis when noninvasive tests of blood, urine, skin, or conjunctiva are uninformative.

(1) The sural and superficial peroneal sensory nerves are the most commonly obtained, often with specimens of underlying soleus and peroneus muscle for analysis of neurogenic changes, or in the case of vasculitis, to maximize the yield of diagnostic lesions.

(2) Motor nerve biopsy is preferable to sensory nerve biopsy in a patient with a motor neuropathy, but it entails more serious operative risk.

Key Tests

- EMG-NCS studies

- Transcranial magnetic stimulation

- Neuroimaging studies

- Blood tests and antibody assays

- Lumbar puncture

- Genetic analysis

- Muscle and nerve biopsy

Bibliography

Younger DS: The diagnosis of progressive flaccid weakness. Semin Neurol 13:241–246, 1993.

Younger DS, Gordon PH: Diagnosis in neuromuscular disease. Neurol Clin 14:135–168, 1996.

Younger DS: Overview. In Younger DS (ed): Motor Disorders. Philadelphia, Lippincott Williams & Wilkins, 1999, pp. 3–17.

8 Gait, Balance, and Falls

William G. Ondo

GAIT AND BALANCE

Gait disorders can be seen in a wide variety of neurologic, musculoskeletal, and medical problems. In all cases careful examination of gait and balance is paramount in obtaining the correct diagnosis. Ancillary gait laboratory analyses are helpful on some occasions. In most cases, treatment depends on the specific diagnosis, although some simple techniques may help poor balance in general. Because treatment is so dependent on the underlying cause, this chapter will mostly concern diagnosis. Furthermore, although gait and balance represent different entities, there is enough overlap that, in this chapter, they will generally be discussed together.

Conceptual Systems Involved in Gait

Afferent

- Vestibular

- Somatosensory

- Visual

Synergistic

- Cerebellum

- Basal ganglia

Efferent

- Entire neurologic axis

- Musculoskeletal system

- Cardiovascular system

Differential Diagnosis

Creating the differential diagnosis of a "gait disorder" is entirely dependent on the clinical assessment and classification of gait phenotype. There are many different ways to classify gait abnormalities; some are based on anatomy, some on severity, and others on physiology. In contrast, the system offered below (see Pathologic Processes Affecting Gait) is designed to facilitate the diagnosis of underlying disease processes.

Pathologic Processes Affecting Gait

Fatiguing

- Medical illnesses (congestive heart failure, pulmonary, arterial insufficiency)

Antalgic

- Orthopedic, arthritic, injury

Spastic (various patterns or combined patterns)

- Hemi-spastic, scissoring, abduction

Parkinsonian

- Parkinson's disease

- Progressive supranuclear palsy

- Cortical basal ganglion degeneration

- Subcortical vascular parkinsonism

- Drug-induced parkinsonism

- Primary gait freezing or gait initiation failure

Frontal Lobe Disorders

- Normal pressure hydrocephalus

- Subcortical vascular disorder

- Primary gait freezing or initiation failure

- Cautious movements

Motor Neuropathy

- Foot drop or flop

Myopathic

- Waddling, hip sway

Dystonic

- Abnormal but patterned excessive movements

Choreatic

- Abnormal and nonpatterned excessive movements

Ataxic

- Cerebellar (wide based, unsteady)

- Vestibular

- Sensory

Psychogenic

• Subjective, unsteady, usually excessive truncal movements

• Fear of walking, usually with clinging

Clinical Evaluation of Gait Disorders

1. Most gait disorders can be diagnosed, or at least classified, on the basis of the patient history and physical examination. Clearly, the most important part of the examination is careful observation of regular gait. Is there hesitation on the initial step, suggesting normal pressure hydrocephalus, gait initiation factor, or possibly other subcortical pathology? Is there reduced arm swing? Reduced unilateral arm swing without overt spasticity is very suggestive of Parkinson's disease (PD). What is the stride length and speed? Is the gait fluid? Is there any asymmetry? Is the patient upright or stooped? How tentative is the motion? Patients with certain pathologies like progressive supra-nuclear palsy (PSP) of Huntington's disease (HD) have particularly cavalier gaits and demonstrate no caution at all, often resulting in falls. Those with PD, frontal lobe disorders, and ataxia may appear more cautious, whereas psychiatric gait disorder patients are the most cautious and often will only ambulate with assistance.

2. Turns are also very revealing. Does the patient make "en bloc" turns that require more than three step, as is seen in PD. Are turns particularly wide based as is seen in ataxic disorders? Do patients turn very quickly and pivot on their heals, as is seen in PSP? Do the feet freeze while turning, as is seen in several frontal lobe and parkinsonian disorders?

3. In some cases, the classification of gait and balance abnormalities can be aided by electrophysiologic testing.

   a. The most common "balance test" is electro-nystagmogram. This test involves placing cool or warm water into the patient's ear canal to elicit an ocululo-vestibular reflex (nystagmus). Therefore, this test is used to evaluate integrity of the peripheral and central vestibular systems.

   b. Computerized posturography testing places patients on a platform and then challenges the balance systems to see how it compensates for changes in visual input and proprioceptive input. A rough anatomic localization of balance deficits can be determined, and several neurodegenerative diseases can be identified from their relatively characteristic patterns of involvement.

   c. Numerous computerized analyses have been developed to help classify gait patterns. Typically, sensors are placed on key body parts and the data are synthesized to report overall gait tendencies. Although promising, gait analysis techniques must be considered investigational.

4. Once a gait pattern is established many ancillary tests may improve specific diagnosis. For example a "frontal lobe" gait pattern would warrant magnetic resonance imaging (MRI) of the brain, whereas a neuropathic or myopathic gait pattern would warrant electromyography.

Examination of Gait/Balance

Balance

• Normal stance

• Tandem stance

• Stand each individual leg

• Normal standing with eyes closed (Romberg)

• Pull testing

Walking/Strength

• Arise from chair without the use of hands

• Arise from chair normally

• Normal walking in open space

• Normal walking in cluttered space, including doorway and turns

• Normal walking with verbal distraction (call the patient's name)

• Walk backwards and in other situations (up or down stairs)

• Walk on toes

Vestibular*

• March in place with eyes closed

• Bárány maneuver

• Walk on foam

*The vestibular examination can be greatly expanded or reduced depending on clinical suspicion of an underlying vestibular disorder.

Clinical: Specific Diseases Associated with Gait Abnormalities

1. The manifestations of gait in **Parkinson's disease** can vary widely, but there are fairly characteristic features. The most common initial sign of gait abnormality in idiopathic PD is reduced unilateral arm swing. This is often not appreciated by the patient. Posture begins to gradually stoop forward, initially at the neck and later in the cervical and lumbar spine. A general reduction in gait speed and stride length then occurs. This is most prominent when the patients turn 180 degrees (en bloc turn). In fact the number of steps required to turn is an easily quantifiable assessment of PD gait. Festination, the appearance that the patient is trying to catch up to the center of gravity, occurs later. Typically, freezing is a later feature. True postural instability and a general poor sense of balance also occur later in the disease. It should be noted that significant gait and balance problems early in the disease course suggest a diagnosis other than idiopathic PD.

   There are no specific medical treatments for PD gait disorders. Some features of PD gait, especially the slowness, arm swing, and stride length will improve with dopaminergic medications. Others, such as forward posture and postural instability, often do not respond to dopaminergic medications. Freezing may respond to visual or audio cueing, or a variety of procedures to change the gait into a more cognitive and less automated paradigm. Examples include stepping over an object or line, walking while bouncing a ball, counting or cadence, exaggerated marching, rocking before taking the initial step, or taking an initial backward step before walking forward.

2. The gait seen in **progressive supranuclear palsy** is much different from that of PD. In general, PSP patients have much worse true balance and fall frequently. Patients are cavalier and don't seem to appreciate their own balance difficulties. Steps are rapid and often of normal size. Arm swing is mostly preserved. Turns are rapid, and patients tend to pivot on a single heel, rather than being slow and "en bloc" as seen in PD. Patients fall forcefully and without bracing themselves, most commonly backwards. Typically after 4 to 5 years of symptoms they become completely unable to walk. It should also be noted that gait abnormalities might presage the characteristic eye findings of PSP by several years.

3. The gait of **normal pressure hydrocephalus** is similar to that of PD, except patients usually have preserved arm swing, and the gait improves after a few steps. The clinical diagnosis of NPH is based on its cardinal features: gait disorder, urine incontinence, and dementia; however, NPH may present with only a single feature, most commonly gait disorder. In fact, gait initiation failure, followed by normal gait once started, may be the only sign in early NPH. MRI of the brain is a good screening test for NPH, but it does not predict response to treatment. Isotope cisternograpy is commonly used to diagnose NPH; however, there are no data to support its use. In fact, the test does not correlate with other predictive tests, nor with surgical shunting outcomes. In contrast, cerebrospinal fluid (CSF) pressure monitoring to assess augmentation of intermittently elevated CSF pressures (B-waves) has been shown to predict a good response to subsequent neurosurgical intervention. Pressure measuring, however, requires invasive and prolonged monitoring techniques, because ultrasound measurements do not seem adequately sensitive. Perhaps the best test for NPH remains CSF drainage through a lumbar puncture needle. With this procedure, 30 to 50 ml of fluid is removed and the gait is reevaluated for improvement. We generally require two consecutive "positive tests" before proceeding to surgical treatment. Ventriculoperitoneal shunt remains the definitive operative procedure for NPH, although lumbar drains are also being used in some centers. The moderate risk of subdural hemorrhage, which is increased in the elderly, must be considered before deciding on this invasive treatment. In some milder cases, serial lumbar punctures may alternatively be considered.

4. The gait of **ataxia** is characterized by a wide base. Normally, the medial malleus of each ambulating foot will converge upon a single line. There is no lateral spread. This rule is usually maintained in parkinsonian gait disorders, even in patients with very poor balance. Patients with ataxic gait, however, abduct their legs and often abduct their arms. They are very conscious of both gait and balance problems. Their gait often appears jerky and seems to require great effort.

   There are hundreds of etiologies that may result in "ataxic" gait, and the diagnosis and treatment depend mostly upon the underlying condition. Many conditions that produce ataxia also have other features that can worsen gait. Therefore it is often necessary to segregate the ataxic component from spasticity, neuropathy, or vestibular confounders. Although several medications have been reported to occasionally help pure ataxic gait (clonazepam, carbamazepam, isoniazid, buspirone), medical management is generally unsatisfactory. Supportive care and gait therapy may benefit some patients.

5. **Acute vestibular disease** can have a profound effect on gait and balance. Most commonly, this results from acute vestibulitis, fistula, Meniere's disease, ischemia, or benign positional vertigo. Patients with these conditions typically have acute true vertigo and may be completely unable to stand. Ambulation classically deviates to the side of the injury, and patients may hyperextend the contralateral leg, thus pushing themselves toward the injured side. To test for less overt vestibular dysfunction, it is useful to have the patient close his or her eyes and march in place (Fukumas test). This will make it possible to observe whether the patient rotates toward the lesioned side. Physiologic testing for vestibular dysfunctions includes an electronystagmogram and computerized posturography. In contrast to acute insults, the body usually compensates for chronic vestibular disease, and gait abnormalities seen in chronic vestibulopathy are often subtle. Therefore, a diagnosis of "vestibular ataxia" is difficult to establish. Patients may have only a sense of poor balance which might be greatly augmented when one of the compensatory balance systems (vision and proprioception) are withdrawn. Therefore, balance problems that present only in the dark or on unsteady surfaces (sand, foam, etc.) suggest vestibular dysfunction.

6. The gait of **motor neuropathy** is usually characterized by foot flop. Weakness in dorsiflexion of the foot causes the anterior foot to touch the ground before the ankle, resulting in two distinct sounds, as if the foot were flopping on the ground. Patients also instinctively raise the leg higher during forward flexion at the hip, which is often referred to as a "steppage" gait. Motor neuropathic gait most commonly results from diffuse motor neuropathies, peroneal neuropathies, or L5 radiculopathies. Specific treatments depend on the underlying pathology; however, the symptom of foot drop may improve with ankle foot orthesis, to maintain a foot position, and gait therapy.

7. In contrast, the gait seen in pure **sensory neuropathy** is less distinct and tends to be ataxic and cautious in nature. Balance difficulties are accentuated when patients close their eyes (Romberg's sign) or walk on unstable surfaces. Sensory loss is likely the most under-recognized contributor to gait disorders and balance problems, especially in the elderly population. It should also be noted that gait disorders might also result from small fiber neuropathies, which are not readily diag-

nosed by standard nerve conduction studies and electromyography. Treatment depends on the underlying etiology.

8. The gait seen in proximal **myopathy** is, classically, waddling. Weakness in the muscles around the pelvic girdle loosens the foundation of the pelvis. Therefore, instead of staying fixed relative to the ground, the ipsilateral side will elevate when that leg pushes off from the ground. The contralateral pelvis will necessarily be depressed, thus resulting in an up and down waddling movement of the hips. Medical management of myopathic gait depends on the underlying pathology.

9. There are several patterns of gait seen in **spasticity**. In all cases the gait appears to be stiff, labored, and usually arrhythmic. Generally, the legs are overextended, such that the toe hits or drags against the ground. Unilateral leg spastic gait is most commonly seen after stroke, head trauma, brain tumor, or other lateralized brain lesions. Classically, the leg circumducts to compensate for the greater functional length caused by decreased knee flexion, hip flexion, and foot dorsiflexion. In contrast, bilateral pediatric spasticity, as seen in static encephalopathy, often has a "scissoring" property. The legs are overly adducted and thus rub against each other. Almost any combination of these abnormal movements is possible. There are many treatments for spastic gait; however, they generally target the underlying spasticity. Numerous muscle relaxant medications, botulinum toxin injections, phenol injection, intrathecal baclofen infusions, and a variety of surgical procedures all play a role in the management of this common condition.

10. The gait seen with **dystonia** is often dramatic, or even bizarre, and can be mistaken as psychogenic in origin. Dystonia gait usually develops indolently in children, although onset can occur in adulthood. The cause may be idiopathic, as seen in a variety of genetic dystonias, or it may be secondary to other neurologic conditions such as Wilson's disease, Hallervorden-Spatz disease, or CNS injury, in which case spasticity may be concurrent. Dystonic gait is patterned. The patient may demonstrate excessive plantar flexion and inversion, excessive hip flexion, or any other stereotyped movement; however that movement will be fairly consistent. Importantly, the gait usually improves when the patient is forced to walk backwards or in an altered environment, such as up stairs. Treatment options are similar to those for spasticity, except that lesioning or deep brain stimulation of the globus pallidus

internus may dramatically improve gait in severe cases.

11. Two different gait patterns might be considered to have a "psychiatric" origin.

   a. Cautious gait of the elderly is best described by picturing someone walking on a slippery surface such as wet ice. The legs and arms are moderately abducted. The body is stiff. The gait is slow and the steps are usually raised slightly so that the feet touch the ground at a more acute angle. Most commonly this is seen in patients who have some minor gait abnormalities or who have fallen, such that they are no longer confident in their balance. In extreme examples, patients develop a true phobia about walking unassisted. They will only stand and walk if they are able to hold onto objects. In the clinic they will be subjectively unable to walk until some assistance is offered. This may be a token assistance such as a single finger that the patient can touch. The patient is then able to walk normally. Little formal data exist on this relatively common problem; however, in our experience this typically occurs in elderly women, often after they have experienced a fall. We have had good treatment success with reassurance and very low doses of benzodiazepines, especially alprazolam.

   b. The second classic psychogenic gait disorder is sometimes referred to as *astasia without abasia*. This is seen in younger patients and seems to reflect either a conversion disorder or malingering. While standing, patients will typically sway back and forth at the hip and trunk, often while only standing on the leg ipsilateral to the side toward which they are leaning. Arms may or may not be abducted but often quickly gyrate. Pull testing typically results in a quick body jerk and more arm gyrating, very different from what would be seen in a parkinsonian condition. The most characteristic feature is that the patients actually demonstrate excellent balance as they maintain the precarious positions that they assume. The typical diagnostic maneuvers used to test features of balance (tandem stance eye closing, etc.) may or may not worsen subjective balance, but they seldom worsen the "objective signs." The gait of these patients is often characterized by irregular leg crossing and knee dipping (flexion at the knee). Patients may fall during gait or balance testing, but these falls are typically controlled and swooning. Treatment can be difficult, but

depends upon resolution of the underlying psychiatric disorder.

12. **Orthostatic tremor** presents with subjective balance problems, which may at first appear psychogenic. Patients report marked difficulties with standing but have difficulty explaining why they feel so unsteady. In contrast, they usually have no problem with walking. Casual examination reveals only a wide-based stance with essentially normal gait. Upon palpation of the calves, one can usually feel a fine high-frequency tremor. This is usually not visible, however, electrophysiology will confirm a 14- to 16-Hz tremor. Patients may have a family history of essential tremor or may demonstrate some arm tremor, but they often have no other feature suggestive of any tremor disorder. Therefore the correct diagnosis often remains cryptic for many years. Treatment options include clonazepam or other benzodiazepines, gabapentin, and phenobarbital. Although these medications are usually initially effective, the tremor often returns over time.

13. The gait seen with **chorea** may also be misdiagnosed as psychogenic. These patients typically have excessive arm movements, characterized mostly by wrist flexion and backward arm deviation rather than abduction. The feet placement is alternatively wide-based, normal, or scissoring. In fact this variability of arm and leg movement is characteristic of choreatic gait. Often the chorea seen in Huntington's disease is first demonstrable during ambulation. Chorea is best pharmacologically treated with dopamine antagonists, tetrabenazine (a dopamine-release inhibitor), or benzodiazepines.

14. Other subcortical abnormalities, most commonly **small-vessel ischemia** can produce varied gait patterns, often similar to NPH. Patients, however, may also have a parkinsonian gait, although they will not usually have such other parkinsonian signs as rest tremor or arm bradykinesia. Small-vessel ischemia is sometimes referred to as *vascular parkinsonism,* or *lower body parkinsonism.* Subcortical ischemia may also mimic PSP or ataxia. Although, this area of research is less well established, it is clear that subcortical white matter changes strongly correlate with gait disorders in the elderly. Our own experience suggests that subcortical ischemia, often in conjunction with arthritic problems, neuropathy, reduced vision, or any other condition that can affect gait, is one of the most common causes of moderate gait disorders in the elderly. Treatment of subcortical ischemia is untested and largely supportive; however, some patients may improve with large-volume CSF removal.

15. This chapter will not cover the gait abnormalities from orthopedic causes. Most hip, knee, and foot problems result in a limp, in which patients clearly seem to volitionally favor one side over the other and have an antalgic component, which is usually absent in neurogenic gait disorders.

Key Parkinsonian Gait Disorders

- Parkinson's disease
- Progressive supranuclear palsy
- Cortical basal degeneration
- Vascular parkinsonism
- Drug-induced parkinsonism
- Gait initiation failure

FALLS

Epidemiology

1. Falls in the elderly represent a major cause of direct morbidity and mortality.
2. Approximately 30% of all people over the age of 65 years fall at least once per year. In 10% of these falls, the patient requires hospitalization, most commonly for fracture. The sequelae of falls constitute the sixth leading cause of death in the elderly, and falls are reported to contribute to nursing home placement in 40% of all cases. Significant psychosocial disability, resulting in social isolation, also complicates falls.
2. The greatest risk factor predicting falls is excessive medication use, especially sedative drugs. Other contributing factors include dementia, medical conditions that impair balance or gait or that cause weakness, and possibly hypotension. Furthermore these risk factors are additive, such that the yearly risk of falls in patients with multiple risk factors may exceed 70%.

Treatment and Prevention

1. Given the severe sequelae of falls in the elderly, preventive measures should be emphasized. Mul-

tiple studies have shown that interventional programs aimed at reducing fall risk factors (reduce sedative medication use, provide gait training and physical therapy, remove environmental risks) do in fact reduce the risk of falls in both community and institutional settings.

2. Specific measures to reduce the risk of injury from a fall can also be used. Recently, a simple hip pad was shown to greatly reduce the incidence of hip fracture after a fall. Treatment of osteoporosis may also reduce fractures.

Causes of Falls in the Elderly

- Medications
  - Benzodiazepines
  - Phenothiazine
  - Antidepressants
- Dementia
- Known disorders of gait/balance/lower limbs
- Hypotension
- Subcortical white matter changes

Bibliography

Kannus P, Parkkari J, Niemi S, et al.: Prevention of hip fracture in elderly people with use of a hip protector. N Engl J Med 23;343:1506–1513, 2000.

Nutt J: Gait and balance disorders: a syndrome approach. In Jankovic J, Tolosa E, (eds): Parkinson's Disease and Movement Disorders. Baltimore, Williams & Wilkins, 1998;687–699.

Stolze H, Kuhtz-Buschbeck JP, Drucke H, et al.: Comparative analysis of the gait disorder of normal pressure hydrocephalus and Parkinson's disease. J Neurol Neurosurg Psychiatry 70:289–297, 2001.

Tinetti M, Speechley M, Ginter S: Risk factors for elderly persons living in the community. N Engl J Med 318:1701–1707, 1988.

Tinetti M, Baker D, McAvay G, et al.: A multifactorial intervention to reduce the risk of falling among elderly people living in the community. N Engl J Med 331:821–827, 1994.

9 Fatigue

Russell C. Packard

Definition

1. Fatigue is defined as an overwhelming sense of tiredness, lack of energy, or feeling of exhaustion. Fatigue is a nonspecific, subjective sensation of ill-being that may reflect emotional, social, or physical dysfunction. There are no specific signs of fatigue.
2. Fatigue should be distinguished from lack of energy associated with depression or generalized weakness.

Etiology

1. Most complaints of fatigue have a nonorganic cause. Depression is the most common diagnosis and occurs in 20% to 30% of cases. Overall, 50% to 60% of cases will be functional or psychological, and 40% to 50% will be physical.
2. Fatigue can be chronic and debilitating in many patients with certain medical or neurologic conditions.
3. Fatigue of recent onset may be an important sign of underlying illness or exacerbation of a known illness.

Key Clinical Features

- Depression is the most common cause.
- Approximately 50% of cases will be functional or psychological.
- Diagnosis is based mainly on history.

Differential Diagnosis

1. Severe anemia
2. Hypothyroidism
3. High or low glucose
4. Electrolyte disturbance.
   a. Low potassium
   b. High calcium
5. Adrenal insufficiency
6. Chronic inflammation
   a. Infection
      (1) Mononucleosis
      (2) Tuberculosis
      (3) Human immunodeficiency virus
      (4) Viral hepatitis
      (5) Lyme disease
   b. Autoimmune
      (1) Giant cell arteritis
      (2) Systemic lupus erythematosus
7. Medication (side effects)
   a. Antihypertensive
   b. Beta blockers
   c. Anticonvulsants
   d. Pain medication
   e. Antidepressants
   f. Benzodiazepines
   g. Other psychiatric medications
8. Occult malignancy
9. Cardiovascular disease
10. Mood disorder: Major depression
    a. Low energy
    b. Early morning awakening
    c. Poor appetite
    d. Stressors
    e. Family history
11. Sleep disorders
    a. Sleep apnea
    b. Excessive daytime sleepiness
12. Chronic Fatigue syndrome
    a. Genuine but poorly understood syndrome
    b. Severe fatigue, generally persistent for at least 6 months
    c. Fatigue interferes with daily function and becomes worse with exertion.
    d. There is an absence of any identifiable medical or psychiatric etiology (although concomitant depression is not unusual).
       (1) Impaired short-term memory
       (2) Unrefreshing sleep
       (3) Headaches, often daily
       (4) Muscle pain/overlapping fibromyalgia
       (5) Sore throat
       (6) Post-exertional malaise
13. Specific neurologic conditions
    a. Multiple sclerosis (MS)
       (1) Fatigue is a problem for 80% to 90% of patients.

(2) Fatigue does not correlate with patient's age, gender, or neurologic impairment.

(3) Fatigue may overlap with depression.

(4) Heat worsens fatigue.

(5) Amantadine or modafinil maybe helpful.

b. Parkinson's disease (PD)

(1) One-third of PD patients report fatigue as the most disabling symptom.

(2) Fatigue doesn't necessarily correlate with disease severity.

(3) Fatigue doesn't vary with time of day.

c. Narcolepsy

d. Chronic daily headache

e. Post-polio syndrome

f. Traumatic brain injury (TBI)

(1) a significant complaint in 60% of patients

(2) fatigue doesn't correlate with location of neuropathology

(3) also seen with mild TBI and/or post-concussive syndrome. Modafinil (Provigil) may be helpful for fatigue associated with TBI.

Neurologic Conditions Associated with Fatigue

• Multiple sclerosis

• Parkinson's disease

• Narcolepsy

• Post-polio syndrome

• Traumatic brain injury

• Chronic daily headache

Laboratory Testing

1. Complete blood test
2. Thyroid function tests
3. Electrolytes
4. Liver function panel
5. Erythrocyte sedimentation rate
6. Antinuclear antibody
7. Urinalysis

Treatment

1. Treatment should be individualized. Many factors may contribute to fatigue, from overwork to a significant medical or neurologic condition. If there is an underlying illness, this should be treated.

2. Listen to the patient; educate, and reassure. Assist the patient to reduce or manage stressors.

3. Psychotherapy or psychiatric consultation may be appropriate.

4. Medication use needs to be assessed and modified (if possible) if fatigue is a side effect.

5. Medication considerations for treatment:

a. Stimulants

(1) Pemoline (Cylert)

(2) Methylphenidate (Ritalin)

b. Antidepressants: Try the least sedating antidepressants first (selective serotonin reuptake inhibitors)

c. Other

(1) Amantadine may be helpful for fatigue associated with MS.

(2) Modafinil is helpful for excessive daytime sleepiness associated with narcolepsy. May be helpful for fatigue related to MS.

Key Treatment

• Help patient to reduce or manage stressors.

• Psychotherapy or psychiatric consultation if appropriate

• Medications (as appropriate): stimulants, antidepressants

Bibliography

American Academy of Disability Evaluating Physicians: Position paper: chronic fatigue syndrome: impairment and disability issues. Disability 8:1–12, 1999.

Chen AL: Fatigue. In Rakel RE (ed): Saunders Manual of Medical Practice. Philadelphia, W.B. Saunders, 2000; pp. 1415–1417.

Elovic E: Use of Provigil for underarousal following TBI. J Head Trauma Rehabil 15:1068–1071, 2000.

Krupp LB, Coyle PK, Sliwinski M: Fatigue. In Sage JI, Mark MH (eds): Practical Neurology of the Elderly. New York, Marcel Dekker, 1996; pp. 377–398.

Rammohan KW, Rosenberg JH, et al.: Provigil (modafinil): Efficacy and safety for the treatment of fatigue with multiple sclerosis. Paper presented at American Academy of Neurology Annual Meeting. San Diego, April 29–May 2, 2000.

10 Memory and Praxis Complaints

David S. Geldmacher

Introduction

At first glance, memory and praxis seem unrelated. However, amnestic disorders can be thought of as a failure of declarative memory (knowing "what"), while apraxia can be conceptualized as a disorder of procedural memory (knowing "how"). Memory disorders tend be associated with bilateral cerebral lesions. Apraxia is more often associated with unilateral hemispheric lesions.

Amnestic Disorders

Most amnestic disorders involve impaired declarative memory. In general "episodic memory," or memory for events directly experienced by the individual is most impaired in people with memory complaints. "Semantic memory"—knowledge of word meanings and facts—tends to be better preserved.

Memories must be formed into a mental representation. This process is known as *encoding*. Subsequently memories are stored, i.e., consolidated and indexed for later use. Retrieval is the process of recalling stored information and bringing it into consciousness when needed. When memory encoding or storage is poor, the period of amnesia progressively increases with the passage of time. This is known as *anterograde amnesia*. An example of anterograde amnesia would be the inability to form new memories after bilateral temporal lobe lesions. Retrograde amnesia is the loss of previously remembered information. This is by necessity a retrieval problem. An example of retrograde amnesia is the loss of memories for events occurring in the month before a serious traumatic brain injury. Retrograde amnesia that is not associated with a period of anterograde amnesia is exceptionally rare in neurologic disorders, and often warrants psychiatric evaluation.

"Short-term memory loss" is a frequent complaint but is somewhat of a misnomer. If an individual fails to encode or store information in memory, then it cannot be recalled in either the short or long term. Lapses in memory, such as forgetting where the car keys are located, could represent deficient encoding, storage, or retrieval and are therefore nonspecific. If the location is susequently remembered, the lapse was due to failed retrieval at the time of the lapse. This is common with mental distraction or other preoccupations at the time

of attempted recall. When intermittent, such lapses are of low clinical significance.

1. Examination
   a. Digit span repetition assesses immediate memory, which is more properly considered attentional capacity. This is a prerequisite for encoding.
   b. Three-word recall after distraction assesses both storage and retrieval.
      (1) Intact recall without cuing represents normal encoding, storage, and retrieval.
      (2) Failure to recall after distraction does not differentiate poor storage from poor retrieval.
      (3) Improved recall with cueing or recognition from lists suggests impaired retrieval.
      (4) Using long and short delays can assess the rate of forgetting.
   c. Most bedside memory testing is verbally mediated. If there is suspicion of nonverbal memory disorder, hide an object (e.g., a reflex hammer) in the examination room while cuing the patient to remember its location. After a delay and distraction (usually other portions of the neurologic exam) ask the patient to recall the location of the hidden object.

Key Clinical Findings

- Digit span repetition assesses immediate memory or attentional capacity.

- Three-word recall after distraction assesses both storage and retrieval.

2. Neuroanatomical localization
   a. Bilateral cerebral hemispheric damage is generally necessary for significant amnesia. Commonly involved areas are the mesial temporal lobes (including the hippocampus and entorhinal cortex), the mammillary bodies, and the fornix. Involvement of the dorsomedial and paramedian thalamic nuclei may also lead to significant amnesia. Anterograde amnesia is

predominant, but there can be retrograde components.

    b. Paramedian basal forebrain damage involving the septal nuclei, nucleus accumbens, substantia innominata, and orbitofrontal areas can also cause an amnestic syndrome.

    c. Unilateral lesions can lead to clinically detectable amnesia, but these tend to be modality specific—e.g., verbal memory deficits with left hemisphere lesions and nonverbal memory difficulties with right hemisphere lesions.

3. Differential diagnosis

    a. Degenerative

      (1) Alzheimer's disease is the most common degenerative dementia. It is associated with extensive bilateral synaptic loss in hippocampal formation structures and association cortices.

      (2) Other forms of degenerative dementia (e.g., frontotemporal degeneration) tend to have prominent nonmemory symptoms early in the course, even though the complaint may be "memory loss."

    b. Epileptic

      (1) Temporal lobe epilepsy is associated with sclerotic changes in hippocampal structures and may result in memory symptoms.

      (2) Generalized seizures disrupt encoding and storage of information. Individuals with generalized seizures are therefore highly unlikely to recall events during their spells. Recall of generalized seizure events is suggestive of psychogenic seizure.

    c. Infectious

      (1) Herpes simplex encephalitis selectively destroys temporal lobe structures. Survivors frequently have severe persistent amnesia.

    d. Metabolic/Nutritional

      (1) The classic metabolic disturbance associated with amnesia is Wernicke-Korsakoff syndrome. Wernicke's encephalitis is caused by thiamine deficiency, often—but not obligately—associated with alcoholism. One late sequela is Korsakoff's psychosis, which represents a dense, permanent anterograde amnesia. Its lesion site is controversial, but it involves mammillary bodies, dorsomedial thalamus, or both.

      (2) A variety of acute metabolic disturbances, ranging from anoxia to uremia, cause acute delirium. Delirium, often called *metabolic encephalopathy* by neurologists, is defined by abnormalities of attention and arousal. These deficits prevent proper encoding and storage of new information, so delirious patients frequently have no recall of the delirious episode or circumstances preceding it. In addition, they may demonstrate poor recall from permanent memory stores during the acute delirium.

      (3) Chronic metabolic abnormalities, such as vitamin B_{12} deficiency or hypothyroidism can cause dementia with memory loss. Other systemic or neuropsychiatric features associated with these deficiencies are almost always present.

    e. Neoplastic

      (1) Intra-axial tumors affecting temporal lobe white matter or thalamocortical pathways can lead to amnesia, but it is not the typical presenting symptom.

      (2) Extra-axial tumors arising from the sphenoid wing (e.g., meningioma) can disrupt the function of mesial temporal lobe structures and lead to memory disturbances.

      (3) Paraneoplastic limbic degeneration has been described as a source of amnesia, but behavioral symptoms, rather than memory loss, typically predominate.

    f. Psychiatric

      (1) Neurologic disorders do not cause amnesia for self-identity while other memories are preserved.

      (2) Patients with dissociative disorders like "fugue states" may appear to be amnestic.

      (3) Depression, mania, and anxiety all reduce attentional function and may result in memory complaints because adequate attention is vital to encoding, storage, and retrieval.

    g. Trauma

      (1) The exact localization of lesions that cause memory loss with brain trauma may be difficult to determine. Closed-head injuries are commonly associated with bilateral frontal and temporal lobe contusions. In addition, diffuse axonal injuries related to shearing forces within the brain can lead to disconnections in memory circuitry. In rare circumstances, penetrating injuries have been known to cause a discrete amnestic disorder.

      (2) Traumatic brain injury causes both anterograde and retrograde amnesia. The duration of retrograde amnesia can provide a surrogate indicator of injury severity.

    h. Vascular

      (1) Infarctions involving the distal territory of

the posterior cerebral arteries and affecting mesial temporal and thalamic structures are the most common vascular cause of persistent memory complaints. Very small, discrete infarctions within the thalamus can cause an amnestic syndrome.

(2) Severe anoxia/hypoxia leads to permanent but selective neuronal loss in the CA1 cell field of the hippocampus, with resultant amnesia. Generally, the severity of anoxia required for this insult will also lead to other neurologic deficits.

(3) Ruptured anterior cerebral or anterior communicating artery aneurysms result in extensive destruction of orbitofrontal cortex and basal forebrain structures, leading to persistent amnesia, often with confabulation.

i. Unknown etiology

(1) Transient global amnesia causes a dense anterograde amnesia, typically 24 hours or less in duration. Recall of remote information (name, family members) is preserved, but formation of new memories is completely obliterated during the spell. Some retrograde amnesia, for items hours to days in the past is common.

Apractic Disorders

Apraxia is defined as a loss of motor skill or gestural communication that is not explained by weakness, ataxia, sensory loss, poor comprehension, or inattention. It is commonly seen in association with aphasia. Several subtypes of apraxia have been described. Distinguishing between them has localizing value.

1. Types

a. *Ideomotor apraxia* is an inability to reproduce specific movements either in response to command or by mimicry. Patients may be able to make the same movements spontaneously. It has been conceptualized as a loss of the "motor engram" or memory trace for learned movements.

b. *Conceptual apraxia* is a term used to describe a loss of tool use and knowledge. Patients with this problem may not, for example, recognize that essential properties of a hammer include a hard, heavy mass at the end of a lever-like handle. This is rarely evaluated in clinical settings.

c. *Ideational apraxia* is seen as a loss of ability to carry out a sequence of movements related to a single larger task, e.g., lighting a cigarette. From the theoretical perspective this is more

appropriately considered a deficit in sequencing or executive function, rather than a loss of skill knowledge.

d. *Limb-kinetic apraxia* involves impaired positioning of the body part in space, like putting an arm into the second sleeve of a garment beyond one's back. Truncal apraxia has been used to describe the same deficit when apparent in the trunk. The deficit is probably not a result of a loss of skill knowledge, but rather represents motor planning problems or deficits in sensorimotor integration.

e. *Constructional apraxia* is a term used to describe poor visuospatial design copying or mimicry of nongestural hand postures. It is not closely related to other apraxias at the conceptual level. Constructional apraxia is better thought of as a dysexecutive state or the end result of a spatial agnosia.

Types of Apraxia

- Ideomotor
- Conceptual
- Ideational
- Limb-kinetic
- Constructional

---

2. Examination

a. Apraxia is assessed by asking the patient to demonstrate everyday activities in pantomime.

b. Different tasks should be used for the dominant and nondominant hand. For example, the patient may be asked to pretend to use a hammer to strike a nail with the dominant hand, and demonstrate the motions of a key opening a lock with the nondominant hand.

c. The spatial integration of motor activity can be assessed by asking that a two-handed task, such as slicing an imaginary loaf of bread, be performed. This task can also be used to evaluate the tool knowledge lost in conceptual apraxia, e.g., the sawing motion needed for cutting bread.

d. Limb-kinetic or truncal apraxia is usually evident as difficulty in positioning body parts during examination.

e. Constructional apraxia is assessed by asking the patient to copy a design like overlapping pentagons or a three-dimensional cube figure.

3. Neuroanatomical localization

a. Ideomotor apraxia represents a loss of the motor engrams or the connections between the engrams and the motor cortex, which will execute the movement. The engrams appear to localize to the region of the supramarginal and angular gyri of the language-dominant hemisphere. The outflow paths traverse to ipsilateral premotor and supplementary motor areas, where they synapse and branch to the same regions contralaterally. Ideomotor apraxia limited to the nondominant limbs may represent a corpus callosum lesion.

b. Conceptual apraxia has not been well localized. It often accompanies ideomotor apraxia with left parietal lesions, and it is sometimes seen in Alzheimer's disease, which frequently affects parietal association cortex.

c. Ideational apraxia, when not caused by conceptual problems, represents a dysexecutive state most likely localizing to frontal-subcortical circuits. Circuits involving dorsolateral frontal-cortex are the most likely to be affected.

d. Limb-kinetic apraxia may be difficult to distinguish from motor deficits. Premotor cortical regions contralateral to the disturbed limb are most likely affected, but somatosensory association cortex may also be involved.

e. Constructional apraxia is generally associated with right hemisphere posterior parietal dysfunction. Depending on the task chosen, left parietal lesions may produce similar deficits.

4. Causes

a. Vascular: An overwhelming majority of acute-onset apraxia is associated with cerebral infarction.

b. Degenerative: Alzheimer's disease can present with a slowly evolving syndrome including multiple apraxia subtypes, even before memory or other cognitive difficulties are evident. Corticobasal degeneration is characterized by prominent ideomotor apraxia.

c. Neoplasm: Primary intraxial brain tumors may undercut parietal cortex or disrupt white matter tracts carrying praxis information from parietal regions to premotor areas.

Bibliography

Bauer RM, Tobias B, Valenstein E: Amnesic disorders. In Heilman KM, Valenstein E (eds): Clinical Neuropsychology, 3rd ed. New York, Oxford University Press, 1993: 523–602.

Devinsky O. Behavioral Neurology: 100 Maxims. St. Louis, Mosby-Year Book, 1992:131–153, 161–166.

Heilman KM, Gonzales Rothi LJ: Apraxia. In Heilman KM, Valenstein E, (eds): Clinical Neuropsychology, 3rd ed. New York, Oxford University Press, 1993:141–164.

Markowitsch HJ: Memory and amnesia. In Mesulam M-M (ed): Principles of Behavioral and Cognitive Neurology, 2nd ed. New York, Oxford University Press, 2000:257–293.

11 Speech Disorders

David B. Rosenfield

Definition

Speech is motor output. *Speech compromise* refers to a deficiency in the way that speech sounds. *Language compromise* involves errors in syntax, word choice, or how the sounds of speech are put together (aphasia). Talking with a paralyzed tongue produces speech compromise. Being unable to put together a sentence with appropriate choice of words and appropriate grammar renders one aphasic.

1. *Communication* versus *Speech* versus *Language*
   a. Animals have a system of communication.
   b. Human beings have a system of language.
   c. Animals lack a generative grammar.
   d. Humans have a generative grammar.
   e. The brain of an animal must learn to control sound output, just as the brain of a human must learn to orchestrate the sounds of language (speech).
2. The speech motor control system in humans is controlled by the brain. It has multiple neuromotor components pertaining to the
   a. Respiratory system
   b. Articulatory system
      (1) Cranial nerve V
      (2) Cranial nerve VII
      (3) Cranial nerve IX
      (4) Cranial nerve X
      (5) Cranial nerve XII
   c. Phonatory system (*phonation* refers to sound production from the larynx.)
      (1) Larynx
      (2) Vagal nerve

Pathophysiology

1. Dysarthria
   a. Implies a problem of articulation only, but can include compromise of phonation or resonance (how sounds are altered in the cavity between the larynx and the vocal fold and the lip/nares; can be hyponasal or hypernasal.)
   b. May involve compromise of brain, brainstem, cerebellum, nerve, neuromuscular junction, or muscle. Any disease affecting these regions can produce dysarthria (see Causes of Dysarthria).

Causes of Dysarthria

- Myopathy
- Myositis
- Myasthenia gravis
- Neuropathy
- Motor neuron disease
- Cerebellar disease
- Tumors of brain and brainstem
- Parkinson's disease
- Other movement disorders

---

2. Speech signs in Parkinson's disease
   a. Weak phonation
   b. Minimal variation in pitch
   c. Low volume
   d. Hoarseness
   e. Accelerated rate
   f. Repetitive dysfluencies
   g. Imprecise consonants
3. Speech signs in cerebellar disease
   a. Phonation may be associated with tremor and variations in loudness.
   b. Irregular articulatory breakdown
   c. Imprecise consonants
   d. Sometimes, excessive and equal stress in all syllables of words
4. Speech signs in motor neuron disease
   a. Strained phonation
   b. Harsh, wet, and sometimes fluttering sounds during vowel prolongation
   c. Hypernasal
   d. Slowed articulation
   e. Imprecise consonants
   f. Short phrases
   g. Distorted vowels
5. The effect of fifth cranial nerve (trigeminal) lesion on speech output
   a. Normal phonation
   b. Normal velopharyngeal function

c. Weak mandibular muscles

d. Imprecise vowels and consonants

6. Lesion of seventh cranial nerve (facial) affecting speech

   a. Normal phonation

   b. Normal velopharyngeal function

   c. Weak orbicularis orbis, causing difficulty in producing /p/ sounds

   d. Imprecise vowels

   e. Imprecise labial consonants (/p/, /b/).

7. Lesion of tenth cranial nerve (vagus) affecting speech

   a. Phonation hoarse and breathy

   b. Volume low

   c. Speech is hypernasal if the lesion is above the pharyngeal branch.

8. Lesion of twelfth cranial nerve (hypoglossal) affecting speech

   a. Normal phonation

   b. Normal velopharyngeal function

   c. Weak tongue on side ipsilateral to lesion, causing lateralization of tongue to side of lesion, atrophy, and fasciculations

   d. Drooling

   e. Imprecise vowels

   f. Imprecise lingual consonants

9. Spasmodic dysphonia

   a. Effortful, strained speech, often associated with a sensation of strain

   b. Can be associated with laryngeal tremor, producing phonatory tremor (demonstrated on sustained vocalization of /ee/ sound), laryngeal dystonia, and other movement disorders

---

Muscles that Abduct Vocal Folds

• Thyroarytenoid

• Interarytenoid

• Lateral cricothyroid

• Lateral cricoarytenoid

• Posterior cricoarytenoid

Causes of Bilateral Abductor Vocal Fold Paralysis

• Thyroidectomy

• Neck malignancy

• Brainstem stroke

• Guillain-Barré syndrome

• Demyelinating disease

---

10. Effect of myopathy/myositis on speech

    a. Hoarse phonatory output

    b. Breathy

    c. Diplophonic

    d. Low volume

    e. Hypernasal vowels; consonants can be compromised

11. Speech characteristics of corticobasal ganglionic degeneration

    a. Dysfluency

    b. Non-fluent-like aphasia

    c. Phonological errors

    d. Oral apraxia

    e. Buccofacial apraxia

12. Dysfluency

    a. Developmental stuttering has an adult prevalence slightly greater than 1%.

       (1) Developmental stutterers are dysfluent at the beginning of sentences and phrases

       (2) Developmental stutterers are more fluent when their speech is markedly slowed. They do not stutter when they sing.

    b. Acquired stuttering

       (1) Occurs with damage to either brain hemisphere in just about any location

       (2) Damage is usually mild.

       (3) May result from stroke, vasculitis, inflection, tumor, or trauma

       (4) Dysfluencies occur throughout the sentence, as opposed to at the beginning of sentences and phrases; stutter when they sing

       (5) Prognosis: good when damage is to one hemisphere; poor, if damage is to both hemispheres.

    c. Cluttering

       (1) Characterized by excessive speed, repetitions, interjections, altered rhythm of

speech, and inconsistent articulatory disturbances

(2) Many have errors in grammar; clutterers are hyperactive, and have poor concentration

(3) The speaker is usually not as distraught by the speech as are listeners.

d. Palilalia

(1) Compulsive repetition of phrases or words with reiteration at increasing speed and with a decrescendo volume

(2) Seen in post-encephalitic Parkinson's disease, idiopathic Parkinson's disease, pseudobulbar palsy

Bibliography

Damasio AR, Damasio AH: Aphasia and the neural basis of language. In Mesulam M-M (ed): Principles of Behavioral and Cognitive Neurology, 2nd ed. New York, Oxford University Press, 2000, pp. 294–315.

Mega MS, Alexander NP, Cummings JL, Benson DF: The aphasias and related disturbances. In Joint RJ, Griggs RC (eds): Baker's Clinical Neurology on CD-ROM. Philadelphia, Lippincott Williams & Wilkins, 2000.

Rosenfield DB, Barroso AO: Difficulties with speech and swallowing. In Bradley WG, et al. (eds): Neurology and Clinical Practice, 3rd ed. Boston, Butterworth-Heinemann, 2000, pp 171–186.

Rosenfield DB: Stuttering. In Schachter SC, Davinsky O (eds): Behavorial Neurology and the Legacy of Norman Geschwind. Philadelphia, Lippincott-Raven, 1997, pp. 101–114.

12 Language Disorders

David B. Rosenfield

Definitions

1. Language: Set of symbols constrained in their interrelationship by perception, production, and central processing rules. Consists of
   a. Semantics (meaning of words)
   b. Phonology (sound of words)
   c. Syntax (rules of grammar)
2. Speech: Neuromechanical process of actual production of sounds. Depends on
   a. Respiratory input
   b. Articulatory input
   c. Phonation
3. Language versus communication: Human beings have a system of language; animals have a system of communication. The "generative grammar" of language is unique to humans. Human brains can generate a grammar, i.e., any of us can utter a sentence that has never before been said, and any of us can understand that it is a true sentence with bona fide meaning.
4. Aphasia: Defined as an acquired disturbance of language. Individuals mentally compromised from birth, and who never developed normal language, are not considered to be aphasic.
5. Handedness and language: Over 90% of human beings state that they are right-handed. However, only 60% of the population uses only the right hand for skilled tasks. Thirty-five percent of the population has a mixed hand preference. Less than 5% use only the left hand for skilled tasks. Over 99% of those who are right-handed have language that "resides" in the left hemisphere of the brain.

Pathophysiology

1. Aphasias—Non-fluent and fluent
   a. Non-fluent
      (1) Impaired articulation
      (2) Impaired melodic production
      (3) Reduced phrase length (five or fewer words per phrase)
      (4) Decreased grammatical complexity
      (5) Patients need not have all elements of non-fluency.
      (6) Broca's aphasia is the most common non-fluent aphasia

Key Symptoms: Non-Fluent Aphasia

- Good comprehension
  - Good repetition > Transcortical motor aphasia
  - Poor repetition > Broca's aphasia
- Poor comprehension
  - Good repetition > Mixed transcortical aphasia
  - Poor repetition > Global aphasia

   b. Fluent
      (1) Usually normal articulation
      (2) Fairly good melodic production
      (3) Phrase length often normal (greater than five words per phrase)
      (4) Grammatical complexity often normal
      (5) Major types are Wernicke's aphasia and Conduction aphasia.

Key Symptoms: Fluent Aphasia

- Good comprehension
  - Good repetition > Anomic aphasia
  - Poor repetition > Conduction aphasia
- Poor comprehension
  - Good repetition > Transcortical sensory aphasia
  - Poor repetition > Wernicke's aphasia

   c. Broca's aphasia
      (1) Non-fluent
      (2) Effortful initiation of speech production
      (3) Poor repetition
      (4) Poor ability to name
      (5) Paraphasic errors (semantic and phonemic)
      (6) Moderately good comprehension but difficulty understanding syntactically complicated sentences
      (7) Often associated with right hemisensory loss, buccofacial apraxia, right hemiparesis, and left ideomotor apraxia

(8) Lesion usually involves left frontal operculum (Brodmann's areas 45 and 44) and deep left frontal white matter.

d. Wernicke's aphasia

(1) Fluent output

(2) Normal sentence length

(3) Good articulation

(4) May have exaggerated prosody

(5) Anomia

(6) Phonemic and semantic paraphasias

(7) Poor auditory and reading comprehension

(8) Impaired repetition

(9) Fluent but empty writing

(10) Lesion usually in left posterior-superior temporal region, including superior and middle temporal gyrus, supramarginal-angular regions. Usually involves posterior portion of Brodmann's area 22.

e. Conduction aphasia

(1) Fluent output

(2) Fairly good comprehension

(3) Poor repetition

(4) Paragrammatic speech

(5) Anomia

(6) Paraphasic errors

(7) Good recitation, good reading aloud

(8) Often associated with agraphia and some degree of limited reading comprehension

(9) Lesion usually involves the left inferior parietal lobe, especially the anterior supramarginal gyrus (part of Brodmann's area 40).

f. Paraphasias: Defined as substitutions within words.

(1) Semantic (verbal) paraphasias: Substitution of one word for another ("green" for "red")

(a) Often, pronouns or prepositions are changed.

(2) Phonemic (literal) paraphasias: Substitution of one sound for another ("hug" for "rug").

g. Global aphasia

(1) Nonfluent

(2) Poor comprehension

(3) Poor repetition

(4) Output often restricted to meaningless speech sounds or stereotypes

(5) Lesions usually involve Broca's area and Wernicke's area. These may be cortical and subcortical, or purely subcortical.

h. Transcortical sensory aphasia

(1) Fluent output

(2) Poor comprehension

(3) Good repetition

(4) Echolalia

(5) Impaired auditory and reading comprehension

(6) Right visual field deficit

(7) Rare motor or sensory deficits

(8) Lesions usually involve left temporal-parietal-occipital junction, posterior to the superior temporal gyrus, and overlapping the posterior portions of Wernicke's area. Some investigators believe that Brodmann's area 37, posterior and inferior temporal gyrus, is the critical lesion.

i. Transcortical motor aphasia

(1) Non-fluent

(2) Good comprehension

(3) Good repetition

(4) Delayed initiation of output

(5) Brief utterances

(6) Semantic paraphasia

(7) Echolalia

(8) Patients usually have normal articulation or dysprosody of the classic non-fluent type (i.e., Broca's aphasia)

(9) Usually lack agrammatical speech output

(10) Lesions can occur in the left frontal lobe, from the operculum to the supplementary motor area.

j. Anomic aphasia

(1) Fluent output

(2) Good comprehension

(3) Good repetition

(4) Word-finding deficit is the only significant impairment.

(5) Lesions usually involve the left temporal-parietal-occipital junction association cortex, Brodmann's areas 37, 39, 40, 19, or 7.

k. Mixed transcortical aphasia

(1) Non-fluent

(2) Poor comprehension

(3) Good repetition

(4) Stock phrases (e.g., "You know," "The thing is")

(5) Considerable echolalia

(6) Lesion overlaps that causing transcortical motor and transcortical sensory aphasias;

left dorsolateral frontal region, anterior to the motor cortex, in the temporal-parietal-occipital junction

(7) Frequently follows anoxia

l. Subcortical aphasia

(1) Set of syndromes occurring in patients primarily with subcortical lesions to the thalamus, basal ganglia, or deep white matter)

(2) Do not produce aphasia as frequently as do cortical lesions

(3) Major types are thalamic and left basal ganglia.

m. Primary progressive aphasia

(1) Progressive deterioration of language; insidious onset and relative absence of decline of other aspects of cognition

(2) Careful neuropsychological testing usually reveals impaired non-language domains.

(3) Pathologic changes in the left temporal lobe

(4) Can be associated with Pick's disease, focal spongiform degeneration, Alzheimer's disease.

2. Alexia

a. Disorder of comprehension of written language—difficulty reading

b. In the United States, generally denotes identified developmental inability to learn to read, due either to inborn deficits or perinatal injury

c. Three types:

(1) Posterior alexia

(2) Central alexia

(3) Anterior alexia

Key Symptoms

Posterior Alexia

- Known as *pure alexia* or *alexia without agraphia*

- Inability to read but ability to write

- 60% of those affected have an associated color anomia

- Often associated with a right homonymous visual field defect

- Lesion usually involves medial aspect of dominant occipital lobe and splenium of the corpus callosum

Central Alexia

- Known as *alexia with agraphia*

- Inability to read or write

- Those affected comprehend spoken language better than written language but have difficulty recognizing words spelled aloud.

- Can neither spell aloud nor produce written language

- Lesion usually involves dominant angular gyrus.

Anterior Alexia

- Usually accompanies classic Broca's aphasia

- Those affected are unable to comprehend grammatically significant relational words, such as prepositions or articles; they may comprehend written substantive words.

- They often fail to read aloud individual letters (*literal alexia*) but may read a word that is a homophone for the latter (i.e., "bear" for "bare")

3. Gerstmann's syndrome

a. Acalculia

b. Agraphia

c. Right/left discrimination

d. Finger agnosia

e. Lesion usually involves dominant angular gyrus

Bibliography

Damasio AR, Damasio AH: Aphasia and the neural basis of language. In Mesulam M-M (ed): Principles of Behavioral and Cognitive Neurology, 2nd ed. New York, Oxford University Press, 2000, pp. 294–315.

Galaburda AM: Anatomy of developmental disorders: Geschwind's last legacy. In Schachter SC, Davinsky O (eds): Behavioral Neurology and the Legacy of Norman Geschwind. Philadelphia, Lippincott-Raven, 1997, pp. 89–100.

Kirshner KS: Aphasia. In Bradley WG, et al. (eds): Neurology and Clinical Practice, 3rd ed. Boston, Butterworth-Heinemann, 2000, pp. 141–160.

Mega MS, Alexander MP, Cummings JL, Benson DF: The aphasias and related disturbances. In Joint RJ, Griggs RC (eds): Baker's Clinical Neurology on CD-ROM. Philadelphia, Lippincott Williams & Wilkins, 2000.

Rosenfield DB, Barroso AO: Difficulties with speech and swallowing. In Bradley WG, et al. (eds): Neurology and Clinical Practice, 3rd ed. Boston, Butterworth-Heinemann, 2000, pp. 171–186.

Ross ED: Effective prosody in the aprosodias. In Mesulam M-M (ed): Principles of Behavioral and Cognitive Neurology, 2nd ed. New York, Oxford University Press, 2000, pp. 316–331.

13 Syncope vs Seizure

Steven C. Schachter

General Principles

1. Syncope is the most common nonepileptic disorder associated with seizures or behaviors that mimic epileptic seizures (see Key Causes of Syncope).

2. Syncope is more frequent than epilepsy; up to 25% of elderly institutionalized patients experience syncope during their lifetimes.

3. Neurologists often evaluate patients who have a witnessed seizure following the abrupt loss of consciousness and must decide whether the event was an epileptic seizure or a syncopal event complicated by an anoxic seizure.

 Key Causes of Syncope

- Vasovagal syncope
- Convulsive syncope
- Syncope in specific situations
  - Micturition syncope
  - Tussive syncope
  - Carotid sinus hypersensitivity
  - Glossopharyngeal neuralgia
- Cardiac syncope
  - Stokes-Adams attack
  - Tachyarrhythmias
  - Prolonged QT syndrome
  - Aortic stenosis
  - Hypertrophic cardiomyopathy
- Orthostatic syncope
  - Idiopathic orthostatic hypotension
  - Shy-Drager syndrome
  - Autonomic neuropathy
- Deliberate syncope (or "fainting lark")

Symptoms and Signs of Syncope

1. The key points of the patient history are the circumstances leading up to the event, the nature of the event-related behavior, and the postictal state (Table 13–1).

2. Pre-syncopal symptoms generally begin gradually and build in intensity. The patient often remembers not feeling well.

3. Similar symptoms in the past that resolved with lying or sitting down with the head bent forward suggest syncope rather than epilepsy.

4. Vasovagal syncope is the most common cause of syncope in young adults and is usually associated with:
   a. A strong emotional stimulus
   b. Fear
   c. Prolonged standing
   d. Dehydration
   e. Warm and crowded environment with poor air circulation
   f. Alcohol ingestion
   g. Diuretics or beta-blockers

5. Less frequent causes of syncope that are suggested by the history
   a. Carotid sinus hypersensitivity
   b. Cough
   c. Glossopharyngeal neuralgia
   d. Aortic stenosis coupled with increased cardiac demand

TABLE 13–1. KEY CLINICAL FEATURES OF SYNCOPE VS. SEIZURE

	SYNCOPE	EPILEPTIC SEIZURES
Precipitating factors	Frequent	None (with the exception of reflex epilepsies)
Premonitory symptoms	Frequent; gradual onset	Occasional; when present, sudden onset and stereotyped
Facial color	Pale, ashen	Flushed
Temporal relation of stiffening and loss of consciousness	Loss of consciousness precedes stiffening by approximately 15 seconds	Synchronous
Duration of loss of consciousness	Usually < 30 seconds	Several minutes
Tongue biting	Rare	Frequent
Postictal confusion	Brief	Brief to prolonged

e. Orthostatic hypotension

f. Micturition

6. Typical premonitory symptoms of syncope are due to global cerebral hypoperfusion and include

a. Lightheadedness or dizziness

b. Warmth, sweating

c. Graying out/blacking out or fading of vision

d. Diminished hearing and tinnitus

e. Nausea or abdominal discomfort

f. Anxiety and palpitations (which should prompt an evaluation for cardiac arrhythmia)

7. Witnesses to a syncopal event often report

a. Pale or ashen facial color (rather than facial flushing as occurs early in a seizure)

b. The patient's eyes remained open and "rolled up" (deviated upward) as consciousness was lost.

c. A groaning sound

d. Patients who remain upright after losing consciousness may become limp or stiffen and have brief myoclonic, clonic, or tonic seizures.

(1) The large majority of syncopal episodes conclude with a seizure.

(2) Stiffening typically occurs 10 to 15 seconds after loss of consciousness, unlike in tonic seizures, where stiffening and loss of consciousness occur simultaneously.

(3) Myoclonic and clonic movements may be restricted, multifocal asynchronous, or generalized.

(4) The change in muscle tone often results in falling to the ground, which terminates the event as cerebral perfusion is restored.

8. Syncopal episodes usually last less than 30 seconds. Similarly, the recovery phase following a syncopal seizure is brief, unlike the postictal state of generalized tonic-clonic seizures, which can last minutes to hours. Patients quickly resume full alertness and awareness, although pre-syncopal symptoms may recur as the patient rises from the supine position.

9. Atypical clinical presentations may be encountered.

a. Not all patients who fall because of syncope completely lose consciousness.

b. Incontinence may occur, especially if the event was triggered by micturition or defecation.

c. Tongue biting and automatisms may be observed.

d. Rarely, partial seizures may cause cardiac arrhythmias that result in syncope.

e. Rarely, epileptic seizures can be triggered from syncope. Such patients require electroencephalographic and electrocardiographic video monitoring for a definitive diagnosis.

Diagnosis

1. Physical examination

a. Cardiovascular function

b. Reactivity of the carotid sinus

c. Evaluation for orthostatic hypotension

2. Laboratory procedures

a. Electrocardiogram

b. Holter monitor

c. Echocardiogram

d. Selected cases: cardiac electrophysiologic testing and tilt table examination

Bibliography

Hopson JR, Kienzle MG: Evaluation of patients with syncope. Separating the 'wheat' from the 'chaff.' Postgrad Med 91:321–338, 1992.

Lempert T, Bauer M, Schmidt D: Syncope: A videometric analysis of 56 episodes of transient cerebral hypoxia. Ann Neurol 36:233–237, 1994.

Lipsitz LA, Wei JY, Rowe JW: Syncope in an elderly institutionalized population. Prevalence, incidence, and associated risk. Q J Med 55:45–55, 1985.

Kapoor WN: Workup and management of patients with syncope. Med Clin North Am 79:1153–1170, 1995.

Vossler DG: Nonepileptic seizures of physiologic origin. J Epilepsy 8:1–10, 1995.

14 Encephalopathies, Coma, Herniation, and Brain Death

G. Bryan Young

ENCEPHALOPATHY

Definition

Encephalopathy means "disease of the brain." In general usage, however, the term is used to indicate a diffuse dysfunction of the cerebral cortex and subcortical systems involved in alertness or awareness. The spectrum of dysfunction ranges from delirium (acute confusional state) to coma.

Etiology

Table 14–1 lists principal causes of encephalopathy. The most common cause of acute brain dysfunction is drug intoxication.

TABLE 14–1. SOME CAUSES OF ENCEPHALOPATHY

Systemic Illnesses	**Withdrawal Syndromes**
Sepsis (septic encephalopathy)	Alcohol
Acute uremia	Drugs
Hepatic failure	
Cardiac failure	**CNS Infections**
Pulmonary disease (especially pneumonia and pulmonary embolism)	Meningitis
	Encephalitis
Electrolyte disturbances	
Hypercalcemia	**Intracranial Lesions**
Porphyria	Head trauma
Carcinoid syndrome	Acute lesions (right parietal, bilateral occipital or mesial frontal)
Endocrinopathies	Subdural hematoma
Thyroid dysfunction	
Parathyroid tumors	**Hypertensive Encephalopathy**
Adrenal dysfunction	Miscellaneous
Pituitary dysfunction	Heat stroke
	Electrocution
Nutritional Deficiencies	Sleep deprivation
Thiamine (Wernicke's encephalopathy)	Psychiatric disorders
	Mania, especially in elderly
Niacin	Schizophrenia
Vitamin B_{12}	Depression—some forms
Folate	
Intoxications	
Drugs (especially anticholinergics in elderly)	
Alcohols	
Metals	
Industrial agents	
Biocides	

Adapted from Cummings JL: Clinical Neuropsychiatry. Orlando, FL: Grune & Stratton, 1985.

Epidemiology

The estimated prevalence of delirium in individuals over 55 years of age living in the community is between 0.1% and 1.1%; from 10% to 15% of patients admitted to acute medical and surgical wards are acutely confused. Diffuse encephalopathies account for approximately two thirds of cases of coma.

Pathophysiology

Encephalopathies most likely relate to a disturbance in the integrated function of the brain structures involved in alertness and attention: the ascending reticular activating system, including the thalamus, the cingulate gyrus, the prefrontal regions, and the parietal cortices. There is probably dysfunction in other regions as well, but these integrated regions are probably the most crucial.

Clinical Features

1. In confusional states a defect of attention is *consistently present*. Attention comprises alertness and the ability to select and focus on a given task or stimulus. Patients show impaired concentration, and other components of cognition are affected as well: perception (including hallucinations), thinking, and memory are all usually impaired to a greater or lesser extent. Patients are often disoriented in time and place, but never to person.
2. The level of alertness often fluctuates between delirium with agitation and lethargy with clouding of consciousness, quiet perplexity, or mild stupor and may progress to coma.
3. Emotional-behavioral disturbances that accompany agitated delirium include rage, combativeness, irritability, fear and apprehension, or euphoria. Conversely, depression or apathy may be found alternating with these or with the quiet confusional state.
4. Cranial nerve findings: The pupils, ocular movements, and respirations are relatively spared in most metabolic encephalopathies. As a corollary, when a patient is deeply comatose, and these cranial nerve functions are spared, one should consider a metabolic or toxic etiology.

5. Motor signs accompanying acute confusion may occur singly or in combination: psychomotor retardation (decreased motor responsiveness without paralysis or profound decrease in conscious level), hyperactivity, asterixis, multifocal myoclonus, *gegenhalten* (see below), and a postural-action tremor. These features are strongly suggestive of a metabolic/toxic/septic encephalopathy as opposed to a structural brain lesion.

Key Clinical Features

- Delirium (earliest manifestation)
- Impaired attention (an essential feature of delirium)
- Features suggestive of a metabolic etiology:
  - Asterixis
  - Tremor
  - Multifocal myoclonus

Laboratory Testing

The history, physical examination, and neurologic examination will likely provide the diagnosis in most cases, but diagnostic procedures are necessary to confirm the clinical suspicions. The following are indicated when specific concerns arise, but many need to be done when the etiological possibilities are wide:

1. Lumbar puncture, especially to exclude meningitis, encephalitis, or subarachnoid hemorrhage

2. Culture blood, urine, sputum, and cerebrospinal fluid (CSF) for systemic or central nervous system infection. A Venereal Diseases Research Laboratory (VDRL) test on serum and/or CSF, for syphilis at least, is probably worth doing, especially when the diagnosis is uncertain.

3. Toxic screen is advisable when there is even a remote possibility of toxicity, or on admission through the emergency department.

4. Metabolic screening for serum concentrations of electrolytes, glucose, urea, calcium, albumin, magnesium, bilirubin, ammonia, aspartate aminotransferase, phosphate, and serum vitamin B_{12} concentrations are useful in most cases.

5. Complete blood count and platelets are advisable for most cases.

6. Blood gases should be measured in most cases.

7. Endocrine studies: thryoid function tests, especially thryoid-stimulating hormone assay in selected cases for hypothyroidism or hyperthyroidism.

8. Electroencephalography (EEG) is used to confirm altered cerebral cortical function, to exclude seizure activity (EEG is the only reliable test for nonconvulsive status epilepticus), and to grade the severity of the encephalopathy. Middle and long latency evoked potentials, including cognitive evoked electrophysiologic responses (e.g., the "P300" response), can be used in the detection of problems in cortical processing.

9. Neuroimaging (e.g., computed tomography [CT] or magnetic resonance imaging [MRI]) is indicated if there are consistent focal signs or if there is a possibility of an extraaxial lesion such as a subdural hematoma or bilateral intracerebral or extraaxial lesions.

Key Tests

- Metabolic screen, including blood gases
- CBC and platelets
- Toxic and drug screen
- Cultures for infection
- CSF analysis when indicated
- EEG
- Neuroimaging only when necessary
- Others when indicated by history or examination

Treatment

See Treatment for Coma, later in this chapter.

Prevention

1. The acute confusional state in the elderly is often prevented by more appropriate use of medications.

   a. Drugs should be used only when necessary, and renal and hepatic function must be considered for the dosage schedule.

   b. Whenever possible, polypharmacy should be avoided.

   c. To prevent drug withdrawal reactions, it is best to taper medications that have been used for some time, especially monoamine oxidase inhibitors, clonidine, narcotics, barbiturates, and antiepileptic drugs.

2. Prompt recognition: Early recognition and prompt investigation and management of the acute confusional state should lessen morbidity and mortality. An acute onset of altered awareness, disorientation, memory impairment, aggressive behavior, and impaired ability to interact

are important indicators. Investigation and supportive and specific therapy follow.

Key Management

- Prevention: Prescribe drugs only when necessary (avoid polypharmacy; taper drugs in chronic use)
- Recognize and investigate confusion promptly.

Bibliography

Cole MG, McCusker J, Dendukuri N, Han L: Symptoms of delirium among elderly medical inpatients with or without dementia. J Neuropsychiatry Clin Neurosci 14:167, 2002.

Engel GL: Delirium. In Friedman AM, Kaplan HS (eds): Comprehensive Textbook of Psychiatry. Baltimore, Williams & Wilkins, 1967, p. 711.

Folstein MF, Bassett SS, Romanski AJ, et al.: The epidemiology of delirium in the community: The Eastern Baltimore Mental Health Survey. Int Psychogeriatrics 3:169, 1991.

Inaba-Roland KE, Maricle RA: Assessing delirium in the acute care setting. Heart Lung 21:48, 1992.

Larson EB, Kukull WA, Buchner D, et al.: Adverse drug reactions associated with global cognitive impairment in elderly persons. Ann Intern Med 107:169, 1987.

Mesulam M-M: Attention, confusional states and neglect. In Mesulam M-M (ed): Principles of Behavior in Neurology. Philadelphia, FA Davis, 1986, pp. 125–168.

Walls RM: Advances in trauma: airway management. Emerg Clin North Am 11:53, 1993.

COMA

Definition

Coma is a state of unarousable unconsciousness in which the patient lies in a sleep-like state, with the eyes closed, but without wake-sleep cycles, spontaneous arousal (eye opening), or arousal following stimulation.

Etiology

Coma relates to a disorder of the ascending reticular activating system (ARAS), especially the brainstem reticular formation rostral to the mid-pons, the nonspecific, midline and reticular thalamic nuclei, and the projection of the thalamus to the cerebral cortex bilaterally.

1. Brainstem: Coma-producing lesions of the midbrain are almost invariably associated with thalamic or pontine tegmental damage, or more widespread damage to the cerebral cortex. Extensive bilateral destructive lesions of the midbrain tegmentum and thalamus, however, consistently eliminate the capacity for alerting.

2. Thalamus: Among patients with thalamic lesions, only those with bilateral dorsal paramedian lesions have shown coma or impaired arousal responses. Conversely, not all patients with bilateral paramedian thalamic lesions are in coma. When coma does occur, it is almost never permanent if the person survives for several weeks or more. Coma-producing lesions often also involve the rostral midbrain, manifested by Parinaud's syndrome or paralysis of vertical gaze, especially upgaze.

3. Cerebral cortex: There is surprisingly inconclusive evidence that diffuse cerebral cortical dysfunction in humans causes coma. In human cases, dysfunction is rarely, if ever, purely cortical. Lesions often involve other sites. In addition, dysfunction of the cortex has profound influences on numerous subcortical regions; loss of this influence may impair their function by "diaschisis."

Epidemiology

Coma is an extremely common medical problem. About 3% of admissions to the emergency rooms of large urban hospitals relate to impaired consciousness.

Pathophysiology

1. Coma relates to dysfunction of the ARAS. The ARAS is not a homogeneous network of interconnected neurons, but consists of varied systems with several neurotransmitters, including cholinergic, dopaminergic, noradrenergic, and serotonergic pathways.

2. Impairment of alertness may affect neuronal transmission involving these systems, due to metabolic, toxic, mechanical (compressive), ischemic, inflammatory, or thermal (elevated or depressed) conditions.

Clinical Findings

1. The history can point to obvious causes; therefore it is important to talk to close associates, and ambulance attendants, and to consult medical records and information on the patient (Medical-alert bracelet or documentation in wallet or purse).

2. Clues often can be found on the general examination: vital signs, evidence of trauma, jaundice, cutaneous bleeding, injection sites, skin color (alcohol, uremia, fetor hepaticus), breath odor, bitten tongue (indicating a convulsive seizure) and fundi (hemorrhages [possible subarachnoid hemorrhage], papilledema [raised intracranial pressure or malignant hypertension], Roth spots [endocarditis, leukemia]).

3. The patient in coma will not show spontaneous

or stimulus-induced arousal, especially eye opening. Some posturing, e.g., decerebrate, decorticate, or even localizing responses are often seen.

4. With purely supratentorial causes of coma (affecting the thalamus and its rostral connections), the pupils and vestibulo-ocular reflexes are intact.

5. With coma-producing brainstem lesions (including transtentorial herniation), the pupillary reactions and extraocular movements are abnormal, as manifested by unilaterally or bilaterally unreactive pupils, gaze palsies, or internuclear ophthalmoplegia with caloric testing. (Think of Wernicke's encephalopathy in the patient with intact pupillary reactions but absent caloric responses.)

Laboratory Testing

1. This should be guided by the history and physical, especially neurological, findings. Neuroimaging with computed tomography is indicated when a structural brain lesion is likely.

2. Metabolic (glucose, blood gases, electrolytes, serum calcium, urea, creatinine, magnesium, ammonia and liver function tests) and drug screening are often necessary for patients in whom a structural lesion is unlikely to be the cause of coma.

3. Drug screens can be narrowed by looking for "toxidromes" (toxic syndromes) with various autonomic, acid-base and osmolar abnormalities (see Gerace, 1998).

4. Cerebrospinal fluid testing to rule out CNS infections, meningeal cancer, subarachnoid bleeding (if scan negative)

Features

- Localize anatomical site producing coma: cerebral hemispheres-thalamus vs. brainstem

- Use historical and physical examinations for clues to etiology

- Tailor investigation (neuroimaging, blood and urine tests and CSF analysis)

Treatment

1. Supportive care: The "ABC" (airway, breathing, and circulation) needs must be met. Ventilatory failure is present when Pa_{CO_2} values are elevated or fail to fall below 40 mm Hg during hypoxemia. Assisted ventilation with endotracheal intubation is indicated in the face of hypoventilation, obstruction of the upper airway, or if there is significant risk of aspiration. Pulse and blood pressure must be assessed promptly, and intravenous access should be obtained immediately. Blood and urine should then be taken for analysis. If the patient is hypotensive or shows evidence of poor tissue perfusion (severe vasoconstriction, elevated serum lactate), the cause is remedied as quickly as possible.

2. Hypoglycemia is a common, correctable cause of impaired consciousness. The serum glucose concentration should be performed immediately in the emergency room. An intravenous bolus of glucose as 50 ml of 50% solution should be given promptly if there is strong suspicion of hypoglycemia or if a spot test shows low serum glucose. Thiamine should be coadministered if there is a possibility of vitamin deficiency.

3. Epileptic seizures should be treated promptly to prevent additional brain damage and to lessen morbidity and mortality.

4. It is wise to protect the patient from vitamin deficiency before glucose is administered by administering thiamine (50 mg intramuscularly). This is also a life-saving, specific therapy for Wernicke's encephalopathy. Naloxone can reverse the sedative effects of opiates and flumazenil counteracts benzodiazepines.

5. Treatment of mass effect (herniation) and markedly raised intracranial pressure: If the patient is deteriorating from increased mass effect, life-saving measures to allow time for more definitive treatment (e.g., a neurosurgical decompressive procedure) can be instituted. Such measures include intravenous mannitol infusion, hyperventilation, raising the head to 30 degrees in a midline position, and, occasionally, barbiturates to reduce cerebral blood volume.

6. Prioritization: It is important to organize and prioritize management steps. Too often comatose patients with metabolic problems or meningitis are sent to the CT suite as an initial step. This wastes valuable time and jeopardizes patient safety and care. Ideally, the essentials of investigation and management can go hand-in-hand with initiation of treatment in the emergency room.

7. Specific therapy for the underlying illness is best instituted promptly; hence the importance of prompt diagnosis.

Key Treatment

- Supportive care: The "ABCs" (airway, breathing, and circulation)

- Hypoglycemia: Intravenous bolus of glucose as 50 ml of 50% solution

- Mass effect: Life-saving measures to allow time for more definitive treatment (e.g., intravenous mannitol infusion, hyperventilation, raising the head to 30 degrees in a midline position)

- It is important to organize and prioritize management steps.

Prevention

See Encephalopathy earlier in this chapter.

Bibliography

Gentilini M, De Renzi E, Crisi G: Bilateral paramedian thalamic artery infarcts: report of eight cases. J Neurol Neurosurg Psychiatry 50:900, 1987.

Gerace RV: Poisoning. In Young GB, Ropper AH, Bolton CF (eds): Coma and Impaired Consciousness: A Clinical Perspective. New York, McGraw-Hill, 1998, pp. 457–467.

Guberman A, Stuss D: The syndrome of bilateral paramedian thalamic infarction. Neurology 33:540, 1983.

Kaada BR, Harkmark W, Stokke O: Deep coma associated with desynchronization in EEG. Electroencephalogr Clin Neurophysiol 13:785, 1961.

Plum F: Coma and related global disturbances of the human conscious state. In Peters A, Jones EG (eds): Cerebral Cortex: Normal and Altered States of Function. New York, Plenum Press, 1991, pp. 359–425.

Zeman A: Consciousness. Brain 124:1263, 2001.

HERNIATION

Definition

Herniations are clinicopathological syndromes that relate to the displacement of part of the brain from one compartment to another, with resultant compression of brain structures. Traditionally, the principal herniation syndromes are subfalcial or transtentorial displacements of supratentorial structures and cerebellar herniations related to displacement of parts of the cerebellum through the tentorium or foramen magnum.

Etiology

Epidemiology: Of 500 cases of coma, the following were likely related to herniation or compression of brain structures:

1. Ninety-nine were supratentorial lesions.

    a. Seventy-six were hemorrhages: 44 intracerebral, 26 subdural, 4 epidural, and 2 pituitary apoplexy.

    b. Nine were hemispheric infarctions with edema.

    c. Seven were tumors.

    d. Six were abscesses.

    e. One was a closed head injury.

2. Twelve were infratentorial compressive lesions: cerebellar hemorrhage tumor, infarct of abscess, and posterior fossa subdural hematoma.

Pathophysiology

Herniation relates to asymmetrical mass lesions and their effect on the ascending reticular activating system. In some cases the process is reversible and in many others it progresses to death.

1. Acute mass lesions and associated acute displacements of brain structures have a more striking effect on level of consciousness than slowly increasing volumes of lesions. Even with slowly evolving mass effect, however, eventually consciousness will be impaired, although a greater amount of displacement may be required.

2. There is a consistent, graded relationship between the horizontal displacement of unilateral, supratentorial, midline structures (e.g., the pineal gland) and the degree of impairment of consciousness/alertness. Drowsiness occurs with a 3-mm shift; stupor, with a 3- to 6-mm shift; coma, after a shift of 9 mm or greater. This relationship is more consistent than downward herniation and, furthermore, impairment of consciousness can occur without *any* downward displacement.

3. Downward herniation with compression of the lower brainstem at the foramen magnum can produce abrupt apnea due to dysfunction of the medullary respiratory center. This, in turn, can cause coma.

4. Brainstem distortion and compression of the rostral brainstem tegmentum (see earlier, under Coma) may also produce coma in some cases. Unfortunately, in many of these cases the damage may be irreversible when such extensive structural damage occurs.

Clinical Features

1. Gradual impairment of level of consciousness is the first abnormality and may fluctuate at first, before progressing to stupor and then coma.

2. With supratentorial lesions, a third cranial nerve palsy on the side of the lesion is common. This is

probably due to stretching of the oculomotor nerve over the clivus rather than to direct compression of the herniating uncus, as was formerly thought. With further herniation, the opposite pupil loses its reactivity, likely as a result of intrinsic brainstem distortion or compression.

3. Hemiplegia contralateral to an intrinsic cerebral lesion is common and expected. With extraaxial lesion, compression of the contralateral cerebral peduncle against the free edge of the tentorium may cause a hemiparesis that is *ipsilateral* to the mass (Kernohan's notch phenomenon).

4. With infratentorial mass lesions, consciousness may be preserved until apnea occurs related to compression of the lower medulla. Alternatively, coma may relate to brainstem compression or to raised intracranial pressure with 4th ventricular obstruction. In these instances, cranial nerve palsies occur pari passu with apnea.

Key Clinical Features

- Gradual impairment of consciousness, followed by stupor and then coma
- Hemiplegia
- Clinical features can usually classify type of herniation: subfalcial, transtentorial, or cerebellar.

Laboratory/Radiologic Testing

Neuroimaging is the test of choice; CT and MRI scans have allowed a better insight into the mechanisms of herniation than were possible with post-mortem examinations. Such scans should be obtained as soon as possible, before irreversible damage has occurred.

Key Tests

- Neuroimaging with CT or MRI must be done promptly for specific diagnosis and planning therapy.

Treatment

1. Extraaxial lesions (e.g., subdural fluid collections, meningiomas) are best treated surgically; complete cure is possible. Edema of the underlying cerebral hemisphere may cause further mass effect, however, and may require therapy to reduce intracranial pressure, at least on a short-term basis (hyperventilation, mannitol, corticosteroids.)

2. Intraaxial lesions can sometimes be managed by steps to reduce intracranial pressure. There is preliminary evidence that hemicraniectomy is helpful for marked mass effect due to edema after unilateral cerebral infarction. The management of intraparenchymal hemorrhage is more controversial, except for cerebellar hemorrhage, where decompression of the clot, with or without edematous brain tissue, can be life-saving. Parenchymal abscesses, when small can sometimes be treated by antibiotics. Larger lesions can be decompressed, sometimes by stereotaxic aspiration.

3. Ventricular drainage for hydrocephalus is sometimes required when ventricular obstruction occurs.

Bibliography

Plum F, Posner JB: The Diagnosis of Stupor and Coma, 3rd ed. Philadelphia, F.A. Davis, 1980.

Riecke K, Schwab S, Krieger D, et al.: Decompressive surgery in space occupying hemispheric infarction. Crit Care Med 9:1576, 1995.

Ropper AH: Transtentorial herniation. In Young GB, Ropper AH, Bolton CF (eds): Coma and Impaired Consciousness. New York, McGraw-Hill, 1998, pp. 119–130.

Steiner T, Ringleb P, Hacke W: Treatment options for large hemispheric stroke. Neurology 57 (Suppl 2): S61, 2001.

BRAIN DEATH

Definition

Brain death is defined as the irreversible loss of the capacity for consciousness combined with the irreversible loss of all brainstem functions including the capacity to breathe. Brain death is equivalent to death of the individual, even though the heart continues to beat and spinal cord functions may persist.

The diagnosis of brain death rests on each of the following factors:

1. An etiology has been established that is capable of causing brain death, and potentially reversible causes have been excluded.

2. The patient is in deep coma and shows no response within cranial nerve distribution to stimulation of any part of the body. No movements such as cerebral seizures, dyskinetic movements, decorticate or decerebrate movements arising from the brain are present.

3. Brainstem reflexes are absent.

4. The patient is apneic when taken off the respirator for an appropriate time.

5. The conditions listed above persist when the patient is reassessed after a suitable interval.

6. There should be no confounding factors for the

application of clinical criteria. Some conditions may mimic brain death, e.g., hypothermia, drug intoxication, the use of neuromuscular blocking or anticholinergic agents, and shock. These should be excluded or reversed before applying the clinical criteria.

7. When clinical criteria cannot be applied, brain death can be confirmed by demonstrating lack of brain perfusion (see below, under Laboratory Features).

Points for the Diagnosis of Brain Death

- Establish etiology and only consider causes that produce neuronal death.

- Brainstem reflexes must be absent, no movements arising from the brain (spontaneous or with stimulation), apnea (proper testing).

- Ancillary tests when clinical criteria cannot be applied. Tests of brain blood flow are the most appropriate.

Special Note: *Neonates and young children.* In children with a conceptional age of 52 weeks or older (more than 2 months post-term) the adult clinical criteria can be applied. Clinical criteria alone are not sufficient in the determination of brain death in infants under this age. The basic tenets accepted in adults that apply to children include:

1. the importance of excluding remediable or reversible conditions, especially toxic and metabolic derangement and the effects of sedative drugs, paralytic agents, hypothermia, and hypotension

2. physical examination criteria must be satisfied (outlined above)

3. irreversibility must be ensured by reevaluation at specified intervals.

   It is recommended:
   a. for term newborns (greater than 38 weeks gestation) and young infants, aged 7 days to 2 months, that the clinical examination and a radionuclide brain flow study be done
   b. for those 2 months to 1 year, a protocol of two examinations and electroencephalograms (EEGs) separated by at least 24 hours has been suggested; a repeat examination and EEG would not be necessary if a concomitant radionuclide angiographic study failed to visualize cerebral arteries
   c. in those over 1 year of age, an observation period of at least 12 hours is recom-

mended. However, in infants comatose due to hypoxic-ischemic encephalopathy, at least 24 hours of observation is suggested. The validity of the application of clinical criteria to preterm infants is still uncertain. Further guidelines are needed. Clearly additional supportive investigative tests—e.g., those of brain perfusion—are needed to substantiate the diagnosis of brain death in this group.

Etiology

Many conditions can cause early or delayed neuronal death. These are not mutually exclusive but share the common feature of arresting circulation to the brain and causing irreversible death of neurons in the brainstem and diencephalon. Causes include:

1. Structural lesions: Trauma, mass lesions (e.g., hemorrhage, tumor, abscess), destructive, infectious or inflammatory ± herniation, and arrest of intracranial circulation

2. Circulatory causes: Basilar artery occlusion, global loss of cerebral perfusion (cardiac arrest or prolonged, sustained hypotension), intracranial hemorrhage with markedly raised intracranial pressure

3. Irreversible cellular poisons/toxins (e.g., cyanide)

4. Brain swelling (various causes) with arrest of intracranial circulation

Pathophysiology

1. The essential component of brain death is death of the brainstem and diencephalon. This precludes alertness, consciousness, respirations, sensory input, motor output, cranial nerve function, homeostatic mechanisms, and other essential brain functions in an irreversible manner.

2. The above-mentioned structures can be destroyed almost simultaneously by some processes (e.g., complete infarction in the vertebrobasilar system, prolonged circulatory arrest or severe trauma), but in others the process depends on a rise in intracranial pressure from brain swelling or an increasing intracranial mass that ultimately causes an arrest of brain perfusion. In other cases, delayed neuronal death may follow a severe insult such as ischemia.

Clinical Findings

Brain death is primarily a clinical diagnosis and relies on the following:

1. Unresponsiveness

a. No motor response of the limbs or grimacing to nail bed and supraorbital pressure

b. No spontaneous movements arising from the brain (e.g., dystonic, decerebrate, or decorticate posturing or seizures)

2. Absence of brainstem reflexes: pupillary light reflex, ocular movements (caloric testing with 50 cc of ice water in each ear independently), facial sensation and movements (corneal reflexes, facial movements), and pharyngeal and tracheal reflexes

3. Apnea testing: pre-oxygenation with 100% oxygen for 10 minutes, then administering 100% oxygen through a tracheal cannula or a cannula inserted to the level of the carina at 6 to 8 liters/minute during disconnection from the ventilator. Respiratory movements are looked for during the time the ventilator is stopped, and a rise of $Paco_2$ to greater than 60 mm Hg is generally accepted as a sufficient stimulus. [Caveats: (a) core temperature should be at least 32.2°C, preferably ≥36.5°C, to allow an adequate rate of rise of $Paco_2$; (b) in chronic retainers of carbon dioxide, the apnea test may not be valid; (c) systolic blood pressure should be ≥90 mm Hg in adults and within normal limits for age in infants and children; (d) the patient should be euvolemic; (e) an initially normal $Paco_2$ before apnea testing is begun (40 ± 5 mm Hg)].

Key Clinical Signs

- No motor response of the limbs or grimacing to nail bed and supraorbital pressure

- No spontaneous movements arising from the brain

- Absence of brainstem reflexes
  - Pupillary light reflex
  - Ocular movements
  - Facial sensation and movements
  - Pharyngeal and tracheal reflexes
  - Apnea

Laboratory Features

Although brain death can be established reliably by clinical criteria alone, special tests can be used to support the clinical diagnosis. This is especially true when the clinical criteria cannot be reliably applied (e.g., trauma to the eyes). Such situations are discussed below. The only tests that are standardized and accepted in most countries as confirmation of brain death when clinical criteria cannot be applied are cerebral angiography and radionuclide scanning.

1. Cerebral angiography: In brain death no intracranial perfusion other than an occasional filling of the superior sagittal sinus is seen.

2. Radionuclide scanning. Two-planar imaging using a radioactively labeled substance that readily crosses the blood–brain barrier (such as technetium 99m hexamthylproplyeneamine-oxime [^{99m}Tc-HMPAO] is recommended. In brain death no uptake is seen in the brain parenchyma. Alternatively, the rapid bolus injection of serum albumin labeled with technetium 99m is given, followed by imaging with a gamma camera. As with cerebral angiography, there should be no vascular component, except for possible filling of the superior sagittal sinus.

3. Potentially useful tests:

a. Transcranial Doppler ultrasonography: The intracranial arteries are insonated bilaterally, including the middle and/or anterior cerebral arteries and the vertebral or basilar artery. The findings of absent diastolic or reverberating flow or small systolic peaks have been reported in brain death. The absence of transcranial Doppler signals cannot be taken as evidence of brain death, as 10% of people do not have temporal insonation windows.

b. Other imaging tests: Although MRI techniques hold promise, they have not been sufficiently studied or validated to be used as the sole confirmatory test. Neuroimaging, e.g., with MRI or computed axial tomography, may help to confirm the structural nature and extent of damage in selected cases.

c. Electroneurophysiologic tests: The EEG does not, however, adequately assess brainstem function and should not be used as the sole confirmatory test for brain death. The use of evoked potentials, including brainstem auditory and somatosensory evoked potential testing, has promise, but these have not been sufficiently validated. Furthermore, they are highly dependent on technical quality and require considerable expertise and experience for reliable performance and interpretation.

d. Atropine test: The absence of an increase in heart rate after the intravenous injection of 2 mg of atropine, is confirmatory of the absence of vagal tone and is helpful in confirming dysfunction of the caudal brainstem. Although helpful, the atropine test is not sufficient as the sole confirmatory test of brain death.

Key Tests

• Cerebral angiography

• Radionuclide scanning

Bibliography

Fishman MA: Validity of brain death in infants. Paediatrics 96:513, 1995.

Medical Consultants on the Diagnosis of Death to the President's Commission: Guidelines for the determination of death. JAMA 246:2184, 1981.

Okamoto K, Sugimoto T: Return of spontaneous respiration in an infant who fulfilled current criteria to determine brain death. Pediatrics 96:518–520, 1995.

Task Force for the Determination of Brain Death in Children: Guidelines for the determination of brain death in children. Arch Neurol 44:587, 1987.

Wijdicks EF: The diagnosis of brain death: N Engl J Med 344:1215, 2001.

Working Group Convened by the Royal College of Physicians: Criteria for the Diagnosis of Brain Stem Death. 29:381, 1995.

15 Neurological Eponyms

Randolph W. Evans, MD

For the neophyte, neurology is a confusing mix of eponyms and neuroscience. Although we learn the disorders behind the eponyms, we seldom learn the stories of the men who described the disorders, and these are often fascinating. An alphabetical list of some key persons follows with a thumbnail sketch of each.

As you read these sketches, you may agree with Samuel Taylor Coleridge (1772–1834): "A dwarf sees farther than the giant when he has the giant's shoulder to mount on. (*The Friend*, Sec. I, Essay 8)." You will also see questions raised about primacy, as in the case of this famous line which echoes these earlier quotations:

- Isaac Newton (1642–1727): "If I have seen further [than you and Descartes] it is by standing on the shoulders of Giants." (In a 1676 letter to Robert Hooke)
- Robert Burton: "Pygmies placed on the shoulders of giants see more than the giants themselves." (*The Anatomy Of Melancholy*, 1621)
- Bernard of Chartres wrote in 1126: "[We are as dwarfs sitting on the shoulders of giants.]"

Two-Word Eponyms Named for a Single Person

Argyll Robertson
Brown-Séquard
Foster Kennedy
Marcus Gunn
Miller Fisher
Ramsay Hunt

Alois Alzheimer (1864–1915)

1. First to reliably describe the histologic alterations in Alzheimer's disease, Pick's disease, Binswanger's disease, Huntington's chorea, and metachromatic leukodystrophy. Key observations made while head of the neuroanatomical laboratory at Emil Kraepelin's psychiatric clinic in Munich.

2. First description of Alzheimer's disease presented at a conference in 1906 (published as an abstract in 1907) from the study of Auguste D, a 51-year-old woman who developed jealousy of her husband, memory loss, paranoia, and auditory hallucinations. When she died after 4½ years, she was stuporous, and her legs were drawn up under her. Microscopic study of the brain demonstrated neurofibrillary tangles and amyloid plaques.

3. Emil Kraeplin (1856–1926) introduced the term "Alzheimer's disease" in his psychiatry textbook in 1910.

4. In 1892, Arnold Pick (1851–1924) described aphasia and apraxia due to circumscribed atrophy of cortical areas but did not realize that he was reporting a new disease. In 1911, Alzheimer described the histologic abnormalities (argentophile inclusions and swollen neurons) in Pick's disease, an eponym suggested by Gans in 1922.

Douglas Moray Cooper Lamb Argyll Robertson (1837–1909)

1. Pioneering Scottish ophthalmic surgeon.

2. In 1869, he reported four cases which ". . . serve well to illustrate the connexion between certain eye-symptoms and a diseased condition of the spinal cord. In all of them there was marked contraction of the pupil . . . in that the pupil was insensible to light, but contracted still further during the act of accommodation for near objects. . . ."

3. In 1933, H. Houston Merritt (1902-1979) and Moore reported that this pupillary abnormality was usually a result of neurosyphilis. Other midbrain lesions and diabetes can cause Argyll Robertson pupils.

Joseph Babinksi (1857–1932)

1. A Parisian of Polish parentage. In 1885, he became Jean-Martin Charcot's *chef de clinique* at the Salpêtrière. In what became a scandal, Babinski was passed over for an academic position by Charles Bouchard (1837–1915; remembered for Charcot-Bouchard aneurysm), who favored his own three pupils, and Babinski went into private practice. In 1914, coined the word *anosognosia* and described the disorder (denial of hemiplegia with a right posterior parietal lesion).

2. Reported the toe sign in an oral communication in1896, which was first termed the "Babinski sign" in 1898 by van Gehuchten

3. The Babinski sign stimulated the search for "new reflexes." Between 1918 and 1935, 76 new pathologic reflexes were reported. This period was referred to as "open season for the hunting of the reflex" by Foster Kennedy. Hoffmann's sign (Johann Hoffmann, 1857–1919) was reported in

1911 in an article by his resident. In 1891, Hoffman and Guido Werdnig (1844–1919) independently described acute infantile spinal muscular atrophy, Werdnig-Hoffmann disease.

Quotation

"In certain pathological states, stimulation of the sole evokes extension of the toes, particularly the great toe. I refer to this modification in the form of the reflex movement as the phenomenon of the toes.

It is not only in the direction of movement that the normal reflex differs from the pathological; usually the extensor response is executed more slowly that the flexor. Furthermore, flexion is ordinarily stronger when one stimulates the inner part of the sole than when the stimulus is applied to the outer part, and it is the opposite with the extensor response. Finally, while flexion predominates generally in the last two or three toes, it is in the first one or two toes that extension is usually the most pronounced."

Translation of Babinski J. Du phénomène des orteils et de sa valeur sémiologique. La Semaine Médicale 18:321–322, 1898.

Charles Bell (1774–1842)

1. Studied medicine in Edinburgh under Alexander Monro (1733–1817; described the interventricular foramen).

2. First description of the clinical signs after loss of function of the facial nerve motor component in 1821. In 1826, he described different causes of facial palsy including the following: a gunshot wound; a facial wound by the horn of an ox; after extirpation of a tumor before the ear; and a physician who had a facial palsy after sleeping with his cheek exposed "at the open window to the east wind." He clearly distinguished lower from upper motor neuron facial weakness.

3. In 1830, described "a very remarkable turning up of the cornea in an attempt to close the eyelids," Bell's phenomenon. In 1811, reported on the motor function of the anterior spinal roots. François Magendie (1783–1855) was the first to prove the function of the anterior and posterior spinal roots, thus the "law of Bell-Magendie."

Charles Bonnet (1720–1792)

1. Swiss lawyer, naturalist, and philosopher. Anticipated Darwin's theory of evolution.

2. Described the Charles Bonnet syndrome (complex visual hallucinations in psychologically normal persons with visual loss) in 1760 in his grandfather. When Charles Bonnet went blind at the end of his life, he also experienced visual hallucinations.

W. Russell Brain (Lord Brain, 1895–1966)

1. Preeminent neurologist in London. Editor of the journal *Brain*.

2. Described carpal tunnel syndrome, dysthyroid ophthalmopathy, complications of cervical spondylosis, unilateral neglect, and more.

3. Unfortunately, he does not really belong in this chapter because he does not have an eponym. However, he was married to the granddaughter of the distinguished London physician, John Langdon Down (1828–1896), who described Down's syndrome in 1865 (the prominent epicanthal folds suggested a mongoloid appearance to him).

4. The word *brain,* of course, is not named after a person but is derived from the Anglo-Saxon word *braegen,* which could have a common root with the Greek *brechmos* ("front part of the head").

Pierre Paul Broca (1824–1880)

1. Described Duchenne's dystrophy in 1851 before Guillaume Benjamin Amand Duchenne (1806–1875) in 1858 (also well-described by Meryon in 1851).

2. In 1861, based on the study of an epileptic patient (Leborgne), described Broca's aphasia (which he termed *aphemia;* the term was changed to *aphasia* by Armand Trousseau [1801–1867] in 1865) and Broca's area (the third frontal gyrus on the left side). The findings were confirmed in the same year with a second clinicopathological correlation of the brain of the patient named Lelong.

3. Published on left cerebral dominance in 1865.

4. Involved in the famous "Broca-Dax controversy" because Marc Dax (1770–1837) had written about but not published several dozen cases with loss of speech and left hemisphere lesions.

Charles-Edouard Brown-Séquard (1817–1894)

1. Born on the isle of Mauritius, a British subject. Son of a merchant sea captain from Philadelphia (Brown), who died before his birth and a French mother (Séquard).

2. Had a transatlantic career: various appointments in the United States (including the Medical College of Virginia and Harvard), London (the National Hospital for the Paralysed and Epileptic where John Hughlings Jackson [1835–1911] was his

assistant. In 1868, Jackson described the "Jacksonian march" of ictal movements through the rolandic cortex.), and Paris.

3. In 1849, he reported his research demonstrating that hemisection of the cord in animals produces sensory loss on the opposite side of the body, which challenged the dominant doctrine of Charles Bell. The Brown-Séquard syndrome results from a unilateral lesion of the spinal cord causing paralysis and abnormal proprioception ipsilateral to the lesion and decreased pain and temperature appreciation (beginning one or two segments below the level of the lesion) contralaterally.

4. As a result of his research on the function of the adrenal glands, testicular and other organ extracts, he is considered a founding father of experimental endocrinology.

Jean-Martin Charcot (1825–1893)

1. Professor at the Salpêtrière in Paris from 1862 until his death. The Salpêtrière was built as a salpeter store in 1634 and was opened as a general hospital in 1657. During Charcot's time, the hospital was mainly a nursing home for some 5000 elderly destitute women.

2. Developed the clinicoanatomic method. He differentiated the clinical picture of multiple sclerosis from Parkinson's disease (tremor can be a feature of both) and reported the features of amyotrophic lateral sclerosis, known to much of the world as Charcot's disease. The relapsing-remitting form of multiple sclerosis is also known as the Charcot variant. The Charcot triad of multiple sclerosis is dysarthria, tremor, and ataxic gait. With Pierre Marie (see below), described peroneal muscular atrophy, which was also reported three months later by Howard Tooth (1856–1926) at Cambridge (thus Charcot-Marie-Tooth disease). Linked the nervous system to joint diseases, Charcot's joints (painless deformity or destruction of joints in tabes dorsalis). Coined the term "ophthalmoplegic migraine" in 1890. Also worked with Henri Parinaud.

3. Studied cerebral localization. Attempted to divide diseases anatomically, focusing on brain and brainstem versus spinal cord and peripheral nerve versus muscle lesions. Coined the term "formes frustes" or "partial expressions." In his later career, he tried to distinguish different types of hysteria. Mental events could act as triggers for hysterical reactions. These ideas had a major impact on the young neurologist Sigmund Freud (1856–1939), who studied with Charcot in 1885

and 1886 and had expected to study neuroanatomy and pathology.

4. His *Leçons du Mardi* or Tuesday lectures attracted an international audience.

John Cheyne (1777–1836) and William Stokes (1804–1878)—Cheyne-Stokes Respiration

1. Cheyne was a Scottish physician and neuropathologist. First author to provide an illustration of subarachnoid hemorrhage. In 1818, in a 60-year-old patient with acute aphasia and hemiplegia, he observed: "For several days his breathing was irregular; it would cease for a quarter of a minute, then it would become perceptible, though very low, then by degrees it became heaving and quick, and then it would gradually cease again. . . ."

2. Stokes was an Irish physician who practiced in Dublin. Described the abnormal respiratory pattern, which he noted had been observed by Cheyne, in 1846. In the same publication, described Adams-Stokes-Morgagni syndrome, syncope of cardiac origin, also described by Dublin physician Robert Adams (1771–1875) and Giovanni Battista Morgagni (1682–1771; provided first account of subarachnoid hemorrhage, and noted that hydrocephalus in children but not in adults caused enlargement of the head).

3. Robert Whytt (1714–1766), a Scottish physician, who had described Cheyne-Stokes breathing previously. In 1751, he was the first to describe the pupillary light reflex and its anatomy. Also described the clinical features of increased intracranial pressure, transient monocular blindness, and diphtheria.

Hans Chiari (1851–1906)

1. Professor of pathology at the University in Prague and then successor to Friedrich Daniel von Recklinghausen in Strassburg.

2. Published on numerous topics including the first report on choriocarcinoma, the first to relate arteriosclerosis of the carotid bifurcation to cerebral embolism, and studies of the pancreas including the concept of self-digestion.

3. In 1891 and 1896, reported four types of malformations. John Cleland (1835–1925) in 1883 and Julius Arnold (1835–1915) in 1894 published on single cases of abnormalities of the hindbrain in cases of spina bifida, discussing them only as side issues. Although the eponym "Arnold-Chiari malformation" is also used, Chiari is deserving of the eponym alone because of his accurate description

of a large number of cases and his theory of pathogenesis.

Hans Gerhard Creutzfeldt (1885–1964) and Alfons Maria Jakob (1884–1931)— Creutzfeldt-Jakob Disease

1. Creutzfeldt studied with Alois Alzheimer. Director of neuropsychiatry at the Christian Albrechts University in Kiel. One of the few academics who refused to join the Nazi party.

2. In 1913, while working at Alzheimer's clinic, Creutzfeldt described the clinical and pathological findings of a "new and unusual type of neurological disease" in a 22-year-old woman. The case was not published until 1920 because of World War I.

3. Jakob studied with Emil Kraepelin (1856–1926), Franz Nissl (1860–1919), and Alzheimer. Worked at the Friedrichsberg State Hospital in Hamburg, which became a center of worldwide fame from his numerous contributions.

4. In 1921, Jakob described cases of what he termed *spastic pseudo-sclerosis.*

5. Carleton Gajdusek transmitted kuru to chimpanzees in 1966, for which he won a Nobel Prize. In 1982, Stanley Prusiner formulated the concept of the prion (from protein and infectious disease), for which he also won a Nobel Prize. Human diseases from prions can be sporadic, infectious, or genetic.

Harvey Williams Cushing (1869–1939)

1. Student of William Halsted (1852–1922). Professor of Neurosurgery at Massachusetts General Hospital in Boston. Difficult man (and boy. His family's nickname for him was "Pepper Pot."). One of his residents, a veteran of World War I, wrote in 1926 "that Gallipoli and the battle of the Marne were as nothing compared to the clinical stress of a year as Cushing's neurosurgical resident."

2. Described the Cushing reflex in 1901 based on his experiments on dogs.

3. Another eponym, Cushing's disease, was incorrectly attributed by him in 1932 to pituitary basophilism rather than adrenal cortex hyperfunction.

4. Founder of modern neurosurgery (silver hemoclip, electrocoagulation, and much more).

5. Won a Pulitzer Prize for the biography of his mentor and friend, Sir William Osler (1849–1919).

Walter Edward Dandy (1886–1946)

1. Trained with William Halsted and Harvey Cushing (later had a longstanding feud with Cushing, and the two men would not speak to each other). Professor of neurosurgery at Johns Hopkins.

2. Introduced pneumoencephalography. Developed a posterior approach for section of the trigeminal nerve for trigeminal neuralgia. First to clip a cerebral aneurysm.

3. With his Hopkins colleague A.E. Walker in 1921, reported Dandy-Walker syndrome (malformation of the fourth ventricle and cerebellum with atresia of the foramina of Luschka and Megendie and failure of development of the midline structures of the cerebellum, which instead form a large cyst obstructing cerebrospinal fluid flow and cause hydrocephalus). J.B. Sutton had previously described this malformation in 1887.

Charles Miller Fisher (1913–   )

1. Trained with Wilder Penfield (1891–1976) and Raymond D. Adams (1911–   ). Long association with Massachusetts General Hospital.

2. Numerous pivotal reports: carotid bifurcation occlusive disease as a cause of stroke and embolism (1951); coined the term "transient global amnesia" in 1953 with Adams; the unique features of thalamic hemorrhage (1959); the vascular pathology underlying lacunar infarcts and described many of the lacunar stroke syndromes (1965, 1967); multi-infarct dementia (1968); and late-life migrainous accompaniments (1980).

3. Described the variant of Guillain-Barré syndrome, Miller Fisher syndrome (ophthalmoplegia, ataxia, and areflexia) in 1956. Also reported Miller Fisher's 1½ syndrome in 1967. (A combined lesion of the ipsilateral medial longitudinal fasciculus and the parapontine reticular formation or the sixth nerve nucleus resulting in a total palsy of ipsilateral lateral gaze and "half" a palsy of contralateral lateral gaze. Etiologies include ischemia, hemorrhage, tumor, trauma, and multiple sclerosis.)

Robert Foster Kennedy (1884–1952)

1. Born in Belfast, trained at the National Hospital, Queen Square, professor at Cornell and chief of neurology at Bellevue Hospital.

2. Published on many topics including shell shock in World War I, epidemic encephalitis, and complications of spinal anesthesia.

3. In 1911, he described unilateral optic atrophy and

contralateral papilledema, commonly with anosmia, typically caused by a tumor of the lesser wing of the sphenoid bone that compresses the first and second cranial nerve and results in contralateral papilledema from raised intracranial pressure. This manifestation had been earlier reported by William Gowers in 1893 and published by Gowers and Paton in 1909, as Foster Kennedy acknowledged in his more complete description.

4. He died shortly after correctly diagnosing Brown-Séquard syndrome in himself due to polyarteritis nodosa.

Georges Gilles de la Tourette (1857–1904)

1. In 1885, at Charcot's request, he published a two-part article describing what he called convulsive tic disease with coprolalia. Charcot gave the eponym of *maladie des tics de Gilles de la Tourette*, now known as *Tourette syndrome*. Also concluded that the "jumping Frenchmen of Maine," latah, and miryachit were identical disorders, excessive startle disorders.

2. In 1887, became Charcot's *chef du clinique* at the Salpêtrière. In 1893, a former patient who claimed that he had hypnotized her against her will, fired three bullets into his head and neck. He survived and went on to write on psychology, physiology, as well as theatrical and social criticism.

William Richard Gowers (1845–1915)

1. Professor at the National Hospital at Queen Square. Had been a junior colleague to John Hughlings Jackson.

2. He wrote influential textbooks: *Manual and Atlas of Medical Ophthalmoscopy, Diagnosis of Diseases of the Spinal Cord, Epilepsy and Other Chronic Convulsive Diseases, Manual of Diseases of the Nervous System* (the bible of neurology for half a century), and *The Border-Land of Epilepsy*.

3. Numerous observations and coining of terms including "knee-jerk" and "fibrositis."

4. First full description of Gower's sign (a child with Duchenne muscular dystrophy and proximal weakness rising from the sitting position by resting on his hands and knees and then "climbing up his legs") and discovery of Gower's tract (the dorsal spinocerebellar tract) with his pupil, the pioneering neurosurgeon Victor Horsley (1857–1916). He also described Gower's maneuver for hysterical paraplegia—pull on the patient's pubic hair and see if the seemingly paralyzed thighs adduct.

Georges Guillain (1876–1961) and Jean-Alexandre Barré (1880–1967)—Guillain-Barré Syndrome

1. Guillain (Gie-yanh), Barré (Bha-ray), and André Strohl (1887–1977) described the syndrome in two French infantry soldiers in 1916. They described, for the first time, the albuminocytologic dissociation (elevated cerebrospinal fluid protein without an elevation in white blood cells). In 1943, A. B. Baker designated the disease *Guillain-Barré syndrome.*

2. The same disorder had been described earlier by Wardrop and Ollivier (1834–1837), Landry (1859), and others including William Osler. Some purists may prefer the eponym "Wardrop-Landry-Guillain-Barré-Strohl syndrome." It may take a village to name a neurologic disorder.

3. Guillain became chair of the neurology service at the Salpêtrière and published a classic biography of Charcot in 1955. Barré, a student of Babinski, became professor of neurology in Strasbourg and published on semiology, neuro-otology, and vestibular syndromes.

Robert Marcus Gunn (1850–1909)

1. Scottish ophthalmologist on the staff of the National Hospital and the Hospital for Sick Children in London.

2. Described the constriction followed by redilation of the pupil with continued exposure to direct light stimulation in an eye with an optic nerve lesion (afferent pupillary defect). Levatin described the swinging flashlight test.

3. In 1883, he described the Marcus Gunn phenomenon or jaw winking in patients with congenital and unilateral ptosis: when the mouth is opened, the lid rises and when the jaw closes, the lid comes down in a wink. The inverted or reversed Marcus Gunn phenomenon, Marin Amat (a Spanish ophthalmologist) syndrome, is eye closure when the jaw is opened wide, which can be congenital or acquired (e.g., following Bell's palsy).

Henry Head (1861–1940)

1. London neurologist. Editor of the journal *Brain* for 15 years.

2. Described Head's areas (or zones), locations of referred pain from visceral organs, in his 1892 M.D. thesis. With Alfred Campbell (1868–1937) in 1900, published a map of the dermatomes from studying the pattern of rashes in patients with herpes zoster.

Johann Friedrich Horner (1831–1886)

1. Born and practiced in Zurich. Mainly worked in his private ophthalmology clinic. Performed an estimated 5000 cataract extractions with a failure rate of only 1%.

2. In 1869, he reported the case of a 40-year-old patient with unilateral ptosis, miosis, enophthalmos, and anhydrosis (Horner's syndrome), which he inferred was due to a lesion of the cervical sympathetic nerve. Horner's syndrome had been described to varying extents by numerous prior investigators going back to 1727. Also described by the French physiologist, Claude Bernard (1813–1878), and is known in the French literature as the syndrome of Claude Bernard or Claude Bernard-Horner.

James Ramsay Hunt (1872–1937)

1. American neurologist, professor at Columbia University College of Physicians and Surgeons.

2. First to describe in detail the effects of internal carotid artery occlusion and of damage to the deep palmar branch of the ulnar nerve.

3. Described Ramsay Hunt paralysis (juvenile parkinsonism syndromes) and three Ramsay Hunt syndromes: dyssynergia cerebellaris myoclonica (an autosomal recessive progressive myoclonic epilepsy with ataxia of multiple etiologies, most commonly mitochondrial encephalomyopathy with ragged red fibers); dentatorubral atrophy; and the most well known, geniculate herpes (painful herpes zoster involvement of the facial nerve with facial paresis and vesicles of the external ear).

George Huntington (1850–1921)

1. Born and raised in East Hampton, Long Island. Attended the College of Physicians and Surgeons of Columbia University.

2. In 1871, while working as an assistant to his physician father, described a hereditary chorea leading to insanity. The disease was termed "Huntington's chorea" by Huber in 1887.

3. Later in 1871, he moved to Pomeroy, Ohio, and was a country doctor. He did not write or do research on any other medical subject.

Ernö (Ernst) Jendrassik (1858–1921)

1. Born in Transylvania. Professor of neuropathology at the Medical University of Budapest.

2. His study of neurodegenerative diseases led to his famous doctrine of "heredodegeneration" before the rediscovery of Mendel's laws in 1900.

3. In 1883, he reported that voluntary muscle contraction anywhere in the body, such as lifting both arms, causes a physiological increase of the tendon reflexes.

4. In 1885, he described Jendrassik's maneuver: "I put the individual, who has no knee jerk with the normal method, on the edge of a table with the legs as relaxed as possible, and while I tap his patellar tendons, I ask him to hook the flexed fingers of the right and left hand in each other, and pull them as hard as possible with the arms extended forward." Reflex reinforcement can occur with other types of muscular contraction such as making one or two fists or merely pressing a button with a thumb. Mental focus, i.e., focusing attention on one extremity, can increase the tendon reflexes in that extremity.

Jean Lhermitte (1877–1959)

1. Clinical director of the Salpêtrière in Paris and one of the founders of modern neuropsychology.

2. Described "Lhermitte's sign" (flexion of the neck produces an electrical sensation running down the spine into the legs and less often also into the arms) in patients with multiple sclerosis. This is not at all a sign but a positive symptom and had previously been described by other physicians including Pierre Marie and Joseph Babinski. In addition to multiple sclerosis, Lhermitte's sign can occur in many other disorders where there is demyelination of the posterior columns including cervical spondylosis and disc disease, cervical radiation myelopathy, and vitamin B_{12} deficiency. Flexion of the neck produces stretching of the ligamenta denticulata and of the abnormal posterior columns, resulting in ectopic impulse generation.

3. Also known for Lhermitte's syndrome, anterior internuclear ophthalmoplegia.

Pierre Marie (1853–1940)

1. Lawyer and then physician in Paris; trained with Jean-Martin Charcot.

2. Charcot-Marie-Tooth disease (see under Charcot). Reported Marie syndrome in 1885 (the association of acromegaly with a pituitary tumor) and Marie ataxia (a dominantly inherited spastic-ataxic syndrome with gaze palsies).

3. Published with Charles Foix (1882–1927) Foix syndrome or red nucleus syndrome. In 1913, they reported an autopsy case of carpal tunnel syndrome and suggested that section of the transverse

carpal ligament could be therapeutic. Also published with Théophile Alajouanine (1869–1959). Marie-Foix syndrome (lateral pontine lesion) and Marie-Foix-Alajouanine syndrome (a sporadic adult-onset cerebellar syndrome with atrophy of the cerebellum and inferior olives).

James Parkinson (1755–1824)

1. His father, grandfather, and great-grandfather were all surgeons-apothecaries. Parkinson was a general practitioner in London.

2. He was also a political reformer who made major scientific contributions in paleontology and geology and published the three quarto volumes, *Organic Remains of a Former World*.

3. In 1817, he reported six cases of the shaking palsy or paralysis agitans including the features of resting tremor, rigidity, and gait disturbance.

4. Jean-Martin Charcot, who added the feature of bradykinesia, introduced the use of the eponym in 1879 when he described a case where "A man aged fifty years was attacked by Parkinson's disease."

Quotation

"The disease is of long duration. . . . It has been seen in the preceding history of the disease . . . that certain affections, the tremulous agitation, and the almost invincible propensity to run, when wishing only to walk, . . . appear to be pathognomonic symptoms of this malady."

Parkinson distinguishes action tremor from Parkinson's tremor as follows: "If the trembling limb be supported, and none of its muscles be called into action, the trembling will cease. In the real Shaking Palsy the reverse of this takes place, the agitation continues in full force whilst the limb is at rest and unemployed; and even is sometimes diminished by calling the muscles into employment."

Parkinson J. An Essay on the Shaking Palsy, 1817.

Moritz Romberg (1795–1873)

1. Professor of pathology at the University of Berlin.

2. Formulated the first blueprint of systematic neurology in his two volume *Lehrbuch der Nervenkrankheiten des Menschen* (1840–1846).

3. In 1853, in the second edition of his textbook, he described Romberg's sign in patients with tabes dorsalis: "[If he is ordered to close his eyes while in the erect position, he at once commences to totter and swing from side to side.]" The test is performed with the patient's feet together. A positive Romberg sign can be present with disorders of proprioception.

Thomas Sydenham (1624–1689)

1. London physician, the "English Hippocrates": recommended careful observation of patients' signs and symptoms and differential diagnoses of seemingly similar conditions.

2. In 1686, described five children with a "curable" chorea (the Greek term for *dance*) under the term, "St. Vitus dance." The Swiss physician Paracelsus (1493–1541) had used the term "St. Vitus dance" after the chapel in Dresselhausen, Swabia, where late fourteenth-century and early fifteenth-century German sufferers of convulsive behaviors made pilgrimages in search of help. Sydenham's chorea is an autoimmune sequela of group A beta-hemolytic streptococcus infection in which autoantibodies cross-react with neuronal cytoplasmic antigens of the caudate and subthalamic nuclei.

Jules Tinel (1879–1952)

1. Department head at the Salpêtrière in Paris. During World War I, he founded a regional neurologic center at the front, where he studied peripheral nerve injuries.

2. In October 1915, on the French side of the front, he described Tinel's sign (digital pressure or a tap over an injured nerve with regenerating nerve fibers produces radiating tingling sensations in the otherwise anesthetic skin area supplied by the nerve).

3. Earlier in 1915, on the German side of the front, Paul Hoffmann (1884–1962) made the same observations. In 1920, he described the H (or Hoffmann) reflex.

4. Neither Hoffmann nor Tinel ever mentioned the most common current application of Tinel's sign, a tool for diagnosing compression neuropathies such as carpal tunnel syndrome or ulnar neuropathy at the elbow. Tinel's sign is present in more than half of carpal tunnel syndrome cases but false-positive results are common in the general population. Tinel's sign for cubital tunnel syndrome has a sensitivity of 0.70 and a specificity of 0.98. George Phalen (American orthopedist, 1911–1998) described Phalen's sign in carpal tunnel syndrome (paresthesias produced by hyperflexion of the wrist for 60 seconds) in 1951.

Robert Bentley Todd (1809–1860)

1. From Dublin, professional career in London. One of the founders of King's College Hospital.

2. Coined the terms "afferent" and "efferent" and published the first account of tabes dorsalis.

3. In 1849, described postictal paralysis following a partial motor seizure, Todd's paralysis, or paresis.

Friedrich Daniel von Recklinghausen (1833–1910)

1. Studied with Rudolf Virchow (1821–1902) of *omnis cellula a cellula* (every cell is the product of another cell) fame. Professor of pathology at the University of Strassburg.

2. Detailed description of neurofibromatosis type 1, von Recklinghausen's disease, in 1882. There had been numerous prior descriptions of neurofibromatosis since 1592. Von Recklinghausen also described osteitis fibrosa cystica, changes in bone accompanying primary hyperparathyroidism.

Adolf Wallenberg (1862–1948)

1. Trained in Heidelberg with Wilhelm Erb (1840-1921; described "delivery paralysis," upper brachial plexopathy in newborns. First to use a hammer to elicit tendon reflexes in 1875.). Practiced in Danzig, Prussia.

2. Described the lateral medullary syndrome (first paper in 1895), Wallenberg's syndrome, which is due to a posterior inferior cerebellar artery lesion. In 1961, Charles Miller Fisher (see earlier) reported the most common cause, vertebral artery occlusion.

Augustus Volney Waller (1816–1870)

1. Born in England and grew up and went to medical school in France. Practiced in London and did research in Germany and France. His son, Augustus (1856–1922), made the first recording of the human electrocardiogram.

2. In 1850, he described sequential degeneration after unilateral sectioning of the glossopharyngeal and hypoglossal nerves of the frog. The term "Wallerian degeneration" has been used since at least 1876.

Carl Wernicke (1848–1905)

1. Studied brain anatomy in 1871 with Theodor Meynert (1833–1892) who described Meynert's basal nucleus (which has an integrative role in the cholinergic forebrain and degenerates in Alzheimer's disease).

2. Professor of psychiatry and neurology in Breslau.

3. In 1874, described the clinical presentation and anatomical substrate (left posterior superior temporal lobe) of Wernicke's aphasia.

4. In 1881 he described the clinical syndrome of "polioencephalitis superior haemorrhagica" also known as "Wernicke's encephalopathy" which is the acute onset of ataxia, ophthalmoplegia, nystagmus, polyneuropathy of the arms and legs, and a global confusional state. In 1887, Sergei Sergeivich Korsakoff (1854-1900), the founder of Russian psychiatry, wrote the first of a series of papers describing Korsakoff's syndrome or psychosis characterized by chronic changes in mental status and memory that often accompanied polyneuropathy. He also commented on the tendency of these patients to confabulate and a typical history of alcohol abuse, although the disorder could occur after prolonged vomiting or intestinal obstruction. These presentations may occur alone or in combination, Wernicke-Korsakoff's syndrome, as a result of thiamine deficiency and direct toxic effects of alcohol on the brain.

Thomas Willis (1621–1675)

1. Student and later Sedleian Professor of Natural History at Oxford

2. His 1664 work, *The Anatomy of the Brain*, was the source for the eponym, "the circle of Willis" first used by Albrecht von Haller in 1774. The first complete illustration of the circle was probably drawn by his collaborator, Christopher Wren, the architect of St. Paul's and many other London churches. Willis also described the eleventh cranial nerve, the ciliary ganglion, thalamus, lentiform body, and intercostal nerves.

3. Described the differentiation between diabetes insipidus and mellitus, meningococcal meningitis, general paralysis, Jacksonian epilepsy, myasthenia gravis, transient ischemic attacks, carotid occlusion with headache (Willis headache), narcolepsy, bipolar disease, migraine, and more. Introduced the doctrine of the gray cortex as the source of cerebral activities and the white matter as a mass of connections.

4. Coined the Greek term "neurologia." Also coined the terms "lobe," "hemisphere," "pyramid," "peduncle," "corpus striatum," and "reflexion" (later changed to "reflex").

5. Willis is buried in Westminster Abbey.

Samuel Alexander Kinnier Wilson (1878–1937)

1. Born in New Jersey and moved to Scotland as a small child. Qualified in medicine at Edinburgh University.

2. Trained at the National Hospital, Queen Square with John Hughlings Jackson, William Gowers, and Victor Horsley.

3. Published his M.D. thesis in 1912, *Progressive Lenticular Degeneration*, describing four cases of Wilson's disease. Kayser-Fleischer rings (corneal copper deposits) described by Bernard Kayser in 1902 and Bruno Fleischer in 1903. In 1948, Cumings was the first to postulate an etiologic role for copper in the disease.

4. Clinical papers on apraxia, aphasia, the epilepsies, epidemic encephalitis, tics, and pathological crying and laughing. His two-volume textbook, *Neurology* (published posthumously in 1940), is considered one of the best.

Space limitations do not permit a more complete listing of eponyms. As much as an honor as it is to have your own eponym, imagine being immortalized by having a part of the brain or nervous system named after you. Key neuroanatomical eponyms are given in Table 15–1.

TABLE 15–1. ADDITIONAL NEUROANATOMICAL NAMES AND EPONYMS

Albert Adamkiewicz (1850–1921)	Adamkiewicz's artery
Vladimir Aleksandrovich Betz (1834–1894)	Betz cells
Korbinian Brodmann (1868–1918)	Brodmann's cortical areas
Claudius Galen (130–200 AD)	great vein of Galen
Herophilus of Chaldecon (335–280 BC)	torcular Herophili
Hubert von Luschka (1820–1875)	foramen of Luschka
François Magendie (1783–1855)f	foramen of Magendie
Georg Meissner (1829–1905)	Meissner's corpuscles and plexus
Alexander Monro "Secundus" (1733–1817)	interventricular foramen of Monro
Jan Evangelista Purkinje (1787–1869)	Purkinje cell
Louis Antoine Ranvier (1835–1922)	node of Ranvier
Luigi Rolando (1773–1831)	Rolandic fissure
Theodor Schwann (1810–1882)	Schwann cell
Sylvius (François de la Boë) (1614–1672)	Sylvian fissure, Sylvian aqueduct
Felix Vicq d'Azyr (1748–1794)	bundle of Vicq D'Azyr (mammillothalamic tract)

Bibliography

Aird RB: Foundation of Modern Neurology. A Century of Progress. New York, Raven Press, 1994.

Finger S: Origins of Neuroscience. New York, Oxford University Press, 1994.

Goetz CG, Bonduelle M, Gelfand T: Charcot. Constructing Neurology. New York, Oxford University Press, 1995.

Koehler PJ, Bruyn GW, Pearce JMS (eds): Neurological Eponyms. New York, Oxford University Press, 2000.

Marshall LH, Magoun HW: Discoveries in the Human Brain. Totowa, New Jersey, Humana Press, 1998.

Pryse-Phillips, W: Companion to Clinical Neurology. Boston, Little, Brown and Company, 1995.

Wilkins RH, Brody IA: Neurological Classics. Park Ridge, IL, American Association of Neurological Surgeons, 1997.

1 Lumbar Puncture and Cerebrospinal Fluid Evaluation

Randolph W. Evans

Basic Principles and Technique

1. Patient positioning is crucial to a successful tap.

   a. For lumbar puncture, place the patient in the lateral decubitus position with flexion of the neck, trunk, hips, and knees and the head resting level on a pillow; shoulders and back perpendicular to edge of bed or table.

   b. If opening pressure is not required or in a difficult puncture, perform with the patient seated on the edge of the bed or examining table, leaning forward over a pillow or a bedside table. If an opening pressure is required, the patient can carefully move from the sitting position to the lateral decubitus position with the needle in place.

2. Select puncture site. Must be below spinal cord which ends at L1–L2 in 94% of cases and at L2–L3 in 6%, except in infants where the cord ends at L3.

   a. Palpate the posterior superior iliac crest. An imaginary line through the two crests intersects approximately at the L3–L4 interspace.

   b. The L3–L4, L4–L5, or L5–S1 interspaces may be used, except in infants where the L4–L5 or L5–S1 interspace should be used.

3. Prepare the skin surface with povidone-iodine. Place sterile drapes if desired. Put on sterile gloves.

4. May use local anesthetic (e.g. 1% lidocaine) infiltrated at the puncture site subcutaneously and then into the deeper tissues.

5. Needle insertion with stylet in place (Fig. 1–1)

   a. In middle of the interspace with an upward angle toward the umbilicus

   b. If a bevel-tipped (Quincke) needle is used, the face or flat portion of the neeedle bevel should be parallel to the long axis of the spine. If performed in the lateral decubitus position, the face of the bevel should point up toward

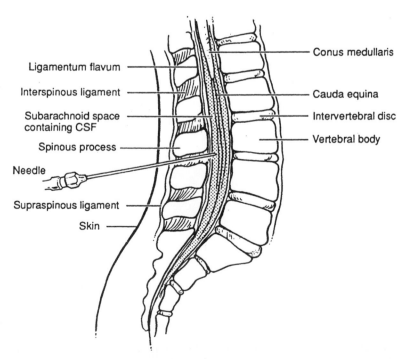

Ligamentum flavum

Interspinous ligament

Subarachnoid space
containing CSF

Spinous process

Needle

Supraspinous ligament

Skin

Conus medullaris

Cauda equina

Intervertebral disc

Vertebral body

Figure 1–1. Sagittal view of the placement of the lumbar puncture needle in the L3–L4 interspace. The needle passes through the supraspinatus ligament, interspinous ligament, and ligamentum flavum before puncturing the dura and entering the subarachnoid space. (From Devinsky O, Feldmann E, Weinreb HJ, Wilterdink JL: The Resident's Neurology Book. Philadelphia, F.A. Davis, 1997, p. 29, with permission.)

the physician. If performed in the sitting position, the face of the bevel should be turned to the left or right.

c. Slowly advance the needle until there is a sudden decrease in resistance as the dura is punctured and the subarachnoid space is entered. Check for cerebrospinal fluid (CSF). If the tap is dry, rotate the needle 90 degrees.

d. If bony resistance is met, withdraw the needle with stylet and try another angle in the midline of the interspace.

e. If the tap is not successful but the patient complains of paresthesias going down one leg, withdraw and redirect the needle to the midline.

f. If lumbar puncture (LP) is not successful, request another more experienced physician to perform the procedure or ask radiologist to perform it with fluoroscopy.

   (1) In some cases (e.g. morbidly obese patient or patient with severe lumbar spondylosis), it may be best to perform LP with fluoroscopy.

   (2) If LP can not be performed or is contraindicated (e.g. skin infection of lower back), a lateral cervical puncture in the C1–C2 interspace (risk of cervical cord damage) or cisterna magna puncture (risk of brainstem or cervical cord damage) can be performed by an experienced physician with fluoroscopy.

6. When the CSF flows, may check the opening pressure with the patient in the lateral decubitus position. The opening pressure cannot be accurately determined in the sitting position.

a. Attach the hub of the manometer to the needle immediately.

b. Allow the CSF to rise in the manometer until a steady state is reached.

   (1) The manometer records the mean intracranial pressure.

   (2) The pressure recorded by the manometer also shows the dampened pulsations synchronous with the pulse of 2 to 5 mm and with respiration of 4 to 10 mm.

   (3) Extend the neck and legs. Falsely elevated pressures can be obtained with coughing, talking, or abdominal straining. Ask the patient to be quiet and relax. Hyperventilation can spuriously decrease CSF pressure.

c. The normal opening CSF pressure varies between 60 and 200 mm H_2O. Normal opening CSF pressure in obese persons can be as high as 250 mm because of increased abdominal venous pressure.

7. Collect 2 ml of CSF in each of 3 or 4 labeled tubes for routine studies (glucose, protein, cell count and, depending on the circumstance, cultures and stains and antigens (e.g., meningitis latex, VDRL). Additional CSF may be necessary for studies such as oligoclonal bands or cytology. Note the general appearance of the CSF (e.g., clear or cloudy).

a. The average adult ventricular system and subarachnoid space contains between 90 and 150 ml of CSF with about 80% in the ventricles.

b. CSF production about 20 ml/hour or 500 ml/day

8. Replace the stylet and withdraw the needle. Apply a bandage to the puncture site.

9. Have the patient stay supine or sitting for a few minutes if there is a risk of a vasovagal reaction. Otherwise the patient may get right back up. The supine position does not reduce the risk of post–lumbar puncture headache.

10. Write your procedure note which may include the patient's position, local anesthetic used, opening pressure (if elevated, note the effect of straightening the legs and neck), volume and appearance of fluid removed (if bloody, indicate if any change in sequential tubes), any complications, and tests ordered.

Indications

1. Absence of contraindications (inappropriate lumbar puncture can kill!)

2. Meningitis and meningoencephalitis

3. Subarachnoid hemorrhage

4. Meningeal cardinomatosis

5. Inflammatory disorders such as multiple sclerosis and Guillain-Barré syndrome

6. Other disorders (pseudotumor cerebri, normal pressure hydrocephalus, etc.)

7. Introduction of diagnostic and therapeutic agents such as contrast media, anesthetics, radionuclides, antibiotics, or chemotherapy.

Indications

- Absence of contraindications

- Meningitis and meningoencephalitis

- Subarachnoid hemorrhage

- Meningeal carcinomatosis

- Multiple sclerosis and Guillain-Barré syndrome

- Pseudotumor cerebri and normal pressure hydro-cephalus

- Introduction of diagnostic and therapeutic agents

Contraindications

1. Increased intracranial pressure from mass lesions such as neoplasm, subdural hematoma, abscess, or parenchymal hemorrhage.
2. Infection in skin or other tissue overlying lumbar puncture site (e.g., cellulitis or epidural abscess).
3. Bleeding disorders
   a. Thombocytopenia: Platelet count should be greater than 50,000 μl. If urgent indication, can perform with platelet count of 20,000 or greater. If platelet count is less or rapidly falling, perform platelet transfusion first.
   b. Coagulopathies such as hemophilia where re-placement therapy is necessary before the pro-cedure
   c. In questionable cases, a platelet count, pro-thrombin time, partial prothrombin time, and semplate bleeding time should be obtained before the lumbar puncture.
4. Anticoagulation therapy
   a. Adequate reversal with protamine for those on heparin and vitamin K or fresh frozen plasma for those on warfarin is mandatory before lumbar puncture.
5. Some cases of meningitis especially in children when focal findings or coma is present (see Complications below)

Contraindications to Lumbar Puncture

- Increased intracranial pressure from mass lesions

- Infection in skin or other tissue overlying puncture site

- Bleeding disorders

- Anticoagulation therapy

- Some cases of meningitis

- Complete spinal subarachnoid block

Normal Findings

1. Clear and colorless; CSF is 99% water
2. Glucose concentration in CSF is normally 60% of the plasma glucose concentration. Typically ranges between 45 and 80 mg/dl in nondiabetics.
3. Total CSF protein level ranges between 15 and 50 mg/dl.
   a. Majority of CSF protein derived from the serum with a CSF to serum albumin ratio of about 1:200
   b. There is a concentration gradient from the lowest levels in the ventricles to the highest level in the lumbar sac.
4. Normal CSF contains no more than 5 lymphocytes or mononuclear cells/mm^3 and 0 red blood cells. Pleocytosis is an abnormal number of white blood cells in the CSF.

Normal Findings

- Clear and colorless

- CSF glucose between 45 and 80 mg/dl in nondia-betics

- Total CSF protein level 15 to 50 mg/dl

- No more than 5 lymphocytes or mononuclear cells/mm^3 and 0 red blood cells

---

Abnormal Findings

1. Protein
   a. May be elevated in numerous conditions, in-cluding infections, brain and spinal cord tu-mors, multiple sclerosis, polyneuropathies (e.g., diabetes and Guillain-Barré syndrome), cere-bral venous thrombosis, cerebral hemorrhage, uremia, myxedema, chronic arachnoiditis, CNS vasculitis, low CSF pressure syndromes, and cerebral trauma. Elevated protein is due to a pathological increase in endothelial cell perme-ability.
   (1) Levels more than 500 mg/dl can be seen in meningitis, spinal block due to cord tumor, arachnoiditis, or with subarachnoid hemor-rhage.

(2) Complete spinal block can lead to Froin's syndrome, with protein concentrations of greater than 1000 mg/dl. The CSF clots due to the presence of sufficient amount of serum fibrinogen.

b. Low CSF protein below 15 mg/dl may be present with CSF leaks or occasionally in pseudotumor cerebri.

c. Increased CSF immunoglobins are indicative of a central nervous system inflammatory response.

  (1) May be seen in immunologic and infectious disorders

  (2) The immunoglobin G (IgG) index,

$$\frac{\text{IgG (CSF)} \times \text{albumin (serum)}}{\text{IgG (serium)} \times \text{albumin (CSF)}},$$

  corrects the CSF level for the entry of immunoglobins from the serum.

    (i) Normal is <0.65.

    (ii) Elevated in 70% to 90% of cases of multiple sclerosis

  (3) Electrophoretic separation of CSF proteins within the gamma region can demonstrate one band (monoclonal), many bands (polyclonal), and two to five bands (oligoclonal).

    (a) A band represents a homogeneous protein secreted by a single clone of plasma cells.

    (b) CSF results need to be compared to serum protein electrophoresis to determine the origin. A normal serum result indicates CNS production.

    (c) CSF oligoclonal bands are usually pathologic but have been reported in 2% of controls.

      (i) Isoelectric focusing with immunofixation is more sensitive than agarose gel electrophoresis.

      (ii) May be present in a variety of inflammatory and infectious diseases including multiple sclerosis (90% of cases; there should be no bands in the serum), subacute sclerosing panencephalitis (100%), CNS lupus, neurosyphilis, and other infections, neurosarcoidosis, Guillain-Barré, Behçet's, meningeal carcinomatosis, and glioblastoma multiforme.

2. Glucose

  a. Increased glucose reflects the presence of hyperglycemia within the 4 hours prior to lumbar puncture.

  b. Low CSF glucose (hypoglycorrhachia) may be present in hypoglycemia, infections (bacterial, fungal, tuberculous, amebic, cysticercosis, mumps, and herpes simplex), meningeal carcinomatosis, meningeal sarcoid, subarachnoid hemorrhage, chemical meningitis, rheumatoid meningitis, and lupus myelopathy.

3. Xanthochromia: a colored CSF supernatant

  a. Red blood cell (RBC) breakdown results in the release of oxyhemoglobin, which is degraded by macrophages and other cells in the leptomeninges to bilirubin by the third to fourth day after a subarachnoid hemorrhage (SAH).

    (1) The CSF supernatant is pink or pink-orange in the presence of oxyhemoglobin, yellow in the presence of bilirubin, and an intermediate color if both are present.

    (2) Although oxyhemoglobin can be detected as early as 2 hours after entry of RBCs into the CSF, xanthochromia is not present in all cases until after 12 hours.

    (3) Absorption spectrophotometry is more sensitive than the naked eye in the detection of xanthochromia. With spectrophotometry, the CSF is xanthochromic afer SAH 100% of the time during the first 2 weeks, >70% at 3 weeks, and >40% at 4 weeks.

  b. Other causes of xanthochromia

    (1) Jaundice, usually with a total plasma bilirubin of 10 to 15 mg/dl

    (2) CSF protein more than 150 mg/dl

    (3) Dietary hypercarotenemia

    (4) Malignant melanomatosis

    (5) Oral intake of rifampin

    (6) Traumatic lumbar puncture

4. Cloudy or turbid appearance of CSF

  a. Usually due to pleocytosis

  b. At least 200 WBC/mm^3 or 400 RBC/mm^3 must be present.

  c. With RBC concentrations between 500 and 6000 cells/mm^3, the unspun CSF is cloudy or pink-tinged. The CSF appears grossly bloody with an RBC count >6000.

5. Traumatic lumbar puncture (also see under Complications)

  a. When the CSF obtained from the first lumbar puncture is bloody, the only certain way to distinguish SAH from a traumatic tap is the presence of a xanthochromic supernatant.

    (1) The supernatant should be checked expediently because even a small number of RBCs can form oxyhemoglobin in vivo. Bilirubin and methemoglobin (a reduction product

of hemoglobin found in encapsulated subdural hematomas and old loculated intracerebral hemorrhages) can only be formed in vitro.

b. Although a decrease in RBCs from the first to the third tube may be present after a traumatic tap, a similar finding can be seen after a SAH. After a traumatic tap, the number of RBCs may stay constant in all three tubes.

c. The presence of crenated RBCs in not a reliable sign of SAH. Crenation occurs very soon after RBCs enter the CSF with a traumatic tap as well.

d. In a traumatic tap, you can calculate the increased number of WBCs over the number in atraumatic CSF if you have the patient's complete blood count.

  (1) Additional WBCs = (peripheral WBCs/peripheral RBCs) × CSF RBCs.

  (2) For example, if the patient's peripheral WBC count is 5,000 cells/mm^3 and RBC count 5,000,000 cells/mm^3, then the ratio 1/1000 multiplied by the number of CSF RBCs provides the excess in CSF WBCs due to the traumatic tap.

e. A traumatic tap also increases the CSF protein level.

  (1) With a normal hemogram and serum protein level, there is an additional 1 mg/100 ml of protein for every 1000 RBCs/mm^3. (The CSF cell count and protein should be checked on the same tube.)

6. Eosinophilia

a. Eosinophils are usually absent in normal CSF, although occasionally a single cell is seen with a normal total cell count.

b. CSF eosinophilia may be present in various diseases.

  (1) Infections of the CNS (especially parasitic but also tuberculous, syphilitic, viral, and fungal)

  (2) Malignancies (e.g., lymphoma, Hodgkin's disease, and leukemia)

  (3) Meningeal irritation (e.g., SAH and myelography)

  (4) Medications (e.g., penicillin, ibuprofen, and intravenous immunoglobin)

  (5) Ventriculoperitoneal shunt complications (infection or obstruction)

7. Infections

a. Acute bacterial meningitis

  (1) Usually elevated opening pressure

  (2) Increased white blood cells of 1000 to 5000 cells/mm^3 with polymorphonuclear predominance but occasionally fewer than 100 cells/mm^3. Initially 10% of patients may show mononuclear predominance.

  (3) Low glucose level (<40 mg/dl or a CSF/serum ratio of <0.3)

  (4) Increased protein level (100 to 500 mg/dl)

  (5) Gram stain positive in over 60% of cases; culture positive in at least 80%

b. Viral meningitis or meningoencephalitis

  (1) Normal to moderate elevation of opening pressure

  (2) Usually elevated white blood cells of 5 to a few hundred with a lymphocytic predominance

  (3) Usually normal but may be reduced in mumps and herpes simplex

  (4) Polymerase chain reaction (PCR) technique can be exceedingly helpful (e.g., highly sensitive and specific in the diagnosis of herpes simplex encephalitis).

c. Tuberculous meningitis

  (1) Usually elevated opening pressure

  (2) Usually 25 to 100 white blood cells, rarely more than 500; lymphocytic predominance in about 70% of cases

  (3) Typically reduced glucose level and elevated protein, usually 100 to 200 mg/dl

d. Cryptococcal meningitis

  (1) Usually elevated opening pressure

  (2) Usually elevated white blood cell count; lymphocytes predominate with an average of 50 and a range of 0 to 800

  (3) Protein level is usually elevated and glucose may be mildly decreased.

  (4) CSF India ink stain is positive in 75%, and cryptococcal antigen is positive in 90% to 100%.

8. Seizures

a. CSF is normal in interictal idiopathic epilepsy.

b. Pleocytosis can be present 72 hours after a seizure(s) with a greater number of WBCs within 12 hours after the seizure.

  (1) Pleocytosis can be due to simple, complex partial, and generalized tonic-clonic seizures.

  (2) Up to 80 WBCs/mm^3 may be present.

  (3) Pleocytosis more likely and greater after repeated or prolonged seizures.

  (4) Benign postictal pleocytosis is a diagnosis of exclusion.

9. Migraine

a. Often indicated for first or worst headaches to rule out SAH or for the evaluation of confusional migraine or some focal neurologic episodes

b. CSF is usually normal (even when migraine is associated with neurologic deficits such as hemiplegic migraine), although protein can rarely be elevated.

c. Episodic headache with neurologic deficit may be due to pseudomigraine, a rare disorder.

   (1) One to twelve episodes of neurologic deficit (usually sensory, aphasia, and motor deficits, less often visual symptoms) with a mean duration of 5 hours and a moderate to severe headache; fever occasionally present

   (2) CSF lymphocytic pleocytosis (10 to 760 cells) and elevated protein present.

   (3) A magnetic resonance imaging study (MRI) will be normal but an electroencephalogram may show focal slowing.

   (4) Twenty-five percent have antecedent viral-like illness up to 3 weeks before onset.

   (5) Benign disorder

Complications

1. Post–lumbar puncture headache (PLPH)

a. Epidemiology and risk factors

   (1) Occurs in up to 40% of patients after diagnostic LP

   (2) Occurs twice as often in women as in men

   (3) Incidence much less in children under the age of 13 years and adults older than 60 years

   (4) Highest incidence in the 18- to 30-year age group

   (5) Incidence greatest is patients with lesser body mass index

   (6) Risk greater in those with prior chronic or recurrent headaches (three times greater) and a prior history of PLPH

b. Pathophysiology

   (1) Not entirely certain: Best explanation is low CSF pressure as a result of CSF leakage through a dural and arachnoid tear produced by the puncture that exceeds the rate of CSF production

   (2) CSF hypotension can produce headache and cranial nerve symptoms.

     (a) Downward descent of the brain and stretching of pain-sensitive structures including the dura, nerves (cranial nerves V, XI, and X and the upper three cervical nerves) and bridging veins

     (b) Secondarily, intracranial venous dilation and increased brain volume occurs as the veins passively dilate in response to decreased extravascular pressure.

c. Clinical features

   (1) Headache begins within 72 hours in 90% of patients but can be delayed for as long as 14 days.

   (2) Duration of headache is less than 5 days in 80% but can persist for 12 months.

   (3) Usually bilateral but may be unilateral

   (4) Often associated with nausea, dizziness, and less often with vomiting

   (5) The headache resolves or decreases when patient lies supine and worsens when upright.

   (6) The longer the patient is upright, the longer it will take for the headache to subside when supine.

   (7) Movement, coughing, straining, sneezing, and jugular venous compression increase the headache.

d. Laboratory findings

   (1) Same findings as in other low CSF pressure disorders (e.g., spontaneous, CSF shunt overdrainage, and traumatic)

   (2) A repeat LP usually demonstrates an opening pressure of 70 cm or less.

   (3) CSF analysis may be normal or can demonstrate a moderate, primarily lymphocytic pleocytosis, the presence of RBCs, and an elevated protein level, which can even be over 500 mg/dL. Abnormalities are probably due to decreased CSF volume and hydrostatic pressure changes resulting In meningeal vasodilatation and vascular leak.

   (4) An MRI scan of the brain may reveal diffuse meningeal enhancement with contrast and less often subdural fluid collections and reversible tonsillar descent. The scan returns to normal with resolution of the headache.

e. Treatment

   (1) Bed rest

   (2) Oral caffeine 300 mg every 4 to 6 hours may reduce the headache albeit transiently.

   (3) A slow intravenous bolus of 500 mg of caffeine sodium benzoate with a second bolus of caffeine after 2 hours if necessary

produces permanent relief in about 50% of patients.

(4) For persistent or severe headaches, a lumbar epidural blood patch is the most effective treatment.

    (a) Performed by slowly injecting 10 to 20 ml of the patient's blood into the same lumbar epidural space or the space before the prior LP.

    (b) After the injection, the patient should stay in the decubitus position for 2 hours to obtain maximal benefit.

    (c) The success rate is about 85% after one injection and nearly 98% after a second.

    (d) Side effects such as pain at the injection site and lower extremity pain or sensory disturbances are usually mild and transient.

f. Prevention

(1) The incidence of PLPH decreases with a smaller diameter of the bevel-tipped or Quincke (traditional) needle.

    (a) However, smaller diameter needles are not practical for diagnostic lumbar puncture.

        (i) The flow rate with a Quincke 20-gauge (G) needle is 133 ml/hour as compared to 10.5 ml/hour with the 25 G.

        (ii) The time to transduce the CSF pressure for manometer reading is about 43 seconds with the 20 G and over 336 seconds with the 25 G.

(2) Parallel insertion of the Quincke bevel (as described above) reduces the risk by 50% or greater.

(3) Pencil-point or atraumatic needles such as the Whitacre and Sprotte (Fig. 1–2) reduce the risk of PLPH to about 5% when using a 21 G or 22 G needle.

    (a) Consider using an atraumatic needle in patients at increased risk of PLPH.

    (b) The decreased risk may be from spreading rather than from cutting the dural fibers.

    (c) Because of the dull tip, it is often easier to perform the puncture when using the Sprotte needle by using a short sharp introducer, which is inserted to two-thirds of its length before the Sprotte needle is placed.

    (d) Replacing the stylet before removing a

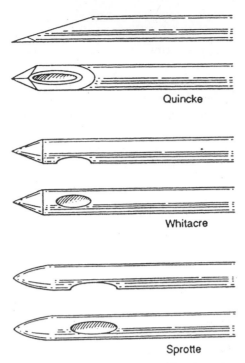

Figure 1–2. Three types of spinal needle tips: the Quincke, Whitacre, and Sprotte. (From Peterman SB: Postmyelography headache rates with Whitacre versus Quincke 22-gauge spinal needles. Radiology 200:771–778, 1996, with permission.)

Sprotte 21 G needle reduces the risk of PLPH from 16% to 5%. This reduced risk might also be present if the stylet is replaced before withdrawing the Quincke needle.

(4) Bed rest for up to 24 hours or various body positions such as prone or head down after the LP do not reduce the risk of PLPH as compared to immediate ambulation.

(5) Intake of oral fluids after the LP does not prevent PLPH.

2. Herniation

a. Uncal or tonsillar herniation leading to neurologic deterioration or death can occur when a LP is performed in the presence of a brain neoplasm, abscess, or hematoma with mass effect.

b. Cerebral or cerebellar herniation can result from a LP performed in children with meningitis and decerebrate or decorticate posturing, focal neurologic signs, or no response to pain, even when a CT scan of the brain is normal.

c. Neurologic deterioration due to spinal coning may occur when a LP is performed below the level of a complete spinal subarachnoid block (usually due to neoplasms).

3. Cranial neuropathies

a. Usually transient dysfunction of cranial nerves III, IV, V, VI, VII, and VIII may occur.

b. Dizziness, tinnitus, clogged up and popping ears, and loss of hearing may accompany the postural headache. Reversible hearing loss may be symptomatic in up to 8% of patients.

c. Abducens paresis may be a complication of 1 in 400 LPs. It usually occurs 4 to 14 days after the procedure and resolves over 4 to 6 weeks.

4. Nerve root irritation and low back pain

a. During the LP, contact with the sensory roots occurs about 13% of the time causing transient electric shocks or dysesthesias.

b. Permanent sensory and motor loss rarely occur.

c. Low back pain is common for several days after the procedure and can occasionally persist for months.

d. Rarely, if the needle is inserted beyond the subararachnoid space, the annulus fibrosis can be damaged and the intervertebral disc can herniate. Discitis is an even rarer complication.

5. Intraspinal epidermoid tumor

a. A rare complication of not using the stylet on insertion of the needle through the skin and subcutaneous tissue

b. The needle without stylet may implant a plug of skin that can grown into this tumor.

6. Infections

a. Bacterial meningitis, discitis, lumbar epidural abscess, and spinal cord abscess are rare complications.

b. Can result from a contaminated needle

(1) Due to respiratory droplets

(2) Disseminating skin flora without adequate disinfection of the skin

(3) LP in the presence of a local infection (e.g., cellulitis, furunculosis, or epidural abscess)

(4) Introducing blood into the subarachnoid space in the presence of bacteremia.

c. In patients with CSF leaks, LP can reverse the flow gradient and produce retrograde spread of organisms from the nasopharynx though the dural leak and result in meningitis.

7. Bleeding complications

a. A unilateral or subdural intracranial hematoma is a rare complication of LP.

(1) Can occur in healthy persons without bleeding disorders

(2) Low CSF pressure can result in traction on the meninges and tearing of dural vesels.

b. Traumatic lumbar puncture

(1) Needle-induced blood in the CSF in 72% of LPs.

(a) 1 to 5 RBCs in 27%, 6 to 50 RBCs in 21%, and >50 RBCs in 24%.

(2) Usually due to puncture of the radicular vessels that accompany each nerve root along the length of its surface and only rarely from the epidural veins.

(3) Occasionally, the radiculomedullary artery of Adamkiewicz and corresponding vein may be present in a lower than usual position and accompany the L3, L4, or L5 nerve roots where puncture could occur.

(4) Spinal hemorrhage

(a) Risk factors include thrombocytopenia, bleeding disorders, anticoagulation, and a difficult or bloody tap.

(b) Spinal subarachnoid and epidural hematomas are a rare complication.

(i) Present with severe low back or radicular pain followed within hours or days by progressive paraparesis, sensory loss, and sphincter disturbances

(ii) May be visualized on MRI scan

(iii) Successful treatments include immediate decompressive laminectomy and hematoma evacuation and percutaneous hematoma aspiration.

8. Other complications

a. Vasovagal syncope, hyperventilation, and rarely cardiac arrest

b. Seizures have been rarely reported in association with PLPH.

c. Incorrect laboratory analysis of various CSF studies can harm the patient.

Complications

- Headache
- Herniation
- Cranial neuropathies
- Nerve root irritation and low back pain
- Intraspinal epidermoid tumor
- Infection
- Bleeding

Bibliography

Evans RW: Complications of lumbar puncture. Neurologic Clinics 16:83–105, 1998.

Evans RW, Armon C, Frohman EM, Goodin DS: Assessment: prevention of post-lumbar puncture headaches: report of the therapeutics and technology assessment subcommittee of the American Academy of Neurology. Neurology 55:909–914, 2000.

Fishman RA: Cerebrospinal Fluid in Diseases of the Nervous System, 2nd ed. Philadelphia, W.B. Saunders, 1992.

Strupp M, Schueler O, Straube A, et al.: "Atraumatic" sprotte needle reduces the incidence of post-lumbar puncture headaches. Neurology 57:2310–2312, 2001.

2 Clinical Electromyography

Bashar Katirji
Kanokwan Boonyapisit

Introduction

1. **Definition:** The designations *electrodiagnostic (EDX) examination, electromyography (EMG) examination*, or *clinical EMG examination* are used interchangeably to describe electrophysiologic studies of the peripheral nervous system. The components of the EDX examination can be divided into several categories.

   a. Nerve conduction studies (NCS), including motor and sensory studies.

   b. Needle EMG examination, also referred to as the *needle electrode examination (NEE)*.

   c. Other special procedures:

      (1) Late responses: H reflexes, F waves, and blink reflexes

      (2) Repetitive nerve stimulation

      (3) Single fiber EMG

2. The final interpretation of the electrodiagnostic studies should be based on the NCS and needle EMG examination results, as well as on the special procedures findings.

3. Value of electrodiagnostic studies: The goals of EDX examination are, first, to localize lesions of the peripheral nervous system and provide further information regarding the underlying pathophysiology, severity, and temporal course of neuromuscular disorders, and then to evaluate the effects of their treatment.

EDX Examination Components

- Nerve conduction studies, including motor and sensory studies

- Needle EMG examination

- Other special procedures:

  - Late responses: H reflexes, F waves, and blink reflexes

  - Repetitive nerve stimulation

  - Single fiber EMG

Nerve Conduction Studies

1. **Basic techniques:** NCS typically are performed by recording action potentials with surface electrodes over the skin.

   a. Motor NCSs are performed by stimulating a motor or mixed peripheral nerve while recording the compound muscle action potential (CMAP) from a muscle innervated by that nerve. The nerve is stimulated distally near the recording electrode and proximally to evaluate its proximal segment.

   b. Sensory NCSs are performed by stimulating a sensory or mixed nerve while recording the sensory nerve action potential (SNAP) over the sensory nerve distally (antidromic studies) or proximally (orthodromic studies).

   c. NCS are planned based on clinical manifestations and suspected diagnosis (Table 2–1).

2. **Parameters.** Several parameters of SNAP and CMAP are recorded whenever sensory and motor NCS are performed (Fig. 2–1).

   a. Amplitude is typically measured from baseline to negative peak and expressed in millivolts for CMAP and microvolts for SNAP.

   b. Duration is the time interval during which the CMAP or SNAP occurs. This is expressed in milliseconds, and typically includes only the initial negative phase of the response.

   c. Area is a function of both the amplitude and the duration of the CMAP. It requires computerized equipment and typically is measured as the negative phase area from the baseline in mVms.

   d. Latency is expressed in milliseconds.

      (1) Distal latency is the interval between the time of distal nerve stimulation and the onset of the CMAP or SNAP.

      (2) Proximal latency is the interval between the time of proximal nerve stimulation and the onset of the CMAP or SNAP.

      (3) SNAP latencies can be measured from either the onset of the SNAP ("onset" or distal latency") or to its peak ("peak latency"), whereas CMAP latencies are always measured from the onset of the response.

TABLE 2–1.   SUGGESTED NERVE CONDUCTION STUDIES FOR COMMON REFERRALS TO THE EMG LABORATORY

Disorder	Nerve Tested (s = sensory, m = motor)*
Cervical radiculopathy	Median (s) Ulnar (s) Radial (s) Median (m) Ulnar (m)
Carpal tunnel syndrome	Nerves tested for cervical radiculopathy plus one or more of the internal hand comparison studies†
Lumbosacral radiculopathy	Sural (s) Peroneal (m) Tibial (m) Bilateral tibial H reflexes
Ulnar neuropathy	Nerves tested for cervical radiculopathy plus Dorsal ulnar (s) Ulnar (m) recording first dorsal interosseous
Peroneal neuropathy	Nerves tested for lumbosacral radiculopathy plus Superficial peroneal (s) Peroneal (m) recording tibialis anterior
Peripheral polyneuropathy	Nerves tested for cervical and lumbosacral radiculopathy
Motor neuron disease	Nerves tested for cervical and lumbosacral radiculopathy
Myopathy	Median (s) Sural (s) Median (m) Tibial (m)

*Nerves should be tested on the symptomatic side. Contralateral studies are recommended for comparison and in patients with bilateral symptoms.
†This may include the mixed median and ulnar plantar study, median and ulnar sensory recording ring finger, or median and ulnar motor recording 2nd lumbrical and 2nd interossei, respectively.
From Katirji, B: The clinical electromyography examination. An overview. Neurol Clin 20:291–303, 2002.

  e. Conduction velocity is obtained by stimulating the nerve at two points along its course. It is expressed in meters per second (m/sec) and is calculated as follows:

$$\text{conduction velocity} = \frac{\text{distance}}{\text{proximal latency} - \text{distal latency}}$$

3. **Nerve conduction studies findings:** The pattern of abnormalities seen on NCS correlates well with the type of peripheral nerve pathology.

  a. *Demyelinating lesion:* When focal injury to myelin occurs, the conduction of the action potentials along the affected nerve fibers is altered. This may result in slowing of conduction or conduction block along the nerve fibers.

  (1) *Focal slowing* of conduction is usually the result of widening of the nodes of Ranvier (paranodal demyelination). This may present in one of two ways:

  (a) Synchronized slowing: When all the large myelinated fibers are slowed to essentially the same degree, there is either a prolongation of distal latency (if the focal lesion is distal) or slowing in conduction velocity (if the focal lesion is proximal). However, the CMAP amplitude, duration, and area are normal and do not change when the nerve is stimulated proximal to the lesion. More than 130% prolongation of the distal latencies and more than 75% slowing of the conduction velocity are common criteria for definite evidence of demyelination.

  (b) Desynchronized slowing (differential slowing): When the speed of impulse transmission is reduced at the lesion site along a variable number of the medium or small nerve fibers (average or slower conducting axons), the CMAPs are dispersed on stimulations proximal to the lesion and have prolonged duration, with normal (nondispersed) responses on distal stimulations. The speed of conduction along the injury site (latency or conduction velocity) is normal because at least some of the fastest conducting axons are spared.

  (c) Synchronized and desynchronized slowing: When the largest (fastest-conducting) axons are also involved and the speed of conduction is reduced at the lesion site along a variable number of the average or slower conducting axons, differential slowing is accompanied by slowing of distal latency or conduction velocity.

  (2) *Conduction block* is caused by interruption of action potential transmission across the nerve lesion.

  (a) Conduction block is usually the result of loss of one or more myelin segments (segmental or internodal demyelination). If enough nerve fibers are affected by conduction block, a significant drop in the CMAP amplitude occurs when the nerve is stimulated proximal to the lesion.

  (b) A nerve lesion manifesting with conduction block is best localized when it can be bracketed by two stimulation points, one distal to the site of injury (resulting in a normal CMAP) and one

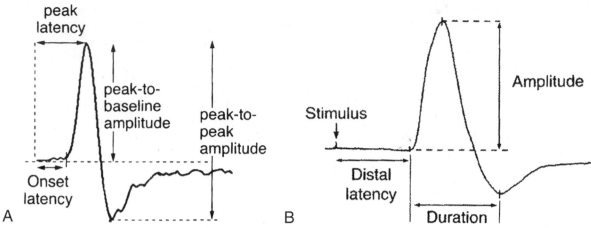

Figure 2–1. Sensory (A) and motor (B) nerve conduction study parameters. (From Levin KH, Lüders HO (eds): Comprehensive Clinical Neurophysiology. Philadelphia, W.B. Saunders, 2000)

proximal (resulting in a partial or complete drop in CMAP).

(c) Conduction block may involve all the myelinated axons (complete) or only some of them, leaving the others normal (partial).

(d) Conduction block is defined as a significant drop of the CMAP amplitude and/or area with stimulation proximal to the injury site, when compared with the CMAP distal to it, without evidence of significant temporal dispersion (i.e, prolongation of CMAP duration). More than 50% decrement of the CMAP amplitude and/or area across the lesion usually is used as the criterion for definite conduction block.

(e) Conduction block may also follow axonal loss before the completion of wallerian degeneration (see b. Axon loss lesion).

b. *Axon loss lesion:* After acute focal axonal damage, the distal nerve segment undergoes wallerian degeneration. If the extent of nerve fiber loss is significant, low CMAP and SNAP amplitudes will be noted on NCS.

(1) NCSs characteristically result in unelicitable or uniformly low CMAP amplitude at all stimulation points. However, there are two exceptions to the above findings, either of which may cause diagnostic confusion:

(a) Although unelicitable or uniformly low CMAP amplitudes are typically seen in cases of axonal degeneration, they may be encountered, occasionally, when there is conduction block (due to

segmental demyelination) situated distally along the nerve, between the most distal stimulating point and the recording site.

(b) After axonal damage, the distal axons undergo degeneration (wallerian degeneration) which is completed in 7 to 11 days. However, soon after a axonal transection, the distal axon remains excitable. Electrophysiologically, the distal CMAP decreases and reaches its nadir within 5 to 6 days, while the distal SNAP lags slightly behind, reaching its nadir in 10 to 11 days (Fig. 2–2). Hence, early after an axon-loss peripheral nerve injury, a pattern of conduction block is common. This is similar to the conduction block pattern seen with segmental demyelination, except that a repeat study (after completion of the period of wallerian degeneration) will reveal a drop in distal CMAP to a value very similar to the proximal CMAP. This type of conduction block has been referred to as *axonal non-continuity conduction block, early axon loss conduction block,* and *axon discontinuity* conduction block. It should be noted that identification of conduction block in the early days of axonal loss is extremely helpful in localizing a peripheral nerve injury, particularly of the closed type where the exact site of trauma is not apparent. Hence, it is important to obtain NCS as soon as the patient seeks medical attention.

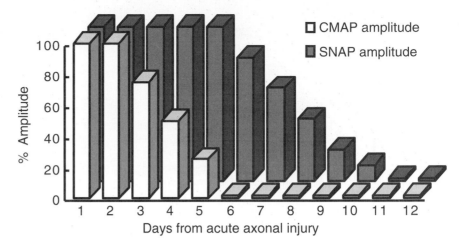

Figure 2–2. Distal CMAP and SNAP decline during wallerian degeneration. (From Katirji B: Electromyography in Clinical Practice: A Case Study Approach. St Louis, C.V. Mosby, 1998)

Waiting for the completion of wallerian degeneration results in diffusely low CMAPs (regardless of stimulation site), which does not allow for accurate localization of the injury site. Needle EMG is useful, but localization by this method is suboptimal because peripheral nerves may not have motor branches from long segments (such as the median and ulnar nerves in the arms).

(2) Axonal loss causes minimal effects on distal latency and conduction velocity. In severe axonal loss, the conduction velocity and distal latency may be slightly slowed secondary to loss of the large fast-conducting axons.

(3) Sensory axonal loss located proximal to the dorsal root ganglion does not affect the SNAP amplitude. This is because the peripheral sensory axons originating from dorsal root ganglion neurons remain intact. Therefore, intraspinal canal lesions (such as radiculopathies) have no effect on SNAP amplitude.

Key Abnormal Findings: Nerve Conduction Studies

Demyelinating Lesion

• Focal slowing of conduction

• Conduction block

Axon Loss Lesion

• Conduction block

• Unelicitable or uniformly low CMAP amplitudes

Late Responses

1. F wave.
   a. Supramaximal stimulation to a motor nerve causes an antidromic action potential that travels toward the alpha motor neurons in the spinal cord. A small percentage (5% to 10%) of the alpha motor neurons then backfire and generate orthodromic action potentials that reach the muscle and are recorded as a low-amplitude motor response that occurs after the initial CMAP (M wave) (Fig. 2–3).
   b. Minimal F-wave latencies are measured, and are 25 to 32 msec in the upper limbs and 45 to 56 msec in the lower limbs, depending on the subject's height.
   c. Because the F wave evaluates the entire length of a motor nerve, an abnormal F wave is a poor localization tool in that it may result from a lesion involving any portion along the entire length of the motor nerve. Prolonged F-wave latencies occur in peripheral polyneuropathies, but their greatest usefulness lies in the early diagnosis of Guillain-Barré syndrome, where prolonged or absent F waves may be the only abnormalities on NCSs. Minimal F-wave latencies may also be abnormal in entrapment neuropathies and radiculopathies, but they have no localizing values.

2. H reflex
   a. Named after Hoffman, the H reflex is a monosynaptic reflex with the Ia sensory fibers from muscle spindles as afferents and the alpha motor neuron and motor axons as efferents (Fig. 2–4).
   b. The tibial H reflex, the only reproducible H reflex in adults, is the electrical equivalent of the Achilles' reflex. Its latency is dependent on

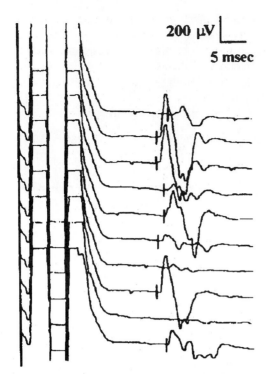

200 μV

5 msec

Figure 2–3. F-wave minimal latency stimulating the median nerve at the wrist while recording from the abductor pollicis brevis. Note the variability in latencies, amplitude, and morphology. (From Preston DC, Shapiro BE: Electromyography and Neuromuscular Disorders. Boston, Butterworth-Heinemann, 1998)

patient height and is approximately 35 msec, with < 3 msec side-to-side difference. Its amplitude varies but usually with less than 50% side-to-side difference. The H reflex may be absent in healthy subjects over the age of 60 years.

   c. The H reflex is prolonged, low in amplitude or absent in peripheral neuropathies, proximal tibial or sciatic neuropathy, lumbosacral plexopathy, or S1 radiculopathy.

3. Blink reflex

   a. The blink reflex, which assesses the trigeminal and facial nerves and their connections in the pons and medulla, is the electrical correlate of the corneal reflex. Similar to the H reflex, the blink reflex represents a true reflex with an afferent limb, mediated by sensory fibers of the supraorbital branch of the ophthalmic division of the trigeminal nerve, and an efferent limb mediated by motor fibers of the facial nerve.

   b. The blink reflex has two components, an early R1 and a late R2 response. The R1 response is usually present ipsilaterally with a di-synaptic pathway between the main sensory nucleus of the Vth cranial nerve in the mid-pons and the ipsilateral facial nucleus in the lower pontine tegmentum. The R2 response is typically present bilaterally with an oligosynaptic pathway

between the nucleus of the spinal tract of cranial nerve V in the ipsilateral pons and medulla, and interneurons forming connections to the ipsilateral and contralateral facial nuclei.

   c. In normal subjects, the absolute R1 latency is <13 msec; the ipsilateral R2 latency, < 41 msec; and the contralateral R2 latency, <44 msec.

   d. The blink reflex is often abnormal in facial and trigeminal neuropathies, but it may be abnormal in brainstem disorders and other central nervous disorders such as Parkinson's disease and stroke.

Repetitive Nerve Stimulation

1. General concepts:

   a. Repetitive nerve stimulation (RNS) aims at recording decremental or incremental responses, useful in the diagnosis of neuromuscular junction (NMJ) disorders.

   b. In a normal NMJ, acetylcholine (Ach) is stored in vesicles in the presynaptic terminals.

     (1) Release of Ach vesicles starts when calcium enters the presynaptic NMJ through voltage-gated calcium channels at the presynaptic terminal. Calcium then initiates Ach vesicle release by interacting with different types of presynaptic proteins. The Ach then diffuses across the NMJ and

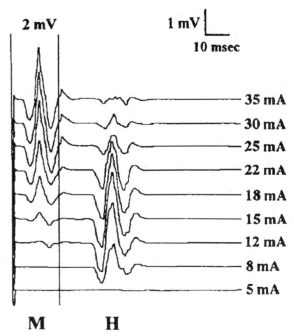

2 mV

1 mV

10 msec

35 mA
30 mA
25 mA
22 mA
18 mA
15 mA
12 mA
8 mA
5 mA

M   **H**

Figure 2–4. Tibial H reflex. Note that the maximal H-reflex response occurs with low stimulation intensities without direct (M) response. With increasing intensities, the M response grows and the H wave diminishes. (From Preston DC, Shapiro BE: Electromyography and Neuromuscular Disorders. Boston, Butterworth-Heinemann, 1998)

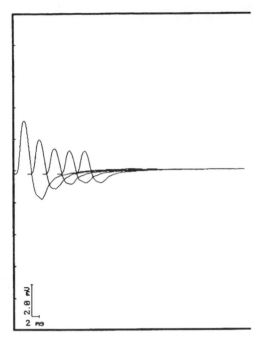

Figure 2-5. CMAP decrement with slow repetitive stimulation (2 Hz) of the median nerve at the wrist while recording from the abductor pollicis brevis. (From Katirji B: Electromyography in Clinical Practice: A Case Study Approach. St Louis, C.V. Mosby, 1998)

binds with the Ach receptors at the postsynaptic membrane. Calcium diffuses slowly out of the presynaptic terminal in 100 to 200 msec.

(2) The safety factor of neuromuscular transmission is the difference between the end plate potential (potential generated at the postsynaptic membrane following a nerve action potential) and the threshold needed for initiating a muscle action potential. In a normal NMJ, the safety factor is about 4, i.e., the number of vesicles released exceeds the number of vesicles required (to generate a postsynaptic membrane potential change required to reach threshold) by a factor of 4.

c. In myasthenia gravis (a postsynaptic disorder), antibodies directed against the Ach receptors at the postsynaptic membrane make it impossible for Ach to bind with the receptors.

d. In presynaptic NMJ disorders, there is disturbance of Ach vesicle release. In Lambert-Eaton myasthenic syndrome (LEMS), the disturbance is caused by antibodies against the voltage-gated calcium channel at the presynaptic membrane, and in botulism it is caused by binding of the toxin to one of the vesicle-docking proteins at the presynaptic terminal.

2. *Slow repetitive nerve stimulation*

a. Slow RNS is usually performed by applying 3 to 5 supramaximal stimuli to a mixed or motor nerve at a rate of 2 to 3 Hz. This rate is low enough to prevent calcium accumulation (which diffuses out in 100 to 200 msec), but high enough to deplete the quanta in the immediately available store before other Ach stores start to replenish it.

b. The choice of nerve to be stimulated depends on the patient's manifestations. Most useful nerves for slow RNS are the median, ulnar, and spinal accessory nerves.

c. In normal NMJ, the number of Ach vesicles released from the presynaptic terminal progressively reduces with each repetitive stimulation, but still exceeds the Ach required to reach action potential threshold.

d. In myasthenia gravis, the postsynaptic terminal requires more Ach to reach the threshold for the action potential, because many Ach receptors are bound to antibodies. This results in a low safety factor and failure of many end plates to reach threshold on subsequent stimuli, resulting in CMAP decremental response (Fig. 2-5). This decrement corrects after a brief exercise *(posttetanic facilitation)*, and worsens 3 to 5 minutes after exercise *(postexercise exhaustion)*.

e. In presynaptic disorders (such as LEMS), there is a decrease in Ach vesicle release from the presynaptic terminal even at baseline, resulting in a low CMAP. Further, progressively decreasing the amount of Ach vesicle released with each stimulation also causes decremental response in LEMS.

f. Decremental response is considered significant when it exceeds 10%. The CMAP decrement is calculated by comparing the lowest (usually the third or fourth) response to the first as follows:

$$\% \text{ decrement} = \frac{\text{amplitude (first response)} - \text{amplitude (third/fourth response)}}{\text{amplitude (first response)}} \times 100$$

g. Certain technical factors increase the sensitivity of the test. These include discontinuation of acetylcholine esterase inhibitors for at least 12 hours before the test, performing the test on clinically weak muscles or proximal muscles, and performing the test before and after exercise.

3. *Rapid repetitive stimulation*

a. Rapid RNS (>10 Hz) causes accumulation of calcium in the presynaptic nerve terminal (because calcium diffuses after 100 to 200 msec) and results in an increase in the amount of Ach released.

b. The optimal frequency is 20 to 50 Hz for 2 to 10 seconds. A typical rapid RNS applies 200 stimuli at a rate of 50 Hz (i.e., 50 Hz for 4 seconds).

c. Significant incremental response of the CMAP amplitude (>100%) occurs in presynaptic disorders, such as LEMS and, to a lesser extent, in botulism. A brief period (10 seconds) of exercise may be used to elicit the incremental response with the same mechanism as in rapid RNS (Fig. 2–6 A & B).

Needle EMG Examination

1. Needle EMG examination is the direct recording of muscle electrical activity. It yields valuable information on the localization and pathophysiology of peripheral nervous system disorders.

2. For each muscle studied, the needle EMG starts by assessing the insertional and spontaneous activities at rest. Then, the examiner asks the patient to slowly contract the muscle and the motor unit action potentials (MUAPs) are evaluated. MUAPs are assessed for duration, amplitude, and number of phases. As the force of contraction is increased,

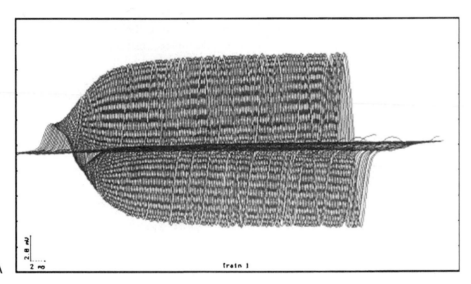

A

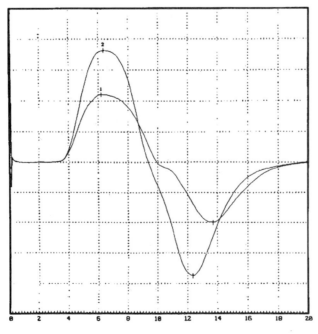

B

Figure 2–6. CMAP increment in a patient with Lambert-Eaton myasthenic syndrome, following brief exercise of the abductor pollicis brevis (A) and rapid repetitive nerve stimulation of the median nerve at 50 Hz (B).

TABLE 2–2. SUGGESTED NEEDLE EMG PROTOCOL FOR COMMON REFERRALS TO THE EMG LABORATORY

DISORDER	MUSCLE EXAMINED
Cervical radiculopathy or carpal tunnel syndrome	First dorsal interosseous Abductor pollicis brevis* Flexor pollicis longus Extensor indices proprius Pronator teres Biceps Triceps Deltoid Mid and low cervical paraspinal muscles
Lumbosacral radiculopathy	Tibialis anterior Medial gastrocnemius Extensor hallucis Flexor digitorum longus Vastus lateralis Gluteus medius Mid and low lumbar paraspinals
Ulnar neuropathy	Muscles tested for cervical radiculopathy plus Abductor digiti minimi Flexor carpi ulnaris Flexor digitorum profundus (ulnar part)
Peroneal neuropathy	Muscles tested for lumbosacral radiculopathy plus Peroneus longus Short head of biceps femoris
Peripheral polyneuropathy	Muscles tested for lumbosacral radiculopathy plus Abductor hallucis Extensor digitorum brevis First dorsal interosseous†
Motor neuron disease	Muscles tested for cervical and lumbosacral radiculopathy in three limbs plus thoracic paraspinals
Myopathy	Tibialis anterior Medial gastrocnemius Vastus lateralis Vastus medialis Gluteus medius Brachioradialis Biceps Triceps Deltoid Mid and low lumbar paraspinals

*Suggested in carpal tunnel syndrome only, because it is extremely painful to sample.
† More proximal muscles should be tested if first dorsal interosseous is abnormal to establish a distal to proximal gradient.
From Katirji, B. The clinical electromyography examination. An overview. Neurol Clin 20:291–303, 2002.

the number of MUAPs and their relationship to the firing frequency (recruitment and activation pattern) are evaluated.

3. The choice of muscles on needle EMG is dependent on the clinical manifestations, neurologic findings, and suspected diagnosis (Table 2–2).

4. Needle EMG examination findings

a. Normal insertional and spontaneous activity: Insertional activity occurs when a needle is quickly moved through the muscle. This creates depolarization of muscle fibers and a brief burst discharge lasting several hundred milliseconds. At rest, normal muscle fibers are silent, with no spontaneous activity except at the end plate region (end plate noise and end plate spikes).

b. Abnormal insertional and spontaneous activity (Table 2–3):

(1) Increased (or decrease) insertional activity

(a) When needle movement results in a waveform lasting longer than 300 msec, it indicates increased insertional activity.

(b) Increased insertional activity may be seen in neurogenic disorders associated with denervation and necrotizing myopathies, mostly the inflammatory myopathies.

(c) Insertional activity is decreased during paralytic phases of periodic paralysis, and when muscle is replaced by fibrous tissue.

(2) Fibrillation potentials

(a) Fibrillation potentials consist of two type of potentials: Brief spikes (brief, regular firing, muscle fiber action potentials) and positive waves (longer duration with initial positive deflection, regular firing, muscle fiber action potentials).

(b) Fibrillation potentials are due to spontaneous depolarization of muscle fibers and are electrophysiologic markers of denervation. They are typically recorded 2 to 3 weeks after denervation in neurogenic disorders (neuropathies, radiculopathies, motor neuron disease, etc.). They may also be seen in muscle disorders, especially the necrotizing myopathies (such as inflammatory myopathies and muscular dystrophies) and are rarely seen in NMJ disorders (such as myasthenia gravis and botulism).

(3) Fasciculation potentials

(a) Fasciculation potentials are random spontaneous discharges of individual motor units. They have simple MUAP morphology or are complex and large.

(b) Fasciculation potentials commonly accompany neurogenic disorders (motor neuron disease, peripheral neuropathies, radiculopathies, or entrapment neuropathies). They are also seen sometimes in normal individuals.

TABLE 2–3. SPONTANEOUS ACTIVITY

POTENTIAL	SOURCE GENERATOR/ MORPHOLOGY	SOUND ON LOUD SPEAKER	STABILITY	FIRING RATE	FIRING PATTERN
End plate noise	MEPP (monophasic negative)	Sea shell		20–40 Hz	Irregular (hissing)
End plate spike	Muscle fiber initiated by terminal axonal twig (brief spike, diphasic initial negative)	Sputtering fat in a frying pan		5–50 Hz	Irregular (sputtering)
Fibrillation	Muscle fiber (brief spike, diphasic or triphasic with initial positive)	Rain on a tin roof or tick/tock of a clock	Stable	0.5–10 Hz (occasionally up to 30 Hz)	Regular
Positive sharp wave	Muscle fiber (diphasic, initial positive, slow negative)	Dull pops, rain on a tin roof, or tick/tock of a clock	Stable	0.5–10 Hz (occasionally up to 30 Hz)	Regular
Myotonia	Muscle fiber (brief spike, initial positive, or positive wave)	Revving engine or dive bomber	Waxing/waning amplitude	20–150 Hz	Waxing/waning
CRD	Multiple muscle fibers time-linked together	Machine	Usually stable, may change in discrete jumps	5–100 Hz	Perfectly regular (unless overdriven)
Fasciculation	Motor unit (motor neuron/axon)	Corn popping		Low (0.1–10 Hz)	Irregular
Myokymia	Motor unit (motor neuron/axon)	Marching soldiers		1–5 Hz (interburst) 5–60 Hz (intraburst)	Bursting
Cramp	Motor unit (motor neuron/axon)			High (20–150 Hz)	Interference pattern or Several individual units
Neuromyotonia	Motor unit (motor neuron/axon)	Pinging	Decrementing amplitude	Very high (150–250 Hz)	Waning

Abbreviations: MEPP = miniature end plate potential; CRD = complex repetitive discharge.
From Shapiro BE, Katirji B, Preston DC: Clinical electromyography. In Katirji B, Kaminski HJ, Preston DC, et al. (eds): Neuromuscular Disorders in Clinical Practice. Butterworth-Heinemann, Boston, 2002.

(4) Complex repetitive discharge (CRD)

(a) CRD is a high-frequency, regular firing, multiserrated repetitive discharge with abrupt onset and termination, that creates a characteristic "machine-liked" sound. It results from the depolarization of a single muscle fiber followed by ephaptic spread to adjacent denervated fibers.

(b) CRDs occur in chronic neuromuscular disorders, but are nonspecific accompanying neurogenic as well as myopathic disorders.

(5) Myotonic discharges

(a) Myotonic discharges are characterized by waveforms with waxing and waning amplitudes and frequencies creating the classic "dive bomber" sounds on the loudspeaker. These discharges are of muscle fiber origin and are usually triggered by needle insertions.

(b) Myotonic discharges are typically seen in the dystrophic and nondystrophic myotonias, and they are more abundant in the latter. They may also accompany hyperkalemic periodic paralysis, acid maltase deficiency, and colchicine, diazocholesterol or clofibrate myotoxicity. They rarely associated with polymyositis and dermatomyositis.

(6) Myokymic discharges

(a) Myokymic discharges are rhythmic, grouped, spontaneous repetitive discharges of the same motor unit.

(b) Facial myokymia is associated with brainstem lesions from multiple sclerosis, brainstem glioma, or vascular disease.

(c) Limb myokymia is classically associated with radiation plexopathy, but it may be seen in Guillain-Barré syndrome, chronic entrapment neuropathy, chronic radiculopathy, and gold toxicity.

(7) Neuromyotonia

    (a) Neuromyotonia consists of a high-frequency (150 to 250 Hz) decrementing, repetitive discharge of a single motor unit that creates a characteristic "pinging" sound on loud speaker.

    (b) Neuromyotonic discharges are associated with the syndromes of continuous motor unit activity such as in Isaac's syndrome, and are occasionally seen in chronic motor neuron diseases (e.g., postpoliomyelitis and spinal muscular atrophy).

(8) Cramp potential

    (a) Muscle cramp is a painful involuntary muscle contraction that tends to occur with muscle in shortened position or contracting. Electrically, cramp potentials are high frequency discharges of motor units.

    (b) Cramps occur commonly in normal individuals, in neurogenic conditions, and metabolic disorders (such as electrolyte imbalance, hypothyroidism, pregnancy, and uremia).

    (c) Cramps should be differentiated from contractures, which are painful, but silent muscle contractures associated with metabolic myopathies such as McArdle's disease.

c. Voluntary motor unit action potentials:

(1) The pattern of MUAP abnormalities allows determination of whether the disorder is a neuropathic or myopathic process and often helps to determine the time course and severity of the lesion.

(2) Assessment of MUAPs can be divided into two parts. The first part is morphology of the MUAPs, which include evaluation of duration, amplitude, and number of phases. The second part of MUAP evaluation is assessment of the number of MUAPs and their relationship to the firing frequency (recruitment and activation pattern).

    (a) MUAP morphology

        (i) *Short duration MUAPs* often have low amplitude. They occur in disorders with loss of muscle fibers in the motor unit. Thus, they are present in myopathic disorders, such as muscular dystrophies, many congenital myopathies, toxic myopathies, and inflammatory myopathies, and in severe NMJ disorders (e.g., botulism). In early reinnervation after severe denervation, in which the newly sprouting axons begin to reinnervate only a few muscle fibers, the MUAP is also small, of short duration, and polyphasic but usually with reduced recruitment ("nascent" MUAP).

        (ii) *Long duration MUAPs* often show high amplitude and are the best indicators of reinnervation. They occur with increased number or density of muscle fibers, or with a loss of synchrony of fiber firing within a motor unit, such as occurs in chronic neuropathic processes—e.g., motor neuron disease, radiculopathies, axonal neuropathies, and entrapment neuropathies.

        (iii) *Polyphasic MUAPs* (five or more phases) may accompany both myopathic and neurogenic disorders. Polyphasia is a measure of synchrony of the firing of muscle fibers within the same motor unit. Polyphasia may be seen in healthy individuals (up to 10% of the MUAPs in distal muscles and up to 20% in proximal muscles).

        (iv) *Unstable MUAPs* fluctuate in amplitude, duration, or morphology from moment to moment. This variation is usually due to blocking of individual muscle fiber action potentials in the motor unit. This may be seen in disorders of neuromuscular transmission, myositis, muscle trauma, reinnervation, and rapidly progressive neurogenic disorders.

    (b) MUAP recruitment and activation

        (i) *Recruitment* refers to the relation of firing rate of individual potentials to the total number of motor units firing. Decreased recruitment (reduction in the number of MUAPs firing with high frequency) occurs when there is decrease in the number of available motor units. Hence, the intact motor units fire at faster frequency to increase the muscle force. Decreased recruitment is associated with disorders causing axonal loss or conduction block. It may occasionally occur in severe myopathies when the entire motor unit territory is lost. Early recruitment (an excess number of MUAPs for a given force) occurs in myopathies. In these situations, the force generated by each individual motor unit is decreased (due to the loss of muscle fibers), and more motor units are recruited to generate the same amount of force.

(ii) *Activation* is the central control of motor units that allows an increase in the firing rate and force. Poor activation of MUAPs (decreased number of MUAPs firing slowly) is generally due to upper motor neuron lesions (such as stroke or myelopathy) or to volitional lack of effort (such as due to pain or with conversion/malingering).

Single Fiber EMG

1. Single fiber EMG (SFEMG) is the selective needle recording of a small number (usually two or three) of muscle fiber action potentials innervated by a single motor unit.

2. Instrumentation for performing SFEMG include
   a. A concentric single fiber needle electrode with a small recording surface (25 μm)
   b. A 500-Hz low-frequency filter to attenuate signals from distant fibers
   c. An amplitude threshold trigger and delay line to allow recording from a single muscle fiber
   d. Computerized equipment for data acquisition and calculation

3. SFEMG is performed using one of two methods.
   a. Voluntary (recruitment) SFEMG is a common method, where the patient activates and maintains the firing rate of the motor unit. This technique is not possible if the patient cannot cooperate (e.g., child, dementia, coma, or severe weakness), and is difficult if the patient is unable to maintain a constant firing rate (e.g., tremor, dystonia or spasticity).
   b. Stimulation SFEMG is performed by inserting a second monopolar needle electrode near the intramuscular nerve twigs, and stimulating at a low current and constant rate. This method does not require patient participation.

4. Neuromuscular *jitter* is defined as the random variability of the time interval between two muscle fiber action potentials (muscle pair) innervated by the same motor unit. With stimulation technique, the jitter reflects the variability of a single fiber in relation to the simulation artifact. In normal subjects, there is a slight variability in the amount of Ach released at the synaptic junction from one moment to another, resulting in a variable end plate action potential slope and slight jitter.

5. Jitter is the mean consecutive difference (MCD) of all interpotential intervals (IPI) recorded of the muscle pair. It is calculated as follows:

$$MCD = \frac{(IPI\ 1 - IPI\ 2) + (IPI\ 2 - IPI\ 3) + \ldots + (IPIN - 1 - IPIN)}{N - 1}$$

Wherein IPI 1 is the interpotential interval of the first discharge, IPI 2 of the second discharge, etc.., and N is the number of discharges recorded. After analyzing 10 to 20 muscle fiber pairs, a mean jitter (MCD) is reported. Normal mean jitter is less than 50 μsec, but values differ between muscles, and tend to increase with age (Fig. 2–7A).

6. Neuromuscular blocking is defined as the failure of transmission of one of the potentials. Blocking represents the most extreme form of jitter.

7. The results of a SFEMG jitter study are expressed by three findings:
   a. The mean jitter of all potential pairs
   b. The percentage of pairs with blocking
   c. The percentage of pairs with normal jitter

8. Jitter is considered abnormal when one or more of the following criteria is met (for individuals above 60 years of age, the first criterion is not used):
   a. Mean jitter value exceeding the normal limit.
   b. More than 10% of pairs have jitter greater than the upper limit of normal.
   c. Blocking is frequently seen in the majority of fiber pairs in a muscle.

9. SFEMG is most useful in the diagnosis of myasthenia gravis (MG). Abnormal jitter values, accompanied by neuromuscular blocking, are common in MG (Fig. 2–7B). SFEMG is the most sensitive diagnostic study in MG, with a sensitivity ranging from 90% to 99%.

10. SFEMG jitter is abnormal in LEMS and botulism, similar to the findings in MG.

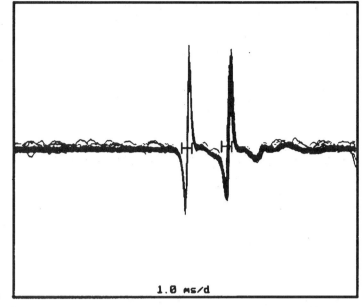

A

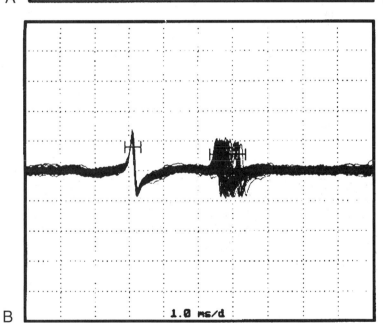

B

Figure 2–7. Single fiber EMG of frontalis muscle. *A.* Normal jitter (MCD 15.8 µsec); *B.* Abnormal jitter (MCD 242.4 µsec and 33% blocking).

11. Stimulation SFEMG technique may help distinguish LEMS from MG. With this method, the jitter may improve significantly with rapid rate stimulation (20-50 Hz) in LEMS, whereas it either will not change or will worsen in MG.

12. Jitter analysis is highly sensitive but not specific. Although it is frequently abnormal in MG and other NMJ disorders, jitter may also be abnormal in a variety of neuromuscular disorders including neuropathies, myopathies, and anterior horn cell disorders. Thus, a diagnosis of MG by jitter analysis alone, has to be considered in the context of the patient's clinical manifestations, laboratory investigations, NCS, and needle EMG findings.

Bibliography

Aminoff MJ: Electromyography in Clinical Practice, 3rd ed. New York, Churchill Livingstone, 1998.

Katirji B: Electromyography in Clinical Practice: A Case Study Approach. St Louis, C.V. Mosby, 1998.

Katirji B. Clinical electrography. Neurologic Clinics. Philadelphia, W.B. Saunders, 2002.

Kimura J: Electrodiagnosis in Disease of Nerve and Muscle. Principles and Practice, 3rd ed. New York, Oxford University Press, 2001.

Oh SJ: Electromyography: Neuromuscular Transmission Studies. Baltimore, Williams & Wilkins, 1988.

Preston DC, Shapiro BE: Electromyography and Neuromuscular Disorders. Boston, Butterworth-Heinemann, 1998.

3 Electroencephalography

Bruce J. Fisch

Indications for EEG Recording

1. Epilepsy—diagnosis and classification: Seizures are classified according to clinical motor, sensory, and autonomic features and ictal and interictal electroencephalographic (EEG) patterns. Accurate seizure classification is necessary for epilepsy syndrome classification (i.e., etiology and prognosis) and for the proper selection of anticonvulsant medications. The EEG is also used to differentiate epileptic disorders from non-epileptic ones, such as psychogenic pseudoseizures.

2. Treatment of status epilepticus: The EEG is used to confirm epileptic status, classify seizure type, and determine when seizure activity has stopped (particularly in patients with impaired consciousness).

3. Intensive care unit patients with impaired consciousness of uncertain origin: The EEG is used to help assess the cause and degree of cerebral dysfunction, prognosis, and to rule out non-convulsive status epilepticus or an epileptic encephalopathic process.

4. Cerebrovascular disease versus Todd's postictal paralysis: The postictal EEG usually contains epileptiform patterns and is unassociated with neuroimaging abnormalities.

5. Coma: The EEG provides information about the severity of cerebral dysfunction and diagnosis and prognosis.

6. Dementia: In the early stages of Alzheimer's dementia the EEG is essentially normal. A moderately or severely abnormal EEG in the first year after onset strongly suggests a different diagnosis. Focal or multifocal abnormalities also indicate a co-existent cerebral disorder or other dementing disorders. The EEG in the pseudodementia of depression is essentially normal. Dialysis dysequilibrium and dementia produces a stereotypical pattern, as does Creutzfeldt-Jakob disease.

7. Organic versus nonorganic disorders: The EEG is normal or very mildly abnormal in common psychiatric disorders. Abnormalities that occur in psychiatric disorders are predominantly reflect CNS medication effects.

8. Encephalitis: In cases of suspected viral encephalitis, a pseudoperiodic epileptiform discharge (PLED) pattern strongly supports the diagnosis and is most often associated with herpes encephalitis.

9. Intraoperative monitoring: The EEG is routinely used to monitor during carotid endarterectomy with light anesthesia to determine if shunting is necessary and to detect cerebrovascular events during anesthesia.

10. Developmental prognosis in the neonatal period and infancy: The EEG can be used to determine gestational and conceptional age, to diagnose epileptic abnormalities, and to specific epileptic syndromes, and to determine prognosis for survival or normal development.

11. Subacute sclerosing panencephalitis produces a nearly pathognomonic EEG pattern.

12. Ceroid lipofuscinosis: The late form, also referred to as the Bielschowsky-Jansky form, produces a characteristic photoparoxysmal response at slow flash frequencies.

Indications

- Seizures
- Altered consciousness
- Development prognosis
- Dementia/Encephalopathy
- Encephalitis
- Intraoperative monitoring

EEG Visual Analysis

1. Routine visual analysis is performed for specific waveforms and for ongoing activity in each of 4 frequency bands: delta <4 Hz, theta 4 to <8 Hz, alpha 8-13 Hz inclusive, and beta >13 Hz. Thus, the frequency bands *have no gaps and no overlap*
2. Visual inspection of the EEG begins with the determination of symmetry of each frequency band and of the peak frequency of the alpha rhythm.

3. The distribution (symmetry and relative amplitudes of frontal temporal-parietal and occipital activity), persistence and amplitude of activity in each frequency band is noted.

4. There are a few distinctive patterns or specific waveforms that are routinely searched for, including the alpha rhythm frequency, photic driving and specific sleep patterns. Otherwise visual inspection is concerned with the search for abnormal waveforms, not the inspection of all normal waveforms.

Basic Principles and Technique

1. Each second of the EEG recording is routinely displayed at 30 mm/second. Slow frequency activity or discontinuous patterns are sometimes more easily seen at more compressed displays of 15 mm/second. Filters are routinely applied to limit the presence of activity below 1 Hz and above 70 Hz. The EEG signal is measured in microvolts, whereas electrocardiographic and electromyographic signals are measured in millivolts.

   a. *Delta* activity refers to waveforms less than 4 Hz (i.e., waveforms with a duration of greater than 0.25 seconds).

   b. *Theta* activity refers to waveforms 4.0 Hz to less than 8.0 Hz (i.e., waveforms with durations $\leq$ 0.25 seconds and $>$ 0.125 seconds).

   c. *Alpha* activity refers to waveforms 8.0 Hz to 13.0 Hz (i.e., waveforms with durations $\leq$ 0.125 seconds and $\geq$ 0.077 seconds).

   d. *Beta* activity refers to waveforms greater than 13.0 Hz (i.e., waveforms with durations $<$ 0.077 seconds).

   e. *Synchrony* refers to waveforms that are spatially independent (usually bihemispheric) that occur simultaneously and in phase with each other.

   f. *Symmetry* refers to left versus right hemisphere amplitude comparisons. Observations regarding symmetry always include the particular waveform (e.g., triphasic waves) or frequency range of the activity being analyzed.

   g. *Morphology* refers to the particular shape of a waveform or waveform complex. *Monomorphic waveforms* are identical in shape.

   h. *Rhythmicity* refers to the appearance of an uninterrupted series of monomorphic waveforms. A sine wave signal at a fixed frequency would be considered perfectly rhythmical as would a more complex waveform that repeats

in an uninterrupted series without changing its shape. *Irregular* patterns consist of waveforms with continuously varying shapes. Patterns that combine varying degrees of rhythmical and irregular activity are refered to as *semirhythmic*.

   i. *Reactivity* refers to the degree of change that occurs in the EEG in response to stimulation. The alpha rhythm is defined, in part, by its attenuation or complete suppression in response to sustained eye opening.

Origins of Scalp EEG

- The scalp-recorded EEG consists of synchronous excitatory and inhibitory postsynaptic potentials arising from the cortex.

- Potentials arising from the gyral cortex near the inner table of the skull covering the convexity of the brain contribute to the EEG.

- Potentials generated in basal cortex, in fissures, in the depths of cortical sulci, in subcortical structures (such as the hippocampus), or in cerebellar cortex do not contribute significantly to the scalp-recorded EEG.

---

2. Origin of the human scalp-recorded EEG

   a. The routine scalp-recorded EEG signal is generated by gyral cortex located over the convexity of the brain. Cortical structures located in the depths of sulci or fissures or the base of the brain do not contribute to the EEG signal recorded at the scalp. Subcortical, cerebellar, and brainstem structures do not produce electrical potentials recorded in the scalp EEG.

      (1) EEG rhythmicity arises from an interaction between thalamic and cortical structures.

      (2) Sleep spindles are generated by the nucleus reticularis of the thalamus.

   b. The scalp-recorded EEG signal consists of cortical inhibitory and excitatory postsynaptic potentials. Most patterns seen at the scalp require approximately 6 cm^2 of synchronous activity arising from convexity cortex. Because of the radial orientation of cortical neuronal cells and the orientation of synapses that generate the signal, inhibitory and excitatory potentials cannot be distinguished in the EEG. Action potentials and glial potentials do not contribute significantly to the EEG.

3. EEG signal propagation
   a. *Volume conduction* consists of the transmission of an electrical current through a conducting volume. Volume conduction travels near the speed of light. The conducting volume of the EEG consists of the substance between the postsynaptic potential and the recording electrode: brain parenchyma, cerebrospinal fluid (CSF), dura, cranial bone, and scalp.
   b. *Transynaptic conduction* refers to the transmission of the EEG signal from one neuron to the next. This may vary from propagation within a gyrus to interhemispheric transmission. Transynaptic conduction occurs at the speed of the axonal conduction velocity plus the synaptic conduction time.
   c. Transynaptic conduction between EEG signals is distinguished from volume conduction by being measurable in milliseconds, whereas volume conduction is instantaneous. When two waveforms appear to occur nearly simultaneously at two separate head regions, the digital screen display can be increased from 30 to 120 to 240 mm/second to determine if they are linked by transynaptic or volume conduction.
   d. Limitations of volume conduction. Impediments to the conduction of the EEG signal include all the tissues between the cortex and recording electrodes, particularly the skull. The EEG signal is usually 1/20 to 1/90 its original cortical amplitude when recorded at the scalp. Therefore, relatively little cortical surface activity is detectable at the scalp.

4. Localization
   a. Amplifier convention. Each amplifier has two electrode inputs. The signal in input 2 is subtracted from input 1. If the signal to input 1 is relatively more negative or less positive than the signal in input 2 then the pen or monitor signal display deflects upward. If the voltage of the signals in inputs 1 and 2 are identical, the signal remains unchanged. If the signal to input 1 is relatively more positive or less negative than the signal in input 2 then the pen deflects downward [if input 1 is −70 μV and input 2 is −50 μV, then the pen or monitor displays an upward deflection of −20 μV; (−70) − (−50) = −20].
   b. *Derivation* refers to the two electrodes selected for each of the two inputs of the EEG amplifer. Fp1-F3 is an example of a derivation (it literally means the Fp1 signal minus the F3 signal). A collection of derivations forms a *montage*. The output of a single amplifier is referred to as a *channel*.
   c. *Bipolar montages* consist of a series of *derivations* that link adjacent electrodes on the scalp. *Longitudinal bipolar montages* link electrodes in an anterior-posterior direction (e.g., Fp1-F3, F3-C3, C3-P3, P3-O1) whereas *transverse bipolar montages* run in a horizontal direction (F7-F3, F3-Fz, Fz-F4, F4-F8). Bipolar montages localize potentials by phase reversal between adjacent channels. If all the waveforms point in the same direction then localization is at one end or the other of the electrode chain.
   d. *Referential montages* consist of a series of derivations in which the same electrode is used in input 2 in all the channels. The electrode in input 2 is referred to as the reference electrode. As long as the *reference electrode* is not near the head region that the signal arises from, localization is determined by amplitude alone.
   e. *Average reference montages* consist of a combination of all available electrodes in input 2 of each channel. Although these montages can sometimes present with a confusing series of opposite deflections, the highest amplitude deflection localizes the scalp region of origin.
   f. *Laplacian montages* consist of a combination of the electrodes that surround the input 1 electrode being placed in input 2. The input 2 electrodes contributing to the total input 2 combination do not have equal representation—the closer the electrode is to the input 1 electrode, the more it contributes to the input 2 signal. A simplistic way of thinking of the input 2 electrodes is that they form a local average reference.
   g. *Spatial filtering*. Bipolar and Laplacian montages filter out widespread waveforms whereas average reference and other references formed by electrodes distant from the input 1 electrode allow widespread waveforms to be seen.

Artifact Identification

- Artifact identification is a substantial part of EEG interpretation

- Artifacts arise from either physiologic potentials generated by muscle, eye movement, cardiac activity, sweat glands, or other sources or from non-physiologic potentials generated by electrical interference from a variety of sources inside and outside of the recording instrumentation.

- A high-amplitude potential that occurs at only one electrode is artifact until proven otherwise.

- Alpha frequency activity that appears prominently and maximally at Fp1 and Fp2 is eye movement artifact until proven otherwise.

5. Artifact identification
   a. *Physiologic artifacts* are produced by electrical potentials arising from the body or movements produced by the body.
      (1) Electrocardiographic artifact appears as a prominent R wave with positivity over the left posterior quadrant of the head and can resemble epileptiform spikes. Premature ventricular contractions usually appear maximally over the occipital head regions and can resemble epileptiform sharp waves.
      (2) Pulse artifact consists of delta waves produced by movement of the electrode with each dilatation of the underlying blood vessels.
      (3) Eye movement artifact consists of a positivity that moves in the direction of eye movement. Vertical eye movement appears maximally in Fp1 and Fp2 whereas horizontal eye movements appear maximally in F7 and F8.
      (4) Muscle artifact appears as apiculate beta activity.
      (5) Respiratory artifact is the most common physiologic artifact in neonatal recordings. It consists of rhythmic delta activity.
      (6) Glossokinetic artifact arises from a resting charge on the tongue. As the tongue moves it produces delta activity over the frontal head regions. In longitudinal bipolar montages delta activity may appear maximally over the anterior and posterior head regions.
      (7) Tremor artifact is sinusoidal at the rate of the body tremor. A parkinsonian tremor typically occurs at 4 to 6 Hz.
      (8) Head movement and cardioballistic artifact produce diffuse or localized delta waves with each head movement.
   b. *Nonphysiologic artifacts* are those produced by electrical sources external to the patient's body.
      (1) Electrical interference typically appears as 60 Hz artifact. It is more likely if an electrode is not attached well to the scalp or if an electrical cable or instrument is near the electrode wires.

(2) Electrostatic artifact produces either very short duration spike-like waveforms usually involving several electrodes or widespread delta waves.

(3) Electrode pop artifact appears as either a single triangular wave or a series of waves in a single electrode sometimes resembling epileptiform spikes. It is caused by poor electrode contact.

Pseudoepileptiform Activity

- Pseudoepileptiform activity includes waveform patterns that contain some features of epileptiform abnormalities but have no association with epilepsy.

- Pseudoepileptiform patterns include wicket spikes, RMTD (psychomotor variant), small sharp spikes (SSS; BETS, benign epileptiform transients of sleep), paroxysmal hypnogogic hypersynchrony, 6 per second phantom spike and wave, 14 and 6 per second positive spikes, subclinical rhythmic EEG discharge of adults (SREDA), triphasic waves (see later under Abnormal EEG, 2c), and asymmetric triphasic waves.

Normal EEG

1. Neonatal EEG: Neonatal patterns change every 2 to 4 weeks from 29 weeks conceptional age until 40 weeks conceptual age.

   a. Discontinuous patterns: until 29 weeks conceptional age the EEG is discontinuous with periods of diffuse inactivity alternating with periods of activity. After that time this discontinuous pattern referred to as *trace discontinu* alternates with periods of prolonged continuous EEG activity. Trace discontinu evolves into trace alternant at 34 to 36 weeks conceptional age, at which time the periods of inactivity grow shorter in duration with less attenuation. The trace alternant pattern gradually loses its periods of diffuse attenuation until it finally disappears at 42 to 44 weeks conceptional age.

   b. Delta brushes; medium to high voltage (25 to 200 μV) 0.3 to 1.5 Hz delta waves with superimposed 10 to 150 μV fast activity (8 to 22 Hz). This pattern first appears at about 26 weeks conceptional age and then begins to appear less frequently until it disappears at term.

   c. Temporal theta bursts, temporal theta rhythm: 4 to < 8 Hz rhythmic sharp wave complexes lasting less than 1 second, maximal over the temporal head regions. This pattern is useful for estimating conceptional age because it rarely occurs before 29 weeks or after 32 weeks conceptional age.

   d. Active sleep: The precursor of rapid eye movement (REM) sleep with more active eye movements, a decrease in muscle tone, and more prolonged periods of irregular respiration.

   e. Quiet sleep: The precursor of non-REM sleep or slow-wave sleep stages III and IV. This is characterized by either continuous high voltage slowing or by trace alternant.

2. Childhood and adolescent EEG: During the first year of life EEG patterns show prominent changes approximately every 3 months. The EEG continues to change at 1- to 3-year intervals until stabilizing at age 22 to 24 for the next 3 to 4 decades.

   a. Alpha activity: The relative amount of alpha increases over all head regions. In most normal individuals the precursor of the occipital alpha rhythm that reacts to eye opening reaches 3 to 4 Hz at 3 to 4 months of age and 5 to 6 Hz at 1 year of age. By 3 years of age the alpha rhythm is usually 8 Hz, and by 9 years of age it is usually 9.5 to 10.5 Hz.

   b. Delta and theta activity are prominent over all head regions throughout childhood. During wakefulness delta activity gradually disappears by ages 13 to 14 and theta activity ceases by ages 16 to 18.

   c. Posterior slow waves of youth: Occipital delta waveforms during wakefulness and eye closure that are formed from the alpha rhythm and therefore are present when the alpha rhythm is present and absent when it disappears. They are often mistaken for abnormal occipital slowing.

   d. Hypnogogic hypersynchrony: Rhythmic, high-amplitude (75 to 200 μV), bisynchronous waveforms, widely distributed, abrupt in onset, lasting several seconds to rarely several minutes during sleep onset (hypnogogic) or awakening from sleep (hypnopompic). This pattern is most common between the ages of 4 months and 2 years of age.

   e. Cone waves: Prominent occipital, negative polarity, delta waveforms during non-REM sleep in childhood up to 5 years of age

   f. Stage I sleep: Slow lateral eye movements, drop-out of the alpha rhythm, vertex waves, and positive occipital sharp transients of sleep

   g. Stage II sleep: Sleep spindles and K complexes. Sleep spindles first appear at 2.5 to 3.5 months of age and consist of 12 to 14 Hz rhythmic waveforms lasting 2 to 4 seconds with maximal amplitude over the central head regions. They increase in duration up to 8 months and become bilaterally synchronous by 2 years of age. K complexes are well seen by 6 to 8 months of age and consist of high-amplitude diphasic waves over the central head regions lasting >0.5 seconds. The appearance of either sleep spindles or K complexes defines stage II sleep.

   h. Stages III and IV sleep (slow-wave sleep, delta sleep): Stage III sleep is defined by the presence of delta activity during 20% to 50% of the recording. Stage IV sleep is defined as delta activity during more than 50% of the recording. Non-REM parasomnias (non-sleep behaviors during sleep) include sleepwalking, night terrors, and confusional arousals.

   i. REM sleep: Rapid eye movements; decreased muscle tone measured by submental electrodes; irregular respiration, blood pressure, and heart rate; poikilothermia. REM parasomnia of REM behavior disorder (i.e., the loss of muscle atonia with acting out of dreams) is rare in childhood but common in the elderly. Narcolepsy is the intrusion of REM sleep during wakefulness (hallucinations, loss of muscle tone—cataplexy) and typically begins in childhood or adolescence.

3. Adult EEG

   a. Delta and theta activity: Absent from the EEG during wakefulness except as posterior slow waves of youth that persist normally in some adults

   b. Alpha rhythm: An alpha rhythm frequency of 8.0 Hz or less is abnormal.

   c. REM sleep occurring during a routine EEG suggests possible narcolepsy. Repeated arousal with snoring during an EEG suggests obstructive sleep apnea.

4. Elderly EEG

   a. Alpha rhythm: The alpha rhythm gradually slows but should remain above 8.0 Hz.

   b. Temporal slowing of the elderly: 1 to 3 second epochs of temporal theta may appear in up to 10% to 12% or temporal delta in 1% to 2% of the recording during apparent wakefulness in clinically normal individuals over the age of 65. For reasons that are unclear, temporal slowing occurs more often on the left.

   c. Slow-wave sleep: The amplitude of slow-wave sleep gradually declines with age. According to sleep-scoring guidelines for amplitude developed in the 1970s it is not unusual for slow-wave sleep to be absent in the elderly.

5. Pseudoepileptiform patterns

   a. Wicket spikes: This EEG pattern consists of a sudden accentuation of a background waveform in the theta or alpha frequency range. It was originally described in adults and localized to the midtemporal head region, but it can occur over any head region at almost any age.

   b. RMTD (psychomotor variant): This pattern occurs during drowsiness, is localized to the temporal head regions, can be unilateral or bilateral or generalized, presents as a 1- to more than 10-second run of sharply contoured notched theta waves, and the frequency of theta is the same at the beginning of the discharge as it is at the end.

   c. Small sharp spikes (SSS; BETS, benign epileptiform transients of sleep) are best seen in referential montages, have single or diphasic or triphasic low amplitude spikes (<60 msec), often demonstrate a longitudinal or interhemispheric dipole configuration, rarely if ever repeat with the same morphology and distribution within a 300 msec period, and tend to have the greatest amplitude over the mid to posterior temporal-parietal head regions.

   d. Paroxysmal hypnogogic hypersynchrony consists of hypnogogic hypersynchrony with low-amplitude spikes that do not maintain a consistent time relationship to the high-amplitude theta/delta waves of the hypnogogic hypersynchrony pattern.

   e. Six-per-second phantom spike-and-wave is clearly benign when it presents as an occipital dominant low-amplitude pattern of 6 Hz spike-and-wave activity usually lasting less than one second. When the pattern is anterior dominant it can be distinguished from abnormal epileptiform patterns by the presence of very low-amplitude frontopolar dominant spikes in combination with high-amplitude slow waves.

   f. 14- and 6-per-second positive spikes are best seen in referential montages, are most common in adolescents, appear as varying combinations of nearly 6 Hz and 14 Hz less than 2-second runs of occipital-parietal-posterior temporal dominant spikes during drowsiness.

   g. Subclinical rhythmic EEG discharge of adults (SREDA) is a pseudoepileptiform electrographic seizure pattern typically lasting 40 to 80 seconds (range <10 seconds to >5 minutes).

In two of every three patients it is bisynchronous and symmetrical; in the third patient it is asymmetrical or unilateral. SREDA occurs most often in elderly individuals, with abrupt onset or brief delay after single wave complex evolving to a sustained theta pattern. It occurs during wakefulness with normal response testing.

   h. Triphasic waves (see Abnormal EEG, 2c). Triphasic waves are occasionally sharply contoured, creating the appearance of an abnormal epileptiform pattern.

   i. Asymmetric triphasic waves. Similar to typical triphasic wave pattern except the triphasic waves have a consistent asymmetry >50%. More easily confused with abnormal epileptiform patterns than generalized triphasic waves. Does not appear as a focal pattern.

6. Activating procedures

   a. Hyperventilation: Performed for 3 to 5 minutes to activate generalized epileptiform patterns, specifically 3 Hz spike-and-wave.

   b. Photic stimulation: Performed at flash frequencies between 4 and 30 Hz to activate epileptiform abnormalities (i.e., photoparoxysmal response)

   c. Sleep: Non-REM sleep activates epileptiform abnormalities, particularly focal spikes.

   d. Sleep deprivation. In patients who fail to be activated by non-REM sleep, sleep deprivation may occasionally be activating.

Abnormal EEG

1. Localized brain dysfunction

   a. Attenuation of all activity always implies the presence of an underlying gross anatomical abnormality. The abnormality may be either a cerebral lesion or an extracerebral fluid accumulation that impedes conduction of the cortical signal, such as a subdural hematoma or scalp edema from a neonatal scalp intravenous line. Because of volume conduction and the spreading of the EEG signal over the scalp by the skull, a complete localized absence of EEG activity is not encountered. However, a greater than 50% reduction in the amplitude of all frequencies compared to the homologous contralateral head region (not due to technical factors) always indicates the presence of a significant cerebral dysfunction.

   b. Delta activity is the most abnormal localized EEG finding after severe attenuation. The more continuous the delta activity and the greater the attenuation of faster frequencies over the same head region, the more likely there is an underlying gross anatomical lesion. Continuous irregular delta activity was formerly referred to as *polymorphic* delta activity. Delta activity indicates a functional or anatomic transection of subcortical white matter. Brainstem lesions that do not interfere with consciousness, and small hemispheric deep white matter lesions do not produce significant EEG changes. Acute hemiparesis due to stroke associated with continuous contralateral delta activity is always a sign of a hemispheric, non-lacunar stroke.

c. Theta activity: As with delta activity, the more continuous the theta activity and the greater the attenuation of faster frequencies, the more likely there is an underlying cerebral dysfunction. Gross anatomical lesions are likely if alpha and beta activity in the same head region are substantially reduced.

d. Beta activity implies the presence of intact cortical function. Therefore focal increased beta amplitude occurs only with skull defects that allow the EEG signal to be conducted easily to the recording electrode. In contrast, localized attenuation of beta activity strongly suggests the presence of an underlying cerebral dysfunction, often associated with a gross anatomic lesion.

2. Generalized brain dysfunction

a. Background slowing: Background activity refers to the predominant sustained rhythmic pattern arising from a given head region. In normal adults background activity during wakefulness over any head region should be greater than 8.0 Hz. Disorders that affect the brain diffusely produce slowing of all background activity. The greater the degree of brain dysfunction, the slower the EEG becomes (see Coma Patterns below).

b. Occipital intermittent delta activity (OIRDA) and frontal intermittent rhythmic delta activity (FIRDA): These patterns consist of medium to high amplitude, 1- to 3-second epochs of rhythmic monophasic delta waves, sometimes with a notched or almost triphasic appearance, with frontal predominance in adults, adolescents, and some children and occipital predominance in many children (a shift to anterior dominance usually occurs at age 7 to 8 years). FIRDA and OIRDA during hyperventilation and well-established stage I sleep may be normal. FIRDA and OIRDA otherwise indicate either a diffuse cerebral dysfunction or deep, midline lesions in the vicinity of the 3rd ventricle.

c. Triphasic waves consist of isolated or rhythmic runs of anterior or posterior dominant waveforms with three phases. Each phase is longer in duration than the preceding phase, and the second phase is relatively positive to the first and third phases. Triphasic waves are age dependent, rarely occurring in individuals under 25 years of age and becoming increasingly common in metabolic toxic encephalopathies with each decade of life. Triphasic wave patterns associated with an absence or severe attenuation of activity in the alpha and beta frequency ranges are most often associated with hepatic, renal, or anoxic encephalopathy.

3. Periodic patterns: These patterns include burst-suppression, bisynchronous symmetric periodic epileptiform discharges (PEDs), and PLEDs (see earlier under Indications for EEG Recording, number 12). Two other forms of clinically distinctive patterns are described below.

a. Spongiform encephalopathy (Creutzfeldt-Jakob disease). Most patients develop a nearly pathognomonic pattern of continuous, highly periodic, often sharply contoured, biphasic and triphasic waves over all head regions within 2 to 3 months of the onset of clinical manifestations. At onset the pattern may be asymmetric or unilateral. If the pattern lacks periodicity it may resemble a triphasic wave pattern (see earlier under Generalized Brain Dysfunction, 2c). Its presence in the setting of subacute dementia and myoclonus is virtually pathognomonic. Other prion diseases (e.g., bovine spongioform encephalopathy or "mad cow disease," familial fatal insomnia, etc.) do not produce this pattern.

b. Subacute sclerosing panencephalitis (SSPE) produces a nearly pathognomonic pattern consisting of high voltage (300 to 1500 uV) generalized 0.5- to 3-second waveform complexes recurring at 3- to 20-second intervals separated by generalized attenuation of all background activity. Rarely, a similar pattern may be seen in patients with tuberous sclerosis.

4. Coma patterns and prognosis

a. Reactivity: A change in the EEG consisting of either attenuation or enhanced electrocerebral activity in any frequency range in response to vigorous (noxious) stimulation is a favorable prognostic sign. The absence of reactivity is a more important indicator of poor outcome in coma than the presence of a specific coma pattern, notable exceptions being the burst-suppression pattern and electrocerebral inactivity.

b. Spontaneous variability: This refers to clear changes in the overall EEG pattern that occur spontaneously (without exogenous stimulation) during the recording. Regardless of the coma pattern (a notable exception being beta coma) an invariant recording in the absence of general anesthesia or hypothermia obtained 6 hours or more after coma onset suggests a poor prognosis for recovery or survival.

c. Beta coma: This pattern consists of predominantly beta activity over all head regions and is a strong predictor of excellent outcome. Beta coma patterns are always due to a medication effect (often in association with drug overdose) caused by benzodiazepines or barbiturates. Beta activity is always a reliable sign of intact cortical function.

d. Alpha coma, theta coma and alpha/theta coma patterns are now considered to have similar prognostic value. Most patients with generalized activity completely restricted to the alpha and theta frequency bands (i.e., there is no intermixed delta or beta activity) that is continous throughout the record and shows no evidence of reactivity do not survive. Other less restricted patterns, particularly those that show spontaneous variability, reactivity and admixtures of other frequency waveforms are not predictive of poor outcome.

e. Burst-suppression

f. ECI

5. Interictal epileptiform patterns

a. Focal patterns: Epileptiform spikes usually indicate that the seizures are focal in onset and that they arise from the underlying cortical area. Focal spikes in neonates do not indicate epilepsy.

b. Multifocal spike and wave activity: Typically associated with underlying cerebral or cortical lesions, multiple seizure types, and medical intractability.

c. Generalized typical spike-and-wave: 3 Hz spike-and-wave associated with impaired consciousness or behavioral arrest if prolonged. The only pattern used to titrate the anticonvulsant response: effective protection is associated with suppression of the epileptiform activity.

d. Generalized atypical spike-and-wave. 4 to 5 Hz spike-and-wave or irregular spike-and-wave. Typically associated with primary generalized epilepsy and convulsive seizures.

e. Generalized slow spike-and-wave: spike-and-wave <2.5 Hz typically associated with Lennox Gastaut syndrome (intractable seizures and mental retardation).

f. Pseudoperiodic lateralized epileptiform discharges (PLEDs): Typically lateralized or unilateral sharp, spike, or multiphasic waveform complexes repeating at 1- to 3-second intervals with suppressed or abnormal surrounding background activity. Most often associated with acute or subacute hemispheric and cortical lesions caused by stroke, trauma, infection, or inflammatory disorders, or as a manifestation of poor seizure control in patients with epilepsy. In patients with suspected encephalitis PLEDs are strongly suggestive of herpes encephalitis.

g. Bilateral pseudoperiodic epileptiform discharges (BiPLEDs): Similar to PLEDs but bilateral and intermittently asynchronous. Often associated with bilateral cerebrovascular (e.g., sickle cell anemia), infectious, or inflammatory disorders, rarely poor seizure control in patients with epilepsy.

h. Pseudoperiodic epileptiform discharges (PEDs) consist of bisynchronous symmetrical sharp, spike, or multiphasic waveform complexes repeating at 1- to 3-second intervals. Usually associated with severe generalized encephalopathies that are metabolic (e.g., anoxia) or inflammatory.

i. Hypsarrythmia: Multiple spikes with shifting foci, high amplitude, generalized asynchronous slow waves with electrodecremental seizure patterns (see Ictal epileptiform patterns, 6e below). Infantile pattern associated with infantile spasms. Poor long-term prognosis in patients with known etiology (caused by a great variety of prenatal, perinatal, or postnatal diffuse, multifocal, or metabolic cerebral disorders). Whereas up to 40% of idiopathic cases do well, approximately 60% of infants with hypsarrhythmia have infantile spasms.

6. Ictal epileptiform patterns

a. Focal patterns: Seizure onset in the brain often precedes the scalp manifestation by 10 to 30 seconds. Scalp localization usually corresponds to underlying localization of the epileptogenic zone.

b. Generalized 3 Hz spike-and-wave: Prolongation of the Interictal pattern with clinical manifestions including behavioral arrest, clonic eyelid contraction, automatisms, and impairment of consciousness.

c. Generalized paroxysmal fast activity: Low- to

medium-amplitude admixture of beta and alpha spike-like waveforms associated with tonic seizures and less often tonic-clonic seizures. Often co-existing neurologic deficits.

d. Generalized tonic-clonic seizures. The EEG is often obscured by muscle and movement artifact that reveals tonic contraction slowly evolving to clonic activity that gradually slows. Abrupt seizure cessation always associated with generalized suppression of all EEG activity.

e. Electrodecremental pattern: Sudden sustained generalized attenuation of amplitude, often preceded by a frontal dominant paroxysmal slow-wave complex or generalized paroxysmal waveforms associated with an infantile spasm.

f. Post-ictal patterns: Localized seizures usually demonstrate postictal localized EEG slowing and suppression in the area of seizure onset. Generalized tonic clonic seizures are clearly identified by severe immediate generalized EEG suppression.

Key Abnormal Findings

- Localized brain dysfunction
- Generalized brain dysfunction
- Periodic patterns
- Coma patterns
- Interictal epileptiform
- Ictal epileptiform

Bibliography

Fisch BJ (ed): Fisch and Spehlmann's EEG Primer. Basic Principles of Digital and Analog EEG. New York, Elsevier Science BV, 1999.

Goldensohn ES, Legatt AD, Koszer S, Wolf SM (eds): In Goldensohn's EEG Interpretation: Problems of Overreading and Underreading. Mt. Kisco, NY, Futura, 1999.

Muscle and Nerve Biopsy

Steven Lovitt
Yadollah Harati

Muscle and nerve biopsy provides objective information about the underlying disease mechanism. However, the biopsy report is sometimes confusing to clinicians because a pathological description is often given instead of a clinical diagnosis. Expectations regarding the results of these tests are therefore sometimes unrealistic. Good communication with the pathology laboratory is required to ensure that the sample is submitted properly. Appropriate screening of patients is critical to maximize the diagnostic yield.

Muscle Biopsy

Factors Increasing the Diagnostic Yield of Muscle Biopsy

1. Patients with signs or symptoms of a myopathic process have a better diagnostic yield:
   a. Weakness, especially proximally
   b. Cramps, fatigue
   c. Elevated creatine phosphokinase (CPK) level
   d. Myopathic features on electromyography (EMG)
2. Obtaining an adequate specimen is important because muscle biopsy can be limited by sampling error. Open biopsy allows for larger specimens to be obtained from different portions of the muscle, lessening sampling error. If only immunohistochemical stains are to be performed, needle biopsy may be adequate.
3. A muscle that has been extensively studied such as the biceps or the quadriceps should be chosen. Although the gastrocnemius is often chosen, it is commonly affected by superimposed radiculopathy complicating interpretation. Also, the orientation of fibers in this muscle make it more difficult to section transversely.
4. The muscle to be sampled should be free of trauma that can cause artifactual changes that might be confused with a primary muscle disease. For example, muscles recently studied by EMG should be avoided. Although the deltoid muscle is easily accessible, it should be avoided because it likely has served as a repository for a lifetime of intramuscular injections.
5. Electrocautery and clamps should never be used to obtain the specimen because they cause severe artifactual changes. The muscle should not be immersed in saline or any other liquid, as this will result in severe separation artifact.

6. In acute myopathy, a significantly weak muscle should be biopsied. However, in chronic myopathic conditions, biopsy of significantly weak muscles may reveal only end-stage changes. In such cases, a mild to moderately weak muscle should be selected.

Disorders in Which Muscle Biopsy May Be Beneficial

1. Inflammatory myopathy
   a. Polymyositis
   b. Dermatomyositis
   c. Inclusion body myositis
2. Noninflammatory myopathy
   a. Muscular dystophy: Genetic testing should be performed when appropriate as this may lead to a diagnosis in a less invasive manner. Because point mutations may not be detected by genetic testing, muscle biopsy with immunostaining or Western blot for affected sarcolemmal proteins may be required if genetic testing is normal
   b. Inclusion body myopathy
   c. Metabolic myopathy: Staining for myophosphorylase, myoadenylate deaminase, and phosphofructokinase can be performed to show enzymatic deficits. Detailed biochemical studies of muscle tissue can reveal enzyme deficits that cannot be tested by routine staining.
3. Systemic disorders with muscle involvement, symptomatically or subclinically
   a. Mitochondrial myopathy
   b. Sarcoidosis
   c. Vasculitits
   d. Amyloidosis
4. Congenital myopathy
   a. Central core disease
   b. Nemaline myopathy
   c. Myofibrillar (desmin) myopathy
   d. Centronuclear myopathy
   e. Multicore disease

When Biopsy Should Not be Performed

1. Disorders diagnosed by EMG
   a. Myasthenia gravis: A 10% decremental response suggests the diagnosis of myasthenia

gravis. An increased acetylcholine receptor antibody titer is diagnostic.

   b. Myotonic disorders

2. Disorders diagnosed by genetic testing

   a. Myotonic dystrophy

   b. Dystrophinopathies: Because point mutations are not detected by genetic testing, muscle biopsy may be required for diagnosis

   c. Fascio-scapulo-humeral muscular dystrophy

   d. Oculopharyngeal muscular dystrophy

   e. Myoclonic epilepsy with ragged-red fibers (MERRF)

   f. Mitochrondrial myopathy, encephalopathy, lactic acidosis, and strokelike episodes (MELAS)

Muscle Biopsy

- The choice of muscle to biopsy should be made by the treating physician.

- The treating physician, surgeon, and pathology laboratory must communicate closely.

- The surgeon and pathology laboratory must have adequate experience in obtaining and preparing muscle to avoid significant artifactual changes.

- Objective clinical findings of a myopathic process greatly increase the diagnostic yield of biopsy.

Nerve Biopsy

The Limitations of Nerve Biopsy

1. In about 30% of cases of neuropathy referred to major medical centers for evaluation of peripheral neuropathy, no cause is found, despite intensive study.

2. Peripheral nerve responds pathologically to insult in a limited number of ways (demyelination, axonal degeneration), regardless of the initial insult; therefore, pathological changes are often nonspecific.

3. Nerve biopsy is not indicated when the diagnosis is apparent on clinical grounds

   a. Diabetic neuropathy

   b. Uremic neuropathy

   c. Alcoholic neuropathy

   d. Guillain-Barré syndrome

   e. Porphyria

4. Nerve biopsy should not be performed if genetic testing is more likely to yield a diagnosis.

5. Because purely sensory nerves are virtually always chosen for biopsy, the yield of such a procedure in patients with significant motor involvement is reduced.

Factors Increasing the Diagnostic Yield of Nerve Biopsy

1. All patients should have a nerve conduction velocity study (especially of the nerve that is to be biopsied) before being considered for biopsy. Patients referred for "neuropathy" are sometimes found to have another cause for their symptoms, such as arthritis, interdigital neuroma, plantar fasciitis, or radiculopathy. Biopsy of an electrically normal nerve is less likely to yield a diagnosis and is more likely to result in painful complications.

2. A pathology laboratory well familiar with preparation of peripheral nerve should be consulted. Improper handling and preparation of the specimen results in severe artifactual changes. Furthermore, preparation of an adequate semithin and teased fiber preparation requires a level of skill that can be obtained only through experience. While routine stains (trichrome or H&E) are sufficient for evaluation of fiber density, myelin digestion chambers, and the presence of inflammation or vasculitis, they cannot reveal underlying pathology (demyelinating vs axonal), which can be revealed only via semithin or teased fiber preparations.

3. The nerve should not be stretched or pulled, as this results in artifactual changes in the semithin section that can be easily be confused with axonal degeneration.

4. The sural nerve is most frequently chosen for its constant location, its protection from mechanical trauma, and the well-standardized normal structure and age-related changes. The physician performing the biopsy should be very familiar with the procedure as the nerve can easily be confused with the saphenous vein, which lies adjacent to it.

5. An adequate length of nerve (at least 5 to 6 cm) should be obtained. Because visualization of foci of inflammation is limited by sampling error, obtaining a larger specimen helps minimize this limitation.

6. Poor wound healing or peripheral edema may complicate sural nerve biopsy. Under these circumstances, another sensory nerve may be chosen. The superficial peroneal nerve is accessible, but it is not found in its expected location in approximately 20% of cases. Nerve conduction studies performed immediately prior to nerve biopsy may help in localizing the position of the nerve. The superficial radial nerve is also accessible, but it is technically more difficult to remove due to its proximity to the tendons of the hand. Although biopsy of motor nerves innervating the anconeus

and gracilis muscles has been performed, removal is technically difficult. In addition, interpretation is limited because of inadequate standardization of normal values for these nerves.

Disorders in Which Nerve Biopsy May Be Helpful

1. Nerve biopsy is commonly requested in patients for whom other diagnostic testing has been unrevealing. However, as the pathological changes in nerve are often not specific, biopsy "as a last resort" is unlikely to lead to a specific diagnosis. Patients should be counseled about this possibility prior to biopsy to avoid unrealistic expectations.

2. If an inherited neuropathy is suspected clinically, but genetic testing is negative, nerve biopsy can provide objective evidence (e.g., onion bulbing) that the neuropathy is indeed from a genetic condition. Clues to an inherited neuropathy include
   a. Pes cavus
   b. Hammer toes
   c. Scoliosis
   d. High arched palate
   e. Minimal or no sensory symptoms
   f. Indolent onset
   g. Marked enlargement of motor unit potentials

3. Vasculitis, may be diagnosed by nerve biopsy [whether systemic or purely neuropathic]. However, because of the potential for poor wound healing, muscle biopsy should be considered in these cases, either instead of or in addition to nerve biopsy, especially if the suspected vasculitis is systemic in nature. In fact, muscle biopsy may have a better diagnostic yield in such cases, although this subject remains somewhat controversial.

4. Nerve biopsy is sometimes performed in suspected cases of chronic inflammatory demyelinating polyradiculoneuropathy, especially if a vasculitic neuropathy is a possibility. Nerve biopsy may also help guide treatment by confirming that the neuropathy is not axonal, especially in patients in whom treatment may be risky. However, nerve biopsy findings are not a criterion for this diagnosis.

5. Amyloid neuropathy may be diagnosed via nerve biopsy, although genetic testing may preclude the need for the invasive procedure. Rectal biopsy or abdominal fat aspirate may be performed if peripheral edema is present, but may not be sufficient to diagnose this condition.

6. Lepromatous neuropathy is commonly diagnosed via nerve biopsy, although skin biopsy may be sufficient.

Approaches to Nerve Biopsy

- The treating physician, surgeon, and pathology laboratory must communicate closely.

- The surgeon and pathology laboratory must have adequate experience in obtaining and preparing nerve to avoid significant artifactual changes.

- Because nerve can respond to insult in a limited number of ways, pathological changes are often nonspecific. Nerve biopsy performed "as a last resort" when another cause for neuropathy is not apparent is therefore unlikely to lead to a specific diagnosis.

- Nerve biopsy is more likely to provide useful information in response to a specific question.

 ## Bibliography

Collins MP, Mendell JR, Periquet MI, et al.: Superficial peroneal nerve/peroneus brevis muscle biopsy in vasculitic neuropathy. Neurology 55:636–643, 2000.

McCleod JG: Sural nerve biopsy. J Neurol Neurosurg Psychiatry 69:431, 2000.

Said G: Indications and value of nerve biopsy. Muscle Nerve 22:1617–1619, 1999.

5 Autonomic Testing

Louis H. Weimer

Basic Principles and Techniques

1. Formal laboratory evaluation of autonomic function is increasingly available because of expanding recognition and need to document suspected autonomic dysfunction as well as standardization of reliable noninvasive testing.

2. Unlike many physiologic measures, most tests do not directly record autonomic signals, but instead measure responses of complex reflex loops after controlled perturbations. A controlled setting is required for reproducible results.

3. Many different tests have been described, but only a few are recognized as suitable for routine clinical application. These are primarily measures of cardiovagal, adrenergic, and sudomotor (sweating) function.

4. There is broad agreement that a battery of individual tests of differing functions under controlled settings is most desirable to produce reliable, clinically relevant results.

Patient Instructions Prior to Autonomic Testing

• Avoid caffeine, nicotine, alcohol, and over-the-counter drugs.

• Avoid heavy exercise.

• Remove compressive garments.

• Ask about which medications to withhold.

---

5. Patient preparation

a. Many endogenous and environmental factors can confound testing and need to be controlled, if possible.

b. The patient should be well hydrated, comfortable, rested, and recuperated from any acute illness. Some but not all labs test only in the morning. Caffeine (6 hours), nicotine (6 hours), alcohol, and vigorous exercise should be avoided before testing.

c. Medications that influence autonomic function, which are numerous, should be avoided preferably for 48 hours unless medically contraindicated (see box Medications that May Confound Autonomic Testing).

d. Compressive garments should not be worn.

Medications that May Confound Autonomic Testing

• Anticholinergics: tricyclic antidepressants, atropine, probanthine, oxybutynin

• Cholinomimetics: pilocarpine, bethanechol, muscarine

• β-Adrenergic blockers: propranalol and others

• α-Adrenergic agonists: phenylpropanolamine, ephedrine (including cold remedies), midodrine, ergot alkaloids

• Ganglionic blockers: guanethidine, hexamethonium, mecamylamine

• α_1-Antagonists: phentolamine, phenoxybenzamine, guanabenz

• α_2-Activity: clonidine, prazosin, alpha methyldopa, terazosin, doxazosin, yohimbine

• Other blood pressure–lowering agents: hydralazine, nitrates, diuretics, acetylcholinesterase inhibitors

• Other: antipsychotics, nonsteroidal anti-inflammatory drugs, antiparkinsonian agents, tyramine, disopyramide, fludrocortisone, monoamine oxidase inhibitors, antihistamines, combination medications, narcotics, anticholinesterases

---

Commonly Used Measures

Cardiovagal (parasympathetic)

1. Heart rate variability to deep breathing (HR_{DB})

a. HR_{DB} is the most common and best validated vagal (parasympathetic) measure. Both afferent and efferent reflex loops are vagally mediated.

b. Heart rate is recorded while the subject breathes cyclically at 6 breaths/ minute. A sinusoidal HR response is produced.

c. There are numerous acceptable ways to evaluate this response. The simplest methods average the magnitude of minimum to maximum HR differences or calculate a ratio of longest to shortest R-R interval. Multiple other statistical measures of HR variation are acceptable methods of analysis and are types of HR time domain analysis. No one measure is considered universally superior in all settings.

d. Responses are influenced by well-described variables, most importantly age.

e. Normal findings. The magnitude of the HR response to deep breathing is evaluated by age range. Maximum-minimum lower limits of normal are as follows: 10–40 years 18; 41–50 years 16; 51–60 years 12; >60 years 8. Statistical measures are generally laboratory specific.

f. Responses are blunted with suboptimal rate and depth of breathing, significant cardiac or pulmonary disease, anticholinergic medications, excessive number of deep breaths, or increased sympathetic tone (anxiety).

g. Abnormal results are concluded when measures are diminished for age and no confounding variables are present.

2. 30:15 ratio. Active standing induces a HR reflex that is more robust than from passive tilt. The HR initially increases and peaks roughly at beat 15; it then reflexively drops, reaching a nadir near beat 30. The ratio of R-R intervals (30/15) is the measure. Normal ratios are age specific and vary by laboratory.

3. Other cardiovagal measures include HR response to cough, facial immersion (diving reflex), and Valsalva ratio (below), and many others. Spectral and complexity analyses of HR (frequency domain) are mainstays in autonomic research but are still of unproven applicability in individual clinical cases.

Most Common and Best-Accepted Autonomic Battery Measures

Cardiovagal

• Heart rate response to deep breathing (HR_{DB})

• Valsalva ratio

• 30:15 ratio with standing

Valsalva Maneuver (VM)

1. Both cardiovagal and adrenergic (sympathetic) data can be gathered if beat-to-beat blood pressure (BP) responses are recorded. Reliable, noninvasive devices of continual BP recording are used in most laboratories.

2. The VM stimulus is achieved by blowing continuously into a tube with a small leak at 40 mm Hg for 15 seconds. HR and BP responses are evaluated.

3. Normal responses demonstrate an initial passive increase in BP (phase I) followed by a decline from a pressure-induced drop in cardiac output. This is the initial stimulus, which stimulates BP recovery and an increase in HR (phase II). After cessation there is a passive BP decline (phase III) then pressure rises again, overshoots baseline (phase IV), and gradually returns to baseline. The HR peaks and then drops to an overshoot bradycardia. A ratio of trough to peak R-R intervals is the Valsalva ratio (VR), which is primarily vagally mediated. Normal VR lower limits are age dependent [20–40 years 1.50; 40–60 years 1.45; and >60 years 1.35].

4. A response is abnormal when phase II recovery or phase IV overshoot is blunted or absent. Phase II recovery is predominantly α-adrenergically mediated and can be blunted in controls with α-blockade and is a marker of peripheral vasoconstriction. Phase IV overshoot can be eliminated by β-blockade.

5. BP waveform abnormalities are often more sensitive than frank orthostatic hypotension to tilt studies or standing. The VR is an additional parasympathetic measure with different physiology than HR_{DB}.

6. The pattern of abnormality can suggest an underlying pathological process.

a. A blunted phase II and normal or augmented phase IV recovery and VR in peripheral length-dependent neuropathies with cardiac sparing.

b. Loss of phase II recovery, phase IV overshoot, and low VR in generalized autonomic failure.

c. Normal BP components with abnormal VR in a restricted cholinergic process.

d. A falsely negative VR can result if the BP waveform is not considered.

Most Common and Best-Accepted Autonomic Battery Measures (Part 1)

Adrenergic

• BP response to Valsalva maneuver

Sudomotor Testing

1. The Quantitative sudomotor axon reflex test (QSART) is an increasingly available and now commercial technique that directly measures dynamic sweat output.

a. A skin patch is chemically stimulated with acetylcholine, causing local sweat glands to initiate a retrograde impulse. The impulse reaches a branch point and may return to stimulate another gland in a separate isolated chamber. The small change in humidity in this chamber is measured and displayed in real time as dynamic sweat output. Typically, four sites are examined.

b. Sweat onset latency and response amplitude are compared to control values.

c. Abnormal patterns include reduced or absent responses signifying hypohidrosis. Other atypical patterns can be seen with pain and primary sweating disorders. Advantages include high reproducibility, dynamic recordings, and isolation of peripheral pathways from central pathways.

2. The thermoregulatory sweat test (TST) is the current evolution of sweat-induced change in an indicator dye. Modern techniques use the somewhat messy powder alizarin red that can be washed away after testing.

a. The indicator is applied to the anterior body surface. Then the body core or oral temperature is raised by a predetermined amount (1°C) in a special chamber. Areas of sweating are visibly contrasted with anhidrotic regions.

b. Clinical patterns are easily surmised, but interpretation can be confounded by a variety of normal variant patterns.

c. When used in combination with other sudomotor tests, some information on central vs. peripheral localization is possible. This distinction is due to a central stimulus with TST and peripheral activation with QSART.

3. The Silastic skin imprint method appears to be equally sensitive to the QSART but is not widely available.

a. Fast-hardening gels are applied after a chemical stimulus. Small dimples from the sweat beads form in the gel that can be manually or automatically counted.

b. A second gel can be applied over the same site after the first hardens.

4. The sympathetic skin response (SSR) is relatively simple to perform but involves complex central and peripheral multisynaptic pathways. This popular test has received undue attention because it is simple to perform and does not require special equipment.

a. The response is best recorded with electrodes over the palm and soles referenced to the back of the hand or foot and recorded simultaneously on four limbs. Electrical activity from sweat glands and local dermal tissues is the generator.

b. Responses are most commonly triggered by noxious electrical stimulation. Other common stimuli include coughing, startle, and inspiratory gasp. The sensitivity approaches that of other sudomotor tests, but the responses are

not highly reproducible and habituate with repeated stimulation.

c. Many other confounding variables hamper reliability. Electrical stimulation may be inadequate in patients with significant large-fiber sensory neuropathy.

d. SSR measures include onset latency and evoked amplitude compared to normal controls. However, there is wide variation of normal ranges between laboratories. Onset latency is insensitive to most peripheral neuropathies but may be prolonged with central demyelination. Some require responses to be absent to be abnormal, limiting sensitivity.

Most Common and Best-Accepted Autonomic Battery Measures

Sudomotor

- QSART
- Thermoregulatory sweat testing
- Silastic skin imprinting
- Sympathetic skin response

Adrenergic Testing

1. Standing and tilt-table testing

a. The physiology of BP maintenance with tilt is not identical to active standing, but it is more readily controlled and more reproducible. The initial decline in systolic BP is greater with standing because of an exercise reflex–induced drop.

b. During passive head-up tilt testing, the patient is tilted to a predetermined angle, typically 60 to 90 degrees with the BP measuring point maintained at heart level. BP and HR are recorded either continually or frequently.

c. A normal response is a small initial decline with return to baseline within 2 minutes with subsequently maintained BP. Study duration for orthostatic hypotension or dysautonomia is generally 10 minutes. Prolonged tilting for 40 to 60 minutes or pharmacologic challenge may be performed for neurocardiogenic (vasovagal) syncope.

d. Abnormal patterns include orthostatic hypotension, defined as a 20 mm Hg decline of systolic BP or 10 mm Hg diastolic BP. Other lesser signs of orthostatic intolerance more difficult to document without beat-to-beat recordings include a large initial decline or delayed BP recovery after initial tilt, wide fluctuations (>40 mm Hg), an excessive HR increase (>30 bpm or 120 bpm), or a delayed fall in BP.

e. Other less standard stressors to BP include lower body negative pressure, sustained hand grip, mental stress, and noxious cold (cold pressor test).

f. Serum catecholamine levels with lying and standing is not highly sensitive or specific in most settings, except the rare disorder dopamine β-hydroxylase deficiency.

g. Other measures are used in individual labs, but most are not as well studied or accepted, have research utility but limited clinical utility, or have other limiting factors.

Most Common and Best-Accepted Autonomic Battery Measures (Part 2)

Adrenergic

• BP response to standing or passive tilt

Indications

1. The primary goals of testing are to establish whether suspected autonomic dysfunction is present, to quantify the severity of involvement, and to characterize the distribution of involvement. Clinical signs may be nondiagnostic or nonspecific especially in the absence of frank orthostatic hypotension.

2. Objective support for generalized autonomic failure is indicated with suspected disorders that carry a poor prognosis such as multiple system atrophy. Alternatively, some benign disorders can mimic life-threatening, generalized disorders and cannot be diagnosed without excluding generalized autonomic failure—e.g., isolated anhidrosis, unusual causes of syncope, or dysfunction restricted to one organ or system.

3. Demonstration of an autonomic component can narrow the differential of a cryptogenic peripheral neuropathy or aid in the detection of mild or restricted autonomic neuropathy. QSART is a useful aid in the diagnosis of difficult to document small-fiber neuropathies.

4. Testing is essential in evaluating and defining syndromes of orthostatic intolerance, which may not include orthostatic hypotension despite persistent postural symptoms.

5. Sequential studies may be useful in evaluating the course of a disorder or treatment response.

6. Individualized studies for atypical patients, such as tilt studies in combination with other modalities including EEG, transcranial Doppler, or cardiac plethysmography.

Complications

1. Significant complications of autonomic testing are extraordinarily rare despite concerns of tilt testing in patients prone to syncope. In large series of thousands of patients no serious complications or lasting sequelae were reported.

2. Older protocols of QSART testing showed a low incidence of skin irritation, but newer protocols have minimized these concerns. Minor skin irritation is reported in 0.1% of patients undergoing TST.

Bibliography

Assessment: Clinical autonomic testing report of the therapeutics and technology assessment subcommittee of the American Academy of Neurology. Neurology 46:873–880, 1996.

Linden D, Diehl RR: Comparison of standard autonomic tests and power spectral analysis in normal adults. Muscle Nerve 19:556–562, 1996.

Low PA: Laboratory evaluation of autonomic function. In Low PA (ed): Clinical Autonomic Disorders, 2nd ed. Philadelphia. Lippincott-Raven, 1997, pp. 179–208.

Ravits JM: AAEM Minimonograph No. 48. Autonomic nervous system testing. Muscle Nerve 20:919–937, 1997.

Stewart JD, Low PA, Fealey RD: Distal small-fiber neuropathy: results of tests of sweating and autonomic cardiovascular reflexes. Muscle Nerve 15:661–665, 1992.

Weimer LH: Autonomic function. In Evans R (ed): Diagnostic Testing in Neurology. Philadelphia, W.B. Saunders, 1999, pp. 337–365.

6 Magnetic Resonance Imaging: Basic Principles and Techniques

Jonathan N. Levine

Basic Principles and Techniques

1. Magnetic resonance imaging (MRI)

   a. The interaction of magnetic field gradients with hydrogen atoms (protons) is manipulated to obtain an image. Protons are used because they yield the strongest signal and are the most abundant isotope in the body.

2. Concept

   a. Place patient in a magnetic field (0.3–3.0 Tesla). [Hydrogen atoms (protons) align themselves in the longitudinal direction.]

   b. A coil surrounding the region of interest is turned on for several milliseconds to produce a radiofrequency pulse to excite the protons.

   c. The radiofrequency pulse is turned off, and the protons return to their lower energy state. As the protons relax, energy is released as signals characteristic of the tissue imaged (the echo).

   d. This is repeated many times, and the data are analyzed by a computer to form an image.

3. The phase, frequency, and slice information are needed to obtain an image.

   a. Spatial localization is achieved by a magnetic gradient across the long axis of the patient (Z-axis). This results in variations of the radiofrequency across the object being imaged.

   b. The frequency of a tissue's radiofrequency response (the larmor frequency) is directly proportional to the precise magnetic field at the location of the individual proton at the time it relaxes. The computer can calculate which frequency comes from what location, as there is a known gradient in the magnetic field.

   c. All of the frequency direction pixel information is acquired during a single repetition at each phase of the signal.

   d. To obtain the entire image

   (1) A repetition is required for each different phase view.

   (2) The number of repetitions depends on the number of views in the phase direction.

   e. Frequency-encoded information is displayed in one direction, often indicated on an MRI image as a lower case "v" with an arrow in that direction.

   f. Phase-encoded direction is displayed orthogonal to frequency direction.

4. When the protons are excited, they are perturbed out of the longitudinal equilibrium alignment to create a transverse component. This transverse component can generate a detectable electrical signal. A longitudinal component may remain, depending on the pulse sequence, but it does not generate a signal.

   a. Different tissues have different rates of hydrogen atom (proton) relaxation, resulting in

   (1) Different signal strength

   (2) Tissue contrast

5. Relaxation time constraints

   a. T1

   (1) After the radiofrequency pulse is turned off, the hydrogen protons are at some magnetic vector at some angle relative to the longitudinal axis (equilibrium state) with longitudinal and transverse components.

   (2) Individual nuclei gradually revert to the longitudinal alignment by losing energy to the thermal environment (spin–lattice interactions).

   (3) T1 is the time for 63.2% recovery of the longitudinal component of the magnetization vector.

   (4) It is relatively larger than T2 (500–2000 ms in the brain).

   b. T2

   (1) After the radiofrequency pulse is turned off, the hydrogen protons are at some magnetic vector at some angle to the longitudinal axis (equilibrium state) with longitudinal and transverse components.

   (2) Nuclei are initially in phase (moving together) after they are excited but immediately start to exchange energy with themselves and their environment, which causes dephasing. They revert to a random

orientation in the transverse plane (spin–spin interactions).

(3) As phase coherence is lost, so is the signal from the transverse plane.

(4) T2 represents the time it takes for the signal in the transverse phase to be reduced to 36.8% of its original value.

(5) It is relatively shorter than T1 (400–100 ms in the brain).

6. If the proton is perturbed 90 degrees away from the longitudinal equilibrium orientation, it lies completely in the transverse phase and, at this time, has the largest signal that can be determined by the MRI apparatus.

   a. Spin echo sequence perturbs protons 90 degrees.

   b. Gradient echo sequence perturbs protons less than 90 degrees.

7. Can modify the effect of T1, T2, or neither (proton density) relaxation characteristics by

   a. Different pulse sequences: Different variations of the magnetic field gradient results in

      (1) Different affects on the proton

      (2) Different signal intensity

   b. Echo time (TE) (Table 6–1): interval between initiating the radiofrequency pulse and measuring the emitted signal

      (1) Short: 10 to 40 ms

      (2) Long: 30 to 200 ms

   c. Repetition time (TR) (Table 6–1): interval between repeated sequences.

      (1) Short: 300 to 600 ms

      (2) Long: 2000 to 4000 ms

   d. T1-weighted images: short TR, short TE (Table 6–1). Short TE minimizes T2 effects.

   e. T2-weighted images: long TR, long TE (Table 6–1). Long TR minimizes T1 effects.

   f. Proton density (PD)-weighted images: long TR, short TE (Table 6–1). This minimizes T1 and T2 effects, giving a picture of the density of the protons.

8. Commonly used MRI sequences

   a. Spin-echo sequence

TABLE 6–1. DETERMINING THE RELAXATION TIME CONSTANT FAVORED BY THE TECHNIQUE BY LOOKING AT THE PARAMETERS ON AN MRI SPIN ECHO SEQUENCE

MRI	TE	TR
T1	Short	Short
T2	Long	Long
PD	Short	Long

Abbreviations: PO, proton density; TE, echo time; TR, repetition time.

      (1) Repeats 90 and 180 degree radiofrequency pulses and measures the signal after the 180 degree pulse.

         (a) The 90 degree pulse energizes the proton completely into the transverse plane and dephases it.

         (b) The 180 degree pulse rephases the signal used for image reconstruction and eliminates the magnetic field inhomogeneous perturbations.

      (2) Disadvantage: long sequence (8–10 minutes)

   b. Fast spin echo sequence

      (1) Images different areas of the brain in one TR. Obtain multiple TEs for one TR.

      (2) Faster sequence (2–3 minutes)

   c. Double echo sequence

      (1) Obtain PD data on first echo and T2-weighted image data on second echo

   d. Inversion recovery (IR) sequences

      (1) Uses an additional 180 degree inverted radiofrequency pulse before a 90 degree pulse. Depending on the timing, it can suppress certain tissues or make certain tissues more prominent.

         (a) Fluid attenuated inversion recovery sequence (FLAIR)

            (i) Suppresses water (cerebrospinal fluid)

            (ii) Essentially a T2-weighted image in which water is dark

            (iii) Sensitive for abnormalities but not specific

         (b) Fat-saturated inversion recovery sequence: suppresses fat

   e. Gradient echo sequence

      (1) Uses a radiofrequency pulse that results in less than 90 degree perturbation of the proton

         (a) Fast imaging time

         (b) Good for detecting hemorrhage but not determining the age of the hemorrhage

         (c) Used for magnetic resonance angiography (MRA) because it is sensitive to flow

   f. Echo planar imaging

      (1) Extremely rapid imaging time (30–40 seconds)

      (2) Poor quality

      (3) Used for diffusion-weighted imaging and functional imaging

TABLE 6–2. KEY NORMAL FINDINGS FOR TISSUE SIGNALS

MRI	PARAMAGNETIC SUBSTANCE*	FAT	PROTEIN	WATER/CSF	CALCIUM/BONE	GRAY MATTER	WHITE MATTER
T1	High	High	High	Low	Low	Intermediate Low	Intermediate High (fat in myelin)
T2	Low†	Low	Low	High	Low	Intermediate High	Intermediate Low

*Paramagnetic substances include contrast and melanin as well as some states of iron.
†Low on T2 if routine spin echo sequence, high on T2 if fast spin echo sequence.

g. Magnetization transfer imaging
   (1) Apply off resonance radiofrequency before the pulse sequence.
       (a) It preferentially saturates bound immobile protons associated with macromolecules such as myelin.
       (b) Bound protons transfer magnetization to mobile protons in free water, which decreases the signal depending on the macromolecule and the strength of the saturation pulse.
   (2) Magnetization transfer ratio (MTR): represents the amount of transferred magnetization.
       (a) Decreased MTR is seen in areas of demyelination, inflammation, wallerian degeneration, brain tumors.
       (b) Reflects the structural integrity of tissues with a large amount of axons and myelin. MTR is decreased in acute multiple sclerosis (MS), but it may increase as the lesion matures.

Normal Findings

1. Tissue signal depends on the sequence and effects of T1 and T2 weighting (Table 6–2). The signal intensities of the brain on axial FLAIR-, T2-, and T1-weighted images are presented in Figure 6–1.
2. Imaging blood depends on the state of the iron content, which depends on the local environment (Table 6–3).

MRI Artifacts

1. Ghost artifacts
   a. Includes artifacts from pulsatile blood and CSF and respiratory motion
   b. Usually occur in the phase-encoded direction, as the sampling rate in this direction is in the range of the pulsation from blood.
   c. Minimized with suppression protocols or by changing the phase-encoded direction
2. Chemical shift artifact

a. Occurs at tissue interfaces, often between fat and water
   (1) Signal emitted by fat protons has a slightly lower frequency than water.
   (2) Spatial mismapping occurs in the frequency-encoded direction.
b. Appears as a black or white band at the interface

3. Susceptibility artifacts
   a. Appears as distortion or a bright band at the interface between substances with different magnetic properties, often at the skull base or near the sinuses and pituitary gland. It is caused by local distortion of the magnetic fields, which causes dephasing and a frequency shift of nearby protons.
   b. Susceptibility effect is responsible for the high sensitivity of gradient echo images for detecting paramagnetic and ferromagnetic substances.

4. Truncation/Gibb's artifact
   a. Secondary to Fourier transformation used to process MRI signal
   b. Cannot be completely eliminated but can be decreased by increasing the number of phase-encoding steps or decreasing the field of view
   c. May see alternating bands of light and dark in the brain periphery or high signal in the cord mimicking a syrinx

Advantages of MRI over CT

1. Better soft tissue contrast
2. Multiplanar imaging
3. Demonstrates physiologic processes
   a. Blood flow: MRA
   b. CSF flow
   c. Water diffusion
   d. Functional MRI
   e. Biochemical makeup of tissues: MR spectroscopy

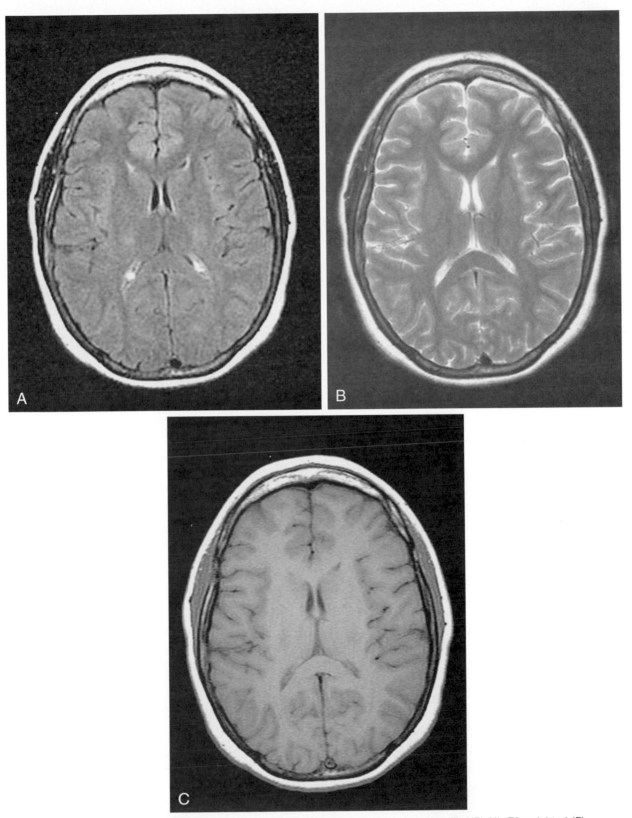

Figure 6–1. Signal intensity of brain on axial fluid attenuated inversion recovery (FLAIR) (*A*), T2-weighted (*B*) (middle), and T1-weighted (*C*) (left) images.

TABLE 6–3. KEY NORMAL FINDINGS FOR BLOOD IMAGING

STATE	IRON STATE	T1	T2	GRADIENT ECHO
Hyperacute (hours)	Oxyhemoglobin	→	↑	↓
Acute (1–3 days)	Deoxyhemoglobin	↓	↓	↓
Subacute (3–21 days)	Intracellular methemoglobin	↑	↓	↓
	Extracellular methemoglobin	↑	↑	↓
Chronic (months)	Hemosiderin, ferritin	↓→	↓	↓

Disadvantages of MRI

1. Long imaging tone: requires more patient cooperation
2. Not available for all patients
   a. About 5% of patients are claustrophobic.
      (1) Open MRI results in poor quality images with less sensitivity for lesion detection and more artifacts.
      (2) Sedation increases examination morbidity and patient discomfort.
   b. Absolute contraindications.
      (1) Cardiac pacemaker
      (2) Most cochlear implants: newer ones supposedly approved
      (3) Older types of aneurysm clips, although many institutions do not image a patient with any type of aneurysm clip
      (4) Metallic foreign body in the eye
      (5) Many types of intravascular stents
      (6) Many types of stimulators
      (7) Many types of metallic devices
   c. Relative contraindication
      (1) Pregnancy. Although no known harmful effects have been demonstrated in humans, fetuses in laboratory animals have possibly been affected.

Contrast MRI

1. The rare earth metal gadolinium is used usually in the form of gadopentate dimeglumine (Gd-DTPA).
   a. It is water-soluble.
   b. It crosses areas of blood-brain barrier breakdown.
      (1) It shortens the T1 and T2 relaxation times.
         (a) This increases the signal on T1-weighted images.
         (b) It decreases the signal on T2-weighted images.
      (2) There are few side effects.
         (a) Allergic reactions are less likely than with CT contrast.

2. Normally enhancing structures include
   a. Vessels
   b. Areas without tight junctions in the vessel wall including the pineal gland, choroid plexus, area postrema, tuber cinereum, paraphysisis, and dura
   c. Sinonasal mucosa
   d. Rectus muscles

3. Contrast MRI is good for imaging tumors, infection, and inflammatory and vascular abnormalities.
   a. Contrast is often not used for imaging patients with chronic debilitating disease, stroke, psychosis, head trauma, or headaches because of the low yield of areas of abnormal enhancement.

4. Triple dose contrast: Give initial contrast dose and image the patient; then give a larger dose and reimage the patient after waiting a variable time.
   a. Metastatic disease: Large number of metastases changes the treatment.
   b. Multiple sclerosis: There may be more areas of enhancement, but this is of questionable significance.

Indications

Select the proper study for a specific clinical scenario.

1. Most patients require routine noncontrast MRI of the brain, which should include a T1-weighted sequence preferably in two planes, a T2-weighted sequence in at least the axial plane, and usually a FLAIR sequence in the axial plane.

2. If infection, tumor, or inflammatory disease is suspected, postcontrast T1-weighted images should be added. At least one sequence of the postcontrast images should be in the same plane as the precontrast T1-weighted images, which is often performed in only the axial plane.

3. Stroke
   a. Obtain diffusion-weighted images and MRA.
   b. Always obtain a T2 sequence at the same levels as the diffusion-weighted images to evaluate for T2 shine-through. Alternatively, if available, images with the T2 signal subtracted or the apparent diffusion coefficient (ADC) map (or both) may be helpful.
4. Trauma or suspected intracranial hemorrhage
   a. Gradient echo images are sensitive for hemorrhage at any stage.
   b. CT, however, is the study of choice for acute hemorrhage.
5. Seizure in a young patient
   a. Add high-resolution coronal T2 and FLAIR images through the temporal lobes to evaluate for mesial temporal sclerosis.
   b. Three-dimensional (3D) T1-weighted gradient echo images are helpful for evaluating the gyri and sulci and to detect subtle gray matter heterotopia.
6. To evaluate the skull base, orbits, temporal bones, and pituitary gland obtain thin section images through these regions.
   a. Precontrast T1-weighted images
   b. Postcontrast T1-weighted images with fat saturation
   c. May want T2-weighted images
7. To evaluate the cochlear nerves or membranous labyrinth, add high-resolution T2-weighted images with a 3D sequence.
8. Multiple sclerosis: may want sagittal T2-weighted images to see plaques in the corpus callosum
9. Presurgical evaluation
   a. MRI with fiducials
   b. Functional MRI to evaluate sensory and motor cortex

Advanced MRI Techniques

1. Perfusion MRI
   a. Need 18-gauge needle for rapid contrast infusion
   b. Best if use T2-weighted echo planar imaging, which is not available at all institutions
2. Diffusion MRI (DWI)
   a. It is usually performed with echoplanar imaging spin echo sequence: images entire brain in less than 1 minute.
   b. Areas of high diffusion of water molecules have low signal.
      (1) Stroke: water molecules show decreased diffusion and therefore an increased signal.

c. ADC map: gives opposite signal compared to diffusion images: inverted diffusion image
   d. T2 shine-through. High signal on diffusion images may be secondary to increased T2 signal. Always need to compare DWI to T2-weighted images obtained at the same level.
   e. Ischemic penumbra: potentially salvageable tissue around an area of stroke—can be imaged by subtracting the diffusion image (infarcted tissue) from the area of decreased perfusion.
3. First-pass bolus tracking technique: evaluates the decrease in T2 signal as contrast goes through the brain, which is plotted against time
4. Spin tagging technique: not often used. Makes use of a radiofrequency pulse to tag red blood cells as they enter the head and evaluates T1 relaxation and flow enhancement
5. Functional MRI
   a. Blood oxygen level-dependent (BOLD) technique is most often used.
   b. Cerebral activation causes increased cerebral blood flow and increased oxygenated blood to a greater extent than the activated area of the brain uses the oxygen in the blood. This results in increased oxyhemoglobin and an increased signal on T2-weighted images.
   c. It is used to assess motor, sensory, and cognitive activation and is helpful for treatment evaluation.
6. MR spectroscopy: can obtain spectrum of metabolites in areas of interest and make judgments about that area based on the levels of the metabolites or spectrum.
   a. Proton spectroscopy is most often used, although phosphorus spectrum is also available.
   b. Can obtain a spectrum on as little tissue as 0.5 cc of tissue.
   c. Poor spectral analysis results if area of interest is located near the bone, sinuses, or ventricles or with patient motion.
   d. Common metabolites imaged with proton spectroscopy
      (1) N-Acetylaspartate (NAA): neuronal marker that is decreased in diseases that destroy or replace neurons
      (2) Choline: cell membrane and myelin marker that is decreased in diseases that destroy myelin and cell membranes
      (3) Creatine: involved with molecular storage of high-energy phosphates
      (4) Lactate: product of anaerobic glycolysis
         (a) Indicator of stressed cells
         (b) By-product of infection

e. Can also measure certain amino acids, *myo*-inositol, lipids, and other metabolites that may become increased in certain diseases

MRI Imaging of the Spine

1. Normal findings (Table 6–4; Fig. 6–2)
2. Indications and techniques

TABLE 6–4. KEY NORMAL FINDINGS FROM IMAGING THE SPINE

MRI	VERTEBRAL BODY	DISC	LIGAMENTS
T1	Increased from fatty marrow	Decreased	Dark
T2	Decreased	Increased from water	Dark

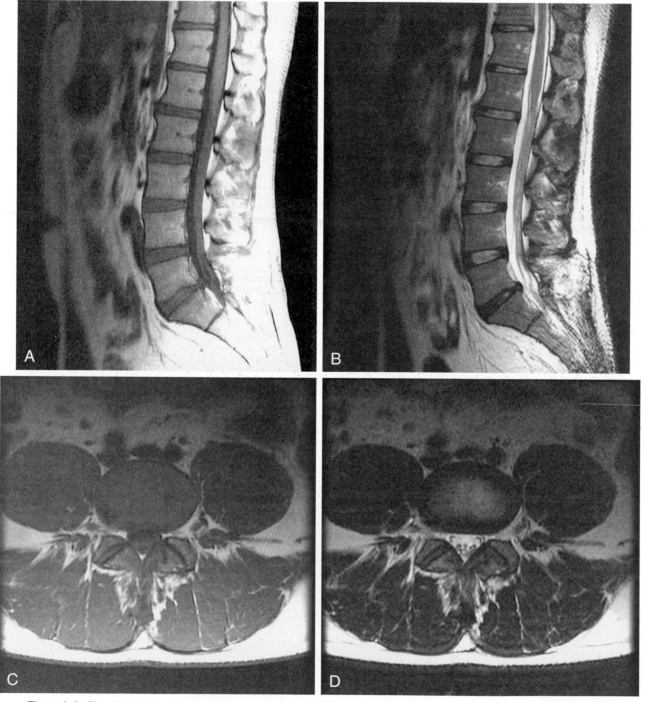

Figure 6–2. Signal intensity of the lumbar spine on midsagittal T1 (*A*), sagittal T2-weighted (*B*), axial T1-weighted (*C*), and axial T2-weighted images (*D*) at the level of the disc.

a. Back pain. MRI is the imaging procedure of choice.

(1) If no prior surgery, contrast is not indicated. Routine sagittal and axial T1 and T2 images, possibly MRI myelogram

(a) Cervical spine: sagittal T1 and T2, axial T1, gradient echo

(b) Thoracic and lumbar spine: sagittal and axial T1 and T2

(2) If prior surgery

(a) Scanning within 3 months after surgery often shows postoperative changes that mimic residual or recurrent disk herniations.

(b) Should always use contrast to evaluate for scar versus disc material. If imaging is delayed, disc herniations can enhance the signal.

b. Tumor, infection, inflammatory and demyelinating disease, vascular malformations, myelopathy. Use contrast MRI. Postcontrast T1-weighted fat-saturated images may be helpful for evaluating soft tissue and bone pathology in patients with tumor or infection.

c. Hemorrhage in the cord. Axial gradient echo images may be helpful.

d. Hemorrhage outside the cord. Use noncontrast MRI.

e. Contraindications are the same as for MRI of the brain.

Bibliography

Ketonen LM, Berz MJ: Clinical Neuroradiology. New York, Oxford University Press, 1997.

Mazziotta JC, Gilmer S: Clinical Brain Imaging. Philadelphia, F.A. Davis; 1992.

Victor M, Ropper AH: Adams and Victor's Principles of Neurology, 7th ed. New York, McGraw-Hill, 2001.

7 Computed Tomography: Basic Principles and Techniques

Jonathan N. Levine

Basic Principles and Techniques

1. X-rays from multiple angles irradiate the area of interest.
   a. Intensity of exiting radiation relative to the incident radiation is measured in small areas called pixels.
   b. Data are interpreted and reconstructed by a computer.
2. Computed tomography (CT) image depends on how much of the original x-ray beam reaches the detector.
   a. CT measures the attenuation of the x-ray beam in units called Hounsfield units and presents them in a gray scale (Table 7–1).
   b. High density = more attenuation = brighter (Table 7–1)
   c. Low density = less attenuation = darker (Table 7–1)
   d. Figure 7–1 (CT scan of the brain) shows different density of normal areas.

Contrast-Enhanced CT

1. Accentuates areas of blood-brain barrier breakdown
   a. Tumor
   b. Infection
   c. Inflammatory disease
   d. Late enhancement for stroke and hematomas
2. Accentuates vessels
   a. Vascular malformations

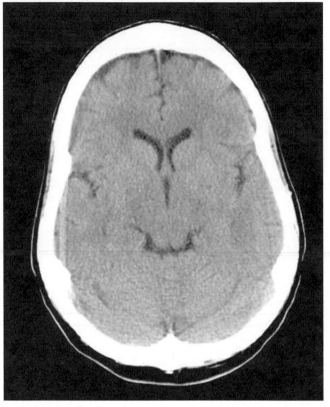

Figure 7–1. Normal CT scan of the brain without contrast demonstrating CSF, gray matter, white matter, bone, and fat in the scalp.

   b. Aneurysms
   c. CT angiography
3. Normal areas that enhance on postcontrast CT
   a. Sinonasal mucosa
   b. Pituitary gland
   c. Area postrema, tuber cinereum, infundibulum
   d. Rectus muscles
   e. Figure 7–2 shows a normal CT scan with contrast.

Contraindications for Contrast CT

1. Renal failure (unless patient undergoes dialysis the same day)
2. Sickle cell disease: increased risk of crisis

TABLE 7–1.   CT DENSITY VALUES

Tissue	Density (Hounsfield) units	Appearance
Metal	1000	Bright
Calcium	100-1000	↑
Blood		
Acute	80-85	↑
Subacute	25-50	↑
Chronic	0-25	↑
Gray matter	35-40	↑
White matter	25-30	↑
Water	0	↑
Fat	−100	↑
Air	−1000	Dark

Relative Contraindications for Contrast CT

1. Prior allergic reaction, allergies, asthma: can premedicate patient usually with a combination of a steroid and antihistamine (given 12 and 24 hours prior to the examination)
2. Heart failure: Contrast may fluid-overload the patient.
3. Diabetes: Patient cannot eat 4 hours prior to study.
4. Pregnancy
   a. Increased risk of abortion from radiation during first trimester
   b. Much lower risk of abnormality after first trimester. Should use lead shield over lower abdomen and pelvis

Types of Contrast

1. Ionic: high osmolar
   a. Increased risk of allergic reaction: 5% of patients have an allergic reaction
   b. Less expensive
2. Nonionic: low osmolar
   a. Decreased risk of allergic reaction: 1.6% of patients have an allergic reaction
   b. More expensive

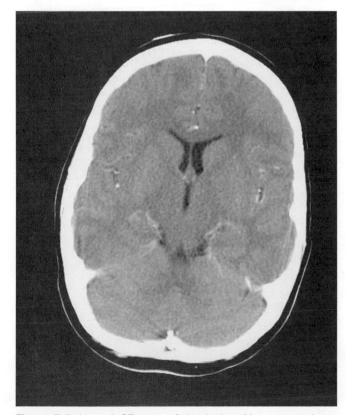

Figure 7–2. Normal CT scan of the brain with contrast shows enhancement of the choroid plexus and vessels.

3. Contrast reaction
   a. Mild: rash, hives, itching, nausea, vomiting
   b. Moderate: mild problems with respiration, retching
   c. Fever: tracheal and bronchiole constriction, low blood pressure, elevated heart rate

Artifacts

1. Motion artifacts
   a. They are decreased with faster techniques, such as helical (spiral) CT.
   b. With helical CT the patient continuously moves forward through CT gantry as the x-ray tube rotates around the patient.
      (1) Computer accesses the data and can reformat for any image plane.
      (2) Fast speed allows CT angiography.
2. Beam hardening artifacts
   a. Lower energy photons are disproportionately attenuated by dense tissue, resulting in a more highly penetrating x-ray beam, which cannot be compensated by the computer software.
   b. They appear as alternating bright and dark lines affecting areas adjacent to bone. They are often seen in the posterior fossa and inferior frontal and temporal lobes and near the cortical–bone interface.
3. Star pattern effect
   a. Cause is similar to that of beam hardening artifacts.
   b. It occurs with metallic objects.
4. Partial volume effect
   a. Occurs when the imaging volume is less than the resolution of the CT scanner
      (1) If two tissues are in the same volume being image (voxel), their density is averaged.
      (2) Effect may be reduced by using a smaller voxel and thinner slice thickness.

Advantages of CT over MRI

1. Safe if metal is present, although there are artifacts if the metal is in the area to be imaged
2. Short examination time
3. Lower cost
4. Easily available
5. Life support monitoring easily accessible

Indications for CT Instead of or Prior to MRI

1. Triage a patient with an acute neurologic abnorality (use noncontrast CT).

   a. Stroke

   b. Subarachnoid hemorrhage (acute headache)

   c. Trauma

   d. Mass with edema, hydrocephalus, mass effect

2. Evaluate ventricular size (use noncontrast CT).

3. Assess bone pathology (use CT with or without contrast, depending on the situation).

   a. Skull base

   b. Temporal bone

   c. Sutures

   d. Erosion

4. Sinus disease (use noncontrast CT unless a mass or an infection)

5. Patient unable to undergo MRI (use CT with or without contrast, depending on the situation)

6. CT angiography (contrast CT)

7. CT perfusion (contrast CT)

8. Pretherapy evaluation (use contrast-enhanced CT)

   a. Functional endoscopic sinus surgery

   b. With fiducials and special head-holders for neurosurgery and irradiation planning

   c. Parkinson's disease: Subthalamic stimulators

9. Pituitary tumor:

   a. If patient is unable to undergo MRI or if evaluation of the thickness of the sella floor is needed for transsphenoidal surgery

   b. Obtain 1 mm thin section pre- and postcontrast coronal images through the sella.

10. CSF leak

    a. Thin section (1 mm) coronal images through area of suspected CSF leak; usually performed after intrathecal injection of contrast

    b. Possibly axial images or sagittal reformatted images

Location of Abnormality: CT versus MRI

The different slice orientation must be taken into account (Figs. 7–3, 7–4).

Specialized CT Techniques

1. Dynamic scanning. Allows measurement of the time–density curve of the enhancing area

   a. The physiologic process of contrast accumulation and vascularity can be recorded.

   b. Highly vascular lesions have rapid wash-in of contrast, high peak, and rapid washout: aneurysm, arteriovenous malformation (AVM), hemangioma, glomus tumor, angiofibroma

2. CT perfusion (can be used for stroke, trauma, cerebral artery bypass surgery, brain death)

   a. Contrast CT perfusion

      (1) May be helpful for acute cerebrovascular accident (CVA), ischemia

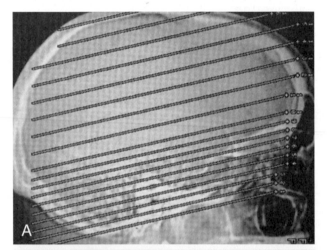
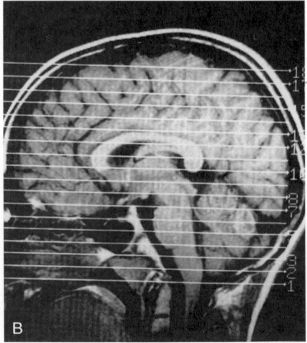

Figure 7–3. Slice variation of a CT scan (*A*) compared with MRI (*B*).

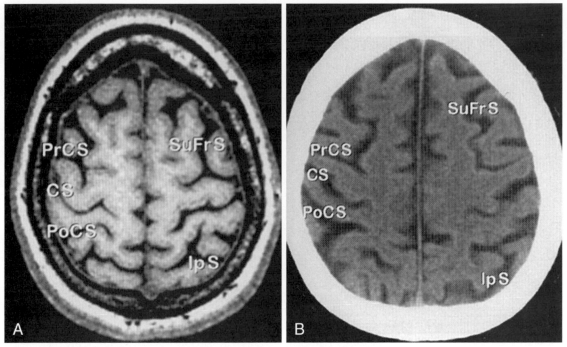

Figure 7–4. Comparison of axial CT (*A*) and MRI (*B*) images through the upper cerebral hemispheres at the level of the superior frontal sutures (SuFrs), precentral sutures (PrCS), central sutures (CS), and posterior central sutures (PoCS). Ips, intraparietal sutures.

(2) To evaluate decreased blood flood to involved area: may have decreased flow before area of infarction is seen on CT

(3) Can obtain CT angiogram at the same time

(4) Need 18-gauge intravenous access and special software

b. Xenon perfusion CT

(1) Xenon is a highly soluble gas that can be used as an x-ray medium.

(2) At steady state, the xenon concentration reflects regional perfusion.

(a) Absolute blood flow can be calculated.

(b) Xenon causes decreased CT attenuation. It is not often used because

(i) Its high anesthetic properties

(ii) Expense of xenon and need for special hardware and software

(iii) Only a limited number of slices through the brain imaged at one time

(iv) Need patient cooperation

3. CT after intrathecal injection of contrast

a. Cerebrospinal fluid (CSF) leak

b. CSF flow dynamics

c. Evaluate for vestibular schwannoma if patient cannot have MRI

d. Was once used to evaluate for arachnoid cyst versus epidermoid tumor

CT Imaging of the Spine

1. Indications

a. Trauma with suspected fracture

(1) Not good for evaluating cord or ligamentous injury

a. Degenerative changes

c. Used with intrathecal injection of contrast

(1) For radiculopathy or stenosis

(2) Evaluate CSF leak or meningocele

d. Postoperative evaluation of the spine

(1) Metallic hardware obscures MRI.

(2) Evaluate fusion.

e. Used if patient cannot have MRI

2. Technique

a. Imaged in the axial plane with or without intrathecal contrast

b. Can also obtain sagittal and coronal reconstruction images

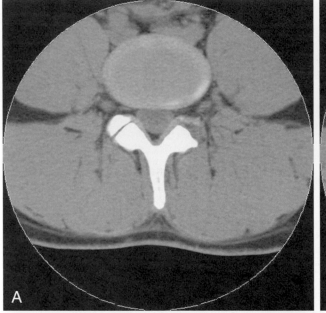

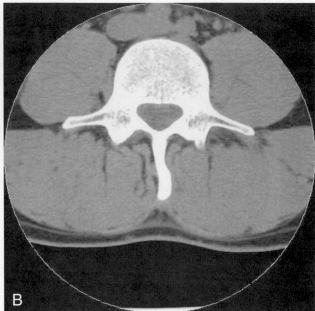

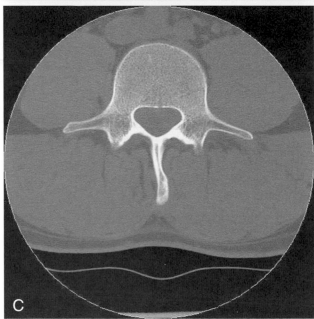

Figure 7–5. Normal anatomy of axial CT of the lumbar spine at the level of the disc (*A*) and vertebral body, in soft tissue windows (*B*) and at the level of the vertebral body in the bone window (*C*).

3. Normal structures (Fig. 7–5)

    a. Bone is dense.

    b. Soft tissue and disc are intermediate hyperdense.

    c. CSF is hypodense.

    d. Fat is extremely hypodense.

 Bibliography

Ketonen LM, Berz MJ: Clinical Neuroradiology. New York, Oxford University Press, 1997.

Mazziota JC, Gilmer S. Clinical Brain Imaging. Philadelphia, F.A. Davis, 1992.

Victor M, Ropper AH. Adams and Victor's Principles of Neurology, 7th ed. New York, McGraw-Hill, 2001.

8 Magnetic Resonance Angiography and Cerebral Angiography

Richard P. Klucznik

MAGNETIC RESONANCE ANGIOGRAPHY

Basic Principles and Techniques

1. The basic principle of imaging flowing blood involves utilizing the signal of fully magnetized spins flowing into a field that has a gradient across it. These fully magnetized spins appear as a bright signal on inflow images. This is the basis of time-of-flight (TOF) imaging. The images are obtained by utilizing the gradient on a high field strength magnet by manipulating the repetition time (TR), the excitation time (TE), and the flip angle (FA) across a certain field of view (FOV).

2. There are two types of TOF imaging: two-dimensional TOF (2-D TOF) and three-dimensional TOF (3-D TOF).

3. 2-D TOF is best utilized for imaging the carotid bifurcation in the neck using a quadrature neck coil. Parameters that may be typical are TR/TE 22/7, FA 68°, with 3 mm thick sections (Fig. 8–1).

4. 3-D TOF is best used for cerebral imaging. Typical parameters are a volume of 20 to 30 cm, TR/TE 45/7, FA 20°, matrix size 512 × 512, voxel size 41 × 41 mm, with a slice thickness of 7 mm (Figs. 8–2, 8–3).

5. In addition, imaging the carotid bifurcation can make use of techniques that, instead of a bright signal, flowing blood is black—the so-called black blood technique.

6. Contrast administration can increase the sensitivity of the scan by using contrast tracking bolus techniques and multiple overlapping, then section acquisition (MOT SA) following a single bolus of gadolinium (Melhem et al., 1999).

7. The third technique for imaging is the "phase contrast" (PC), either 2-D (2-D PC) or 3-D (3-D PC). It involves the use of bipolar gradients that cancel any nonmoving objects in a given volume (e.g., normal gray and white matter). This technique is sensitive, but the velocity of flowing spins must be taken into account, as it is the velocity of the flowing blood. Therefore the sensitivity depends on setting the proper velocity encoding

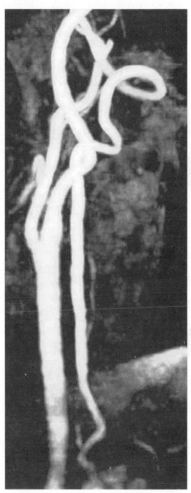

Figure 8–1. Lateral view of a normal two-dimensional time-of-flight magnetic resonance angiographic (MRA) examination of a normal carotid bifurcation.

(VENC). Typical parameters are TR/TE 20–40/6–9, excitation FA 20°, FOV 20 to 30 cm, matrix 512 × 512, and VENC 30 to 60 cm/s.

Indications

Magnetic resonance angiography (MRA) is an excellent screening tool for evaluating stenoses, aneurysms, vascular malformations, and especially the acute stroke situation (Figs. 8–4, 8–5, 8–6). Indications include

1. Acute stroke (Fig. 8–7)

2. Transient ischemic attacks (TIAs)

127

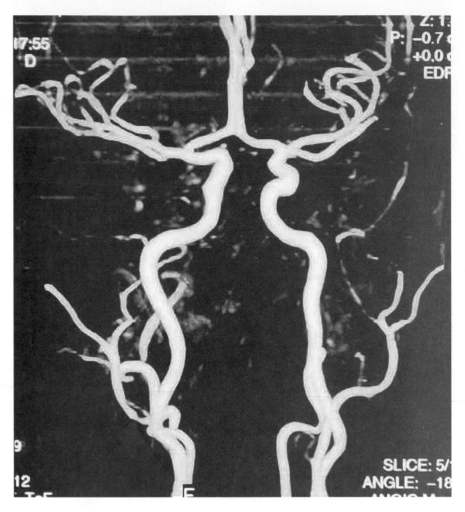

Figure 8–2. Example of a normal MRA examination of the superior cervical carotids and circle of Willis territory, showing the normal anterior and middle cerebral artery branches.

3. Carotid bifurcation stenoses (Fig. 8–4)

4. Intracerebral stenoses

5. Vertebrobasilar insufficiency

6. Arteriovenous malformations (AVMs) (Fig. 8–8)

7. Aneurysms (Figs. 8–9, 8–10)

8. Vasculitis

Contraindications

1. Placing a patient with an aneurysm clip into a magnetic resonance imaging (MRI) unit is controversial. Only the most current surgical clips made of titanium or alloys may be compatible. It is safer to consider the presence of any aneurysm clip a contraindication to MRI. One must also consider that in some cases of surgical resection of AVMs aneurysm clips are used to control bleeding.

2. Platinum coils used for endovascular treatment of aneurysms (Guglielmi detachable coils, Boston Scientific) are MRI-compatible.

Key Contraindication

• Patient with an aneurysm clip

Abnormal Findings

1. It is the imaging of carotid stenoses that brings MRA to the forefront. It may be important not only to measure the degree of stenoses but to examine plaque morphology. In 50% of TIAs there are stenoses of more than 70%. The risk of stroke may depend on ulceration, hemorrhage, or the lipid morphology of the plaque. It has been stated that a large lipid core with a thin overlying fibrous cap is a feature of plaque vulnerability (Kallmes et al., 1996).

2. There are variable ways to image the carotids. The routine sequences are described under Basic Principles and Techniques (above). To look at plaque morphology, T1-weighted axial images after contrast can detect inflammatory changes in the wall.

Axial T2-weighted images can distinguish the lipid core from fibrous tissue. "Black blood imaging" is used to subtract the flowing blood (usually imaged as bright blood) to allow visualization of the arterial wall.

Abnormal Findings (Artifacts)

1. There are imaging or flow artifacts associated with all techniques utilized, especially the TOF techniques.

    a. Turbulent signal loss at bifurcation points or vessel tortuosity

    b. Overestimation of stenoses due to turbulence

    c. Lack of flow related enhancement (FRE) in slow-flow areas

    d. Saturation of in-phase flow

    e. Phase incoherence due to overlying bone

    f. Overall specificity reported in the literature is 16% to 90%, but the real specificity may be closer to 75% (Chung et al.; 1999; Jager et al., 2000).

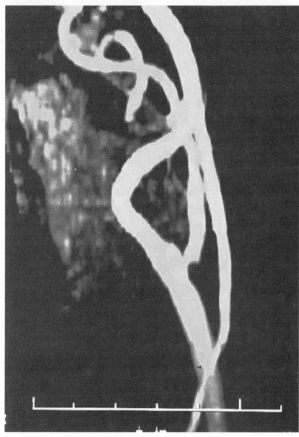

Figure 8–4. This lateral view of the carotid bifurcation shows atherosclerotic narrowing at the origin of the internal carotid artery. Note that the external carotid artery has normal caliber but appears to have the same luminal diameter as the normal internal carotid artery.

Key Abnormal Findings

- Turbulent signal loss at bifurcation points or vessel tortuosity

- Overestimation of stenoses due to turbulence

- Lack of flow-related enhancement in slow-flow areas

- Saturation of in-phase flow

- Phase incoherence due to overlying bone

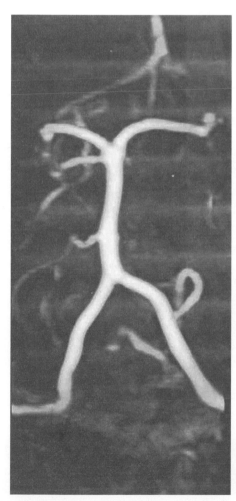

Figure 8–3. Normal distal vertebral and basilar MRA examination.

2. Abnormal findings in a few specific areas are noted.

    a. Aneurysms (Figs. 8–8, 8–10, 8–11, 8–12)

    (1) Even with the present imaging quality, MRA cannot detect an aneurysm smaller than 3 mm. It is an excellent screening tool but cannot replace catheter angiography for the evaluation of subarachnoid hemorrhage (SAH) because of its 3 mm

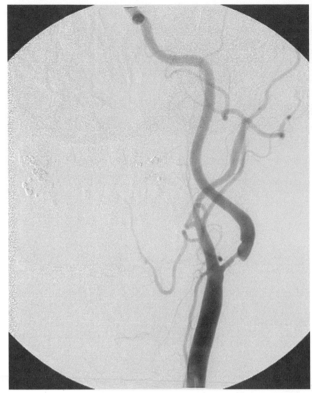

Figure 8–5. Single frontal projection of digital subtraction catheter angiography, showing approximately 90% stenosis, with some poststenotic dilatation with associated atherosclerotic calcified plaque.

limitation. Small aneurysms can still rupture with significant SAH (Griffiths et al., 2000).

(2) MRA is inferior to intraarterial digital subtraction angiography (DSA) for detecting aneurysms but can provide ancillary data about the intraluminal thrombus that DSA may not.

(3) 3-D TOF can be supplemented with newer techniques, such as isosurface rendering.

(4) Techniques used included 3-D TOF 30/4–6, FA 20° with section interpolation technique, FOV 20 to 30, 512 × 512 matrix (Heiseman et al., 1994).

(5) MRA can be used to follow patients treated via an endovascular approach with platinum coils, as they are MR compatible, to evaluate for possible recanalization (Fig. 8–11).

(6) Giant and fusiform aneurysms can be eloquently demonstrated because of the multiplanar capabilities and the relation of the aneurysm to surrounding structures can be shown.

b. AVMs

(1) MRI/MRA can detect the presence of AVMs; but unless newer techniques are

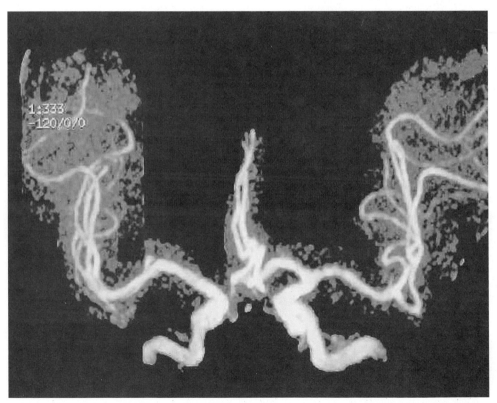

Figure 8–6. Single frontal view of an MRA examination, showing a hypoplastic right A1 segment.

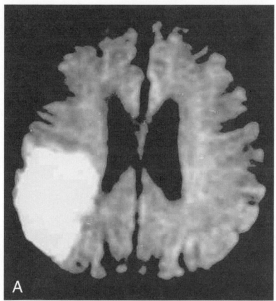

Figure 8–7. *A,* Single diffusion weighted image showing abnormal signal intensity within the right parietooccipital lobes in the posterior division of the middle cerebral artery. *B,* Associated MRA examination showing occlusion of the right distal M1 segment, with some faint opacification of the anterior division of the middle cerebral artery. The quality is somewhat degraded owing to patient motion.

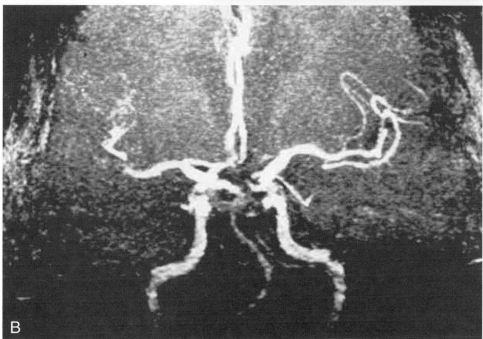

used (e.g., dynamic MR-DSA with contrast bolus) the flow dynamics of the AVM cannot be fully appreciated (Fig. 8–8).

(2) There is current work that includes combining 3-D DSA, MRA, and functional MRI to allow evaluation of eloquent regions of the brain and their relation to the nidus, which is important for preoperative management of these cases.

c. Intracranial stenoses

(1) With improving stent technology, more patients will be candidates for angioplasty and stenting.

(2) Present technology allows only the use of coronary stents [which are not presently Food and Drug Administration (FDA)-approved for intracranial use], which may not reach critical stenoses of the M1 segment.

d. Pulsatile tinnitus

(1) Paragangliomas

(2) Aberrant carotids

(3) Vessel tortuosity

(4) Jugular bulb variants

e. Other abnormalities

(1) Vasospasm

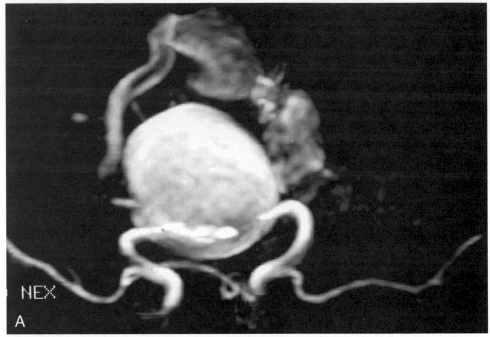

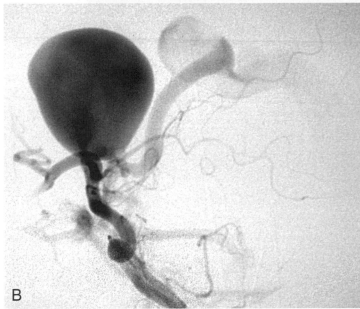

Figure 8–8. *A,* Three-dimensional time-of-flight MRA examination in a newborn, showing a large aneurysmal dilatation associated with an arteriovenous fistula, representing a variant of the vein of Galen fistula. *B,* Associated frontal projection of catheter digital subtraction angiography delineates the arteriovenous fistula with a large aneurysmal dilatation and slow opacification of the vein of Galen.

   (2) Moyamoya
   (3) Sturge-Weber syndrome
   (4) Carotid cavernous fistula

CEREBRAL ANGIOGRAPHY

Basic Principles

1. Angiography is an invasive procedure involving access to the arterial system, usually by a transfemoral route (Seldinger approach).
2. A catheter (usually 4.0F to 5.5F) is maneuvered under fluoroscopic guidance selectively and se-

quentially into the carotid and vertebral arteries. Ionic isoosmolar contrast is injected while filming.
3. Current technology routinely uses biplane DSA with a 1024 × 1024 matrix.
4. For aneurysms or stenoses, we also routinely use 3-D rotational angiography.

Indications

1. Cerebral aneurysms
2. Carotid and cerebral stenoses
3. AVMs
4. Vasculitis

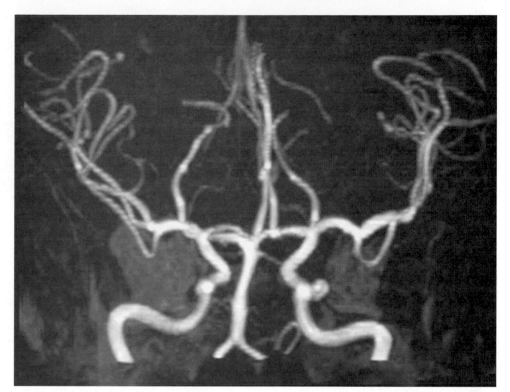

Figure 8–9. Single frontal view of a three-dimensional MRA examination of the circle of Willis showing a left carotid cave aneurysm projecting laterally.

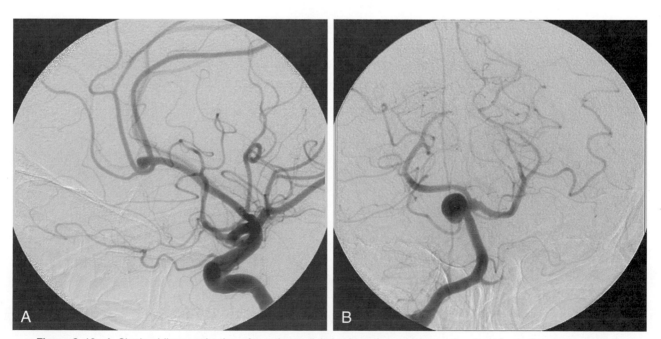

Figure 8–10. *A,* Single oblique projection of a catheter digital subtraction angiogram showing a pericallosal aneurysm. *B,* The patient also harbors a larger right superior cerebellar artery aneurysm, with origin of the right superior cerebellar artery from the aneurysm base.

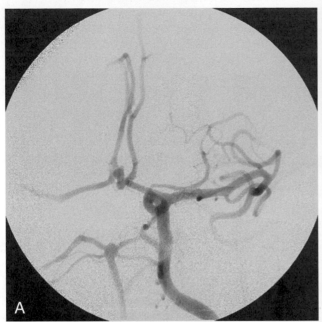

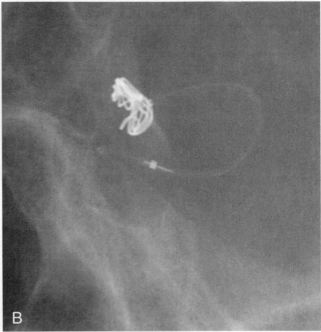

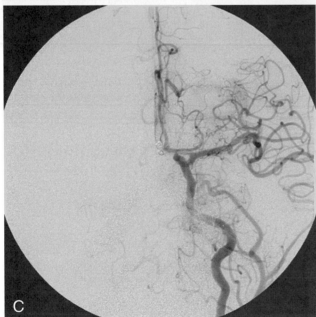

Figure 8–11. This case demonstrates the endovascular treatment of intracerebral aneurysms. *A,* Pretreatment frontal projection of a left internal carotid injection, identifying a bilobed anterior communicating artery aneurysm. *B,* Microcatheter is in place within the aneurysm fundus, delivering Guglielmi detachable coils. *C,* Posttreatment internal carotid examination, showing complete obliteration of the aneurysm with preservation of the anterior cerebral artery.

5. Tumors
6. AV fistulas
7. Vein of Galen malformations
8. Pulsatile tinnitus

Normal Findings

1. Catheter angiography (CA) is the most sensitive test for the detection and now endovascular treatment of cerebral aneurysms (Figs. 8–10, 8–11, 8–12).
2. The sensitivity and specificity are 100%.
3. Typical "four-vessel" cerebral angiography may

consist of both carotids and one vertebral artery (three-vessel) if there is sufficient reflux to see both posterior inferior cerebellar arteries.

Important Questions Answered by CA

1. Exact location of aneurysm and relation to surrounding vessels
2. Size of the dome
3. Size of the neck and relation to vessels
4. Fundus/neck ratio
5. Lobulation or site of rupture
6. Size

7. For carotid bifurcation examination, it is still the gold standard for evaluating the percent of stenosis, keeping in mind that other modalities (MRA, ultrasonography) may provide information about the wall architecture (Fig. 8–5).

8. CA is the only method that can examine the microarchitecture of AVMs, especially during preoperative embolization procedures where a microcatheter is situated in the nidus. Important aspects of AVM architecture can be detected.

a. "Training" aneurysms on vessels supplying the AVM

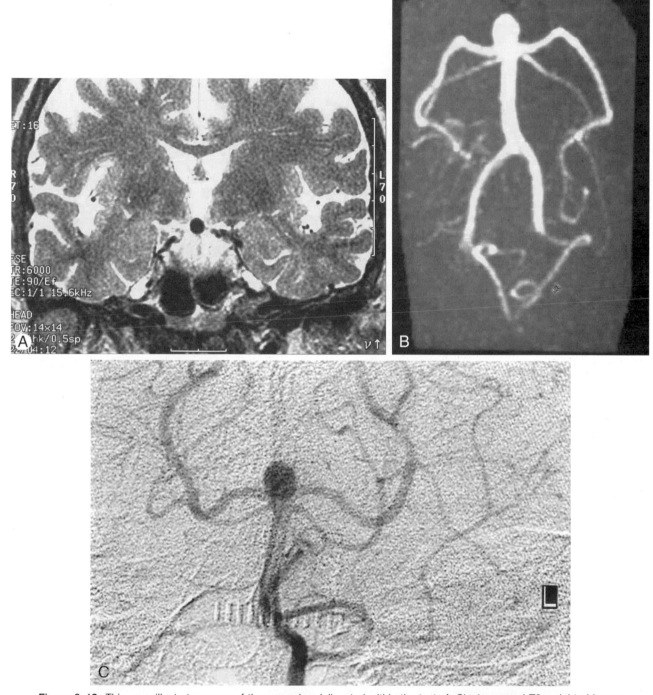

Figure 8–12. This case illustrates many of the examples delineated within the text. *A,* Single coronal T2-weighted image shows a flow void in the region of the basilar tip, suggestive of aneurysm. *B,* Three-dimensional time-of-flight MRA examination delineates the basilar tip aneurysm. *C,* Catheter angiography shows the basilar tip aneurysm and its relation to the origin of the posterior cerebral arteries.

Illustration continued on following page

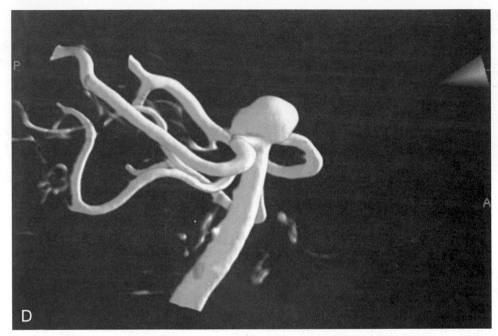

Figure 8–12. *Continued D,* Three-dimensional rotational angiographic representation best delineates the true size of the aneurysm, the architecture, the size of the neck, and its relation to the origin of the P1 segments.

b. Intranidal aneurysms

c. Venous aneurysms

d. Venous strictures

e. Intranidal fistulas

Complications

1. Hematoma
2. Damage to femoral or other vessels
3. Stroke
4. Dissection
5. Contrast reaction
6. Oversedation
7. Infection
8. Overall complication ratio is 1% to 2% with 0 to 5% persistent neurologic deficit.

THREE-DIMENSIONAL ROTATIONAL ANGIOGRAPHY

Principles

1. Probably the most exciting recent advance in imaging is the 3-D capability.
2. By combining an intra-arterial injection of contrast while the image intensifier moves in a 200° arc, images are obtained that can be computer-rendered using a standard maximum intensity projection technique to provide true 3-D images.

3. These images are displayed as surface images or typically volume-rendered images (Fig. 8–12D).

Indications

1. Aneurysms. 3-D angiography is the most sensitive technique for evaluating aneurysms. All information concerning the architecture, including the size and relation of the neck, the neck ratio, and the fundus size, can be evaluated while rotating the 3-D image in real time in any plane. True length measurements can be detected directly on the monitor. Using techniques for further subtraction of metal, 3-D angiography is extremely useful for posttreatment analyses following endovascular coil placement or surgical clipping.
2. Stereo angiography. With specialized viewing glasses that direct images sequentially to either eye while viewing images on a computer screen, true stereo imaging of the aneurysm is possible that allows a sense of depth.
3. AVMs. Combining the data from 3-D angiography, MRA, and functional MRI makes it possible to evaluate eloquent areas of movement and speech in relation to the AVM nidus for preendovascular and surgical/irradiation planning.
4. Carotid stenoses. In addition to the surface rendered images, a "fly through" technique allows one to pass through the lumen of the vessel as if floating or flying inside the lumen. This is particularly useful in patients who have undergone carotid stenting or postoperative endarterectomy.

Bibliography

Chung TS, Joo JY, Lee SK, et al.: Evaluation of cerebral aneurysms with high-resolution MR angiography using a section-interpolation technique: correlation with digital subtraction angiography. AJNR Am J Neuroradiol 20: 229–235, 1999.

Griffiths PD, Hoggard N, Warren DJ, et al.: Brain arteriovenous malformations: assessment with dynamic MR digital subtraction angiography. AJNR Am J Neuroradiol 21: 1892–1899, 2000.

Heiseman JE, Dean BL, Hodak JA, et al.: Neurological complications of cerebral angiography. AJNR Am J Neuroradiol 15:1401–1407, 1994.

Jager HR, Ellamushi H, Moore EA, et al.: Contrast-enhanced MR angiography of intracranial giant aneurysms. AJNR Am J Neuroradiol 21:1900–1907, 2000.

Kallmes DF, Omary RA, Dix JE, et al.: Specificity of MR angiography as a confirmatory test of carotid artery stenosis. AJNR Am J Neuroradiol 17:1501–1506, 1996.

Melhem ER, Caruthers SD, Faddoul SG, et al.: Use of three-dimensional MR angiography for tracking a contrast bolus in the carotid artery. AJNR Am J Neuroradiol 20:263–266, 1999.

9 Molecular Genetic Testing

Katie Plunkett
Tetsuo Ashizawa

Mutations

1. DNA testing has become available for many inherited neurologic disorders. There are different types of mutations.
   a. Point mutation: Substitution, deletion, or insertion of a single nucleotide
   b. Deletion/duplication/inversion: When a larger segment of DNA, several kilobytes (kb) is involved
   c. Aneuploidy or segmental aneuploidy: The entire chromosome or a part of chromosome may be duplicated.
   d. Tri-tetra.-, and pentanucleotide repeat: A group of degenerative neurologic disorders has been identified to be caused by a novel class of mutations involving expansions of short tandem repeat sequences.
2. Different techniques are used to detect different types of mutations. When ordering DNA testing, knowing the techniques behind the analysis is helpful for understanding their limitations and advantages.
3. Technology advances are expected to change the DNA tests, particularly with inventions of new high-throughput assays.
4. The most commonly used assays in DNA diagnostic testing today include polymerase chain reaction (PCR), Southern analysis, pulsed-field gel electrophoresis, and fluorescence in situ hybridization. These techniques can detect deletions, insertions, duplications, and amplifications of the sequences within the DNA fragment of interest.

Techniques/Tests

1. Polymerase chain reaction
   a. Polymerase chain reaction amplifies a DNA segment of interest defined by two PCR primer sequences, using a DNA polymerase.
   b. A short time (hours) and a small quantity (nanograms) of the DNA sample required for this assay make PCR the preferred test.
   c. The limitation of PCR is that the targeted DNA fragment must be relatively small (usually shorter than a few kb).
2. Southern analysis
   a. Southern analysis is a more complex and time-consuming technique that is useful in determining the size of larger specific DNA fragments in the 0.5 to 50 kb range.
   b. DNA samples undergo a restriction enzyme digest (for several hours), agarose gel electrophoresis (for several hours to overnight), and then a transfer from the gel to a membrane ("Southern blot"; for 4 hours to overnight), followed by crosslinking of the DNA to the membrane matrix by baking or an ultraviolet exposure.
   c. The DNA fragment of interest is distinguished from numerous other DNA fragments on the membrane by hybridization using a denatured radiolabeled DNA probe that shares a specific sequence with the target DNA fragment.
   d. After washing the blotted membrane to remove unbound probes, the DNA fragment of interest in the blot is detected by exposure of an x-ray film overlaid on the blot.
   e. The hybridization, washing, and autoradiographic procedures take several hours to several days.
3. Pulsed-field gel electrophoresis
   a. Pulsed-field gel electrophoresis (PFGE) allows for the separation of large DNA molecules, >50 kb.
   b. Instead of using one uniform electrical field, perpendicularly oriented alternate pulses of electric current are used to keep the DNA fragment moving in a straight line and migrating according to size within the gel.
   c. Once the PFGE is finished, Southern analysis and hybridization can be performed in the usual manner. Performing this technique requires practice and an experienced laboratory.
4. Fluorescence in situ hybridization
   a. Fluorescence in situ hybridization (FISH) involves the hybridization of a probe with specific DNA sequences in situ to cells.
   b. This testing has various uses including determination of aneuploidies in amniotic fluid and the direct determination of duplications and deletions of specific genes.
   c. Depending on the use, fluorescence-tagged DNA probes specific to the target chromosome or gene are hybridized to tissues or cells fixed, in most cases, to a microscope slide.

d. After post-hybridization washes, the hybridized sequences are detected under a fluorescence microscope.

e. FISH analysis usually takes from 6 hours to overnight.

Key Tests

- PCR: fast, simple, only for a short segment of DNA (<2 to 3 kb)

- Southern blot analysis: slow, complex, for a 0.5 to 50 kb segment

- PFGE: slow, complex, technically demanding, for a segment >50 kb

- FISH: fast, simple, for a large rearrangement of DNA

Indications

1. Guidelines for DNA testing have been developed for a limited number of disorders such as Huntington's disease and myotonic dystrophy type 1. However, specific guidelines are not available for the great majority of genetic neurologic disorders. The indications below provide guidance for these disorders.

   a. Confirmatory DNA testing

      (1) Most DNA testing is performed to confirm a clinical diagnosis of an inherited disorder, especially when there is a family history of the disease.

      (2) However, neurologists often order DNA testing as part of a work-up for broader differential diagnoses, even in sporadic cases.

      (3) Neurologic disorders for which DNA testing is commercially available are listed in Table 9–1.

      (4) When a specific genetic disorder is strongly suspected, genetic counseling may become an important consideration.

         (a) The results of genetic testing usually have serious medical, social, psychological, and legal implications for the patient and the family.

         (b) Geneticists and genetic counselors are professionals who are best trained to address these complicated issues.

   b. Presymptomatic testing

      (1) Many neurologic conditions do not present until adulthood, raising the question of presymptomatic and juvenile testing.

TABLE 9–1. NEUROLOGIC DISORDERS FOR WHICH DNA TESTING IS COMMERCIALLY AVAILABLE

Amyloidosis type 1
Amyotrophic lateral sclerosis
Ataxia telangiectasia
Early-onset familial Alzheimer's disease
Late-onset familial Alzheimer's disease
Becker muscular dystrophy
Charcot-Marie-Tooth type 1A
Charcot-Marie-Tooth type 1B
Charcot-Marie-Tooth type 1D
Charcot-Marie-Tooth type 2E
Charcot-Marie-Tooth type 4B
Charcot-Marie-Tooth type 4E
Charcot-Marie-Tooth type 4F
Charcot-Marie-Tooth type X
Congenital muscular dystrophy with merosin deficiency
Dentatorubral-Pallidoluysian atrophy
Duchenne muscular dystrophy
Early-onset primary dystonia
Emery-Dreifuss muscular dystrophy
Episodic ataxia type 1
Episodic ataxia type 2
Facioscapulohumeral muscular dystrophy
Familial dysautonomia
Friedreich's ataxia
Hereditary neuropathy with liability to pressure palsies
Huntington's disease
Myotonia congenita, dominant
Myotonia congenita, recessive
Myotonic dystrophy type 1
Myotonic dystrophy type 2
Oculopharyngeal muscular atrophy
Progressive dystonia with diurnal variation
Progressive myoclonus epilepsy type 1
Spinal and bulbar muscular atrophy
Spinal muscular atrophy
Spinocerebellar ataxia type 1
Spinocerebellar ataxia type 2
Spinocerebellar ataxia type 3
Spinocerebellar ataxia type 6
Spinocerebellar ataxia type 7
Spinocerebellar ataxia type 8
Spinocerebellar ataxia type 10
Spinocerebellar ataxia type 12
Spinocerebellar ataxia type 17
X-linked myotubular myopathy

      (2) For presymptomatic testing of progressive untreatable disorders, a multidisciplinary approach involving varied specialists is recommended.

         (a) Pretest education and counseling should be provided to ensure that the subject understands the natural history of the disease, the accuracy of the testing, and the predictive value of the testing.

         (b) Motivation for taking the test and readiness to receive a result should also be explored.

      (3) Issues of confidentiality should also be addressed prior to testing.

         (a) Individuals need to be informed of the possibility of discrimination in the workplace and in obtaining insurance if they test positive for the abnormal gene.

(b) Many people choose to pay for presymptomatic DNA testing with cash so that insurance companies will not be involved.

(4) Once informed consent has been obtained and the individual has had testing, the results should be provided in person.

(a) Follow-up counseling for both medical and psychological issues should be made available.

(b) The counseling is best provided by geneticists and genetic counselors.

(5) Keep in mind the limitations of DNA testing in predicting the age of onset and prognosis in presymptomatic individuals who are diagnosed as having an abnormal gene.

(6) In just about every DNA test currently available, including the tests for trinucleotide repeat expansions, such predictions are not recommended because there are significant determinants in addition to the mutant genotype itself that influence these clinical parameters.

(7) A clinical diagnosis can only be made by a clinician familiar with the symptoms; in other words, individuals do not have a disease until they show clinical signs. Stressing this point is important for social, legal, and psychological reasons.

c. DNA testing for juvenile subjects

(1) The presymptomatic testing of children and adolescents for adult-onset conditions has been cause for a great deal of discussion.

(2) If early or preventive treatment is available for the condition, as in familial adenomatous polyposis, testing is generally encouraged.

(3) For adult-onset disorders in which no treatment is available, such as Huntington's disease, testing asymptomatic children and adolescents is usually not done.

(4) The consensus stands at letting people decide for themselves, once they have reached the legal age of maturity in their country, whether or not they wish to pursue presymptomatic testing.

(5) For juvenile subjects in whom the clinical diagnosis of a specific disorder has been established, DNA testing can be done as a confirmatory test.

d. Prenatal DNA testing

(1) Prenatal testing is done by either chorionic villus sampling (CVS) or amniocentesis.

(2) For autosomal dominant disorders, most couples choosing this option already know that one of them has an abnormal gene for the adult-onset disorder from a clinical diagnosis or presymptomatic testing.

(3) In the autosomal recessive conditions, most couples will have had a previously affected child or know they are both carriers from prior DNA analysis.

(4) Because testing of minors is not recommended for the adult-onset disorders, prenatal diagnosis should not be performed unless the couple has indicated that they intend to terminate the pregnancy if the fetus has the affected allele.

(5) Without such an intention, the couple should be counseled that prenatal diagnosis for adult-onset disorders is not recommended.

e. Preimplantation genetic diagnosis

(1) A newer option for couples is preimplantation genetic diagnosis (PGD).

(a) In PGD, genetic testing is performed on the embryo prior to implanting in the uterus.

(b) In theory, only unaffected embryos would be put back into the uterus.

(2) This testing is currently being performed at a handful of centers in the United States.

(3) Problems include misdiagnosis and a decreased pregnancy rate.

(4) The cost of the testing is also a limiting factor because in vitro fertilization is required.

(5) For couples at risk for genetic disease who want children and do not believe in termination of pregnancy, PGD may be a real option.

Indications for Testing

• Confirmatory testing: Genetic counseling is recommended when a specific genetic disorder is strongly suspected.

• Presymptomatic testing: If it is for a progressive and nontreatable disease, extensive counseling is a must.

• Juvenile testing: For progressive and nontreatable conditions, presymptomatic juvenile testing should be avoided.

• Prenatal testing: Determination of parental geno-types is recommended. If abortion of a mutation-positive fetus is not planned, prenatal testing for adult-onset disorders should be avoided.

Finding a Laboratory

1. Commercial testing

   a. As genetic testing is made available for a growing number of diseases, finding a laboratory to do the test is becoming more complicated.

   b. An invaluable resource is GeneTests, a free online directory that includes a Medical Genetics Laboratory Directory, a Genetics Clinic Directory, and a Genetic Testing Resource.

   c. GeneTests is a free service supported by grants from the National Library of Medicine of the National Institutes of Health and the Maternal Child Health Bureau of the Health Resources and Services Administration.

   d. GeneTests can be accessed via the internet at *www.genetests.org*

2. Other DNA testing

   a. For uncommon conditions, finding a laboratory to do a DNA test may be more difficult.

   b. The first question is whether the gene for the particular condition has been discovered.

      (1) If the gene has been discovered but there is not a listing in GeneTests, geneticists and genetic counselors often know where to go or whom to ask to learn if testing is available.

      (2) Commercial laboratories shy away from testing for low volume conditions.

   c. Another option is to contact the researchers who discovered the gene. They may be willing to accept samples on a research basis. GeneTests also lists laboratories that are doing research for certain conditions.

   d. Before sending a sample, clarify whether the research results will be reported to the referring physician and family.

      (1) In some studies, the results are not for use in clinical situations and the results are not reported.

      (2) Ask for a copy of the laboratory's consent form, which should list the details of the study.

Key Tips for Finding a Laboratory

• GeneTests *(www.genetests.org)* is a useful public domain information site.

• Noncommercial tests may be done case by case at a research laboratory.

• The consent form should be carefully examined prior to sending samples.

Common Forms of Gene Mutations

1. Expanded trinucleotide and other short tandem repeat sequences

   a. Over the last decade, expanded trinucleotide repeats have been found to cause an increasing number of neurologic conditions.

   b. Except for Friedreich's ataxia whose mutation is an expansion of GAA repeats, most other diseases caused by trinucleotide repeat expansion involve CAG/CTG repeats or CCG/CGG repeats (Table 9–2).

   c. In normal individuals these repeats vary in number (i.e., repeat length polymorphism); however, once the repeat size goes over a certain number, the disease is expressed.

   d. The extent of repeat expansion that is required to cause a disease phenotype varies from disease to disease.

   e. In some conditions, a pre-mutation range exists and individuals with a specific number of trinucleotide repeats will not develop symptoms of the disease but may have children who have the disease (Table 9–2).

   f. Expansions at the lower end of the disease range may be associated with reduced penetrance in some diseases such as Huntington's disease.

   g. Besides trinucleotide repeat disorders, myotonic dystrophy type 2 (DM2), spinocerebellar ataxia type 10 (SCA10) and progressive myoclonus epilepsy type 1 (EPM1, also known as myclonic epilepsy of Unverricht and Lundborg) are caused by tetranucleotide, pentanucleotide and dodecanucleotide repeat expansions, respectively.

   h. Depending on the size of the trinucleotide repeat, either PCR or Southern analysis is used by laboratories to determine the number of repeats in a particular condition.

TABLE 9–2. COMMON FORMS OF GENE MUTATIONS

Disease	Repeat Sequence	Normal Range	Premutation Range	Disease Range	Main Clinical Features	Pattern of Inheritance
HD	CAG	26 and less	27–35	36 and greater	Chorea, psychological/psychiatric problems, dementia	Autosomal dominant
SCA1	CAG	39 and less, 40–44 if interrupted by 1 or 2 CAT repeats		39 and greater	Ataxia, pyramidal and extrapyramidal features	Autosomal dominant
SCA2	CAG	31 and less	32–35	36 and greater	Ataxia, slow saccade, areflexia	Autosomal dominant
SCA3/MJD	CAG	40 and less		55 and greater	Ataxia, protruded eyes, facial fasciculations	Autosomal dominant
SCA6	CAG	20 and less		21 and greater	Relatively pure ataxia	Autosomal dominant
SCA7	CAG	19 and less	28–35	37 and greater	Ataxia, macular dystrophy	Autosomal dominant
SCA8*	CTG	91 and less		100 and greater	Ataxia, nystagmus, diminished vibration perception	Autosomal dominant
SCA10	ATTCT	22 and less		800 and greater	cerebellar ataxia and seizures	Autosomal dominant
SCA12	CAG	28 and less		55 and greater	Ataxia, hyperreflexia, dementia, upper extremity tremors	Autosomal dominant
SCA 17	CAG	44 and less		50 and greater	Ataxia, dystonia	Autosomal dominant
DRPLA	CAG	35 and less		49 and greater	Progressive myoclonus, seizures, ataxia, dementia	Autosomal dominant
SBMA	CAG	34 and less		36 and greater	Proximal muscle weakness and atrophy, fasciculations, androgen insensitivity	X-linked recessive
DM	CTG	37 and less	40–49	50 and greater	Myotonia, weakness, multisystem abnormalities	Autosomal dominant
EPM1	D(C4gC4GCG).d(CGCG4CG4)	3 and less		40 and greater	Myoclonus, seizures, cerebellar ataxia	Autosomal recessive
FRDA	GAA	27 and less, 28–36—must be interrupted by (GAGGAA) to remain stable	28–36 uninterrupted GAA repeats leads to unstable alleles	66 and greater	Ataxia, dysarthria, pyramidal signs, sensory loss, cardiomyopathy, diabetes	Autosomal recessive
FRAX	CGG	5-43 44-54 – most stable but can expand in some instances	55-199	200 and greater	Mental retardation, dysmorphic features	X-linked recessive
DM2	CCTG	74 or less		75 and greater	Myotonia, weakness, multisystem abnormalities	Autosomal dominant

Abbreviations: HD = Huntington's disease; SCA = spinocerebellar ataxia; MJD = Machado-Joseph disease; DRPLA = Dentatorubral-Pallidoluysian atrophy; SBMA = Spinal and bulbar muscular atrophy; DM = Myotonic dystrophy type 1; EPM1 = progressive myoclonic epilepsy type 1; FRDA = Friedreich's ataxia; FRAX = Fragile X syndrome; DM2 = Myotonic dystrophy type 2.
*Expanded SCA8 CTG repeats have been reported in some individuals with neither clinical evidence of ataxia nor family history of ataxia, raising a question regarding the specificity of the test.

i. The larger the expansion, the less likely PCR will be able to pick it up.

j. Many DNA laboratories group the DNA tests into a panel for a group of related disorders, such as the spinocerebellar ataxias, so that the patient is screened for all of the types at once.

2. Deletions and duplications

a. Charcot-Marie-Tooth type 1A (CMT1A)

(1) Most cases of CMT1A (>98%) are due to a duplication in the *PMP22* gene.

(2) Two methods, PFGE and FISH, are reliable in detecting this duplication.

(3) A deletion of the same region of *PMP22* duplicated in CMT1A causes the condition hereditary neuropathy with liability to pressure palsies in 70% to 80% of families diagnosed with the condition.

b. Spinal muscular atrophy (SMA)

(1) SMA is a group of clinically heterogeneous neuromuscular disorders characterized by degeneration of the anterior horn cells in the spinal cord.

(2) Studies have documented that approximately 90% to 95% of patients with the different forms of childhood-onset SMA are homozygously deleted for the survival motor neuron (SMN^T) gene.

c. Duchenne and Becker muscular dystrophy (DMD and BMD)

(1) DMD and BMD are caused by mutations in the same gene, *DMD,* coding for dystrophin.

(2) Various studies have shown that 60% to 65% of individuals with DMD/BMD have a deletion in the gene and approximately 6% have a duplication.

(3) In males, mutation analysis for DMD/BMD is typically performed in two steps: a multiplex PCR analysis and Southern analysis.

(a) The multiplex PCR analysis takes advantage of the location of the deletions and duplications clustering within two regions of the gene; simultaneous PCR amplification of the two regions detects up to 98% of deletions.

(b) If a deletion is detected and the beginning and end points are clear from the multiplex PCR, Southern analysis is not necessary.

(c) However, if the beginning or end points cannot be determined or the multiplex analysis is normal, Southern analysis must be performed. Southern analysis for DMD/BMD is a labor-intensive process using cDNA (complementary DNA) probes that cover the entire gene.

(4) The genetic testing is complemented by immunohistologic studies of muscle biopsy specimens for dystrophin.

3. Single nucleotide alterations (point mutations)

a. Many gene mutations are caused by a single change in one nucleotide that causes a nonfunctioning gene or a gene of aberrant functions.

b. Whether or not testing is available for point mutations varies from gene to gene. For example, the 30% to 40% of men with DMD/BMD who do not have a deletion or duplication are believed to have point mutations in the gene. Testing for point mutations is now available and they are found in approximately 75% of individuals who were not found to have a large deletion.

c. DNA analysis for two other forms of CMT, CMT1B and CMTX, is currently performed by sequencing the genes and searching for point mutations.

Conclusion

1. The list of DNA tests is expected to grow longer as novel mutations are discovered for inherited neurologic disorders.

2. New high-throughput technologies, such as DNA chip arrays and denaturing high-performance liquid chromatography, may allow for routine analyses of a wide variety of mutations including point mutations.

3. Completion of the Human Genome Project provides an enormous amount of new information useful for neurologic diagnosis.

a. For example, single nucleotide polymorphisms (SNPs) may be useful for assessing the susceptibility for many neurologic disorders. The *ApoE* alleles in Alzheimer's disease are a prelude to such applications.

b. Although the usefulness of the *ApoE* alleles in risk assessment for Alzheimer's disease is limited, analyses of compound alleles of several susceptibility loci may provide better predictive values, and a similar approach may be applicable to many other neurologic disorders.

4. Thus, we should anticipate the increasing importance and complexity of DNA testing in neurologic practice.

Bibliography

The American College of Medical Genetics/American Society of Human Genetics Huntington Disease Genetic Testing Working Group: ACMG/ASHG statement. Laboratory guidelines for Huntington disease genetic testing. Am J Hum Genet 62:1243–1247, 1998.

The International Myotonic Dystrophy Consortium (IDMC): New nomenclature and DNA testing guidelines for myotonic dystrophy type 1 (DM1). Neurology 54:1218–1221, 2000.

Tan E, Ashizawa T: Genetic testing in spinocerebellar ataxias: defining a clinical role. Arch Neurol 58:191-195, 2001.

10 Neuropsychological Testing

Ola A. Selnes

Basic Principles and Techniques

1. Cognitive deficits are manifestations of brain dysfunction that cannot be observed directly, but rather are inferred from behavioral changes.

2. Neuropsychological testing is among the most sensitive and reliable methods for quantifying such changes.

3. The testing typically includes assessment of the principal domains of cognition, including attention, language, memory, and visuospatial, executive, and motor functions.

4. It differs from *psychological* testing in that the focus is on specific cognitive functions, rather than on personality, mood, or anxiety.

5. It differs from *mental status* and intelligence testing in that neuropsychological testing provides detailed information about the specific *nature* of the cognitive impairment, rather than a summary number or index of *degree* of impairment.

6. As with other diagnostic tests, the results of neuropsychological tests should be interpreted in the context of the patient's history and other clinical and laboratory information.

7. There are two major approaches to neuropsychological testing.

   a. One method relies on a fixed battery of tests, regardless of the question to be answered by the testing. Examples of this type of neuropsychological testing include the Halstead-Reitan neuropsychological test battery and the Luria-Nebraska neuropsychological test battery.

   b. The second, and more commonly used approach is to select individual tests appropriate for the referral question, the patient's premorbid level of functioning, and the degree of cognitive impairment.

   c. In practice, many neuropsychologists combine the two approaches and use a core battery of tests that is always administered, supplemented by individual tests specifically targeting the patient's cognitive symptoms and the referral question.

8. A number of neuropsychological tests are now available for computerized administration.

   a. These are appropriate, particularly for detection of mild impairments of attention and psychomotor speed in high-functioning individuals.

   b. Computerized testing is generally reliable and repeatable and can therefore be used to measure subtle fluctuations in cognitive performance, such as those associated with side-effects of drugs.

9. The cognitive domains typically assessed during a clinical neuropsychological exam and their associated tests are listed in Table 10–1.

10. Test batteries such as the Wechsler scales (Wechsler Adult Intelligence Scale and the Wechsler Memory Scale) were formerly administered in their entirety and were the core of a neuropsychological evaluation.

    a. For the revised versions of these batteries, the total administration time can be close to 3 hours, however, making it impractical to give the entire batteries.

    b. Instead, only certain subtests from these batteries are now typically included.

TABLE 10–1. STANDARDIZED TESTS COMMONLY USED FOR ASSESSMENT OF THE PRINCIPAL DOMAINS OF COGNITION

COGNITIVE DOMAIN	NEUROPSYCHOLOGICAL TEST
Attention	Digit Span
	Spatial (pointing) Span
	Reaction Time
	Paced Auditory Serial Addition Test (PASAT)
Language	Boston Naming Test
	Token Test
	Boston Diagnostic Aphasia Exam
Memory	Rey Auditory Verbal Learning Test
	Recognition Memory Test
	Rey 15-item Memory Test
Visuospatial	Rey Complex Figure Copy
	Block Design (WAIS-III)
	Hooper Visual Organization Test
Executive functions	Wisconsin Card Sorting Test
	Stroop Test
	Shipley-Hartford Abstraction
	Verbal Fluency
Psychomotor speed	Grooved Pegboard
	Symbol Digit Substitution
	Trail Making Test A & B
General intellectual abilities	Shipley Hartford
	Raven's Standard Progressive Matrices
	New Adult Reading Test

11. Like other diagnostic tests in neurology, such as electroencephalogram (EEG) and magnetic resonance imaging (MRI), neuropsychological tests are typically administered by a trained technician, whereas the results of the tests are interpreted by a person with specific training and experience in clinical neuropsychology.

Indications

1. Neuropsychological testing is indicated for detection of cognitive impairment in a variety of disorders with known or suspected central nervous system involvement.

2. Dementia

    a. Because neuropsychological tests can measure subtle cognitive impairments, they are particularly useful for *early* diagnosis of primary degenerative dementias such as Alzheimer's disease.

    b. Careful evaluation of the pattern of cognitive impairment revealed by the neuropsychological testing can be useful to differentiate between Alzheimer's disease and so-called focal dementias, such as primary progressive aphasia, frontal lobe dementia, and posterior cortical degeneration.

    c. A pattern of significant psychomotor slowing but preserved cortical function, is typical for conditions with subcortical involvement and can thus contribute to the early diagnosis of subcortical dementias such as normal pressure hydrocephalus, HIV-related dementia, and progressive supranuclear palsy.

    d. The term *mild neurocognitive disorder* (DSM-IV diagnostic code 294.9) has been proposed to describe mild cognitive deficits that are not necessarily progressive.

        (1) Certain autoimmune disorders (Sjögren's disease, systemic lupus erythematosus), infections (Lyme disease), trauma (closed-head injury), metabolic disorders (vitamin B_{12} deficiency, thyroid disease), and hypoxia (sleep apnea, chronic obstructive pulmonary disease) can be associated with mild cognitive impairment.

        (2) The severity of the cognitive symptoms may correlate with the severity of the underlying disease and often involves attentional changes rather than primary memory disturbance.

3. Neuropsychological testing is increasingly used to establish a baseline for measuring functional recovery.

    a. After closed-head injury, stroke, and other neurologic injuries.

    b. For some patients undergoing surgical therapies, such as corticectomies, aneurysm clippings, and pallidotomies, baseline cognitive assessment is also becoming a standard of care.

    c. Neuropsychological testing can also aid in establishing cognitive side effects associated with new drug therapies.

4. Forensic evaluations to assess whether impairment is present in tort proceedings (after head injury, toxin exposure, hypoxic/hypotensive insults), disability claims, and competency issues.

Key Indications

- Diagnosis of cognitive disorders
- Baseline assessment
- Forensic evaluations

Contraindications

1. Severe medical illness or delirium may make formal neuropsychological testing impossible. Otherwise, there are very few specific contraindications.

2. Like other tests, such as MRI and EEG, a basic level of cooperation is required, however. A very low level of education, a non-native language background, and severe visual and or hearing deficits can make certain neuropsychological test results difficult to interpret.

Normal Findings

1. The evaluation of neuropsychological test findings is made with reference to normative data sets that should be adjusted for both age and education.

    a. Experienced neuropsychologists will also rely on qualitative features of a patient's test performance for their interpretation.

    b. Such qualitative features are important for evaluating the validity of a patient's neuropsychological test profile.

    c. If there is a high index of suspicion for suboptimal effort or deliberate poor performance, more formal measures of malingering may be required.

2. A neuropsychological test profile that is within normal limits for the patient's age and education does not necessarily rule out an underlying problem.

a. Mild frontal lobe or executive type deficits can be quite difficult to detect using standardized tests, particularly in more educated patients.

b. Contrary to traditional teaching, however, patients with above average intelligence do not necessarily have above average memory performance.

c. Significant discrepancies between Verbal and Performance IQ scores on the Wechsler scales can occur in neurologically normal individuals, and therefore should not, by themselves, be taken as direct evidence for impaired functioning.

Abnormal Findings

1. Abnormalities of possible clinical significance are established by reference to external norms *and* internal consistencies of the neuropsychological testing profile.

2. Like other laboratory tests, such as serum vitamin B_{12} or 20–20 visual acuity, the standards for what constitutes "normal" cognitive performance are somewhat arbitrary.

3. Clinical judgment and experience is therefore required to relate neuropsychological test findings to clinical observations and other laboratory findings.

4. In general, abnormalities on a single test should be interpreted with caution.

   a. Abnormalities on several tests relevant to one or more cognitive domains provide convergent evidence of possible clinical significance.

   b. Patterns of abnormalities within a single cognitive domain, such as memory, can also carry diagnostic implications. For example, subcortical disease is often associated with deficits of immediate memory as well as spontaneous retrieval of information, while recognition memory is either mildly impaired or normal.

5. Thus, the overall pattern of preserved versus impaired performance carries more information than individual test abnormalities.

   a. Very mild cognitive impairment cannot always be reliably detected by a single, cross-sectional assessment.

   b. If the mild impairment is secondary to progressive disease, longitudinal follow-up can usually establish decline in performance.

Complications

Other than occasional boredom and frustration, neuropsychological testing is a safe procedure with no known adverse effects.

Bibliography

American Academy of Neurology: Neuropsychological testing of adults. Considerations for neurologists. Report of the Therapeutics and Technology Assessment Subcommittee of the American Academy of Neurology. Neurology 47:592–596, 1996.

Dodrill CB: Myths of neuropsychology. Clin Neuropsychologist 11:1–17, 1997.

Lezak M: Neuropsychological Assessment, 3rd ed. New York, Oxford University Press, 1995.

Mitrushina M, Boone K, D'Elia L: Handbook of Normative Data for Neuropsychological Assessment. New York, Oxford University Press, 1999.

1 Localization in Neurovascular Disease

Marc Fisher
Erdem Orberk
Muhammad Ramzan

The clinical examination with neurovascular syndromes uses the principles of lateralization and localization adapted from general neurology. For example, crossed findings consisting of contralateral long tract signs and ipsilateral cranial nerve deficits point to the brainstem. Of additional help, however, is the non-congruence of anatomical organization in vascular distributions, which leads to specific neurovascular syndromes. The posterior cerebral artery for example, supplies upper brainstem as well as thalamus and occipital lobe.

Localization of neurovascular lesions is relevant for treatment as well as for prognosis. Because time is crucial in neurovascular diseases (most urgent in ischemic strokes but also important in subarachnoid hemorrhage and, to a lesser degree, in intracerebral hemorrhage), familiarity with the major neurovascular syndromes is important. Otherwise valuable time may be lost.

1. Large vessel syndromes: The blood supply of the brain is generally divided into two territories.

   a. The anterior circulation consists of the internal carotid artery (ICA) and its branches. The main branches are the anterior cerebral artery (ACA) and the middle cerebral artery (MCA), the largest cerebral artery.

      (1) A typical ACA syndrome consists of contralateral hemiparesis and/or hemihypesthesia that affect the leg more than the arm or face, combined with incontinence or personality changes. In patients where the ACA of both sides is fed by one ICA, occlusion of the ACA ipsilateral to the feeding ICA can result in paraparesis and abulia.

      (2) The MCA syndrome consists of contralateral hemiparesis and/or hemihypesthesia affecting the face and arm more than the leg. Cortical functions such as graphesthesia and stereognosis may be the sole deficit. Higher cortical function loss depends on the side of the brain: Left MCA syndromes can include aphasia (disorders of language, in contrast to dysarthria, disorders of articulation) and apraxia (disorders of execution of movements beyond paresis, sensory loss, aphasia, or incoordination), when the left hemisphere is dominant. The dominant hemisphere is defined as the side subserving language and is the left side in almost all right-handed patients and in most left-handed individuals as well. With involvement of the right MCA, hemi-inattention is often found. Hemi-inattention can be divided into *neglect*, best tested by simultaneous bilateral stimulation, and *extinction*, defined as lack of responsivity to stimuli on one side of the body in the absence of sensory or motor deficit severe enough to account for the interception. Another common finding with non-dominant MCA stroke is anosognosia (unawareness of illness). Less often, constructional apraxia and disorders of spatial localization (loss of topographic memory leading to an inability of the patient to orientate himself or herself in familiar environments), dysarthria, dyscalculation, or confabulation occur. MCA syndromes on both sides usually also include homonymous contralateral visual field defects, either as quadrant anopsia or hemianopsia, depending on the size of the lesion. Furthermore with large MCA infarcts, a gaze preference toward the side of the infarct, away from the paretic/hypesthetic side, occurs, in extreme cases with a forced deviation of eyes and head and inability to move past the midline.

      (3) Smaller arteries coming off the ICA proximal to the two main branches are the inferior hypophyseal artery, supplying the hypophysis; the ophthalmic artery, supplying the eye; the posterior communicating artery, supplying anterior and medial parts of the thalamus; and the anterior choroidal artery, supplying the hippocampus, part of the basal ganglia, and the internal capsule.

   b. The posterior circulation consists of both vertebral arteries (VA), whose main branch is the posterior inferior cerebellar artery (PICA).

      (1) Either VA or PICA infarct can lead to the most frequent brainstem syndrome, the dorsolateral medulla oblongata syndrome, also known as the Wallenberg syndrome.

      (2) Distal to the PICA both VA form the

basilar artery (BA). Several small branches from the BA supply the brainstem, the largest arteries being the anterior inferior cerebellar artery and the superior cerebellar artery (SCA). BA syndromes can include varying degrees of mid- or upper brainstem deficits, depending upon which of its branches is affected and on the degree of collateral flow.

(3) Typical brainstem symptoms include the six Ds: diplopia, dizziness, dysarthria, dysphagia, dysmetria-dyssynergia with involvement of cerebellar pathways. Classically, contralateral to the brainstem deficits, somatic findings such as long tract signs (sensory or motor) can be found. If the long tracts are involved bilaterally, quadriparesis can evolve. With lower and middle brainstem function loss, the result can be a locked-in syndrome.

(4) A red flag for BA syndromes is impairment of the degree of consciousness, which can include coma.

(5) Further distally, the BA separates into its main branches, the posterior cerebral arteries (PCA). The PCA supply the occipital lobes, parts of the thalamus, and to varying degrees the middle temporal lobes. Typically, PCA syndromes include hemianopia or quadrantanopia in incomplete cases, sometimes with sparing of central vision because of perfusion of the corresponding cortex by MCA collaterals. Occasionally hemihypesthesia or hemiparesis can occur with involvement of the thalamus or the internal capsule.

Key Brainstem Symptoms

"Six D's"

- Diplopia
- Dizziness
- Dysarthria
- Dysphagia
- Dysmetria-dyssynergia with involvement of cerebellar pathways

2. Small vessel syndromes: Lead to smaller infarcts called *lacunes*. They typically do not affect the visual pathways except with lacunes in the territory of the anterior choriodal artery. Hence there is no clinically significant hemianopia or quadrantanopia. Gaze preference is not part of lacunar syndromes. With lacunes affecting the brainstem, crossed findings are rare. Depressed level of consciousness is NOT associated with brainstem lacunes. Patients with lacunar syndromes may have a stuttering course and generally have had fewer previous TIAs. They usually have a good spontaneous prognosis. Sites of the lacunar syndromes include

a. Pure motor hemiparesis (the most common) with a lesion in the posterior limb of the internal capsule, corona radiata, pons, or medulla

b. Pure sensory stroke: Mostly in the ventral posterior thalamus or thalamocortical projections.

c. Sensorimotor syndrome: Thalamus

d. Ataxic hemiparesis: Pons, arguably also the internal capsule.

e. Dysarthria-clumsy hand syndrome: Anterior limb of the internal capsule, rarely the basis pontis.

f. Dystonia and hemiballismus/hemichorea: Basal ganglia, mostly head of caudate nucleus, thalamus, and subthalamus.

3. Hemodynamic infarcts: In contrast to large-vessel and small-vessel infarcts, hemodynamic infarcts occur not because of embolization in the vessel supplying the infarct site but because of more proximal stenosis or occlusion with secondary perfusion failure. They affect the border zones between end vessels. A typical clinical picture is the man-in-the-barrel syndrome [1], which presents like a man standing with a barrel covering his trunk. The proximal limb movements are much more impaired than the distal ones.

4. Dissections: Infarcts secondary to dissections of the ICA can be misleading. Hemodynamic infarcts, as well as embolic large vessel infarcts on the side of the dissection, will have contralateral deficits (hemiparesis/paresthesia/anopia) combined with an ipsilateral Horner's syndrome, which is usually a sign of posterior circulation impairment in the Wallenberg syndrome. The distinction of central Horner's or Wallenberg's syndrome from the peripheral Horner's of ICA-dissection can be made by pharmacological tests. Furthermore ICA dissections can also show ipsilateral lower brainstem cranial nerve deficits, which may mimic, together with contralateral long tract deficits, the pattern of crossed findings typical of brainstem stroke.

PEARLS

Horner syndrome: Always ipsilateral to lesion

Bilateral homonymous hemianopia (BHL): Bilateral occipital infarcts

Sensori or motor hemi-syndromes with homonymous hemianopia: Almost always large-vessel disease

Crossed findings: Brainstem diplopia, dizziness, dysarthria, dysphagia, dysmetria-dyssynergia: often brainstem.

Impairment of the level of consciousness: Posterior circulation event until proven otherwise

Bibliography

Benito-Leon J, Munoz A, Ruiz J, Gomez-Fuentes JR: 'Man-in-the-barrel' syndrome: MRI and SPECT imaging. Eur J Radiol 24: 260–262, 1977.

Hess DC, Sethi KD, Nichols FT: Carotid dissection: A new false localising sign. J Neurol Neurosurg Psychiatry 53: 804–805, 1990.

Schievink WI: Spontaneous dissection of the carotid and vertebral arteries. N Engl J Med 344: 898–906, 2001.

Silverman IE, Liu GT, Volpe NJ, Galetta SL: The crossed paralyses. The original brainstem syndromes of Millard-Gubler, Foville, Weber, and Raymond-Cestan. Arch Neurol 52: 635–638, 1995.

Marc Fisher
Erdem Orberk
Muhammad Ramzan

2 Transient Ischemic Attacks

Definition

1. Transient ischemic attacks (TIAs) are defined as focal neurologic symptoms of an ischemic origin lasting less than 24 hours.

2. They are sudden in onset, and the typical duration is 5 to 30 minutes. TIAs lasting longer than 1 hour are usually embolic in nature.

3. The frequency varies from one to several in a day.

4. It is estimated that about 50,000 Americans suffer from TIAs every year, and one third of these culminate in stroke. Two thirds of those affected are men.

5. TIAs are an important harbinger of stroke and allow physicians the possibility to intervene before a stroke occurs.

6. Focal neurologic deficits may be caused by many other neurologic conditions (e.g., focal seizures, complicated migraine, syncope, neoplasm, subdural hemorrhage, hypoglycemia or hyperglycemia); it is imperative to diagnose TIAs correctly.

7. The risk of stroke is approximately 4% to 8% in the first month after a TIA, and it is recommended that each patient with a TIA be completely evaluated.

8. Crescendo TIAs are characterized by episodes that are uniform and multiple, with increasing duration and severity. They are a true medical emergency and signify impending vascular occlusion.

9. TIAs may originate from either the carotid system or the vertebrobasilar system. In general 90% of TIAs are related to carotid circulation; 7%, to vertebrobasilar circulation; and 3%, to both.

Clinical Features

1. Symptoms depend on the artery involved and the territory affected. Thus, they can be described as involving either the anterior circulation or the posterior circulation.

1. Anterior circulation
   a. TIAs in the anterior circulation may affect either the eye or the brain.
   b. Transient monocular blindness (amaurosis fugax): This is secondary to ischemia of the central retinal artery, a branch of the ophthalmic artery, which in turn is a branch of the internal carotid artery.
      (1) It lasts from seconds to minutes and usually is characterized by blurring or foggy vision.
      (2) The patient may describe it as a shade or a curtain falling along the line of sight.
      (3) The embolic particles such as cholesterol crystals (Hollenhorst plaques) can be seen in retinal artery branches on ophthalmoscopy. These are more stereotypic than hemispheric TIAs and usually have a benign course.
   c. Transient hemispheric attacks: The symptoms include aphasia, contralateral motor or sensory deficits, hemineglect, homonymous hemianopia, irregular arm shaking (limb shaking TIAs), and confusion.
   d. Lacunar TIAs: These are due to the involvement of penetrating lenticulostriate arteries. Stuttering lacunes with intermittent episodes may in fact be a TIA. One such phenomenon was described as the "capsular warning syndrome," in which there are escalating episodes of weakness in face, arm, and leg, culminating in a lacunar infarction involving the internal capsule.

Key Signs: Anterior Circulation TIAs

Transient Mononuclear Blindness

- Lasts from seconds to minutes

- Blurred or foggy vision

- "A shade or a curtain falling along the line of sight"

- Embolic particles, such as cholesterol crystals (Hollenhorst plaques), in retinal artery branches

Transient Hemispheric Attacks

- Aphasia, contralateral motor or sensory deficits, hemineglect, homonymous hemianopia, irregular arm shaking (limb-shaking TIAs), and confusion

Lacunar TIAs

- "Capsular warning syndrome": escalating episodes of weakness in face, arm, and leg

2. Posterior circulation

 a. TIAs of the posterior circulation may be more likely to result in stroke than anterior circulation TIAs.

 b. They are usually prolonged and less stereotyped.

 c. Homonymous hemianopia and hand and arm paresthesias may suggest stenosis of the posterior cerebral artery.

 d. Other features of posterior circulation involvement include vertigo, cranial nerve abnormalities—e.g., dysarthria, dysphagia, hearing deficits, pupillary change, ptosis, tunnel vision, and unsteadiness.

 e. Headache is not a common feature, and isolated episodes of loss of consciousness, diplopia, vertigo, wooziness, and light-headedness are rarely attributable to TIAs.

Key Signs: Posterior Circulation TIAs

- Homonymous hemianopia
- Hand and arm paresthesias
- Vertigo
- Cranial nerve abnormalities (e.g., dysarthria, dysphagia, hearing deficits, pupillary change, ptosis, tunnel vision, and unsteadiness)

Etiology/Mechanism

1. The most common cause of TIAs is atherothrombotic disease with ulceration and stenosis of extracranial vessels. These TIAs are usually brief in nature.

2. The next most common etiology is embolic, in which a blood clot can be either from an ulcerated aortic plaque (artery to artery) or proximally from the heart. These emboli are composed of fibrin and platelet-rich material. Embolic TIAs are generally of a longer duration (more than 1 hour).

3. Other postulated mechanisms are lacunar events (small penetrating arteries), hypotension (more common in the vertebrobasilar distribution), cardiac arrhythmias, vasospasm, vasculitis, hyperviscosity syndromes (macroglobulinemia, polycythemia), hematologic abnormalities (clotting disorders, sickle cell disease, thrombocytosis), and

metabolic abnormalities (hypoglycemia or hyperglycemia).

Diagnosis/Evaluation

1. The history is the most important part of the evaluation, because the neurologic examination is often normal. Unfortunately, the symptoms may be vague and the patient may not be able to provide details, especially if the nondominant hemisphere is involved.

2. Physical examination in some case may be helpful, for example by revealing emboli in the retinal vessels on funduscopic examination, a cervical (carotid stenosis) or supraclavicular (subclavian steal) bruit and cardiac murmur or arrhythmias on auscultation, a discrepancy in blood pressure when measured in both arms (subclavian steal), or an irregular pulse (atrial fibrillation).

3. Laboratory investigations

 a. Initial evaluation includes routine blood tests—i.e., complete blood count, blood chemistry, coagulation studies, erythrocyte sedimentation rate, lipid profile, syphilis serology—and electrocardiogram, chest x-ray, and carotid ultrasound.

 b. Neuroimaging studies may include head computerized tomography (CT), magnetic resonance imaging (MRI) of the brain, and magnetic resonance angiography. Sometimes small infarcts may clinically manifest as TIAs and be visible on CT or MRI. In addition, imaging may help to exclude causes like tumors, vascular malformations, and subdural hematoma.

 c. Further work-up in selected cases may require echocardiography, either by the transthoracic or the transesophageal method, Holter monitoring, screening for hypercoagulable state, cerebrospinal fluid examination, or even a conventional angiogram.

Differential Diagnosis

1. The differential diagnosis of TIAs includes focal seizures, complicated migraine, syncope, drop attacks, transient global amnesia, metabolic abnormalities such as hypoglycemia or hyperglycemia, tumors, subdural hemorrhage, primary eye or ear disease, and conversion disorder or malingering.

2. Marching of symptoms (i.e., different parts of body are affected in succession) may indicate an epileptic or migrainous etiology.

3. Positive symptoms like flashing lights, scintillation, seeing colors, and strong family history are more suggestive of migraine

Treatment / Management

The goal of therapy is to prevent the occurrence of stroke. This can be accomplished to a reasonable extent by adopting the following measures:

1. Risk factor modification: Control of blood pressure, cessation of smoking, use of statins as lipid-lowering agents, and exercise are established factors to reduce the risk of stroke.

2. Antiplatelet agents

   a. Aspirin (acetylsalicylic acid-ASA) acts by inhibiting the enzyme cyclooxegenase, resulting in decreased production of thromboxane A_2, a potent inducer of platelet aggregation. The effect is immediate, irreversible, and lasts for the life of platelets—i.e., 7 to 10 days.

      (1) The current recommended dose range is 50–325 mg, and current evidence suggests relatively similar benefits throughout this range.

      (2) Side effects include epigastric pain, erosive gastritis, ulcers, and gastrointestinal bleeding and are more common with increasing doses.

      (3) Using an enteric coated form of ASA and other medications such as sucralfate, H_2-receptor blockers, or proton pump inhibitors can minimize these side effects. ASA remains the first line of therapy. It reduces the relative risk of stroke by 15% to 20%.

   b. Ticlopidine: Acts by irreversibly inhibiting adenophosphate-induced platelet aggregation. The effect appears after 3 to 4 days of treatment and remains for the life of platelets. Side effects include abdominal pain, diarrhea, skin eruptions, thrombotic thrombocytopenic purpura, and neutropenia. The incidence of neutropenia is 0.9% and requires frequent hematologic monitoring. For these reasons the use of Ticlopidine is now very limited.

   c. Clopidogrel: Its mechanism of action is similar to Ticlopidine, but has a better side effect profile. The efficacy is similar to aspirin and the dose is 75 mg per day.

   d. Extended-release dipyridamole and aspirin combination: The most recent addition to the antiplatelet aggregation armamentarium. The formulation contains dipyridamole 200 mg in the extended-release form, together with aspirin 25 mg and is administered twice a day. The side effects include headache and gastrointestinal upset. It should be prescribed with caution in patients with active coronary artery disease. According to available data, the efficacy appears to be superior to the other antiplatelet agents.

3. Anticoagulation: The role of anticoagulation with warfarin is limited to atrial fibrillation, antiphospholipid antibody syndrome, and other inherited abnormalities of coagulation factors. Administration of intravenous heparin in patients with TIAs is not substantiated by any studies and is falling out of favor.

4. Carotid Endarterectomy

   a. Data from the North American Symptomatic Carotid Endarterectomy Trial (NASCET) and the European Carotid Surgery Trial (ECST) provide significant support of surgery for symptomatic high-grade (70% to 99%) carotid artery stenosis as opposed to medical treatment.

   b. The NASCET study also showed beneficial effects of surgery in cases of moderate carotid artery stenosis (50% to 69%) among males.

   c. Current recommendations are to consider carotid endarterectomy in most TIA patients with high-grade stenosis and in selected patients with moderate stenosis.

5. Angioplasty: The role of angioplasty and stenting is not yet well established. The data from the Carotid and Vertebral Artery Transluminal Angioplasty Study (CAVATAS) trial show the results to be comparable with those of carotid endarterectomy.

 Key Treatment

- Goal of therapy is to prevent stroke

Risk Factor Modification

- Controlling blood pressure
- Cessation of smoking
- Lipid-lowering agents
- Exercise

Antiplatelet Agents

- Aspirin
- Ticlopidine
- Clopidogrel
- Dipyridamole and aspirin

Surgery

- Carotid endarterectomy

Prognosis

1. The risk of stroke is increased in patients with a history of TIA and ranges from 24% to 29% over first 5 years.

2. The risk is higher in patients with high-grade carotid stenosis and hemispheric TIAs and is estimated to be 40% over 2 years. Of all the patients with TIAs who develop stroke, 20% will have stroke within 1 month after TIA, and 50% will experience stroke within the first year.

Bibliography

Adams HP Jr, Davis PH: Management of transient ischemic attacks. Comprehensive therapy 21:355–361, 1995.

American Heart Association Medical/Scientific Statement: Guidelines for the management of transient ischemic attacks. Stroke 25:1320–1335, 1994.

Barnett HJ, Meldrum HE: Carotid endarterectomy: a neuro-threrapeutic advance. Arch Neurol 57:40–45, 2000.

Brown MM: Carotid angioplasty and stenting: are they therapeutic alternatives? Cerebrovasc Dis 11(Suppl 1): 112–118, 2001.

Hennessy MJ, Britton TC: Transient ischemic attacks: evaluation and management. Int J Clin Pract 54:432–436, 2000.

Johnston SC, Gress DR, Browner WS, Sidney S: Short-term prognosis after emergency department diagnosis. JAMA 284;2901–2906, 2000.

Acute Ischemic Stroke

Marc Fisher
Erdem Orberk
Muhammad Ramzan

Etiology

1. Definitions: Acute ischemic stroke (AIS) is the most common cerebrovascular disorder and also the most frequent inpatient problem seen in a typical general hospital. AIS occurs as a consequence of disruption of the blood supply to an area of the brain, leading to ischemic injury and focal brain infarction.

2. Epidemiology
   a. AIS represents about 85% of the acute cerebrovascular disease population, estimated to be in excess of 700,000 per year in the United States.
   b. The three main subtypes of AIS are related to large-vessel atherosclerosis, small-vessel disease (lacunar stroke), and cardioembolism. The three main AIS subtypes each comprise approximately 25% to 30% of the total AIS population.
   c. More uncommon stroke pathophysiological subtypes include arterial dissection, hypercoagulable disorders, aortic arch emboli, arteritis, and infectious etiologies.
   d. Stroke incidence increases with age, and with the aging of the population there will be an increase of AIS incidence in the twenty-first century.
   e. Common modifiable, potentially modifiable, and nonmodifiable risk factors associated with AIS are outlined in Table 3–1.

3. Pathophysiology
   a. Interruption of the blood supply to a brain region initiates a complex cascade of cellular events that, if left unimpeded, result in focal infarction.
   b. The rapidity of the evolution of the ischemic cascade toward infarction is related to the severity of the blood flow decline and the underlying metabolic milieu. Both factors vary among individual AIS patients, leading to variation of the therapeutic window and potential outcome.
   c. Ischemic but still potentially viable brain tissue is known as the *ischemic penumbra,*

and there is mounting evidence to confirm its existence in animal stroke models and stroke patients.

Symptoms

1. Symptoms seen in individual AIS patients reflect the brain region affected by the ischemic injury.

2. A multitude of symptoms may occur in association with AIS (see Table 3–2) and are typically divided into those occurring in the posterior circulation and those in the anterior circulation.

Clinical Findings

1. Abnormal findings on the neurologic exam, like the symptoms, reflect the brain region affected by the ischemic event (see Table 3–2).

2. Careful interpretation of symptoms and signs allows for accurate localization of the focal ischemic brain region and, with the past medical history, general physical examination, and laboratory testing, reliable stroke subtyping is possible in 80% to 90% of cases.

TABLE 3–1.   AIS RISK FACTORS

Potentially Modifiable Factors
- Hypertension
- Cigarette smoking
- Diabetes
- Elevated cholesterol
- Hyperhemocysteinemia
- Atrial fibrillation
- Transient ischemic attack
- Elevated hematocrit

Nonmodifiable Factors
- Age
- Sex
- Season and climate

Potentially Modifiable Factors
- Obesity
- Inactivity
- Prescription and illicit drug use
- Elevated fibrinogen
- Hypercoagulability

TABLE 3–2. COMMON AIS SYNDROMES AND THEIR CLINICAL MANIFESTATIONS

1. Dominant middle artery syndrome: Aphasia (expressive, receptive, or global), hemiparesis, hemisensory loss, homonymous hemianopsia, limb apraxia, neglect (all typically involve the right side)
2. Nondominant middle cerebral artery syndrome: hemiparesis, neglect, homonymous hemianopsia (all typically involve the left side), failure to recognize faces, objects
3. Anterior cerebral artery syndrome: contralateral leg > arm weakness, incontinence, personality change
4. Posterior cerebral artery (PCA) syndrome: contralateral homonymous hemianopsia, alexia without agraphia if left PCA infarct
5. Common lacunar syndromes (with anatomic localization): Pure motor stroke internal capsule, basis pontis), pure sensory stroke (lateral thalamus), clumsy hand dysarthria syndrome (internal capsule), unilateral ataxia > hemiplegia (basis pontis, internal capsule)
6. Basilar artery syndrome: Depressed level of consciousness, bilateral extremity weakness, cranial nerve deficits
7. Lateral medullary syndrome: Contralateral loss of arm-leg pain-temperature sensation with ipsilateral facial loss, ipsilateral limb ataxia, ipsilateral Horner's syndrome, ipsilateral facial weakness

Laboratory Tests

1. Brain imaging should be performed routinely.
2. Computed tomography (CT) is the most widely available and most commonly employed brain imaging modality in AIS patients. It is most useful for excluding primary intracerebral hemorrhage, although susceptibility-weighted magnetic resonance imaging (MRI) is also useful.
3. Subtle, early signs of ischemic injury are being increasingly recognized with modern CT imaging techniques, but the sensitivity and reliability of early CT signs (sulcal effacement, hypodensity, loss of insular ribbon) remain controversial.
4. Standard T_1 and T_2 MRI scans are not more sensitive than CT in the first 6 to 12 hours after stroke onset.
5. The new techniques of diffusion and perfusion MRI provide easily identifiable imaging confirmation of hyperacute, focal ischemic brain injury and are being employed with increasing frequency.
6. Magnetic resonance and CT angiography are other new imaging techniques that provide important information about the vasculature in AIS patients.
7. Carotid and transcranial ultrasound are noninvasive techniques that also provide valuable information about the vasculature.
8. Cardiac evaluation with transthoracic and/or transesophageal echocardiography provide information about potential cardiac and aortic stroke sources.

9. Blood fasting for evidence of an antiphospholipid antibody or hypercoagulability should be considered in selected AIS patients.

Key Tests

- Computed tomography, magnetic resonance imaging-arteriography/magnetic resonance ventriculography
- Transesophageal and transthoracic echocardiography
- Coagulopathy evaluation
- Cerebral angiography (selected cases)
- CT
- Diffusion-perfusion MRI
- CT and MRA
- Transthoracic and transesophageal echocardiography
- Carotid and transcranial ultrasound

When Indicated

- CT scan or MRI of the head
- Electroencephalography
- Electronystagmography
- Audiogram
- Visual fields
- Neuropsychological testing

Differential Diagnosis

1. Patients presenting with the abrupt onset of focal neurologic symptoms are very likely to have either AIS or an intracerebral hemorrhage. Acute brain imaging can reliably distinguish the two.
2. Rapidly resolving focal signs may be associated with complicated migraine or postictal episode.
3. Patients presenting with a depressed level of consciousness and focal signs are unlikely to have an AIS syndrome. Cerebral hemorrhage, trauma, or an atypical metabolic encephalopathy are much more likely.

Treatment

1. The only clearly established therapy for AIS to improve outcome is intravenous thrombolysis

with recombinant tissue plasminogen activator initiated within 3 hours of stroke onset, using a dose of 0.9 mg/kg as a 10% bolus and the remainder over 1 hour.

2. Emergent CT scanning must be done to exclude an intracerebral hemorrhage or early infarct signs in more than one third of the middle cerebral artery territory. Patients with very mild strokes should not be treated, and patients with very severe strokes should be treated with caution because of an increased risk of intracerebral hemorrhage.

3. Recent evidence suggests that intravenous rt-PA has less efficacy the later in the 3-hour window therapy is begun.

4. Intraarterial treatment with ProUrokinase improved outcome when initiated a median time of 5.3 hours after stroke onset in a population with fairly severe AIS. An additional, larger study will be required for regulatory approval.

5. Secondary prevention after AIS is important because there is a high recurrence risk.

6. Antiplatelet agents such as aspirin, clopidogrel, and sustained-release dipyridamole plus low-dose aspirin are commonly used. Current evidence suggests that sustained-release dipyridamole plus low-dose aspirin is the most effective antiplatelet regimen available. A recent study suggests that warfarin is not superior to aspirin in noncardioembolic stroke patients.

7. For cardioembolic AIS patients, especially those with atrial fibrillation, rheumatic valvular disease, prosthetic valves, and mural thrombi, long-term oral anticoagulation is commonly used.

8. Emerging evidence suggests that several statins (pravastatin, simvistatin) and angiotensin converting enzyme inhibitors (ramipril, perindopril) reduce secondary stroke risk beyond their effects on lipids and blood pressure. Secondary stroke prevention may, therefore, be enhanced by using a "cocktail" of various drugs.

Key Treatment

- Secondary prevention
- Antiplatelet agents
- Identify and treat risk factors: blood pressure, lipids, homocysteine, diabetes
- Intravenous rt-PA within 3 hours
- Anticoagulation with warfarin
- Statins and angiotensin converting enzyme inhibitors

Follow-Up

1. Patients should be encouraged to continue treatment of modifiable stroke risk factors and to take antithrombotic drugs.

2. Patients should be encouraged to alter deleterious dietary habits and receive regular follow-up care with their primary care physician.

3. The prognosis for AIS varies considerably and is primarily dependent on the extent, location, and initial severity of the stroke.

4. There is some indication that rehabilitation can improve outcome.

Bibliography

Cucchiara BL, Kasner SE: Atherosclerotic risk factors in patients with ischemic cerebrovascular disease. Curr Treat Options Neurol 4:445–453, 2002.

Fisher M, Schaebitz W: An overview of acute stroke therapy. Arch. Intern. Med. 160:3196–3206, 2000.

Gorelick PB, Sacco RL, Smith DB, et al.: Prevention of a first stroke. JAMA 281:1112–1120, 1999.

Hossman R-A: Viability thresholds and the penumbra of focal ischemia. Ann Neurol 36:557–565, 1994.

Neumann-Haeflin T, Moseley ME, Albers GW: New magnetic resonance imaging methods for cerebrovascular disease: emerging clinical applications. Ann Neurol 47:559–570, 2000.

Onal MZ, Fisher M, Bogousslavsky J: Clinical evaluation of stroke. In Current Review of Cerebrovascular Disease, vol. 4. Philadelphia, Current Medicine, 2000, pp. 102–114.

4 Spontaneous Intracerebral Hemorrhage

Marc Fisher
Erdem Orberk
Muhammad Ramzan

Definition

Spontaneous intracerebral hemorrhage (ICH) is non-traumatic hemorrhage into the brain parenchyma, which may extend into the ventricles and from there to the subarachnoid space.

Etiology

1. Hypertensive bleeding accounts for 50% to 60% of all ICH.

2. Amyloid angiopathy is the most frequent cause of lobar ICH. Amyloid angiopathy rarely occurs before age 55, but it steadily becomes more frequent with age. It is found in 8% of ICH patients in the seventh decade of life and approximately 40% of those in the eighth decade.

3. In young patients, illicit drugs (cocaine, amphetamines) are a frequent cause of ICH, leading to 40% of lethal ICH.

4. Coagulopathies can cause ICH with a rate of 0.3% to 1% per year in patients older than 60 years of age and account for approximately 10% of ICH.

5. Vascular pathologies, including arteriovenous malformations (AVM) or cavernous malformations, account for 5% of ICH but occur more often in the third and fourth decades of life.

6. Brain tumors occasionally (2% in autopsy series, 6% in clinical radiology series) present initially through bleeding into the mass.

7. Septic aneurysms (called "mycotic aneurysms") are an infrequent source of ICH.

Epidemiology

1. ICH has an overall incidence of 10 to 20/100,000, affecting 30,000 to 60,000 U.S.-Americans each year.

2. The incidence increases considerably with age, being as low as 0.3/100,000 in people younger than 35 years of age. Because of the increasing age of the U.S. population, the numbers are expected to double over the next several decades.

3. 10% to 15% of all strokes are ICH. The mortality is as high as 40%.

4. The incidence rate for Asians and African Americans is more than two times higher than among Caucasians.

5. ICH occurs more frequently in men than in women.

6. Annual recurrence rate of hypertensive ICH is low at 2% to 4%; 5%, with cavernous malformation; higher in amyloid angiopathy, with 11% and 18% of those with AVM. Recurrent bleeding is almost always at a location different from previous sites, except in cases of underlying vascular pathology.

Pathophysiology

1. ICH can occur from rupture of arteries secondary to longstanding hypertension or to sudden blood pressure peaks with hypertensive crisis. Histopathology studies often show lipohyalinosis of the ruptured small penetrating arteries.

2. Typical locations for hypertension-related ICH are, in descending order of frequency, the basal ganglia, thalamus, cerebellum, and pons. In contrast, amyloid angiopathy-related ICH usually spares the basal ganglia, is lobar, and can be multilocal.

3. Underlying vascular anomalies may be congenital or progressively acquired over years.

4. ICH is associated with hypocholesterolemia, but the molecular pathophysiology of this relationship is speculative.

Clinical Findings

1. The variety of clinical signs is more a function of ICH localization than of the type of lesion.

2. The sudden onset of a focal deficit is typical for ICH, subarachnoid hemorrhage, and ischemic stroke. The velocity of development of other signs and symptoms can indicate the type of cerebrovascular disease.

3. ICH is more often associated with headache than ischemic stroke, and will lead more often to early (less than one day) deterioration of consciousness and vomiting because of raised intracranial pressure (ICP). It is also likely to cause a midline shift of brain tissue secondary to continuation of bleeding for several hours after onset.

4. Ischemic strokes usually need more than a day of swelling to raise ICP. Subarachnoid hemorrhage patients may or may not develop raised ICP, but eventually they will have signs of meningeal irritation, which generally occurs later, if at all, with ICH. It is important to recognize, however, that it is not possible, on clinical grounds alone, to make a reliable distinction between these three major entities of cerebrovascular disease.

Key Signs

• Headache, nausea, and focal deficits together with quickly evolving signs of raised ICP

Radiographic Changes

1. ICH will be demonstrable immediately after bleeding as a bright (hyperdense) round to ovoid space-occupying lesion. As long as the blood is fluid, a meniscus forms between sedimented erythrocytes at the dependent part of the hematoma and the less hyperdense plasma part above. With blood resorption over the ensuing 2 to 3 weeks, the hyperdense center shrinks. At the same time a hypodense rim develops, presumably delineating the area of brain edema. After 2 to 3 weeks, the edema resolves and a slit-like defect persists.

2. The course of MRI findings is more complex: After a few minutes the extravasated hemoglobin becomes deoxygenated at the periphery of the hematoma, and this gives the magnetic properties of the blood a paramagnetic character. With susceptibility-weighted MRI sequences, paramagnetic, deoxygenated blood can be shown as early as 30 minutes after bleeding as a hypointense region around a center of blood. Because the blood at the center stays oxygenated longer than that at the periphery, it will appear isointense to hyperintense. Over a few days, progressive enlargement of the hypointense periphery toward the center occurs. Also after a few days, deoxyhemoglobin is transformed to methemoglobin, which will last up to several weeks, showing as hyperintensity in T1-weighted sequences. Finally methemoglobin disappears and residual hemosiderin will be seen on T2-weighted images as an area of hypodensity for many years.

3. ICH at locations other than the typical sites of hypertensive bleeding, or in patients without hypertension who are younger than 45 years of age, should be followed a few weeks after onset by further imaging (MRI and MRA) to rule out underlying vascular anomalies or brain tumor.

Laboratory Findings

Lumbar puncture is rarely needed and often is dangerous in patients with ICB. Leucocytosis in the peripheral blood may be seen.

Key Tests

• CT or MRI of the brain

Treatment

1. Surgical treatment of ICH is controversial except for larger cerebellar hematomas.

2. Early (before signs of brainstem compression) decompressive surgery, consisting of widening the foramen magnum by partial removal of the occipital bone, together with cerebellar clot removal, is safe and significantly improves survival and independence rate.

3. In all ICH patients, frequent neurochecks and close blood pressure control is standard medical therapy, together with osmotherapy (mannitol) and hyperventilation as needed. The mean arterial blood pressure should be kept below 130 mm Hg, and cerebral perfusion pressure above 70 mm Hg.

4. Developing hydrocephalus is treated early by extraventricular drainage (EVD). The combination of EVD with application of intraventricular thrombolytics is under investigation.

5. Underlying vascular anomalies as well as brain tumors are treated accordingly.

Key Treatment

• Early decompressive surgery for cerebellar ICH

• Osmotherapy (mannitol) and hyperventilation for hypertension

 ## Bibliography

Broderick JP, Adams HPJ, Barsan W, et al.: Guidelines for the management of spontaneous intracerebral hemorrhage: A statement for healthcare professionals from a special writing group of the Stroke Council, American Heart Association. Stroke 30:905–915, 1999.

Linfante I, Llinas RH, Caplan LR, Warach S: MRI features of intracerebral hemorrhage within 2 hours from symptom onset. Stroke 30:2263–2267, 1999.

McEvoy AW, Kitchen ND, Thomas DGT: Lesson of the week: Intracerebral haemorrhage in young adults: The emerging importance of drug misuse. BMJ 2000 320:1322–1324, 2000.

Qureshi AI, Tuhrim S, Broderick JP, et al.: Spontaneous intracerebral hemorrhage. N Engl J Med 344:1450–1460, 2001.

5 Subarachnoid Hemorrhage and Saccular Aneurysm

Marc Fisher
Erdem Orberk
Muhammad Ramzan

Definition

Subarachnoid hemorrhage (SAH) occurs most commonly secondary to the rupture of intracranial aneurysms of extraparenchymal arteries. These run in the cerebrospinal fluid confined by the arachnoidal membrane.

Etiology

1. Aneurysmal bleeding accounts for 85% of SAH.
2. Perimesencephalic SAH occurs in another 10%.
3. The remaining 5% are attributable to A-V-malformations, hypocoaguability, and other unusual causes.

Epidemiology

1. SAH has an incidence of approximately 10/100,000 affecting 30,000 Americans each year. Only 3% of all strokes are SAH.
2. However, SAH causes one fourth of the loss of potential life before age 65 secondary to strokes. The peak incidence occurs in the fifth to sixth decades of life.
3. The incidence rate for African Americans, Asians, and Hispanics is about two times higher than among Caucasians. Although in the past it was shown that SAH occurred more frequently among women, this finding was not reproduced in a multinational study.
4. Eleven percent to 14% of all patients with subarachnoid hemorrhage die before admission to the hospital. Death from SAH reaches 40% in the first month. Most patients die in the first 24 hours.

Pathophysiology

1. The exact cause of aneurysm formation is unknown. Most are saccular aneurysms, which occur most often at bifurcation points at the circle of Willis or its major branches. Rare forms include fusiform, mycotic, traumatic, or dissecting aneurysms.
2. In a minority (<5%) of patients with SAH, genetic comorbidities present are autosomal dominant polycystic kidney disease, Ehlers-Danlos syndrome type IV, and neurofibromatosis type 1. In addition, first-degree relatives of SAH patients have a 4–7-fold increased risk for SAH.
3. In autopsy series of children saccular aneurysms are seldom found, but they represent 2% of adult autopsies. Therefore beyond genetic factors, age and other acquired risk factors contribute to the development of aneurysms. Modifiable risk factors include alcohol or cocaine use, smoking, and hypertension.

Clinical Findings

1. Before rupture, most aneurysms are clinically silent. Exceptions are large aneurysms pressing on adjacent nerve structures.
2. The physical examination findings after rupture range from completely normal (especially after a sentinel bleed) to deeply comatose with brainstem signs. Signs of meningeal irritation often need several (3 to 12) hours to develop and may be absent in two thirds of patients at presentation. Therefore, the history may be more important than the physical examination findings. In a prospective study almost 20% of patients complaining of "the worst headache in my life" had proven SAH.
3. Minor headaches should be taken seriously: sentinel bleeds are reported in 15% to 20% of SAH, often considered innocuous by the patient. Red flags for complicated minor headaches are sudden (<2 minute) onset, any episode of impaired consciousness, amnesia, Valsalva maneuver shortly before onset, associated seizure, or focal deficits (especially of the cranial nerves).

Key Sign

- Any severe headache of sudden onset or complicated minor headache should be regarded as possible SAH until proven otherwise.

Radiographic Changes

1. The first step in the diagnosis of SAH is computed tomography (CT) of the head without contrast. Subarachnoidal blood will show up as bright

white (hyperdense) areas around the central nervous system surfaces and/or in the ventricles (white sediment line in the occipital horn). The sensitivity of current CT scanners can be as high as 97%, but it declines quickly with time down to 88% at day 3, 50% on day 7, 20% on day 9, and almost zero at day 10.

2. In subacute SAH, FLAIR-MRI (fluid attenuated inverse recovery sequences-magnetic resonance imaging) is more sensitive than CT and may show SAH, in most cases, up to 18 days after onset.

3. Determining the type of SAH by radiologic methods is essential for the prognosis. Aneurysm rebleeding has a mortality of 50%. Rebleeding can only be prevented by detection and subsequent elimination of the aneurysm. Distribution of blood can sometimes but not always indicate the location of the ruptured aneurysm.

4. Digital subtraction angiography (DSA) is the "gold standard" for aneurysm detection. The combined risk of permanent and transient neurologic complication secondary to angiography is, however, significant at about 2%.

5. CT angiography (CTA), being noninvasive, does not have the inherent risk of DSA. The ability to reconstruct the CTA images in any of the three-dimensional planes can increase sensitivity and facilitate planning of surgical approach.

6. Magnetic resonance angiography (MRA) shares the same advantages with CTA but may be less suitable than CTA for the critically ill, unstable SAH patient. The acquisition time with current MR scanners is longer than CTA. MRA is more susceptible to movement artifacts.

7. In cases of perimesencephalic distribution of blood, in 99% of cases CTA is sufficient to rule out a basilar artery aneurysm. Perimesencephalic SAH has an excellent prognosis without intervention.

8. If the blood distribution is non-perimesencephalic, repeat imaging after initial negative angiography is mandatory: Up to 13% of patients may have an aneurysm found at the second study.

9. Serial CT or MRI will detect enlargement of the ventricles as sign of hydrocephalus.

Laboratory Findings

1. An indication for lumbar puncture in SAH is the CT-negative patient with clinically suspected SAH. Decrease in red cells in consecutive tubes of cerebrospinal fluid (CSF) occurs more often in traumatic tap, but it does not definitively distinguish traumatic tap from real SAH.

2. Xanthochromic CSF is an unequivocal sign of

SAH. However testing the CSF after centrifugation for xanthochromia with the naked eye is not as sensitive as spectrophotometry. CSF is positive for xanthochromia between 6 and 12 hours after hemorrhage, Xanthochromia stays positive in almost all patients up to 2 weeks after hemorrhage; in 70%, after 3 weeks; and in 40%, after 4 weeks.

Key Laboratory Findings

- Xanthochromic CSF—detected best by spectrophotometry—is the only unequivocal finding of SAH.

- Normal CSF 12 hours after onset of headache effectively rules out SAH.

Treatment

1. The main focus of treatment is prevention of rebleeding, hydrocephalus, and vasospasm. Very early rebleeding (24 hours after first SAH) may occur in up to 17% of patients. Without elimination of the aneurysm, about 40% of initial SAH survivors suffer a rebleeding within 1 month of the initial SAH, with subsequent fatality up to 50%. Two features associated with early rebleeding are high systolic blood pressure and angiography in the first 6 hours after SAH.

2. Early surgery with clipping of the aneurysm in patients in Hunt and Hess Stages I–III has therefore been the standard treatment. Timing of surgery in stages IV–V is, however, still controversial because of high perioperative risk.

3. Endovascular intervention (coiling) had originally been an alternative, mainly for patients with high perioperative risk. Short-term and midterm (up to 1 year) follow-up comparing conventional aneurysm clipping and endovascular treatment (coiling) have shown no significant difference. Long-term efficacy of endovascular treatment in preventing rebleeding is not yet known.

4. The incidence of hydrocephalus after SAH is significantly higher with age (even after mild SAH) symptomatic vasospasm, and intraventricular hemorrhage, and in those with vertebro-basilar artery aneurysms. The mainstay of treatment of hydrocephalus is extraventricular drainage in the acute phase, changed to permanent shunt implant if needed.

5. Vasospasms leading to ischemic infarcts, usually occur in 30% of survivors of SAH and typically develop on days 4 to 12. Treatment of vasospasm may include early clot removal and intracisternal

Key Treatment

- Surgical clipping of the aneurysm (Hunt and Hess Stages I–III)

- Coiling

- Hydrocephalus: Extraventricular drainage

- Vasospasm:

  - Clot removal

  - Intracisternal fibrinolysis

  - Nicardipine, nimodipine, or tirilazad

  - "Triple H therapy": hemodilution, hypertension, hypervolemia

fibrinolysis. Pharmacological treatments include nicardipine, nimodipine, or tirilazad.

6. Because autoregulation of brain perfusion may be disturbed, blood pressure should be lowered only very cautiously once the aneurysm is eliminated. The "triple H therapy" (hemodilution, hypertension, hypervolemia) is widely used in the prevention and/or treatment of cerebral vasospasm. When other measures fail, angioplasty, sometimes combined with intraarterial papaverine, is applied, although the effect seems to be short-lived.

7. Elimination of the aneurysm is the most important step. Complications can occur up to 2 weeks after successful aneurysm treatment.

Bibliography

Cloft HJ, Joseph GJ, Dion JE: Risk of cerebral angiography in patients with subarachnoid hemorrhage, cerebral aneurysm, and arteriovenous malformation: a meta-analysis. Stroke 30:317–320, 1999.

Dovey Z, Misra M, Thornton J, et al.: Guglielmi detachable coiling for intracranial aneurysms: the story so far. Arch Neurol 58:559–564, 2001.

Johnston SC, Selvin S, Gress DR: The burden, trends, and demographics of mortality from subarachnoid hemorrhage. *Neurology* 50:1413–1418, 1998.

Treggiari-Venzi MM, Suter PM, Romand JA: Review of medical prevention of vasospasm after aneurysmal subarachnoid hemorrhage: a problem of neurointensive care. Neurosurgery 48:249–261, 2001.

Van Gijn J, Rinkel GJ: Subarachnoid haemorrhage: diagnosis, causes and management. Brain 124:249–278, 2001.

6 Spinal Cord Stroke

Marc Fisher
Erdem Orberk
Muhammad Ramzan

Etiology

1. Spinal cord stroke is an uncommon clinical disorder that occurs secondary to ischemic injury to the spinal cord.

   a. The clinical syndrome will reflect the location of the infarct in a rostral-caudal direction in the spinal cord and the extent of the cross-sectional injury at that level.

   b. The anterior spinal artery supplies the anterior two-thirds of the spinal cord and the posterior spinal cord supplies the remaining posterior one-third.

   c. A few penetrating radicular arteries supply a large portion of the blood supply to the spinal cord, and the thoracolumbar spinal cord receives a large proportion of its blood flow from the artery of Adamkiewicz. Occlusion of this artery or another major penetrator can lead to an extensive spinal cord infarction.

2. Spinal cord infarcts can develop in relationship to many mechanisms. The most common etiology is profound hypotension superimposed on atherosclerosis in the aorta or penetrating arteries that supply the spinal cord.

Epidemiology

The precise incidence of spinal cord infarction is not established. However, a busy general hospital may encounter one or two cases per year.

Pathophysiology

1. Hypotension superimposed on atherosclerotic compromise of blood vessels supplying the spinal cord can lead to local areas of ischemic injury at a particular spinal cord level.

2. Aortic dissection can similarly impair blood flow at the level of the dissection.

3. An embolic occlusion of a spinal radicular artery may rarely occur.

4. Vascular malformations most commonly located extradurally can cause chronic ischemia by reducing perfusion and increasing venous pressure.

Symptoms

Symptoms reflect the location and transverse extent of the spinal cord ischemia. The most common clinical syndromes associated with spinal cord infarction are outlined below (see Key Symptoms).

Key Symptoms

- Leg and arm weakness
- Bladder and bowel disturbance
- Pain over the spine or radiating to the limbs
- Loss of feeling below the level of infarction
- Flushing of the skin

Clinical Findings

1. Total transverse infarction of the spinal cord is associated with paraplegia or quadriplegia, if the upper cervical spinal cord is the region infarcted. Other signs include loss of bladder and bowel function, a sensory level reflecting the level of ischemic injury, and initial loss of reflexes below the level of the ischemic injury ("spinal shock") followed by hyperreflexia and spasticity. Bilateral Babinski signs will commonly be present initially.

2. The findings with anterior spinal artery infarction are similar to those with total transverse infarction, but there is dissociated sensory loss. Pain and temperature sensations are lost below the level of the ischemic injury, but vibration and joint position sensation are spared.

3. Posterior spinal artery infarction is rare. Pain is common and is associated with loss of vibratory and position sensation below the level of the ischemic injury.

Laboratory Testing

1. T1- and T2-weighted magnetic resonance imaging (MRI) provides the best available visualization of the intrinsic spinal cord injury associated with infarction. The clinician should guide the radiologic assessment by careful clinical localization.

2. Spinal fluid examination should be considered in selected cases to exclude any infectious cause such as neurosyphilis.

3. Spinal angiography may also be considered in occasional patients to evaluate localized injury.

Key Tests

- MRI

- Spinal angiography

- Spinal fluid examination

Differential Diagnosis

The abrupt onset of a spinal cord syndrome raises the possibility of other acute processes affecting the spinal cord.

1. The most important other acute cause of spinal cord dysfunction is a compressive lesion related to tumor, abscess, or disc herniation. MRI should distinguish all of these possibilities from the intrinsic pattern seen with infarction.

2. Transverse myelitis may also develop rather quickly, and MRI findings may mimic those of infarction. Spinal fluid should show evidence of an inflammatory process, and there should be no cardiovascular compromise with this disorder.

Treatment

There is no specific treatment available for patients with spinal cord infarction. Management of bladder and bowel dysfunction and skin breakdown is important to prevent complications. It is unclear what if any role antithrombotic therapy plays in secondary prevention.

Key Treatment

- Manage medical complications.

- Rehabilitation

Follow-up

The long-term prognosis will reflect the severity of the initial injury in most cases. Patients with complete transverse infarction have the most unfavorable outlook. The more caudal the level of infarction and the smaller the amount of tissue infarcted, the better the long-term outlook. Acute and long-term rehabilitation are useful. The risk for recurrence is unclear.

Bibliography

Cheschire WP, Santos CC, Massey EW, Howard JP: Spinal cord infarction: etiology and outcome. Neurology 47:321–330, 1996.

Kareki M, Inoue K, Shimzu T, Manmen T: Infarction of the unilateral posterior horn and lateral column of the spinal cord with sparing of posterior columns; demonstration by MRI. J Neurol Psychiatry 57:629–631, 1994.

Kouchoukos NT: Spinal cord ischemic injury: is it preventable? Semin Thorac Cardiovasc Surg 3:323–328, 1991.

Leys D, Weerts JGE, Pruvo JP: Spinal ischemic strokes. In Ginsburg MD, Bogousslavsky J (eds): Cerebrovascular Disease. Malden, MA, Blackwell Science, 1998, pp. 1560–1568.

Pelfer H, VanGijn J: Spinal infarction. A follow-up study. Stroke 24:896–898, 1993.

7 Stroke in Younger Adults

Marc Fisher
Erdem Orberk
Muhammad Ramzan

Definition

Stroke in the young can arbitrarily be defined as stroke occurring before the age of 45 (range 15 to 45) years. This constitutes approximately 5% to 10% of all strokes, and the causes are heterogeneous and different from the causes of stroke in older patients. The cause of stroke may remain uncertain despite a thorough diagnostic evaluation. Most cases are due to ischemic stroke, but brain hemorrhages also occur.

Causes

The causes of ischemic stroke in young adults can be categorized into five major subgroups:

1. Vascular
2. Embolic
3. Hematologic
4. Miscellaneous
5. Cryptogenic

VASCULAR

Arterial Dissection

Arterial dissections cause 10% to 20% of the strokes in young adults.

1. Dissections are produced by subintimal penetration of blood in the vessel wall. This results in the formation of an intramural hematoma, causing narrowing or occlusion of the involved vessel. It can affect the carotid system as well as vertebrobasilar system.

2. The most commonly affected vessels are the extracranial internal carotid arteries. The recurrence rate is 1% per year and may be even higher in patients with a positive family history or in very young patients.

3. Dissections may be traumatic or spontaneous, and are associated with fibromuscular dysplasia, Marfan syndrome, moyamoya disease, α_1-antitrypsin deficiency, and Ehlers-Danlos syndrome.

4. The presence of an ipsilateral Horner's syndrome, head or neck trauma in cervical manipulation, and facial or neck pain preceding the stroke are suggestive of carotid or vertebral artery dissection.

Key Clinical Signs

- Face or neck pain
- Evidence of head or neck trauma
- Ipsilateral Horner's syndrome

5. Diagnosis: Magnetic resonance arteriography (MRA) or conventional arteriography can be used to establish the diagnosis. The characteristic features are a string sign or double-lumen sign.

6. Treatment: Anticoagulation with heparin and warfarin; 85% of patients have an excellent recovery.

Key Treatment

- Heparin and warfarin

Migraine

Also known as *complicated migraine* or *migrainous infarction.*

1. This condition occurs only in patients with a history of migraine with aura, and should be diagnosed only when infarction occurs during the course of a typical migraine attack.

2. The most common symptoms are aphasia, hemiparesis, and vertebrobasilar insufficiency. The posterior cerebral artery territory is more commonly affected than the anterior circulation.

Key Clinical Signs

- Aphasia
- Hemiparesis
- Vertebrobasilar insufficiency

3. Treatment: Treatment includes migraine control, and the goal is to prevent vasospasm. Triptans and other vasoconstricting agents should be avoided. If

patients are taking an oral contraceptive pill, it should be discontinued.

Key Treatment

- Treatment includes migraine control; the goal is to prevent vasospasm.

Vasculitis

Vasculitis should be considered in patients with recurrent stroke, or stroke associated with encephalopathy, multifocal neurologic symptoms, fever, seizures, and systemic findings of skin involvement, kidney disease, and a high erythrocyte sedimentation rate (ESR).

Key Clinical Signs

- Recurrent stroke

- Stroke associated with encephalopathy, multifocal neurologic symptoms, fever, seizures, and systemic findings of skin involvement, kidney disease, and a high ESR

1. The most common entities include, polyarteritis nodosa, Wegener's granulomatosis, systemic lupus erythematosus (SLE), rheumatoid arthritis, Sjögren's syndrome, giant cell arteritis, infectious vasculitis, and isolated central nervous system angiitis.

2. The diagnosis requires an angiogram, which will show areas of narrowing and irregularity of the vessel wall lumen. In some cases it may be necessary to perform a brain and leptomeningeal biopsy to establish the diagnosis.

3. Corticosteroids are the mainstay of therapy, but chemotherapy can also be used in refractory cases. Surgery may be the best option in cases with Takayasu arteritis

Key Treatment

- Corticosteroids are the preferred treatment.

- Chemotherapy can be used for refractory cases.

- Surgery may be the option for Takayasu arteritis.

Premature Atherosclerosis

This is usually seen in patients with diabetes, hypertension, and hyperlipidemia who have a history of smoking. Treatment: These patients are treated the sameway as older stroke patients, and the therapeutic modalities include antiplatelet agents, anticoagulation, carotid endarterectomy (CEA), and lipid-lowering agents.

Key Treatment

- Antiplatelet agents

- Anticoagulation agents

- Carotid endarterectomy

- Lipid-lowering agents

Others

Other causes include, hypertensive encephalopathy, toxemia of pregnancy, moyamoya disease, and venous infarcts.

EMBOLIC (13% TO 35%)

Cardiac Arrhythmias

Cardiac arrhythmias are not as common in the young as in the older population; they include atrial fibrillation and, rarely, sick sinus syndrome. Management is the same for either age group—i.e., either anticoagulation or pacemaker insertion.

Valvular Heart Disease

Cardiac valve disease can be due to rheumatic fever, bacterial endocarditis, marantic endocarditis, mitral annulus calcification, prosthetic valves, or congenital abnormalities such as bicuspid aortic valve, and mitral valve prolapse (MVP).

Causes of Valvular Heart Disease

- Rheumatic fever

- Bacterial endocarditis

- Marantic endocarditis

- Mitral annulus calcification

- Prosthetic valves

- Congenital abnormalities

1. Rheumatic fever is a common cause of valvular heart disease (most commonly mitral stenosis) worldwide, but especially in developing countries.

2. Cardioembolic cerebral ischemia occurs in 60% to 75% of patients with mitral stenosis. The risk of embolism is increased in the presence of atrial fibrillation.

3. Mechanical prosthetic valves are associated with higher risk of embolism than are biological prosthetic heart valves. The estimated risk of systemic thromboembolism in patients with a mechanical prosthetic valve and receiving anticoagulation therapy is 2% per year for the aortic position and 4% per year for the mitral position.

4. Embolic vegetations can also be seen in patients with acute and subacute bacterial endocarditis. Very rarely, these patients present with mycotic aneurysms caused by septic emboli. Nonbacterial thrombotic or marantic vegetations are a common source of emboli in patients with malignancy or SLE.

5. MVP is not an established source of embolic stroke. It affects 10% to 15% of the population and is more common in women. A mid-systolic click can be heard on cardiac auscultation.

6. Diagnosis: Cardiac examination, blood cultures, and transesophageal echocardiography

Key Tests

- Cardiac examination
- Blood cultures
- Transesophageal echocardiography

7. Treatment: Antibiotics, antiplatelet agents, and anticoagulation

Key Treatment

- Antibiotics
- Antiplatelet agents
- Anticoagulation agents

Patent Foramen Ovale

The incidence of patent foramen ovale (PFO) in the general population is approximately 15% to 20%. PFO as such is not emboligenic, but paradoxical emboli with right-to-left shunting may occur in the setting of peripheral venous thrombosis. Usually the stroke is triggered by a Valsalva maneuver, e.g., while defecating or with vigorous coughing.

PEARL

- PFO is usually triggered by a Valsalva maneuver.

1. Diagnosis: Echocardiogram with bubble study or saline injection with Doppler studies of the carotid and intracranial arteries

Key Tests

- Echocardiogram with bubble study
- Saline injection with Doppler studies of the carotid and intracranial arteries

2. Treatment: Antiplatelet agents, anticoagulation, or surgery

Key Treatment

- Antiplatelet agents
- Anticoagulation agents

Others

Other causes of cardioembolic stroke include acute myocardial infarction, atrial myxoma, cardiomyopathies, atrial septal aneurysms, and endocardial fibrosis.

HEMATOLOGIC DISORDERS

Hyperviscosity Syndromes

Sickle Cell Anemia

The symptoms of sickle cell anemia, an important cause of stroke in the African American population, are seen in patients with sickle cell disease and not the sickle cell trait. They include premature atherosclerosis and watershed infarcts.

Key Clinical Signs

- Premature atherosclerosis
- Watershed infarcts

1. Diagnosis: Hemoglobin electrophoresis
2. Treatment: Intravenous hydration, blood transfusions, and hydroxyurea to increase the synthesis of fetal hemoglobin

Key Treatment

- Intravenous hydration
- Transfusions
- Hydroxyurea

Polycythemia Vera

Polycythemia vera is a myeloproliferative disorder characterized by increased hematocrit and blood volume. There is increased blood viscosity, decreased blood flow, and engorgement of vessels, resulting in thrombosis. Hyperviscosity can also be seen in conditions like Waldenstrom's macroglobulinemia.

Key Indications

• Increased hematocrit and blood volume

1. Diagnosis: Complete blood count
2. Treatment: Phlebotomy

Key Treatment

• Phlebotomy

Primary Hypercoagulable (Hereditary) State

A family history of thrombotic events, recurrent deep venous thrombosis, or thrombosis at unusual sites—e.g., in the arm—are suggestive of a primary hypercoagulable state. This condition may account for 2% to 7% of strokes.

Summary

Multiple coagulation defects are associated with ischemic strokes and include inherited or acquired (e.g., in nephrotic syndrome) deficiencies of naturally occurring anticoagulants (protein C and S, antithrombin III), or a disturbance of the clotting system such as resistance to activated protein C (Factor V Leiden mutation), elevated plasma fibrinogen, abnormalities of fibrinolysis, and prothrombin mutation. These disorders are usually associated with venous thrombosis, but arterial thrombosis and strokes also occur.

Antiphospholipid Antibodies (Lupus Anticoagulant)

The presence of lupus anticoagulant should be considered in women with recurrent fetal loss as well as in patients with thrombocytopenia or a history of SLE.

Key Indications

• Recurrent fetal loss

• Thrombocytopenia

• History of SLE

1. Diagnosis: The hematologic evaluation should include anticardiolipin antibodies (IgG and IgM) as well coagulation testing to screen for a circulating lupus anticoagulant.

2. Treatment: Anticoagulation with warfarin or heparin

Key Treatment

• Warfarin or heparin

Secondary Hypercoagulable (Acquired) State

Hypercoagulable or thrombophilic states can be seen in association with use of oral contraceptive pill, as well as in many systemic conditions like ulcerative colitis, regional enteritis, or cancer (prothrombic state or marantic/nonbacterial thrombotic endocarditis). Other causes include thrombotic thrombocytopenic purpura, disseminated intravascular coagulation, and paroxysmal nocturnal hemoglobinuria.

MISCELLANEOUS

Drug Abuse

Cocaine or amphetamines may cause cerebral hemorrhage. Intravenous drug abuse may cause bacterial endocarditis, leading to bacterial or fibrinolytic emboli, or to mycotic aneurysms. Acute alcohol intoxication has also been reported as a cause of stroke.

• Diagnosis: Clinical history and toxicology screening

Homocysteinuria

An aminoaciduria, homocysteinuria is inherited in autosomal recessive fashion. It is characterized by an increased level of homocysteine in blood, CSF, and urine. Three different enzymatic defects have been identified: cystathione synthase, 5,10 methyltetrahydrofolate reductase, and homocysteine methyltransferase. The brain infarcts can be either thrombotic or embolic.

1. Diagnosis: High levels of homocysteine in blood, with or without a methionine load

2. Treatment: Pyridoxine, vitamin B_{12}, and folic acid supplementation.

Others

Other disorders include Fabry disease (galactosidase-A deficiency), sulfite oxidase deficiency, and mitochondrial disorders (MELAS—mitochondial encephalomyopathy with lactic acidosis and stroke-like episodes; MERRF—myoclonic epilepsy with ragged red fibers; Kearns-Sayre syndrome).

CRYPTOGENIC STROKE (7% to 40%)

The cause of cryptogenic stroke remains unknown, even after a detailed and thorough work-up.

INTRACERBERAL HEMORRHAGE

Intracerebral hemorrhage is not as well studied as ischemic stroke in young adults. It may account for 40% to 45% of stroke cases. The most common site is lobar, and the commonest causes are arteriovenous malformation, aneurysms, hypertension, and cocaine and amphetamine abuse.

Bibliography

Biller J: Strokes in the young. In Toole JF, Murros K and Veltkamp R (eds): Cerebrovascular disorders, 5th ed. Philadelphia, Lippincott Williams & Wilkins 1999;283–316.

Bogousslavsky J, Pierre P: Ischemic stroke in patients under age 45. Neurol Clin 10:113–124, 1992.

Catto A, Grant P: Risk factors for cerebrovascular disease and the role of coagulation and fibrinolysis. Blood Coagul Fibrinol 1995;6:497–510.

Homma S, Sacco RL, Di Tulio MR, et al.: Effect of medical treatment in stroke patients with patent foramen ovale: patent foramen ovale in Cryptogenic Stroke Study. Circulation 105:2625–2631, 2002.

Schievink WI, Mokri B, Piepgras DG. Spontaneous dissection of cervicocephalic arteries in childhood and adolescence. Neurology 44:1607–1612, 1994.

Toffol GJ, Biller J, Adams HP Jr. Nontraumatic intracerebral hemorrhage in young adults. Arch Neurol 44:483–485, 1987.

8 Cerebral Venous Thrombosis

Marc Fisher
Erdem Orberk
Muhammad Ramzan

Definition

Cerebral venous thrombosis (CVT) occurs secondary to an occlusion of the dural venous sinuses, the superficial cortical veins, or the deep veins of the brain.

Etiology

1. The majority of predisposing factors for peripheral venous thrombosis also apply for CVT. See also Parts XX, XXIII, XIV.

2. Autoimmune and inflammatory diseases have been described as risk factors in 30% of the largest case series (160 patients). In a Middle Eastern (Saudi Arabian) population, Behçet's disease was the single most common cause.

3. Pregnancy and oral contraceptive use have each been associated with approximately 12% of patients with CVT.

4. In developing countries, generalized or local infections are reportedly often the cause, whereas in Europe only 6% of cases have been attributed to infection.

5. Hemato-oncologic or hemostasisologic risk factors are leukemia, thrombocythemia, red blood cell disorders (sickle cell disease), and coagulation abnormalities. Adjacent space-occupying lesions can mechanically impair blood flow. In at least 30% of patients, however, no underlying cause is found.

Epidemiology

CVT is more often found in women (1.5:1) than in men, which may reflect the gender specificity of the puerperium and oral contraceptives. In can occur at any age. The true incidence of CVT is unknown. In a retrospective study in Saudi Arabia in two tertiary referral centers, the hospital frequency was 7 per 100,000 patients, and the relative frequency versus arterial strokes was 1:62.5 reaching a ratio of 1:8.5 in stroke patients aged 15 to 45 years.

Pathophysiology

Virchow's triad (changes in the vascular wall, stasis of blood flow and hypercoagulability) applies to CVT as well as to peripheral venous thromboses.

Clinical Findings

1. CVT is a chameleon among neurovascular disorders. First it is highly variable in its clinical spectrum. Headache, the most frequent complaint, is nonspecific. In 5% of patients it is the sole complaint with a nonfocal exam. One third of CVT cases mimic pseudotumor cerebri. Slowly progressing cognitive deficits as the main manifestation have been described as well. At the other end of the clinical spectrum the patient can be in deep coma.

2. In addition to the clinical variability, the onset of symptoms is highly variable. In contrast to the typical acute onset of other stroke types, symptoms of CVT develop subacutely (2 days up to 2 months) in 50% of cases and are slowly progressive in 20% of cases. Because of this great variability, there is no reliable clinical syndrome. Therefore imaging is the only definitive way to prove the diagnosis.

Key Signs

- Headache or blurred vision with a prominent optic disc, focal deficits, seizures and/or altered level of consciousness

Radiographic Changes

1. Unenhanced computed tomography (CT) can be normal in 50% of the patients. A thrombus in the superior sagittal sinus above the sinus confluens can sometimes be seen as dense triangle sign. Contrast-enhanced CT can detect the absence of contrast in that sinus, the so-called empty delta sign. CT arteriography (CTA) and magnetic resonance arteriography (MRA) are able to delineate all of the venous sinuses. A pitfall is the physiologic variant of left transverse and sigmoid sinus hypoplasia; inability to visualize flow there does not prove sinus venous thrombosis. Magnetic resonance imaging (MRI) detection of the thrombus itself, and not only absence of flow, is often necessary. The signal intensity of the thrombus is, however, time dependent. Therefore the combination of MRI and MRA is advisable. The inner cerebral veins are visualized by venous MRA, and sometimes by CTA. Cortical vein occlusion may

escape MRA but can be proven by conventional angiography.

2. Indirect signs of CVT include hematoma, infarcts, and edema. Especially when those do not follow an arterial distribution, CVT should be ruled out. Diffusion-weighted MRI can distinguish between vascular and cytotoxic edema.

Laboratory Findings

Testing for hypercoagulability: Factor V Leiden mutation; prothrombin 20210 G→A mutation; deficiencies of antithrombin III, protein C, and protein S; or antiphospholipid antibody tests are positive in 15% of CVT cases. Cerebrospinal fluid (CSF) is abnormal in 45% of patients, showing an elevated white cell count, red cell count, or protein. Opening pressure is elevated above 200 mm Hg in approximately three fourths of the patients.

Key Laboratory Findings

- Hypercoagulability tests positive

- Elevated opening pressure with lumbar puncture

- Imaging findings not following an arterial distribution pattern

- MRI and venous MRA proving occlusion of intracranial venous vessels

Treatment

1. Effective anticoagulation, initially with heparin, later with warfarin, is the generally accepted treatment. It has been proven to be safe, even in the presence of multiple intracerebral hemorrhages. Although the degree of benefit is disputed, meta-analysis has shown anticoagulation to be superior to placebo.

2. Intra-arterial thrombolysis, sometimes combined with rheolytic thrombectomy, has been applied in several cases but needs further evaluation. In a few cases with massive CVT, decompressive craniectomy has been performed.

3. Seizures can be treated symptomatically with anti-epileptic drugs, but eliminating the cause by reopening the occluded vessel is best.

4. Autoimmune inflammatory diseases, tumors, or infections leading to CVT have to be treated appropriately.

5. Prognosis for patients with CVT, when treated before consciousness deteriorates, is excellent.

Key Treatment

- Anticoagulation agents (heparin followed by warfarin) are the mainstay of therapy.

Bibliography

Biousse V, Ameri A, Bousser MG: Isolated intracranial hypertension as the only sign of cerebral venous thrombosis. Neurology 53:1537–1542, 1999.

Bousser MG: Cerebral venous thrombosis: diagnosis and management. J Neurol 247:252–258, 2000.

de Bruijn SF, de Haan RJ, Stam J: Clinical features and prognostic factors of cerebral venous sinus thrombosis in a prospective series of 59 patients. For the Cerebral Venous Sinus Thrombosis Study Group. J Neurol Neurosurg Psychiatry 70:105–108, 2001.

de Bruijn SF, Stam J: Randomized, placebo-controlled trial of anticoagulant treatment with low-molecular-weight heparin for cerebral sinus thrombosis. Stroke 30:484–488, 1999.

Einhaupl KM, Villringer A, Meister W, et al.: Heparin treatment in sinus venous thrombosis. Lancet 338:597–600, 1991.

Teasdale E: Cerebral venous thrombosis: making the most of imaging. J R Soc Med 93:234–237, 2000.

Stroke in Pregnancy and the Postpartum Period

Marc Fisher
Erdem Orberk
Muhammad Ramzan

Etiology

1. The occurrence of an ischemic stroke, intracerebral hemorrhage, or cerebral venous sinus thrombosis during or shortly after pregnancy represents, by definition, a cerebrovascular event in a young, exclusively female patient. Many of the causes of cerebrovascular events temporally related to pregnancy are identical to those considered in all younger stroke patients. There are, however, a few unique etiologies during or shortly after pregnancy such as eclampsia, amniotic fluid embolism, and postpartum cerebral angiopathy, that must occasionally be considered. Additionally, pregnancy-associated hypercoagulability and hemodynamic changes should also be considered.

2. Epidemiology: A wide range of ischemic stroke rates during pregnancy and shortly after have been reported. In developed countries the risk approximates 4 to 8 per 100,000 deliveries. The risk of intracerebral hemorrhage is approximately the same. Cerebral venous thrombosis (CVT) is less well characterized, but appears to have a higher incidence, occurring in approximately 10 to 20 per 100,000 deliveries. In developing countries, the risk for all three types of cerebrovascular events appears to be substantially greater.

Ischemic Strokes

1. Pathophysiology: Hypercoagulability, cardiac emboli, vascular disorders (i.e., dissection, fibromuscular dysplasia, arteritis)

2. Symptoms: Based on location of ischemic injury (as described in Section 3, Neurovascular Disorders)

3. Clinical findings: Also reflect location of ischemic injury (as described in Section 3, Neurovascular Disorders)

4. Timing: Most occur during pregnancy or within 1 week of delivery

5. Laboratory testing: Brain imaging with computed tomography (CT) or magnetic resonance imaging (MRI) is mandatory. CT may be done during pregnancy with abdominal shielding. MRI and MR arteriography are also relatively safe. Transthoracic and transesophageal echocardiography can both be done safely. Blood tests should be performed to evaluate hypercoagulability. Specific consideration should be given to exclude an antiphospholipid antibody syndrome, deficiency of protein C, protein S, antithrombin III, and the Factor V Leiden mutation.

Key Tests

- CT during pregnancy with abdominal shielding
- MRI
- Transthoracic and transesophageal echocardiography

6. Differential diagnosis: In postpartum patients, exclude CVT: differential diagnostic considerations of arterial ischemic stroke as shown in Table 9–1

7. Treatment: Typical supportive measures as for stroke unrelated to pregnancy. Tissue plasminogen activator is probably contraindicated during and shortly after pregnancy. If anticoagulation is required, warfarin should not be used during pregnancy because of its teratogenic effects. Standard or low molecular weight heparin can be used. If antiplatelet therapy is warranted, low-dose aspirin (81 to 162 mg) is probably safe during the second and third trimesters. It is uncertain if clopidogrel or dipyridamole can be given safely during pregnancy. Postpartum, all of the commonly used antithrombotic agents are probably safe to employ.

Key Treatment

- Heparin (standard or low molecular weight) for anticoagulation
- Aspirin (81–162 mg) for antiplatelet therapy

TABLE 9–1. DIFFERENTIAL DIAGNOSIS OF ISCHEMIC STROKE DURING AND SHORTLY AFTER PREGNANCY

Cardioembolic Sources
Atrial fibrillation
Cardiomyopathy: specifically peripartum
Ischemic heart disease
Paradoxical embolus: patent foramen ovale, atrial septal defect
Rheumatic valvular disease
Prosthetic heart valve
Endocarditis
Cardiac tumor

Hematologic Disorders
Antiphospholipid antibody syndrome
Protein C, protein S, antithrombin III deficiency
Factor V Leiden mutation
Prothrombin mutation
Thrombotic thrombocytopenic purpura or disseminated
  intravascular coagulation

Cerebral or Extracerebral Vasculopathy
Dissection
Fibromuscular dysplasia
Vasculitis
Premature atherosclerosis, hemocysteinuria, familial dyslipidemia
Postpartum cerebral angiopathy
Eclampsia

Key Tests

• CT is the preferred imaging modality.

• MRA and/or standard angiograms when an aneurysm or arteriovenous malformation is suspected

6. Differential diagnosis: Is the hemorrhage parenchymal or subarachnoid? Is it related to eclampsia or a ruptured vascular malformation?

7. Treatment: Same as for parenchymal or subarachnoid hemorrhage in nonpregnant patients. Delivery may be affected and cesarean section should be considered if the hemorrhage occurs near the time of delivery.

Key Treatment

• Nonpregnant patients: Same as for parenchymal or subarachnoid hemorrhage

• Pregnant patients: Consider cesarean section if hemorrhage occurs near the time of delivery.

8. Follow-up: The same recommendations as in nonpregnant patients

Cerebral Venous Thrombosis

1. Pathophysiology: Must consider an underlying coagulopathy or venous anomaly

2. Symptoms: Similar to non-pregnancy-related CVT, i.e., headache, visual disturbance, and focal neurologic deficits. Seizures may be a manifestation.

Key Signs

• Headache

• Visual disturbance

• Focal neurologic deficits

• Seizures

3. Clinical findings: May be obscure. Papilledema with headache in the peripartum period is strongly suggestive of stroke. Venous infarcts may cause sensory or motor disturbances.

4. Timing: Typically occur in the second and third week postpartum, but may occur at the end of pregnancy or shortly after delivery

5. Laboratory testing: MRI and MR venography are very helpful. Occasional patients may require catheter angiography and venograms. CT may suggest diagnosis, i.e., high convexity hemorrhagic infarcts, delta sign.

8. Follow-up: Patients receiving heparin need careful monitoring to avoid excessive anticoagulation. Pregnancy-related stroke patients without an obvious cause should be periodically assessed to determine if the cause becomes apparent. Those receiving warfarin will need periodic international normalized ratio (INR) monitoring. It is unclear what the stroke risk may be in subsequent pregnancies, but it is likely higher in patients with an underlying coagulopathy.

Intracerebral Hemorrhage

1. Pathophysiology: May be related to the hypertensive crisis of eclampsia, rupture of an aneurysm, or vascular malformation

2. Symptoms: The same as in the nonpregnant patient: intracerebral hemorrhage; headache, focal neurologic deficits, nausea-vomiting, and depressed level of consciousness

3. Clinical findings: Reflect hematoma location, as in primary intracerebral hemorrhage

4. Timing: More likely at the end of pregnancy or early in the postpartum period

5. Laboratory testing: CT is preferred imaging modality, but susceptibility-weighted MRI also appears to accurately diagnose intracerebral hemorrhages. MR arteriography and/or standard angiograms are needed when an aneurysm or arteriovenous malformation is suspected.

6. Differential diagnosis: Other causes of headache (i.e., migraine, post lumbar puncture headache) or acute focal symptoms (arterial stroke).

7. Treatment: Heparin is widely recommended and used. Oral anticoagulation is then employed for several months, typically until the obstructed vein recanalizes. Oral anticoagulation may be continued indefinitely in patients with an underlying coagulopathy.

Key Treatment

• Heparin, then warfarin

8. Follow-up: Consider avoiding further pregnancies or use prophylactic anticoagulation with standard or low molecular weight heparin in CVT patients who become pregnant again.

Other Pregnancy-Specific Cerebrovascular Disorders

1. Eclampsia: Can occasionally be related to the development of diffuse cerebral edema. This can cause headache, visual blurring, focal neurologic deficits, impaired consciousness, and seizures. The edema is readily demonstrated on CT or MRI, and it is most common in the occipital and posterior-temporal regions. The pathogenesis is likely related to disruption of the blood–brain barrier. Early and rapid blood pressure lowering is mandatory. If increased intracranial pressure develops, hyperventilation and hyperosmotic agents are useful.

2. Postpartum cerebral angiopathy: A rare syndrome that typically presents with headaches, seizures, and focal neurologic signs. Angiography (standard or MRA) demonstrates multiple segmental narrowing. The etiology is uncertain, but the prognosis is favorable, as spontaneous recovery usually occurs. Therapy for headache and seizures is indicated. Some clinicians have tried steroids.

Bibliography

Digre KB, Varnum MW, Oswald AM, et al.: Cranial magnetic resonance imaging in severe pre-eclampsia vs eclampsia. Arch Neurol 1993;50:399–406.

Donaldson JO, Lee NS: Arterial and venous stroke associated with pregnancy. Neurologic Clinics. Neurologic Complications of Pregnancy. Philadelphia, W.B. Saunders, 1994, 583–599.

Mas JL, Lamy C: Stroke in pregnancy and the postpartum period. In Ginsburg MD, Bogousslavsky J (eds): Cerebrovascular Disease, Malden MA, Blackwell Science, 1998,1684–1697.

Shashan T, Lamy C, Mas JL: Incidence and causes of stroke associated with pregnancy and puerperium. Stroke 1995; 26:930–936.

Weibeir DO: Ischemic cerebrovascular complications of pregnancy. Arch Neurol 1985;42:1106–1113.

10 Neurorehabilitation

David S. Kushner

Introduction

1. Definition: Neurorehabilitation is a process that encompasses medical, physical, social, educational, and vocational interventions that can be provided in a variety of institutional and community settings to facilitate a person's functional recovery after the onset of disablement resulting from a neurologic disease.

2. Terms
   a. *Disablement* is described by the World Health Organization in terms of a conceptual model involving disease, impairment, disability, and handicap.
   b. *Disease* is an underlying condition or process that results in an impairment.
   c. *Impairment* is a partial or complete loss of physical or psychological capacity.
   d. *Disability* is the limitation an impairment places on a person's ability to perform a functional activity.
   e. *Handicap* is the social disadvantage that may result from disabilities that prevent a person from fulfilling his/her expected role in a society (handicap is influenced in a society by physical, social, and cultural barriers).

3. Neuropathology of disablement
   a. A neurologic disease may be static or progressive and can occur at any point during a person's lifetime. It can result from developmental, hereditary, infectious, autoimmune, metabolic, degenerative, vascular, neoplastic, or traumatic causes.
   b. Pathology involving any part of the nervous system from the central nervous system to the peripheral nervous system and muscle may result in neurologic impairments affecting strength, endurance, balance, coordination, mobility, cognition, perception, and emotion.
   c. Impairments may be partial or complete, and reversible or irreversible, depending on the pathologic process and the regions of the nervous system involved.
   d. Disabilities result from neurologic impairments affecting cognition, communication, the loss of mobility, the loss of the ability to perform basic self-care tasks (such as self-feeding, grooming, dressing, toileting, and bathing), and the loss of

the ability to perform the more complex tasks of independent living (such as banking, shopping, homemaking, working, and driving). (See Key Features.)

Key Features: Disabilities and Related Neurologic Impairments

Impaired Mobility/Self-Care
- Abnormal muscle strength/tone
- Loss of joint range of motion
- Psychomotor delay
- Abnormal muscle synergy/sequencing
- Abnormal coordination/balance
- Loss of endurance
- Sensory impairments/pain
- Abnormalities of cognition

Impaired Cognition
- Poor concentration/attention
- Disorientation
- Impaired memory, perception, executive function
- Fatigue/apathy/sedation
- Emotional dysfunction
- Distracters (pain, diplopia, anxiety, etc.)

Impaired Communication
- Aphasias
- Right-hemispheric language disorders
- Dysarthrias

4. Objectives of neurorehabilitation
   a. Functional disabilities are the focus of medical, physical, restorative, adaptive, environmental, and social interventions.
   b. Patient needs are matched with the capability of available programs.

5. Goals of neurorehabilitation include the prevention of secondary complications (such as pneumonia, contractures, or deep vein thrombosis); treatment to reduce neurologic impairments when possible; compensatory strategies for permanent

residual disability; patient/caretaker education; and interventions to promote the long-term maintenance of function.

6. Neurorehabilitation professionals include specialized physicians, nurses, therapists, psychologists, social workers, dieticians, and orthotists.

Assessment in Neurorehabilitation

1. Patient evaluation throughout the neurorehabilitation process involves physical examination and the use of well-validated standardized measurement instruments and scales that complement the physical examination in evaluating functional recovery; facilitate reliable documentation of functional disability severity; help to increase the consistency of treatment decisions; facilitate communication between therapists; and provide a reliable basis for monitoring progress.

2. Goals of patient assessment change over the clinical course of rehabilitation from the acute hospitalization, to the transfer to a rehabilitation program, to the transition back into the community.

3. Objectives of neurorehabilitation assessment during acute care include documentation of the diagnoses, the impairments, and the disabilities; identification of treatment needs; documentation of response to acute care interventions; determination of any changes in neurologic or medical status; identification of medically stable patients who will benefit from further rehabilitation; and determination of a setting for the post-acute rehabilitation process.

4. Upon admission to a neurorehabilitation program assessment is performed to develop a rehabilitation management plan with realistic goals and to document a baseline level of function for monitoring progress. Then weekly or bi-weekly evaluations allow progress to be monitored, treatment regimens to be adjusted, and discharge planning to be facilitated.

5. Objectives of assessment after discharge include evaluation of patient adjustment to the discharge setting; determination of further rehabilitation and medical needs; and assessment of caretaker burden and patient home management needs.

Neurorehabilitation During Acute Care

1. Priorities
   a. Neurorehabilitation interventions should begin during an acute hospitalization once a patient's condition has been stabilized and a diagnosis has been established.

   b. Acute care neurorehabilitation interventions include prevention of secondary complications; maintenance of homeostasis; promotion of early mobilization; and promotion of early return to self-care.

2. Prevention includes active interventions and regular patient monitoring for secondary complications of neurologic conditions that may include deep vein thrombosis and pulmonary embolism; skin breakdown; spasticity, joint contractures, and heterotropic ossification; pneumonia; falls, fractures and joint dislocations; known complications of specific neurologic disorders (i.e., dysautonomia in spinal cord injury and recurrent stroke in ischemic vascular disease); volume depletion and malnutrition; and orthostasis and syncope.

3. Maintenance of homeostasis involves routine monitoring of basic health functions and health indicators including vital signs, nutrition and hydration status, bladder and bowel function, sleep adequacy, and pain.

4. Early mobilization and return to self-care.
   a. Early patient mobilization helps to prevent deep vein thrombosis, skin breakdown, pneumonia, joint contractures, and constipation; and promotes early ambulation, orthostatic tolerance, and the return to self-care.

   b. Early participation in self-care increases strength, endurance, balance, coordination, awareness, communication, cognition, and social activity.

   c. Early mobilization is delayed or approached with caution in patients with coma, obtundation, evolving neurologic signs, intracranial hemorrhage, deep vein thrombosis, or persistent orthostasis.

   d. Early mobilization may be passive or active at first, depending on a patient's condition.

Determination of Rehabilitation Needs and Settings

1. Patient criteria for determination of neurorehabilitation services and settings include neurologic condition, extent of functional disabilities, medical comorbidities, the ability to tolerate physical activity, and the ability to learn.

2. Rehabilitation services after discharge from acute care can be provided at the rehabilitation unit of an acute care hospital, a free-standing inpatient rehabilitation hospital, a nursing home facility, the patient's home, or an outpatient rehabilitation facility.

3. Rehabilitation program criteria
   a. Threshold criteria for admission to any active

inpatient or outpatient rehabilitation program include medical stability, the ability to learn, and the endurance to sit supported for at least 1 hour per day.

b. Candidates for rehabilitation in a supported living setting or nursing facility do not meet criteria for active comprehensive rehabilitation programs.

c. Candidates for outpatient programs include patients with limited functional deficits of mobility or self-care.

d. Candidates for interdisciplinary inpatient rehabilitation include those who require total to moderate assistance with mobility or self-care tasks and those who can tolerate at least 3 hours of active daily therapy.

e. Patients with complex medical problems are candidates for inpatient rehabilitation programs with full-time medical supervision.

The Rehabilitation Management Plan

1. A patient management plan is formulated on admission to a neurorehabilitation program. It includes a clear description of patient impairments, disabilities, and strengths. Included are explicit short-term and long-term functional goals that should be realistic in terms of patient potential; overly modest goals can limit a patient's potential for recovery, and overly ambitious goals can set up the patient for failure. Treatment strategies are tailored to a patient's specific impairments and disabilities (Table 10–1).

2. The management plan is regularly reevaluated by the interdisciplinary rehabilitation team based on patient progress, and may be adjusted to suit patient needs and to facilitate discharge planning.

Discharge Follow-up

1. Goals of discharge follow-up include assessment of health status, safety at home and in the community, and maintenance of functional abilities. Areas of concern include medical, physical, cognitive, social, and emotional function.

2. Adequacy of family or caregiver interventions should be assessed. The full impact of a disability may first become apparent to the patient/family after discharge home. Changes in traditional family roles may have profound social and emotional consequences (support groups or psychotherapy may be useful in some circumstances).

3. Deterioration of functional abilities may result from exacerbation of co-morbid medical conditions, exacerbation of the neurologic disorder, or

from poor stimulation, poor self-confidence, or suppression of initiation by overprotective caregivers. The need for continued or additional rehabilitation services must be considered; goals may include the return to work or school.

4. Functional capacity assessments are available at most large rehabilitation programs to assist with decision making regarding a person's ability to return to driving a car or working at a particular vocation.

TABLE 10–1. KEY TREATMENTS

Management of Impaired Mobility
Remediation/facilitation: (volitional movement present)
  Traditional exercises
  Resistive training
  Forced sensory stimulation
Compensatory strategies: (volitional movement absent)
  Use of unaffected limbs
  Use of orthotics or braces
  Use of adaptive equipment
Task-specific retraining: (motor apraxias)
  Components of the above strategies
  Environmental cues to enhance performance
Pharmacologic interventions

Management of Impaired Cognition/Perception
Identify/treat causal factors (i.e., sedation)
Cognitive retraining
Substitution of intact abilities
Compensatory strategies
Pharmacologic interventions

Management of Communication Disorders
Aphasias
  Target problems of comprehension/expression
  Compensatory strategies
  Adjustment issues
  Caregiver/patient communication issues
Right-hemisphere language disorders
  Increase awareness of deficits
  Reinstate pragmatics of communication
  Compensatory strategies
Dysarthrias
  Oral motor exercises
  Manipulation of vocalization/articulation/respiration/prosody

Management of Emotional Dysfunction
Identify cause and treat
Psychotherapy
Maladaptive behavior modification
Pharmacologic intervention

Management of Pain
Identify cause and treat
Pharmacologic interventions
Physical interventions
Psychotherapy/biofeedback
Education

Bibliography

American Physical Therapy Association: Standards for tests and measurements in physical therapy practice. Phys Ther 71:589–622, 1991.

Gresham GE, Duncan PW, Stason WB, et al.: Poststroke rehabilitation: Clinical practice guideline. Rockville, MD, US Department of Health and Human Services (Agency for Healthcare Policy and Research), 1995.

Johnston MV, Kieth RA, Hinderer SR: Measurement standards for interdisciplinary medical rehabilitation. Arch Phys Med Rehabil 73 (suppl 12 S): S3-S23, 1992.

Kirby RL: Impairment, disability and handicap. In Delisa JA, Gans BM (eds): Rehabilitation Medicine Principles and Practice, 3rd ed. Philadelphia, Lippincott-Raven, 1998; pp. 55–60.

Kushner D: Principles of neurorehabilitation. In Weiner WJ, Goetz CG (eds): Neurology for the non-neurologist, 4th ed. Philadelphia, Lippincott Wiliams & Wilkins, 1999, pp. 453–466.

Stineman MG, Hamilton BB, Goin JE, Granger CV, et al.: Functional gain and length of stay for major rehabilitation impairment categories: Patterns revealed by function related groups. Am J Phys Med Rehabil 75:68–78, 1996.

1 Dementia Overview

David S. Geldmacher

Definition

1. Dementia is commonly defined as persistent (>6 to 12 months) impaired memory with a loss of other cognitive abilities or change in personality sufficiently severe to interfere with previously achieved levels of daily function.

   a. Formally, *dementia* is a description of a clinical state and does not imply cause or course. In common use, however, *dementia* is frequently used to describe the underlying brain disease as well as its clinical manifestation.

   b. Differentiating the clinical state of dementia from the causative dementing illness becomes important when planning treatment approaches.

      (1) Treatments might improve the symptoms but not affect the underlying disease process (e.g., cholinesterase inhibitors in Alzheimer's disease).

      (2) Similarly, some treatments alter progression of the dementia but do not affect the symptoms already present (e.g., secondary stroke prevention in vascular dementia).

2. Cognitive decline in late life has been recognized throughout history.

   a. *Senility* has long been a synonym for the loss of cognitive abilities in old age that we now call *dementia*. Senility, however, means only the state of being old and should no longer be used.

   b. Other synonyms for dementia have also been superseded and should not be used.

      (1) *Cerebral atherosclerosis* and its lay equivalent, "hardening of the arteries" should be avoided. These terms were based on the mistaken impression that cognitive impairment was due to a chronic state of oxygen starvation and brain hypoperfusion.

      (2) Another obsolete term for dementia is "organic brain syndrome." This diagnosis is important historically because it acknowledged that late-life dementia was of neurologic (organic) rather than psychiatric origin.

Epidemiology

1. There is wide variation in the incidence rates reported for dementia.

   a. Methodologic and cultural differences, as well as variability in diagnostic schema, account for more of the variation in reported incidence rates than intrinsic differences in the populations under study.

   b. At age 65, dementia incidence is about 0.5 new cases per 1000 population per year. It increases dramatically with age, reaching 65 to 100 new cases per 1000 population per year by age 90.

2. Broad measures of dementia prevalence in developed countries suggest an overall rate of 5% to 10% over age 65, but these figures do not account very well for mild cases that have not come to medical attention or formal diagnosis.

   a. One useful model is to consider dementia prevalence to be about 1% at age 60, and to double every 5 years.

   b. Prevalence of dementia may exceed 50% in people over the age of 90.

Clinical Features

1. Diagnostic criteria
   The American Academy of Neurology practice guidelines (Knopman et al, 2001) recommend the use of the DSM-III-R (American Psychiatric Association, 1987) criteria for diagnosing dementia.

   a. Impaired memory function is required.

      (1) It should represent a loss of abilities, rather than poor development or achievement.

      (2) Because of individual differences in life-long memory skills and achievements, there are no specific scores on tests like the Mini-Mental State examination for defining poor memory.

   b. In addition to poor memory, at least one other cognitive or behavioral change should be present, such as:

      (1) Poor abstract thinking

      (2) Impaired judgment evident in interpersonal, family, and job-related interactions

      (3) Disturbed higher cortical functions like

179

aphasia, apraxia, agnosia, or visuospatial problems

(4) Personality changes

c. These deficits must be sufficiently severe to interfere with usual activities and relationships (American Psychiatric Association, 1987).

2. Clinical approach

a. By definition, persons with dementia will forget things. Consequently, they are poor informants.

(1) It is therefore necessary to seek corroborating evidence from family members if dementia is suspected because of inconsistencies or vagueness in patient responses to questioning.

(2) Family members may also be poor at identifying changes in function as indicative of disease, instead suggesting depression or loss of physical capacity as the source of the complaints.

b. Identification of poor judgment or personality change generally requires questioning someone familiar with the patient, such as a spouse or child. This is best done away from the patient.

c. Bedside screening can assess for the key cognitive elements of the dementia criteria.

(1) Memory and abstract thinking may be screened with a simple question such as, "Can you tell me how you like to spend your free time?"

(2) Responding meaningfully to this question requires recall of broad categories of activity and the formulation of abstract categories.

(3) Memory can be assessed more directly.

(a) Memory questions should focus on what the patient has been following in the news or sports, i.e., items that the examiner can corroborate.

(b) Unverifiable information, such as what the patient ate for breakfast, is less useful because it is subject to confabulation.

(4) Focal cortical function can also be assessed directly.

(a) Ask the patient to name everyday items, especially parts of an item, e.g., jacket: lapel, pocket, sleeve.

(b) Ask the patient to draw a clock from memory, or copy a three-dimensional cube figure.

(c) Should these screening tests raise suspicions of clinically significant or functionally impairing cognitive deficits, then standardized instruments like the Mini-Mental State exam are useful for quantifying the deficit.

Key Signs

- Persistent decline from prior levels of mental ability

- Disordered memory

- At least one other deficit, such as

  - Poor abstract thinking

  - Reduced judgment

  - Focal cortical deficit

  - Personality change

- Deficits severe enough to interfere with normal daily function

- Deficits not resulting from acute illness (e.g., delirium)

Differential Diagnosis

More than 60 causes of dementia have been identified. Differentiation between primary neurologic causes is discussed in subsequent chapters in this section. However, it remains important to identify clinical states associated with cognitive impairment that may not meet full dementia criteria, or that arise from systemic conditions affecting the brain secondarily.

1. Cognitive changes with aging
There are losses in thinking and memory associated with the healthy aging process, sometimes known as "Aging-Associated Cognitive Decline" (AACD).

a. AACD typically involves reports of memory impairment accompanied by mild changes on objective memory testing and slowed information processing.

b. AACD typically includes insidious onset of cognitive decline with a duration of at least 6 months and impairment in memory, language, attention, concentration, thinking, or visual functioning.

c. Scores on standardized neuropsychological testing should be at least one standard deviation below age-corrected norms in at least one of these realms.

d. The impairment does not significantly reduce daily function, and it is generally not progressive.

e. Prevalence rates vary widely with the methods and criteria used to study the problem. About 25% of the older adult population has complaints consistent with AACD.

2. Mild cognitive impairment
A more ominous situation is the increasingly

recognized condition known as "Mild Cognitive Impairment" (MCI).

   a. Like AACD, the bedside findings are typically restricted to memory, but in MCI the deficits are clearly evident on bedside testing.

   b. MCI may represent a very early stage of dementia; about 50% of affected individuals will progress into dementia, usually Alzheimer's disease, over a 3-year period.

   c. Current practice guidelines suggest serial and systematic follow-up of these patients to determine whether the condition is progressing into Alzheimer's disease (Petersen et al., 2001)

3. Dementia vs depression
The differential diagnosis of degenerative dementia vs cognitive impairment resulting from depression can be problematic.

   a. In depression, the patient most often notices and complains about cognitive difficulties. In dementia (especially Alzheimer's disease), it is usually a relative who brings the patient to the physician because the patient has reduced awareness of illness.

   b. The duration of depression is shorter at the time care is sought, often weeks or a few months, and it typically has a more discrete onset than most causes of dementia.

   c. A personal or family history of depression also increases the likelihood of depression as a cause of cognitive difficulty.

   d. It is unusual for first-ever depression to present after the age of 60 in the absence of a clear precipitant like grieving.

   e. Confirming a low mood directly with the patient is important. Family members often report "depression" based on low activity levels or motivation related to dementia-induced apathy.

   f. Patients with depression typically demonstrate psychomotor slowing and produce incomplete answers with poor effort on testing (e.g., "I don't know").

   g. Even when a patient's cognitive function improves with treatment of depression, there is high risk for developing irreversible dementia over the next several years.

4. Dementia vs delirium

   a. Delirium is typically acute, reversible, and metabolically induced.

      (1) Fluctuating consciousness is the key clinical observation in delirium.

      (2) Focal neurologic causes are identified in less than 10% of delirium in older patients, leading many neurologists to use the term "metabolic encephalopathy" synonymously with delirium.

      (3) The distinction between delirium and dementia may be hindered by the fact that delirium is a common complication of chronic dementia.

   b. Frequent causes of delirium in the elderly are fluid and electrolyte derangement, cerebral hypoperfusion, pain, and infections.

   c. Medications are the most common cause of reversible cognitive impairment in late life, including delirium (see Section XXIV, Chapter 3, Cognitive Side Effects of Medications).

      (1) Consider alcohol and drug use (over-the-counter, prescriptive, and illicit) as potential contributors.

      (2) Unintended polypharmacy is common when a person receives care from multiple providers.

      (3) Anticholinergic drugs for gastrointestinal or genitourinary complaints are common contributors to reduced cognition.

      (4) Anxiolytics, sedative/hypnotics (including over-the-counter products), and low potency opioid analgesics like propoxyphene are frequently problematic.

PEARLS

Simple age-related memory deficits are distressing, but do not interfere with normal everyday function.

Mild cognitive impairment is often the prodrome of progressive dementia.

Drug effects and depression are the most common reversible causes of cognitive impairment suggesting dementia.

Low mood or low self-worth are typical when depression is the cause of cognitive decline.

Laboratory Evaluation

Recommendations for laboratory evaluation of dementia have been developed for the American Academy of Neurology (Knopman et al, 2001).

1. Blood studies should include chemistry panel, complete blood count, thyroid function, and vitamin B_{12} level.

2. All patients with suspected dementia should be evaluated for potential depression.

3. Other tests, such as electroencephalography and lumbar puncture should not be considered routine, although they may be useful in some clinical situations.

Key Tests: Blood Studies

- Chemistry panel

- Complete blood count

- Thyroid function

- Vitamin B$_{12}$ level

- Others, when clinically indicated (e.g., syphilis, serology, heavy metals, sedimentation rate)

Radiologic Features

1. Structural imaging with cranial computed tomography (CT) is useful to identify surgically correctable lesions causing dementia such as subdural hematoma, neoplasm, or hydrocephalus.

2. Caution must be exercised in interpreting nonspecific white matter changes on magnetic resonance imaging (MRI). There is an association between nonfocal white matter change and cognitive state on CT, but this is much less clear for MRI.

3. Imaging findings suggestive of ischemic change should not be a determining factor in treatment. Treatment for stroke risk factors should be initiated on clinical grounds alone.

Treatment

1. Therapy in dementia is based on the underlying cause and the symptoms expressed. There are no blanket therapies useful in all cases.

   a. If depression is suspected, therapeutic trials of serotonin selctive reuptake inhibitor antidepressants are warranted.

   b. If delirium is suspected, underlying causes should be treated.

2. Cognitive dysfunction in several forms of dementia has now been shown to respond to cholinesterase inhibitor drugs (e.g., donepezil, galantanine, rivastigmine).

3. Behavioral disturbances are common to many forms of dementia, and their expression is nonspecific. They are treated with conventional psychotropic agents, but these are most effective when combined with nonpharmacologic approaches and caregiver education.

   a. Antidepressants are effective for depressive symptoms and nonpsychotic agitation.

   b. Atypical antipsychotic agents (olanzepine, quetiapine, risperidone) are effective for psychosis with agitation.

   c. Chronic benzodiapine use is not recommended.

   d. Antiepileptic agents may be useful for chronic

suppression of nonpsychotic anger and agitation.

   e. The Alzheimer's Association (1-800-272-3900 or *www.alz.org*) is an important resource for caregiver education to reduce behavioral difficulties.

Key Treatment

- Therapy is based on the underlying cause and symptoms.

- Cholinesterase inhibitors

- Antidepressants

- Atypical antipsychotics such as olanzepine, quetiapine, risperidone

- Antiepileptics

Key Resource

- Alzheimer's Association (1-800-272-3900 or *www.alz.org*) for caregiver education

Prognosis and Prevention

Prognosis in dementia is determined solely by the underlying causes as described in subsequent chapters in this section. Likewise, for prevention see specifics later in this section.

Bibliography

American Psychiatric Association: Diagnostic and Statisical Manual for Mental Disorders (DSM-III-R), 3rd ed., revised. Washington, DC, American Psychiatric Association, 1987.

Costa PT Jr, Williams TF, Somerfeld M, et al.: Early Identification of Alzheimer's Disease and Related Dementias. Clinical Practice Guideline, Quick Reference Guide for Clinicians, No. 19. Rockville, MD: U.S. Department of Health and Human Services, Public Health Service, Agency for Health Care Policy Research AHCPR Publication No. 97-0703. November, 1996.

Doody RS, Stevens JC, Beck C, et al.: Practice parameter: management of dementia (an evidence-based review). Report of the Quality Standards Subcommittee of the American Academy of Neurology. Neurology 56:1154–1166, 2001.

Knopman DS, DeKosky ST, Cummings JL, et al.: Practice parameter: diagnosis of dementia (an evidence-based review). Report of the Quality Standards Subcommittee of the American Academy of Neurology. Neurology 56: 1143–1153, 2001.

Petersen RC, Stevens JC, Ganguli M, et al.: Practice parameter: early detection of dementia: mild cognitive impairment (an evidence-based review). Report of the Quality Standards Subcommittee of the American Academy of Neurology. Neurology 56:1133–1142, 2001.

2 Alzheimer's Disease

David S. Geldmacher

Definition

1. Alzheimer's disease (AD) is the prototypical and, by far, the most common form of dementia.
2. Clinically, it is characterized by a gradual decline in cognitive, social, or occupational function from a previously higher level. Short-term memory loss is the dominant feature reported by patients and families, though the actual cognitive deficits are far more pervasive.
3. Pathologically, AD is characterized by extracellular plaques of β-amyloid protein and intraneuronal accumulations of hyperphosphorylated *tau* protein, known as neurofibrillary tangles.
4. AD is a major public health problem. It is the third most expensive illness to the U.S. economy, with a total annual cost estimated at over $100 billion.

Epidemiology and Risk Factors

1. AD is the most common late life neurodegenerative disease, occurring approximately 10 times as frequently as Parkinson's disease. It occurs in all regions of the world and in all ethnic groups, although there is variability in its prevalence across groups.
   a. Alzheimer's disease, either alone or in combination with other pathologies, accounts for up to 90% of dementia cases in the United States.
   b. Incidence rates for AD increase with age from about 0.5% per year at age 60 to 65 years, to approach 10% per year by age 85 to 88 years.
   c. Epidemiologic estimates suggest 4 million cases of AD in the United States. The prevalence among people aged 65 or older is 8% to 10%. Above age 80, prevalence estimates range from about 30% to 45%.
   d. The number of AD cases is expected to triple over the next 50 years with the continued aging of the population.
2. Risk factors
   a. Increasing age is the principal risk factor for AD.
   b. Family history of dementia contributes to risk.
      (1) Most familial AD is not explained by known mutations.
         (a) Individuals with an affected first-degree relative, but not an autosomal dominant family history, have a two-

fold to fourfold increase in their age-adjusted risk for developing Alzheimer's disease.
         (b) An individual with two or more first-degree relatives affected with dementia has dramatically increased risk (10–40×)
      (2) About one half of early-onset familial AD is associated with autosomal dominant mutations on chromosomes 21, 14, or 1
      (3) Apolipoprotein-E (APOE) allelic variation modifies the risk for late-onset AD.
         (a) The ε4 allele confers increased risk in most populations and is associated with younger age at symptom onset
         (b) The ε2 allele is associated with reduced risk of AD
         (c) APOE testing is not sufficiently specific and sensitive to recommend for routine clinical use
   c. Other risk factors
      (1) Strongly supported
         (a) Female gender
         (b) Brain trauma
      (2) Less well supported
         (a) Low educational achievement
         (b) Cardiovascular disease and associated risks
         (c) Occupational heavy metal exposure
         (d) Less intellectually or physically active lifestyle
   d. Down syndrome
      (1) 100% of individuals with Down syndrome (DS) develop AD pathology by the fifth decade of life.
      (2) Family history of DS may be a risk factor for AD.

Risk Factors

- Age
- Family history of dementia
- Gender (female)
- Brain trauma
- Down syndrome

Etiology and Pathophysiology

The pathophysiologic basis for neuronal death in Alzheimer's disease is not known. Synaptic dysfunction and loss are the probable basis for the clinical signs, but the links between the pathological features and mechanism of neuronal failure are not well understood.

1. Pathological features
   a. Senile, neuritic, plaques are composed of neuronal and glial processes, as well as extracellular amyloid.
      (1) Plaques range in diameter from 15 μm to 100 μm, and are distributed throughout the cortex and hippocampus.
      (2) The primary component of plaques is aggregated β-amyloid protein. The β-peptide is derived from a larger protein known as *amyloid precursor protein* encoded on chromosome 21. The precursor protein undergoes proteolysis by normal constitutively expressed enzymes known as α-, β-, and γ-secretases.
      (3) The combined action of β- and γ-secretase creates the insoluble β-amyloid, which is deposited extracellularly in plaques.
      (4) Plaques appear normally in aging, but AD plaques are characterized by activation of macrophage-like microglial cells.
   b. Neurofibrillary tangles are intracellular collections of abnormal filaments, and they have a distinctive paired helical structure in Alzheimer disease.
      (1) Tangles accumulate throughout cortex, hippocampus, and subcortical nuclei with increasing AD severity.
      (2) Clinical AD severity correlates more closely with tangle density than with plaque burden.
   c. Neuronal loss in cortex and subcortical regions, granulovacuolar degeneration, and Hirano bodies are also found in AD brains.
2. Neurotransmitter changes are important in AD. There are losses of acetylcholine, monoamines (dopamine, norepinephrine), and intrinsic cortical neurotransmitters. These losses relate closely to the clinical expression of AD and provide targets for symptomatic drug therapies.

Clinical Features

1. Cognitive deficits
   a. Memory dysfunction is usually the first AD symptom recognized by clinicians.
      (1) The typical memory impairment in AD involves difficulties with learning new information, but memory for remote factual information is usually preserved until later in the course.
      (2) Loss of semantic knowledge, e.g., memory related to word meanings, is a pervasive but subtle early deficit.
      (3) Generic knowledge, such as how many days are in a year, begins to be lost early in the disease course.
      (4) Late-stage AD is associated with severe memory loss, extending to forgetting the names of children or spouse.
   b. Disorientation for time, then place, is universal as the disease progresses.
   c. Language disturbances are common, even early in the disease course
      (1) Anomia, or word-finding difficulty characterized by long pauses in speech is typical.
      (2) Speech patterns and vocabulary become simpler. Excessive use of pronouns and clichéd phrases is common.
   d. Apraxia most often develops later in the disease course and may result in loss of the ability to dress or use silverware. It can be an early sign in a small number of patients.
   e. Visual and spatial difficulties, like getting lost while driving and problems with reading or depth perception, are frequent, despite preserved visual acuity
   f. Problems with judgment, problem solving, planning, and abstract thought are common in early AD. These represent losses of mental executive function, but they are difficult for families to distinguish from pure memory loss.
2. Noncognitive symptoms
   a. Many patients with AD do not recognize that they are impaired. This can range from mild denial of functional impairment to complete anosognosia (unawareness of illness). In effect, the patients forget that they forget things. This makes them poor reporters of the medical history and current health status.
   b. Apathy is a lack of motivation or behavioral initiation that is not attributable to disordered consciousness or emotional distress. It is a pervasive problem throughout the course of AD, and is perhaps the most common adverse behavior in the illness, with prevalence rates estimated as high as ~90%.
   c. Passivity, withdrawal, as well as reduced affectionate behaviors and verbalizations are seen in a large proportion of patients with mild AD. Passive personality change often predates frank

dementia, but AD is not recognized until the full symptom pattern emerges.

d. Depressive symptoms occur in most AD patients, but major depression is rare. Depression does not tend to increase with disease severity. Anxiety is a common concomitant of depression in AD, occurring in up to 40% of patients

e. Psychosis and agitation are characteristic later in the disease course. Delusions affect up to 50% of patients, and hallucinations occur in about 25%.

f. Sleep disruptions are common, resulting from distorted circadian rhythms and exacerbated by lack of daytime mental and physical activity.

3. The general neurologic exam is nearly always normal early in the course. Parkinsonism may evolve in one third of patients late in the illness.

Key Signs

- Insidious onset
- Progressive decline
- Loss of daily functional ability (dysexecutive state)
- Memory/Learning deficits
- Vague, empty speech
- Preserved social skills early in course
- Usually poor insight into deficits

Differential Diagnosis

AD can be distinguished from other dementing disorders by clinical features and course.

1. If motor signs or gait disturbances are evident early in the course, consider cerebrovascular disease, dementia with Lewy bodies, progressive supranuclear palsy, corticobasal degeneration, or normal pressure hydrocephalus.

2. If social behavior is more impaired than cognitive ability, consider frontotemporal degeneration, e.g., Pick's disease.

3. If there is a rapid decline, i.e., evident within weeks, consider prion disease, uncontrolled cerebrovascular disease, or cerebral vasculitis.

4. Depression rarely leads to focal cognitive deficits like aphasia, apraxia, and agnosia. The depressed patient generally puts forth poor effort or cooperation on cognitive testing.

5. Drug effects are a common cause of cognitive difficulties among older adults.

6. Hypothyroidism and hyperthyroidism can lead to cognitive and behavioral changes that resemble

AD. Physical signs of thyroid dysfunction are usually present when thyroid abnormalities cause dementia-like symptoms.

7. Vitamin B_{12} deficiency is associated with dementia, but other neurologic abnormalities, specifically neuropathy or myelopathy, typically accompany the cognitive losses.

Laboratory Testing

1. AD is not associated with any abnormalities on routine laboratory testing.

2. Testing to exclude metabolic or nutritional causes of cognitive decline should include

a. Routine blood chemistry (electrolytes, glucose, and renal and liver function panels)

b. Complete blood count

c. Thyroid function tests

d. Vitamin B_{12} level

3. Genetic or other biomarker testing is not recommended for routine use. Testing for mutations in presenilin-1, presenilin-2, and amyloid precursor protein may be of value in cases associated with family history of early-onset AD following an autosomal dominant pattern. This should be accomplished only with appropriate genetic counseling.

Radiologic Features

There are no routine imaging findings specific for AD. Cerebral atrophy and ventricular enlargement are typical. Periventricular white matter change on CT or MR imaging does not exclude AD. Hippocampal complex atrophy is strongly associated with AD.

Treatment

Optimal management of AD includes both pharmacological and nonpharmacological approaches.

1. Drug treatment in AD is focused on three goals:

a. Improving or maintaining cognitive abilities

b. Reducing behavioral disturbances

c. Slowing neuronal loss

2. Acetylcholinesterase inhibitors (AChEI) are the mainstay of therapy.

a. AChEI provide meaningful benefit to patients and families:

(1) Improve or maintain cognitive status for about 1 year

(2) Maintain functional ability for about one year

(3) Delay emergence of, or improve, difficult behaviors

(4) Delay nursing home placement

b. Gastrointestinal side effects are most common with AChEI drugs, but they vary in frequency and severity across available agents. Currently marketed agents are not associated with hepatotoxicity.

3. Behavioral disturbances are treated with conventional psychotropic agents, but these are most effective when combined with nonpharmacological approaches and caregiver education.

a. Antidepressants are effective for depressive symptoms and nonpsychotic agitation. Anticholinergic antidepressants should generally be avoided.

b. Atypical antipsychotic agents (olanzepine, quetiapine, risperidone) are effective for psychosis with agitation.

c. Chronic benzodiapine use is not recommended.

d. Antiepileptic agents may be useful for chronic suppression of nonpsychotic anger and agitation.

e. The Alzheimer's Association (1-800-272-3900 or *www.alz.org*) is an important resource for caregiver education to reduce behavioral difficulties.

4. Vitamin E 2000 IU daily (usually dosed as 1000 IU twice a day) appears to delay the time to reach clinical end points such as nursing home placement, loss of basic activities of daily living, progression to severe AD, and death.

Key Treatment

Cholinesterase Inhibitors

• Donepezil 5–10 mg daily

  • Starting dose 5 mg daily

• Galantamine 8–12 mg twice a day

  • Starting dose 4 mg bid × 2 to 4 weeks

• Rivastigmine 3–6 mg twice a day

  • Starting dose 1.5 mg twice a day × 2–4 weeks

Note: Efficacy is similar across agents

• Vitamin E 2000 IU daily may delay progression of disease.

Antidepressants (for common behavioral symptoms)

• Serotonin reuptake inhibitors (e.g., sertraline, citalopram)

  • For depressive symptoms, anxiety, nonpsychotic agitation

• Trazodone 25–150 mg at bedtime

  • For sleep initiation and nocturnal agitation (sundowning)

Antipsychotics (for psychotic agitation; atypical antipsychotics are preferable)

• Olanzepine

  • 2.5–10 mg at bedtime

• Quetiapine

  • 25–100 mg daily, single or divided doses

• Risperidone

  • 0.25–3.0 mg daily, single or divided doses

Antiepileptics (for resistant, difficult behaviors; dosing titrated to efficacy or toxicity)

• Valproic acid

• Lamotrigine

Prognosis and Complications

AD invariably follows a progressive course.

1. Plateau periods, with temporarily slowed or arrested progression, are common.

2. Mean survival is about 8 years, but individual life expectancy varies widely.

3. Complications of other age-related illnesses and AD-related immobility and malnutrition are the most common causes of death.

Prevention

There are no known preventions for AD. Several potential protective factors have been identified.

1. Regular nonsteroidal anti-inflammatory drug use conveys a strong protective effect against AD.

2. Postmenopausal estrogen replacement therapy in women may have a protective effect.

3. The "statin" class of cholesterol-lowering drugs may provide a mild protective effect.

4. The risk–benefit ratio of these "protective" factors is not understood sufficiently to recommend their routine use. Clinical trials are planned, and some are under way to determine relative efficacy and safety.

5. Agents with protective effects may have no impact on cases with established clinical disease.

PEARLS

· Patients with true AD almost never spontaneously complain of memory loss.

· Insidious onset and progressive course of dementia is AD, unless

Motor signs are present early

· Consider vascular or parkinsonian disorders, normal pressure hydrocephalus

Daily behavior is worse than measured cognition

· Consider fronto-temporal dementia (Pick's disease), depression

Hallucinations are present with mild dementia

· Consider dementia with Lewy bodies

Course is very rapid (normal to debilitated over months)

· Consider Creutzfeldt-Jakob disease

· The presence of cerebrovascular disease does not imply the absence of Alzheimer's disease.

Bibliography

American Psychiatric Association: Practice guideline for treatment of patients with Alzheimer's disease and other dementias of late life. Am J Psychiatry 54(Suppl 5):1–39, 1997.

Doody RS, Stevens JC, Beck C, et al.: Practice parameter: management of dementia (an evidence-based review). Report of the Quality Standards Subcommittee of the American Academy of Neurology. Neurology 56:1154–1166, 2001.

Geldmacher DS: Contemporary diagnosis and management of Alzheimer's disease. 1st ed. Newtown, Pennsylvania, Handbooks in Health Care, 2001.

Knopman DS, DeKosky ST, Cummings JL, et al.: Practice parameter: diagnosis of dementia (an evidence-based review). Report of the Quality Standards Subcommittee of the American Academy of Neurology. Neurology 56: 1143–1153, 2001.

Small GW, Rabins PV, Barry PB, et al.: Diagnosis and treatment of Alzheimer disease and related disorders: consensus statement of the American Association of Geriatric Psychiatry, The Alzheimer's Association, and the American Geriatrics Society. JAMA 278:1363–1371, 1997.

3 Vascular Dementia

Ron Tintner

Definition

1. Vascular dementia (VaD) is cognitive impairment severe enough to disrupt daily life, which is attributable to cerebrovascular disease.

2. The diagnosis is made by establishing the presence of both these conditions and a causal link. Dementia is established by mental status or neuropsychological tests and a change in cognitive function by the history. Cerebrovascular disease is inferred from clinical and radiologic evidence of strokes, or the presence of peripheral cardiovascular disease.

3. VaD is not a unitary syndrome but consists of several subtypes, which can be grouped by their underlying pathology and clinical features.
   a. Multi-infarct dementia (involving both cortical and subcortical regions)
   b. Strategic single-infarct dementia
   c. Small-vessel disease with dementia
   d. Hypoperfusion
   e. Hemorrhagic dementia
   f. Combinations of the above lesions and other yet-unknown factors.

4. VaD is also part of a spectrum of vascular brain insult and thus co-exists with other signs of neurologic dysfunction. Cerebrovascular disease causes neurologic deficits or syndromes depending on the location of lesions.

5. Recently, the term *vascular cognitive impairment* (VCI) has been proposed to emphasize the concept that vascular disease may produce a range of cognitive deficits from mild to severe, and that early recognition of a deficit allows the clinician to intervene before the dementia occurs.

Clinical Features

1. Multi-infarct dementia (MID) can result in either a cortical or subcortical pattern of dementia, depending on the location of the lesions.
   a. Cortical lesions
      (1) Typical cognitive deficits include aphasia, agnosia, amnesia, apraxia, and neglect
      (2) Other cortical neurologic deficits are common, e.g. visual field loss, hemiparesis, hemihypaesthesia.
      (3) Presents more as obvious "multiple strokes"
      (4) Typically associated with
         (a) Large-vessel ischemic disease such as occlusions of main trunks or branches of anterior, middle, and posterior cerebral arteries
         (b) Cortical vascular malformations, usually resulting in hemorrhagic disease
         (c) Occlusion of the internal carotid and/or vertebral arteries, or the aorta, or global hypoxia/ischemia of arteries may cause watershed ischemia between major vascular territories resulting in cortical plus white matter infarctions with similar cognitive impairments.
   b. Multiple subcortical (lacunar) infarctions. This is the syndrome classically thought of as MID and described by Hachinski, Lassen, and Marshall (1974):

      Multiple small infarcts in association with hypertension is one of the commonest causes of vascular dementia. It is characterized by abrupt episodes, which lead to weakness, slowness, dysarthria, dysphagia, small-stepped gait, brisk reflexes and extensor plantar reflexes. All these signs are usually present by the time that mental deterioration occurs. Pathological laughing and crying are common.

      (1) The Hachinski ischemia score is a useful way to differentiate this type from degenerative dementias (primarily AD) (See Table 3–1).

2. Strategic infarct dementia
   Cases in which a single stroke presents with a clearly documented temporal relationship to the onset of dementia. The most common sites seen with this are the angular gyrus, thalamus, and deep subcortical white matter.

3. Small-vessel disease with dementia (chronic microvascular encephalopathy)
   a. The penetrating vessels of the subcortical white matter are vulnerable to pathological changes. These are long penetrating end arterioles, and their area of perfusion is then prone to ischemia, causing neurologic impairment, including cognitive, dysfunction, without frank infarction.
   b. The end product of this chronic ischemia is Binswanger's disease—a controversial en-

TABLE 3–1. HACHINSKI ISCHEMIA SCORE (HIS) AND MODIFIED ISCHEMIA SCORES (MIS)

FEATURE	HIS	MIS
Abrupt onset	2	2
Stepwise deterioration	1	1
Fluctuating course	2	
Nocturnal confusion	1	
Relative preservation of personality	1	1
Depression	1	
Somatic complaints	1	1
Emotional incontinence	1	1
History of hypertension	1	1
History of strokes	2	2
Evidence of associated atherosclerosis	1	
Focal neurologic symptoms	2	2
Focal neurologic signs	2	2
CT low density areas		
Isolated		
Multiple		
Maximum score	18	13
Vascular dementia	7–18	4–13
Degenerative dementia	0–4	0–3

tity—and the entity *senile dementia of the Binswanger type* has been proposed (see Table 3–2). Loeb (2000) has proposed that this is part of a spectrum of chronic microvascular leukoencephalopathy, which has several causes including cerebral autosomal dominant arteriopathy with subcortical infarct and leukoencephalopathy (CADASIL) (see below under Epidemiology and Risk Factors).

 Key Signs: Multi-Infarct Dementias

History

• Sudden onset of neurologic deficits, a stepwise deterioration, a fluctuating course, and hypertension

Examination

• Cognitive impairment—more executive dysfunction and functional problems in everyday activities than memory and language deficits

• Focal neurologic signs

• Slowness

• Small-stepped gait

Epidemiology and Risk Factors

1. VaD is widely reported to be the second leading cause of dementia, after AD, estimated to account for approximately 15% to 20% of cases of dementia, but there are conflicting studies about the prevalence of vascular dementia because of methodologic difficulties. In autopsy series from university centers, vascular dementia is very rare,

which may reflect an ascertainment bias. On the other hand, in Japan, China, and Russia vascular dementia may in fact be more common than Alzheimer's disease.

2. The prevalence of VaD doubles with every 5.3 years of age, and the estimated lifetime risk of VaD is 34.5% for men and 19.4% for women. In community-based studies, the incidence of VaD has ranged from 0.17 to 0.71 per 100 person-years.

3. Stroke is a major risk factor for VaD. After an acute stroke, dementia was diagnosed in over 25% of patients at 2 to 3 months, and the incidence of VaD was estimated to be 8.4 per 100 person-years. Therefore it is reasonable to expect that risk factors for stroke would also increase the risk of VaD.

4. Increasing size and number of strokes increases the risk of dementia. Prevention of further stroke with appropriate medical or surgical therapy is crucial, as evidence of a prior ischemic stroke on brain imaging has been associated with a ninefold increase in the development of dementia.

   a. It used to be claimed that MID required more than 100 ml tissue loss; less, if thalamus was involved. The issue of absolute volume of tissue loss requirement has been left unsettled.

5. Stroke location is a risk factor for VaD.

   a. Left hemisphere strokes are more likely than right to produce severe cognitive impairment

   b. Infarction of certain strategic areas may be crucial (e.g., deep frontal white matter, dominant thalamus, and angular gyrus).

   c. VaD may occur in the absence of strokes, and this is usually associated with periventricular white matter lesions or lacunes and silent infarcts

6. Risk factors for dementia

7. Age > 60

8. Hypertension

TABLE 3–2. CRITERIA FOR THE CLINICAL DIAGNOSIS OF SENILE DEMENTIA OF THE BINSWANGER'S TYPE

1. Dementia confirmed by clinical examination
2. At least two of the following must be present:
   a. Hypertension or known systemic vascular disease (for example, coronary artery disease, peripheral vascular disease)
   b. Evidence of cerebrovascular disease (for example, stroke)
   c. Subcortical brain dysfunction (for example, abnormal gait, muscular rigidity, neurogenic bladder)
3. Bilateral subcortical leukoaraiosis (attenuation of white matter) on CT or MRI
NOTE: Criteria are not valid if: Multiple cortical lesions on CT or MRI or severe dementia (MMSE score <10).

From Bennett DA, Wilson RS, Gilley DW, Fox JH: Clinical diagnosis of Binswanger's disease. J Neurol Neurosurg Psychiatry 53:961–965, 1990.

9. Risk factors for stroke (not shown directly for VaD)

   a. Hypercholesterolemia

   b. Race/ethnicity—Asian, African American

   c. Sex—male

   d. Coronary artery disease

   e. Diabetes mellitus

   f. Cigarette smoking

   g. Fibrinogen, obesity

   h. Other cardiovascular disease

      (1) Atrial fibrillation

      (2) Valvular heart disease, including mitral valve prolapse

      (3) Peripheral vascular disease

   i. Genetics—rare; e.g., CADASIL

Etiology and Pathophysiology

1. Vascular pathology (varied)

   a. Atherosclerosis

   b. Arteriosclerosis

   c. Lipohyalinosis

   d. Amyloid angiopathy

   e. Senile arteriolar sclerosis

   f. Other angiopathies (arteiovenous malformations, cavernous angiomas, aneurysms)

2. Systemic causes of thromboembolism

3. Inflammatory diseases (e.g., systemic lupus erythematosus, polyarteritis nodosa, sarcoidosis)

4. Hyperviscosity syndromes (e.g., polycythemia vera, sickle cell anemia)

5. Embolic disorders (e.g., atrial fibrillation, myocardial infarction with mural thrombus, congenital heart disease, as well as septic, air, or fat emboli).

6. Concomitant Alzheimer-type changes

   a. 10% to 20% of patients with dementia are classified clinically and pathologically as having both AD and VaD.

   b. VaD is known to promote the clinical expression of AD.

Differential Diagnosis: The Problem of Diagnosis of VaD

1. There are two common diagnostic scenarios:

   a. The patient who comes with dementia or cognitive decline, without an obvious source, and some evidence of vascular disease

   b. The patient with prominent vascular disease, who becomes demented, and the question becomes, "is there another explanation?"

2. In practical clinical terms, the diagnostic issue is trying to determine the existence and severity of the cerebrovascular disease and whether this is causally related to the cognitive decline. Numerous criteria for VaD have been established. A recent, relatively well-accepted set, which has greater than 90% specificity, is from NINDS-AIREN (see Table 3–3).

3. Mixed dementia, which is combined vascular and Alzheimer's dementia, is very difficult to differentiate from vascular dementia.

4. Deficits in several domains of cognitive function constitute dementia, but patterns of dysfunction can be highly variable. Because of this variability a reliance on memory problems or the Mini-Mental State Exam can be insensitive. In the early stages of dementia there is much less involvement of memory in vascular dementia than in Alzheimer's disease, but there is more executive dysfunction.

5. The differential diagnosis consists primarily of the same entities that cause dementia, primarily degenerative disease. Care must be taken to ensure that the dementia is not merely concomitant with mild cerebrovascular disease (i.e., not causally related) so as not to miss the opportunity to uncover the true cause, which may be reversible.

6. Dementia with Lewy bodies, which is associated with transient alterations of consciousness, is often mistaken for vascular dementia.

Laboratory Testing

1. Complete blood count

2. Glucose

3. Serum lipid profile

4. Erythrocyte sedimentation rate, antinuclear antibodies, and tests for collagen-vascular disease

5. Specific treponemal antibody test (for syphilis)

6. Vitamin B_{12} level

7. Thyroid function tests

8. Hemoglobin A1c

9. Carotid ultrasound

10. Echocardiography

Radiologic Features

1. Site

   a. Large-vessel strokes in several areas

      (1) Bilateral anterior cerebral artery

      (2) Posterior cerebral artery

      (3) Parietotemporal and temporo-occipital association areas

TABLE 3–3. CRITERIA FOR PROBABLE VASCULAR DEMENTIA ACCORDING TO NINDS-AIREN CRITERIA

I. Criteria for the clinical diagnosis of PROBABLE vascular dementia include *all* of the following:

1. *Dementia* defined by cognitive decline from a previously higher level of functioning and manifested by impairment of memory and of two or more cognitive domains (orientation, attention, language, visuospatial functions, executive functions, motor control, and praxis), preferably established by clinical examination and documented by neuropsychological testing; deficits should be severe enough to interfere with activities of daily living not due to physical effects of stroke alone.

   Exclusion criteria: cases with disturbance of consciousness, delirium, psychosis, severe aphasia, or major sensorimotor impairment precluding neuropsychological testing. Also excluded are systemic disorders or other brain diseases (such as AD) that in and of themselves could account for deficits in memory and cognition.

2. *Cerebrovascular disease*, defined by the presence of focal signs on neurologic examination, such as hemiparesis, lower facial weakness, Babinski's sign, sensory deficit, hemianopia, and dysarthria consistent with stroke (with or without history of stroke), and evidence of relevant CVD by brain imaging (CT or MRI) *including multiple large-vessel infarcts or a single strategically placed infarct* (angular gyrus, thalamus, basal forebrain, or PCA or ACA territories), as well as *multiple basal ganglia and white matter lacunes* or *extensive periventricular white matter lesions,* or combinations thereof.

3. A *relationship between the above two disorders,* manifested or inferred by the presence of one or more of the following: (a) onset of dementia within 3 months of a recognized stroke; (b) abrupt deterioration in cognitive functions; or fluctuating, stepwise progression of cognitive deficits.

II. Clinical features consistent with the diagnosis of PROBABLE vascular dementia include the following:

1. Early presence of a gait disturbance (small-step gait or marche à petits pas, or magnetic, apraxic-ataxic or parkinsonian gait)
2. History of unsteadiness and frequent, unprovoked falls
3. Early urinary frequency, urgency, and other urinary symptoms not explained by urologic disease
4. Pseudobulbar palsy
5. Personality and mood changes, abulia, depression, emotional incontinence, or other subcortical deficits including psychomotor retardation and abnormal executive function

III. Features that make the diagnosis of vascular dementia uncertain or unlikely include

1. Early onset of memory deficit and progressive worsening of memory and other cognitive functions such as language (transcortical sensory aphasia), motor skills (apraxia), and perception (agnosia), in the absence of corresponding focal lesions on brain imaging
2. Absence of focal neurologic signs, other than cognitive disturbance; and absence of cerebrovascular lesions on brain CT or MRI

From Roman GC, Tatemichi TK, Erkinjuntti T, et al.: Vascular dementia: diagnostic criteria for research studies. Report of the NINDS-AIREN International Workshop. Neurology 43, 250–260, 1993.

(4) Superior frontal and parietal watershed territories

b. Small-vessel disease

(1) Basal ganglia and frontal white matter lacunes

(2) Extensive periventricular white matter lesions

(3) Bilateral thalamic lesions

2. Severity

a. Large-vessel lesions of the dominant hemisphere

b. Bilateral large-vessel hemispheric strokes

c. Leukoencephalopathy involving at least 25% of the total white matter

d. Also called *leukoaraiosis* (Greek: *leuko* = white, *araiosis* = rarefaction), seen as increased white matter signal (magnetic resonance imaging—MRI)/attenuation (computed tomography—CT).

 Key Radiologic Findings

- Multiple large-vessel infarcts
- **or** a single strategically placed infarct (angular gyrus, thalamus, basal forebrain, or posterior cerebral artery or anterior cerebral artery territories)
- **or** multiple basal ganglia and white matter lacunes
- **or** extensive periventricular white matter lesions
- **or** combinations thereof

Treatment

1. The goal is prevention—i.e., preventing progression of the underlying disorders causing vascular disease.

   a. Anti-platelet agents

   b. Statins

   c. Blood pressure control (Be careful not to cause hypotension in patients already manifesting VaD, as this may worsen symptoms.)

   d. Carotid endarterectomy for greater than 70% stenosis

   e. Normoglycemia

   f. Warfarin for atrial fibrillation

2. Anticholinesterases may improve dementia in isolated vascular dementia.

3. Behavioral abnormalities. Depression is common and responds to treatment with usual antidepressants (e.g., selective serotonin release inhibitors, tricyclic antidepressants)

Key Treatment

- Treat underlying vascular risk factors.
  - Blood pressure control (but avoid hypotension)
  - Statins (3-hydroxy-3-methylglutaryl coenzyme A reductase inhibitors)
  - Normoglycemia
  - Warfarin for atrial fibrillation
  - Carotid endarterectomy
- Treat depression if present.
- Anticholinesterases if patient has Alzheimer's disease

Prognosis and Complications

1. Prognosis for patients with vascular dementia is worse overall than that for AD patients: the 3-year mortality rate in patients over the age of 85 years is quoted at 67%, as compared to 42% in AD, and 23% in non-demented individuals.

2. Outcome is ultimately dependent, however, on the underlying risk factors and mechanism of disease, and further studies taking these distinctions into account are warranted.

3. The cognitive disorder is not necessarily a relentless progressive course, as in AD, because VaD may have a stable, ameliorating, or progressive course.

Prevention

Prevention involves those medicine and lifestyle changes that prevent cerebrovascular disease, especially lowering blood pressure.

Bibliography

Chui HC: Dementia due to subcortical ischemic vascular disease. Clinical cornerstone 3; 40–51, 2001.

Chui HC, Wendy W, Jackson JE, et al.: Clinical criteria for the diagnosis of vascular dementia. A multicenter study of comparability and interrater reliability. Arch Neurol 57: 191–196, 2000.

Erkinjuntti T, Kurz A, Gauthier, et al.: Efficacy of galantamine in probable vascular dementia and Alzheimer's disease combined with cerebrovascular disease: a randomised trial. Lancet 359:1283–1290, 2002.

Hachinski V, Lassen N, Marshall J: Multi-infarct dementia. A cause of deterioration in the elderly. Lancet 2:207–210, 1974.

Loeb C: Binswanger's disease is not a single entity. Neurol Sci 21:343–348, 2000.

McPherson S, Cummings J: Neuropsychological aspects of vascular dementia. Brain and cognition 31:269–282, 1996.

4 Subcortical Dementia

Ron Tintner

Definition

1. Subcortical dementia (SD) is a syndrome associated with a characteristic pattern of neuropsychological deficits typically seen with subcortical lesions.

2. The typical neuropsychological pattern of subcortical dementia was defined by Albert et al. (1974) as an association of some form of memory defect, a general slowing of intellectual activity, alterations of personality, and impaired ability to manipulate acquired knowledge in patients with progressive supranuclear palsy (PSP).

3. This neurobehavioral pattern includes
   a. "Forgetfulness" due to memory disturbances involving deficits of retrieval more than encoding
   b. Slowed thought processes (bradyphrenia)
   c. Disturbance of mood and affect, especially apathy, depression, and irritability
   d. Visuospatial abnormalities
   e. Executive control dysfunction: Problems with planning, organizing, sequencing, and abstracting.
      (1) Difficulty with complex intellectual tasks such as strategy generation and problem solving
      (2) Impaired ability to manipulate acquired knowledge
   f. Motor system abnormalities are also frequently seen, which are usually not apparent in the cortical dementias

4. The syndrome of SD can be produced by a variety of underlying disorders with diverse pathology (see below).

5. The usefulness in differentiating a cortical pattern from subcortical pattern is in working through the differential diagnosis. Most reversible dementias are subcortical.

Epidemiology and Risk Factors

1. Subcortical, or mixed cortical–subcortical dementias account for 35% to 50% of patients with dementia, depending on the nature of the epidemiologic study.

2. The most common SD is due to vascular disease and may represent up to 30% of patients with dementia.

3. Dementia with Lewy bodies is a mixed cortical–subcortical form that may represent up to 10% of patients with dementia.

Etiology and Pathophysiology

1. This pattern is seen with pathological involvement of subcortical structures, such as the basal ganglia (particularly the striatum), brainstem, thalamus, and central white matter; however, these subcortical structures are closely linked with the frontal cortex, and lesions of this cortical area can also produce this syndrome.

2. The term *subcortical* is controversial because the classic cortical dementias have been shown to involve subcortical structures pathologically, and, at the same time, most subcortical dementias have at least secondary metabolic effects on the cortex.

3. The term *cortical dementia* has really been used to differentiate dementias that affect principally "higher cortical functions"; practically speaking,
   a. Aphasia, apraxia, agnosia, in the case of posterior cortical dementias (primarily Alzheimer's disease)
   b. Behavioral disinhibition, apathy, or muteness, in the case of the anterior cortical dementias (primarily frontotemporal dementia)
   c. In these disorders, the fundamental neurologic exam (i.e. cranial nerves, motor system, sensory, coordination, gait and station, reflexes) is normal.

Clinical Features (see Table 4–1)

1. Neuropsychological abnormalities
   a. The Mini-Mental State Exam is relatively insensitive to the deficits of SD; the Mattis Dementia Rating scale is much more sensitive.
   b. Typical abnormalities are seen in tests often called "frontal lobe" tests.
      (1) Tower of London
      (2) Stroop Intereference Test
      (3) Wisconsin Card Sorting Test
      (4) Trail Making Test
      (5) Verbal fluency (letter > category)

193

TABLE 4–1. CLINICAL CHARACTERISTICS OF CORTICAL AND SUBCORTICAL DEMENTIAS

CHARACTERISTIC	CORTICAL	SUBCORTICAL
Verbal output		
Language	Aphasic	Normal
Speech	Normal	Abnormal (hypophonic, dysarthric, mute)
Mental status		
Memory	Amnesia (learning deficit)	Forgetful (retrieval deficit)
Cognition	Abnormal (acalculia, poor judgment, impaired abstraction)	Abnormal (slowed, dilapidated)
Visuospatial	Abnormal	Abnormal
Affect	Abnormal (unconcerned or disinhibited)	Abnormal (apathetic or depressed)
Motor system		
Posture	Normal	Abnormal
Tone	Normal	Usually increased
Movements	Normal	Abnormal (tremor, chorea, asterixis, dystonia)
Gait	Normal	Abnormal

    c. Short-term memory recall is impaired, but it is markedly aided by cueing.

Key Signs: Subcortical Dementia

- Apathy, withdrawal
- Decreased executive control functions
- Memory impairment improved with cueing
- Mental slowness (bradyphrenia)
- Gait abnormalities

    d. Three brief tests are sensitive to the deficits found in SD and are easily administered at the bedside.
       (1) Addenbrooke's Cognitive Evaluation (ACE) (Mathuranath, 2000)
       (2) Frontal Assessment Battery (FAB)
       (3) CLOX executive clock-drawing task

Key Tests: Subcortical Dementia

- Addenbrooke's Cognitive Evaluation
- Frontal Assessment Battery
- CLOX executive clock-drawing task

  2. Neurologic examination reveals slow gait, bradykinesia, rigidity, and increased and primitive reflexes

  3. Frontal cortical dementias can have similar neuropsychological findings, but the neurologic exam (other than the mental status examination) is usually normal.

Key Radiologic Findings: Subcortical Dementia

- Magnetic resonance imaging (MRI) and computed tomography (CT): Vary in different entities
- All patients tend to have relatively decreased frontal cortex metabolism/cerebral blood flow on positron emission tomography/single photon emission CT (PET/SPECT)

DIFFERENTIAL DIAGNOSIS

See also Table 4–2 and refer to specific chapters in this volume.

Parkinson's Disease (PD)

Clinical

  1. The characteristic motor findings are (asymmetric) rest tremor, rigidity, and bradykinesia. Balance and autonomic dysfunction generally deteriorate after several years.

TABLE 4–2. CLASSIFICATION OF DEMENTIA BASED ON CORTICAL OR SUBCORTICAL DYSFUNCTION

Cortical Dementias	Dementias with Combined Cortical and Subcortical Dysfunction
Alzheimer's disease	Multi-infarct dementias
Frontal temporal dementias	Prion diseases
Pick's disease (frontotemporal variant)	Syphilis (general paresis)
Semantic dementia (temporal variant)	Toxic/metabolic encephalopathies
Progressive nonfluent aphasia	Systemic illnesses
	Endocrinopathies
Subcortical Dementias	Deficiency states (vitamin B_{12})
Dementia with parkinsonism	Drug intoxications
Parkinson's disease	Heavy metal exposure
Huntington's disease	Industrial dementias
Progressive supranuclear palsy	Miscellaneous dementia syndromes
Multiple system atrophies	Posttraumatic
Neurodegeneration with brain iron accumulation	Postanoxic
Hydrocephalus	Neoplastic
Dementia syndrome of depression	Mass lesions
White matter diseases	Paraneoplastic
Multiple sclerosis	Corticobasal degeneration
HIV encephalopathy	Dementia with Lewy bodies
Vascular dementias	
Subcortical ischemic vascular disease	
Lacunar state	
Binswanger's disease	
CADASIL	
Radiation-induced leukoencephalopathy	

Abbreviations: HIV = human immunodeficiency virus; CADASIL = cerebral autosomal dominant arteriopathy with subcortical infarcts and leukoencephalopathy.

2. Dementia occurs late (up to 1 to 3 years after onset of motor symptoms). The earliest cognitive dysfunction is diminished verbal fluency and set-shifting.

3. True dementia is rare in younger PD patients, but is common in the elderly.

4. If dementia is marked early in the course of PD, the diagnosis is more likely dementia with Lewy bodies or Alzheimer's disease (AD) with PD.

Key Signs: Parkinson's Disease

- (Asymmetric) rest tremor

- Rigidity

- Bradykinesia

- Balance and autonomic dysfunction generally occur after several years.

Imaging

1. Normal CT/MRI

2. (Putamen > caudate) decreased striatal uptake of dopamine transporter ligands and dopamine precursors

Treatment

1. L-DOPA and dopamine agonists help motor dysfunction but not cognitive dysfunction; these agents as well as amantadine and anticholinergics may worsen hallucinations.

2. Anticholinesterases may help cognition.

Key Treatment: Parkinson's Disease

- L-DOPA and dopamine agonists for motor functions

- Anticholinesterases for cognition

Dementia with Lewy Bodies

Clinical Features

1. Dementia, visual hallucinations, fluctuations of consciousness, parkinsonism (with less rest tremor), REM behavior disorder. Very sensitive to neuroleptic extrapyramidal symptoms.

2. Dementia occurs early (prior to or < 1 year after onset of motor symptoms). Visuospatial abnormalities are prominent.

3. Pathology
   a. Lewy bodies in cortex, limbic system; more variably in substantia nigra and autonomic system

b. Half also have pathologic changes of AD (plaques > tangles).

c. More severe cortical cholinergic loss than AD.

4. Controversial entity: One form of PD? Mixed PD and AD?

Key Signs: Dementia and Lewy Bodies

- Dementia

- Visual hallucinations

- Fluctuations of consciousness

- Parkinsonism (with less rest tremor)

- Recent event memory behavior disorder

Imaging

1. As for PD, except some patients have mild temporal lobe atrophy

2. Decreased occipital uptake on metabolic/regional cerebral blood flow PET/SPECT

Treatment

1. Dementia may respond to anticholinesterases.

2. Avoid neuroleptic antipsychotics if possible; clozaril best for psychosis

3. Parkinsonism responds to dopaminergic agents, but with a high risk of hallucinations.

Key Treatment: Dementia with Lewy Bodies

- Anticholinesterases for dementia

- Clozaril for psychosis

- Dopaminergic agents for parkinsonism

Progressive Supranuclear Palsy (PSP)

Clinical Features and Imaging

1. Early balance problems; axial > limb rigidity; very early balance problems; supranuclear gaze dysfunction (especially vertical)

2. The pattern of cognitive deficits in PSP consists of slowing of thought processes and impaired executive functions, with preservation of instrumental activities. Generally speaking, the dysexecutive syndrome of PSP is much more severe than that observed in other subcortical disorders, and the memory deficit is dramatically improved, or even normalized, in conditions that facilitate retrieval processing such as cued recall and recognition.

3. Imaging studies reveal midbrain atrophy.

Key Signs: PSP

- Axial > limb rigidity
- Supranuclear gaze dysfunction (especially vertical)
- Slowing of thought processes and impaired executive functions

Treatment

L-DOPA sometimes helps motor dysfunction; no treatment for dementia.

Key Treatment: PSP

- L-DOPA sometimes helps motor dysfunction.
- No treatment for dementia

Corticobasal Degeneration (CBD)

Clinical Features and Imaging

1. CBD is a mixed cortical-subcortical pattern of cognitive dysfunction.
2. Typically defined by unilateral rigidity of one arm with apraxic disorders. In addition, dysarthric disorders, speech apraxia, increased and primitive reflexes, and alien limb phenomeon.

Key Signs: PSP

- Unilateral rigidity of one arm with apraxic disorders

3. Imaging: CT/MRI show parietal atrophy

Multiple System Atrophy (MSA)

Clinical Features and Imaging

1. There are three types of MSA: Parkinsonism with akinesia, rigidity, early balance and voice problems, anterocollis (striatonigral degeration), dysautonomia (Shy-Drager syndrome) or ataxia olivopontocerebellar atrophy (OPCA)
2. Cognitive problems are usually very mild, but with a subcortical pattern

Key Signs: Multiple System Atrophy

- Three types
  - Parkinsonism with akinesia, rigidity, early balance and voice problems
  - Anterocollis (striatonigral degeration)
    - Dysautonomia (Shy-Drager syndrome) or ataxia olivopontocerebellar atrophy (OPCA)
- Mild cognitive problems of subcortical pattern

3. Imaging: Increased signal on T2-weighted MRI ("hot cross bun" sign)

Huntington's Disease

Clinical Features

1. Cognitive changes occur early in the course of the disease—even before the choreic movements in some cases—and are consistently found with the passage of time.
2. The cognitive changes consist of disorders of memory and executive functions; however, visuospatial perception is unusual in that there is poor right-left personal orientation or performance on a road-map test but constructional skills are relatively normal.
3. Cognitive changes more apparent in patients with bradykinesia.
4. Psychiatric symptoms are also characteristic of the disease.
   a. Irritability and apathy, anxiety, depression, peculiarities of thought, and interpersonal difficulties
   b. Schizophreniform disorders with persecutory delusions and auditory or visual hallucinations (rarely)
5. Neurologic exam: Chorea, saccadic slowing, increased reflexes

Key Signs and Symptoms: Huntington's Disease

- Disorders of memory and executive functions
- Psychiatric symptoms:
  - Irritability and apathy, anxiety, depression, peculiarities of thought, and interpersonal difficulties
  - Schizophreniform disorders
- Neurologic exam
  - Chorea, saccadic slowing, increased reflexes

Imaging and Laboratory Studies

1. Caudate atrophy on CT/MRI
2. Decreased striatal metabolism
3. Key lab study: Increased (>39) CAG repeats in *huntingtin* gene.

Prognosis and Treatment

1. Progressive downhill course: Disease duration is 15 to 30 years
2. Depression responds to selective serotonin re-uptake inhibitors (SSRIs)
3. Delusions and chorea respond to antipsychotics.

Key Treatment and Prognosis: Huntington's Disease

- SSRIs for depression
- Antipsychotics for delusions and chorea
- Disease gets progressively worse
- Disease duration is 15 to 30 years.

SUBCORTICAL VASCULAR ISCHEMIC SYNDROMES (CHRONIC MICROVASCULAR LEUKOENCEPHALOPATHIES)

Multiple Sclerosis

Clinical Features

1. Cognitive impairment occurs in 40% to 60% of MS patients; severe in some. Subtle abnormalities may already be present in those with clinically isolated syndromes, but impairment tends to be more severe as the disease progresses.
2. Difficulties with memory, information processing, and executive functions are frequent.

Key Signs: MS

- Cognitive impairment (40% to 60% of patients)
- Difficulties with memory, information processing, and executive functions

Imaging
Loss of brain parenchyma (atrophy) predicts cognitive decline better than other MRI indices (T2 lesion load).

Prognosis and Treatment

1. Cognitive deterioration is not universal in the early stages of the disease; over two thirds remain stable or improved over a 2 year period.
2. Immunotherapy reduces cognitive decline.
3. There is some evidence that anticholinesterases are helpful in improving cognition.

Key Treatment: MS

- Immunotherapy for cognitive decline
- Anticholinesterases may improve cognition.

Normal Pressure Hydrocephalus

Clinical Features

1. Gait disturbance early; disinhibited urinary detrusor reflex causing urgency and possibly incontinence
2. Cognitive decline in subcortical pattern with true dementia late.

Key Signs: Normal Pressure Hydrocephalus

- Early gait disturbance
- Disinhibited urinary detrusor reflex causing urgency and, possibly, incontinence
- Cognitive decline in subcortical pattern with true dementia late

Etiology

1. About half idiopathic
2. Others associated with subarachnoid hemorrhage, head trauma, infection, etc.

Imaging

1. Ventriculomegaly
2. Other findings: Cerebrospinal fluid (CSF) flow void, periventricular attenuation, decreased isotope disposition on radioisotope cisternogram, variably and not necessarily predictive of shunt response

Treatment and Prognosis

1. If there is a known cause for the hydrocephalus, about 90% improve with shunt; if not, about 60%.
2. Shunt has a 40% overall complication rate (shunt failure, infection, "shunt ventricles," intracerebral bleeds)
3. Gait usually responds well to shunt; dementia is poorly responsive
4. Improvement with "CSF tap test," large-volume lumbar puncture (~50 ml) is strongly predictive of shunt response.
5. Other CSF tests, capacitance, continuous CSF pressure monitoring are only available in more specialized centers and are more controversial.

Key Treatment: Normal Pressure Hydrocephalus

- Shunt

AIDS Dementia Complex

Clinical Features

1. Mildly cognitively impaired AIDS patients, characterized by bradyphrenia, inattention, deficits in conceptualization and initiation and memory impairment. As this progresses to AIDS dementia, bradykinesia and impaired free recall are more severe.

2. Behavioral or affective changes are seen in about one third of patients. Apathy and social withdrawal (more than irritability or emotional lability) are less common. In the later stages of the disease, patients seem quietly confused and indifferent to their illness or their surroundings.

3. Motor changes are also present early during the course of the disease; loss of balance and leg weakness, loss of motor coordination, a deterioration in handwriting, or tremor.

4. Opportunistic infections, especially progressive multifocal leukoencephalopathy, toxoplasma; cytomegalovirus can also occur and cause rapid deterioration. These are treatable.

Key Signs and Symptoms: AIDS Dementia Complex

Mild Cognitive Impairment

- Bradyphrenia
- Inattention
- Deficits in conceptualization and initiation
- Memory impairment
- Apathy, withdrawal

Motor Impairment

- Loss of balance and leg weakness, loss of motor coordination, a deterioration in handwriting, or tremor

Epidemiology and Risk Factors

1. Approximately 95% of AIDS patients' brains show signs of damage, and 60% of patients develop some degree of dementia.

2. In one study over one half of the patients developed severe global mental impairment within 2 months of the onset of symptoms.

Imaging

1. Atrophy; ventriculomegaly

2. White matter lesions, bright on MRI T2-weighted images (can also be PML).

3. SPECT/PET: Decreased cortical metabolism; increased striatal metabolism

Dementia Syndrome of Depression

Clinical Features

1. Particular problems with selective attention, working memory, verbal long-term memory, and verbal fluency.

2. Lots of "I don't know" as answers, rather than near-misses.

3. Fundamental neurological exam is normal.

Key Signs: Dementia Syndrome of Depression

- Problems with selective attention, working memory, verbal long-term memory, and verbal fluency
- Fundamental neurologic exam is normal.

Imaging

1. Normal CT/MRI; may have increased incidence of white matter hyperintensities on MRI.

2. SPECT/PET: Global hypometabolism, decreased cerebral blood flow

Treatment

1. Antidepressants

2. Electroconvulsive therapy

Key Treatment: Dementia Syndrome of Depression

- Antidepressants
- Electroconvulsive therapy

Vascular Dementia (see Part IV, Chapter 3, Vascular Dementia)

Bibliography

Albert ML, Feldman RG, Willis AL: The "subcortical dementia" of progressive supranuclear palsy. Neurol Neurosurg Psychiatry 37:121–130, 1974.

Bret P, Guyotat J, Chazal J: Is normal pressure hydrocephalus a valid concept in 2002? A reappraisal in five questions and proposal for a new designation of the syndrome as "chronic hydrocephalus." J Neurol Neurosurg Psychiatry 73:9–12, 2002.

Cummings JL (ed): Subcortical Dementia, Oxford, Oxford University Press, 1990.

Dubois B, Slachevsky A, Litvan I, Pillon B: The FAB: A Frontal Assessment Battery at bedside. Neurology 55: 1621–1626, 2000.

Filley CM: The behavioral neurology of cerebral white matter. Neurology 50:1535–1540, 1998.

Landrø NI, Stiles TC, Sletvold H: Neuropsychological function in nonpsychotic unipolar major depression. Neuropsychiatry, Neuropsychol Behav Neurol 14: 233–240, 2001.

Mathuranath PS, Nestor PJ, Berrios GE, et al.: A brief cognitive test battery to differentiate Alzheimer's disease and frontotemporal dementia. Neurology 55:1613–1620, 2000.

Royall DR, Cordes JA, Polk M: CLOX: An executive clock drawing task. J Neurol Neurosurg Psychiatry 64:588–594, 1998.

Savage CR: Neuropsychology of subcortical dementias. Psychiatric Clin North Am 20:911–931, 1997.

Vanneste JAL: Diagnosis and management of normal-pressure hydrocephalus. J Neurol 247:5–14, 2000.

5 Transient Global Amnesia and Other Amnestic Disorders

William G. Ondo

Amnestic Disorders

1. Amnesia is often part of other neurologic conditions, such as dementia, delirium, seizures, and sleep disorders, that result in altered mental status. This chapter will discuss specific conditions that result in isolated, or nearly isolated, amnesia without other alterations in cognitive functioning.

2. Amnesia is segregated into retrograde and anterograde amnesia. Retrograde amnesia is the loss of memory prior to a certain point in time, but without an inability to incorporate new memories. Conversely, anterograde amnesia is the inability to incorporate new memories. Past memory may be intact. Often both forms of amnesia will be present, but typically one is prominent.

3. Retrograde amnesia is further segregated into global or semantic memory (all memory) and episodic or personal memory (memory of the individual's personal experiences, as opposed to factual information). This is sometimes further segregated into autobiographical when referring to knowledge of self-identity.

Acute Amnesia Associated with Relatively Preserved Cognition

- Transient global amnesia
- Head trauma
- Drug-induced (ethanol) amnesia
- Structural lesions
- Korsakoff's syndrome
- Paraneoplastic
- Psychiatric (fugue states)

Transient Global Amnesia

Epidemiology
Transient global amnesia (TGA) is defined by relatively isolated and significant anterograde amnesia and variably severe retrograde amnesia.

1. In several well-designed trials, the annual incidence consistently ranges between 6 and 10/100,000. This is greater than the number of patients who present for medical evaluation.

2. There is no pronounced gender preference, and the age at symptom onset varies widely, from the teens through old age.

3. Although there are several associated medical conditions (see below), there is no consistent demographic risk factor for TGA.

Clinical Features
The symptoms of typical TGA are usually quite characteristic and diagnostic.

1. Patients have the acute onset of inability to incorporate new knowledge (anterograde amnesia). They have varying degrees of retrograde amnesia. This is almost always autobiographical rather than factual, such that they will be able to state current events from several days ago, but not what they themselves did. Other aspects of cognition will be only minimally effected. Speed of processing appears slower, but this may result from the patient's confusion about current surroundings. Likewise, some researches have found mild language or praxis deficits, but these are seldom meaningful.

2. The affect of these patients is also quite characteristic. They appear quietly confused. They will repeatedly ask questions about their current circumstances and will often have a perplexed expression, but are usually not panicked or agitated. In fact, the subdued and almost apologetic nature of their questioning is particularly characteristic.

3. The duration of TGA is typically 12 to 36 hours, although cases as short as 1 hour or as long as several days have been reported. If recovery has not began by 48 hours, additional investigation should be pursued. The recovery process usually occurs over a 12-hour period but this may also vary. A specific pattern of memory recovery has been proposed; however, this is not consistently observed. Upon recovery, patients will have a complete retrograde amnesia covering the duration of their TGA episode.

4. About 10% to 18% of patients with TGA will have at least one additional episode. Otherwise the prognosis is excellent. Patients have essentially

normal memory function within days to weeks of the episode. There may be some subtle changes on neuropsychiatric testing, especially in those with multiple TGA episodes. Importantly, TGA patients do not have any increased risk of cerebrovascular events, seizures, sudden death, or any shortening of the life span.

Key Signs

- Acute onset of inability to form new memories (mostly autobiographical)

- Confusion

- Duration: Typically 12 to 36 hours

Precipitating Events

Precipitating events are present in up to 84% of cases. Significant and acute psychologic stressors commonly precipitate TGA, and the condition was thus initially thought to be "functional." In reality, any event that can effect autonomic homeostasis, or cause a vasovagal reaction, appears potentially culpable. Classically, these include swimming in cold water and lifting heavy objects. High altitude, sexual intercourse, and several medical procedures, especially angiography, are also commonly cited. The later is proposed to occur secondary to cerebral vasospasm. Rarely, structural lesions seen on imaging are felt to be culpable. In reality, however, it appears that any psychiatric or physical stressful event can precipitate TGA. The clinical course does not depend on whether a precipitating event was identified.

Conditions Associated with Transient Global Amnesia

- Migraine

- Patent foramen ovale

- High altitudes

- Cold water

- Psychological stressors

- Possible seizures

Etiology

The pathology of TGA has been debated since its initial description more than 30 years ago. Three distinct theories have been most widely suggested: ischemic, seizure, and migraine variant.

1. Ischemic: There is little evidence to support a traditional thromboembolic mechanism for TGA.

Patients do not have residual evidence for ischemia on clinical or radiographic grounds. They have fewer cardiovascular risk factors than patients with typical transient ischemic attacks (TIA) and do not appear to be at higher cardiovascular risk than age-matched controls. TGA patients do have a higher percentage of patent foremen ovale than normal controls; however, this has been postulated to affect hemodynamic stability rather than create a source of paroxysmal emboli.

2. Epileptic: After reports of several isolated cases of TGA in patients with seizure disorders, it was speculated that many episodes of TGA are in fact deep or atypical seizure activity. A large number of studies, however, have failed to show any clear seizure focus. About 10% of TGA patients are noted to have some electroencephalographic (EEG) slowing during their episodes; however, the significance of this is not clear. Even patients with short-duration (less than 1 hour) episodes of TGA have failed to show physiologic evidence of seizure or an increased risk for developing subsequent seizures.

   Clearly epilepsy can result in anterograde amnesia (pure amnestic seizure; PAS). This, however, is almost always accompanied by other seizure manifestations. It is postulated that amnestic epilepsy results from either isolated bitemporal seizures or a previous structural lesion on one temporal lobe and seizure activity in the other. In one series, six of eight patients with PAS had a structural lesion on one or both hippocampi. All eight, however, also had additional seizure types. PAS can therefore be clinically distinguished from TGA based a shorter duration of amnesia, the history of other seizure symptoms, and typically, more impaired interaction with the patients' environment.

3. Migraine: Reported series of TGA, including several well-documented epidemiologic studies, have shown that patients with TGA have a higher than predicted frequency of migraine. Nevertheless, most do not have migraine, and the TGA attack itself is not temporally related with migraine headaches. It is likely that some underlying tendency predisposes to both conditions, but TGA should probably not be considered a "migraine variant."

Etiology (Laboratory)

Routine serologic, electrophysiologic, and imaging assessments are usually normal in TGA. Magnetic resonance imaging (MRI) sequences are almost always normal; however diffusion-weighted MRI is reported by some to show patchy abnormal areas including the mesial temporal lobes. Those results, however, have not been consistently observed. Functional imaging including single photon emission tomography (SPECT) and positron emission tomography (PET) have also been inconsistent, but they usually show reduced activity in a single or both mesial temporal lobes (amygdala and hippocampus). More diffuse tracer hypoperfusion in both the anterior and posterior circulation is also sometimes reported. Hypoperfusion could result from either a primary reduction in blood flow to the area or reduced blood flow secondary to reduced metabolic demand. Therefore, physiologic studies have demonstrated the anatomy of TGA but not the primary etiology.

Evaluation

No evaluation is clearly indicated for a typical case of TGA. Nevertheless it could be argued that both imaging (preferably MRI with diffusion-weighted images) and electroencephalogram (EEG) should be obtained to assess for ischemic disease or seizure.

Treatment

No treatment is clearly indicated for TGA. However, education and reassurance for the patient and family is very important. Given the dramatic symptomatology, it is reasonable to admit the patients overnight for observation, although this is unlikely to affect outcome.

Key Treatment

- Educating and reassuring patient and family about symptoms

Traumatic Amnesia

Head trauma resulting in amnesia is almost always accompanied by some alteration in consciousness. Nevertheless, both an anterograde and retrograde amnesias are often the most prominent features. Blunt head trauma resulting in concussion most often causes amnesia; interestingly, more severe penetrating head injuries usually do not. Typically, patients experience an anterograde amnesia that lasts from minutes to days. In most cases, alertness is also reduced. Most patients will also report a retrograde amnesia for up to 30 minutes prior to the trauma. The duration of retrograde amnesia roughly correlates with the severity of head trauma.

Key Signs

- Anterograde amnesia that lasts from minutes to days
- Reduced alertness

- Retrograde amnesia
  - Up to 30 minutes prior to the trauma in most patients
  - Duration roughly correlates with the severity of head trauma

Etiology

The pathogenesis of amnesia in blunt trauma is not known but likely results from global cerebral dysfunction.

Assessment

Patients with head trauma–associated amnesia always warrant imaging with CT of MRI to evaluate for edema, hemorrhage, or other focal lesions. Cervical imaging is also usually necessary. Otherwise, the assessment will depend on the extent of the injury.

Treatment

There is no specific treatment for trauma-induced amnesia. Treatment depends on the extent of head trauma.

Key Treatment

- Treatment depends on the extent of head trauma.

Korsakoff's Amnesia

Korsakoff's syndrome is a condition in which memory is lost out of proportion to other cognitive features. Although it is usually associated with alcoholism, a variety of structural and metabolic conditions affecting the limbic system can cause identical clinical features. Anatomical lesion amnesia will be discussed later. Korsakoff's syndrome often follows the symptoms of Wernicke's encephalopathy, such that the combined symptom complex is commonly referred to as Wernicke-Korsakoff syndrome; however, each can occur in isolation.

Epidemiology

1. The incidence of Korsakoff's syndrome from alcoholism is probably declining secondary to vitamin supplementation of thiamine in bread and other basic foods.
2. Nevertheless autopsy series consistently demonstrate that pathologic Wernicke-Korsakoff syndrome far exceeds the frequency reported in clinical series, suggesting under-recognition.

Clinical Features

Korsakoff's amnesia affects both anterograde and retrograde memory for both personal and factual information. Patients may have almost no ability to form new memories and can only recall distant past memories. Confabulation can often be elicited by asking leading questions, e.g., "Tell me about the book that you wrote." Wernicke's encephalopathy often precedes Korsakoff's syndrome. The classic triad of general encephalopathy, truncal ataxia, and ophthalmoplegia is not consistently present. More commonly patients have nystagmus. The threshold for suspecting Wernicke-Korsakoff syndrome should be low.

Key Signs

- Both anterograde and retrograde memory are affected.

- Almost no ability to form new memories

- Only distant past memories are recalled.

- Nystagmus

Etiology and Pathophysiology

1. Wernicke-Korsakoff syndrome is caused by thiamine deficiency. Although poor nutrition secondary to alcoholism is the best known precipitant, any nutritionally deficient state can be culpable.
2. The pathology includes small hemorrhages, atrophy, and gliosis of the paraventricular areas, especially the mammillary bodies.

Diagnosis

The diagnosis of Wernicke-Korsakoff syndrome should be made on clinical grounds. MRI may show enhancement, atrophy, or hemorrhage of the mammillary bodies.

Treatment

The treatment consists of intravenous thiamine, typically 100 mg/day. High-dose oral supplementation is not adequate because gastroenteric absorption is poor. Prognosis with treatment is good in isolated Wernicke's encephalopathy if the duration is relatively short. The prognosis is much worse if significant amnesia or confabulations are present.

Key Treatment

- Intravenous thiamine, typically 100 mg/day

Structural Amnesias

Relatively isolated amnesia may occur with structural lesions within the brain. The most commonly involved structures are the hypothalamus, thalamus, and medial temporal lobes. Various lesion etiologies have been reported; however microvascular ischemia as is seen in neurosyphilis, and space-occupying lesions appear to be most frequently culpable.

Severe anterograde amnesia and variable degrees of retrograde amnesia may develop after lesions in the bilateral anterior thalamus. The most common cause is ischemia, although trauma and neoplasm are occasionally implicated. The anterior nucleus of the thalamus subserves the major hippocampus output via the mammillothalamic tract (Papez circuit). The diagnosis is typically made on imaging studies. Prognosis is quite variable, and depends on the severity of the underlying etiology. Treatment depends on the underlying lesion.

Paraneoplastic Amnesia

Paraneoplastic limbic encephalitis can occasionally result in isolated amnesia. Small-cell lung cancer is most commonly responsible; however amnesia symptoms may presage diagnosis of the cancer. Functional imaging may show reduced temporal lobe activity. The amnesia may improve with treatment of the underlying tumor.

Dissociative States

Patients may occasionally have amnestic states resulting from severe psychiatric illness. As a group, DSM-4 refers to these as *dissociative disorders*.

Psychiatric Disorders Causing Amnestic States

- Situational amnesia

- Fugue state

- Multiple personality disorder

- Posttraumatic stress disorder

- Severe depression

Epidemiology

There are few good epidemiologic data on dissociative disorders. Posttraumatic stress disorder is likely the most common cause, but amnesia of the event is not consistent and usually is not an isolated symptom. Situation amnesia may also occur commonly, but its epidemiology is greatly debated. Although examples of fugue states and multiple personality disorders are well publicized, they are rare.

Clinical Features

Classically, patients will transform into another state. Upon return to their original person, they are amnestic or almost amnestic to the events that occurred during that transformation.

1. Situational amnesia usually results from an extremely traumatic event. Although severe sympathetic discharge, as would be experienced in most traumatic events, normally worsens memory in all people, patients with situational amnesia lack any recall of the event. Memory before the event is variably present and there is no anterograde amnesia after the event. "Suppressed memories" are currently controversial. Although situational amnesia clearly exists, "false suppressed memories" may result from overaggressive psychological analysis. Situational amnesia may also occur within the spectrum of posttraumatic stress disorder.

2. Fugue states usually involve wandering away from one's life. Upon completion of the fugue state, which may last hours to years, the patient is amnestic to that time. During the fugue, patients are able to interact correctly with their environment. There is usually no amnesia from before or after the fugue state.

3. In multiple personality disorder, a single personality may have some insight into or knowledge of the actions or characteristics of other personalities. Otherwise, the patient is amnestic to personal memory while another personality is in control.

4. The memory loss or pseudodementia associated with severe depression is neither a dissociative state nor a true isolated amnesia, because other psychological and apparent cognitive features are invariably present. Patients with severe depression do have poor true memory capabilities; apparently this will be augmented by poor effort on recall tests. For example, these patients typically will answer "I don't know" to memory test items without giving any effort.

Key Signs and Symptoms

- Failure to recall a traumatic event
- Fugue states

Etiology and Pathophysiology
The specific etiology of these disorders is not known. Various psychological theories advocate variations on the theme that the conscious mind will suppress memories that are severely in contrast to its own set of mores. A consistent biological basis has not been established.

Treatment
The treatment of these disorders is variable; it usually involves extensive psychological therapy. Antidepressant medications are advocated for posttraumatic stress disorder and depression.

Key Treatment

- Psychological therapy
- Antidepressant medications for PTSD and depression

Ethanol Blackouts

Ethanol-induced blackouts are probably the most common form of retrograde amnesia.

1. Between 20% and 30% of all young men experience at least one episode between the ages of 18 and 35. The incidence in women is somewhat lower.

2. Ethanol blackouts are associated with excessive ethanol intake, an earlier age of ethanol intake, and binge drinking behavior. Although almost all alcoholics have experienced ethanol-induced amnesia, there is no evidence that ethanol amnesia is an independent risk factor for the development of alcoholism.

Bibliography

Anthenelli RM, Klein JL, Tsuang JW, et al.: The prognostic importance of blackouts in young men. J Stud Alcohol 55:290–295, 1994.

Hodges JR, McCarthy RA: Autobiographical amnesia resulting from bilateral paramedian thalamic infarction. A case study in cognitive neurobiology. Brain 116:921–940, 1993.

Jovin TG, Vitti RA, McCluskey LF: Evolution of temporal lobe hypoperfusion in transient global amnesia: A serial single photon emission computed tomography study. J Neuroimaging 10:238–241, 2000.

Lewis SL: Aetiology of transient global amnesia. Lancet 352:397–399, 1998.

Pantoni L, Lamassa M, Inzitari D: Transient global amnesia: A review emphasizing pathogenic aspects. Acta Neurol Scand 102:275–283, 2000.

Strupp M, Bruning R, Wu RH, et al.: Diffusion-weighted MRI in transient global amnesia: Elevated signal intensity in the left mesial temporal lobe in 7 of 10 patients. Ann Neurol. 43:164–170, 1998.

Zorzon M, Antonutti L, Mase G, et al.: Transient global amnesia and transient ischemic attack. Natural history, vascular risk factors, and associated conditions. Stroke. 26:1536–1542, 1995.

1   Parkinson's Disease

Alireza Minagar
Lisa M. Shulman
William J. Weiner

Definition

Parkinson's disease (PD) is an age-related, common progressive neurodegenerative disease. James Parkinson in 1817 originally described the disease in his monograph on the shaking palsy. Other common neurodegenerative diseases with parkinsonian features include progressive supranuclear palsy (PSP) and multiple system atrophy (MSA).

Epidemiology and Risk Factors

1. The exact incidence and prevalence of PD is unknown. Estimates of the prevalence (number of existing cases) in the United States varies from 300,000 to 1 million individuals. The incidence ratio (the number of new cases) ranges from 4.5 to 21.0 per 100,000 population.
2. Most cases of PD start between 50 and 70 years of age, with a peak age of onset at 60 years old.
3. A number of factors possibly associated with an increased risk of PD are presented below under Factors Associated with Risk of PD.
4. Other factors, such as cigarette smoking and caffeine intake, maybe associated with decreased risk for PD.
5. PD appears to be slightly more common in men than women, and it may be less prevalent in China, Asian countries, and among African Americans.

Factors Associated with Risk of PD

- Aging
- Gender (male)
- Race (whites)
- Farming
- Rural residence
- MPTP (1-Methyl-4-phenyl-1,2,3,6-tetrahydropyridine) and MPTP-like compounds
- Infectious agents
- Pesticide and herbicide exposure

This work was supported in part by the Rosalyn Newman Foundation.

Etiology and Pathogenesis

1. The precise cause of PD is unknown.
2. The discovery of several genes that are linked to familial parkinsonism has resulted in renewed interest in a genetic etiology, but the exact role of genetics in sporadic Parkinson's disease is unknown.
3. Advances in the understanding of mitochondrial genetics may clarify the role of genetically determined alterations in the mitochondrial respiratory chain and detoxification pathways in the pathogenesis of PD.
4. Recent studies support the role of excitotoxic processes and perhaps nitric oxide in the pathogenesis of PD. There appears to be a defect in complex I activity of the electron transport chain, and this impairment of oxidative phosphorylation enhances the potential for excitotoxicity.

Genetics

1. Existence of genetic susceptibility factors is strongly suspected. In the past few years, well-documented pedigrees with mendelian dominant inheritance have been reported, but this pattern is clearly exceptional.
2. One large pedigree of familial parkinsonism has been linked to a mutation of alpha-synuclein. Two genes alpha-synuclein and ubiquitin carboxy-terminal hydrolase L1 (Leroy, 1998), and two gene loci on chromosomes 2p13 and 4p14-16.3 have been implicated in the pathogenesis of PD (Gasser, 1998; Farrer, 1999).
3. Mutations in another gene designated *Parkin* have been identified in multiple families with relatively early onset Parkinsonism (Lucking, 2000).

Neuropathology

1. The histopathologic findings of PD consist of selective and severe degeneration of pigmented neurons of the pars compacta of the substantia nigra and moderate degrees of gliosis involving the locus coeruleus and dorsal vagal nucleus, with variable involvement of the nucleus basalis of Mynert.
2. Lewy bodies, the pathognomonic hallmark of

Parkinson's disease, are concentric hyaline intracytoplasmic inclusions observed in monoaminergic and other subcortical nuclei, the spinal cord, sympathetic ganglia, and occasionally the cerebral cortex.

Clinical Features

1. PD is a clinical diagnosis based on the major signs of resting tremor, bradykinesia, rigidity, and loss of postural reflexes. Other less frequent clinical manifestations of PD include dystonia, cognitive decline, psychiatric disorders, sleep disturbances, sensory symptoms, akathesia, restless legs syndrome and autonomic dysfunction.

2. Resting tremor is the most easily recognized sign of PD. Tremor is the presenting symptom in 70% of patients and usually begins unilaterally, and as the disease progresses becomes bilateral. The frequency of parkinsonian tremor is slow, typically in the 4 to 6 Hz range.

3. Bradykinesia or slowness of movement is the most disabling motor abnormality in PD. Difficulties performing daily activities such as writing, shaving, combing hair, and beating eggs may occur.

4. Muscle tone is increased in both flexor and extensor muscles of parkinsonian patients, providing a constant resistance to passive motion of the joints. Rigidity underlies the characteristic stooped posture, anteroflexed head, and flexed knees and elbows of the patients with PD.

5. Dystonia is a rare motor manifestation of PD. Dystonia presents as a sustained muscle contraction resulting in an abnormal posture. Dystonia in PD may be a feature of the disease process or a complication of drug treatment.

6. Approximately one third of PD patients have depression.

7. Dementia occurs in approximately 25% of PD patients after disease of long duration. Hallucinations and psychotic behavior resulting from drug treatment are not uncommon.

Key Signs and Symptoms

- Tremor

- Rigidity

- Bradykinesia

- Loss of postural reflexes

- Hypomimia, micrographia, impaired blinking

- Monotonous speech, reduction in speech volume

- Autonomic abnormalities

- Dysphagia, gait abnormalities, sleep dysfunction

Differential Diagnosis

1. Essential tremor (ET) is most frequently confused with PD.

2. Other parkinsonian syndromes that can be mistaken for PD include PSP, MSA (which includes olivopontocerebellar atrophy, Shy-Drager syndrome, and striatonigral degeneration), cortical basal ganglionic degeneration, hemiparkinsonism-hemihypertrophy, diffuse Lewy body disease, drug-induced parkinsonism, and Western Pacific amyotrophic lateral sclerosis (ALS)-parkinsonism-dementia complex.

Laboratory Testing

1. The current laboratory evaluation of PD is limited. Brain imaging studies and the electroencephalogram are typically normal in patients with PD.

2. Positron emission tomography with a fluorinated dopa ligand provides additional diagnostic information but is not readily available.

Treatment

Treatment of PD is symptomatic and must be individualized. The available therapeutic measures include nonpharmacologic and pharmacologic treatments, and surgical procedures.

1. Nonpharmacologic interventions are fundamental elements of the overall management of patients with PD.
   a. Education regarding PD
   b. Support strategies
   c. Exercise

2. Available drug treatment: Various classes of drugs are available for the treatment of PD (Table 1–1).
   a. Anticholinergics (benztropine, trihexyphenidyl, procyclidine, and biperiden). Anticholinergics are often effective for the symptomatic treatment of tremor. These agents are useful because the striatum contains high levels of both dopamine and acetylcholine, and the dopamine deficiency state in the striatum of patients with PD produces a relative cholinergic hyperactivity. Anticholinergics exert their useful effect by partially correcting this apparent cholinergic excess. Their adverse effects include blurred vision, constipation, urinary retention, memory impairment, cognitive deterioration, confusion, and delirium. Anticholinergics must be used with caution in older patients.
   b. Amantadine is an antiviral agent with antiparkinsonian activity that is useful in the treatment of early PD. It is believed that its predominant pharmacological effect is in blocking N-methyl-

TABLE 1–1. ANTIPARKINSONIAN MEDICATIONS

MEDICATION	DAILY DOSE (MG)
Anticholinergics	
Trihexylphenidyl	4–10
Benztropine	0.5–8.0
Amantadine	100–300
Dopamine agonists	
Bromocriptine	7.5–40.0
Pergolide	1.5–6.0
Pramipexole	0.75–4.5
Ropinirole	9–24
Levodopa/carbidopa	300–2000
(10:100; 25:250; 25:100)	(expressed as levodopa)
Levodopa/carbidopa	25/100; 50/200
(controlled released formulation)	
Selegiline	10
COMT inhibitors	
Tolcapone	300–600

D-aspartate (NMDA). It can improve akinesia and rigidity, but has only mild effects on the tremor. Amantadine may also improve dyskinesia for 6 to 12 months. Common side effects include lower limb edema and livedo reticularis; it may also produce psychiatric complications similar to those caused by anticholinergics.

c. Dopamine agonists (bromocriptine, pergolide, pramipexole, and ropinirole). Dopamineric agents activate dopamine receptors directly and are useful in the treatment of PD. There are multiple dopamine receptors; however, pharmacologic concerns are focused on D1 and D2 receptors for antiparkinsonian effects. The most recent dopamine agonists pramipexole and ropinirole, also stimulate D3 receptors. Oral dopamine agonists are effective in early PD. There is evidence to suggest that pramipexole and ropinirole when used as monotherapy in the early treatment of PD will result in fewer and less severe complications than levodopa alone. However, agonist monotherapy also produces less robust motor changes than levodopa. Side effects of dopamine agonists include nausea and vomiting, orthostatic hypotension, cardiac arrhythmia, sedation, somnolence, headache, and dopaminergic psychosis. Sudden irresistible sleep episodes are an uncommon but significant side effect of the dopamine agonists.

d. Levodopa (carbidopa-levodopa) remains the most effective drug in the treatment of PD, and patients who fail to respond to high doses of levodopa are unlikely to respond to other dopaminergic agents. Levodopa markedly improves rigidity, tremor, and bradykinesia but ultimately is limited by motor fluctuations, dyskinesia, and neuropsychiatric complications. Levodopa is usually administered orally in three or four divided doses. Generally, it is better to start with lower doses of levodopa and increase the dose slowly to minimize the risk of acute side effects like nausea and hypotension. Levodopa in combination with the decarboxylase inhibitor carbidopa is most commonly prescribed. Dosage strengths of 10/100, 25/100, and 25/250 are available, with the first number representing the carbidopa dosage and the second number the levodopa dosage. Sustained-release formulations of levodopa/carbidopa (Sinemet CR) are also marketed in the United States. It is convenient to start with low doses of levodopa (25/100 twice a day) and slowly titrate the dosage upward at weekly intervals until symptomatic relief is achieved. Although levodopa is the most potent antiparkinsonian drug, chronic administration of levodopa is associated with adverse effects in most patients; anorexia, nausea, orthostatic hypotension, somnolence, insomnia, motor fluctuations, dyskinesias, and neuropsychiatric disorders may develop. With disease progression, other features also develop; falling, postural instability, freezing, autonomic abnormalities, and dementia manifest and are unresponsive to levodopa treatment. Motor fluctuations and dyskinesias associated with levodopa treatment are a particular problem in younger patients. Most PD patients develop motor fluctuations after 5 to 10 years of treatment. These motor complications may initially be mild, but they progress over time and become a major cause of disability. The pathogenesis of motor complications in levodopa-treated PD patients remains to be established; however, pulsatile stimulation of dopamine receptors has been implicated.

e. The adverse psychiatric effects of long term dopaminergic treatment include altered sleep patterns, vivid nightmares, auditory and visual hallucinations, paranoia, and psychosis. These drug-related complications can be ameliorated by reduction of antiparkinsonian medications. Quetiapine (Seroquel), a new selective antipsychotic agent, can be useful in management of psychosis without worsening the parkinsonian features. Quetiapine can be started at a dose of 12.5 mg at bedtime and titrated at 3- to 5-day intervals until favorable response is observed or side effects emerge. Olanzepine (Zyprexa), another selective neuroleptic with dopamine- and serotonin-blocking properties, can be prescribed at low doses for psychosis in PD patients. Olanzepine in high doses is a D2-blocker and can worsen parkinsonian features; it should be initiated at a dose of 2.5 mg at bedtime.

f. Selegiline (Eldepryl) causes irreversible inhibition of monoamine oxidase-β (MAO-β inhibitor). The drug has a mild symptomatic effect and can reduce levodopa-induced motor fluctuations. It is not neuroprotective. Selegiline can be used in early PD in combination with levodopa to reduce the need for increased doses of levodopa. Selegiline is given twice daily, 5 mg early in the morning and again at lunchtime. Administering selegiline in the evening may cause insomnia.

g. The COMT (catechol-O-methyltransferase) inhibitors entacapone (Comtan) and tolcapone (Tasmar) have been used as adjunctive therapy with levodopa in the treatment of PD. COMT metabolizes levodopa and dopamine to 3-O-methyldopa (3-MT) and 3-methoxytyramine (3-MT), respectively, in both the peripheral and central nervous systems. Tolcapone and entacapone both are reversible inhibitors of COMT (Piccini, 2000). Entacapone is a peripheral inhibitor of COMT because it poorly enters the brain. Tolcapone is active in the periphery and in the brain in animal studies, but at the doses used in PD patients, PET studies provide no evidence of central inhibition of COMT by this medication. The clinical effects of both medications are thought to be mainly mediated by their peripheral actions on levodopa metabolism. They increase the bioavailability of levodopa and increase the availability and transfer of levodopa in the brain. Clinically, the COMT inhibitors potentiate the antiparkinsonian effects of levodopa in both fluctuating and nonfluctuating patients. Addition of a COMT inhibitor as an adjunct to levodopa can significantly decrease "off" time and increase "on" time in patients with "wearing off" episodes. The COMT inhibitors are associated with an increased incidence of dopaminergic adverse effects (such as dyskinesia and neuropsychiatric disorders), which may require a reduction in levodopa dose of 20% to 30%. Tolcapone has been associated with liver toxicity and death, so close surveillance of hepatic function is necessary. Entacapone has not been associated with serious hepatic damage.

3. Symptomatic drug treatment: All medications currently used to manage PD provide symptomatic relief and do not alter the underlying pathogenesis of the disease; in other words, the natural progression of PD continues despite treatment. The treatment of each PD patient should be highly individualized to provide acceptable symptomatic relief. If a patient's symptoms are very mild and do not interfere with the activities of daily living, delay of treatment may be the appropriate decision. When patients' symptoms produce functional impairment, however, symptomatic treatment should be initiated for PD. Levodopa or a dopamine agonist can be used. Levodopa produces a better motor response and also improves functional abilities more than dopamine agonist treatment, but it is associated with motor fluctuations and dyskinesia. The choice of agent to begin treatment must be individualized.

4. Surgical procedures. The potential of surgical procedures to provide benefit for PD patients who can not be satisfactorily managed with available pharmacologic treatment is evident. There are currently three brain regions considered as targets for functional neurosurgery for PD.

   a. The ventral intermediate nucleus of the thalamus (Vim)

   b. The internal segment of the globus pallidus (GPi)

   c. The subthalamic nucleus (STN)

   Deep brain stimulation (DBS) of Vim nucleus can be used to treat PD tremor. DBS of Vim nucleus does not ameliorate rigidity, bradykinesia, or gait dysfunction. DBS of GPi simulates the beneficial effects of pallidotomy, which includes amelioration of bradykinesia and rigidity, reduction of dyskinesia, and to a lesser degree improvement of tremor. DBS of STN improves tremor, bradykinesia, rigidity, dyskinesia, and to a smaller degree gait disorder in PD patients.

   Ablative central nervous system lesions such as thalamotomy, pallidotomy, or subthalamic nucleus lesions or implants of chronic stimulating electrodes at these sites (DBS) are currently being used.

   There has been interest in the role of fetal tissue transplantation as a treatment for PD based on the concept that embryonic dopaminergic neurons implanted into the denervated striatum can survive and compensate for lost substantia nigra (pars compacta) neurons. Although there have been reports that some PD patients have improved following transplant, there are also reports of inducing uncontrollable dyskinesias and of producing little or no effect.

Key Treatment

Nonpharmacologic Interventions

• Education regarding PD

• Support strategies

• Exercise

Medications

Drug	Initiating Dose (mg)
Bromocriptine	1.25 bid-tid
Pergolide	0.05 qd
Pramipexole	0.125 tid
Ropinirole	0.25 tid
Levodopa/carbidopa	25/100 bid

Surgery (patients who cannot be satisfactorily managed with medications)

- The ventral intermediate nucleus of the thalamus (Vim)

- The internal segment of the globus pallidus (GPi)

- The subthalamic nucleus

- Deep brain stimulation of Vim nucleus

Drug-Induced Parkinsonism

A number of drugs that interfere with central dopaminergic transmission can induce parkinsonism. Drugs that deplete central dopamine (e.g., reserpine) or block the dopamine receptors (e.g., neuroleptics, metoclopramide) often cause parkinsonian symptomatology, which can simulate all of the features observed in idiopathic PD. Akinesia is the most common manifestation, and resting tremor is observed less often. Other features that may distinguish drug-induced parkinsonism form PD include a clear history of ingestion of a compound known to interfere with central dopaminergic activity, bilateral manifestation instead of unilateral manifestation, and the presence of other drug-related motor disorders (e.g., tardive dyskinesia). The diagnosis of drug-induced parkinsonism demands a high index of suspicion. Once the diagnosis is reached, treatment should be directed to discontinue the insulting drug. In almost all patients with this syndrome, the parkinsonism will resolve. If active therapy is required, anticholinergic agents, amantadine, and levodopa can be used. In those cases in which drug-induced parkinsonism does not resolve, idiopathic PD may have been unmasked.

Bibliography

Farrer M, Gwinn-Hardy K, Muenter M, et al.: A chromosome 4p haplotype segregating with Parkinson's disease and postural tremor. Hum Mol Genet 8:81–85, 1999.

Gasser T, Muller-Myshok B, Wszolek ZK, et al.: A susceptibility locus for Parkinson's disease maps to chromosome 2p13. Nat Genet 18:262–265, 1998.

Leroy E, Boyer R, Auberger G, et al.: The ubiquitin pathway in Parkinson's disease. Nature 395:451–452, 1998.

Lucking CB, Durr A, Bonifati V, Vaughan J, et al.: Association between early-onset Parkinson's disease and mutations in the PARKIN gene. N Engl J Med 342:1560–1567, 2000.

Piccini P, Brooks DJ, Korpela K, Pavese N, Karlsson M, Gordin A: The catechol-O-methyltransferase (COMT) inhibitor entacapone enhances the pharmacokinetic and clinical response to Sinemet-CR in Parkinson's disease. J Neurol Neurosurg Psychiatry 68:589–594, 2000.

2 Progressive Supranuclear Palsy

Alireza Minagar
Lisa M. Shulman
William J. Weiner

Definition

Parkinsonian symptoms and signs are occasionally the manifesting features of a group of neurologic conditions that together are known as parkinsonism-plus syndromes. These syndromes are differentiated form idiopathic Parkinson's disease by the presence of additional neurologic signs and symptoms. Among these signs and symptoms are impairment of extraocular movements; spinocerebellar, corticospinal, and autonomic nervous system dysfunction; motor neuron degeneration; peripheral neuropathy; and dementia. There are many syndromes that manifest as parkinsonism; in this chapter we consider progressive supranuclear palsy (PSP).

1. PSP, the most common parkinsonism-plus syndrome, is characterized by the presence of extensor rigidity of the axial muscles, lack of tremor, and impairment of extraocular movements.
2. PSP is frequently misdiagnosed as Parkinson's disease. Like Parkinson's disease, it results in rigidity, bradykinesia, postural instability, dysarthria, dysphagia, and, in many patients, dementia.

Epidemiology and Risk Factors

1. The age-adjusted prevalence of PSP is about 5% of the prevalence of Parkinson's disease (Schrag, 1999).
2. Men are slightly more affected than women.
3. Approximately half of the patients with PSP experience the initial symptoms during their 60s.

Neuropathology

1. PSP is a neurologic syndrome associated with neurofibrillary degeneration.
2. The histopathologic findings include neuronal loss, gliosis, and flame-shaped and globose neurofibrillary tangles composed of paired helical filaments and straight filaments of tau protein. The tangles are similar to those in Alzheimer's disease, except for the *tau* protein (Chambers, 1999).
3. PSP is not associated with amyloid deposition or apolipoprotein E allelic association.
4. The pathology is most prevalent in the substantia nigra, subthalamic nucleus, globus pallidus, superior colliculus, pretectal area, and substantia innominata.
5. Dopaminergic, cholinergic, and adrenergic neurotransmitter systems are affected.

Clinical Features

1. PSP usually begins with disturbance of posture and gait. Many patients complain of difficulty with posture and slowed gait. Early in the disease, falling is common.
2. Hypokinesia and rigidity of the axial and limb muscles are characteristic.
3. Impaired ocular pursuit movements, especially in the downward direction, are usually present at the time of the first visit to a neurologist. The paresis can be overcome by passive head movement activating the oculocephalic reflexes (hence the designation "supranuclear").
4. Associated ocular findings are horizontal square-wave jerks, slow and hypometric saccades, and paresis of upward gaze. Lateral gaze paresis may occur late in the disease course.
5. "Apraxia" of lid movement and blepharospasm are common among PSP patients.
6. Unlike Parkinson's disease, tremor is rare in PSP.
7. Mental disturbance is a common feature of PSP, often presenting as personality change, emotional incontinence, or depression. The dementia is usually similar to that of frontal lobe disease.
8. The combination of dysarthria, dysphagia, and profound disability may result in death from aspiration.
9. PSP patients show a poor therapeutic response to levodopa.

Key Signs

- Hypokinesia and rigidity of axial and limb muscles
- Lack of tremor
- Impairment of extraocular movements, especially in downgaze
- Frequent falls
- Horizontal square-wave jerks; slow and hypometric saccades

This work was supported in part by the Rosalyn Newman Foundation.

- Apraxia of lid movement and blepharospasm
- Poor therapeutic response to levodopa

 Key Caveat

- PSP is frequently misdiagnosed as Parkinson's disease.

Differential Diagnosis

1. PSP should be differentiated from idiopathic Parkinson's disease. This may be difficult in those PSP patients in whom eye movements are still intact.
2. Other disorders that should be differentiated from PSP include corticobasal degeneration, parkinsonism-dementia-amyotrophic lateral sclerosis complex of Guam, Whipple's disease, neuroacanthocytosis, and motor neuron disease.

Laboratory Testing

1. Brain magnetic resonance imaging (MRI) can be useful in patients thought to have PSP. MRI can exclude multi-infarct dementia or hydrocephalus. Disproportionate atrophy of the midbrain may be present on MRI.
2. Single photon emission computed tomography (SPECT) and positron emission tomography (PET) scans using deoxyglucose can reveal prefrontal hypoactivity in PSP.

 Key Tests

- MRI of the brain
- SPECT and PET scans using deoxyglucose

Treatment

1. Treatment of PSP remains unsatisfactory. In one third of patients levodopa may improve the bradykinesia and rigidity; an effect that is often short-lived. If no motor improvement is noted with levodopa, there is no need to continue the drug.
2. Amantadine and amitriptyline may occasionally be useful, but their adverse effects limit their use.
3. Zolpidem may ameliorate the imbalance and eye movement abnormalities (Daniele, 1999).
4. Speech therapy should be begun for management of the dysarthria and dysphagia. Feeding gastrostomy should be discussed with the patient and family after the first confirmed episode of aspiration or of aspiration pneumonitis.
5. Blepharospasm responds well to botulinum toxin injection. Dry eyes from infrequent blinking can be treated with topical lubricants.

 Key Treatment

- Treatment is limited and unsatisfactory
- Levodopa for bradykinesia and rigidity
- Amantadine and amitriptyline (although adverse effects limit their use)
- Zolpidem for imbalance and eye movement abnormalities
- Speech therapy
- Botulinum toxin injection for blepharospasm
- Topical lubricants for dry eyes caused by infrequent blinking

 Bibliography

Chambers CB, Lee JM, Troncoso JC, et al.: Overexpression of four-repeat *tau* mRNA isoforms in progressive supranuclear palsy but not in Alzheimer's disease. Ann Neurol 46:325–332, 1999.

Daniele A, Moro E, Bentivoglio AR: Zolpidem in progressive supranuclear palsy. N Engl J Med 341:543–544, 1999.

Schrag A, Ben-Shlomo Y, Quinn NP: Prevalence of progressive supranuclear palsy and multiple system atrophy: A cross-sectional study. Lancet 354:1771–1775, 1999.

3 Huntington's Disease

Alireza Minagar
Lisa M. Shulman
William J. Weiner

Definition

Huntington's disease (HD) is a dominantly inherited progressive neurodegenerative disorder that typically manifests in mid-adult life (although about 10% of patients have onset of HD before age 20 and another 10% after age 55). Clinical manifestations of HD include a characteristic movement disorder (usually chorea), progressive cognitive decline, and varying degrees of psychiatric and behavioral dysfunction.

Epidemiology and Risk Factors

1. Approximately 30,000 individuals in North America are affected with HD and another 150,000 unaffected individuals are at 50:50 risk for developing the disease because they have an affected parent.
2. HD occurs with a worldwide prevalence of 5 to 10 per 100,000 population.
3. Most patients have onset of their symptoms around the age of 39 years.

Etiology and Pathophysiology

HD results form an expanded and unstable trinucleotide repeat in IT15 gene on the short arm of chromosome 4. This gene produces a protein called huntingtin (Huntington's Disease Collaborative Research Group, 1993).

1. People without HD may have as many as 35 repetitions of the CAG trinucleotides in the HD gene. Patients with HD have a CAG repeat of more than 39, and people with 36 to 39 repeats are regarded as "indeterminate" and may or may not develop HD (Nance, 1996).
2. CAG repeat length is the major determinant of age at onset for HD, with larger expansions responsible for earlier onset of disease.
3. Patients with juvenile-onset HD have greater expansions, with as many as 80 CAG repeats. Most of these patients have inherited HD from an affected father.
4. Marked expansion of CAG repeat length most likely occurs during spermatogenesis.

Neuropathology

1. The neurodegeneration in HD affects the caudate and putamen primarily, and brain weight is decreased.
2. Cortical and brainstem neuronal loss occurs.
3. Neuronal intranuclear inclusions have recently been described in a mouse model transgenic for the HD mutation (Davies, 1997). Postmortem histopathologic study of brain tissue from HD patients revealed similar neuronal intranuclear inclusions containing huntingtin (DiFiglia, 1997).

Clinical Features

1. The clinical manifestations of HD comprise a characteristic extrapyramidal movement disorder, subcortical dementia, and various degrees of psychiatric and behavioral abnormalities. The onset of illness is insidious.
2. The major motor manifestation of HD is chorea. *Chorea* derives from the Greek word *choros* meaning "to dance." Patients develop excessive spontaneous movements that are irregularly timed, nonrepetitive, randomly distributed, and abrupt in character.
3. With further progression and worsening of HD, chorea may be replaced by dystonia and parkinsonian features such as rigidity, postural instability, and bradykinesia.
4. The subcortical dementia of HD is characterized by bradyphrenia and attention and sequencing impairments without the presence of apraxia, agnosia, or aphasia. Registration of new information and immediate memory recall are relatively intact, while retrieval of recent and remote memories is impaired.
5. Psychiatric and behavioral abnormalities of HD can include psychosis with visual or auditory hallucinations, mania, apathy, obsessive behavior, and depression.

Key Signs

- Chorea
- Subcortical dementia
- Psychiatric and behavioral disorders

This work was supported in part by the Rosalyn Newman Foundation.

Differential Diagnosis

1. A wide range of metabolic and infectious processes may precipitate chorea and dystonia, and some are associated with dementia.
2. Neuroacanthocytosis, a very rare disorder, maybe confused with HD as it causes dementia, involuntary movements, and caudate atrophy. However, the presence of abnormal red blood cell morphology, neuropathy, myopathy, epilepsy, and self-mutilation differentiates neuroacanthocytosis form HD.
3. Tardive dyskinesia, a choreodystonic movement disorder, is a complication of neuroleptic use. The patient may have a behavioral or psychiatric history and chorea. This can be differentiated from HD on the basis of the history of neuroleptic use and no family history.
4. Other disorders with chorea include Sydenham's chorea, chorea gravidarum, systemic lupus erythematosus, Wilson's disease, and side effects of medications such as phenytoin and amphetamines.

Laboratory Testing

1. HD genotyping is available.
2. Computed tomography and magnetic resonance imaging (CT/MRI) may show remarkable caudate atrophy but is not diagnostic.
3. Presymptomatic detection of the HD gene should only be undertaken at centers that provide the appropriate psychological and genetic counseling.

Laboratory and Radiologic Findings

• More than 39 CAG repetitions

• Caudate atrophy on MRI

• Caudate and cortical atrophy

Treatment

Treatment of HD is individualized.

1. Depression can be treated with antidepressants.
2. Carbamazepine or valproate may help patients with manic disorder.
3. Neuroleptics decrease chorea but may worsen cognitive problems associated with HD.

Key Treatment

• Antidepressants

• Carbamazepine or valproate for manic disorder

• Neuroleptics for chorea

Prognosis

HD is a progressive neurodegenerative disease that is fatal. Death is most often caused by aspiration pneumonia and injuries secondary to falls. Additional factors affecting prognosis of HD are the length of CAG repeat and its relationship to age of onset.

Bibliography

Davies SW, Turmaine M, Cozens B, et al.: Formation of neuronal intranuclear inclusions underlies the neurological dysfunction in mice transgenic for the HD mutation. 90:537–548, 1997.

DiFiglia M, Sapp E, Chase KO, et al.: Aggregation of huntingtin in neuronal internuclear inclusions and dystrophic neuritis in brain. Science 277:1990–1993, 1997.

Huntington's Disease Collaborative Research Group: A novel gene containing a trinucleotide repeat that is expanded and unstable on Huntington's disease chromosomes. Cell 72: 971–983, 1993.

Nance MA: Invited editorial: Huntington's disease—another chapter rewritten. Am J Hum Genet 59:1–6, 1996.

4 Dystonia

Alireza Minagar
Lisa M. Shulman
William J. Weiner

Definition

Dystonia is a common neurologic disorder characterized by involuntary, sustained, patterned, and frequently repetitive contractions of antagonist muscles resulting in abnormal movements and postures. Dystonia is classified according to etiology, age of onset, and anatomic distribution. Dystonia may be of no identifiable cause (idiopathic or primary dystonia) or a symptom of an underlying neurologic disease (secondary dystonia). Primary dystonia can be either familial or sporadic. The earlier the age of onset, the more likely that dystonia will become more severe and involve several body parts. Dystonia can be focal, segmental, generalized, multifocal, or hemidystonia (Table 4–1).

Etiology

1. Primary dystonia may be sporadic or hereditary. Hereditary primary dystonia manifests in childhood with a progressive pattern. It usually begins in one leg prior to spreading to the trunk or other limbs.

2. Focal dystonia is usually of adult onset with little or no progression.

3. Metabolic or structural insults to brain, particularly if affecting the putamen, basal ganglia, rostral brainstem, or upper cervical spinal cord have been associated with dystonia. Secondary dystonia can manifest in association with Wilson's disease, Huntington's disease, infection, stroke, focal brain lesions, cerebral hemiatrophy, multiple sclerosis, and progressive supranuclear palsy.

4. About 40% of patients with dystonia are initially misdiagnosed as having psychogenic illness, but fewer than 5% have psychogenic disease. Psychogenic dystonia is characterized by the presence of incongruous movements and postures, inconsistent weakness and sensory deficits, fluctuating or intermittent dystonia, response to placebo or suggestion, distractibility, and self-inflicted injuries.

5. Drug-induced dystonia is related to the use of the dopamine receptor blocking agents (e.g., the major tranquilizers, metocloperamide) which can cause either an acute transient dystonic reaction or a permanent tardive dystonia.

6. Dopa-responsive dystonia (DRD) typically manifests in children between infancy and adolescence as postural abnormalities in the legs. Symptoms most often occur while walking, and falls are frequent. Diurnal fluctuation of dystonia may be present. DRD may be associated with parkinsonian features and characteristically improves with low-dose levodopa. All patients with childhood-onset dystonia should have a therapeutic trial of levodopa.

Epidemiology and Risk Factors

1. The incidence has been estimated at 2 per million population per year for generalized dystonia and 24 per million per year for focal dystonia.

2. The prevalence of generalized dystonia is 3.4 per 100,000 and prevalence of focal dystonia is 29.5 per 100,000.

3. There is a higher prevalence of dystonia in Ashkenazi Jewish populations.

Genetics

1. Idiopathic torsion dystonia (ITD) is most frequently caused by an autosomal dominant gene or genes with reduced penetrance. The *DYT1* gene has been reported to be responsible for early-onset ITD in Ashkenazi Jewish families, and in one large non-Jewish family. This gene has been mapped to chromosome 9q32-34. However, in patients without a family history of dystonia, the frequency of detecting *DYT1* gene mutation is less than 5% (Brassat, 2000). The *DYT1* gene encodes a 332-amino acid protein called torsin A (Ozelius, 1997). The mutation causing early onset generalized dystonia has been identified as the deletion of a single GAG triplet in a novel gene coding for an ATP-binding protein termed *torsin A* (Kelin, 1998). Mapping of *DYT1* mRNA in postmortem studies of normal human brain has revealed abundant expression related to the dopaminergic system. The disturbance of dopaminergic function has been implicated as a contributing mechanism in the development of early-onset torsion dystonia.

2. A sex-linked inheritance form of idiopathic torsion dystonia has been well described in the Philippines. The X-linked torsion dystonia gene has been assigned to chromosome Xq21 by linkage analysis.

This work was supported in part by the Rosalyn Newman Foundation.

214

TABLE 4–1. CLASSIFICATION OF DYSTONIA BY ANATOMICAL DISTRIBUTION

Focal: Blepharospasm, oromandibular dystonia, spasmodic dysphonia, cervical dystonia, writer's cramp
Segmental: Several related sets of muscles such as neck and trunk (axial); one arm and one shoulder, or both shoulders, neck and trunk (brachial); one or both legs and trunk (crural)
Multifocal: Two or more unrelated parts of the body
Generalized: Combination of crural dystonia and any other segment
Hemidystonia: Arm and leg

Neuropathology

Autopsy studies of brains of patients with primary dystonia have not revealed any specific abnormalities.

Clinical Features

1. Primary focal dystonia may involve the face, neck, or limb. Various types of focal dystonia include blepharospasm, oromandibular dystonia, spasmodic dysphonia (laryngeal dystonia), spasmodic torticollis (cervical dystonia), and limb dystonia.

   a. Adult-onset dystonia affecting the upper parts of the body is usually sporadic and tends to remain focal. Idiopathic focal dystonias almost always occur in adulthood and affect women more than men. In the first 1 or 2 years of illness, spontaneous resolution may occur and can last weeks or months, but generally the dystonia recurs. In some patients, focal dystonia may become generalized, but even in such cases, disability is less than that occurring in generalized childhood dystonia, when patients are commonly wheelchair-bound.

   b. Patients with dystonia show other types of involuntary movements such as tremor or myoclonus. Various sensory tricks such as tactile or proprioceptive stimuli can ameliorate dystonic spasms. The mechanism(s) by which such tricks improve dystonia is unknown. Dystonic spasms can also be influenced by other factors such as stress and emotional tension.

   c. Infrequently, adult-onset focal dystonia may be associated with known causes such as structural lesions of the spinal cord, thalamus, globus pallidus, or putamen.

   d. Patients with blepharospasm have intermittent or sustained bilateral eyelid closure due to involuntary contractions of the orbicularis oculi muscles. The combination of blepharospasm and oromandibular dystonia is known as Meige's syndrome. Eye closure spasms are commonly aggravated by stress and resolve during sleep. Blepharospasm may also worsen upon exposure to bright light, looking upward, walking, reading, and less frequently, driving, watching television, or looking downward.

   e. Oromanibular dystonia manifests with spasms in the jaw, lower face, and mouth. Involvement of masticatory muscles commonly causes spasms of jaw closure or opening, jaw protrusion, or lateral deviation. Jaw closure spasms may be associated with trismus and bruxism. Platysmal contractions are also common.

   f. Spasmodic dysphonia affects more women than men and usually occurs between 30 and 50 years of age. Two types of spasmodic dysphonia exist: the adductor type, which is caused by irregular hyperadduction of the vocal cords, and the abductor type, caused by contraction of the posterior cricoarythnoid muscles during the action of speaking, resulting inappropriate abduction of the vocal cords. Those affected with adductor spasmodic dysphonia have a choked, strained, or strangled voice quality with abrupt initiation and termination of voicing. Abductor spasmodic dysphonia is less frequent than the adductor type and results in a whispering voice.

   g. Spasmodic torticollis affects the neck muscles and results in abnormal head and neck posture. Patients with spasmodic torticollis have sustained muscular contractions that cause repetitive, involuntary movements of head and neck muscles resulting in abnormal postures. Spasmodic torticollis is the most frequent form of dystonia. The head and neck may move in any combination of directions: lateral rotation (torticollis), forward rotation (antecollis), or backward rotation (retrocollis). Commonly, the shoulder is raised on the side toward which the chin is directed. In one third of patients dystonia involves contiguous body parts including the oromandibular region, shoulder, and arms. Spasmodic torticollis may be associated with head and hand tremor. Unlike other focal dystonias, the incidence of pain in cervical dystonia is very high and pain contributes to disability. Sensory tricks or "geste antagonistique" such as touching the face, chin, or occiput are used by some patients to reduce the severity of their spasms.

   h. Limb dystonia manifests with involuntary contraction of limb muscles that results in twisting and repetitive movements or abnormal postures. Limb dystonia can affect the arm or the leg, as in writer's cramp, or be segmental in distribution, involving the arm and the neck (brachial) or the leg and the trunk (crural).

2. Generalized dystonia manifests with crural and any other segment involvement. Idiopathic torsion

dystonia, the most common form of generalized dystonia, begins with limb dystonia and then spreads to the trunk or the other leg and eventually involves other body sites. Idiopathic torsion dystonia usually affects children below age 20. These children are typically normal in their development. The dystonia spreads to involve the proximal lower limbs, trunk, upper limbs, neck, and cranial structures in varying degrees. A family history suggesting autosomal dominant inheritance may be obtained in the majority of patients with childhood-onset idiopathic torsion dystonia and in some with adult-onset idiopathic torsion dystonia.

a. Patients with generalized dystonia have an abnormal gait. They also can have dystonic tremor of the affected limb, but cognitive function, postural reflexes, extraocular movements, and the rest of the neurologic examination are normal.

b. Classic childhood-onset generalized idiopathic torsion dystonia is an autosomal dominant disorder, and the gene has been mapped to the long arm of chromosome 9. A summary of genetically defined primary dystonias is presented in Table 4–2.

c. Childhood-onset dystonia with marked diurnal fluctuations is a levodopa-responsive condition. Other characteristic features of this dystonic disorder include concurrent or subsequent development of parkinsonian features, favorable therapeutic response to low doses of levodopa, diurnal fluctuations, worsening with exercise and improvement with sleep, and a autosomal dominant pattern of inheritance.

Key Signs

- Blepharospasm
- Tremor
- Spasms in the jaw, lower face, and mouth
- Choked, strained, or strangled voice quality
- Whispering voice quality
- Abnormal head and neck posture
- Abnormal gait
- Twisting and repetitive movements

Differential Diagnosis

1. Drug-induced dystonia should be considered in all patients with dystonia, and any history of exposure to neuroleptics should be explored.

2. In all patients younger than 40 years with dystonia, Wilson's disease should be excluded. Wilson's disease is a treatable condition in which early therapeutic intervention may arrest and reverse progression of the disease.

3. Homocystinuria can manifest with progressive dystonia and should be ruled out.

4. Metabolic disorders that may manifest with dystonia include mitochondrial disorders, GM1 and GM2 gangliosidosis, metachromatic leukodystrophy, glutaric acidemia, Lesch-Nyhan syndrome, and triosephosphate isomerase deficiency.

5. Dystonic syndromes may occur in association with neurodegenerative diseases such as Leigh disease, Fahr's disease, ceroid lipofuscinosis, ataxia-telangiectasia, neuroacanthocytosis, Hallervorden-Spatz disease, and Hartnup disease.

Laboratory Testing

For children and adolescents suspected of having primary torsion dystonia, magnetic resonance imaging (MRI) of brain, slit-lamp examination, serum ceruloplasmin level, serum antinuclear antibody titer, routine blood chemistry, and a uric acid test should be requested.

Key Tests

- MRI of the brain
- Slit-lamp examination
- Serum ceruloplasmin
- Serum antinuclear antibody titer
- Routine blood chemistry
- Uric acid test

Treatment

Available treatments for dystonias are medical and surgical.

1. Anticholinergics (trihexyphenidyl) have been useful in the treatment of generalized dystonia.

2. Other medications such as muscle relaxants, clonazepam, diazepam, and spasmolytics have been used with little efficacy. Levodopa is very effective in the management of dopa-responsive dystonia. Intramuscular injection of botulinum toxin (BTX) often provides dramatic amelioration of dystonias. Proper selection of the involved muscles is the most important determinant of response to BTX treatment. BTX causes presynaptic neuromuscular blockade and induces weakness of the dystonic

TABLE 4–2. A SUMMARY OF GENETICALLY DEFINED DYSTONIAS

DYSTONIA TYPE	DESIGNATION	MODE OF INHERITANCE	CHROMOSOMAL LOCATION
DYT1	Early-onset torsion dystonia	AD	9q34
DYT2	Autosomal recessive torsion dystonia	AR	unknown
DYT3	X-linked dystonia, parkinsonism "Lubag"	XR	Xq13.1
DYT4	Non DYT1 torsion dystonia	AD	unknown
DYT5a	Dopa-responsive dystonia, parkinsonism	AD	14q22.1-q22.2
DYT5b		AR	11p15.5
DYT6	Adolescent-onset torsion dystonia	AD	8p21-8p22
DYT7	Adult-onset focal torsion dystonia	AD	18p
DYT8	Paroxysmal dystonia choreoathetosis	AD	2q33-q35
DYT9	Paroxysmal choreoathetosis with episodic ataxia and spasticity	AD	1p21-p13.3
DYT10	Paroxysmal kinesigenic choreoathetosis	AD	unknown
DYT11	Myoclonus–dystonia	AD	11q23
DYT12	Rapid onset dystonia–parkinsonism	AD	19q

muscles. The therapeutic effects of each injection usually last 3 to 4 months. Side effects include injection site pain, hematoma, irritation of greater occipital nerve and brachial plexus, dysphagia, weakness of neck muscles in cases of cervical dystonia, and, uncommonly, generalized weakness.

3. Surgical options include thalamotomy, myotomy and rhizotomy, and selective rhizotomy; however, these are often unsuccessful. Another surgical approach is selective peripheral denervation with section of the nerve twigs innervating the dystonic muscles. The use of deep brain stimulation is also being explored.

4. Supportive therapy such as physiotherapy and occupational therapy are important aspects of management.

Key Treatment

- Anticholinergics for generalized dystonia

- Levodopa for dopa-responsive dystonia

- Botulinum toxin is the treatment of choice for many types of dystonia.

Bibliography

Brassat D, Camuzat A, Vidailhet M, et al.: Frequency of the DYT1 mutation in primary torsion dystonia without family history. Arch Neurol 57:333–335, 2000.

Klein C, Brin MF, de Leon D, et al.: De novo mutations (GAG deletion) in the DYT1 gene in two non-Jewish patients with early-onset dystonia. Hum Mol Genet 7:1133–1136, 1998.

Ozelius LJ, Hewett JW, Page CE, et al.: The early-onset torsion dystonia gene (DYT1) encodes an ATP-binding protein. Nat Genet 17:40–48, 1997.

5 Tourette's Syndrome

Alireza Minagar
Lisa M. Shulman
William J. Weiner

Definition

Tourette's syndrome (TS) is characterized by the presence of waxing and waning motor tics plus at least one vocal tic. Age of onset is usually between 5 and 20 years. The presence of behavioral abnormalities is not required for the diagnosis of TS; however, the clinical impact of such abnormalities is often more significant to patients than the tics.

Epidemiology and Risk Factors

1. TS is one of the most frequent movement disorders. However, an accurate lifetime prevalence rate for TS has not been established.

2. In an epidemiology study of a school district, 26% of children requiring special education had tics, versus 6% of children in regular classroom programs (Kurlan, 1994).

3. Males consistently outnumber females in large studies by a ratio as great as 4:1.

Etiology and Pathophysiology

1. Biochemical, imaging, neurophysiology, and genetic studies support the concept that TS is an inherited, developmental disorder of synaptic neurotransmission resulting in the disinhibition of the cortico-striatal-thalamic-cortical circuitry.

2. Although neuropathology studies of the brains of TS patients have not revealed any specific pathologic abnormalities, the basal ganglia, particularly the caudate nucleus and the inferior parietal cortex, have been implicated in the pathogenesis of TS, as well as in that of behavioral abnormalities of TS.

3. The potential role of antecedent infection with group A beta-hemolytic streptococcus and the consequent presence of antineuronal antibodies have been investigated in TS. Evidence in favor of the immunologic theory of TS includes elevated titers of antistreptococcal antibodies in some patients and increased levels of antineuronal antibodies against putamen in patients with TS.

Clinical Features

1. Tics
   a. Tics are brief, sudden, irregularly occurring, repetitive movements or sounds. Two major categories of tics are *motor* and *vocal*. Each category is further subdivided into *simple* and *complex*.

   b. Simple motor tics are abrupt, purposeless, and isolated movements involving individual muscle groups. Shoulder shrugs, eye blinking, and head jerks are examples.

   c. Some simple motor tics appear as slower, sustained, and tonic movements (e.g., neck twisting, abdominal tightening) that resemble dystonia and are therefore termed *dystonic tics*.

   d. Complex motor tics consist of coordinated, sequenced movements resembling normal motor acts or gestures that are inappropriately intense and timed. Touching, throwing, hitting, and jumping are examples. Other examples of complex motor tics are grabbing or exposing one's genitalia (copropraxia) or imitating gestures (echopraxia).

   e. Phonic tics are noises that can be produced from mouth, throat, and nose, whether vocal cords are involved or not.

   f. Simple phonic tics are inarticulate noises, while complex phonic tics include words, word fragments, or musical elements.

   g. Obscene speech (coprolalia) affects only a minority of TS patients.

   h. Motor and phonic tics may persist during all stages of sleep.

2. Behavioral disturbances
   a. Behavioral abnormalities of TS include obsessive-compulsive disorder (OCD), obsessive thoughts, compulsive rituals, attention deficit hyperactivity disorder (ADHD), dyslexia, depression, phobias, antisocial behavior, and personality disorders.

   b. Obsessions are defined as recurrent ideas, thoughts, images, or impulses that intrude on conscious thought and are persistent and unpleasant. Obsessive-compulsive symptoms may manifest several years after the onset of the tics. Obsessive symptoms may include feelings of incompleteness and need for symmetry; fears or

This work was supported in part by the Rosalyn Newman Foundation.

images of one's family being harmed, of contamination with dirt or germs, and of being responsible for the misfortune of others; or doubt that one has said or performed an action even though "reason" indicates that it has been done.

c. Compulsions are repetitive, purposeful behaviors performed in response to an obsession, or according to certain rules, or in a stereotyped fashion. Common compulsive symptoms include ordering and arranging habits, frequent counting, rituals for checking (locks, doors, or stove) and repeated hand washing.

d. Obsessive-compulsive symptoms (also called obsessive-compulsive behaviors) become OCD when activities are sufficiently severe to cause marked distress, consume more than 1 hour per day, or have a significant impact on normal routine, function, or social activities.

e. Nearly half of TS patients have some degree of OCD. However, there are differences between obsessive-compulsive symptoms among TS patients and primary OCD patients. Certain types of compulsive behavior such as touching and need for symmetry occur more frequently in TS patients than in patients with OCD but without TS.

f. TS is different from primary OCD in the triggers of compulsive behavior. Patients with primary OCD report anxiety as the trigger for performance of compulsions. In contrast, patients with TS report feelings of escalating tension, not anxiety, associated with both their compulsions and their tics. This tension is followed by a sense of release after the act (tic or compulsion) is performed.

g. It has been hypothesized that simple tics, complex tics, and compulsions may represent a continuous spectrum of symptoms in TS, and that the obsessive-compulsive symptoms seen in TS may actually be more phenomenologically related to tics themselves than to the types of obsessive-compulsive symptoms seen in primary OCD.

h. One distinction between the tics and compulsions observed in TS is in their response to medication, which indicates differences in the biological bases of the two. Tics are often treated with D2 antagonists whereas OCD symptoms are most responsive to serotonin reuptake inhibitors. Serotonin reuptake inhibitors are not as effective in treating OCD associated with TS or other tic disorders.

i. ADHD manifests with impulsivity, hyperactivity, and a decreased ability to maintain atten-tion, particularly during nonpreferred tasks. The diagnosis of ADHD requires an age of onset before 7 years, the presence of symptoms in two or more settings, and "clear evidence of clinically significant impairment in social, academic, or occupational functioning" (American Psychiatric Association, 1994).

j. Many researchers believe that ADHD symptoms are due to a decreased ability for behavioral inhibition (Barkley, 1994; Pennington, 1996) providing an interesting parallel to tics, which may be secondary to decreased inhibition of specific motor pathways.

k. ADHD typically begins at about age 4 to 5 years, and in TS usually precedes the onset of tics by 2 to 3 years. ADHD is reported to affect about 50% of referred TS cases. Its appearance is not associated with the concurrent severity of tics, although ADHD is frequently observed in TS patients with more severe tic symptomatology.

 Key Signs

- Simple or complex motor tics
- Phonic tics
- Obsessive-compulsive disorder
- Obsessive thoughts
- Compulsive rituals
- Attention deficit hyperactivity disorder
- Onset before age of 21 years

Differential Diagnosis

1. Tics should be differentiated from dystonia, chorea, myoclonus, and hyperexplexia.

2. Transient tic disorder, which affects 2% of children, is differentiated from TS by its short duration of less than 1 year.

3. Chronic motor tic disorder manifests with only one type of motor or vocal tic for life.

4. Chronic multiple tic disorder patients demonstrate either motor or vocal tics, but not both.

5. Tics may be observed in association with a variety of neurologic disorders such Huntington's disease, Parkinson's disease, startle disorders, and early developmental disorders.

6. Some tic disorders may have an autoimmune basis. Cases of OCD or tic disorder with acute onset, or sudden exacerbations have shown an association with group A beta-hemolytic streptococcal infec-

tion; it has been hypothesized that these cases represent a new syndrome designated as PANDAS (pediatric autoimmune neuropsychiatric disorders associated with streptococcal infection) (Swedo, 1998). This is a controversial hypothesis.

Laboratory Testing

1. TS is a clinical diagnosis.
2. Neuroimaging and other diagnostic studies are usually not required.
3. Neuropsychiatric evaluation and assessments with standardized neuropsychologic measures of attention and obsessive-compulsive behavior, may be valuable in characterizing associated behavioral abnormalities.

Treatment

1. Treatment of tics
   a. The goal of medical treatment of tics is to achieve maximum control with the fewest side effects.
   b. All medications should be initiated at low doses and gradually increased until sufficient benefit is obtained, or until intolerable side effects supervene (Table 5–1).
   c. Clonazepam may be used as once-a-day medication, because it may relax the patient and ameliorate concomitant emotional and behavioral abnormalities.

TABLE 5–1. DRUG TREATMENT OF TOURETTE'S SYNDROME

Drug	Starting Dose (mg/day)
Dopamine-receptor blockers for tics	
Fluphenazine	1.0
Pimozide	2.0
Haloperido	0.5
Risperidone	0.5
Ziprasidone	20.0
Thiothixene	1.0
Trifluperazine	1.0
Molindone	5.0
CNS stimulants for ADHD	
Methylphenidate	5.0
Pemoline	18.7
Dextroamphetamine	5.0
Noradrenergic drugs for impulse control and ADHD	
Clonidine	0.1
Guanfacine	1.0
Serotonergic drugs for OCD	
Fluoxetine	20.0
Clomiperamine	25.0
Sertraline	50.0
Paroxetine	20.0
Fluvoxamine	50.0
Venlafaxine	25.0

d. Clonidine has tic-suppressing effects and may be useful in children with associated ADHD. Clonidine is available as a weekly patch, but this formulation often causes hypersensitivity reactions.
e. The most effective agents for tics are dopamine receptor blockers that include fluphenazine, pimozide, haloperidol, thiothixene, trifluperazine, and molindone. The full spectrum of drug-induced movement disorders, from acute dystonic reactions to tardive syndromes, may complicate the use of these agents. Tardive disorders appear to be relatively rare in the TS population, but tardive dystonia may be more common than believed.
f. Flufenazine is the most effective and least sedative anti-tic drug. Pimozide is effective and less sedative than haloperidol, but it can cause prolongation of the Q-T interval and other changes on the ECG. Haloperidol is another effective anti-tic drug, but it can cause sedation, depression, weight gain, and school phobia.
g. The development of atypical neuroleptics such as olanzapine and quetiapine may make it possible to avoid the undesirable side effects of older neuroleptics.
h. Botulinium toxin injected in the area of tics can reduce their intensity and frequency. The benefits last 3 to 4 months, and are usually free from serious complications. Botulinium therapy ameliorates both the involuntary movements and premonitory sensory component associated with the tics.
i. A variety of behavioral techniques including psychotherapy, habit reversal, and hypnosis have been employed in the treatment of tics. In one case, complete abolition of tics was achieved with bilateral thalamic stimulation (Vandewalle, 1999).

2. Treatment of behavioral disorders
   a. A number of antidepressant medications, most notably serotonin-specific reuptake inhibitors, appear to have specific effects on obsessive-compulsive symptoms.
   b. Fluoxetine (20 to 60 mg/day), sertraline (50 to 200 mg/day), paroxetine (20 to 60 mg/day), fluvoxamine (50 mg/day and up), and venlafaxine (25 mg/day) may all improve obsessive-compulsive symptoms without affecting tic severity. The effectiveness of these drugs is likely dose-dependent, and doses higher than standard antidepressant ones are often required.
   c. Clomipramine is equally effective but has

anticholinergic, cardiotoxic, and seizure-potentiating effects.

d. Other pharmacologic agents for obsessive-compulsive symptoms include tryptophan, monoamine oxidase inhibitors, mianserin (a selective serotonin antagonist), and benzodiazepines.

e. A few TS patients have undergone successful surgery for obsessive-compulsive symptoms. Neurosurgery procedures used for this indication include thalamotomy, subcaudate tractotomy, cingulotomy, limbic leucotomy, and capsulotomy.

3. Education

Proper education of patients and their family members, as well as correction of misconceptions regarding TS and its behavioral complications, are significant parts of management of these patients. Parents should be informed that their child has a limited capacity to control the tics, which will be most prominent when the child feels his or her tics are unobserved or unlikely to provoke a negative social response, such as at home. Parents should tell the child's teachers of the diagnosis and of any medication. National and local support groups, such as the Tourette Syndrome Association (*http://www.tsa-usa.org*), can provide additional information and can serve as a valuable resource for patients and their families.

Key Treatment

- Dopamine-receptor blockers for tics
- Dopamine-depleting agents for tics
- Central nervous system stimulants for ADHD
- Noradrenergic drugs for impulse control and ADHD
- Serotonergic drugs for OCD

Bibliography

American Psychiatric Association: Diagnostic and Statistical Manual of Mental Disorders, 4th ed. Washington, DC, American Psychiatric Association, 1994.

Barkley RA: Impaired delayed responding. In Routh DK (ed): Disruptive behavior disorders in childhood: Essays honoring Herbert C. Quay. New York, Plenum, 1994, pp. 11–57.

Jankovic J: Tourette's syndrome. N Engl J Med 345:1184–1192, 2001.

Kurlan R, Whitmore D, Irvine C, et al.: Tourette's syndrome in a special education population: A pilot study involving a single school district. Neurology 44:699–702, 1994.

Pennington BF, Ozonoff S: Executive functions and developmental psychopathology. J Child Psychol Psychiatry 37:51–87, 1996.

Swedo SE, Leonard HL, Garvey M, et al.: Pediatric autoimmune neuropsychiatric disorders associated with streptococcal infections: Clinical description of the first 50 cases. Am J Psychiatry 155:264–271, 1998.

Vandewalle V, van der Linden C, Groenewegen HJ, Caemaert J: Stereotactic treatment of Gilles de la Tourette syndrome by high frequency stimulation of thalamus [letter]. Lancet 353:724, 1999.

6 Essential Tremor

Alireza Minagar
Lisa M. Shulman
William J. Weiner

Definition

Essential tremor (ET) is a monosymptomatic (tremor) disorder that occurs in a sporadic or familial form. Tremor results from simultaneous or alternating contraction of agonist and antagonist muscle groups. ET is a slowly progressive disorder that remains stable in some patients for prolonged periods of time. ET can interfere with performance of activities of daily living such as writing and eating.

Epidemiology and Risk Factors

1. ET is probably the most common movement disorder.
2. As many as 13% of individuals older than 65 years may have ET.
3. ET occurs equally in men and women.

Etiology and Pathophysiology

The pathophysiologic mechanisms of ET remain to be established. A disturbance of olivocerebellar rhythmicity is currently the most cited hypothesis for the etiology of ET.

Genetics

1. ET in some families is an autosomal dominant disorder. 60% of patients have a clear familial component.
2. During a genome investigation for familial forms of ET in 16 Icelandic kindreds with 17 affected members, investigators identified linkage to chromosome 3q13.1 (Glucher et al., 1997). The gene was designated *FET1*.
3. A second study evaluated a large American kindred of Czech descent in whom ET affected 18 of 67 family members. In this kindred, a gene for ET (*ETM2*) was mapped to chromosome 2p22-p25 (Higgins et al., 1997).

Neuropathology

Histopathologic examinations of patients with ET have not revealed any distinctive abnormalities.

This work was supported in part by the Rosalyn Newman Foundation.

Clinical Features

1. Diagnostic criteria for diagnosis of ET are presented under Core and Secondary Criteria (Findley, 1995; Deuschl, 1998; Bain, 2000).
2. The mean age of onset of ET is 45 years.
3. Tremor may be unilateral or bilateral at onset.
4. Tremor may spread to head and neck; approximately 50% to 60% of patients with ET have head involvement.
5. Voice tremor occurs in 30% of patients with ET and is characterized by rhythmic alterations in intensity at the same frequency as the hand tremor.
6. Less commonly, tremor may involve the trunk and legs.
7. Tremor tends to progress with age.
8. Alcohol improves tremor in 70% of patients with ET. In many patients ingestion of small amount of alcoholic beverages lessens the tremor for 30 to 45 minutes. ET is absent during sleep.

Core and Secondary Criteria for Diagnosis of Essential Tremor*

Core Criteria	Secondary criteria
Bilateral kinetic tremor of the hands and forearms	Long duration (>3 years)
Absence of other neurologic signs, with the exception of the cogwheel phenomenon	Positive family history
May have isolated head tremor with no signs of dystonia	Beneficial response to alcohol

*Adapted from Findley (1995), Deuschl (1998), Bain (2000).

Differential Diagnosis

1. The most common misdiagnosis of ET is Parkinson's disease. However, the two conditions can be differentiated by careful history and physical examination. Tremor of Parkinson's disease occurs at rest, whereas the tremor of ET is postural and kinetic. In addition Parkinson's disease is associated with bradykinesia, rigidity, shuffling gait,

TABLE 6–1. DOSES AND SIDE EFFECTS OF MEDICATIONS FOR ESSENTIAL TREMOR

MEDICATION	STARTING DOSE	THERAPEUTIC DOSE	ADVERSE EFFECTS
Propranolol	30 mg/day	160 to 32 mg/day	Fatigue, impotence, headache, depression, breathlessness, bradycardia
Primidone	12.5 to 25 mg/day	62.5 to 350 mg/day	Sedation, nausea, vomiting
Gabapentin	300 mg/day	1200 to 3600 mg/day	Drowsiness, fatigue, nausea, dizziness, imbalance
Alprazolam	0.75 mg/day	0.75 to 2.75 mg/day	Sedation, fatigue, tolerance
Topiramate	25 mg/day	100 to 300 mg/day	Paresthesias, weight loss, kidney stones
Nimodipine	120 mg/day	120 mg/day	Orthostatic hypotension
Theophylline	150 to 300 mg/day	15 to 300 mg/day	Insomnia, restlessness, headache

hypophonia, hypomimia, and a pill-rolling rest tremor.

2. Other neurologic conditions associated with tremor include multiple sclerosis, Wilson's disease, Huntington's chorea, and cerebellar degenerative diseases. In addition, drugs, toxins, and systemic illness can precipitate tremor. Occasionally ET may be misdiagnosed as anxiety disorder. In each of these cases, careful history, neuroradiologic examinations, and laboratory tests can differentiate ET.

Laboratory Testing

There are no specific laboratory tests for the diagnosis of ET.

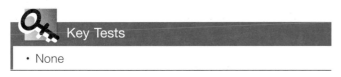

Key Tests

- None

Treatment

1. Propranolol (and other β-adrenergic blockers) and primidone are two medications that have been shown to be effective in suppressing ET. It is unclear which should be the drug of first choice.

2. Propranolol and primidone both reduce tremor amplitude but not tremor frequency.

3. Propranolol at a dose of at least 120 mg/day results in a significant reduction in the severity of ET.
   a. Peripheral β-adrenergic receptors probably mediate the effects of propranolol, although central mechanisms may be involved as well.
   b. Relative contraindications of propranolol include asthma, congestive heart failure, diabetes mellitus, and atrioventricular block.

4. Primidone is generally well-tolerated, but acute side effects such as vertigo, nausea, and unsteadiness may occur in 20% to 30% of patients.
   a. Primidone is started at a low dose, such as 25 mg/day or less to avoid the risk of acute side effects.
   b. The dosage may be titrated upward by 25 mg or 50-mg increments until efficacy or a dose of 250 to 350 mg/day is achieved. Administering primidone at night may increase compliance and minimize the sedative effect of the drug (Table 6–1) (Louis, 2001).

5. In cases of propranolol and primidone failure, alprazolam, gabapentin, topiramate, nimodipine, or theophylline as second-line agents can be tried (Table 6–1). Botulinum toxin A appears to possess some efficacy for ET of the head, voice, and hand.

6. Two surgical treatments for ET include continuous deep brain stimulation through an electrode implanted in the ventral intermediate nucleus of the thalamus and surgical lesioning of this nucleus (thalamotomy) contralateral to the more disabled arm.

Bibliography

Bain P, Brin M, Deuschl G, et al.: Criteria for the diagnosis of essential tremor. Neurology 54(Suppl 4):S7, 2000.

Deuschl G, Bain P, Brin M, et al., and an Ad Hoc Scientific Committee: Consensus statement of the Movement Disorder Society on tremor. Mov Disord 13(Suppl 3):S2–S23, 1998.

Findley LJ, Koller WC: Handbook of Tremor Disorders. New York, Marcel Dekker, 1995.

Glucher JR, Jonsson P, Kong et al.: Mapping of a familial essential tremor gene, FET1, to chromosome 3q13. Nature Genet 17:84–87, 1997.

Higgins JJ, Pho LT, Nee LE: A gene (ETM) for essential tremor maps to chromosome 2p22-p25. Mov Disord 12:859–864, 1997.

Louis ED: Essential tremor. N Engl J Med 345:887–891, 2001.

7 Wilson's Disease

Alireza Minagar
Lisa M. Shulman
William J. Weiner

Definition

Wilson's disease (WD) is a rare autosomal recessive neurologic disorder of copper metabolism that causes massive deposition of copper in the liver, cornea, kidneys, and nervous system. The exact cause of tissue damage remains an enigma, but the primary defect of copper transport is thought to be in the liver. When the copper storage capacity of the liver is exceeded the brain, kidneys, and other organs become secondarily involved.

Epidemiology and Risk Factors

1. Hall (1921) identified WD as a hereditary process.
2. A prevalence figure of 30 cases per million is most frequently quoted (Saito, 1981).
3. In northern Europe, calculations of WD gene frequency range from 0.34 to 0.53.

Etiology and Pathogenesis

1. WD is an autosomal recessive disorder of hepatocyte copper trafficking caused by impaired function of a P-type adenosine triphosphatase (Bull, 1993; Tanzi, 1993; Yamaguchi, 1993).
2. The gene for WD is located on chromosome 13 at q14.3. More than 25 gene mutations of the *WD* gene have been identified. The full-length DNA sequence reveals a length of 1411 amino acid protein.
3. The abnormal protein leads to failure of the liver to excrete copper into the bile. This copper excretion is mandatory to maintain a neutral copper balance.
4. Ceruloplasmin is a copper-containing molecule synthesized by the liver and may be the copper-packaging, protease resistant molecule that is excreted into the bile to eliminate excess copper via stool.

Neuropathology

1. The lenticular nuclei are affected bilaterally. The lesions range from softening and discoloration to frank cavitation.
2. Other regions with less involvement include the subcortical white matter, cerebellum (most commonly the dentate nucleus), and other basal ganglia nuclei.
3. Neuronal loss is commonly observed in both basal ganglia and the cerebral cortex.
4. Other microscopic alterations include diffuse proliferation of Alzheimer's type II cells in the basal ganglia, and Opalski cells in association with cavitary sites.

Clinical Features

1. Clinically, WD may manifest as an isolated hepatic syndrome, particularly in childhood up to 8 to 12 years of age. Neurologic presentations with hepatic cirrhosis are more common during the late teenage years.
2. The hepatic presentation can vary in its mode of onset from a syndrome similar to chronic active hepatitis to acute fulminant hepatic failure.
3. Tremor is the most frequent neurologic manifestation in WD, occurring in approximately 50% of individuals. The tremor may be resting, postural, or kinetic. WD tremor can be asymmetric and may be proximal or distal. A proximal component of tremor in the arms may give it a "wing-beating" appearance.
4. Other common neurologic symptoms of WD are dysarthria, dystonia, rigidity, and abnormalities of posture, gait, and facial expression. Drooling is common.
5. Intellect and sensory perception are intact.
6. Approximately one third of patients with WD initially present with psychiatric symptoms including depression, irritability, loss of temper, manic behavior, and sexual disinhibition.
7. Other systemic non-neurologic manifestations of WD include abnormalities of renal tubular function (including Fanconi's syndrome), Kayser-Fleischer ring, sunflower cataract, osteoporosis, renal stones, and gallstones.

Key Signs

- Acute hepatitis, chronic active hepatitis, cirrhosis
- Tremor, dysarthria, incoordination
- Parkinsonism, dystonia
- Depression, emotionality, bizarre behavior

This work was supported in part by the Rosalyn Newman Foundation.

TABLE 7–1.   KEY ANTICOPPER AGENTS FOR WILSON'S DISEASE TREATMENT

Drug	Mechanism of Action	Toxicity
Zinc acetate	Blockade of copper absorption	Abdominal discomfort
D-penicillamine	Chelation and urinary excretion of copper	Acute hypersensitivity subacute effects on bone marrow or kidney chronic effects on collagen and the immune system
Trientine	Chelation and urinary excretion of copper	Similar subacute and chronic toxicities as penicillamine, but with lower frequency
Tetrathiomolybdate	Copper/protein complex formation with prevention of copper absorption and detoxification of circulating copper	Copper deficiency anemia

Differential Diagnosis

WD must be distinguished from other juvenile genetic extrapyramidal disorders such as Huntington's disease, Hallervorden-Spatz disease, idiopathic torsion dystonia, and chorea-acanthocytosis.

Laboratory Testing

1. The most frequent screening method for WD is serum ceruloplasmin level, which usually is low in WD patients. However, in 10% of WD patients it may be normal or near normal.

2. The other useful screening test for WD is a 24-hour urine copper test. The 24-hour urine copper is always elevated.

3. Slit-lamp ocular examination for Kayser-Fleischer rings is very useful.

4. The gene for WD has been cloned, and this fosters hope for the development of a direct DNA test. This approach may not be practical, however, because of the large number of mutations that may cause WD.

5. Brain magnetic resonance imaging (MRI) scans are generally informative in patients with neurologic or psychiatric symptoms. The most common findings are abnormal hyperintense signals on T2-weighted images in the lentiform and caudate nuclei, thalamus, brainstem, and white matter. Brain scans are often negative in patients with only hepatic disease.

6. The definitive diagnostic test for WD is liver biopsy with quantification of hepatic copper.

Key Tests

- Serum ceruloplasmin level

- Twenty-four hour urine copper test (always elevated to a value of 100 µg/per 24 h in WD)

- Slit-lamp examination for Kayser-Fleischer rings

- Elevated hepatic copper value (in untreated WD > 200 µg/g dry weight of tissue)

- DNA analysis

Treatment

1. WD is a treatable disorder, and once a diagnosis is made therapy should be initiated without delay. Available pharmacologic agents are zinc acetate, D-penicillamine, trientine, and tetrathiomolybdate. Mechanisms of action and toxicity of these agents are presented in Table 7–1.

2. Zinc (50-200 mg three times a day) acts by inducing intestinal cell metallothionein which binds copper in the GI tract.

3. D-penicillamine (1–3 g/day, orally in four divided doses) acts by chelation of copper and mobilizes large amounts of copper, particularly from liver.

4. Trientine (600 mg 3 times daily) is a chelator and induces urinary excretion of copper. It may be a substitute in patients intolerant of D-penicillamine.

5. Tetrathiomolybdate is an experimental drug and not commercially available.

6. There is currently a controversy surrounding initial treatment of Wilson's disease. D-penicillamine has been the initial choice of therapy; however, there is growing concern that penicillamine may induce permanent neurologic deterioration in a significant number of patients. Some suggest zinc therapy as the initial treatment of choice.

Bibliography

Bull PC, Thomas GR, Rommens JM, et al.: The Wilson's disease gene is a putative copper transporting P-type ATPase similar to the Menkes gene. Nature Genet 5:327–337, 1993.

Hall HCL: La degenerescene hepato-lenticulaire: Maladie de Wilson pseudosclerose. Paris, Paul Masson, 1921.

Saito T: An assessment of efficiency in potential screening for Wilson's disease. J Epidemiol Community Health 35:274–280, 1981.

Tanzi RE, Petrukhin K, Chernov I, et al.: The Wilson disease gene is a copper transporting ATPase with homology to the Menkes disease gene. Nature Genet 5:44–50, 1993.

Yamaguchi Y, Heiny ME, Gitlin JD: Isolation and characterization of a human liver cDNA as a candidate gene for Wilson disease. Biochem Biophys Res Commun 197:271–277, 1993.

8 Multiple System Atrophy

Alireza Minagar
Lisa M. Shulman
William J. Weiner

Definition

Multiple system atrophy (MSA) is a neurodegenerative syndrome occurring sporadically. It is characterized by parkinsonism, cerebellar dysfunction, and dysautonomia. In this section three syndromes, MSA with olivopontocerebellar degeneration, MSA with dysautonomia, and MSA with striatonigral degeneration are described.

1. When one encounters the combination of parkinsonism in association with ataxic gait, limb dysmetria, and cerebellar dysarthria, the diagnosis of MSA with olivopontocerebellar degeneration should be considered.

2. Orthostatic hypotension frequently occurs in patients with parkinsonism. It is commonly drug induced, but in many patients it is an integral part of their idiopathic Parkinson's disease. In some patients, orthostatic hypotension and other dysautonomic features are severe and precede the parkinsonian symptoms; in such cases MSA with dysautonomia should be considered.

3. Parkinsonism with no or minimal tremor and that is mostly unresponsive to levodopa maybe striatonigral degeneration.

Epidemiology and Risk Factors

The exact incidence and prevalence of MSA is unknown, and obtaining accurate information is difficult because the disorder is frequently misdiagnosed.

1. Based on a large referral center experience of 100 patients with MSA, the reported median age of onset was 53 years (range, 33 to 76 years) (Wenning, 1994).

2. Quinn (1996) and Rajput (1991) have reported that MSA accounts for 8% to 22% of brains in parkinsonian brain banks.

3. Both sexes are affected equally.

4. The incidence in the 50- to 99-year age group has been measured at 3.0 new cases per 100,000 person-years, and the prevalence in a medically based series in London was 4.4 per 100,000 population (Schrag, 1999), about 3% of that of Parkinson's disease.

This work was supported in part by the Rosalyn Newman Foundation.

Etiology and Pathophysiology

The etiology and pathophysiology of these syndromes are unknown.

Neuropathology

1. Pathologically, the olivopontocerebellar degeneration is marked by various degrees of cell loss in basal ganglia, substantia nigra, Purkinje's cell layer of the cerebellum, dentate nucleus, pontine nuclei, and inferior olivary nuclei.

2. Striatonigral degeneration is characterized pathologically by marked neuronal loss and gliosis in the putamen, globus pallidus, and substantia nigra. Macroscopically, there is a brownish discoloration of putamen with significant atrophy.
   a. The caudate may appear normal or somewhat shrunken without discoloration.
   b. The substantia nigra exhibits hypopigmentation.
   c. Microscopically, severe neuronal loss, gliosis, and loss of myelinated fibers are evident in the putamen. The posterior two thirds and the dorsolateral regions are most affected.

Clinical Features

1. MSA with olivopontocerebellar degeneration
   a. Cerebellar ataxia, especially gait ataxia, is the initial manifestation in 73% of patients. The presence of dysmetria, limb ataxia, and cerebellar dysarthria is characteristic. Other initial symptoms consist of rigidity, hypokinesia, fatigue, disequilibrium, involuntary movements, visual changes, spasticity, and mental deterioration.
   b. With further progression, cerebellar impairments remain the most outstanding clinical features, affecting 97% of familial olivopontocerebellar atrophy patients and 88% of sporadic olivopontocerebellar atrophy patients.
   c. Dementia is the next most frequent manifestation of familial olivopontocerebellar atrophy and is present in 60% of the patients. Dementia occurs in 35% of sporadic olivopontocerebellar atrophy patients.
   d. Neuropsychological test scores on frontal lobe functions (hand sequencing and verbal reason-

ing) and parietal lobe functions (visual-spatial memory) are lower in olivopontocerebellar atrophy patients. Personality changes, such as emotionality, anxiety, and a tendency toward depression, are also present.

e. In sporadic olivopontocerebellar atrophy, parkinsonian features such as rigidity and akinesia appear as the second most frequent findings, being present in 57% of the patients, while occurring in only 35% of familial olivopontocerebellar atrophy patients. Abnormal movements usually appear late, and may include myoclonus, spasmodic torticollis, blepharospasm, choreoballism, and choreiform or athetoid dyskinesias.

f. Pyramidal signs, such as hyperreflexia or extensor plantar responses, develop relatively early and are found in half the patients. Later in the course of the disease, reflexes may become depressed or absent.

g. Supranuclear ophthalmoplegia (less commonly internuclear or nuclear) and visual defects, including macular degeneration, diffuse pigmentary degeneration, optic atrophy, and cataracts, are more typical in familial olivopontocerebellar atrophy.

2. MSA with dysautonomia

a. These patients have orthostatic hypotension, sometimes so severe that patients may lose consciousness on standing.

b. Bowel and bladder control are lost, and impotence is common in male patients.

c. Patients with MSA and dysautonomia may be further subdivided into two groups: those with only parkinsonism and autonomic insufficiency and those with cerebellar or pyramidal or lower motor neuron abnormalities.

d. In the latter group, dysautonomia is the presenting manifestation, and parkinsonism may not develop until 4 to 6 years after the onset of the illness.

e. Ataxia and atrophy of distal musculature with fasciculations are frequent.

f. Mental decline is rare.

3. MSA with striatonigral degeneration

a. Patients with striatonigral degeneration initially present with rigidity, hypokinesia, and unexplained falling.

b. The symptoms may be symmetrical or asymmetrical at onset.

c. The course is progressive, with a duration ranging from 2 to 10 years. Eventually, patients are severely disabled by marked akinesia, rigid-

ity, dysphonia or dysarthria, postural instability, and autonomic dysfunction.

d. Mild cognitive decline and affective changes with difficulties in executive functions, axial dystonia with anterocollis, stimulus-sensitive myoclonus and pyramidal signs such as hyperreflexia and extensor plantar responses may be present.

e. Resting tremor is uncommon and cerebellar signs are typically absent.

f. Most of patients with striatonigral degeneration do not respond to levodopa. However, early in the course, some patients may transiently respond to levodopa in high doses.

 Key Signs

Olivopontocerebellar Degeneration

• Cerebellar ataxia, especially gait ataxia

• Dysmetria, limb ataxia, and cerebellar dysarthria

• Dementia

• Parkinsonian features such as rigidity and akinesia

• Personality changes

Dysautonomia

• Orthostatic hypotension

• Incontinence

• Impotence in males

• Ataxia and atrophy of distal musculature

Striatonigral Degeneration

• Rigidity, hypokinesia, and unexplained falling

Differential Diagnosis

MSA syndromes should be differentiated from idiopathic Parkinson's disease, progressive supranuclear palsy, multi-infarct states, and corticobasal degeneration.

Laboratory Testing

1. All routine laboratory tests are normal in MSA.

2. Brain magnetic resonance imaging (MRI) scan can be used to exclude multi-infarct state or normal pressure hydrocephalus as causes of dopa-unresponsive parkinsonism and to exclude any cerebellar abnormalities. MRI can also demonstrate cerebellar and brainstem atrophy in MSA with olivopontocerebellar degeneration.

3. In patients with MSA, iron deposition in the posterolateral putamen may occur. It presents with a hypointense signal on T2-weighted MRI scans (Kraft, 1999).

4. In a large proportion of patients with MSA, striatonigral degeneration type, gliosis manifests as a hyperintense "slit" at the posterolateral border of the putamen on T2-weighted images.

5. Nerve conduction and EMG studies may demonstrate subclinical polyneuropathy in multiple system atrophy. External urethral sphincter EMG reveals denervation in almost all patients with MSA, but not usually in Parkinson's disease or in other forms of cerebellar degeneration.

Radiologic Findings

Olivopontocerebellar Atrophy

- Cerebellar and brainstem atrophy on MRI

Striatonigral Degeneration

- Hypointense signals in putamen on T2-weighted images

- Gliosis, seen in T2-weighted MRI as a hyperintense "slit" in the posterolateral border of the putamen

---

Treatment

Limited symptomatic treatment is available for parkinsonism and autonomic disturbances, but no specific therapy is available for the cerebellar abnormalities. More than two thirds of patients with MSA fail to respond to levodopa. Treatment may be initiated with levodopa/carbidopa 25/100 ½ to 1 tablet twice daily and escalated to efficacy or toxicity. Patients with MSA may require and tolerate far larger dosages than do patients with Parkinson's disease, but because some are quite sensitive to dopaminergic side effects, particularly nausea and dyskinesias, treatment should begin cautiously.

1. Symptomatic orthostatic hypotension can be managed with sodium and volume replacement, unless the patient is at risk of congestive heart failure or renal failure.

2. Patients should be instructed to avoid extreme heat with its reflex peripheral vasodilation and to avoid overeating and straining at stool, which increases vagal activity.

3. The mineralocorticoid fludrocortisone (Florinef) may be started at 0.1 mg daily and increased to a maximum of four tablets per day in two divided doses, given with fluid repletion. Midodrine (ProAmatine), an α-adrenergic agonist, is a suitable alternative. Treatment starts with 2.5 mg three times a day increasing to 10 mg three times a day.

4. Urinary frequency or incontinence may respond to a peripherally acting anticholinergic such as oxybutynin (Ditropan) 5 to 10 mg at bedtime, tolterodine (Detrol) 2 mg at bedtime, or propantheline (Pro-Banthīne) 15 to 30 mg at bedtime if the mechanism is detrusor hyperreflexia.

5. Anticholinergic treatment may worsen the constipation of MSA. This may be overcome by traditional stool softeners and bulk forming agents. The impotence of multiple system atrophy may respond to yohimbine (Yohimex, Yocon).

 Key Treatment

- Initial treatment: Levodopa/carbidopa 25/100 ½ to 1 tablet bid (dosage can increased every few days for efficacy)

- Most patients do not show response to levodopa/carbidopa

- Sodium and volume repletion for orthostatic hypotension

- Fluorocortisone and midodrine (an α-adrenergic agonist) for orthostatic hypotension

---

 # Bibliography

Kraft E, Schwarz J, Trenkwalder C, et al.: The combination of hypointense and hyperintense signal changes on T2-weighted magnetic resonance imaging sequences: A specific marker of multiple system atrophy? Arch Neurol 56:225–228, 1999.

Quinn NP, Wenning G. Multiple system atrophy. In Battistin L, Scarlatto G, Caraceni T, Ruggieri S (eds): Advances in Neurology, vol. 69. Philadelphia, Lippincott-Raven, 1996; pp. 413–419.

Rajput AH, Rozdilsky B, Rajput A: Accuracy of clinical diagnosis in parkinsonism: A prospective study. Can J Neurol Sci 18:275–278, 1991.

Schrag A, Ben-Shlomo Y, Quinn NP: Prevalence of progressive supranuclear palsy and multiple system atrophy: A cross-sectional study. Lancet 354:1771–1775, 1999.

Wenning GK, Ben Shlomo Y, Magalhaes M, et al.: Clinical features and natural history of multiple system atrophy: An analysis of 100 cases. Brain 117:835–845, 1994.

9 Myoclonus

Alireza Minagar
Lisa M. Shulman
William J. Weiner

Definition

Myoclonus is defined as sudden, short, jerky, shock-like, involuntary movements caused by abrupt muscular contraction (positive myoclonus) or sudden cessation of muscle contraction for a silent period of electromyographic (EMG) discharges (negative myoclonus). Myoclonic jerks arise from the central nervous system and involve the limbs, face, and trunk. Myoclonus may be classified in various ways.

1. On the basis of distribution, myoclonus can be *focal, segmental,* or *generalized.*

2. Neurophysiologic studies have demonstrated the existence of several types of myoclonus: *cortical; brainstem;* and *spinal.*

3. The temporal distribution of myoclonus can be irregular, rhythmic, or oscillatory. Myoclonus may be present at rest or manifest during performance of voluntary movements or the maintenance of a posture (action myoclonus).

4. Reflex or stimulus-sensitive myoclonus is precipitated by peripheral somatosensory or auditory stimuli.

5. Marsden and colleagues (1981) classified myoclonus as (i) physiologic; (ii) essential; (iii) epileptic; and (iv) symptomatic (Table 9–1).

   a. Physiologic myoclonus (PM) consists of sudden and isolated jerks of the entire body that occur upon falling asleep or during sleep, particularly as part of an arousal response to an external stimulus. PM occurs after prolonged exercise or during intense emotional stress. Hiccup is regarded as physiologic myoclonus.

   b. Essential myoclonus (EM) begins in the first or second decade of life, affects both sexes equally, causes mild functional impairment, and is not associated with any neurologic or systemic disturbances. EM may occur spontaneously or during voluntary action. It usually disappears during sleep and is exacerbated during emotional stress.

   c. Epileptic myoclonus: A host of myoclonic phenomena accompany epilepsy, particularly childhood epilepsies. Focal myoclonus is observed in patients with epilepsia partialis continua. Progressive myoclonic epilepsies include a heterogenous group of disorders associated

TABLE 9–1. OTHER ETIOLOGIES OF MYOCLONUS

Drug-induced myoclonus
  Anticonvulsants
  Levodopa
  Lithium
  Fentanyl
  Clozapine
  Penicillin
  Vigabatrin
  Cyclosporin
  Tricyclic antidepressants
  Serotonin-reuptake inhibitors
  Monoamine oxidase inhibitors
Opsoclonus-myoclonus syndrome
  Viral infections
  Ovarian cancer
  Melanoma
  Lymphoma
  Non-ketotic hypoglycemia
Asterixis
  Metabolic encephalopathies such as hepatic encephalopathy
  Lesions of the thalamus, putamen, and the parietal lobe
Cortical myoclonus
  Tumors
  Angiomas
  Encephalitis
Palatal myoclonus
  Idiopathic
  Stroke
  Multiple sclerosis
  Neurodegenerative disorders
Spinal myoclonus
  Inflammatory myelopathy
  Cervical spondylosis
  Tumors
  Ischemic myelopathy
Postanoxic encephalopathy
Progressive myoclonic ataxia (Ramsay Hunt syndrome)
Gender (male)
Race (white)
Trauma
Metals (manganese, iron)
Farming
Rural residence
MPTP and MPTP-like compounds
Infectious agents

with multifocal or generalized myoclonus and epileptic seizures. Progressive myoclonic epilepsies are identified by epileptic seizures and progressive neurologic symptoms such as dementia, ataxia, spasticity, and hearing loss. Unverricht-Lundborg disease, Lafora body disease, myoclonic epilepsy–ragged red fibers syndrome (MERRF), Kufs' disease, and sialodosis are examples of these progressive myoclonic epilepsies.

   d. Symptomatic myoclonus is associated with a variety of infective, degenerative, metabolic, and toxic encephalopathies.

This work was supported in part by the Rosalyn Newman Foundation.

Key Signs

- Sudden, short, jerky, shock-like involuntary movements

- Movements can be focal, segmental, or generalized

Epidemiology and Risk Factors

The only available study, from Olmstead County, Minnesota (Caviness, 1999), revealed an average annual incidence of 1.3 cases per 100,000 patient years. The rate increased with advancing age and was consistently higher among men.

Etiology and Pathophysiology

1. Cortical myoclonus is due to focal activity in the sensorimotor cortex, and the abnormal cortical discharges are propagated via the corticospinal pathways to the spinal cord.

   a. Focal cortical lesions including tumors, angiomas, and encephalitis, may be associated with focal cortical myoclonus. Epilepsia partialis continua can occur in the context of focal encephalitis as in Rasmussen's syndrome, stroke, tumors, and, rarely, in multiple sclerosis. Occasionally, subcortical abnormalities may be associated with myoclonic jerks; examples include Parkinson's disease, multiple system atrophy, and cortical-basal ganglionic degeneration.

   b. Cortical myoclonus manifest spontaneously, during voluntary movements or somatosensory stimulation.

   c. The EMG bursts of myoclonus are of short duration, lasting 10 to 30 milliseconds. The EEG recording may reveal simultaneous spike or spike and wave. Cortical somatosensory evoked potentials (SEPs) are enlarged in many of these patients, and normal SEPs do not exclude a cortical origin for myoclonus.

2. Brainstem myoclonus is typically generalized and manifests in response to auditory or sensory stimulation of the head and neck area.

   a. It may represent an exaggeration of the normal brainstem startle response and activates the sternocleidomatoid muscles first, followed by the facial muscles, the masseter muscles, and the trunk and limb muscles.

   b. This muscular activation progresses up the brainstem and down the spinal cord. The bilateral and predominantly proximal pattern of muscle recruitment suggests efferent spinal conduction in reticulospinal pathways.

   c. EMG recording reveals bursts of muscle activity of 100 milliseconds duration.

   d. Electroencephalography may demonstrate generalized spike discharges.

3. Spinal myoclonus originates from abnormal discharge of spinal motoneurons.

   a. In spinal segmental myoclonus, muscle jerks are repetitive, rhythmic, and confined to adjacent spinal segments; they persist during sleep at a frequency of 0.5 to 2.0 Hz.

   b. It is thought that spinal segmental myoclonus arises from enhanced anterior horn cell excitability.

4. Palatal myoclonus results from a lesion interrupting the Guillain-Mollaret triangle, which consists of the dentate nucleus, the contralateral central tegmental tract, and the inferior olive.

   a. Autopsy studies have revealed hyperplasia of the inferior olivary nucleus, particularly in the symptomatic (secondary) form of palatal myoclonus (Deuschl, 1990).

   b. There is hypermetabolism of the inferior olive by positron emission tomography scanning.

   c. In unilateral palatal myoclonus the lesion involves the contralateral central tegmental tract or the olivary nucleus or the ipsilateral dentate nucleus.

Genetic Factors

1. Unverricht-Lundborg disease and the Mediterranean and Baltic forms are linked to chromosome 21q (locus EMP1). The pattern of inheritance is autosomal recessive. The EMP1 locus has been identified with the gene coding for cystatin B.

2. Myoclonic dystonia is a dominantly inherited disorder, and the linkage analysis has shown a 23-centimorgan region on chromosome 11q23 that cosegregates with the disease state. This region contains an excellent candidate gene, i.e., the D2 dopamine receptor gene (Klein, 1999).

3. The underlying gene for Lafora's progressive myoclonic epilepsy maps to chromosome 6q23-25. There are mutations in the protein tyrosine phosphatase gene. However, some families do not show linkage to this area, suggesting genetic heterogeneity.

4. The MERRF syndrome is typically associated with point mutations in the mtDNA *tRNALys* gene. However, double mutations may be observed (Arenas, 1999).

5. In multiple symmetrical lipomatosis and myoclo-

nus and ataxia, mitochondrial DNA mutations may be seen.

6. Essential myoclonus has a dominant mode of inheritance with a variable degree of clinical severity.

Clinical Features

1. EM may be focal, segmental, or generalized. Onset is usually in the first two decades of life. Men and women are equally affected.

2. Progressive myoclonic epilepsy is a progressive disease with frequent generalized seizures, myoclonus, and dementia commonly caused by neurodegenerative storage disorders. These include gangliosidosis, neuronal ceroid lipofuscinosis, sialidosis, and Lafora body disease.

3. Palatal myoclonus may be idiopathic or it may be associated with various neurologic disorders such as stroke, tumors, multiple sclerosis, trauma, and neurodegenerative disorders.

4. Spinal myoclonus is associated with inflammatory myelopathy, cervical spondylosis, tumors, trauma, and ischemic myelopathy.

5. Multifocal and generalized myoclonus occur in association with spinocerebellar degenerations, mitochondrial disease (myoclonus epilepsy with ragged-red fibers), storage diseases such as GM2 gangliosidoses, ceroid lipofuscinosis, sialidosis, and dementias including Creutzfeldt-Jakob disease and Alzheimer's disease. Viral and postviral syndromes may cause myoclonus. Multifocal myoclonus is frequently due to metabolic causes including hepatic failure, uremia, hyponatremia, hypoglycemia, and nonketotic hyperglycemia. Toxic encephalopathies causing myoclonus include bismuth, methyl bromide, and toxic cooking oil. Lance-Adams syndrome refers to action myoclonus occurring after hypoxic brain injury with associated asterixis, seizures, and gait problems.

Differential Diagnosis

1. The differential diagnosis of an isolated myoclonic jerk includes chorea and tic.

2. Choreic movements are not stimulus sensitive and are slower than myoclonic jerks.

3. Tics may be simple or complex and in contrast to myoclonic jerks may be preceded by premonitory sensations and can be voluntarily delayed or suppressed.

Laboratory Tests

1. EMG is useful to determine the sequence of contractions and identify the origin of the myoclonus.

2. Somatosensory evoked response to search for giant SEPs

3. Magnetic resonance imaging (MRI) of brain and spinal cord to detect focal lesions

4. Electron microscopic study of skin, conjunctiva, and muscle specimens can assist diagnosis of Lafora body disease, neuroaxonal dystrophy, and mitochondrial disorders.

Laboratory Findings

- EMG may reveal the sequence of contractions and the origin of the myoclonus.

- SSEP studies may show giant somatosensory evoked potentials

- MRI of brain and spinal cord can detect focal lesions

- Electron microscopic study of skin, conjunctiva, and muscle can assist diagnosis of Lafora body disease, neuroaxonal dystrophy, and mitochondrial disorders

---

Treatment

1. Characterize the type of myoclonus.

2. Identify the underlying cause of the myoclonic syndrome. Metabolic disorders and other underlying causes, if identified, must be rectified.

3. Control symptomatic myoclonic jerks with appropriate drug therapy. The most effective drugs are clonazepam (4 to 10 mg/day) and sodium valproate (250 to 4500 mg/day). Other less effective drugs are lisuride, acetazolamide, carbamazepine. In posthypoxic myoclonic syndrome (Lance-Adams syndrome) a combination of 5-hydroxytryptophan and carbidopa can be effective.

4. Progressive myoclonic epilepsy may be worsened by phenytoin, and acetazolamide may be useful in treatment of Ramsay Hunt syndrome.

5. Spinal myoclonus may improve with removal of the compressing lesion.

6. Negative myoclonus (asterixis) often resolves with the correction of the responsible metabolic insult, and ethosuximide may be useful in the symptomatic management.

 Key Treatment

- Sub-classify the type of myoclonus

- Clonazepam (4 to 10 mg/day) or sodium valproate (250 to 4500 mg/day)

- 5-hydroxytryptophan and carbidopa for posthypoxic myoclonus

- Negative myoclonus may resolve with the correction of the metabolic insult.

B Bibliography

Arenas J, Campos Y, Bornstein B, et al.: A double mutation (A8296G and G8363A) in the mitochondrial DNA tRNA (Lys) gene associated with myoclonus epilepsy with ragged-red fibers. Neurology 52:377–382, 1999.

Caviness J, Alving L, Maraganore D, et al.: The incidence and prevalence of myoclonus in Olmsted County, Minnesota. Mayo Clin Proc 74:565–569, 1999.

Deuschl G, Mischke G, Schenck E, et al.: Symptomatic and essential rhythmic palatal myoclonus. Brain 113:1645–1672, 1990.

Klein C, Brin MF, Kramer P, et al.: Association of a missense change in the D2 dopamine receptor with myoclonic dystonia. Proc Natl Acad Sci USA 6:5173–5176, 1999.

Marsden CD, Hallett M, Fahn S: The Nosology and Pathophysiology of Myoclonus. In CD Marsden, Fahn S, (eds): Movement Disorders 2. London: Butterworth, 1981, p. 196.

1 **Multiple Sclerosis**

Alireza Minagar
William A. Sheremata

Definition

Multiple sclerosis (MS) is clinically characterized by relapsing remitting or progressive neurologic deficits reflecting lesions in multiple areas of the central nervous system (CNS) over time.

Epidemiology and Risk Factors

1. MS is the most common cause of chronic neurologic disability in young adults. There are at least 250,000 to 300,000 patients diagnosed with MS in the United States (Noseworthy, 2000).

2. MS is more common in northern regions of Europe and the United States, with a prevalence as high as 1 per 1,000 population.

3. Epidemiologic studies suggest that the risk of MS is related in part to geographic location in temperate zone during childhood years: Individuals born or migrating to low-risk areas before the age of 15 appeared to have reduced risk.

4. Migration, ethnic, and twin studies suggest that both genetic and environmental factors are involved in pathogenesis of MS.

   a. The risk of developing MS in identical twins where one twin has clinically definite MS is about 30%.

   b. Siblings of MS patients have a risk of about 2.6%; parents, a risk of about 1.8%; children, a risk of about 1.5%.

5. MS is more common in women (M:F ratio 2:1) with a peak incidence at age 24.

   a. Symptoms rarely begin before the age of 10 years or after the age of 60 years.

   b. About 70% have symptoms from 21 to 40 years; 12%, ages 16 to 20; 13%, ages 41 to 50.

Etiology and Pathophysiology

1. The etiology of MS remains to be established. The CNS pathology involves white matter: immune-mediated destruction of myelin sheaths with relative preservation of axons. Viruses that have been hypothesized to be involved in the etiology of MS include influenza, measles, canine distemper, human T- cell lymphocytotropic virus (HTLV-1), and, most recently, human herpessimplex virus-6 (HHSV-6).

2. Numerous studies have revealed altered immune responses in MS. Lymphocytes are frequently present in moderate numbers (<50 mm^3) in the cerebrospinal fluid (CSF).

3. Histopathologic specimens containing MS plaques contain both helper (CD4+) and suppressor/cytotoxic (CD8+) T cells, as well as macrophages, which are primarily responsible for myelin destruction.

4. The inflammatory reaction resolves in 2 to 6 weeks, presumably suppressed by endogenous CNS and immune mechanisms, such as production of the cytokines IL-4, IL-10, transforming growth factor-beta (TGF-β), prostaglandin E; a rise in cortisol; and apoptosis of invading cells. Astrocytic reaction and gliosis follow the initial inflammatory reaction.

5. Demyelination results in conduction block as a result of exposure of fast-conducting K$^+$ channels and increased energy cost resulting from the loss of saltatory conduction.

Neuropathology

1. MS is an inflammatory demyelinating disease affecting CNS white matter. Inflammatory cells, mainly activated lymphocytes and monocytes, cross the blood–brain barrier in the white matters surrounding blood vessels, destroying myelin with relative sparing of axons.

2. Individual lesions are termed *plaques,* and with time, perivenular lesions may coalesce, forming plaques that measure several centimeters.

3. These plaques have a predilection for periventricular white matter, particularly that adjacent to the frontal and occipital horns of the ventricular system. Other areas of involvement are spinal cord, especially the cervical region; optic nerve; periaqueductal gray matter; and corpus callosum.

4. Electron microscopic studies have revealed the active role of invading macrophages in myelin destruction. These changes are accompanied by swelling of the astrocyte foot processes and interstitial edema.

5. The traversing axons are decreased in number and

may disappear entirely. Axonal loss occurs in MS as a consequence of an inflammatory reaction to severe and chronic weakness (Trapp, 1998).

Clinical Features

1. Onset of MS is typically acute or subacute over several days and is only rarely sudden.

2. Motor symptoms are prominent initial manifestations of MS, with weakness often affecting the legs and sometimes the arms. Commonly, a young woman complains that she cannot walk down a sidewalk without tripping over the curb or uneven sections of pavement. Patients may also report stiffness and present with foot-drop. Corticospinal tract involvement in MS occurs in 32% to 41% of patients during the initial attack and manifests in 62% of patients with chronic illness.

3. Sensory symptoms are an early hallmark of MS and include tingling, "pins and needles," numbness, a tight band around the torso, "a dead feeling," or "ice inside the legs." Sensory complaints are present in 21% to 55% of MS patients, and during the course of the disease they manifest in 52% to 70% of patients. Patients often use strange metaphors to describe their sensory aberrations.

4. The cerebellum and its connections are involved in 50% of MS patients by the end of their clinical illness. Patients may present with symptoms such as limb tremor, ataxia, scanning speech, and head or trunk titubation. Charcot's triad, consisting of intention tremor, dysarthria, and nystagmus, is a well recognized but rare presentation.

5. Optic neuritis and retrobulbar optic neuritis are associated with blurring or obscuration of vision, scotomas, decreased color perception, and occasionally flashes. Pain often occurs with movement of the affected eye. Optic neuritis is one of the most common initial manifestations of MS, occurring in 14% to 23% of patients.

6. Diplopia occurs in 12% to 22% of MS patients and is caused by pontine demyelinating plaques involving the intramedullary portions of the sixth and third cranial nerves or the medial longitudinal fasciculus (MLF). In 13% of patients MLF involvement causes internuclear ophthalmoplegia (INO), which is pathognomonic sign of MS. Lesions are often not visualized in magnetic resonance imaging (MRI) scans. Nystagmus, frequently on horizontal axis, manifests with a frequency as high as 40% to 70%.

7. Trigeminal neuralgia is uncommon in MS, and only 1% of patients present with the characteristic severe momentary lancinating pain in the distribution of the maxillary or mandibular divisions of cranial nerve V. However, the appearance of trigeminal neuralgia in a young adult is highly suggestive of MS.

8. Facial myokymia affecting the lower face is an uncommon but important finding in MS patients. These wormlike movements of the muscles are frequently unilateral and occasionally are difficult to observe. They are pathognomic of MS.

9. Vertigo occurs in at least 15% of MS patients and may be associated with diplopia. Severe disabling vertigo happens in 5% of MS patients, abating after a few days, more often noted early in the clinical course.

10. Paroxysmal symptoms that may last only seconds to hours occur, often early in the course of the disease. Most commonly recognized is paroxysmal dystonia, which is characterized by tonic seizures. They may occur in one fourth of the patient population during their illness.

11. The neurobehavioral aspects of MS consist of both cognitive dysfunction and neuropsychiatric disorders. Cognitive difficulties occur in 45% to 60% of MS patients; occasionally, they will be the initial manifestation. They include memory retrieval, mental processing speed, reasoning and goal-oriented behavior, verbal fluency, and visuospatial skills. Neuropsychiatric disturbances are mainly mood disorders. The neurobehavioral aspects of multiple sclerosis may be present in either relapsing attacks or in a chronic progressive course. Mood disorders occur more frequently in MS than in other chronic disabilities. Collectively, major depression, bipolar illness, and dysphoria occur in the majority of MS patients, with severe depression occurring in 37% to 54%.

12. A relatively common sensory complaint in MS patients is sudden electric-like sensation radiating down the spine and frequently extending into the limbs as well (Lhermitte's sign).

13. MS patients may experience sudden and transient neurologic deterioration, often due to elevated body temperature. This temporary worsening that is frequently associated with febrile illnesses also may manifest during physical exercise. Blurring of vision is the most commonly reported transient neurologic symptom that is aggravated or precipitated by even moderate exercise (Uhthoff's phenomenon).

14. Impairments of defecation and, especially, urination are common in MS, occurring in up to 78% of MS patients during the course of the illness. Sexual dysfunction is common among MS patients. Men often experience erectile dysfunction

as well as problems with ejaculation. Women commonly complain of difficulty reaching orgasm and problems with lubrication.

15. Paroxysmal symptoms may last only seconds to hours and often occur early in the course of the disease in more than 34% of patients. Paroxysmal dystonia (tonic spasms) of MS can be similar to the muscle spasms, tetany, and paresthesia of hyperventilation syndrome. The episodes consist of brief, recurrent, often painful abnormal posturing of 1 or more limbs without alteration of consciousness, loss of sphincter control, or clonic movements. Other paroxysmal symptoms include blurred vision, dysarthria, ataxia, falling, akinesia, and paresthesia.

16. Diagnostic criteria for MS are presented in (Table 1–1) (McDonald, 2001).

17. Four characteristic clinical courses of MS are recognized for the purposes of study: relapsing-remitting, secondary progressive, primary progressive, and relapsing-progressive (Table 1–2).

Laboratory Tests

1. Brain and spinal cord MRI with gadolinium infusion plays an important role in diagnosis of MS. Typical features of MS on MRI are bright lesions on T_2-weighted images, especially in a periventricular location and the corpus callosum. Lesions are characteristically ovoid or linear and are at right angles to the ventricular surfaces. A lesion larger than 5 mm and lesions below the tentorium, especially in the cerebellar peduncle, help confirm the diagnosis. Usually, T_1-weighted images are less sensitive in detecting plaques than T_2-weighted images. However, when there is active breakdown of the blood–brain barrier, the lesions enhance with gadolinium infusion. Newer

TABLE 1–1.   NEW DIAGNOSTIC CRITERIA FOR MULTIPLE SCLEROSIS

CLINICAL PRESENTATION	ADDITIONAL DATA NEEDED FOR MS DIAGNOSIS
Two or more attacks; objective clinical evidence of 2 or more lesions	None[a]
Two or more attacks; objective clinical evidence of 1 lesion	Dissemination in space, demonstrated by MRI[b] or Two or more MRI-detected lesions consistent with MS plus positive CSF[c] or Await further clinical attack implicating a different site
One attack; objective clinical evidence of 2 or more lesions	Dissemination in time, demonstrated by MRI[d] or Second clinical attack
One attack; objective clinical evidence of 1 lesion monosymptomatic presentation; clinically isolated syndrome)	Dissemination in space, demonstrated by MRI[b] or Two or more MRI-detected lesions consistent with MS plus positive CSF[c] and Dissemination in time, demonstrated by MRI[d] or Second clinical attack
Insidious neurological progression suggestive of MS	Positive CSF[c] and Dissemination in space, demonstrated by 1) nine or more T2 lesions in brain or 2) 2 or more lesions in spinal cord, or 3) 4–8 brain plus 1 spinal cord lesion or abnormal VEP[e] associated with 4–8 brain lesions, or with fewer than 4 brain lesions plus 1 spinal cord lesion demonstrated by MRI and Dissemination in time, demonstrated by MRI[d] or Continued progression for 1 year

If criteria indicated are fulfilled, the diagnosis is multiple sclerosis (MS); if the criteria are not completely met, the diagnosis is "possible MS"; if the criteria are fully explored and not met, the diagnosis is "not MS."

[a]No additional tests are required; however, if tests [magnetic resonance imaging (MRI), cerebral spinal fluid (CSF)] are undertaken and are *negative,* extreme caution should be taken before making a diagnosis of MS. Alternative diagnoses must be considered. There must be no better explanation for the clinical picture.

[b]MRI demonstration of space dissemination.

[c]Positive CSF determined by oligoclonal bands detected by established methods (preferably isoelectric focusing) different from any such bands in serum or by a raised IgG index.

[d]MRI demonstration of time dissemination.

[e]Abnormal visual evoked potential of the type seen in MS (delay with a well-preserved wave form).

TABLE 1–2. CLINICAL COURSES IN MULTIPLE SCLEROSIS

CLINICAL COURSE	DEFINITION
Relapsing-remitting	Episodes of acute worsening with recovery and a stable course between relapses
Primary progressive	Gradual, nearly continuous neurologic deterioration from the onset of symptoms
Secondary progressive	Gradual neurologic deterioration with or without superimposed acute relapses in a patient who previously had relapsing-remitting multiple sclerosis
Progressive-relapsing	Gradual neurologic deterioration from the onset of symptoms, but with subsequent superimposed relapses

From Lublin FD, Reingold SC: Defining the clinical course of multiple sclerosis: Results of an international survey. In National Multiple Sclerosis Society (USA) Advisory Committee on Clinical Trials of New Agents in Multiple Sclerosis. Neurology 46:1907, 1996.

neuroimaging techniques such as fluid-attenuated-inversion-recovery (FLAIR) provide increased sensitivity and specificity for the diagnosis and treatment of MS. FLAIR is perhaps the most sensitive imaging sequence for white matter abnormalities; it detects two to three times the number of lesions observed on T_2-weighted imaging.

2. *N*-acetylaspartate (NAA), a marker for neuronal and axonal function, can be measured by MR spectroscopy. NAA levels are decreased not only in MS plaques, but also in apparently unaffected areas of white matter. This finding suggests the presence of axonal damage.

3. Analysis of CSF obtained by lumbar puncture provides significant information in the evaluation of patients. Elevated IgG index, presence of oligoclonal bands (OCBs), and increased myelin basic protein, all support the diagnosis of MS. In general, OCBs are found in over 90% of MS patients. However, their presence is not specific for MS and OCBs are found in 30% of CNS inflammatory and infectious disease controls, and in 5% to 10% of other, noninflammatory neurologic diseases. Elevated CSF protein may be observed in 40% of MS patients, and values >100 mg/dL are rare. The number of cells in the CSF of MS patients is increased, and in one third of cases a pleocytosis in the range of 10 to 20 mononuclear cells per cubic millimeter is noted. CSF leukocyte counts of >50 mm^3 are uncommon in MS, and >100 mm^3 should raise doubt about the diagnosis of MS.

4. Visual evoked responses are performed using a light and dark checkerboard pattern reversal stimulus. Computer averaging of occipital scalp electrode potentials normally reveals a major

positive wave (P100) with a latency of about 100 msec, which varies with patient age and the stimulus variables for each laboratory. Prolonged latencies of the P100 wave are abnormal and, if monocular, specifically indicate prechiasmal involvement. Abnormal findings are more prevalent with increased duration of MS, ultimately observed in more than 75% of patients.

Key Tests

- Brain MRI with gadolinium
- Brain spectroscopy
- Evoked responses
- Lumbar puncture
- Neuropsychological testing

Differential Diagnosis

1. MS is one among many demyelinating disorders
   a. Autoimmune: acute disseminated encephalomyelitis and acute hemorrhagic leukoencephalopathy
   b. Toxic/metabolic: carbon monoxide poisoning, vitamin B_{12} deficiency, alcohol/tobacco amblyopia, central pontine myelinolysis, Marchiafava-Bignami disease, and hypoxia.
   c. Infection: subacute sclerosing panencephalitis and progressive multifocal leukodystrophy

2. Postinfectious encephalomyelitis and disseminated encephalomyelitis are acute neurologic syndromes with disseminated CNS demyelination and MRI abnormalities similar to MS. However, they are usually monophasic and are preceded by a febrile illness. In case of progression or recurrence of the signs, a diagnosis of MS should be considered.

3. Retrobulbar or optic neuritis must be differentiated from ischemic optic neuropathy, vitamin B_{12} deficiency, vasculitis (giant cell arteritis), and viral infection. Optic neuritis is frequently the first manifestation of MS, and most patients with optic neuritis eventually develop MS. Some clinical features of vitamin B_{12} deficiency are similar to MS, including myelopathy, neuropathy, and dementia. However, vitamin B_{12} deficiency is usually chronic and progressive and can be excluded by measurement of serum vitamin B_{12} levels and a search for megaloblastic anemia.

4. Compressive myelopathy is a major consideration in the differential diagnosis of MS. The cord lesion in MS presents as increased T_2 signal on MRI,

with or without enhancement, and is often partial, patchy, and asymmetric.

5. Tropical spastic paraparesis/human T-cell leukemia virus associated myelopathy (TSP/HAM), is caused by the human T-cell lymphocytotropic virus HTLV-1. TSP/HAM is prevalent in the Caribbean region and manifests as an indolent progressive myelopathy with paraparesis, bladder dysfunction, and sexual dysfunction in men. Serologic testing discloses antibody to HTLV-1. MRI scans are usually negative except in Haitians, in whom rapidly progressive disease is common.

6. Lyme disease and neurosyphilis are infectious diseases that can mimic MS and present with a multifocal nervous system disease. The clinical course, as well as CSF antibody studies can differentiate both conditions from MS. In neurosyphilis, however, oligoclonal bands may be present.

7. Devic's disease is clinically characterized by attacks of optic neuritis and necrotizing myelitis without clinical or MRI evidence of brain involvement or presence of oligoclonal bands in the CSF. Normal brain MRI scans, normal CSF IgG synthesis, and the absence of oligoclonal bands will differentiate Devic's disease from MS (Minagar, 2000).

8. Dysmyelinating disease such as adrenoleukodystrophy (ALD), adrenomyeloneuropathy (AMN), metachromatic leukodystrophy (MLD), Krabbe's disease, van Bogaert's disease, Canavan's disease, and Pelizaeus-Merzbacher disease.

Treatment

Treatments for MS can be divided into two categories: disease modifying and symptomatic. The former category includes various therapies designed to modulate or suppress the immune response or its inflammatory end results.

1. Disease-modifying agents include:

    a. Adrenocorticotropic hormone (ACTH) is the only agent approved for the management of exacerbations of MS. Infusions of ACTH lasting 8 to 10 hours a day over periods of up to 3 weeks shorten exacerbations significantly. The drug is obtained with difficulty.

    b. Intravenous corticosteroids are frequently used to treat clinical exacerbations of MS to hasten recovery. The most common treatment plan is intravenous methylprednisone (Solumedrol) in doses of 500 to 1000 mg daily for 3 to 5 days. After intravenous corticosteroid infusion, a tapered course of oral prednisone over 1 to 3

weeks is usually described. Aseptic necrosis of the hip and other joints is an important complication.

2. Immunomodulating agents are used to modify the course of MS. For relapsing-remitting MS, four FDA-approved drugs have been shown to decrease the relapse rate and may also affect disease progression. Three of these agents (Avonex, Rebif, and Betaseron) are interferons, while Copaxone is a synthetic polypeptide, glatiramer acetate. Betaseron (interferon-β1b) has three molecular differences with human β-interferon: it is not glycosylated, there is an amino acid substitution at position 17, and there is no "N-terminal" methionine.

    a. There are two types of recombinant β-interferon: Avonex and Rebif. Interferon β-1a (Avonex) is administered 30 μg intramuscularly injection once per week. A randomized, double-blind trial has shown that initiating treatment with interferon beta-1a at the time of a first demyelinating event is beneficial for patients with at least two brain lesions on magnetic resonance imaging, which indicates a high risk of clinically definite multiple sclerosis (Jacobs, 2000).

    b. Rebif (interferon β-1a) is administered 22 μg and 44 μg subcutaneously three times a week. In a 2-year clinical trial (PRISMS Study Group 1998) (n = 560), both a low (22 μg, 6 MIU) and a high (44 μg, 12 MIU) dose of Rebif administered three times weekly reduced the number of clinical relapses and were associated with an increased proportion of relapse-free patients compared with placebo after 2 years of study.

    c. Interferon β-1b (Betaseron) is injected 8 MIU subcutaneously once every other day. Betaseron reduces the exacerbation rate of MS by 34%.

    d. All of these three drugs are usually well tolerated, although side effects are more prominent with Betaseron: fever and flu-like symptoms and fatigue. Pre-medication with nonsteroidal anti-inflammatory agents such as acetaminophen or ibuprofen may lessen the severity and duration of flu-like symptoms.

    e. Glatiramer acetate (Copaxone, Copolymer-1) is injected 20 mg subcutaneously daily. Glatiramer acetate reduces the exacerbation rate of MS by 29%. Side effects include injection reactions and an acute anxiety-like reaction, with flushing and chest tightness.

3. Immunosuppressive agents with modest efficacy in preventing disease exacerbations include mitoxantrone (Novantrone), cyclophosphamide, imu-

ran, and methotrexate. Only mitoxantrone is approved by the FDA for patients with chronic progressive MS. Mitoxantrone is an anthracenedione antineoplastic agent that intercalates with DNA and suppresses humoral immunity, reduces T cell number, abrogates helper cell activity, and enhances suppressor function (Lubin, 1987; Edan, 1997). The greatest potential risk of mitoxantrone is a toxic cardiomyopathy, which limits its use in MS patients. Mitoxantrone and methotrexate, as well as Imuran, should be used only by physicians experienced and familiar with their use.

 Key Treatment: Disease-Modifying Agents

- ACTH

- Intravenous corticosteroids: methylprednisone

- Immunomodulating agents: Avonex, Rebif, Betaseron, Copaxone

- Immunosuppressive agents: mitoxantrone, cyclophosphamide, Imuran, methotrexate

Symptomatic Treatment

1. Physical and emotional rest are important strategies in the management of MS.
2. Fatigue can be improved with amantadine. Provigil (modafinil) 100–200 mg per day may be of value. Amantadine (Symmetrel) 100–200 mg per day has been reported to improve fatigue in MS, but the benefit frequently is not sustained. Anecdotal reports suggest that fluoxetine (Prozac) may be effective in treatment of fatigue in MS patients.
3. Spasticity can be relieved by a small dose of diazepam at bedtime, or multiple doses of baclofen, or tizanidine alone or in combination. Because patients' response to baclofen varies, an initial dose of 5 mg 3 times daily should tried. The recommended maximum dose of tizanidine is 36 mg in 3 divided doses daily. Gabapentin (Neurontin) is also helpful for spasms and can be used in MS, usually at doses of 2000 mg daily.
4. Carbamazepine, or other anticonvulsants, can alleviate paroxysmal dystonia or other paroxysmal manifestations.
5. Bladder dysfunction is common among MS patients, and acute urinary retention can often be relieved by intermittent catheterization. Anticholinergics such as oxybutynin (Ditropan, 5 mg two or three times daily), tolterodine (Detrol, 2 mg twice day), and amitriptyline (Elavil, 25 mg at bedtime) may be useful in controlling nocturia.

6. Constipation may be treated with adequate fluids and fiber intake including supplemental fiber such as psyllium (Perdiem). Occasional patients will benefit from suppositories and enemas.
7. Sexual dysfunction in men is often the result of spinal cord disease and psychological factors. New oral pharmacologic approaches such as sildenafil citrate (Viagra) may improve erectile function.
8. Physical therapy and regular exercise can improve gait and general level of functioning.

 Key Treatment: Symptomatic Therapy

- Physical and emotional rest

- Amantadine or modafinil for fatigue

- Baclofen or tizanidine—alone or combined—or Neurontin for spasticity

- Carbamazepine for paroxysmal dystonia or other paroxysmal manifestations

- Intermittent catheterization for acute urinary retention

- Anticholinergics for controlling nocturia

- Adequate fluids and fiber intake for constipation

- Sildenafil citrate for sexual dysfunction

- Physical therapy and regular exercise for improving gait and general level of functioning

Pregnancy and MS

The exacerbation rate declines during pregnancy (Confavreux, 1998); however, the relapse rate increases significantly 3 to 6 months postpartum, and the attacks are more severe. Multiple sclerosis is less likely to appear de novo during pregnancy, and pregnancy decreases the risk of a progressive course. The decline in exacerbations during pregnancy is presumably from immunosuppressive factors that prevent rejection of the placenta and fetus. The progesterone/17-beta-estradiol ratio falls during the third trimester of pregnancy, when clinical activity is low. However, the ratio increases during the luteal phase of the menstrual cycle and corresponds to higher MRI activity (Pozzilli, 1999). There is a rebound in immune function after delivery that may boost disease activity.

 Bibliography

Confavreux C, Hutchinson M, Hours MM, et al.: Rate of pregnancy-related relapses in multiple sclerosis. N Engl J Med 339:285–291, 1998.

Edan G, Miller D, Clanet M, et al.: Therapeutic effect of mitoxantrone combined with methylprednisolone in multiple sclerosis: A randomized multicenter study of active disease using MRI and clinical criteria. J Neurol Neurosurg Psychiatry 2:112–118, 1997.

Jacobs LD, Beck RW, Simon JH, et al.: Intramuscular interferon beta-1a therapy initiated during a first demyelinating event in multiple sclerosis. CHAMPS Study Group. N Engl J Med 343:898–904, 2000.

Lublin FD, Lavasa M, Viri C, Knobler RI: Suppressions of acute and relapsing experimental allergic encephalomyelitis with mitoxantrone. Clin Immunol Immunopathol 45: 122–128, 1987.

McDonald WI, Compston A, Edan G, et al: Recommended diagnostic criteria for multiple sclerosis: guidelines from the International Panel on the diagnosis of multiple sclerosis. Ann Neurol 50:121–127, 2001.

Minagar A, Sheremata WA: Treatment of Devic's disease with methotrexate and prednisone. Int J MS Care [serial on-line]. 2(4), 2000.

Noseworthy JH, Lucchinetti C, Rodriguez M, Weinshenker BD: Multiple sclerosis. N Engl J Med 343:938–952, 2000.

Pozzilli C, Falaschi P, Mainero C, et al.: MRI in multiple sclerosis during the menstrual cycle: Relationship with sex hormone patterns. Neurology 53:622–624, 1999.

PRISMS Study Group: Randomised, double-blind, placebo-controlled study of interferon beta-1a in relapsing/remitting multiple sclerosis. PRISMS (Prevention of Relapses and Disability by Interferon beta-1a Subcutaneously in Multiple Sclerosis) Study Group. Lancet. 352:1498–1504, 1998.

Rammohan KW, Rosenberg JH, Lynn DJ, et al.: Efficacy and safety of modafinil (Provigil) for the treatment of fatigue in multiple sclerosis: a two centre phase 2 study. J Neurol Neurosurg Psychiatry. 72:179–183, 2002.

Trapp BD, Peterson J, Ransoholl RM, et al.: Axonal transection in the lesion of multiple sclerosis. N Engl J Med 338:278–285, 1998.

2 Acute Disseminated Encephalomyelitis

Alireza Minagar
William A. Sheremata

Definition

Acute disseminated encephalomyelitis (ADEM) and its hyper-acute form, acute necrotizing hemorrhagic encephalopathy (ANHE), are thought to be forms of immune-mediated inflammatory demyelination. ADEM manifests as an acute, uniphasic syndrome occurring often in association with an immunization, vaccination, or systemic viral infection. ADEM and ANHE differ from MS. Importantly, either illness is typically uniphasic and has a favorable long-term prognosis. In contrast, MS is, by definition, relapsing and chronically progressive. At present there are no generally accepted diagnostic criteria for ADEM; therefore, differentiation of ADEM from the first episode of MS is not possible. Moreover, cases of recurrent and multiphasic ADEM have been described.

Epidemiology and Risk Factors

1. ADEM occurs as a postinfectious complication in 1:400 to 1:2000 measles, 1:600 mumps, 1:10,000 varicella, and 1:20,000 rubella cases. It has also been reported as a postvaccination complication in 1:63 to 1:300,000 of vaccinia, as well as following other immunizations. It was relatively common after rabies vaccination until the new "diploid vaccines" were produced (Johnson, 1994; Johnson, 1985; Scott, 1967).

2. ADEM has also been reported after diphtheria/tetanus, pertussis, and rubella.

Etiology and Pathophysiology

1. ADEM is a T cell–mediated autoimmune disease targeted at a myelin/oligodendrocyte antigen, probably myelin basic protein. Proposed mechanisms for ADEM include:

   a. Molecular mimicry in which certain peptide, carbohydrate, or lipid epitopes on an infecting virus or other antigen are similar to epitopes on myelin or oligodendrocytes.

   b. Nonspecific activation of T cells by viruses or other antigens. The activated T cells expand clonally, migrate across the blood–brain barrier, and upon identifying recognizable epitopes, trigger an inflammatory process within the central nervous system.

   c. Downregulation of CD4+ suppressor T cells by viral infections, which would permit activation of myelin-reactive T-helper cells.

Neuropathology

1. The neuropathology of ADEM consists of perivenular inflammatory myelinopathy. Grossly, the brain appears swollen, with engorgement of veins in the white matter.

2. Microscopically, there is perivascular edema with intense mononuclear infiltration, mainly composed of lymphocytes and macrophages.

3. The salient histopathologic feature of ADEM is demyelination, with relative axonal sparing. Demyelination occurs around small veins.

Clinical Features

1. ADEM is characterized by a monophasic illness, often with multifocal neurologic manifestations and involvement of the brainstem, spinal cord, optic nerves, cerebrum, and/or cerebellum.

2. Neurologic symptoms appear abruptly 1 to 3 weeks after the viral infection. Typically, systemic symptoms dominate the clinical presentation, including headache, nausea, vomiting, confusion, delirium, obtundation, and coma. In milder cases these symptoms may be minimal.

3. Often superimposed on this multisymptomatic syndrome are focal neurologic abnormalities such as hemiparesis, hemisensory loss, ataxia, optic neuritis, and transverse myelitis. After mumps, ADEM tends to present with a cerebellar ataxia.

4. Seizures, myoclonus, and memory loss have been reported.

Key Clinical Features

- Monophasic illness, often with multifocal neurological manifestations and involvement of the brainstem, spinal cord, optic nerves, cerebrum, and/or cerebellum

- Neurologic symptoms appear abruptly 1 to 3 weeks after the viral infection.
- Focal neurologic abnormalities such as hemiparesis, hemisensory loss, ataxia, optic neuritis, and transverse myelitis
- Seizures, myoclonus, and memory loss

Differential Diagnosis

1. ADEM should be differentiated from MS because it characteristically occurs as a single episode with acute onset and is accompanied by fever and headache. A history of antecedent viral infection or vaccination further supports the diagnosis of ADEM. The magnetic resonance imaging (MRI) lesions of both ADEM and MS are similar; however, in ADEM lesions frequently are synchronously enhancing, a finding that is rare in MS. Perhaps in 25% of patients, ADEM, may evolve into MS, and MS may rarely manifest with synchronus enhancing lesions. Long-term follow-up with clinical examinations and brain MRI with gadolinium should differentiate ADEM as a monophasic disorder from MS with its characteristic relapsing or progressive course.

2. When ADEM presents with optic neuritis or acute myelopathy, it must be distinguished from other disorders that may have similar presentations, such as syphilis, acute viral infections, HIV-1 infection, HTLV-I/II, and systemic collagen vascular diseases.

3. Acute viral meningoencephalitis is another condition that should be distinguished from ADEM. A clear period of well being after a febrile illness, benign cerebrospinal fluid (CSF), and negative cultures, all suggest ADEM rather than direct infection. Brain biopsy is not needed to make this distinction and is rarely justifiable.

Laboratory Testing

1. The diagnosis of ADEM rests on the clinical picture of a uniphasic presentation and, except for brain biopsy, there are no definite laboratory tests for its diagnosis. When brain biopsy is performed, lymphoblastic transformation in response to myelin basic protein is typically present in ADEM but not in MS. CSF findings are frequently abnormal but nonspecific in ADEM. CSF shows a mononuclear pleocytosis, with a mildly elevated protein level. However, the cell count and protein concentration may be within normal limits in one third of patients.

2. Brain MRI reveals hyperintense signals in white matter on T2-weighted images and proton density images and gadolinium enhancement on T1-weighted images. Abnormal areas may be observed in the cortex and basal ganglia. The lesions on MRI vary in size and, because of surrounding edema, tend to be larger than the pathologic lesions. In acute transverse myelitis, cord enlargement may appear in the absence of hyperintense signals on T2-weighted images.

Key Tests

- Brain MRI with gadolinium
- Evoked responses
- Lumbar puncture

Treatment

There are no specific therapies for ADEM, and management is primarily supportive and symptomatic. In severe cases, maintenance of vital functions, preservation of fluid and electrolyte balance, and avoidance of pneumonia, urinary tract infections, and decubiti are crucial.

1. Corticosteroids: High doses of intravenous corticosteroids are usually used in ADEM; however, definite information on their efficacy is lacking. Many neurologists treat patients with ADEM with methylprednisolone 1000 mg/day × 5 days, followed by oral prednisone (on a slow tapering schedule over 7 to 10 days). When available, adrenocorticotropin hormone (ACTH) is effective.

2. Plasmapheresis: A favorable therapeutic response to plasmapheresis in patients with ADEM has been reported. However, some of these patients were treated simultaneously with corticosteroids and cyclophosphamide, so a delayed response to corticosteroids or spontaneous improvement cannot be excluded.

3. There are case reports of improvement of patients with ADEM after treatment with intravenous immunoglobulin (IVIG). However, controlled clinical trials are needed to confirm the efficacy of these treatments.

Key Treatment

- Supportive and symptomatic treatment
- Corticosteroids
- Plasmapheresis
- IVIG

Prognosis

As many as one fourth to one third of patients initially diagnosed with ADEM relapse during long-term follow up. If relapse occurs, a diagnosis of MS is often made; however, some patients who experience relapse early after disease onset do not exhibit relapsing illness on follow-up. There are no useful diagnostic criteria to differentiate uniphasic ADEM from the first episode of MS (Hartung, 1994; Schwartz, 2001). In recent studies indicate that mono-symptomatic illness (optic neuritis, isolated brainstem syndromes, or transverse myelitis) accompanied by MRI scans demonstrating two or more brain lesions will relapse within 1 year in 50% of cases.

References

Hartung HP: ADEM: Distinct disease or part of MS spectrum? Neurology 56:1257–1260, 2001.

Johnson RT: The virology of demyelinating diseases. Ann Neurol 36:S54–60, 1994.

Johnson RT, Griffin DE, Gendelman HE: Postinfectious encephalomyelitis. Semin Neurol 5:180–190, 1985.

Schwarz S, Mohr A, Knauth M, Wildemann B, Storch-Hagenlocher B: Acute disseminated encephalomyelitis: A follow-up study of 40 adult patients. Neurology 56:1313–1318, 2001.

Scott TH: Postinfectious and vaccinal encephalitis. Med Clin North Am 51:701–717, 1967.

Part VII   Epilepsy

1   Etiology and Manifestations

Steven C. Schachter

Etiology

1. Seizures are symptoms, not a pathological process; therefore it is important for the physician to determine if the seizures are idiopathic or symptomatic of an underlying condition.

2. Less than one-half of patients with epilepsy have an identifiable cause.

3. Among the remaining cases, causes of epileptic seizures include

   a. Congenital brain malformations

   b. Inborn errors of metabolism

   c. High fevers

   d. Head trauma

   e. Brain tumors

   f. Stroke

   g. Intracranial infection

   h. Cerebral degeneration

   i. Withdrawal states

   j. Iatrogenic drug reactions (see Section XXIV, Chapter 5, Iatrogenic Seizures)

4. In elderly patients, vascular, degenerative, and neoplastic etiologies are more common than in younger adults and children.

5. A higher proportion of epilepsy in children is due to congenital brain malformations than in other age groups.

Manifestations

1. Definitions

   a. A seizure is a sudden change in behavior that is the consequence of brain dysfunction.

      (1) Epileptic seizures result from electrical hypersynchronization of neuronal networks in the cerebral cortex.

      (2) Epilepsy is characterized by recurrent epileptic seizures due to a genetically determined or acquired brain disorder.

         (i) Approximately 0.5% to 1% of the population has epilepsy.

         (ii) Incidence is highest in early childhood and among those aged 65 and older.

   b. Non-epileptic seizures (NES) are sudden changes in behavior that resemble epileptic seizures but are not associated with the neurophysiological changes that characterize epileptic seizures.
   NES are subdivided into two major types: physiologic and psychogenic.

      (1) Physiologic NES are caused by a sudden alteration of neuronal function caused by metabolic derangement or hypoxemia, including

         (a) Hyper- and hypothyroidism

         (b) Hypoglycemia

         (c) Nonketotic hyperglycemia

         (d) Hyponatremia

         (e) Hypocalcemia

         (f) Hypomagnesemia

         (g) Renal failure

         (h) Disorders of porphyrin metabolism

         (i) Cerebral anoxia

      (2) Psychogenic NES are thought to result from stressful psychological conflicts or major emotional trauma and rarely occur de novo in patients without a significant psychiatric history.

   c. Seizure precipitants or triggers are particular environmental or physiologic factors that immediately precede seizures.

      (1) Some patients with epilepsy tend to have seizures under particular conditions (see Common Seizure Triggers). Most patients with epilepsy have no identifiable or consistent trigger to their seizures; triggers are the sole cause of epileptic seizures in only a very small percentage of epileptic patients.

      (2) Triggers may also precipitate physiologic NES; for example, coughing may bring on a syncopal seizure (see Section I, Chapter 13, Syncope vs Seizure).

Common Seizure Triggers

- Fever
- Menstrual period
- Flashing lights
- Lack of sleep
- Stress
- Strong emotions
- Intense exercise
- Loud music

---

2. Seizure classification: Generalized or partial

a. Generalized seizures originate virtually in all the regions of the cortex. Subtypes include

(1) Absence seizures

(a) Usually occur during childhood and typically last between 5 and 10 seconds. If an absence seizure lasts for 10 seconds or more, there may also be eye blinking and lip smacking.

(b) Frequently occur in clusters and may occur dozens or even hundreds of times a day

(c) Atypical absence seizures usually begin before 5 years of age and are associated with mental retardation and a tendency for multiple seizure types. They last longer than typical absences and are often associated with a slackening or stiffening of the muscles.

(2) Generalized tonic-clonic seizures (also called grand mal seizure, major motor seizure, or convulsion)

(a) Begin with an abrupt loss of consciousness, often in association with a scream or shriek

(b) Muscles of the arms and legs as well as the chest and back become stiff (tonic phase), and the patient may begin to appear cyanotic.

(c) After approximately 1 minute, muscles begin to jerk and twitch for an additional 1 to 2 minutes (clonic phase). The tongue may be bitten and frothy; bloody sputum may be seen coming out of the mouth.

(d) Once the twitching movements end, the post-ictal phase begins. The patient is initially in a deep sleep, breathing deeply, and then gradually wakes up, often complaining of a headache.

(3) Clonic seizures: Rhythmic jerking muscle contractions that usually involve the arms, neck, and face

(4) Myoclonic seizures

(a) Characterized by sudden, brief muscle contractions that may occur singly or in clusters and that can affect any group of muscles, though typically the arms are affected

(b) Consciousness is usually not impaired.

(5) Tonic seizures: Cause sudden muscle stiffening, often associated with impaired consciousness and falling to the ground

(6) Atonic seizures (also known as *drop seizures* or *drop attacks*): Produce the opposite effect of tonic seizures—a sudden loss of control of the muscles, particularly of the legs, that results in collapsing to the ground and possible injuries

b. Partial seizures begin in a focal brain region. Subtypes are

(1) Simple partial seizures

(a) "Simple" means that consciousness is not impaired.

(b) May be referred to by patients as the *warning* or *aura*.

(c) Specific symptoms of simple partial seizures depend on where the seizure originates in the brain.

(d) Common simple partial seizures are

(i) Jacksonian seizures

(ii) Olfactory hallucinations

(iii) Fear and panic

(iv) Déjà vu

(v) Rising epigastric sensation

(2) Complex partial seizures (CPS) (previously called *temporal lobe seizures* or *psychomotor seizures*)

(a) "Complex" means that consciousness and awareness of the surroundings are lost.

(b) The most common type of seizure in epileptic adults. The presentation under Differential Diagnosis Of Complex

Partial Seizures (below) shows other disorders to be ruled out.

(c) Patients appear to be awake but are not in contact with others in their environment and do not respond normally to instructions or questions. They often seem to stare into space and either remain motionless or engage in repetitive behaviors, called automatisms, such as facial grimacing, gesturing, chewing, lip smacking, snapping fingers, repeating words or phrases, walking, running, or undressing. If physically restrained during complex partial seizures, patients may become hostile or aggressive.

(d) CPS typically last less than 3 minutes and may be immediately preceded by a simple partial seizure. Afterward, the patient enters the post-ictal phase, often characterized by somnolence, confusion, and headache for up to several hours. The patient has no memory of what took place during the seizure other than, perhaps, the aura.

Differential Diagnosis of Complex Partial Seizures

- REM behavior disorder

  - Parasomnia that consists of sudden arousals from REM sleep immediately followed by complicated, often aggressive, behaviors that the patient does not remember

  - Diagnosed by overnight sleep testing (polysomnography)

- Transient ischemic attack

- Transient global amnesia

- Migraine

Bibliography

Commission on Classification and Terminology of the International League Against Epilepsy: Proposal for revised clinical classification of epileptic seizures. Epilepsia 22: 489–501, 1981.

Hauser WA, Annegers JF, Kurland LT: Incidence of epilepsy and unprovoked seizures in Rochester, Minnesota: 1935–1984. Epilepsia 34:453–468, 1993.

Sander JWAS, Shorvon SD: Epidemiology of the epilepsies. J Neurol Neurosurg Psychiatry 61:433–443, 1996.

2 Epilepsy Syndromes

Steven C. Schachter

Definition and Classification

1. Defined by a characteristic cluster of features (see Features of Epilepsy Syndromes)

Features of Epilepsy Syndromes

- Age of onset of seizures
- Associated neurologic symptoms and signs
- Seizure type(s) (e.g., benign rolandic epilepsy, juvenile myoclonic epilepsy)
- Family history of epilepsy
- Prognosis

---

2. Epilepsy syndromes are divided into those with generalized seizures (generalized epilepsies) and those with partial-onset seizures (localization-related or focal epilepsies) (Table 2–1).

3. They are further divided into *idiopathic* (primary, cryptogenic) syndromes (those with no identifiable cause) and *symptomatic* (secondary) syndromes when the cause is known.

4. Determining that a patient has a particular epilepsy syndrome has implications with regard to
   a. Genetic risk/counseling
   b. Treatment (see Section VII, Chapter 3, Medical Treatment, for discussion of therapy for specific seizure types)
   c. Prognosis

Common Epilepsy Syndromes

1. Benign rolandic epilepsy (benign childhood epilepsy with centrotemporal spikes)
   a. Age of onset from 3 to 13 years; peak incidence around age 8
   b. Normal cognitive function and normal neurologic examination
   c. Nocturnal seizures are typically generalized with probably focal onset and include excessive salivation, gurgling or choking sounds, and clonic mouth contractions
   d. Daytime seizures (which occur in the minority of children) involve tonic and/or clonic movements of one side of the body (especially the face) and speech arrest

Key Signs: Benign Rolandic Epilepsy

- Age of onset from 3 to 13 years; peak incidence around age 8

Nocturnal Seizures

- Excessive salivation
- Gurgling or choking sounds
- Clonic mouth contractions

Daytime Seizures

- Tonic and/or clonic movements of one side of the body
- Speech arrest

---

   e. The electroencephalogram (EEG) shows high-amplitude midtemporal-central spike and sharp waves, mainly during light sleep.
   f. Prognosis is excellent; seizures are readily controlled with anti-epileptic drugs (AEDs), and remission is the rule.

Key Treatment: Benign Rolandic Epilepsy

- Anti-epileptic drugs

---

2. Juvenile myoclonic epilepsy
   a. Usually begins during teenage years
   b. Normal cognitive function and normal neurologic examination
   c. Myoclonic jerks, tonic-clonic seizures, clonic-tonic-clonic seizures, or absence seizures
      (1) Typically occur within the first few hours after awakening
      (2) Myoclonic seizures are usually mild, bilateral, and involve the upper limbs.

Key Signs: Juvenile Myoclonic Epilepsy

- Usually begins during teenage years
- Myoclonic jerks or seizures (tonic-clonic, clonic-tonic-clonic, or absence) usually occur within the first few hours after awakening.

---

   d. EEG shows characteristic 3.5 to 6 Hz spike-

TABLE 2–1.   INTERNATIONAL CLASSIFICATION OF EPILEPSIES AND EPILEPSY SYNDROMES

Localization-Related (focal, local or partial) Epilepsies and Syndromes
- Idiopathic epilepsy with age-related onset
  - Benign childhood epilepsy with centrotemporal spikes
  - Childhood epilepsy with occipital paroxysms
- Symptomatic epilepsy

Generalized Epilepsies and Syndromes
- Idiopathic epilepsy with age-related onset listed in order of age
  - Benign neonatal familial convulsions
  - Benign neonatal non-familial convulsions
  - Benign myoclonic epilepsy in infancy
  - Childhood absence epilepsy
  - Juvenile absence epilepsy
  - Juvenile myoclonic epilepsy
  - Epilepsy with generalized tonic-clonic seizures on awakening
- Other idiopathic epilepsies
- Idiopathic or symptomatic epilepsy
  - West's syndrome (infantile spasms)
  - Lennox-Gastaut syndrome (childhood epileptic encephalopathy)
  - Epilepsy with myoclonic-astatic seizures
  - Epilepsy with myoclonic absence seizures
- Symptomatic epilepsy
  - Nonspecific etiology
    - Early myoclonic encephalopathy
  - Specific etiology
    - Epileptic seizures may complicate many disease states.

Epilepsies and Syndromes Undetermined as to Whether They are Focal or Generalized
- With both generalized and focal seizures
  - Neonatal seizures
  - Severe myoclonic epilepsy in infancy
  - Epilepsy with continuous spike waves during slow-wave sleep
  - Acquired epileptic aphasia (Landau-Kleffner syndrome)
- Without unequivocal generalized or focal features

Special Syndromes
- Situation-related seizures
  - Febrile convulsions
  - Seizures related to other identifiable situations, such as stress, hormonal changes, drugs, alcohol withdrawal, or sleep deprivation
- Isolated, apparently unprovoked epileptic events
- Epilepsies characterized by specific modes of seizure precipitation

From Commission on Classification and Terminology of the International League against Epilepsy: Proposal for revised classification of epilepsies and epileptic syndromes. Epilepsia 30:389–399, 1989.

and-wave pattern; polyspike-and-waves that are induced by photic stimulation and sleep deprivation.

   e. Seizures respond well to AEDs; relapse upon AED withdrawal is highly likely.

Key Treatment: Juvenile Myoclonic Epilepsy
- Anti-epileptic drugs

   f. Family history is often positive.
3. Febrile seizures
   a. Usually occur between age 3 months and 5 years in approximately 4% of children
   b. Neurologic examination is usually normal.
   c. Generalized seizures with or without focal onset

Key Signs: Febrile Seizures
- Generalized seizures with or without focal onset

   d. Treatment includes reducing fever and giving rectal diazepam in children with fever and previous history of febrile seizures. Long-term AED prophylaxis is generally not recommended if seizures are strictly generalized and last under 15 minutes.

Key Treatment: Febrile Seizures
- Reduce fever
- Diazepam

   e. Family history of epilepsy may be present
   f. Up to 5% of affected children develop chronic epilepsy. Predictive factors include
     (1) Seizures that have focal features or that last longer than 15 minutes
     (2) Focal neurologic abnormalities
     (3) Family history of afebrile seizures
4. Infantile spasms
   a. Typically begin by age 1, particularly between the ages of 4 and 6 months; rare for spasms to develop after 18 months of age
   b. Affected infants usually have West's syndrome.
     (1) Infantile spasms
     (2) Mental retardation
     (3) Hypsarrhythmia on waking EEG (high-voltage diffuse spike-and-slow waves su-

perimposed on a disorganized, slow background)

c. Often associated with cerebral malformations or perinatal/postnatal brain damage

d. Seizures are characterized by sudden, brief tonic flexor spasms of the waist, extremities, and neck that may occur hundreds of times each day in clusters.

Key Signs: Infantile Spasms

- Spams typically begin by age 1, particularly between the ages of 4 and 6 months

- West's syndrome

- Sudden, brief tonic flexor spasms of the waist, extremities, and neck; may occur hundreds of times each day in clusters

e. Prognosis is poor.
   (1) Mortality rate is 20%.
   (2) Most survivors are mentally retarded and have chronic epilepsy.

5. Lennox-Gastaut syndrome

a. Devastating epilepsy syndrome that begins in childhood

b. Cognitive deficits antedate seizures in most children, and the majority have abnormal neurologic examinations and behavioral disorders.

c. Seizures are axial tonic (typically activated by

sleep), tonic-clonic, atypical absence, myoclonic and atonic (head drops or falls) that may occur hundreds of times daily.

Key Signs: Lennox-Gastaut Syndrome

- Seizures begin in childhood

- Cognitive deficits antedate seizures

- Seizures are axial tonic (typically activated by sleep), tonic-clonic, atypical absence, myoclonic, and atonic (head drops or falls)

d. EEG characteristically shows slow (<2.5 Hz) spike-and-wave pattern.

e. Prognosis for seizure control is poor.

Bibliography

Beaumanoir A, Ballis T, Varfis G, et al.: Benign epilepsy of childhood with rolandic spikes: a clinical, electroencephalographic, and telencephalographic study. Epilepsia 15: 301–315, 1974.

Commission on Classification and Terminology of the International League against Epilepsy: Proposal for revised classification of epilepsies and epileptic syndromes. Epilepsia 30:389–399, 1989.

King DW, Dyken PR, Spinks IL, et al.: Infantile spasms: ictal phenomena. Pediatr Neurol 1:213–218, 1985.

Kurokowa T, Goya N, Fukuyama Y, et al.: West syndrome and Lennox-Gastaut syndrome: a survey of natural history. Pediatrics 65:81–88, 1980.

3 Medical Treatment

Steven C. Schachter

Goals of Treatment

1. Complete freedom from seizures
2. No bothersome side effects

General Principles of Medical Treatment

1. Determine the patient's seizure type(s) (see this section, Chapter 1, Etiology and Manifestations)
2. Start anti-epileptic drug (AED) therapy if a patient is at increased risk for recurrent seizures (see this section, Chapter 7, Starting and Stopping Medications).
3. Maximize the likelihood of successful AED treatment.
   a. Teach the patient and his or her family about epilepsy.
   b. Discuss the importance of compliance and what to expect from treatment. Written instructions on how and when to take AEDs should also be provided, along with potential adverse effects or drug–drug interactions.
      (1) Calcium-based antacids may impair drug absorption.
      (2) Drugs that inhibit hepatic enzymes such as propoxyphene, erythromycin, verapamil, and cimetidine may increase the concentrations of hepatically metabolized AEDs.
   c. Patients should be warned not to stop taking an AED and to avoid letting a prescription run out.
   d. Encourage patients to report seizures and possible medication-related side effects, and to avoid seizure triggers such as stress and sleep deprivation.
   e. Slowly titrate the dosage of an AED to that which is maximally tolerated. Patients with infrequent seizures can more safely start a drug with a slow loading or dose initiation schedule than patients with frequent seizures.
4. Monotherapy vs combination therapy
   a. Monotherapy is generally preferred.
      (1) The likelihood of compliance is increased.
      (2) The therapeutic window is wider.
      (3) Treatment with one agent is more cost-effective than combination drug treatment.
      (4) There are fewer side effects, idiosyncratic

reactions, and teratogenic effects associated with single-drug therapy.
   b. Complete seizure control with minimal side effects is achievable with single-drug therapy in 50% to 60% of patients with partial seizures; this goal is achievable in an additional 10% to 15% of patients with multiple drug therapy.
   c. A second AED should be prescribed if the initial AED is judged ineffective; the second drug is titrated to a therapeutic level before tapering off the original agent unless there is significant morbidity from the first drug.
   d. The duration of epilepsy predicts success of AED treatment; the longer patients continue to have seizures, the less likely their seizures will be controlled.
5. Oral contraceptive therapy
   a. Failure rates for hormonal contraceptive therapy are increased in women who take AEDs that induce hepatic enzymes.
   b. Breakthrough bleeding is a sign of oral contraceptive failure.
   c. Patients must be made aware of this so that unwanted pregnancies do not occur while on AED therapy.
   d. Women on enzyme-inducing AEDs who want to take oral contraceptives should receive a preparation with at least 50 µg of the estrogen component.

TABLE 3–1. RECOMMENDED AEDs FOR DIFFERENT SEIZURE TYPES

Seizure Type	Initial Therapy	Second-Line or Adjunctive Therapy
Primary generalized tonic-clonic seizures	Valproate Phenytoin Oxcarbazepine	Lamotrigine Carbamazepine Topiramate
Partial seizures with or without secondary generalization	Carbamazepine Phenytoin Oxcarbazepine	Valproate Gabapentin Lamotrigine Tiagabine Topiramate Levetiracetam Zonisamide
Absence seizures	Valproate	Lamotrigine Ethosuximide
Myoclonic seizures	Valproate	Lamotrigine
Mixed seizures (myoclonic and tonic-clonic)	Valproate	Lamotrigine Topiramate

TABLE 3–2. AEDs: LOADING AND INITIAL DOSING, AND MECHANISM OF ACTION

DRUG	TRADE NAME	INTRAVENOUS LOADING DOSE	ORAL LOADING AND MAINTENANCE DOSE	MECHANISM OF ACTION
Phenytoin	Dilantin	15 mg/kg (not more than 50 mg/min)	15 mg/kg in 3 divided doses over 9–12 hours; 5 mg/kg/day maintenance	Blocks sodium-dependent action potentials; reduces neuronal calcium uptake
Carbamazepine	Tegretol, Carbatrol	N/A	Start at 2–3 mg/kg/day in 2 divided doses; increase dose every 3–5 days to 10 mg/kg/day in 3 divided doses; dose may need to be further increased to 15–20 mg/kg/day after 2–3 months because of hepatic autoinduction	Blocks sodium-dependent action potentials; reduces neuronal calcium uptake
Valproate	Depakote	N/A	15 mg/kg/day in 3 divided doses; increase by 5–10 mg/kg/day every week as needed and tolerated	Reduces high-frequency neuronal firing; (?) blocks sodium-dependent action potentials; enhances GABA effects on CNS
Gabapentin	Neurontin	N/A	300 mg first day, 300 mg bid second day, 300 mg 3 times daily third day; increase as needed to 1,800 mg/day in 3 divided doses	Unknown
Ethosuximide	Zarontin	N/A	20–40 mg/kg/day in 1–3 divided doses	Modifies low-threshold or transient neuronal calcium currents
Phenobarbital		90–120 mg every 10-15 minutes as needed to maximum of 1,000 mg	1–5 mg/kg/day	Prolongs GABA-mediated chloride-channel openings; decreases CNS excitability
Lamotrigine	Lamictal	N/A	For patients taking and enzyme-inducing AED: 25 mg twice a day titrated upward by 50-mg increments every 1–2 weeks as needed. For patients taking VPA: 25 mg every other day with increases of 25–50 mg every 2 weeks as needed to a maximum of 300–500 mg/day. The maximum dosage used in U.S. open-label drug trials is 700 mg/day.	Inhibition of voltage-dependent sodium channels, resulting in decreased release of the excitatory neurotransmitters glutamate and aspartate
Tiagabine	Gabitril	N/A	4–10 mg/day; increase 8–12 mg/day every 4 weeks until 20–60 mg/day maintenance in 2–4 divided doses is reached	Inhibits neuronal and glial reuptake of GABA
Topiramate	Topamax	N/A	25–50 mg/day; increase 25–50 mg/day every 1–2 weeks until 100–1000 mg/day maintenance in 2 divided doses is reached	Blocks sodium-dependent action potentials; attenuates kainite-induced responses; enhances GABAergic transmission
Oxcarbazepine	Trileptal	N/A	150–300 mg/day; increase 300 mg/day every 3–5 days until 900–2700 mg/day maintenance in 2–3 divided doses is reached	Blocks sodium-dependent action potentials; reduces neuronal calcium uptake
Levetiracetam	Keppra	N/A	1000 mg/day; increase by 1000 mg/day every 2 weeks until 1000–4000 mg/day in 2 divided doses is reached	Not known
Zonisamide	Zonegran	N/A	100 mg/day; increase by 100 mg/day every 2 weeks until 400–600 mg/day in 1–2 divided doses is reached	Blocks voltage-dependent sodium and T-type calcium channels; inhibits release of excitatory neurotransmitters

Abbreviations: GABA = gamma aminobutyric acid; CNS = central nervous system

6. Noncompliance
   a. Up to 50% of patients with epilepsy do not take their medications as directed.
   b. Most patients with epilepsy evaluated in emergency departments for recurrent seizures have been noncompliant.
   c. Clinicians should suspect noncompliance if a patient
      (1) Denies the diagnosis of epilepsy
      (2) Has limited financial means to pay for AEDs
      (3) Has difficulty tolerating side effects

(4) Forgets when or how to take medication because of frequent seizures or memory impairment.

d. Compliance diminishes when intervals between office visits grow longer and when medication regimens grow increasingly complex.

e. Noncompliance may resolve by improving the patient's understanding of the disorder and the need for regular intake of medications.

 Key Treatment

- Determine seizure type.
- Start antiepileptic drug therapy if there is an increased risk of recurrent seizures.
- Discuss importance of compliance and what to expect from treatment.
- Slowly titrate AED dosage.

Selecting Antiepileptic Drugs

1. Recommended initial treatment for the different types of seizures is shown in Table 3–1.

   a. The AEDs differ in how easily and rapidly a loading dose can be administered, as shown in Table 3–2, which also gives the likely mechanism of action for each AED.

   b. Table 3–3 gives pharmacokinetic information for adults, including frequency of dosing, number of days needed to achieve steady state, and frequency of initial monitoring (serum levels, liver function tests, renal function tests, and complete blood counts).

2. Side effects of AEDs

   a. Table 3–4 shows the common and rare side effects of the most prescribed AEDs.

   b. Systemic toxicity and neurotoxicity are as much responsible for AED failure during the first 6 months of treatment as lack of efficacy.

TABLE 3–3. PHARMACOKINETIC INFORMATION FOR AEDs

Drug	Percent Bound to Plasma Protein	Elimination Half-Life (h)	Time to Steady State (days)	Frequency of Dosing	Frequency of Initial Monitoring	Therapeutic Level (μg/mL)
Phenytoin	90	15-30	5-15	qd or bid	2–3 weeks	10–20
Carbamazepine	70–80	11–17 (chronic therapy)	3–10	bid, tid, or qid	3, 6, 9 weeks	4–12
Valproate	60–95 (decreases with serum levels over 100 μg/ml)	6–18	2–4	bid or tid	1–2 weeks	50–150
Felbamate	25	20–23	5–10	bid or tid	See package insert for detailed instructions	32–137
Gabapentin	0	5–7; increases with decreased creatinine clearance (see prescribing information)	1–2	tid	None	2–3
Ethosuximide	0	40–50	6–12	qd, bid, or tid	2–3 weeks	40–100
Phenobarbital	40–60	30–50	16–21	qd or bid	3–4 weeks	10–40
Lamotrigine	50–55	10–15 with enzyme-inducing AEDs*; 40–60 with VPA	5–15	bid	None	Not established
Tiagabine	96	5–9	3	bid, tid, qid	None	Not established
Topiramate	9–17	20–24	5–7	bid	None	Not established
Oxcarbazepine	40	8–10	3–4	bid, tid	None (except sodium every 2–4 weeks in patients at risk for hyponatremia)	Not established
Levetiracetam	< 10	7–8	3–4	bid	None	Not established
Zonisamide	40–60	50–68	12–14	qd, bid	None	Not established

Abbreviations: qd = daily; bid = twice a day; tid = three times a day
*such as carbamazepine, phenytoin, and phenobarbital

TABLE 3–4. COMMON AND RARE SIDE EFFECTS OF ANTIEPILEPTIC DRUGS

Drug	Trade Name	Systemic Side Effects	Neurotoxic Side Effects	Rare Idiosyncratic Reactions
Phenytoin	Dilantin	Gingival hypertrophy, body hair increase, rash, lymphadenopathy	Confusion, slurred speech, double vision, ataxia, neuropathy (with long-term use)	Agranulocytosis, Stevens-Johnson syndrome, aplastic anemia, hepatic failure, dermatitis/rash, serum sickness
Carbamazepine	Tegretol, Carbatrol	Nausea, vomiting, diarrhea, hyponatremia, rash, pruritus, fluid retention	Drowsiness, dizziness, blurred or double vision, lethargy, headache	Agranulocytosis, Stevens-Johnson syndrome, aplastic anemia, hepatic failure, dermatitis/rash, serum sickness, pancreatitis
Valproate	Depakote	Weight gain, nausea, vomiting, hair loss, easy bruising	Tremor	Agranulocytosis, Stevens-Johnson syndrome, aplastic anemia, hepatic failure, dermatitis/rash, serum sickness, pancreatitis
Felbamate	Felbatol	Nausea, vomiting, anorexia, weight loss	Insomnia, dizziness, headache, ataxia	Aplastic anemia, hepatic failure
Gabapentin	Neurontin	None known	Somnolence, dizziness, ataxia	Unknown
Primidone, Phenobarbital	Mysoline	Nausea, rash	Alteration of sleep cycles, sedation, lethargy, behavioral changes, hyperactivity, ataxia, dependence	Agranulocytosis, Stevens-Johnson syndrome, hepatic failure, dermatitis/rash, serum sickness
Ethosuximide	Zarontin	Nausea, vomiting	Sleep disturbance, drowsiness, hyperactivity	Agranulocytosis, Stevens-Johnson syndrome, aplastic anemia, dermatitis/rash, serum sickness
Lamotrigine	Lamictal	Rash, nausea	Dizziness, somnolence	Stevens-Johnson syndrome, hypersensitivity syndrome
Tiagabine	Gabitril	N/A	Dizziness, weakness, ataxia nervousness, tremor, somnolence	N/A
Topiramate	Topamax	Anorexia, weight loss	Confusion, cognitive slowing dysphasia, dizziness, fatigue, paresthesias	Nephrolithiasis
Oxcarbazepine	Trileptal	Nausea, vomiting, hyponatremia, rash	Drowsiness, dizziness, headache, double vision, ataxia	N/A
Levetiracetam	Keppra	Anorexia	Somnolence, dizziness, headache, nervousness	N/A
Zonisamide	Zonegran	Anorexia	Dizziness, ataxia, fatigue, somnolence, confusion	Nephrolithiasis

c. Serum concentrations that are associated with neurotoxicity vary from patient to patient and may occur even when measured levels are within the appropriate therapeutic range.

d. Serum drug concentrations may fluctuate in compliant patients because of laboratory error or drug interactions.

Bibliography

Elwes RD, Johnson AL, Shorvon SD, et al.: The prognosis for seizure control in newly diagnosed epilepsy. N Engl J Med 311:944, 1984.

Kwan P, Brodie MJ: Early identification of refractory epilepsy. N Engl J Med 342:314, 2000.

Pellock JM: Standard approach to antiepileptic drug treatment in the United States. Epilepsia 35:S11–S18, 1994.

Schachter SC: Update in the treatment of epilepsy. Compr Ther 21:473, 1995.

4 Status Epilepticus

Steven C. Schachter

Definition

1. Convulsive status epilepticus (SE) is a life-threatening medical emergency that is usually defined as convulsive seizure activity persisting for 30 minutes (some authorities say 5 minutes) or two seizures without return of consciousness in between.

2. Other types of status epilepticus include absence status epilepticus, myoclonic status epilepticus, tonic status epilepticus, complex partial status epilepticus, nonconvulsive status epilepticus, and electrographic status epilepticus.

Epidemiology and Risk Factors

1. The incidence of convulsive SE is estimated at approximately 60,000 cases per year in the United States; half are children.

2. Two thirds of cases occur in patients without a previous history of seizures.

3. Approximately 1% of patients with epilepsy will have an episode of SE in a given year.

Etiology

1. In patients with a history of epilepsy
   a. Noncompliance with medication
   b. Recent change in treatment
   c. Barbiturate or benzodiazepine withdrawal
2. In patients without a history of epilepsy
   a. Recent stroke, hemorrhage or cerebral ischemia
   b. Meningo-encephalitis
   c. Acute head trauma
   d. Cerebral neoplasm
   e. Metabolic disorders
   f. Iatrogenic (drug-induced)
   g. Alcohol withdrawal
   h. Arteritis
   i. Unknown/idiopathic

Clinical Features

1. Usually begins with a generalized tonic-clonic seizure, though it may start with a partial seizure.

2. Convulsions recur, most lasting less than 2 minutes, along with intervals of persistent unresponsiveness.

3. Less often, convulsions are continuous, manifesting as clonic movements eventually replaced by repetitive jerking movements of the facial muscles, sometimes with intermittent limb jerking.

4. Convulsive SE can be associated with numerous complications.
   a. Cardiac: Hypertension, tachycardia, arrhythmias, cardiac arrest
   b. Pulmonary: Apnea, respiratory failure, hypoxia, neurogenic pulmonary edema, aspiration pneumonia
   c. Autonomic: Increased circulating catecholamines, fever, sweating, tracheobronchial hypersecretion, vomiting
   d. Metabolic: Hyperkalemia, hyperglycemia then hypoglycemia, volume depletion, venous stasis, possible thrombosis
   e. Endocrine: Increased prolactin and cortisol
   f. Cerebral: Neuronal damage (similar to hypoxic injury), hyperthermia, cerebral edema, raised intracranial pressure, cortical vein thrombosis
   g. Other: Leukocytosis, cerebrospinal fluid pleocytosis, vertebral and other fractures, physical injury, rhabdomyolysis, renal failure, disseminated intravascular coagulation

5. Electroencephalograms (EEGs) show typical sequence of patterns—discrete seizures, merging seizures, seizures interrupted by flat periods, and finally periodic discharges.

 Key Signs

- Usually begins with generalized tonic-clonic seizure; however, partial seizure is possible

- Recurring convulsions recur–most lasting less than 2 minutes–with intervals of persistent unresponsiveness.

Treatment

1. Most important aspect of treatment for convulsive status epilepticus is to have an established protocol

254

that all members of the team (emergency medicine technicians, neurologists, emergency room physicians and nurses, and intensive care unit physicians and nurses) are familiar with.

2. The goals are to stop the convulsions and to interrupt continuing EEG discharges.

3. One suggested protocol is

   a. Establish airway and ensure adequate respiration.

   b. Start intravenous line. Draw blood for metabolic studies, AED levels, and toxic screens.

   c. Give thiamine and a bolus of 50% glucose.

   d. Monitor electrocardiogram for arrhythmias and cardiac ischemia.

   e. Start search for underlying cause.

   f. Arrange for EEG monitoring.

   g. Phenytoin 50 mg/minute maximum intravenously in saline with attention to heart rate and blood pressure to a dose of 15–20 mg/kg.

      (1) Watch for cardiac arrhythmias.

      (2) Instead of phenytoin, an alternative is fosphenytoin in any intravenous fluid up to 150 mg/minute.

   h. Besides phenytoin or fosphenytoin, intravenous phenobarbital may be given 10–20 mg/kg, up to 100 mg/minute, with attention to blood pressure and respiration.

   i. If necessary, give lorazepam at 0.1–0.2 mg/kg, <2 mg/minute. Other possible alternatives are propofol and midazolam.

   j. If SE continues, and after intubation, give pentobarbital 3–5 mg/kg until epileptiform activity is eliminated on the EEG.

      (1) Maintenance doses are 1–5 mg/kg/hour as necessary.

      (2) Watch for respiratory depression, hypotension, and hypothermia.

      (3) Consider discontinuing pentobarbital after 24 to 48 hours if clinical and electrographic seizures have stopped and anti-epileptic drugs (AEDs) are at high serum concentrations.

   k. Monitor and treat potential complications of SE; i.e., normalize blood pressure, volume status, temperature, ventilation, and oxygenation.

4. Ongoing reassessment of the patient's clinical condition and EEG findings are necessary.

Key Treatment

- All team members should be familiar with an established protocol for SE (see text for suggested protocol).

Prognosis and Complications

Mortality ranges from 10% to 50% and increases with age, peaking in elderly patients.

1. Mortality and morbidity arise from the underlying cause(s) of the SE and the physiologic effects of convulsions listed above, particularly autonomic dysfunction and cardiac arrhythmias. Other poor prognostic indicators are shown under Key Poor Prognostic Factors. NOTE: SE in patients with a previous history of epilepsy, or due to alcohol or drug withdrawal, has a better prognosis.

2. Delay in starting treatment worsens the prognosis and increases the likelihood that general anesthesia will be necessary.

   a. Particularly true for patients whose EEG patterns show the later states of SE.

Poor Prognostic Factors

- Advanced age
- Duration of SE
- Anoxia
- Stroke
- Drug toxicity
- Central nervous system infection
- Severe metabolic derangements
- Hypotension
- Renal or hepatic failure
- Intracranial hypertension

Bibliography

DeLorenzo RJ, Pellock JM, Towne AR, et al.: Epidemiology of status epilepticus. J Clin Neurophysiology 12:316–325, 1995.

Drislane FW: Status epilepticus. In Schachter SC, Schomer DL (eds): The Comprehensive Evaluation and Treatment of Epilepsy. San Diego, Academic Press, 1997, pp. 149–172.

Shorvon S: Tonic-clonic status epilepticus. J Neurol Neurosurg Psychiatry 56:125–134, 1993.

Working Group on Status Epilepticus: Treatment of convulsive status epilepticus. JAMA 270:854–859, 1993.

5 Surgical Treatment

Steven C. Schachter

When to Consider Surgery

Surgical therapy for epilepsy should be considered for patients with medically refractory seizures, particularly when seizures significantly affect their lives.

1. Definition of medical refractoriness generally means failure of seizures to respond to trials of 3 or more anti-epileptic drugs (AEDs) used at maximally tolerated doses in compliant patients.

2. Patients with operable structural brain lesions that are shown to correlate in location with seizure onset should be evaluated for surgery earlier.

3. The indications and types of surgery for epilepsy are shown in Table 5-1.

Brain Surgery

1. Evaluation process

   a. Thorough review of the patient's seizure history and prior trials of AEDs to ensure medical refractoriness

   b. Seizure localization with ictal electroencephalographic (EEG) recordings

   c. Magnetic resonance imaging (MRI) scans

   d. Functional imaging (when necessary)

   e. Neuropsychological testing to identify any cognitive deficits that have localizing significance.

TABLE 5-1. INDICATIONS AND TYPES OF SURGERY FOR EPILEPSY

Procedure	Indication
Cranial surgery	
Focal (lobar) resection	• Partial-onset seizures arising from resectable cortex
Corpus callosotomy	• Tonic, atonic, or tonic-clonic seizures with falling and injury • Large nonresectable lesions • Secondary bilateral synchrony
Hemispherectomy	• Rasmussen's encephalitis • Other unilateral widespread hemispheric pathology in association with a contralateral hand that is functionally impaired
Subpial transection	• Partial-onset seizures arising from unresectable (eloquent) cortex
Extracranial surgery	
Vagus nerve stimulator implantation	• Partial-onset seizures

2. Ictal monitoring with invasive electrodes (grids, strips, depth electrodes) should be considered if

   a. Scalp EEG data do not clearly identify the seizure focus

   b. Neuroimaging or neuropsychological test results are inconsistent with the EEG seizure localization

3. Lobar excision may be carried out with a high probability of improvement when

   a. Ictal recordings show that the onset for the patient's typical seizures is consistently from the same portion of one lobe (for example, frontal or temporal)

   b. MRI, functional imaging, and neuropsychological testing are consistent with the ictal EEG seizure localization

   c. The brain tissue can be removed safely without risk of permanent cognitive, sensory, or motor deficits

4. Lobar excision should not be carried out if a patient's seizures arise from different sides or lobes, or if seizures prove to be generalized in onset.

5. Outcomes from lobar surgery

   a. Success rates are high when patients are carefully screened.

   b. Best results are seen in patients with seizure localized to the anterior temporal lobe and MRI evidence of mesial temporal sclerosis ipsilateral to the seizure focus.

   c. Overall proportions of patients who become seizure free are shown under Seizure-Free Rates and Types of Focal Resection.

Seizure-Free Rates and Types of Focal Resection

• Temporal lobectomy—70% to 85%

• Frontal lobectomy—30% to 40%

• Lesional neocortical resection—50% to 70%

• Nonlesional neocortical resection—35% to 45%

---

6. Corpus callosotomy

   a. Atonic seizures benefit most, although procedure is palliative at best.

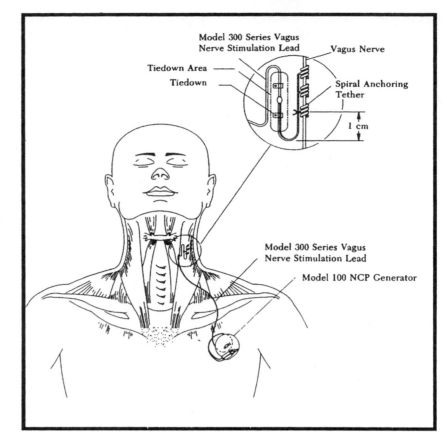

Figure 5-1. VNS components. Courtesy of Cyberonics, Inc.

b. Partial seizures may worsen in frequency.

c. No improvement in cognitive function is likely.

Vagus Nerve Stimulation (VNS)

1. VNS was approved by the FDA in 1997 for use as adjunctive therapy for adults and adolescents over 12 years of age with medically refractory partial seizures. It may also be effective for generalized seizures, and should be considered an option for patients with atonic seizures.

2. The system (Fig. 5–1) consists of

   a. A programmable signal generator that is implanted in the patient's left upper chest

   b. A bipolar lead that connects the generator to the left vagus nerve in the neck

   c. A programming wand that uses radiofrequency signals to communicate noninvasively with the generator

   d. A hand-held magnet used by the patient or carer to turn the stimulator on or off

3. Mechanism of action of VNS is unknown

4. Implantation procedure

   a. Lasts approximately 1 hour

   b. Typically performed under general anesthesia

   c. Side effects are transient and include incisional pain, coughing, voice alteration, chest discomfort, and nausea; 0.1% of patients have asystole during the lead test in the operating room.

      (1) There have been no reported asystolic events outside of the operating room.

      (2) All patients fully recovered.

5. Treatment protocols

   a. Within the first 2 postoperative weeks, increasing the output current is initiated by the physician and adjusted to patient tolerance.

   b. Typical settings are 30-Hz signal frequency with a 500-microsecond pulse width for 30 seconds of on time and 5 minutes off time.

   c. Once programmed, the generator delivers intermittent stimulation at the desired settings. Battery life is typically 8 to 10 years.

   d. The patient or companion may activate the generator by placing the hand-held magnet over it for several seconds; in some patients, on-demand activation aborts or shortens the seizure.

6. Outcome

    a. In studies of long-term effects, approximately 37% of patients have at least a 50% reduction in seizures within the first year of stimulation. Improvement appears to continue, and possibly increase, over time.

    b. Side effects of stimulation, which are usually mild and resolve with adjustment in the settings, include hoarseness, throat pain, coughing, dyspnea, and paresthesias.

Bibliography

Lesser RP, Fisher RS, Kaplan R: The evaluation of patients with intractable complex partial seizures. Electroencephalogr Clin Neurophysiol 73:381–388, 1989.

Polkey CE: Surgical treatment of epilepsy. Lancet 336:553–555, 1990.

Schachter SC, Saper CB: Vagus nerve stimulation. Epilepsia 3:677–686, 1998.

Sperling MR, O'Connor MJ, Saykin AJ, et al.: Temporal lobectomy for refractory epilepsy. JAMA 276:470–475, 1996.

6 Epilepsy and Pregnancy

Steven C. Schachter

Overview

1. The fertility rate for women with epilepsy (WWE) is up to 33% lower than expected. Factors affecting fertility may include psychosocial issues, menstrual irregularities, and reproductive endocrine disorders, such as polycystic ovarian syndrome.

2. More than 90% of WWE who become pregnant will have uneventful pregnancies and will give birth to healthy normal babies.

3. WWE are at greater risk than women without epilepsy of bearing babies with birth defects and of experiencing complications associated with pregnancy and labor.

   a. The incidence of major congenital malformations is 4% to 6%, approximately double the risk in the general population.

      (1) Common major malformations include orofacial clefts, cardiac abnormalities, and neural tube defects.

      (2) All commonly used anti-epileptic drugs (AEDs) have been associated with congenital malformations. The teratogenic risks of the newer AEDs are not yet known. The risk of neural tube defects, in particular spina bifida, in WWE taking valproic acid is 1% to 2%; the risk with carbamazepine is 0.5%.

      (3) Family history of birth defects is a risk factor.

   b. Up to 10% of babies born to WWE may have minor malformations, including hypertelorism, epicanthal folds, shallow philtrum, and distal digital hypoplasia. Risk factors besides epilepsy and AED treatment are other medications and excessive alcohol use.

   c. The rate of prenatal (especially after 20 weeks gestation), neonatal, and infant mortality is increased in the children of WWE; risk factors are not well known.

Points

- Fertility rate for women with epilepsy is lower than expected.

- More than 90% of women with epilepsy have uneventful pregnancies and give birth to healthy normal babies.

- Women with epilepsy are at greater risk than women without epilepsy of bearing babies with birth defects and of experiencing pregnancy and labor complications.

Prenatal Management

1. Caution patients to avoid unplanned pregnancies when possible.

   a. Enzyme-inducing AEDs (carbamazepine, oxcarbazepine, phenytoin, phenobarbital, primidone, and topiramate) may reduce the potency of hormonal contraceptives by increasing their metabolism; for example, estrogen concentrations may be reduced up to 50%.

   b. WWE should consider a barrier method of contraception to supplement hormonal contraceptives.

2. Minimize the risk of birth defects in WWE who intend to become pregnant

   a. Folic acid supplementation: Doses of 0.4 to 4.0 mg daily prior to conception and through at least the first trimester are recommended to lower the risk of neural tube defects.

   b. Use the lowest doses and the fewest number of AEDs possible—ideally a single AED—prior to conception and through at least the first trimester.

      (1) The risk of birth defects increases with AED polypharmacy and higher serum concentrations of AEDs.

      (2) The goal of treating seizures in WWE who plan to conceive is to achieve complete control of seizures that could pose a health risk to the mother or developing child.

         (a) Generalized tonic-clonic seizures, atonic seizures, and complex partial

259

seizures may result in maternal or fetal injury secondary to falls, fetal hypoxia and acidosis, and miscarriage. Convulsive status epilepticus during pregnancy is associated with high maternal and fetal mortality.

(b) Complete eradication of simple partial seizures may not be necessary if risk to the fetus from AEDs outweighs the potential benefit to mother and child.

(c) Withdrawal of AEDs should be considered if the patient has been free of seizures for at least 2 years; ensure a sufficiently long observation period off AEDs prior to conception to determine whether seizures are likely to recur.

(d) As in every clinical situation, the physician must weigh the risk–benefit ratio for treating epilepsy in a pregnant woman.

c. Counsel the patient

(1) Discuss the importance of AED compliance during pregnancy and the need for frequent monitoring to lower the potential hazards of seizures to mother and developing child.

(2) Explain the risks of birth defects and the need for folic acid prior to conception.

(3) Discuss the chance that the baby will develop epilepsy.

(4) Encourage the patient to enroll in a pregnancy registry (call 800-EFA-1000 or visit *www.epilepsyfoundation.org* for more information).

(5) Help the patient identify an obstetrician who has expertise in managing high-risk pregnancies. WWE have a higher-than-expected incidence of premature labor, failure to progress, and cesarean sections.

(6) Discuss the issues outlined under Parenting Issues and Concerns.

Key Management: Prenatal Care

- Unplanned pregnancies should be avoided.

- Risk of birth defects should be minimized.

  - Folic acid supplementation

  - Lowest doses and fewest number of AEDs prior to conception and through at least the first trimester

- Issues—such as birth defects and baby developing epilepsy—should be discussed with the patient.

Parenting Issues and Concerns

- Breast-feeding

  - Concentrations of AEDs in breast milk are too low to affect the baby except for phenobarbital and primidone, which may result in irritability or sedation.

- Transporting the baby

  - Avoid papoose or backpack type carriers if there is a history of falling with seizures.

  - Minimize stair climbing.

- Bathing

  - The child should be bathed when others are present.

- Adequate sleep to avoid sleep deprivation seizures

Management during Pregnancy

1. Minimize seizures: Anticipate changes in AED concentrations and dosage adjustments

   a. Up to one-third of WWE who are compliant with their AED regimen have an increased frequency of seizures during pregnancy. Factors include

      (1) Changes in AED concentration as a consequence of decreased AED protein binding, increased AED clearance, and increased maternal plasma volume

      (2) Sleep deprivation associated with the discomfort of pregnancy

      (3) Stress

   b. Monitor AED concentrations (including unbound concentrations of phenytoin and valproate) and seizure occurrence frequently, and make AED changes as necessary.

2. Working in conjunction with the obstetrician, monitor fetal development. Measure plasma alpha-fetoprotein levels (to screen for neural tube defects) and obtain level II ultrasonography at 18 to 22 weeks of gestation (to screen for a variety of major malformations).

3. Anticipate complications of pregnancy

   a. Hyperemesis gravidarum

   b. Vaginal bleeding

   c. Anemia

4. Administer oral vitamin K (10 mg per day) during the last month of pregnancy. Up to 7% of children born to WWE taking AEDs (phenobarbital, primidone, phenytoin, and possibly others) are at risk of

a hemorrhagic disorder during the first 24 hours of life.

a. Maternal AEDs inhibit transport of vitamin K across the placenta; the infant has prolonged prothrombin and partial thromboplastin times.

b. Risk increases with AED polypharmacy and is reduced by vitamin K supplementation.

Postpartum Management

1. Monitor AED levels during first 2 postpartum months because serum AED concentrations commonly rise in the early postpartum period
2. Readdress the need for adequate sleep, AED compliance, and safe parenting.

Key Management

During Pregnancy

- Anticipate changes in AED concentrations and dosage adjustments to minimize seizures.
- Monitor fetal development with obstetrician.
- Anticipate complications of pregnancy.
- Administer oral vitamin K (10 mg per day) during the last month of pregnancy.

Postpartum

- Monitor AED levels during the first 2 months after birth.
- Readdress the need for adequate sleep, AED compliance, safe parenting.

Bibliography

Brodie MJ: Management of epilepsy during pregnancy and lactation. Lancet 336:426–427, 1990.

Bruno MK, Harden CL: Epilepsy in pregnant women. Curr Treat Options Neurol 4:31–40, 2002.

Delgado-Escueta AV, Janz D: Consensus guidelines: Preconception counseling, management, and care of the pregnant woman with epilepsy. Neurology 42:149–160, 1992.

Yerby M: Treatment of epilepsy during pregnancy. In Wyllie E (ed): The Treatment of Epilepsy, 2nd ed. Baltimore, Williams & Wilkins, 1997, pp. 785–798.

7 Starting and Stopping Medications

Steven C. Schachter

General Principles of When to Start Medical Treatment

1. Chronic anti-epileptic drug (AED) therapy is not necessary if a first seizure is provoked by a time-limited factor, such as transient hypotension, hypoglycemia, or an iatrogenic drug reaction.

2. Chronic AED therapy should be considered in patients with seizures caused by a structural abnormality or neurologic insult, who are more likely to develop refractory epilepsy than patients with idiopathic disease.

   a. Factors contributing to the risk of recurrent seizures include

      (1) A history of brain insult (e.g., head injury with loss of consciousness)

      (2) A lesion revealed by brain computed tomography or magnetic resonance imaging studies

      (3) Focal abnormalities detected during the neurologic examination

      (4) A record of cognitive impairment

      (5) A partial seizure as the first seizure

      (6) An abnormal electroencephalogram (EEG) (particularly epileptiform abnormalities)

      (7) In addition, certain seizure types are more prone to recurrence, particularly absence seizures and myoclonic seizures.

   b. AED treatment is generally started after the second seizure, because recurrence proves that the patient has a propensity for repeated seizures. However, it may be appropriate to initiate AED therapy after the first seizure if the patient is considered at high risk for recurrence based upon the above factors.

   c. Other factors that must be considered when deciding whether to start AED therapy include the potential occupational and psychological consequences of suffering a recurrent seizure. An adult who operates heavy machinery or drives may be more likely to choose drug therapy. In contrast, treatment for most children who experience a single unprovoked seizure may not be necessary.

General Principles Guiding When to Stop Medical Treatment

1. In general, approximately 60% of patients with perfectly controlled seizures over a long period (2 to 5 years) will remain seizure free, at least for several years, after withdrawal of AEDs.

2. In a patient treated with AEDs whose seizures are completely controlled, the risks of continued treatment versus the benefit should be weighed.

   a. Possible risks of continued treatment include side effects of AEDs, potential teratogenesis in women of childbearing potential, and the stigma of taking pills for epilepsy.

   b. The principal disadvantage of discontinuing drug therapy is the possibility of recurrent seizures. The psychosocial implications of recurrent seizures are particularly significant for adults who are employed or who drive, and whose lifestyle would be adversely affected by recurrent seizures.

   c. Decisions to taper AEDs should be made on an individual basis.

3. There is no way to prospectively identify patients who will remain seizure free after they discontinue AEDs.

   a. Associated risks of seizure recurrence off drug therapy is described under Factors Associated with Increased Risk of Seizure.

Factors Associated with Increased Risk of Seizure after Discontinuation of AEDs

- Readily identifiable brain disease (e.g., brain tumor, congenital anomaly, cerebral contusion)

- Seizure onset after 12 years of age

- Severe epilepsy before the start of drug therapy

- Specific epilepsy syndromes (especially juvenile myoclonic epilepsy)

- Abnormal electroencephalograms (particularly in children with idiopathic epilepsy)

- Multiple types of seizure occurring in the same patient

---

b. Ameliorating factors are shown under Factors Associated with Decreased Risk of Seizure. Patients with benign epilepsy of childhood with rolandic spikes and benign familial neonatal convulsions tend to do well after AED withdrawal.

Factors Associated with Decreased Risk of Seizure after Discontinuation of AEDs

• Relatively few seizures before and after starting AED therapy

• Seizures that were completely controlled with a single AED

• No seizures during treatment for many years

• Normal neurologic examination

• No structural brain lesion

---

c. Even patients who have been seizure free for a number of years and who have no risk factors for seizure recurrence have a higher risk of seizure recurrence than the general population. Because this risk cannot be known exactly for any given patient, and because the timing of seizure recurrence cannot be predicted, many patients elect to continue AED therapy.

AED Discontinuation Strategies

1. If the decision is made to withdraw therapy, central nervous system depressants such as phenobarbital and the benzodiazepines, as well as carbamazepine, should be discontinued gradually over many weeks to months to minimize the likelihood of withdrawal seizures. Other drugs may be tapered over days to weeks.

2. There are no general guidelines about driving restrictions during and after AED taper. Many clinicians suggest that patients refrain from driving until they have been seizure free without treatment for the same amount of time required by state law to be seizure free with treatment.

Bibliography

Hart YM, Sander JW, Johnson AL, Shorvon SD: National General Practice Study of Epilepsy: Recurrence after a first unprovoked seizure. Lancet 336:1271–1274, 1990.

Hauser WA, Rich SS, Lee JR, Annegers JF, et al.: Risk of recurrent seizures after two unprovoked seizures. N Engl J Med 338:429–434, 1998.

Medical Research Council Antiepileptic Drug Research Group: Randomised study of antiepileptic drug withdrawal in patients in remission. Lancet 337:1175–1180, 1991.

Shinnar S, Berg AT: Withdrawal of antiepileptic drugs. Curr Opin Neurol 8:103–106, 1995.

Specchio LM, Tramacere L, La Neve A, Beghi E: Discontinuing antiepileptic drugs in patients who are seizure free on monotherapy. J Neurol Neurosurg Psychiatry. 72:22–25, 2002.

Tennison M, Greenwood R, Lewis D, Thorn M: Rate of taper of antiepileptic drugs and the risk of seizure recurrence in children. N Engl J Med 330:1407–1410, 1994.

8 Driving and Other Restrictions

Steven C. Schachter

Overview

1. For some patients, the psychosocial problems associated with epilepsy may have a greater impact on quality of life than the seizures themselves.

2. Limitations on driving and other activities reinforce the stigma and loss of independence felt by many patients. Physicians must therefore balance the need for patient and public safety with the patient's need for maintaining as normal a lifestyle as possible.

Driving

Every state differs in driver licensing requirements for patients with epilepsy or episodes of loss of consciousness.

1. Most states require patients to be seizure free for a specified period of time, typically 3 to 12 months, and to submit a physician's evaluation of their ability to drive safely.

   a. The time period varies state to state.

   b. Seizures that are attributable to temporary illness or related to an isolated event that is unlikely to recur (for example, not having access to anti-epileptic drugs–AEDs) may not require any driving restriction at the discretion of the physician and/or state authorities.

   c. When patients can drive after discontinuation of an AED is not usually well defined by state regulations (see this section, Chapter 7, Starting and Stopping Medications).

2. Some states require physicians to report patients with epilepsy to the appropriate authorities.

3. Physicians are expected to know their obligations and may be liable for failing to advise patients of their responsibilities as drivers or for failing to report patients.

4. Physicians should advise patients not to drive if their cognitive and neurologic function is affected by AEDs sufficiently to affect driving ability.

5. Discussions with patients regarding driving should be carefully documented in the patient's chart.

Points Regarding Driving

- Most states require patients to be seizure free for 3 to 12 months and to submit to a physician's evaluation of their ability to drive safely.

- Some states require reporting epileptic patients to the appropriate authorities.

- Physicians are expected to know their obligations and could be liable for failing to advise patients of their responsibilities as drivers.

- Patients adversely affected by AEDs should be advised not to drive.

- Discussions regarding driving should be carefully documented in the patient's chart.

Other Lifestyle Modifications

1. Patients should be counseled about lifestyle modifications that help to prevent injury to themselves or others, that minimize seizure precipitants, and that enhance their sense of control and independence.

   a. Bathing safety is important to prevent accidental drowning and burns.

      (1) Tubs should be filled no more than 3 inches high for baths.

      (2) Drains must function properly.

      (3) An upper limit to water temperature should be set, or the hot water thermostat should be kept below scalding temperature.

      (4) A family member or carer should be nearby.

   b. Kitchen safety is important to prevent burns and injuries

      (1) Sharp utensils should be kept away

      (2) A microwave oven should be used when possible rather than a stove

   c. Recreation should be encouraged with common-sense restrictions

      (1) Patients should never swim alone.

      (2) Certain activities that would put the patient in imminent danger if a seizure occurred should be avoided (see Potentially Hazardous Activities)

Potentially Hazardous Activities

- Scuba diving

- Skydiving

- Hang gliding

- Rock climbing

- Bike riding if seizures are frequent

- Camping around an open fire

---

2. Seizure control may be improved by measures to reduce stress at home, in the workplace, or at

school; strategies can be employed to increase sleep and enhance compliance with AEDs.

Bibliography

Berg AT, Vickrey BG, Sperling MR, et al.: Driving in adults with refractory localization-related epilepsy. Multi-Center Study of Epilepsy Surgery. Neurology. 54:625–630, 2000.

Krass GL, Ampaw L, Krumholz A: Individual state driving restrictions for people with epilepsy in the US. Neurology. 57:1780–1785, 2001.

Krauss GL, Krumholz A, Carter RC, et al.: Risk factors for seizure-related motor vehicle crashes in patients with epilepsy. Neurology. 52:1324–1329, 1999.

1   Epidemiology and Pathophysiology in Neuro-oncology

Morris D. Groves

Introduction

Neuro-oncology is a relatively new subspecialty within neurology and has three main areas of focus. These include the clinical management, and clinical and basic research concerning patients with (1) primary central nervous system (CNS) tumors, (2) non-CNS cancers directly (metastatic) or indirectly (paraneoplastic) affecting the nervous system, and (3) toxic nervous system effects of cancer therapies.

Epidemiology

1. Primary brain tumors: The combined annual incidence of primary brain tumors in the United States is 11 to 12 per 100,000 population. Approximately 20,000 patients per year are newly diagnosed with a primary brain tumor.

2. Approximately 30% of patients with cancer will develop some sort of neurologic complication from their cancer, either metastases or neurologic toxicity from therapy. This includes patients who develop metabolic encephalopathy, neuropathies, psychosis, cerebellar dysfunction, and leukoencephalopathy.

3. Metastatic disease to the nervous system: Annually in the United States, 100,000 and 150,000 patients per year are diagnosed with parenchymal brain metastases, 30,000 to 40,000 are diagnosed with metastases to the meninges or spinal fluid, and 25,000 to 30,000 develop spinal cord compression from metastatic disease.

4. Toxic effects from radiation and chemotherapy are evident in nearly all patients with cancer. Somewhere between 5% and 10% of patients develop frank radiation-induced CNS necrosis of either the brain or spinal cord. A large percentage (in some studies, even up to 100%) of patients who have received radiotherapy to the brain develop some degree of neurocognitive decline.

5. The chemotherapies most likely to cause peripheral neuropathy include platinum-based therapies, vinca alkaloids, and taxanes.

6. Paraneoplastic syndromes: Those affecting the nervous system are rare, with well-defined syndromes affecting less than 5% of patients with cancer. However, patients with systemic cancer report a number of nonspecific neurologic symptoms, including weak muscles, generalized fatigue, and neuromyopathy.

Annual Incidence in the United States

- Primary brain tumors: 20,000

- Metastatic brain tumors: 100,000 to 150,000

- Neoplastic meningitis: 30,000 to 40,000

- Spinal cord compression: 25,000 to 30,000

Pathophysiology

The pathophysiology underlying each of these clinical problems is different. Genetic alterations that allow for uncontrolled cellular proliferation, such as the malfunction of tumor suppressor genes, are commonly involved in the development of primary CNS tumors. Also, amplification or overexpression of growth factor receptors that promote cellular proliferation are well known in primary CNS malignancies. Specific mutations have been identified in various tumors, and those will be discussed in succeeding chapters in this section.

The specific pathophysiologic cause of symptoms in patients with primary CNS tumors is usually due to tumor cell proliferation, invasion, tissue destruction, and resulting cerebral edema. These processes interfere with normal neuronal interconnections, resulting in nervous system dysfunction. The mechanisms by which tumor cells invade and proliferate are still being unraveled.

1. Metastatic tumors to the nervous system: Metastatic tumors to the nervous system, both parenchymal and nonparenchymal, are the most common brain tumors. They usually reach the nervous system by hematogenous dissemination, but they can also reach the CNS by direct extension. Specific genetic changes that give rise to nervous

system metastases have not been well characterized, although DNA gains on chromosomes 1q23, 8q24, 17q24-q25, 20q13, and 7p12 and DNA losses at 4q22, 4q26, 5q21, and 9p21 have been identified as common abnormalities in a variety of tumors metastatic to the brain. Symptoms, signs, and pathophysiology are due to tumor location, degree of invasion and edema, and blockage of normal information routes and spinal fluid flow pathways.

2. The pathophysiology of radiation-induced nervous system damage is believed to involve inflammatory mechanisms, autoimmune mechanisms, and vascular endothelial proliferation and subsequent ischemia.

3. The pathophysiology of chemotherapy-induced nervous system toxicity is also specific to the particular therapeutic agents and often has to do with injury to axonal transport and interference with normal protein syntheses within nervous system cellular components.

4. Pathophysiology of paraneoplastic syndromes is specific for each syndrome and is due to the production of antibodies, the most commonly known being anti-Hu, anti-Yo, and anti-Ri, and the reaction to these antibodies with receptors of the specific neurons. In the Anti-Yo syndrome, near complete destruction of the cerebellar Purkinje cells can occur.

Ways Tumor Cells Gain Access to the CNS

- Direct extension

- Perineural spread

- Hematogenous spread

- Perivenous spread

- Intraoperative spread

Bibliography

Kaye AH, Laws Jr ER (eds): Brain Tumors. An Encyclopedic Approach. 2nd ed., London, Churchill Livingstone, 2001.

Kleihues P, Cavenee W (eds): WHO Classification Tumors of the Nervous System. Lyon, France, IARC Press, 2000.

Levin V, Leibel S, Gutin P: Neoplasms of the central nervous system. In DeVita V, Hellman S, Rosenberg S (eds): Cancer: Principles and Practice of Oncology, 6th ed. Philadelphia, Lippincott Williams & Wilkins, vol. 2, 2001, pp. 2100–2160.

Posner JB: Neurologic Complications of Cancer. Philadelphia, F.A. Davis, 1995.

Definitions

1. Brain tumors cause focal and generalized neurologic symptoms. Elevated intracranial pressure (ICP) causes generalized symptoms that include headache, nausea and vomiting, sixth-nerve palsies, and mental status changes.
2. Tumor location, invasiveness, and growth rate determine clinical features.

Epidemiology and Risk Factors

1. Annually in the United States, 20,000 persons are diagnosed with primary brain tumors. Approximately 12,000 die from tumor complications.
2. Between 100,000 and 150,000 persons will be diagnosed with metastatic tumors to the CNS.
3. In children, primary brain tumors comprise 22% of all cancers; most arise below the tentorium.
4. The incidence of primary and metastatic brain tumors is approximately 46 per 100,000.
5. Prior cranial radiation is a risk factor for the development of primary brain tumors.

Pathophysiology

1. The Monro-Kellie hypothesis states that the three main constituents of the cranium (brain, 1400 cc; cerebrospinal fluid, 140 cc; blood, 150 cc) are incompressible. For one to increase in volume (as in the case of a brain tumor), the others must decrease or the overall pressure must increase.
2. Brain edema occurs due to leakiness of capillary endothelial cells, enhanced by vascular endothelial growth factor, which can be released by tumors.
3. Common herniation syndromes
   a. Subfalcine herniation occurs when the cingulate gyrus is forced under the falx. This often causes no symptoms.
   b. Temporal lobe, uncal herniation occurs when the temporal lobe is forced medially into the tentorial opening and pushes the mesencephalic structures contralaterally. Signs of this include
      (1) False localizing ipsilateral hemiparesis
      (2) Ipsilateral pupillary dilation
      (3) When severe, elevated blood pressure, bradycardia, Cheyne-Stokes respirations, stupor and coma, and dilated fixed pupils

      (4) Occipital and thalamic strokes due to compression of the posterior cerebral arteries between the temporal lobe and tentorium.
   c. Cerebellum–foramen magnum herniation is due to downward displacement of the cerebellar tonsils, through the foramen magnum, posterior to the cervical spinal cord. Clinical manifestations include aching and stiffness of the neck, shoulder paresthesias, back and neck extension, internal arm and leg rotation, and respiratory and cardiac abnormalities. Medullary compression can cause death from respiratory arrest.

Clinical Features

1. Papilledema
   a. A genuine direct effect of elevated ICP.
   b. Symptoms include transient visual obscuration, especially with postural change.
   c. The incidence has become lower as brain tumors are diagnosed earlier with neuroimaging (8% of patients with malignant gliomas have papilledema).
2. Headaches
   a. Headache is the presenting symptom in 35% of patients and develops during the course of the disease in 40% to 70%.
   b. Usually dull, nonthrobbing. Mimics tension headache. Occasionally can mimic migraine or even cluster headaches
   c. Supratentorial tumors produce headache in the frontal region; posterior fossa tumors produce pain in occiput and neck.
   d. Clinical features that increase possibility of tumor as cause include awakening with headaches at night; worse on waking and improve over the course of the day; headaches exacerbated by postural change or exertion; presence of nausea or vomiting, papilledema or focal neurologic signs.
   e. Neuroimaging indicated if change in character or severity of patient's usual headaches
3. Altered mental status
   a. Changes in mentation common in frontal lobe tumors, with increased ICP, and in gliomatosis cerebri
      (1) Subtle problems include difficulty with

concentration, memory, affect, personality, initiative, and abstract reasoning.

(2) Severe cognitive problems and confusion can occur.

b. Elevated ICP causes drowsiness and eventually stupor and coma if treatment is not initiated urgently.

4. Seizures

a. Presenting symptoms in one third of patients with brain tumors; present at some stage of the illness in 40% to 60%.

b. Slow-growing tumors more likely to cause seizures

c. 10% to 20% of adult patients with new-onset seizures have brain tumors, so neuroimaging should be part of their initial evaluation.

d. 50:50 focal:secondarily generalized seizures

5. Focal neurologic symptoms and signs

a. Postictal paralysis may indicate tumor location.

b. Enlarging frontal lobe tumors may cause personality changes, urinary frequency and urgency, gait difficulty, motor weakness, aphasia, seizures, gaze preference, primitive reflexes, and anosmia.

c. Temporal lobe tumors often cause seizures, memory disturbances, visual field defects, language disorders.

d. Parietal lobe tumors can cause contralateral sensory loss, apraxias, hemineglect, anosognosia, homonymous visual field defects, apraxia, and sensory seizures.

e. Occipital lobe tumors cause homonymous visual field defects, prosopagnosia, Balint's syndrome, and visual seizures.

f. Thalamic tumors can cause obstructive hydrocephalus, contralateral sensory loss, hemiparesis, cognitive impairment, visual field defects, and aphasia.

g. Brainstem tumors produce cranial neuropathies, weakness, numbness, ataxia, vertigo, nausea, vomiting, and hiccups.

h. Pineal region tumors produce hydrocephalus by third ventricular or aqueductal compression. Midbrain compression causes Parinaud's syndrome (upgaze impairment, convergence-retraction nystagmus, and dilated pupils with light-near dissociation, lid retraction).

i. Third ventricle tumors produce hydrocephalus related to Valsalva, positional changes resulting in episodic leg weakness and syncope, hypothalamic and autonomic dysfunction, and memory impairment.

j. Cerebellar tumors cause headache, nystagmus, hypotonia, cranial nerve abnormalities, and corticospinal tract signs. Midline lesions cause truncal ataxia, and hemispheric lesions cause appendicular ataxia.

6. Cranial nerve involvement

a. Meningiomas of the olfactory groove: Anosmia

b. Optic nerve glioma or meningioma: Unilateral visual loss

c. Pituitary adenoma or suprasellar tumors: Bitemporal hemianopia

d. Cavernous sinus or brainstem gliomas: Extraocular eye movement weakness

e. Vestibular schwannomas: Hearing loss; peripheral facial nerve weakness

f. Brainstem or posterior fossa tumors: Lower cranial nerve deficits

g. Leptomeningeal metastasis: Multiple cranial nerve palsies

7. False localizing signs

a. Herniating uncus producing ipsilateral hemiparesis due to compression of the contralateral cerebral peduncle against the tentorium.

b. Elevated ICP can compress the abducens nerve as it passes over the petrous ligament.

8. Vascular effects of brain tumors

a. Brain tumors can present with spontaneous hemorrhage, sudden neurologic deficit, and progressive decrease in consciousness.

b. Glioblastoma, oligodendroglioma, and mixed gliomas are the most common primary brain tumors to bleed.

c. Subarachnoid hemorrhage is more common in meningiomas than in intra-axial tumors.

d. Pituitary apoplexy is acute hemorrhagic infarction of a pituitary tumor that often requires urgent surgical intervention. The clinical syndrome consists of acute headache, meningismus, visual impairment, ophthalmoplegia, and alterations in consciousness. Severe, life-threatening hypopituitarism occurs and requires rapid hormone replacement.

e. Metastatic tumors most prone to hemorrhage include melanoma, choriocarcinoma, renal cell carcinoma, and bronchogenic carcinoma.

f. Primary brain tumors can mimic ischemic cerebrovascular syndromes by direct vascular occlusion or arterial steal.

g. Postradiation arteriopathy can present with stroke.

h. Brain tumor patients are at high risk of thromboembolic events, including deep vein thrombosis and pulmonary embolus.

i. Hemangioblastomas release erythropoietin and can cause polycythemia.

PEARLS

- Frontal/temporal tumors often are silent.

- Need tissue for diagnosis

- Primary brain tumors rarely metastasize outside the central nervous system.

- Primitive neuroectodermal tumor (PNET), medulloblastoma, pineoblastoma, and oligodendrogliomas can seed the CSF

Key Symptoms: Brain Tumor

- Headaches

- Seizures

- Focal neurologic deficits

- Nausea and vomiting

- Altered mental status

- Cranial nerve deficits

Frequency of Seizures by Tumor Histology

- Oligodendroglioma: 75% to 79%

- Astrocytoma: 65% to 70%

- Meningioma: 39% to 57%

- Glioblastoma multiforme: 30% to 57%

- Metastases: 10% to 30%

Laboratory Testing

1. Magnetic resonance imaging (MRI) is the most informative test.

2. Other tests are sometimes useful.

   a. Visual field perimetry

   b. Electroencephalography (EEG)

   c. Evoked potentials

   d. Cerebrospinal fluid (CSF) analysis. Avoid in patients with increased ICP or mass lesions.

      (1) In AIDS-related primary central nervous system lymphoma (PCNSL), CSF should be screened for Epstein-Barr virus DNA and JC virus polymerase chain reaction.

      (2) Useful in pineal region tumors for diagnosis, important in postoperative staging (> 2 weeks after surgery) of patients with medulloblastoma and primitive neuroectodermal tumor (PNET), diagnosis of neoplastic meningitis in metastatic brain tumors and rarely useful in initial diagnosis of gliomas.

      (3) Biological markers, alpha-fetoprotein, beta subunit of human chorionic gonadotropin, and placental alkaline phosphatase help in diagnosis and subsequent follow-up of germ cell tumors.

   e. Audiometry: Useful in acoustic schwannoma evaluation

   f. Endocrine evaluation for tumors of pituitary and hypothalamus.

Radiologic Features

1. Computed tomography (CT) scans less sensitive but useful initial test (calcium in tumor suggests oligodendroglioma).

2. MRI with gadolinium enhancement is the test of choice for diagnosis of brain tumor.

3. Angiography is occasionally used for preoperative evaluation of vascular anatomy (sphenoid wing meningioma relationship to carotid artery, patency of venous sinuses in falx meningioma) or embolizing large tumors.

4. Ultrasound screening is the procedure of choice for fetal and infant tumors.

Key Tests

- MRI

- Visual field tests

- EEG

- CSF if safe to acquire

- Audiometry

- Endocrinologic tests

- Neuropsychological tests

Treatment

1. Corticosteroids are used to control cerebral edema; often, dexamethasone 10- to 50-mg bolus followed by 4 to 10 mg every 6 hours until stable.

2. Osmotic diuretics (mannitol) and endotracheal intubation and hyperventilation can be used in critical cerebral edema.

3. Specific treatments for each tumor type are cov-

ered in the chapters on gliomas, meningiomas, embryonal and pineal region tumors, skull based and sellar region tumors, and metastatic tumors, but usually treatment entails resection, often radiotherapy, and occasionally chemotherapy and/or biologic therapy.

Bibliography

Antinori A, De Rossi G, Ammassari A, et al.: Value of combined approach with thallium-201 single photon emission computed tomography and Epstein-Barr virus DNA polymerase chain reaction in CSF for the diagnosis of AIDS-related CNS lymphoma. J Clin Oncol 17:554–560, 1999.

Berger MS, Ghatan S, Geyer JR, et al.: Seizure outcome in children with hemispheric tumors and associated intractable epilepsy: The role of tumor removal combined with seizure foci resection. Pediatr Neurosurg 17:185–191, 1991–92.

DeAngelis, Lisa M: Medical progress: Brain tumors. N Engl J Med 344:114–123, 2001.

Levin VA: Neuro-oncology: An overview. Arch Neurol 56:401–404, 1999.

Kleihues P, Cavenee WK (eds): Pathology and genetics of tumours of the nervous system. World Health Organization Classification of Tumours. Lyon, France, IARC Press, 2000.

3 Glial Tumors

Sigmund Hsu

Definition

1. Glial tumors (gliomas) are primary tumors of the central nervous system, derived either from astrocytes, oligodendrocytes, or ependymocytes, and include astrocytoma, oligodendroglioma, ependymoma, as well as mixed tumors such as the oligoastrocytoma.

2. The World Health Organization (WHO) schema characterizes tumors by describing the histology and grading the degree of malignancy on a scale from I to IV. Grading criteria include overall cellular architecture, individual cellular morphology (nuclear atypia, mitotic activity), and presence of secondary structures (endovascular proliferation, necrosis). Tumors are graded according to the highest degree of malignancy present in the sample. The WHO grading of gliomas is depicted in Table 3–1.

Epidemiology

1. The annual incidence of primary brain tumors in the United States is 11 to 12 per 100,000. Gliomas comprise approximately 60% of primary brain tumors and 25% of primary spinal tumors.

2. The incidence of gliomas is increasing, especially among those over 75 years old, probably as a consequence of improved imaging sensitivity.

3. The most common glioma in the brain is glioblastoma multiforme, accounting for 15% of all brain tumors and 50% of all gliomas, followed by anaplastic astrocytoma.

4. Anaplastic glial tumors (WHO grade III) comprise 10% to 30% of all glial tumors.

5. Low-grade, slow-growing tumors (WHO grades I and II) comprise approximately 20% of all glial tumors.

6. In the spine the most common glioma is ependymoma, followed by astrocytoma.

7. The peak incidence for gliomas is from 65 to 75 years of age, as reflected by the large contribution of high-grade tumors. The peak incidence of lower grade tumors is from 35 to 45 years of age.

8. The childhood annual incidence of primary brain tumors is 3 to 4 per 100,000. In children, brain tumors (all types) account for 25% of all cancer deaths.

Risk Factors

1. Irradiation is the strongest causative agent of gliomas. Prophylactic cranial irradiation of children with acute lymphoblastic lymphocytic leukemia resulted in a 2.5% prevalence of glial tumors, a 22-fold increased risk. Exposure risk has resulted from therapeutic irradiation of other brain tumors (pituitary adenoma, craniopharyngioma) and from low-dose irradiation for tinea capitis.

2. No specific chemical or occupational exposure has been definitively linked to human brain tumors. There are suspicions, however, that vinyl chloride production and pesticide manufacturing are associated with brain tumors, and the petrochemical industry exposure is controversial. There have been no proven associations with brain tumors from exposure to electromagnetic radiation.

3. Germ line mutations that cause gliomas (among a spectrum of other tumors) include Li-Fraumeni (*p53* gene), neurofibromatosis (NF1 and NF2 genes), and Turcot syndrome (APC and hMLH1 genes).

Etiology and Pathophysiology

1. Gliomas likely result from an accumulation of genetic disturbances involving DNA damage, cell proliferation and migration, intracellular signaling pathways, and genetic stability, which ultimately result in uncontrolled cell growth. The genes involved include oncogenes, tumor suppressor genes, and genes that control cell death. Table 3–2

TABLE 3–1. WHO GRADING OF GLIAL TUMORS

GRADE	TUMOR TYPE
I	Pilocytic astrocytoma, myxopapillary ependymoma, subependymoma
II	Diffuse astrocytoma, pleomorphic xanthoastrocytoma, oligodendroglioma, oligoastrocytoma, ependymoma
III	Anaplastic astrocytoma, anaplastic oligodendroglioma, anaplastic oligoastrocytoma, gliomatosis cerebri, anaplastic ependymoma
IV	Glioblastoma, giant cell glioblastoma, gliosarcoma

TABLE 3–2. IMPORTANT GENETIC DEFECTS IN GLIOMAS

Type of Gene Altered	Specific Genes
Growth factors	PDGF (platelet-derived growth factor), vEGF (vascular endothelial growth factor), overexpression of EGF receptor, mutant EGF receptor
Tumor suppressor genes and cell cycle regulators	*p53, p21, RB* gene, cyclins, cyclin-dependent kinases, *PTEN* gene
Apoptosis pathway genes	*bcl-2* gene, *myc, bax*
Chemotherapy-resistant genes	Production of AGT (O-6-alkyl-guanine-DNA alkyltransferase) reverses the effects of nitrosourea-based chemotherapy (production of DNA adducts)

depicts some of the important genetic defects involved.

2. Glial tumors are infiltrative.

a. Gliomas produce an extracellular matrix that facilitates invasion through production of multiple proteins (tenascin, vitronectin, fibronectin), receptors (integrin, CD44, RHAMM, versican, NCAM), and enzymes that degrade neighboring extracellular matrix (metalloproteases).

b. Tumor cells can be isolated from areas of edema as far as 4 cm away from the enhancing lesion of a high-grade glioma.

3. Gliomas are heterogeneous with areas of high-grade tumor interspersed between areas of low-grade tumor. This degree of heterogeneity exists between tumors of similar grade and even within the same tumor, both morphologically and molecularly. This heterogeneity may help explain the resistance of gliomas to therapy.

4. Models of glioma progression are presented in Table 3–3, but are far from comprehensive and are limited by tumor heterogeneity.

Clinical Features

1. Symptoms on presentation depend on tumor location.

2. Low-grade tumors may be asymptomatic for years and can be found incidentally; they often present with seizure.

3. High-grade tumors often present with neurologic deficits and increased intracranial pressure (ICP) with headache, nausea, and vomiting. Focal neurologic signs include weakness, personality change, and short-term memory loss and executive dysfunction.

4. High-grade lesions are extremely aggressive and usually recur despite the best therapy. Initial sites of recurrence are typically within 2 cm of the surgical resection.

5. Glial tumors spread locally throughout the central nervous system (CNS), including the leptomeninges, but they usually do not metastasize to distant organs.

6. Ependymomas often line the cerebrospinal fluid pathways and present with signs of increased ICP from outflow obstruction.

 Key Signs

Low-Grade Tumors
- Can be stable for years
- Usually present with seizures

High-Grade Tumors
- Present with focal neurologic deficits or increased intracranial pressure
- Usually recur despite the best therapies

TABLE 3–3. MODELS OF GLIOMA PROGRESSION

Progression Model	Tumor Grade	Genetic Changes
Astrocytoma to glioblastoma	Low-grade astrocytoma	*p53* mutation, PDGF-A overexpression
	Anaplastic astrocytoma	Loss of heterozygosity 19q, *RB* alteration
	Secondary glioblastoma	Loss of heterozygosity 10q, *PTEN* mutation, loss of expression DCC, *PDGFR*-alpha amplification
De novo glioblastoma	Glioblastoma	EGFR amplification or overexpression, *MDM2* amplification or overexpression, p16 deletion, loss of heterozygosity 10p and 10q, *PTEN* mutation, *RB* alteration
Oligodendroglioma to anaplastic oligodendroglioma	Oligodendroglioma	Loss of heterozygosity 1p, 19q, 4q, overexpression EGFR, PDGF, PDGFR
	Anaplastic oligodendroglioma	Loss of heterozygosity 9p, 10q, deletion CDKN2A (p16 and p14^{ARF}), mutation/deletion CDKN2C, vEGF overexpression

Abbreviations: PDGFR: platelet derived growth factor receptor; PDGF-A: platelet-derived growth factor A; PDGFR-alpha: platelet-derived growth factor receptor alpha; DCC: deleted in colorectal cancer; MDM2: Murine Double Minute chromosome clone number 2.

Differential Diagnosis

Differential diagnosis of primary CNS neoplasms includes abscess, demyelinating disease, metastatic disease, primary CNS lymphoma, progressive multifocal leukoencephalopathy, and encephalitis.

Laboratory Testing

1. Magnetic resonance imaging (MRI) with and without contrast
2. Chest radiograph, computed tomography (CT) of the chest, abdomen, and pelvis (C/A/P) if metastatic lesion is a possibility
3. Complete blood count, basic metabolic panel
4. Biopsy, resection

Radiologic Features

1. Infiltrative lesions with ill-defined borders (butterfly glioma crossing the corpus callosum)
2. Low-grade tumors are usually nonenhancing.
3. Oligodendrogliomas are often more circumscribed and can have areas of calcification or cyst formation.
4. High-grade enhancing tumors are typically associated with edema, areas of necrosis with irregular enhancing borders, and may contain regions of hemorrhage and be multifocal.

Radiologic Findings

- Infiltrative on MRI

- Low-grade tumors: little edema

- High-grade tumors: heterogeneous enhancement, edema, necrosis, hemorrhage

---

Treatment

1. Overview
   a. Accurate diagnosis requires biopsy or resection.
   b. The best treatment (surgery, radiation, chemotherapy, observation) depends on the tumor classification and risks and benefits to the patient of each treatment.
   c. Because of the frequent lack of effectiveness of standard treatment modalities, consider experimental treatments as early as possible.
2. Low-grade tumors
   a. Treatment is controversial, ranging from observation to surgical resection to radiation and, only rarely, chemotherapy.
   b. A general strategy for treatment would be

observation until the tumor has been demonstrated to grow or the patient becomes symptomatic (difficult seizure control or neurologic dysfunction).
   c. Proponents of observation argue that no treatment has been proven to improve survival for these patients, and the risks of surgery outweigh any benefit.
   d. Radiation therapy for low-grade tumors has been shown to prolong time to relapse but not to lengthen overall survival.
   e. WHO grade I lesions may be cured by complete resection alone.
   f. Proponents of surgery argue that (1) accurate pathology, which could alter treatment strategy, may not be possible without adequate sampling, and (2) the natural history of these tumors is known, and ultimately these patients will relapse with higher grade tumors; if the tumor can be "completely" resected, there will is less residual available for further malignant transformation.
3. Anaplastic gliomas
   a. Ideal treatment consists of a gross total surgical resection, typically followed by radiation and chemotherapy.
   b. The extent of surgical resection can be proven prospectively to affect outcome as long as resection is followed by radiation therapy.
   c. The timing of chemotherapy is controversial; some advocate using chemotherapy early, others use chemotherapy only on recurrence.
   d. The benefit of adjunct chemotherapy is best proven for anaplastic oligodendroglioma where the loss of heterozygosity at the 1p/19q chromosome is a marker for chemosensitivity and response.
   e. The recommended chemotherapy regimen is typically based on alkylating agents BCNU (carmustine) or procarbazine.
   f. Temozolomide is a new oral agent approved for treatment of anaplastic gliomas.
4. Glioblastoma
   a. The best therapy includes aggressive surgical resection followed by radiation therapy.
   b. Chemotherapy shows uneven benefit, with optimal response rates only 30% to 40% at best, although most long-term survivors have received a gross total resection, full-dose radiation therapy (54 to 60 Gy), and chemotherapy.
   c. BCNU wafers implanted at surgery for recurrence provide minimal progression-free survival benefit.
   d. These patients should be considered for partic-

ipation in clinical trials because current therapy offers only marginal benefit.

e. New investigational agents include inhibitors of signal transduction pathways, gene therapy, and often combination therapy with standard cytotoxic chemotherapy.

5. Ependymoma

a. The primary therapy for ependymoma is surgery.

b. Unlike other glial tumors, these tumors often recur with the same tumor grade as opposed to malignant transformation.

c. When malignant transformation occurs, these tumors are often resistant to radiation and chemotherapy.

d. Ependymomas can seed the CSF pathways with malignant cells, and work-up requires complete cranial-spinal imaging.

 Key Treatment

- Accurate pathology
- Maximal surgery
- Conformal radiation
- Chemotherapy
- Clinical trials
- Multidisciplinary team interaction

Prognosis

1. Low-grade tumors: The overall prognosis for low-grade tumors is a median survival time of 4 to 7 years, with some studies reporting a 10-year median survival. Prognostic factors for prolonged survival include younger age and oligodendroglial histology.

2. Anaplastic tumors: The median survival time for anaplastic gliomas ranges from 3 to 5 years, with improved survival for younger patients with anaplastic oligodendroglioma, no preoperative neurological impairment, and gross total resection.

3. Glioblastoma: Despite the best therapy, median survival ranges from 9 to 14 months, with a 5-year survival rate of less than 5%. Prognostic factors include age and preoperative neurologic function.

4. Ependymoma: Five-year survival ranges from 50% to 80%. Myxopapillary ependymoma and subependymoma have especially good prognosis, with survival usually greater than 10 years.

Complications of Treatment and Tumor Progression

1. Radiation somnolence: During radiation therapy, many patients complain of overwhelming fatigue and sleepiness, which seems to be cumulative and may not begin to lift until months after completion of therapy. Psychostimulants such as methylphenidate may help.

2. Radiation necrosis: After the completion of radiation therapy, patients may develop areas of necrosis within the radiation field not related to tumor progression. This is a late complication of therapy and is more common with high-dose irradiation. It can often be confused with tumor progression, and can be just as debilitating.

3. Cognitive decline: Cognitive decline is a common symptom in brain tumor patients. The causes are multifactorial and include tumor progression, side effects of radiation and chemotherapy, and exacerbation by systemic illness. Psychostimulants may help.

4. Long-term corticosteroid use: Complications of steroids, often necessary to control cerebral edema, include myopathy, psychosis, and increased risk for opportunistic infections (*Pneumocystis carinii*).

5. Seizure control: Focal and generalized seizures can be difficult to control despite therapeutic anticonvulsant levels. Reducing edema through use of steroids and primary treatment of the tumor often help control. Drugs that utilize similar hepatic enzyme metabolic pathways may interact with each other, including chemotherapy.

6. Drug rash: Severe drug rash, including Stevens-Johnson syndrome, may develop and be exacerbated by prolonged use of the offending drug because of masking from use of corticosteroids. The most severe reactions may involve synergy from concomitant radiation therapy, steroid use, and anticonvulsants.

Pregnancy

1. No specific contraindications to pregnancy; however brain tumor management raises numerous issues regarding management of intracranial pressure, chemotherapy effects on the fetus, and seizure control.

2. Anticonvulsants increase risk of fetal malformations. Valproic acid is strongly associated with neural tube defects.

3. Chemotherapy usually causes loss of fertility. Patients planning to have a child should consider

banking of sperm and ovum prior to chemotherapy.

Bibliography

Bernstein M, Rerger M (eds): Neuro-Oncology: The Essen-
tials. New York, Thieme Medical Publishers, 2000.
Greenberg H, Chandler W, Sandler H: Brain Tumors. New
York, Oxford University Press, 1999.

Kleihues P, Cavenee W (eds): WHO Classification Tumors
of the Nervous System. Lyon, France, IARC Press,
2000.
Levin V, Leibel S, Gutin P: Neoplasms of the central nervous
system. In DeVita V, Hellman S, Rosenberg S (eds): Cancer:
Principles and Practice of Oncology, 6th ed. Philadelphia,
Lippincott Williams & Wilkins, vol. 2, 2001, pp. 2100–
2160.
Louis D, Cavenee W: Molecular biology of the central
nervous system neoplasms. In DeVita V, Hellman S,
Rosenberg S (eds): Cancer: Principles and Practice of
Oncology, 6th ed. Philadephia, Lippincott Williams &
Wilkins, vol. 2, 2001, pp. 2091–2100.

4 Meningiomas

Howard Colman

Definition

Meningiomas are intracranial or spinal tumors arising from arachnoid cap cells. Most are benign and slow growing, but higher grade lesions, and some lower grade lesions, have a high rate of recurrence and behave more aggressively.

Epidemiology and Risk Factors

1. Meningiomas comprise approximately 20% of primary intracranial tumors (13% to 40%).
2. Overall incidence is approximately 2.5 per 100,000 persons.
3. The incidence increases with age.
4. Incidence is higher in women (up to 2:1), especially in middle age.
5. The best-characterized risk factors for meningioma formation are prior cranial irradiation (low or high dose) and neurofibromatosis type 2. Evidence for prior head trauma and the role of estrogen and progesterone as risk factors are controversial.

Etiology and Pathophysiology

1. Meningiomas arise from neoplastic transformation of arachnoid cap cells.
2. Approximately 91% to 94% of meningiomas are benign (World Health Organization [WHO] grade I), 5% to 7% are atypical (WHO grade II), and 1% to 2% are anaplastic (WHO grade III).
3. The most common sites of meningioma formation are parasagittal, followed by cerebral convexity, sphenoid ridge, suprasellar, posterior fossa, olfactory groove, middle cranial fossa, and ventricular. Rarely, meningiomas can develop intraparenchymally.
4. A number of genetic and biochemical alterations are implicated in meningioma formation and progression including alterations in the *NF2* gene on chromosome 22, expression of progesterone receptors, expression of vascular endothelial growth factor (VE6F), and the expression of platelet-derived growth factor (PDGF) and PDGF receptor. Other cytogenetic alterations include changes on chromosomes 1, 6, 9, 10, 12, 14, 15, 17, 18, and 20.

Clinical Features

1. The presenting symptoms of meningioma depend on tumor location.
2. The most common presenting symptoms include headache, focal weakness, behavioral change, and seizures.
3. Autopsy studies and more recent imaging studies suggest that a significant number of meningiomas can be asymptomatic, especially in older patients.

Key Signs

- Depend on tumor location, with the most common being headache, focal weakness, behavioral change, and seizures

---

Caveat

- Autopsy studies and more recent imaging studies suggest that a significant number of meningiomas can be asymptomatic, especially in older patients.

Radiologic Features

1. Generally isodense or slightly hyperdense on precontrast computed tomography (CT) with strong, homogeneous contrast enhancement.
2. Usually isointense or hypointense on T_1-weighted magnetic resonance imaging (MRI) sequences with isointense or hyperintense signal on T_2-weighted sequences. Usually strong, homogeneous enhancement on postcontrast T_1-weighted MRI sequences.
3. Margins of tumor are usually well defined, except in some high-grade lesions.
4. Dural tail is often visible on postcontrast images (MRI more sensitive than CT).
5. Hyperostosis or lysis of overlying bone may be seen in some cases.
6. Calcification, hemorrhage, or cystic changes may be present.
7. Extent of surrounding edema is variable.
8. MR angiography or conventional angiography may be employed in some cases to evaluate for preoperative embolization.

Radiologic Findings

- Homogeneously contrast-enhanced lesion attached to the dura
- Dural tail often visible
- Usually well-defined margins
- Variable edema of adjacent brain

Pathology

1. The WHO grading system separates meningiomas into three grades, with a number of different histologic subtypes (Table 4–1).

2. Atypical meningiomas have increased mitotic activity or several features such as increased cellularity, high nucleus-to-cytoplasm ratio, sheetlike growth, and foci of necrosis.

3. Anaplastic (malignant) meningiomas have histologic features of malignancy in excess of those abnormalities seen in atypical meningiomas, such as very high mitotic rate or histologic appearance similar to sarcoma or carcinoma.

Treatment

1. Complete surgical resection is the initial treatment of choice for symptomatic meningiomas. Tumor location significantly affects the probability for complete resection, with lesions in the cerebral convexities, lateral sphenoid wing, cerebellar convexities, olfactory groove, and spinal canal generally more accessible for complete resection.

2. Involvement of cranial nerves, venous sinuses, cavernous sinus, and eloquent brain parenchyma can limit extent of resection.

3. External-beam radiation therapy after surgery significantly reduces recurrence rates in subtotally

TABLE 4–1. WORLD HEALTH ORGANIZATION (WHO) CLASSIFICATION OF MENINGIOMAS

GRADE I	GRADE II	GRADE III
Meningothelial	Atypical	Anaplastic (malignant)
Fibrous (fibroblastic)	Clear cell	Rhabdoid
Transitional (mixed)	Chordoid	Papillary
Psammomatous		
Angiomatous		
Microcystic		
Secretory		
Lymphocyte-rich		
Metaplastic		

resected lesions. Radiation therapy is also effective in reducing recurrence rates of high-grade lesions after complete resection and for improving progression-free survival in recurrent lesions of all grades.

4. Stereotactic radiosurgery and gamma knife radiosurgery have shown promise for improving local control of some unresectable lesions.

5. Dexamethasone is effective for reducing symptoms of peritumoral edema.

6. Anticonvulsants are often necessary to control seizures secondary to meningiomas.

7. Chemotherapy and hormonal therapy have generally been of little benefit in meningiomas that continue to progress after maximal surgery and radiation. However, several small series have reported some efficacy with various drugs, including hydroxyurea or interferon-alpha as single agents, and with the combination of cyclophosphamide, adriamycin (doxorubicin), and vincristine.

8. Treatment of asymptomatic meningiomas in elderly patients is controversial because many of these lesions may remain indolent or progress very slowly.

Key Treatment

- Complete resection is the best treatment.
- External beam radiation
- Focal radiation
- Dexamethasone for edema
- Anticonvulsants
- Observation of asymptomatic benign meningiomas in the elderly is reasonable.

Prognosis and Complications

1. Prognosis and risk of recurrence is related to tumor grade and extent of resection.

2. Recurrence rates for benign menigiomas after complete resection have been reported between 7% and 19%. The recurrence rate for atypical meningiomas is between 30% and 45%. Anaplastic meningiomas have recurrence rates of 60% to 70%.

3. Recurrence rates of subtotally resected benign meningiomas can be as high as 60% after surgery alone, and approximately 30% with the addition of radiation therapy.

4. High-grade lesions, and some low-grade tumors, can behave very aggressively, with resultant morbidity and mortality.

5. The significance of brain invasion is controversial, with some authors believing that evidence of brain invasion alone indicates an anaplastic grade, whereas others favor an atypical grade without other histologic features of anaplasia.

6. Metastasis of meningiomas outside the central nervous system is rare but has been reported, most commonly to the lungs with high-grade tumors.

Bibliography

Kaye AH, Laws ER (eds): Brain Tumors: An Encyclopedic Approach. London, Churchill Livingstone, 2001, pp. 719–750.

Kleihues P, Cavanee WK (eds): Pathology and Genetics of Tumours of the Nervous System. Lyon, France, IARC Press, 2000, pp. 175–184.

Simpson D: The recurrence of intracranial meningiomas after surgical treatment. J Neurol Neurosurg Psychiatry 20:22–39, 1957.

Stafford SL, Perry A, Suman VJ, et al.: Primarily resected meningiomas: Outcome and prognostic factors in 581 Mayo Clinic patients, 1978 through 1988. Mayo Clin Proc 73:936–942, 1998.

MEDULLOBLASTOMA

Definition

A malignant embryonal tumor usually originating in the cerebellum.

Epidemiology

1. The annual incidence is about 0.5 per 100,000 children under the age of 15 years.

2. Rare in adulthood, particularly beyond the fifth decade of life.

3. A male preponderance is seen in medulloblastoma (65% of patients).

Clinical Features

1. Symptoms: Early symptoms reflect increased intracranial pressure secondary to 4th ventricle obstruction (headache, vomiting), cerebellar dysfunction (ataxia, falls), or both.

2. Signs: papilledema, truncal ataxia, nystagmus, head tilt. Patients may have signs of meningeal seeding (e.g., leg weakness).
   See Table 5–1 for key symptoms and signs, key tests, key treatments, and germ cell tumor marker profiles for all tumor types discussed in this chapter.

Laboratory Tests

1. Magnetic resonance imaging (MRI) of the brain with contrast reveals a contrast-enhancing lesion in the posterior fossa with projection into the 4th ventricle. Obstructive hydrocephalus is often also present.

2. MRI of the spine is necessary at presentation given the high incidence of "drop" metastases to the spinal leptomeninges.

3. Lumbar puncture with cerebrospinal fluid (CSF) cytology for meningeal seeding (if lumbar puncture is performed after surgery, should wait at least 2 weeks to allow postoperative cells to clear).

4. Bone scan for bone metastases.

Treatment

Surgery, radiation, and chemotherapy: Extensive surgery has been associated with improved survival. Chemotherapy is used with radiation treatment, particularly in high-risk patients (age <3 years, metastatic disease, residual postoperative disease, and supratentorial disease). Chemotherapy without radiation has also been used in attempts to spare the central nervous system the effects of radiotherapy.

Differential Diagnosis: Medulloblastoma

- Ependymoma

- Cerebellar astrocytoma

SUPRATENTORIAL PRIMITIVE NEUROECTODERMAL TUMOR (PNET)

Definition

An embryonal tumor composed of poorly differentiated neuroepithelial cells usually developing in the cerebrum or suprasellar region.

Epidemiology

Supratentorial PNETs are rare tumors; they usually occur in the first decade of life and are twice as common in males.

Clinical Features

1. Symptoms: Headache, vomiting from increased intracranial pressure. Seizures or focal symptoms (weakness, numbness) in cerebral lesions.

2. Signs: Papilledema, enlarging head circumference in infants, focal weakness, or numbness.

Laboratory Tests

MRI of the brain with contrast is the imaging modality of choice. PNETs usually appear as well-circumscribed, heterogeneous masses, denoting necrotic change, calcification, and hemorrhage. Spinal MRI is necessary for possible "drop" metastases.

TABLE 5–1. KEY SYMPTOMS AND SIGNS, KEY TESTS, KEY TREATMENTS, AND TUMOR MARKERS OF EMBRYONAL AND PINEAL REGION TUMORS

Tumor Type	Key Symptoms and Signs	Key Tests	Key Treatments	Germ Cell Tumor Marker Profile*
Medulloblastoma	Papilledema, truncal ataxia, nystagmus, head tilt Increased ICP (headache, vomiting), cerebellar dysfunction (ataxia, falls), or both Leg weakness: meningeal seeding	Contrast brain MRI Spinal MRI LP with CSF cytology Bone scan	Extensive surgery Chemotherapy with radiotherapy in high-risk patients Chemotherapy alone in attempt to spare CNS effects of radiotherapy	N/A
PNET	Symptoms of increased ICP: headache, vomiting; seizures or focal symptoms (weakness, numbness) in cerebral lesions Papilledema, enlarging head circumference in infants, focal weakness or numbness	Contrast brain MRI Spinal MRI	Surgical resection Often followed by radiotherapy and chemotherapy	N/A
Pineocytoma	Headache, nausea, vomiting; visual disturbances (e.g., diplopia) Papilledema; vertical gaze paralysis, limited convergence with nystagmus, lid retraction (Parinaud's syndrome)	Contrast brain MRI	Surgical resection	N/A
Pineoblastoma	ICP symptoms: headache, vomiting, lethargy; visuomotor disturbances Papilledema Parinaud's syndrome Limited convergence Lid retraction Impaired upgaze Delayed or precocious puberty	Contrast brain MRI Spinal MRI LP with CSF cytology	Aggressive multimodality treatment: surgical debulking, radiotherapy, chemotherapy	N/A
Germinoma	Symptoms of increased ICP: headache, vomiting, and visual disturbances; growth failure Papilledema, changes in mental status, Parinaud's syndrome	Contrast brain MRI LP with CSF cytology Serum analysis	Radiation therapy: germinomas are very radiosensitive. Chemotherapy is sometimes also used to reduce total radiation dose.	hGC, + LD, ++ PAP, ++
Embryonal carcinoma	Symptoms of increased ICP or tectal plate invasion with diplopia and upgaze paralysis Examination may show papilledema, eye movement abnormalities (Parinaud's syndrome), and delayed or precocious puberty.	Contrast brain MRI Biopsy a must for definitive diagnosis LP with CSF cytology Serum analysis	Multimodality: surgical resection plus chemotherapy, then radiotherapy, then chemotherapy (sandwich therapy)	AFP, + hGC, ++
Yolk sac tumor	Symptoms of increased ICP pressure and visual disturbances Papilledema, eye movement abnormalities (Parinaud's syndrome), and delayed or precocious puberty	Contrast brain MRI Spinal MRI LP with CSF cytology Serum analysis	Aggressive multimodality treatment	AFP, +++
Teratoma	Symptoms of increased ICP pressure or midbrain compression Papilledema, eye movement abnormalities (Parinaud's syndrome), and delayed or precocious puberty.	Contrast brain MRI LP with CSF cytology Serum analysis	Complete surgical excision followed by radiotherapy and chemotherapy	AFP, +/–
Choriocarcinoma	Symptoms of increased ICP: headache, nausea, vomiting, visual disturbances; maybe delayed puberty Papilledema, abnormal eye movements (such as restricted upward gaze); delayed puberty	Contrast brain MRI LP with CSF cytology Serum analysis Full endocrine profile with signs of delayed puberty	Surgery, radiotherapy, and platinum-based chemotherapy Success with stereotactic radiosurgery has been reported.	hGC, +++

Abbreviations: ICP: intracranial pressure; MRI: magnetic resonance imaging; LP: lumbar puncture; CSF: cerebrospinal fluid; PNET: primitive neuroectodermal tumor; N/A: Not applicable; hGC: human chorionic gonadotropin; LD: lactate dehydrogenase; PAP, placental alkaline phosphatase; AFP, alpha-fetoprotein.

Treatment

Surgical resection is often followed by radiation and chemotherapy treatment.

PINEOCYTOMA

Definition

A tumor arising in the pineal region composed of cells that resemble pineocytes. Usually slow-growing, well-differentiated neoplasms.

Epidemiology

Pineocytomas are most common in young adults (25 to 35 years of age) and show no sex predilection.

Clinical Features

1. Symptoms: Headache, nausea, and vomiting from increased intracranial pressure. Visual disturbances (e.g., diplopia) from dorsal rostral midbrain compression.
2. Signs: Papilledema. Vertical gaze paralysis, limited convergence with nystagmus and lid retraction (Parinaud's syndrome).

Laboratory Tests

MRI of the brain with contrast shows a well-circumscribed pineal region tumor, usually with decreased signal on T_1-weighted sequences and increased signal on T_2-weighted images.

Treatment

Surgical resection helps relieve obstruction, improve prognosis, and differentiate pineocytomas from other pineal region tumors.

PINEOBLASTOMA

Definition

A primitive, malignant embryonal tumor of the pineal region.

Epidemiology

1. Rare tumors with a peak incidence in the first two decades of life.
2. Incidence is greater in males than in females.

Clinical Features

1. Symptoms: Often present with symptoms of increased intracranial pressure (headache, vomiting, lethargy) because they grow more rapidly than other pineal tumors. Visuomotor disturbances also occur.
2. Signs: Papilledema, changes in mental status, Parinaud's syndrome

Laboratory Tests

1. MRI of the brain with contrast usually shows contrast-enhancing lesions in the pineal region. Associated hydrocephalus is common.
2. MRI of the spine and lumbar puncture with CSF analysis for leptomeningeal disease

Treatment

Aggressive multimodality treatment with surgical debulking, radiation, and chemotherapy

GERMINOMA

Definition

Germinoma is a germ cell tumor that may arise in the CNS, typically in the pineal or suprasellar region.

Epidemiology

1. Very rare tumors in the Western hemisphere; germinomas (and other germ cell tumors) are more common in Asia, particularly Japan.
2. All germ cell tumors are more common in children (peak incidence in the second decade of life).
3. Male:female ratio is 2:1.

Clinical Features

1. Symptoms: headache, vomiting, and visual disturbances from increased intracranial pressure. Children may present with growth failure caused by pituitary dysfunction with large suprasellar tumors.
2. Signs: Papilledema, changes in mental status, Parinaud's syndrome

Laboratory Tests

1. MRI of the brain with contrast usually shows a contrast-enhancing mass in the pineal or suprasellar region.
2. Serum and CSF analysis for beta-human chorionic

gonadotropin (β-hCG) and placental alkaline phosphatase.

Treatment

Germinomas are very radiosensitive. Chemotherapy is sometimes also employed to reduce total radiation dose.

EMBRYONAL CARCINOMA

Definition

Embryonal cell carcinomas are composed of large, totipotential, undifferentiated embryonal-type epithelial cells, usually arising in midline structures, such as the pineal region.

Epidemiology

Embryonal carcinomas are rare tumors, usually occurring in children and with a male preponderance.

Clinical Features

1. Symptoms: As with other pineal region and midline tumors, symptoms reflect increased intracranial pressure or tectal plate invasion with diplopia and upgaze paralysis.

2. Signs: Examination may show papilledema, eye movement abnormalities (Parinaud's syndrome), and signs of delayed or precocious puberty.

Laboratory Tests

1. MRI of the brain with contrast is sensitive for tumor size, midbrain involvement, and pituitary or optic tract compression in suprasellar tumors. Like other germ cell tumors, however, embryonal carcinoma has no specific MRI characteristics, and biopsy is necessary for definitive diagnosis.

2. Serum and CSF levels of hCG and alpha-fetoprotein (AFP) are elevated.

Treatment

Embryonal carcinoma has a much poorer prognosis than germinoma. The 5-year survival for patients with malignant intracranial non-germinomatous germ cell tumors is less than 25% after partial resection and radiation. Improved survival (74% at 5 years) has been reported with radical surgery, and multimodality "sandwich" therapy (chemotherapy–radiation–chemotherapy).

YOLK SAC TUMOR

Definition

A germ cell tumor composed of epithelial cells with a primitive morphology and often located in midline CNS structures (e.g., pineal).

Epidemiology

1. Yolk sac tumors are rare, as are other germ cell tumors.

2. More common in males.

Clinical Features

1. Symptoms of increased intracranial pressure occur with large midline tumors, and visual disturbances may be secondary to obstruction or direct pressure on midbrain structures.

2. Examination may show papilledema, eye movement abnormalities (Parinaud's syndrome), and delayed or precocious puberty.

Key Tests

- MRI of the brain with contrast
- MRI of the spine for metastases
- CSF and serum AFP and hCG

Treatment

Aggressive multimodality treatment is recommended for all non-germinomatous germ cell tumors (see Treatment under Embryonal Carcinoma, above).

TERATOMA

Definition

Teratomas are germ cell tumors that contain elements of ecto-, meso- and endodermal origin such as such as hair, teeth, and cartilage.

Epidemiology

1. As with other germ cell tumors, a male preponderance is noted.

2. Occurrence is typically in the first or second decade of life.

Clinical Features

1. Symptoms: As with the other germ cell tumors, teratomas often occupy a midline location and symptoms result from aqueductal obstruction with increased intracranial pressure or midbrain compression.
2. Signs: Examination may show papilledema, eye movement abnormalities (Parinaud's syndrome), and delayed or precocious puberty.

Laboratory Tests

1. MRI of the brain with contrast defines size and location. Heterogeneity of signal and variable enhancement are typical and result from the various components of the tumor.
2. CSF and serum oncoproteins.

Treatment

1. Complete excision of mature teratomas gives good results.
2. Radiation and chemotherapy usually administered after surgery

CHORIOCARCINOMA

Definition

A germ cell tumor characterized by cytotrophoblastic and syncytiotrophoblastic elements.

Epidemiology

1. Choriocarcinoma is more common in males.
2. Typical occurrence is the first or second decade of life.

Clinical Features

1. Symptoms: Patients may present with headaches, nausea, vomiting, and visual disturbances from increased intracranial pressure. Cases of delayed puberty have also been reported.

2. Signs: Papilledema, abnormal eye movements (such as restricted upward gaze). Signs of delayed puberty may be present.

Laboratory Tests

1. MRI of the brain with contrast is the imaging investigation of choice.
2. CSF and serum β-hCG levels are elevated.
3. A full endocrine profile is warranted in patients with evidence of dysfunction such as pubertal delay, menstrual irregularities, and the like.

Treatment

Surgery, radiation, and platinum-based chemotherapy are usually employed. Success with stereotactic radiosurgery has been reported.

PEARLS

- The combination of upgaze paralysis, limited convergence, convergence-retraction nystagmus, lid retraction, and light-near dissociation (Parinaud's syndrome) is indicative of dorsal rostral midbrain dysfunction and is most commonly seen in cerebrovascular disease and pineal region tumors.

- Head tilt in children may be indicative of a posterior fossa lesion such as medulloblastoma.

- Investigation of medulloblastoma and non-germinomatous germ cell tumors should always include spinal imaging.

Bibliography

Kleihues P, Cavenee WK: Pathology and Genetics Tumors of the Nervous System. World Health Organization Classification of Tumors. International Agency for Research on Cancer. Lyon, France, IARC Press, 2000.

Robertson PL, DaRosso RC, Allen JC: Improved prognosis of intracranial non-germinoma germ cell tumors with multimodality therapy. J Neuro-Oncol 32:71–80, 1997.

Skull-Based and Sellar Region Tumors

Pierre Giglio

ACOUSTIC NEURINOMA (VESTIBULAR SCHWANNOMA)

Definition

A schwann cell tumor arising from the vestibular division of the eighth cranial nerve and growing to occupy the cerebellopontine angle.

Epidemiology

1. The annual incidence is about one per 100,000.

2. Occur in neurofibromatosis type 1 (unilateral) or more commonly, type 2 (bilateral).

3. Usually sporadic. Chromosome 22 mutations have been reported.

4. Female:male ratio 60:40.

5. Sporadic cases occur in middle age; neurofibromatosis-associated cases present in the third decade. In children the tumor is rare and no sex preponderance is seen.

Clinical Features

1. Symptoms: Early symptoms are caused by pressure effects on cranial nerves V, VII, and VIII. Hearing loss is the most common presenting symptom. Patients may also complain of balance problems; tinnitus; pain in or behind the ear; and facial numbness, weakness, or both. Headache and facial pain are also common.

2. Some patients present with a triad of vertigo, nausea and vomiting, and hearing difficulty, suggesting Ménière's disease.

3. Signs: Sensorineural hearing loss is present in most patients at presentation. Facial sensory loss and facial weakness may also be present. Cerebellar compression in larger tumors may cause limb incoordination; brainstem compression may cause hydrocephalus and signs of increased intracranial pressure.

Key Signs

- Triad of vertigo, nausea and vomiting, and hearing difficulty, suggesting Ménière's disease.
- Sensorineural hearing loss
- Facial sensory loss and facial weakness
- Cerebellar compression in larger tumors may cause limb incoordination.
- Brainstem compression may cause hydrocephalus and signs of increased intracranial pressure.

Differential Diagnosis

See Table 6–1.

Laboratory Tests

1. Magnetic resonance imaging (MRI) of the brain with contrast is the most sensitive test.

2. Audiometry is used to document degree of hearing loss prior to surgery.

Key Tests

- Contrast-enhanced MRI of the head
- Pure tone and speech audiometry
- Brainstem-evoked responses

Treatment

Surgical excision with intraoperative monitoring of the facial and auditory nerves (electromyography and brainstem auditory evoked response). Preservation of facial nerve function depends on tumor size and surgical approach but is possible (70% to 90%). Preservation of hearing ranges from 3% to 50% in surgeries planned to preserve function.

TABLE 6–1. DIFFERENTIAL DIAGNOSIS OF ACOUSTIC NEURINOMAS

Condition	Distinguishing Features
V, VII neurinomas and epidermoid cyst	Facial pain, numbness, or weakness occur earlier than in acoustic neuromas
Cerebellopontine angle meningioma	May have an identical presentation; imaging may distinguish a meningioma by its being dural based (tail-sign)
Glomus jugulare tumor	Imaging helpful; skull films may show erosion of jugular foramen
Meniere's disease	Symptoms are intermittent and imaging is normal; persistent (as opposed to episodic) vertigo, hearing loss, or tinnitus must be investigated with imaging

Key Treatment

- Surgical excision with intraoperative monitoring of the facial and auditory nerves

CHORDOMAS AND CHONDROSARCOMAS

Definition

1. Chordomas are tumors that arise from embryonic notochord remnants, usually in the clivus or sacrococcygeal region. They are slow growing but have a high propensity for local invasion and recurrence. Metastases are rare.
2. The basic neoplastic tissue of chondrosarcomas is cartilage, and it is made up of large cells with mucin within and around the cells.

Epidemiology

1. Both chordomas and chondrosarcomas are rare tumors, constituting less than 0.5% of all intracranial tumors.
2. Chondrosarcoma is more common in men.
3. Peak presentation is between the third and fifth decades of life.

Clinical Features

1. Symptoms: headache, diplopia, dysphonia, and dysphagia (VII, IX, and X cranial nerve involvement). Local invasion and cerebellar/brainstem compression may cause focal weakness, numbness, or ataxia.

2. Signs: Lateral rectus palsy, palatal weakness; in advanced cases, cerebellar ataxia, focal weakness, or numbness.

Key Signs and Symptoms

- Headache, diplopia, dysphonia, dysphagia
- Local invasion and cerebellar or brainstem compression may cause focal weakness, numbness, ataxia.
- Lateral rectus palsy, palatal weakness
- In advanced cases, cerebellar ataxia, focal weakness, numbness

Differential Diagnosis

See Table 6–2.

Laboratory Tests

1. Contrast-enhanced brain MRI is the best diagnostic test.
2. Computed tomography (CT) scan may be useful in defining the degree of bone destruction.
3. With more laterally placed chordomas (often chondrosarcomas), auditory testing is necessary.
4. Biopsy may be necessary.

Key Tests

- Contrast-enhanced MRI of the brain
- CT scan for defining degree of bone destruction
- Auditory testing
- Biopsy

TABLE 6–2. DIFFERENTIAL DIAGNOSIS OF CHORDOMAS

Condition	Distinguishing Features and Comments
Petroclival meningioma	Bone invasion prominent in chordoma; MRI enhancement more variable than in meningiomas.
Nasopharyngeal carcinoma	Chordomas and chondrosarcomas may invade the nasopharynx, causing nasal symptoms and even dysphagia. Biopsy usually required for differentiation from nasopharyngeal carcinoma.
Craniopharyngioma	Chordomas have a decreased to normal signal on T_1-weighted MR sequences; craniopharyngiomas may have increased signal intensity on T_1-weighted sequences (caused by high cholesterol content)

Treatment

1. Surgical removal (sometimes multiple-staged surgeries)
2. Residual disease treated with external beam irradiation, radiosurgery, or proton beam irradiation.

Key Treatment

- Removal, which may require multiple-staged surgeries
- External beam irradiation, proton beam irradiation, or radiosurgery for residual disease

Prognosis

This has improved dramatically with improved surgical approaches and radiation techniques. Chordomas are considered to be potentially curable tumors. Tumor-free survival rates exceed 70% at 5 years. Prognosis is less favorable for chondrosarcomas.

CRANIOPHARYNGIOMA

Definition

1. A tumor originating in the remnants of Rathke's pouch, usually at the junction of the pituitary stalk with the adenohypophysis. Rathke's cleft cysts share a common origin with craniopharyngioma.
2. Craniopharyngiomas often develop a cyst filled with calcium deposits, cholesterol crystals (giving the tumor a characteristic increased signal on T_1-weighted images), and proteinaceous fluid. The solid parts of the tumor consist of epithelioid cells.

Epidemiology

1. In the adult population, craniopharyngiomas represent 1% to 4% of all intracranial tumors.
2. The annual incidence is about 1 to 2 cases per million population.
3. There is a slight male preponderance in most series.
4. Peak incidence is seen at ages 5 to 10 years and again at 50 to 60 years.

Clinical Features

1. Signs: On examination, patients may have visual field deficits, papilledema, and optic atrophy. Children may have evidence of growth failure or delayed puberty.

2. Symptoms: Patients may present with symptoms of increased intracranial pressure (headaches, vomiting, and visual disturbances) or symptoms referable to hypothalamic-pituitary axis dysfunction (diabetes insipidus, thermoregulatory insufficiency, menstrual disturbances, and loss of libido). Children may present with delayed physical and mental development.

Key Signs and Symptoms

- Visual field deficits, papilledema, and optic atrophy. Children may have growth failure or delayed puberty.
- Increased intracranial pressure or hypothalamic-pituitary axis dysfunction. Children may have delayed physical and mental development.

Differential Diagnosis

Craniopharyngioma must be distinguished from chordoma, pituitary adenoma, sellar/parasellar meningioma, metastases, and suprasellar arachnoid cyst.

Laboratory Tests

Testing has two main purposes in the craniopharyngioma syndrome: defining the extent of local pressure on neighboring structures (such as the optic pathway) and quantifying hypothalamic and pituitary dysfunction (see the later section on pituitary tumors in this chapter).

Key Tests

- MRI, with contrast, of the head
- Visual acuity and visual field mapping
- Endocrine profile

Radiologic Features

Increased signal on T_1-weighted MRI related to the high cholesterol content of the tumor cyst. High calcium content in some tumors results in decreased and increased signal on T_2- and T_1-weighted MRI, respectively.

Treatment

1. Complete resection is curative. Microsurgery has improved the outlook in these tumors and has

reduced postoperative complications (endocrinopathies, hypothalamic dysfunction, sleep disorders, appetite changes).

2. External beam radiation, brachytherapy, and radiosurgery are used to treat residual or recurrent tumor.

Key Treatment

- Complete resection is curative.

- External beam radiation, brachytherapy, and radiosurgery for residual or recurrent tumor

Prognosis

Survival rates of 90% at 10 years are achieved with good surgical resection and adjuvant radiation treatment in incomplete resections.

PITUITARY TUMORS

Definition

Tumors arising from the anterior lobe of the pituitary. Conventionally classified as *chromophobe, acidophil,* or *basophil* adenomas, based on affinity for staining methods. Current classifications stress importance of size (macroadenoma compared with microadenoma), and hormone product of the tumor (e.g., prolactinomas compared with growth hormone secreting tumors).

Epidemiology

1. Inclusion of asymptomatic cases in autopsy series: up to 25% occurrence of pituitary tumors.

2. Annual incidence rates of 14 per 100,000 population have been reported.

3. Incidence increases with age.

4. Overall female preponderance.

Clinical Features

Clinical presentation depends on the size and hormone product of tumor.

Differential Diagnosis

Endocrine syndromes with typical abnormalities in the sella turcica or parasellar region on imaging make for a straightforward diagnosis. However, up to one third of tumors are composed of nonsecretory cells. Such tumors present with pressure effects and may be quite large at presentation. In such cases, the differential diagnosis includes meningiomas, chordomas, metastases, craniopharyngiomas, Rathke's cleft cysts, suprasellar arachnoid cysts, and lipomas.

Laboratory Tests

1. Serologic testing is as outlined in Table 6–3.

2. MRI is the imaging modality of choice. Homogeneous enhancement is usually noted in macroadenomas, as well as extension above or below the

TABLE 6–3.   CLINICAL PRESENTATION OF PITUITARY ADENOMAS

Pituitary Adenoma	Symptoms	Signs	Serum Test
Prolactinoma (prolactin secreting)	Galactorrhea and menstrual abnormalities in females; headache, visual disturbances and impotence in males (amenorrhea/galactorrhea syndrome)	Galactorrhea, bitemporal hemianopia	Serum prolactin level; chlorpromazine test (administration causes increase in prolactin in normal; this is suppressed in prolactinomas)
Gonadotroph adenoma (GH secreting)	Headache, jaw and acral growth. Gigantism in tumors before puberty (acromegaly/gigantism)	Prognathism, coarse facial features, visual field deficits	GH levels; failure of GH levels to increase on administration of glucose or TRH
Corticotroph adenoma (ACTH secreting)	Obesity, weakness, hirsutism, menstrual abnormalities, behavior changes (Cushing's disease)	Hypertension, muscle weakness, abdominal striae	Serum cortisol, urinary steroids, dexamethasone suppression test, glucose levels
Thyrotroph adenoma (TSH secreting)	Tremor, palpitations, sweating, weight loss, anxiety (hyperthyroidism)	Tremor, tachycardia, sweaty palms	TSH, TRH, T_4
Gonadotroph adenoma (FSH, LH secreting)	Menstrual irregularities, subfertility		FSH, LH, estradiol, testosterone levels

Abbreviations: GH: growth hormone; TRH: thyrotropin-releasing hormone; ACTH: adrenocorticotropic hormone; TSH: thyroid-stimulating hormone; FSH: follicle-stimulating hormone; LH, luteinizing hormone; T_4: thyroxine.

sella turcica and, in some cases, invasion into the cavernous or sphenoid sinuses. Microadenomas usually have decreased signal intensity on T_1-weighted sequences and increased signal on T_2-weighted sequences.

Key Tests

• Blood tests

• MRI is the modality of choice.

Treatment

1. Transsphenoidal surgery: Most adenomas are resected via this approach; mortality and morbidity are low.

2. Dopamine agonists: bromocriptine inhibits prolactin secretion.

3. Growth-hormone inhibitor hormone analogues: inhibit growth hormone secretion.

4. Radiation treatment is less commonly used. Damage to optic pathways and hypopituitarism are potential complications. It may be necessary in some recurrent tumors.

5. Hormone deficiency in cases presenting with hypopituitarism.

Caveat

• Pituitary adenomas may present with hypersecretion or deficiency of one or more hormones.

• Surgery is the treatment of choice in most tumors.

• Microadenomas and some macroadenomas may require only pharmacotherapy.

• Radiation therapy plays a minor role in the management of pituitary adenomas.

RATHKE'S CLEFT CYST

Definition

An intrasellar cyst resulting from persistence of the lumen of Rathke's pouch (an invagination of the roof of the oral cavity in the embryo).

Epidemiology

Symptomatic Rathke's cleft cysts are uncommon and account for less than 1% of brain tumors. Usually become symptomatic in adults.

Clinical Features

1. Symptoms: Headache and visual disturbances
2. Signs: Visual field deficits, hypopituitarism

Differential Diagnosis

Consider arachnoid cyst, pituitary adenoma, and craniopharyngioma.

Laboratory Tests

1. MRI of the brain.
2. Tests for pituitary dysfunction.

Treatment

Surgical excision or drainage is the treatment of choice.

Bibliography

Gsponer J, De Tribolet N, Deruaz J-P, et al.: Diagnosis, treatment and outcome of pituitary tumors and other abnormal intrasellar masses: Retrospective analysis of 353 patients. Medicine 78:236–269, 1999.

Macfarlane R, King TT: Acoustic neurinomas (vestibular schwannomas). In Kaye AH, Laws ER Jr. (eds): Brain Tumors. New York, Churchill Livingstone, 1995.

Sen C, Triana A: Cranial chordomas. In Issues in Neuroscience. Continuum Health Partners, Inc., Continuum Neurosciences, Spring 2001.

7 Other Tumors

Ivo W. Tremont-Lukats

HEMANGIOBLASTOMA

Definition

A benign, vascular tumor composed of stromal cells and capillaries. It can be sporadic or a major constituent of von Hippel-Lindau disease (VHL), an autosomal dominant disease with capillary hemangioblastomas of the central nervous system (CNS), retinal angiomas, renal cell carcinoma, pheochromocytomas, and pancreatic cysts. This section will focus on hemangioblastomas associated with VHL.

Epidemiology and Risk Factors

1. The incidence is approximately 1:35,000 population. There is no ethnic or gender preponderance. The peak age at diagnosis is 20 to 39 years. Hemangioblastoma represents 2% of all primary brain tumors and 7% to 10% of all posterior fossa tumors.
2. Location: cerebellum (80% to 85%), spinal cord (3% to 13%), medulla (2% to 3%); supratentorial lesions are rare.

Key Factors

- Most common location: posterior fossa
- Most frequent cause of death in von Hippel-Lindau disease
- Most affected: 20 to 39 years of age

Etiology and Pathophysiology

1. A germ line mutation of the VHL tumor suppressor gene in chromosome 3p25-26 is responsible for sporadic and VHL-associated cases.
2. This missense mutation inactivates the gene, which normally inhibits tumor development and growth. Inheritance is autosomal dominant with high penetrance. Phenotypic expression only occurs if the nonmutated allele is inactivated.

Clinical Features

1. Hemangioblastomas can be asymptomatic and found incidentally, or during VHL work-up.

2. Headaches, nausea and vomiting, and disequilibrium are the most frequent presenting symptoms (50%, 30%, and 53%, respectively, in one series).
3. Examination may reveal papilledema, ataxia, dysarthria, and nystagmus. Brainstem or spinal lesions can cause cranial nerve and spinal cord signs.

Key Signs

- Papilledema
- Gait ataxia, appendicular ataxia
- Nystagmus
- Cranial nerve palsy

Key Symptoms

- Headache
- Nausea and vomiting
- Unsteady gait
- Slurred speech

Differential Diagnosis

Symptoms of CNS hemangioblastoma can be confused with those of any primary or metastatic CNS tumors in the posterior fossa. A positive family history or coexistence of extracranial VHL disease should differentiate hemangioblastoma from other tumors. Magnetic resonance imaging (MRI) appearance and tumor location are suggestive of hemangioblastoma.

Laboratory Diagnosis

The best test to confirm VHL and sporadic hemangioblastoma is chromosomal analysis demonstrating the 3p25-26 mutation. In sporadic cases without the mutation, diagnosis relies on the surgical specimen.

Radiologic Features

1. Computed tomography (CT): Hypodense, often with cyst, intensely enhancing mural nodule.
2. MRI shows mural nodule (hypointense on T_1-

weighted sequences, hyperintense on T_2-weighted sequences), which strongly enhances.

Treatment

1. Surgical resection. Up to 33% of patients may need multiple surgeries because resection was partial or because there is new tumor growth.

2. In selected cases, when surgery is not indicated because of tumor inaccessibility or the patient's general condition, endovascular embolization and radiosurgery are reasonable alternatives.

Prognosis and Complications

1. The most common cause of death in VHL patients is untreated CNS hemangioblastoma.

2. Surgical morbidity is low.

3. Symptom resolution or local control at 1 year occurs in about 90% of patients.

4. Recurrence from partial resections occurs in 20% of patients.

Prevention

In VHL, genetic counseling is important, but prevention is possible only if the affected carrier decides not to have children. Some authors recommend MRI screening for detection of asymptomatic cases and early surgical treatment.

PRIMARY CENTRAL NERVOUS SYSTEM LYMPHOMA

Definition

Primary central nervous system lymphoma (PCNSL) is an extranodal lymphoma of the CNS. Most CNS lymphomas are of B cell origin but about 5% can be of T cell lineage.

Epidemiology and Risk Factors

1. PCNSL accounts for 6% to 7% of all primary CNS tumors. The incidence is 30 cases per million population, a 10-fold increase in 20 years due to the acquired immune deficiency syndrome (AIDS) pandemic. In AIDS patients, the incidence is 4.7 per 1000 person-years, with 2% to 10% of AIDS patients ultimately developing PCNSL.

2. In immunocompetent patients, the peak incidence is 60 to 69 years, with a 3:2 male-to-female ratio.

3. In immunodeficient patients, the peak incidence is 10 years for patients with primary immunodeficiencies, and 35 to 40 years for transplant and AIDS patients. In AIDS patients, the male-to-female ratio is 9:1

Etiology and Pathophysiology

1. Primary and secondary immunodeficiencies predispose to PCNSL. In patients with acquired immunodeficiency, the Epstein-Barr virus plays a major role in the development of PCNSL. Its role in immunocompetent patients is less clear.

2. In some non-AIDS patients, chromosomal translocations and clonal abnormalities have been found.

3. Neoplastic cells usually accumulate in the vascular adventitia and then can infiltrate the brain.

Clinical Features

1. 60% of PCNSL are supratentorial; of these, half are solitary lesions. In AIDS patients, multiple lesions are more frequent (65% to 85%). The overall distribution is frontal (15%), posterior fossa (13%), basal nuclei (10%), temporal lobe (8%), leptomeninges (8%), parietal lobe (7%), occipital lobe (3%) and spinal cord (1%).

2. Secondary meningeal involvement from PCNSL is reported in 40% of cases, and ocular involvement is noted in 20% of cases.

3. Common presenting symptoms include confusion, personality changes, headaches, visual changes, focal neurologic deficits, and seizures. Exceptional presentations mimic diabetes insipidus, subdural hematoma, optic neuropathy, dementia, narcolepsy, pseudotumor cerebri, parkinsonism, and trigeminal neuropathy

 Key Signs

- More than half are supratentorial, and half of those are solitary lesions.

- Multiple lesions occur more often in AIDS.

- Secondary meningeal involvement

- Ocular involvement

- Presenting symptoms: Confusion, personality changes, headaches, visual changes, focal neurologic defects, seizures

Differential Diagnosis

Other primary brain tumors, brain metastases, pyogenic abscess, toxoplasmosis, and multiple sclerosis. Consider underlying human immunodeficiency virus (HIV) infection.

Laboratory Testing

1. Cerebrospinal fluid (CSF) pleocytosis occurs in 35% to 60% of patients, but cell count can be normal. CSF protein is usually markedly elevated, and glucose may be low.

2. Cytology is diagnostic in 25% of cases; flow cytometry and tumor marker analysis can enhance sensitivity.

3. Slit-lamp eye examination is needed (20% patients have ocular involvement).

Radiologic Features

1. CT shows solitary (two thirds of patients) or multiple, hyperdense or isodense lesions, usually solid, and occasionally cystic. On contrast MRI, lesions usually solidly and intensely enhance; however, central necrosis and ring enhancement can mimic a glioblastoma multiforme.

2. Most tumors are located periventricularly, in the corpus callosum, thalamus, or basal nuclei. The location of metastatic lymphoma to the CNS is different, and includes the subdural, subarachnoid, and epidural spaces and the spinal cord.

Key Tests

- CSF protein is usually markedly elevated, and glucose may be low.

- Cytology, flow cytometry, tumor marker analysis

- Slit-lamp eye examination

- Neurologic imaging

Treatment

1. Presurgical steroids can induce temporary resolution of the lesions.

2. Surgery for PCNSL is limited to diagnostic biopsy or, occasionally, emergency debulking to prevent life-threatening herniation.

3. Chemotherapy is the treatment of choice for PCNSL. Most effective regimens include intravenous methotrexate. Other regimens effective for systemic lymphoma are also useful.

4. Response to radiotherapy is greater than 80%. It is the treatment of choice for those patients who refuse or cannot receive chemotherapy.

Key Treatment

- Presurgical steroids

- Intravenous methotrexate

- Radiation therapy

Prognosis and Complications

1. Without treatment, median survival is 3 months. Radiation increases median survival to anywhere from 10 to 40 months. Because of the risk of cognitive decline after radiotherapy (especially in the elderly), radiation is usually reserved for patients with tumor refractory to chemotherapy.

2. With combined-modality treatment, immunocompetent patients with favorable prognostic factors (Karnofsky performance status above 70 simple score, age below 60 years, and a single lesion) have a median survival of 20 to 45 months, with a 5-year overall survival of 25% to 45%. In similarly-treated AIDS patients, median survival is 13.5 months.

3. PCNSL can respond spectacularly to steroids, and in a few cases this response can be sustained. Spontaneous remissions rarely occur.

Caveats

- The incidence of primary central nervous system lymphoma is 30 cases per million, but it has increased tenfold in 20 years as a consequence of AIDS.

- Emergency debulking to prevent life-threatening herniation may be needed for patients with primary central nervous system lymphoma.

PARAGANGLIOMAS, CENTRAL NEUROCYTOMA, CHOROID PLEXUS TUMORS, AND COLLOID CYSTS

Definition

1. Paragangliomas are neuronal or mixed neuronal–glial neoplasms from the neural crest.

2. Central neurocytomas are tumors of neuronal differentiation and low-grade histology; classically, they are located in the lateral or third ventricles; less commonly, in brain parenchyma.

3. Choroid plexus tumors (CPTs) are neoplasms from the epithelium of the choroid plexus of the ventricles. They are divided into two categories:

choroid plexus papilloma (benign, slow-growing tumor, surgically curable), and choroid plexus carcinoma (malignant, with frequent CSF metastases).

4. Colloid cysts are surgically curable benign tumors that originate in the roof of the 3rd ventricle. They represent the most common tumor in the 3rd ventricle.

Epidemiology

1. CNS paragangliomas are rare. Cauda equina tumors are the most frequent, followed by jugulotympanic (also known as *glomus jugulare tumors*) and carotid body paragangliomas (also known as *chemodectomas* or *carotid body tumors*). The peak age of presentation is the fifth decade with a slight predominance for men (1.4:1), with the exception of jugulotympanic paragangliomas, which are more frequent in women (4:1).

2. Central neurocytomas represent 0.25% to 0.5% of all intracranial tumors. The most affected group is between 20 and 29 years of age, without gender preponderance.

3. Choroid plexus tumors make up <1% of all intracranial tumors, 2% to 4% of brain tumors in children, and 10% to 20% of brain tumors in the first year of life. Half of these tumors are in children younger than 2 years of age. The annual incidence is 0.3 per 1 million population. The papilloma-to-carcinoma ratio is 5:1. These tumors may occur in association with Sturge-Weber syndrome.

4. Colloid cysts are 0.3% to 0.5% of all brain tumors. Most cases present in patients between 20 and 50 years of age, but any age can be affected. There is no gender predominance, and there are no familial cases nor any inheritance pattern.

Etiology and Pathophysiology

1. The etiology of paragangliomas, choroid plexus tumors, neurocytomas, and colloid cysts is unknown.

2. Carotid body paragangliomas can show clustering in families, with an autosomal dominant inheritance pattern. However, sporadic and familial cases seem to share a common genetic defect, a mutation in chromosome 11q13 or 11q22-23.

3. Symptoms in paragangliomas can occur from extrinsic compression of adjacent structures. In CPT, neurocytomas, and colloid cysts, symptoms are due to CSF flow obstruction.

Clinical Features

1. Paragangliomas of the filum terminale cause a cauda equina syndrome. Jugulotympanic and carotid paragangliomas cause dysfunction of the V, VII-XII cranial nerves. Neurosecretory activity can cause autonomic symptoms (palpitations, flushing, explosive diarrhea, headaches, and sweating). Large jugulotympanic paragangliomas can present with intracranial hypertension.

2. Neurocytoma, CPT in older children and adults, and colloid cysts: Most patients present with symptoms of elevated ICP (headaches, visual obscurations, nausea and vomiting). The classic presentation of colloid cyst is paroxysmal headache after a change in head position. Some cases present with sudden leg weakness, causing falls but not loss of consciousness. Progressive headache with raised ICP is a common presentation. Progressive dementia, with gait apraxia and urinary incontinence, can also occur. Many cysts are asymptomatic and can be found incidentally. Sudden death can occur.

3. CPT in the pediatric population: because of overproduction of CSF by the tumor, or because of CSF flow obstruction, signs of hydrocephalus occur in 80% to 90% of infants: head enlargement, tense fontanel, emesis, lethargy, and irritability. Less common signs of high ICP in infants include head tilt, titubation, developmental delay, and seizures. Posterior fossa lesions can present with cranial nerve dysfunction and cerebellar signs. Tumors in the 3rd ventricle can present with endocrine disturbances. The duration of symptoms is from weeks to months.

Differential Diagnosis

1. Paragangliomas in the filum terminale can be confused with ependymomas, meningiomas, and non-Hodgkin's lymphoma. Jugular and carotid paragangliomas must be distinguished from other tumors located in the cerebellopontine angle, such as vestibular shwannomas, meningiomas, or hemangioblastomas.

2. CPT: Consider oligodendroglioma, ependymoma, pineocytoma, dysembryoplastic neuroepithelial tumor (DNT), ependymoma, teratoma, subependymal giant cell astrocytoma, and metastatic carcinoma

3. Central neurocytoma: Consider oligodendroglioma, ependymoma, pineocytoma, DNT, choroid plexus papilloma, teratoma, and subependymal giant cell astrocytoma. Synaptophysin immunochemistry and electron microscopy can differentiate central neurocytoma from the other tumors.

4. Colloid cysts: Ependymoma, metastasis, meningioma, primitive neuroectodermal tumor (PNET), astrocytoma, germinoma, and teratoma

Radiologic Features

1. Paragangliomas present as hypointense to isointense lesions on T_1-weighted MRI, hyperintense on T_2-weighted sequences, and enhance after gadolinium. Carotid paragangliomas can be seen on carotid Doppler ultrasound. CT scan is useful to evaluate bone invasion.

2. In CPT: the CT scan shows an isodense contrast-enhancing mass that can contain calcifications and cysts. Hydrocephalus may be present. MRI: Normal appearance to hyperintensity on T_1- and T_2-weighted sequences, with enhancement after contrast.

3. In neurocytomas, the CT scan can reveal an isodense contrast enhancing mass with calcifications and cysts. Hydrocephalus may be present. MRI: Normal appearance to hyperintensity on T_1- and T_2-weighted sequences with enhancement after contrast.

4. For colloid cysts, CT scans show a hyperdense (70%), isodense (25%), or hypodense (5%) ovoid lesion in the anterior 3rd ventricle with noncontrast images. Contrast enhancement occurs in 12% to 55% of cases. MRI: The cyst location suggests the diagnosis, and signal intensity is variable (Table 7–1).

Treatments

1. The appropriate management of paragangliomas hinges on a careful evaluation of symptoms, clinical aggressiveness of the tumor, patient age, and performance status. In cauda equina paragangliomas: Surgery, with total excision as the goal. The recurrence rate is around 5%. In head and neck paragangliomas: Surgery, radiation therapy, and stereotactic radiosurgery are modalities that can be used alone or combined. Persistent disease and relapse rates are 6% to 11% and 7% to 8%, respectively. Radiosurgery is playing an increasing role in the treatment of these tumors.

2. In central neurocytoma, complete surgical resection is the treatment of choice. The benefit of adjuvant radiotherapy is not known. The current trend is to use radiotherapy if there is recurrence, if the MIB-1 labeling index is >2%, or if the tumor is not completely resected.

3. For CPT and colloid cysts, complete resection is the best treatment. For recurrent CPTs, occasionally x-ray radiation treatment or chemotherapy is used (Table 7–2).

Prognosis and Complications

1. If treated adequately, paragangliomas can be controlled with little or no morbidity. In 5% of cases, the tumor behaves aggressively, eroding adjacent structures and causing metastases (malignant paragangliomas). Other paragangliomas are locally invasive and either cannot be resected totally or recur after every resection.

2. In CPT, total resection has a good prognosis. Total resection cures choroid plexus papilloma, with a 5-year survival of 100%. Choroid plexus carcinoma has a 5-year survival of 40%; CSF seeding and distant metastases occur.

3. With total resection of a central neurocytoma, prognosis is good. Recurrence is more likely (63%) with an MIB-1 labeling index >2%. Periventricular location seems to be a poor prognostic factor. Incomplete resection can result in hydrocephalus by obstruction of CSF flow to the 3rd ventricle from the lateral ventricles.

4. Given the unpredictable course of colloid cysts, surgical excision is advocated whenever possible in asymptomatic patients. Mental decline and hydrocephalus indicate the need for urgent ventricular drainage. Patients with headaches or dementia should receive a shunt.

TABLE 7–1. KEY SIGNS AND SYMPTOMS

Location of Paraganglioma	Symptoms	Signs
Filum terminale	Low back pain, diffuse or radicular	Cauda equina syndrome, with sensorimotor and autonomic deficits
Jugulotympanic	Hearing loss, otic fullness, otorrhea, dizziness, vertigo, tinnitus (sometimes pulsatile), double vision, facial droopiness, hoarseness, shoulder weakness	Deficits in cranial nerves VII to XII in isolation or combined. High-pitched bruit over the mastoid bone.
Carotid body	A painless, slow-growing neck mass, especially in the anterior triangle	Fontaine's sign: carotid body tumor can be displaced laterally but not vertically. With larger tumors, a tonsilar bulge is apparent.

TABLE 7–2. KEY TESTS AND TREATMENTS

TUMOR TYPE	TESTS	TREATMENTS
Paraganglioma	Hypointense to isointense lesions on T_1-weighted MRI, hyperintense on T_2-weighted, and enhanced after gadolinium. Carotid paragangliomas: carotid Doppler ultrasound; CT scan to evaluate bone invasion	First, careful evaluation In cauda equina paragangliomas: Surgery, with goal of total excision In head and neck paragangliomas: Surgery, radiation therapy, and stereotactic radiosurgery alone or combined.
Central neurocytoma	CT scan MRI	Surgery Radiotherapy for recurrence
Choroid plexus tumor	CT scan MRI	Complete resection is the best treatment. Occasionally, radiotherapy or chemotherapy for recurrence
Colloid cyst	CT scan MRI	Complete resection is the best treatment. Occasionally, radiotherapy or chemotherapy for recurrence

B Bibliography

DeAngelis LM: Primary CNS lymphoma: Treatment with combined chemotherapy and radiotherapy. J Clin Oncol 43:249–257, 1999.

Giannella-Borradori A, Zeltzer PM, et al.: Choroid plexus tumors in childhood. Response to radiotherapy, chemotherapy, and immunophenotypic profile using a panel of monoclonal antibodies. Cancer 69:809–816, 1992.

Kaye AH, Laws ER Jr (eds): Brain Tumors. An Encyclopedic Approach, 2nd ed. London, Churchill Livingstone, 2001.

Kleihues P, Cavenee WK (eds): World Health Organization Classification of Tumors of the Nervous System. IARC Press, Lyon, 2000.

Nasir S, DeAngelis LM: Update on the management of primary CNS lymphoma. Oncology 14:228–234, 2000.

Definition

Neoplasms originating in the spinal canal can be extradural or intradural. Intradural tumors can be extramedullary or intramedullary. Intradural, extramedullary tumors usually arise from meninges, nerve roots, connective tissue, or blood vessels and include meningiomas, neurofibromas, lipomas, dermoids, hemangiomas, and often metastatic tumors. Intramedullary tumors are usually glial, ependymal, or vascular.

Epidemiology

1. Primary spinal cord tumors account for 4% to 10% of central nervous system (CNS) tumors; 30% to 35% are malignant; 23% of primary spinal cord tumors are gliomas.
2. Most primary spinal cord tumors are intradural.
3. Spinal cord tumor locations: Thoracic, lumbar, cervical: 50%, 30%, 20%
4. In adults, 25% of intraspinal neoplasms are intramedullary; in children, most spinal cord tumors are intramedullary.
5. The most common intramedullary spinal cord tumors are gliomas. Common types are astrocytoma, ependymoma, and ganglioglioma; less common tumors include hemangioblastoma and primitive neuroectodermal tumors.
6. Ependymomas make up about 60% of intramedullary spinal cord tumors. Astrocytomas make up about 25%.
7. Astrocytomas are distributed throughout the spinal cord.
8. Most ependymomas involve the conus medullaris or cauda equina.
9. In children younger than 10 years old, intramedullary spinal cord tumors above the conus are either astrocytomas or gangliogliomas 75% of the time; 10% are ependymomas.
10. If the patient is at least 20 years old and the tumor is above the conus, 60% are ependymoma.

Etiology and Pathophysiology

The cause of primary spinal cord tumors is unknown. However, ependymomas are associated with neurofibromatosis type 2 and have chromosomal abnormalities in chromosome 22 (monosomy, deletions, translocations). Less common chromosomal changes are found on 9q, 10, 17, 13, 7, and 10. Some have p53 tumor suppressor gene mutations.

Clinical Features

1. Many patients are aware of the problem before objective signs develop; onset of symptoms is usually gradual, evolving over weeks to months.
2. Low-grade tumors can cause symptoms for months or years, whereas malignant tumors often become symptomatic over a period of weeks.
3. Patients with low-grade tumors and relatively trivial symptoms often have massive spinal cord expansion, whereas patients with high-grade malignant tumors, with a rapidly occurring disability, often have a less dramatic expansion of the spinal cord.
4. Segmental sensory changes, motor changes, and tenderness of the spinous processes are seen in 50% of patients with spinal cord tumors.
5. Signs, symptoms, and clinical manifestations that help differentiate extramedullary from intramedullary tumors and further localize spinal cord tumors are listed in Tables 8–1 and 8–2.
6. The most common early symptom is spine pain (70% patients), often noted at night and worse when supine. Other symptoms include weakness, radicular pain (10% cases), paresthesias or dysesthesias (10% cases), and bladder or bowel control difficulty. A dissociation of thermal, pain, and tactile sensory loss over different spinal segments on the trunk is indicative of an intramedullary lesion.
7. In children, there may be an increase of falling, walking on the heels or toes, or a history of being late-walkers or motor regression.
8. Spinal cord tumor presentation can be varied.
    a. *Sensory-motor spinal tract syndrome:* Patients often present with back pain, later asymmetric motor and sensory disturbances. When lesions are near the cervical spinal cord, symptoms can progress from one arm to the ipsilateral leg, the contralateral leg, and lastly to the remaining arm, generating a windmill, or around-the-clock pattern of progression.
    b. *Painful radicular spinal cord syndrome* occurs because of external compression or infiltration of the spinal cord roots. Pain is knifelike or

TABLE 8–1. CLINICAL FEATURES OF INTRAMEDULLARY AND EXTRAMEDULLARY TUMORS

CLINICAL FEATURE	EXTRAMEDULLARY	INTRAMEDULLARY
Pain	Occurs early, radicular quality	Poorly localized, burning
Sensory changes	Contralateral loss of pain and temperature, ipsilateral loss of proprioception	Patchy sensory loss and dissociation of sensation
Lower motor neuron changes	Segmental	Prominent, atrophy, fasciculations
Upper motor neuron changes	Occurs early, prominent	Late, minimal
Reflexes	Increased	Minimal changes
Corticospinal tract signs	Early	Late
Spinal subarachnoid block and CSF changes	Early, prominent	Late, less prominent

Adapted from Haerer AF, DeJongs The Neurologic Examination, 5th ed. Philadelphia, Lippincott Williams & Wilkins, 1995, pp. 588.

dull, with occasional sharp stabs exacerbated by the Valsalva maneuver.

c. In the *central syringomyelic syndrome,* pain is the most common symptom, often in tumors of the filum terminale.

Key Signs

- Nighttime back pain
- Truncal radicular pain
- Leg weakness
- Bladder control problems
- Cervical lesions cause windmill syndrome
- Partial Brown-Séquard syndrome

Differential Diagnosis

1. Consider diseases of the gallbladder, internal abdominal organs, and pleura, which can be difficult to distinguish from spinal cord manifestations. Once the focus is narrowed to the spinal cord, magnetic resonance imaging (MRI) scan is the best diagnostic tool.
2. For extradural tumors, the differential diagnosis includes cervical spondylosis, tuberculosis, chronic granulomatous lesions, sarcoidosis, lipomas, ruptured discs, and dural tears.
3. Differential for intradural, extramedullary lesions includes meningioma, neurofibroma, and meningeal carcinomatosis.

4. When intramedullary lesions are encountered, one must distinguish glioma, vascular malformation, metastatic carcinoma, multiple sclerosis, or postinfectious spinal cord enhancement.

Laboratory Tests

Spinal fluid, computed tomographic (CT) myelography, and spinal MRI are the most useful tests in evaluating patients with spinal cord lesions. Cerebrospinal fluid (CSF) can show elevated protein and xanthochromia, and occasionally neoplastic cells. Care should be taken when obtaining CSF from patients with spinal cord tumors because a partial block can be transformed into a complete CSF block and complete paralysis can result.

TABLE 8–2. SIGNS AND SYMPTOMS OF SPINAL CORD TUMORS

LOCATION	SIGNS AND SYMPTOMS
Foramen magnum	Posterior head and neck pain, stiffness; weakness of neck extensors, ipsilateral arm and hand; 11th and 12th cranial nerve palsies; cerebellar ataxia; quadriparesis
Cervical	Neck pain, arm weakness, then ipsilateral leg and later opposite arm; wasting and fibrillation of ipsilateral neck, shoulder, and arm; decreased pain and temperature sensation in upper cervical region; head tilt, torticollis
Thoracic	Unilateral radicular pain; abdominal muscle weakness with sparing of arms; sensory level
Thoracolumbar junction	Produces spasticity, and cauda equina symptoms and sensory loss. Babinski reflex suggests cord involvement above L5 cord segment
Lumbosacral	Root pain in groin or sciatic distribution; impotence; bladder paralysis; decreased patellar, increased ankle reflexes
Conus medullaris	Pain not common or severe, but if present usually bilateral, symmetric; in perineum or thighs; sensory loss saddle-like, onset can be sudden and bilateral; pain and back stiffness can precede sensory abnormalities, which often precede motor and reflex abnormalities. Back pain worse when supine; improved after sitting up. Early, marked bladder and rectal symptoms; erection and ejaculation impaired; Dissociation of sensation; mild symmetric motor loss, occasionally weak legs; fasciculations; loss of ankle jerks; sensory changes over the sacral dermatomes, loss of anal and bulbocavernous reflexes
Cauda equina	Unilateral back and leg pain (bilateral if tumor is large); radicular sensory loss and bowel and bladder sphincter abnormalities; bilateral asymmetric atrophy and paralysis; areflexia

Adapted from DeVita V, Hellman S, Rosenberg SA (eds), Cancer: Principles and Practice of Oncology, 6th ed. Philadelphia, Lippincott Williams & Wilkins, 2001, pp. 2100–2160.

Radiologic Features

1. MRI can reveal intramedullary cysts above and below the tumor.

2. Contrast enhancement of the MRI may reveal high-grade tumor. Ependymomas tend to enhance brightly and homogeneously, whereas gliomas may enhance heterogeneously.

3. Focal spinal cord expansion favors ependymoma over astrocytoma. Diffuse widening of the spinal cord suggests astrocytoma.

Treatment

1. Surgery

   a. Tumors are usually removed from the inside out through a midline myelotomy overlying the tumor. Ultrasonic aspiration devices, laser, and the operating microscope are used for spinal cord surgery. Ependymomas often have clear margins around the tumor. Motor evoked potentials from transcortical stimulation and somatosensory evoked potentials are helpful in monitoring the integrity of the motor and sensory pathways intraoperatively.

   b. Surgical complications

      (1) Patients with malignant tumors have a greater risk of intraoperative neurologic damage than those with low-grade tumors.

      (2) Postoperative spine deformity: More common following surgery in children than adults; the spine deformity itself can occasionally cause cord compression.

      (3) Hydrocephalus can occur in cervical cord tumors, either from obstruction of the foramen of Luschka, or from extreme elevations of CSF protein levels proximal to the tumor resulting in slow CSF flow and communicating hydrocephalus.

2. Radiation

   a. Radiation therapy is recommended for intramedullary tumors that cannot be completely removed. Dose is between 45 and 54 Gy.

   b. Occasionally, for tumors that tend to spread via the spinal fluid (ependymoma), radiation is delivered to the entire thecal sack.

   c. For totally resected ependymomas, no radiation therapy is needed. Radiation improves tumor control and disease-free survival in patients whose ependymomas are not completely resected.

3. Chemotherapy: There are no controlled trials of chemotherapy in spinal cord tumors; however, drugs used for intracranial tumors of similar histologies are used in spinal cord tumors.

Key Diagnostics and Treatment

- MRI is essential
- Surgery
- Radiation therapy
- Occasionally chemotherapy

Prognosis and Complications

1. Leptomeningeal dissemination is common with spinal axis tumors.

2. Intradural, extramedullary tumors, such as meningiomas and schwannomas, can be cured with surgery alone.

3. Astrocytomas that recur usually recur within 3 years after treatment. Approximately, 50% to 65% of astrocytomas are locally controlled.

4. 5- and 10-year survival rates for patients with low-grade astrocytoma of the spinal cord range from 60% to 90% and 40% to 90%, respectively. 5- and 10-year relapse-free survival rates range from 66% to 83% and 53% to 83%, respectively.

5. Anaplastic astrocytoma and glioblastoma multiforme have shorter survivals, in the range of 8 to 10 months.

6. Ependymoma recurrence can be delayed as long as 12 years. 5- and 10-year survival rates for ependymoma patients that receive radiation range from 60% to 100% and 68% to 95%, respectively. 10-year relapse-free survival rates in ependymoma patients that are irradiated vary from 43% to 61%.

7. Histology affects outcome in ependymomas. Well-differentiated tumors have a 5-year cause-specific survival rate of 97%, compared with 71% for intermediate or poorly differentiated tumors. Myxopapillary ependymomas arising in the conus medullaris have an excellent prognosis.

Bibliography

Balmaceda C: Chemotherapy for intramedullary spinal cord tumors. J Neurooncol 47:293–307, 2000.

Levin VA, Leibel SA, Gutin PH: Neoplasms of the central nervous system. In DeVita V, Hellman S, Rosenberg SA (eds): Cancer: Principles and Practice of Oncology, 6th ed. Philadelphia, Lippincott Williams & Wilkins, 2001, pp. 2100–2160.

Rodrigues GB, Waldron JN, Wong CS, Laperriere NJ: A retrospective analysis of 52 cases of spinal cord glioma managed with radiation therapy. Int J Radiat Oncol Biol Phys 48:837–842, 2000.

Schild SE, Nisi K, Scheithauer BW, et al.: The results of radiotherapy for ependymomas. The Mayo Clinic experience. Int J Radiat Oncol Biol Phys 42:953–958, 1998.

Metastatic Brain Tumors

Morris D. Groves

Definition

Metastasis occurs when systemic neoplasms spread to the brain parenchyma, intracerebral blood vessels, dura, dural sinuses, or cranial nerves.

Epidemiology and Risk Factors

1. Most common cause of brain tumors in adults, 24% cancer patients with intracranial metastases at autopsy.
2. In the United States, 100,000 to 150,000 new cases per year
3. Incidence increases with age; male:female ratio 1.36:1
4. In adults, most common tumors causing brain metastases: lung (50% all cases), breast (20%), unknown primary (10%), melanoma (10%), colon (5%); less common, choriocarcinoma and renal cell cancer
5. In children, the most common sources of brain metastases are sarcomas, neuroblastomas, and germ cell tumors.
6. Tumors that almost never metastasize to the brain include those of the esophagus, oropharynx, prostate, and nonmelanoma skin cancer.

Etiology and Pathophysiology

1. Most common mechanism of spread to brain is hematogenous.
2. Usually located at gray–white junction and arterial border zones (80% lesions) where vessels narrow and trap floating tumor cells. Cells can also come to rest in preexisting lesions (e.g., infarcts, arteriovenous malformations).
3. Distribution of brain metastases within the brain: cerebral hemispheres, 80%; cerebellum, 15%; brainstem, 5%
4. Pelvic tumors (prostate, uterus) often metastasize to posterior fossa.
5. The ratio of single:multiple metastases is 50:50. Single are more common in breast, colon, renal, prostate, and uterine cancers; multiple metastases more frequent in melanoma, lung, and unknown primary tumors.
6. Little is known about the genetic reasons for metastasis to the brain. Recent studies show

central nervous system (CNS) metastases to have DNA gains at chromosomes 1q23, 8q24, 17q24-25, and 20q13 (>80% cases) and DNA losses at chromosomes 4q22, 4q26, 5q21, and 9p21 (>70% cases).

Most Common Tumors to Metastasize to Brain

- Lung cancer
- Melanoma
- Unknown primary site
- Breast cancer
- Renal
- Colorectal
- Sarcoma
- Thyroid

Most Common Metastatic Tumors to Cause Bleeding into Brain

- Lung cancer
- Renal
- Melanoma
- Choriocarcinoma
- Thyroid cancer

Clinical Features

1. During the course of the illness two thirds of patients have neurologic symptoms
2. Neurologic dysfunction is caused by tumor mass, edema, or hydrocephalus.
3. Clinical presentation of brain metastases includes headaches, focal deficits or cognitive dysfunction, and seizures.
4. Headaches occur in 40% to 50% of patients.
   a. Occur more commonly with multiple or posterior fossa metastases.
   b. Usually dull, nonthrobbing; often associated with nausea, transient visual obscuration; can resemble tension headaches.

c. Usually ipsilateral to tumor

d. Papilledema present in <10% patients at presentation

5. Focal neurologic dysfunction presenting symptom in 20% to 40% of patients

6. Cognitive dysfunction and memory, mood, and personality changes are presenting symptoms in one third of patients.

7. Present with acute-onset seizures: 10% to 20%

8. Present with acute strokelike syndrome: 5% to 10%

 Key Signs

- Neurologic symptoms and dysfunction

- Headaches, focal deficits or cognitive dysfunction, seizures

Differential Diagnosis

1. If diagnosis is in doubt, biopsy must be performed.

2. Differential diagnosis includes primary brain tumors, abscesses, demyelination, strokes, intracranial bleeds, progressive multifocal leukoencephalopathy, radionecrosis.

3. Eleven percent of patients thought to have single brain metastasis will have an alternative diagnosis (primary brain tumor, infection).

4. In those with no known primary tumor who present with brain metastasis, a lung primary or lung metastases is found in 60%; melanoma and colon cancer also contribute. In 25% to 30%, the primary remains unknown.

Radiologic Features

1. Best diagnostic test is contrast-enhanced magnetic resonance imaging (MRI) scan.

2. MRI imaging features of metastases: 50% single, well-circumscribed lesions, gray–white junction location, prominent vasogenic edema

Imaging Features

- Contrast-enhanced lesion on CT or MRI

- Edema prominent relative to lesion size

- Often multiple

- Often round

- Near gray–white junction

Treatment

1. Corticosteroids

   a. Dexamethasone reduces capillary permeability and edema. Load with 10 to 50 mg, then 4 mg every 6 hours; higher steroid doses of 100 mg/day may help refractory disease.

   b. Tapering steroids as soon as feasible reduces long-term toxicity.

   c. Trimethoprim-sulfamethoxazole prophylaxis may help prevent *Pneumocystis carinii* pneumonia.

2. Anticonvulsants

   a. During the course of the illness, 20% of patients present with seizures and 40% have seizures.

   b. Corticosteroids can reduce anticonvulsant levels.

   c. Without seizure history, it is unclear if patients should receive anticonvulsants. At least one study showed no benefit to prophylactic anticonvulsant treatment.

3. Surgery

   a. The best treatment for a particular patient depends on size, location, and number of brain metastases; the patient's age; overall performance status and neurologic condition; extent of cancer; and potential for the cancer to respond to additional treatments.

   b. Surgery can provide immediate relief of symptoms.

   c. Multiple technological advances including computer-assisted surgery, intraoperative mapping and ultrasonography, and functional and operative MRI have improved surgical outcomes. Extracranial tumor burden is the most important factor when considering surgery.

   d. Single brain metastases

      (1) In patients with single brain metastases, surgery plus whole brain radiotherapy (WBRT) vs biopsy and then WBRT results in fewer local recurrences (20% vs 52%, respectively), improves survival (40 weeks vs 15 weeks, respectively), and quality of life. Median time to recurrence after surgery plus WBRT is more than 59 weeks compared with 21 weeks if patients receive WBRT alone.

      (2) Factors associated with increased survival are surgery, absence of or controlled extracranial disease, increased time to the development of brain metastases, and younger age.

   e. Multiple brain metastases

(1) Undiagnosed lesions or large masses causing significant symptoms are removed. If all visible lesions are removed, survival is about the same as for patients with single brain metastases.

(2) Some series suggest that patients with multiple brain metastases have worse survival than patients with single brain metastases.

(3) Median survival is 17 months compared with 3.1 months for those with controlled versus active systemic disease.

f. Recurrent brain metastases

(1) Median survival is 10 to 11.5 months after a second operation.

(2) Second operations improve symptoms in 75% of patients.

(3) Patient survival is negatively affected by presence of systemic disease, Karnofsky performance status score lower than 80, time to recurrence less than 4 months, age older than 39 years.

(4) The faster the recurrence after an initial resection, the less likely repeat operation will provide significant survival.

4. Radiotherapy

a. Primary radiotherapy

(1) Radiation palliates symptoms and decreases risk of neurologic death. Overall survival is determined by activity/extent of extracranial disease, not control of the brain metastases.

(2) The most common schedule is 30 Gy in 10 fractions over 2 weeks.

(3) Radiosensitizers do not benefit patients with brain metastases.

(4) Response rate to radiation is between 50% and 85%.

b. Postoperative radiotherapy

(1) The goal is to destroy microscopic residual cancer cells. WBRT decreases the likelihood of brain failure at the original sight of disease from 70% to 18% and other areas of the brain from 37% to 14%. WBRT postsurgery does not improve overall survival (approximately 48 weeks). When treated with surgery alone or no WBRT, 37% of patients fail in other sites within the brain.

(2) Complications of radiotherapy include leukoencephalopathy, brain atrophy, neurocognitive deterioration, brain necrosis, and neuroendocrine dysfunction. The risk for late complications from WBRT is re-

lated to total dose, fraction size, patient age, extent of disease, and neurologic impairment at presentation.

(3) Repeat radiation can be delivered with a response rate of 42% to 75% and median survival between 3.5 and 5 months.

Caveats

• Radiosensitizers are of no benefit for brain metastases.

• Chemotherapy is generally not used for brain metastases.

---

c. Stereotactic radiation (STR)

(1) STR is delivered by linear particle accelerators, gamma-knife, or charged particles; it aims to decrease toxicity to normal tissue with a significant falloff of radiation dose at the edge of the target volume.

(2) STR may be useful in relatively radioresistant (melanoma, renal cell) or surgically inaccessible tumors.

(3) STR can result in local control in 73% to 94% of patients. Median survival of patients receiving STR ranges from 6 to 15 months.

(4) It is not clear yet whether WBRT plus STR is better than STR alone in controlling a tumor or in overall survival.

(5) Complications of STR include seizures in 2% to 6%, headaches, exacerbation of preexisting neurologic deficits, nausea, and occasional hemorrhage. Radiation necrosis can occur in 16% of patients.

(6) The best patients for STR are young, with good performance status, limited extracranial disease, and one or two small lesions. Poor prognostic factors include poor performance status, progressive systemic disease, large tumor size, and three or more metastases.

5. Chemotherapy

a. Chemotherapy is generally not used for brain metastases.

b. Some tumors can respond to chemotherapy, including breast cancer, choriocarcinoma, ovarian cancer, small-cell lung cancer, and germ cell tumors.

c. Breast cancer patients who have not previously been exposed to chemotherapy and have brain metastases can have up to a 50% response rate; median response duration is 10 months.

Key Treatment

- Resection of fewer than three lesions
- Whole-brain irradiation
- Stereotactic radiation

Prognosis and Complications

1. In patients treated only with steroids, median survival is 1 to 2 months.
2. Conventional WBRT increases median survival to 3 to 6 months.
3. Patients with single brain metastases who undergo surgery and WBRT have a median survival of 10 to 16 months.
4. Favorable prognostic factors include absence of systemic disease, age younger than 60 years, good performance status, increased time to the development of brain metastases, surgical resection, and two or fewer brain metastases.
5. Patients with unknown primary site cancer have a median survival of 10.4 months after diagnosis of brain metastases.
6. Breast cancer patients have a better prognosis and colon cancer patients have a worse prognosis than other cancer patients with brain metastases.
7. Patients with cerebellar metastases have a worse prognosis than patients with supratentorial metastases.

Prevention

In small-cell lung cancer, early treatment of brain metastases with radiotherapy has not been shown to significantly improve patient survival, probably because of the effect of systemic failure on survival.

Bibliography

Patchell RAF, Tibbs PAF, Regine WFF, et al: Postoperative radiotherapy in the treatment of single metastases to the brain: a randomized trial. JAMA 280:1485–1489, 1998.

Patchell RAF, Tibbs PAF, Walsh, JWF, et al: A randomized trial of surgery in the treatment of single metastases to the brain. N Engl J Med 322:494–500, 1990.

Posner JB: Neurologic Complications of Cancer. Philadelphia, F.A. Davis Company, 1995.

Sawaya R, Bindal RK: Metastatic brain tumors. In Kaye AH, Laws ER (eds): Brain Tumors. Edinburgh, Churchill Livingstone, 1995, pp. 923–946.

Zimm SF, Wampler GLF, Stablein DF, et al: Intracerebral metastases in solid-tumor patients: natural history and results of treatment. Cancer 48:384–394, 1981.

10 Meningeal and Spinal Metastases

Morris D. Groves

Definition

1. Meningeal metastases occur when cancer disseminates to the pia or arachnoid mater, subarachnoid space, or cerebrospinal fluid (CSF).
2. Spinal metastases occur when cancer disseminates to the spinal cord, either intra- or extra-axially. Bony spinal metastases also cause spinal symptoms.

Epidemiology and Risk Factors

1. In neoplastic meningitis (NM), most patients have widespread cancer at diagnosis, although 25% to 30% have no identifiable active disease outside the nervous system.
   a. Six percent to 38% of patients have no known history of malignant disease.
   b. One third of patients with NM have evidence of metastatic spread to other areas of the nervous system, such as the brain, spine, or epidural space.
   c. Up to 19% of cancer patients who undergo autopsy and have had a history of neurologic symptoms have evidence of meningeal involvement of their tumor.
   d. The most common tumors to spread to the meninges include breast cancer (5%), small cell lung cancer (11%, up to 25% at 3-year survival), non—small-cell lung cancer (5%), melanoma (up to 23%), lymphoma (6%), and leukemia (10%).
2. Twenty-five percent to 70% of patients with metastatic cancer have spine involvement.
   a. 5% of cancer patients who die each year have spinal cord compression (SCC). SCC is the second most frequent neurologic complication of metastatic cancer.
   b. Rarely, SCC can be the first sign of cancer.
   c. Clinically symptomatic spinal tumor locations occur in the ratio of 4:2:1 thoracic:lumbosacral:cervical, respectively.
   d. Prostate, renal, and gastrointestinal (GI) cancers more commonly affect the thoracolumbar spine.
   e. In adults, the most common cancers to result in

SCC are breast cancer (22%), lung cancer (15%), prostate cancer (10%), lymphoma (10%), sarcoma (9%), renal (7%), GI tract (5%). In children, SCC is most often due to neuroblastoma, Ewing's sarcoma, Wilms' tumor, sarcomas, lymphoma, and leukemia.
   f. Less than 5% of all metastatic spinal cord tumors are intradural or intramedullary.
   g. Tumors causing intramedullary spinal cord metastases include lung, breast, GI malignancies, melanoma, lymphoma, and renal tumors.

Etiology and Pathophysiology

1. The blood–brain barrier may protect tumor cells in the cerebrospinal fluid (CSF) from chemotherapy.
   a. Malignant cells gain access to the meninges and spinal fluid by several paths.
      (1) Direct extension from central nervous system (CNS) parenchymal or epidural metastases
      (2) Direct extension from primary tumors that develop in close proximity to the spinal fluid pathways (ependymoma, pineoblastoma, medulloblastoma)
      (3) Direct extension from parameningeal, non-CNS foci of cancer
      (4) Spread along cranial or spinal nerves
      (5) Hematogenous spread via arachnoid vessels, spinal veins, or choroid plexus
   b. Once tumor cells reach the CSF, disease progresses by
      (1) Direct tumor cell migration along and through the meninges
      (2) Tumor cell dis-attachment, flotation in the CSF, and reimplantation in other areas of the CNS (gravity results in accumulation of tumor cells in dependent areas such as the basal cisterns, posterior fossa, and cauda equina).
   c. Tumor cells in the meninges and CSF can form subarachnoid nodules or sheets of tumor. Occasionally, tumor cannot be seen with neuroimaging tests.

Caveat

• Occasionally, tumor cannot be seen on neuro-imaging.

2. Spinal metastases

a. Epidural SCC causes neurologic signs through direct compression, ischemia, and edema.

b. Epidural metastases are usually located anterior or anterolateral to the spinal cord. Those located anterior or posterior to the cord can occlude blood vessels to the center of the cord, resulting in spinal cord infarction.

c. Edema is due to direct pressure on the cord or venous congestion by compression of the epidural venous plexus.

d. Intramedullary metastases arise from growth of subarachnoid tumor or by hematogenous spread to spinal cord parenchyma.

e. Intramedullary tumors are often located in the ventral posterior horn and medial lateral column (these areas correspond to the terminal blood supply of the central artery).

f. Of patients with intramedullary spinal cord metastases, 50% and 25% will be found to have parenchymal brain and leptomeningeal metastases, respectively.

Clinical Features

1. Symptoms and signs of NM are referable to specific structures involved by tumor and are categorized by cerebral, cranial nerve, and spinal symptoms (Table 10–1).

2. Spinal metastases

a. Pain is the earliest, most common symptom of SCC and is caused by distortion of periosteum, soft tissues, and dural nerves, and by compression of nerve roots.

(1) Treatment is most effective when pain is the only symptom.

(2) Local pain is exacerbated by the Valsalva maneuver or body movement, is usually worse when supine (due to venous-plexus distention), and is often nocturnal, associated with tenderness over the vertebral body, occasionally exacerbated with neck flexion and straight leg raising.

(3) Radicular pain is present in 80% of patients with cervical lesions, 55% with thoracic cord compression, and 90% with lumbar spine metastases.

(4) Referred pain: Cervical cord compression can cause leg pain simulating sciatica, or bandlike pain or paresthesias around the chest or abdomen. Lumbar root compression can mimic symptoms of vascular insufficiency.

b. Weakness is the second most common finding in SCC, often associated with spasticity, hyperreflexia, and extensor plantar responses.

(1) Leg weakness, an early sign of SCC, is

TABLE 10–1. SYMPTOMS AND SIGNS OF NEOPLASTIC MENINGITIS AT PRESENTATION

Neuraxis Level	Symptoms	Patients Affected (%)	Signs	Patients Affected (%)
Cerebral	Headache	51–66	Altered mental status	27–62
	Mental changes	26–33	Seizures/syncope	11–18
	Gait difficulty	27	Papilledema	11
	Nausea/vomiting	22–34	Diabetes insipidus	4
	Incoordination	20	Hemiparesis	2
	Loss of consciousness	4	Cerebellar signs	15
	Dizziness	4		
Cranial nerve	Diplopia	20–36	III, IV, VI	5–36
	Visual loss	9–10	II	6–19
	Facial numbness	10	V	6–10
	Tinnitus/hearing loss	10–14	VII	10–30
	Hypogeusia	4	VIII	7–18
	Dysphonia/dysphagia	2–7	IX/X	2–6
	Vertigo	2	XII	5–10
Spinal	Lower motor neuron weakness	34–46	Nuchal rigidity	9–13
	Paresthesias	33–42	Weakness	73
	Radicular pain	26–37	Sensory loss	32
	Back/neck pain	31–37	Straight leg raise test positive	15
	Bowel/bladder dysfunction	16–18	Anal sphincter dysfunction	5–14

usually more notable in the proximal than the distal muscles and can be asymmetric. Patients report difficulty standing from a chair or climbing stairs, and knee buckling.

    (2) Sudden-onset SCC causes flaccid leg weakness and areflexia.

    (3) Lower motor neuron weakness occurs in cauda equina involvement from metastases; characterized by hypotonia, atrophy, fasciculations, and hyporeflexia. Can see foot drop, difficulty descending stairs.

  c. Sensory loss usually accompanies weakness and pain.

    (1) Symptoms usually begin in the toes and ascend in a stocking-like fashion.

    (2) Loss of light touch or pinprick one to five levels below the actual site of SCC.

    (3) Sacral sparing occurs in 20% of patients with SCC.

    (4) Cauda equina compression causes sacral root dermatomal sensory loss.

  d. Autonomic symptoms are common. Bowel and bladder dysfunction occurs in 50% of patients at the time of SCC or cauda equina compression. Common complaints are impotence, constipation, urinary urgency, urinary retention, incontinence. Sweat level at the level of cord compression or a Horner syndrome can also occur. Anal sphincter laxity or loss of anal reflex points toward the cauda equina or conus medullaris.

  e. Ataxia can persist after restoration of strength and sensation.

  f. Unusual signs and symptoms of SCC include hydrocephalus, nystagmus, facial weakness, double vision, lower limb fasciculations, pseudoclaudication, tongue numbness, and the syndrome of painful legs and moving toes.

Key Signs and Symptoms: Spinal Cord Compression

- Pain
- Weakness
- Autonomic dysfunction
- Sensory changes
- Ataxia

Findings in Neoplastic Meningitis

- Multiple levels of neuroaxis involvement
- Malignant cells in CSF
- Elevated protein level
- Low CSF glucose level
- CSF lymphocytic pleocytosis
- Nodular or "sugar-coating" enhancement on magnetic resonance imaging (MRI)

Differential Diagnosis

1. Multifocal neurologic symptoms suggest neoplastic meningitis. Alternative diagnoses to consider include

  a. Multiple brain or epidural metastases

  b. CNS infections; especially mycobacteria, epidural abscess, treponematosis, candidiasis, and aspergillosis

  c. Inflammatory or neoplastic disorders such as neurosarcoidosis, rheumatoid arthritis, Wegener's granulomatosis, idiopathic hypertrophic pachymeningitis, intracranial hypotension, meningeal melanoma, and en plaque meningioma

2. Differential diagnostic concerns in patients with spinal metastases include primary cord tumor, epidural abscess or hematoma, cord infarct, radionecrosis, chemotherapy injury, and paraneoplastic disorder, syrinx, schwannoma, neurofibroma, meningioma, arteriovenous malformation, postinfectious myelopathy.

Laboratory Testing

1. Neoplastic meningitis

  a. Tumor cells in the CSF are the *sine-qua-non* of this diagnosis.

  b. Sensitivity of the single spinal fluid analysis can be as low as 45%.

  c. Repeating CSF analysis increases sensitivity above 75%.

  d. Abnormal imaging increases likelihood of positive cytology to more than 60%.

  e. If imaging is negative, the odds of obtaining a positive CSF cytology 25%.

  f. CSF opening pressure above 150 mm H_2O, cell count more than 5, protein above 50 mg/dL, and CSF glucose lower than 60 mg/dL, all support diagnosis of NM.

2. MRI is the best test to evaluate patients with myelopathy and suspected spinal cord lesions. Bony metastatic lesions are often noncontiguous and multiple so the entire spine requires imaging to search for silent areas that may need treatment or close observation.

Radiologic Features

In NM, imaging of the entire neuraxis is necessary. Imaging abnormalities suggestive of NM include leptomeningeal, subependymal, dural, cranial nerve, and superficial cerebral enhancement, and communicating hydrocephalus. In patients with known NM, solid tumors are more likely to cause imaging abnormalities than hematologic malignancies—90% vs 55%, respectively. Depending on location, spinal metastases can have varying imaging characteristics. Bony spine metastases can cause lucency on plain spinal radiographs. T_1 weighted MRI shows hypointense vertebral body lesions. Epidural tumors can be isointense with soft tissues and can enhance. Intramedullary spinal metastases usually enhance with contrast and occasionally cause syrinx formation.

Treatment

1. The treatment of NM is controversial. Because of the associated poor prognosis, some physicians do not treat this condition, although there are patients who benefit from treatment.
    a. Focal radiation is delivered to nodular symptomatic disease and areas of CSF flow obstruction (identified by indium CSF flow testing). Radiotherapy often re-opens CSF flow, which improves patient survival and allows for better distribution of intrathecally administered chemotherapy.
    b. Tumor cells floating in the CSF can be treated with intrathecal chemotherapy. Standard intrathecal chemotherapies include methotrexate, cytarabine, liposomal cytarabine, and thiotepa. Systemic therapies used in NM include high-dose methotrexate and hormonal therapy.
2. Spinal metastases
    a. Steroids relieve pain and improve function for patients with spinal cord compressive symptoms. For some tumors, steroids can be antineoplastic.
    b. Radiotherapy is used for SCC caused by radio-sensitive tumors (breast cancer, lymphoma), and should be administered as soon as the diagnosis is established because patients may deteriorate rapidly.

    c. Vertebral body resection is performed in some patients. Indications include unknown diagnosis, spinal instability, post- or intra-radiation progression of SCC, rapid decline in neurologic status, radio-resistant tumors.
    d. Chemotherapy may play a role in pediatric SCC patients with chemosensitive tumors, or as adjunctive or recurrent therapy in adults.

Prognosis and Complications

1. Multiple complications can occur while treating NM. Intraventricular reservoir placement can result in infections and necessitate removal. Intrathecal chemotherapy can result in brain injury, brain necrosis, nausea, vomiting, mental status changes, and, occasionally, myelosuppression. Radiation therapy to the brain after intrathecal methotrexate can be associated with severe brain necrosis.
2. Treatment of NM stabilizes or improves neurologic symptoms in 45% of patients.
3. Without therapy, patients have a poor prognosis and survival in the 3- to 6-week range, with death usually from progressive neurologic dysfunction (Table 10–2).
4. Table 10–3 lists factors that predict improved survival and response to therapy.
5. More than 95% of patients with SCC who are ambulatory at the onset of radiotherapy will maintain ambulation. The degree of pretreatment neurologic dysfunction is the strongest predictor of treatment outcome.
6. Patients who are paraplegic for up to 10 days occasionally regain ambulation.
7. The slower the rate of development of paralysis the better the eventual recovery; 40% to 50% of patients, who are weak but unable to walk prior to either radiation or surgery will be able to walk after the radiation or surgical intervention.
8. Systemic infections are common after radiation or surgery for SCC.

TABLE 10–2. MEDIAN SURVIVAL TIME (WEEKS) OF PATIENTS WITH NEOPLASTIC MENINGITIS BY HISTOLOGY

HISTOLOGY	SURVIVAL MEAN OF STUDIES IN WEEKS (RANGE)	NO. OF STUDIES
Breast	16.5 (5–38)	13
Lung	15 (8–22)	3
Small-cell lung cancer	8.6 (4–15.5)	4
Non—small-cell lung cancer	13 (9–20)	3
Lymphoma	16 (8.8–32)	9

TABLE 10–3. FACTORS PREDICTIVE OF SURVIVAL OR RESPONSE IN NEOPLASTIC MENINGITIS

Parameter	Impact on Survival or Response*
Clear CSF of cells with IT chemotherapy	+, +, +
No CSF block or CSF block cleared	+, +
Controlled systemic disease	+
History of intraparenchymal tumor	+
KPS ≥ 70	+
Longer duration of neurologic symptoms	+
Concomitant systemic plus IT chemotherapy	+
Treatment with IT chemotherapy	+
Female sex	+
Negative neuroimaging	+
Longer pretreatment duration of CSF disease	+
Spinal involvement	+
Long delay from diagnosis to neurologic symptoms	+
Low CSF protein	+
Elevated CSF protein	+, −, 0, −
Low CSF glucose	−, 0
Cerebral involvement	−, −
ECOG > 3	−
Cranial nerve deficit	−
Progressive systemic disease at study entry	−

Abbreviations: +: Positive impact on survival or response; −: Negative impact on survival or response; 0: No impact on survival or response; CSF, cerebrospinal fluid; IT, interthecal; KPS, Karnofsky performance status; ECOG, Eastern Cooperative Oncology Group.
*Each +, −, or 0 represents one paper which discusses a factor and suggests a positive, negative, or neutral impact.

9. Median survival for patients with intramedullary spinal cord metastases treated with radiotherapy is 4 months.

Bibliography

Posner JB: Neurologic Complications of Cancer. Philadelphia, F.A. Davis, 1995.

Schiff D, O'Neill BP: Intramedullary spinal cord metastases: clinical features and treatment outcome. Neurology 47: 906–912, 1996.

Ushio, Y, Posner R, Kim JH, et al: Treatment of experimental spinal cord compression caused by extradural neoplasms. J Neurosurg 47:380–390, 1977.

Wasserstrom WR, Glass JP, Posner, JB: Diagnosis and treatment of leptomeningeal metastases from solid tumors: experience with 90 patients. Cancer 49:759–772, 1982.

11 Paraneoplastic Neurologic Syndromes

Josep Dalmau

Definition and Epidemiology

1. Paraneoplastic neurologic syndromes (PNS) are disorders of the nervous system unrelated to metastases or any of the following complications of cancer: coagulopathy and cerebrovascular disorders, infections, metabolic and nutritional deficits, or the effects of cancer treatment.

2. Between 10% and 50% of cancer patients develop mild PNS or abnormalities in electromyographic (EMG) and nerve conduction studies that are unrelated to cancer therapy, weight loss, or metabolic abnormalities.

3. In contrast, the incidence of PNS with severe symptoms that affect quality of life is probably less than 3% for all types of cancers, and 30% for patients with thymoma.

4. The importance of identifying PNS

   a. PNS may involve any part of the central or peripheral nervous system and can mimic many cancer-related or unrelated neurologic complications (Table 11–1).

   b. In about 60% of the patients, the PNS develops before the presence of a tumor is known. Therefore, recognition of a disorder as paraneoplastic avoids unnecessary diagnostic tests and often leads to an earlier tumor diagnosis.

   c. Prompt diagnosis and treatment of the tumor is the best approach to improve or stabilize the PNS.

Concepts: Importance of Paraneoplastic Neurologic Syndromes

- Affect any part of the nervous system
- Often precede diagnosis of the tumor
- Treatment of the tumor is a priority in the management of PNS
- Most PNS appear to be immune mediated.

Etiology and Pathophysiology

1. Most PNS appear to be immune mediated, and are characterized by the presence of distinct antibodies in the serum or cerebrospinal fluid (CSF) (Table 11–2).

   a. These antibodies react with proteins expressed by neurons, peripheral nerve or neuromuscular junction, and also by the associated cancer.

   b. For most PNS, the role of the antibodies in the pathogenesis of the disorder is unknown, but their detection serves as a useful diagnostic marker of paraneoplasia.

   c. In the Lambert-Eaton myasthenic syndrome (LEMS), myasthenia gravis, and neuromyotonia, the corresponding antibodies are pathogenic.

   d. The absence of paraneoplastic antibodies does not rule out that a disorder is paraneoplastic.

      (1) There are several PNS for which there is no evidence of immune-mediated mechanisms.

      (2) For some of these PNS, other mechanisms have been identified, including cytokine-related symptoms (i.e., tumor necrosis factor-α, interleukin-1, and interleukin-6, in cachectic myopathy), ectopic secretion of hormones by the tumor (i.e., parathyroid hormone, adrenocorticotropic hormone, antidiuretic hormone resulting in encephalopathy), and competition for a substrate between cancer and the nervous system (i.e., hypoglycemia resulting in encephalopathy).

Clinical Features

1. Approach to the diagnosis

   a. Most PNS develop acutely or subacutely, sometimes resembling a viral process. Symptoms evolve over weeks or months and then stabilize, differentiating them from the more chronic degenerative diseases of middle age and adulthood.

   b. Diagnostic awareness depends on the type of syndrome. Some syndromes have a paraneoplastic origin more frequently than others. For example, LEMS is paraneoplastic in about 60% of cases, whereas subacute sensory neuronopathy is paraneoplastic in less than 20% of patients.

   c. In addition, the age of the patient should be

309

TABLE 11–1. PARANEOPLASTIC SYNDROMES OF THE NERVOUS SYSTEM

Central Nervous System
Limbic encephalitis
Cerebellar degeneration
Encephalomyelitis
Sensory neuronopathy
Opsoclonus-myoclonus
Stiff-man syndrome
Motor neuron syndrome and motor neuronopathy (*)
Necrotizing myelopathy (*)

Peripheral Nervous System
Chronic sensorimotor neuropathy
Acute sensorimotor neuropathy (Guillain-Barré, plexitis) (*)
Vasculitis of the nerve and muscle
Neuropathy associated with malignant monoclonal gammopathies
Neuromyotonia
Autonomic neuropathy
Lambert-Eaton myasthenic syndrome
Myasthenia gravis (*)
Polymyositis/Dermatomyositis
Acute necrotizing myopathy
Cachectic myopathy (*)
Carcinoid myopathy (*)
Myotonia (*)

(*) Not discussed in the current chapter

considered. The development of subacute cerebellar degeneration in a middle-aged or elderly patient should suggest paraneoplasia, while in children similar symptoms are usually related to viral or metabolic disorders.

2. Paraneoplastic syndromes of the central nervous system (CNS)
   a. Paraneoplastic limbic encephalitis (PLE)
      (1) Characterized by depression, irritability, seizures, and short-term memory loss

(2) Neurologic symptoms usually develop in days or weeks, and stabilize, leaving the patient with severe memory loss or dementia.
(3) The tumor most frequently involved is lung cancer, usually small-cell lung cancer (SCLC).
(4) Pathology findings include perivascular and interstitial inflammatory infiltrates, neuronal loss, and microglial proliferation that predominate in the limbic system (hippocampus, amygdala, hypothalamus, and insular and cingulate cortex). Most patients have variable involvement of other areas of the nervous system, mainly the brainstem.

Key Signs
- Depression
- Irritability
- Seizures
- Short-term memory loss

b. Paraneoplastic cerebellar degeneration (PCD)
   (1) The presenting symptoms of this disorder are dizziness, nausea, blurry or double vision, oscillopsia, and gait difficulties.
   (2) In association with these symptoms, or after a few days, the patient develops truncal and limb ataxia, dysarthria, and dysphagia.

TABLE 11–2. ANTIBODIES ASSOCIATED WITH PARANEOPLASTIC NEUROLOGIC SYNDROMES

Antibody	Associated Cancer	Syndrome	Immunohistochemical and Western Blot Reactivity
Anti-Hu	SCLC, other	Encephalomyelitis, sensory neuronopathy	All neuronal nuclei; 35–40 kDa
Anti-Yo	Gynecological, breast	Cerebellar degeneration	Cytoplasm Purkinje cells; 34, 62 kDa
Anti-Ri	Breast, gynecological, SCLC	Cerebellar ataxia, opsoclonus	Neuronal nuclei of the CNS; 55, 80 kDa
Anti-Tr	Hodgkin's lymphoma	Cerebellar degeneration	Cytoplasm neurons, Purkinje spiny dendrites
Anti-CV2 (or anti-CRMP1, 3, 5)	SCLC, other	Encephalomyelitis Cerebellar degeneration	Neuronal and glial; 66 kDa
Anti-Ma proteins[a]	Testicular germ-cell tumors and other neoplasms	Limbic, brainstem encephalitis, cerebellar degeneration	Neuronal nuclei and cytoplasm; 39, 41 kDa
Anti-amphiphysin	Breast	Stiff-man syndrome	Synaptic vesicle protein; 128 kDa
Anti-VGKC[b]	Thymoma, others	Neuromyotonia	Several VGKC
Anti-VGCC[b]	SCLC	LEMS	Presynaptic P/Q type VGCC
Anti-acetylcholine receptor[b]	Thymoma	Myasthenia gravis	Postsynaptic acetylcholine receptor

Abbreviations: VGKC: voltage-gated potassium channels; VGCC: voltage-gated calcium channels; SCLC: small cell lung cancer; LEMS: Lambert-Eaton myasthenic syndrome.
[a]Antibodies limited to Ma2 (also called anti-Ta antibodies) usually associated with limbic and brainstem encephalitis and germ-cell tumors. Antibodies directed to Ma1, Ma2, and Ma3 usually associated with brainstem encephalitis, cerebellar degeneration, and several types of cancer (lung, breast, ovary, etc).
[b] These antibodies are also identified in the non-paraneoplastic form of the syndrome.

(3) The examination may show down-beating nystagmus.

(4) There is a strong association between certain antineuronal antibodies and the type of associated tumor.

(5) As with any other PNS, PCD may occur without antineuronal antibodies, in which case the tumors more frequently involved are non-Hodgkin's lymphoma and lung cancer.

(6) Pathology studies show diffuse loss of Purkinje cells, degeneration of the deep cerebellar nuclei, and sometimes of the olivary nuclei and spinocerebellar tracts of the spinal cord. Inflammatory infiltrates may be absent, mild, or prominent.

 Key Signs

- Dizziness
- Nausea
- Blurry or double vision
- Oscillopsia
- Gait difficulties
- Truncal and limb ataxia, dysarthria, and dysphagia

c. Paraneoplastic encephalomyelitis (PEM)

(1) Describes patients with cancer who develop multifocal neurologic deficits and signs of inflammation involving multiple areas of the nervous system, resulting in a mixture of symptoms derived from limbic encephalitis, cerebellar degeneration, brainstem encephalitis, myelitis, and autonomic dysfunction.

(2) Because the tumor most frequently involved is a SCLC, the detection of anti-Hu antibodies is frequent. Patients with anti-Hu associated PEM usually develop sensory neuronopathy secondary to dorsal root ganglionitis. Other associated antineuronal antibodies (sometimes in combination with anti-Hu) are shown in Table 11–2.

 Key Signs

- Multifocal neurologic deficits
- Signs of inflammation involving multiple areas of the nervous system

d. Paraneoplastic sensory neuronopathy (PSN)

(1) Characterized by progressive sensory loss involving lower and upper limbs, trunk, and face.

(2) At presentation, vibration and joint position sensations may be more affected than nociceptive sensation. The sensory loss causes ataxia and pseudoathetoid movements. Sensorineural hearing loss can occur.

(3) Nerve conduction studies demonstrate small-amplitude or absent sensory nerve action potentials. Motor nerve and F-wave studies are usually normal, with no signs of denervation unless there is involvement of the spinal motor neurons in the setting of PEM.

(4) In more than 80% of the patients, PSN precedes the diagnosis of the tumor, usually a small cell lung cancer.

(5) The detection of anti-Hu antibodies is highly specific for PSN.

(6) Pathology studies show an inflammatory degeneration of the neurons of the dorsal root ganglia, atrophy of the posterior nerve roots, axonal degeneration, and secondary degeneration of the posterior columns of the spinal cord.

 Key Signs

- Progressive sensory loss involving lower and upper limbs, trunk, and face

e. Paraneoplastic opsoclonus-myoclonus (POM)

(1) Usually affects infants younger than 4 years of age and is associated with hypotonia, ataxia, and irritability.

(2) Nearly 50% of children with POM have neuroblastoma.

(3) POM frequently responds to treatment of the tumor, steroids, and intravenous immunoglobulin (IVIg), but neurologic relapses are frequent, often as a result of intercurrent infection. About 65% of patients are left with deficits, including psychomotor retardation and behavioral abnormalities.

(4) In adults, POM develops in association with truncal ataxia. The tumor most frequently involved is a SCLC. Patients with breast cancer may harbor anti-Ri antibodies. The clinical course of POM is worse than that of idiopathic opsoclonus.

Key Signs

- Usually affects children younger than 4 years of age
- Hypotonia, ataxia, and irritability

---

   f. Paraneoplastic stiff-man syndrome

     (1) Characterized by fluctuating rigidity of the axial musculature with superimposed spasms that are precipitated by emotional upset and auditory or somesthetic stimuli.

     (2) Symptoms resolve during sleep or following local or general anesthesia.

     (3) Rigidity primarily affects the lower trunk and legs, but it can extend to the shoulders, the upper limbs, neck, and face. Symptoms may be limited to one limb (stiff-limb syndrome).

     (4) Electrophysiologic studies show continuous activity of motor units in the stiffened muscles that improves after treatment with diazepam.

     (5) The disorder is caused by autoimmunity directed to three target molecules (glutamic acid decarboxylase, amphiphysin, gephyrin) present in GABA/glycine inhibitory synapses of spinal cord interneurons.

     (6) The idiopathic form of the disorder is associated with glutamic acid decarboxylase antibodies and is often accompanied by diabetes and other endocrine abnormalities.

     (7) Paraneoplastic stiff-man syndrome usually associates with immunity to amphiphysin.

Key Signs

- Rigidity of the lower trunk and legs
- Rigidity can extend to the shoulders, the upper limbs, neck, and face in some cases
- Symptoms may be limited to one limb (stiff-limb syndrome)

---

3. Paraneoplastic syndromes of the peripheral nervous system

   a. Paraneoplastic sensorimotor neuropathy

     (1) Many patients with advanced malignancy develop a mild peripheral neuropathy that has little impact on quality of life.

     (2) The cause of these neuropathies is multifactorial, including metabolic and nutritional deficits and perhaps, cytokines produced by the tumor or the immunologic system.

     (3) There is a group of sensorimotor neuropathies that usually develop before or by the time the malignancy is discovered, and that are very debilitating. Symptoms may present in a subacute or acute fashion and are usually progressive, although some patients have relapsing and remitting symptoms.

     (4) Pathology studies usually show axonal degeneration with frequent inflammatory infiltrates, and sometimes demyelinating findings. Patients with signs of demyelinating neuropathy may improve with steroids or IVIg.

   b. Paraneoplastic vasculitis of nerve and muscle

     (1) A nonsystemic vasculitic neuropathy that involves nerve, muscle, or both.

     (2) The tumors more frequently involved are SCLC and lymphoma.

     (3) Patients develop a painful symmetric or asymmetric subacute sensorimotor polyneuropathy, and less frequently a multiple mononeuropathy.

     (4) Electrophysiologic studies show axonal degeneration equally involving motor and sensory nerves.

     (5) Typically, the erythrocyte sedimentation rate is elevated and the CSF shows a high protein content.

     (6) Nerve and muscle biopsies show intramural and perivascular inflammatory infiltrates composed of CD8+ T cells.

   c. Peripheral neuropathy associated with malignant monoclonal gammopathies

     (1) Multiple myeloma: May develop a mild sensorimotor axonal neuropathy, a pure sensory neuropathy, or a subacute monophasic or relapsing and remitting neuropathy with evidence of demyelination on electrophysiologic and morphologic studies. There is no specific treatment for these neuropathies.

     (2) Osteosclerotic myeloma

       (a) An unusual form of myeloma characterized by single or multiple plasmacytomas involving ribs, vertebrae, pelvic bones, or proximal long bones.

       (b) More than 50% of patients develop a peripheral neuropathy that resembles a chronic demyelinating polyradiculoneuropathy with motor predominance and high CSF protein content.

       (c) All or some features of the POEMS syndrome (*p*olyneuropathy, *o*rganomegaly, *e*ndocrinopathy, *M* component, and *s*kin changes) can be present.

(d) The neuropathy often improves with treatment of the plasmacytoma.

(3) Waldenström's macroglobulinemia

(a) Peripheral neuropathy occurs in 5% to 10% of these patients.

(b) The neuropathy may result from antibody activity of the IgM M-protein against myelin-associated glycoprotein or against various gangliosides. It is characterized by a progressive distal symmetric sensorimotor polyneuropathy with predominant involvement of large sensory fibers (in particular, vibration sense).

(c) Treatment should be directed at the Waldenström's macroglobulinemia.

d. Paraneoplastic neuromyotonia (Isaacs' syndrome)

(1) Characterized by spontaneous and continuous muscle fiber activity of peripheral nerve origin.

(2) Symptoms include muscle cramps, weakness, and sometimes excessive sweating. The involved muscles show undulating myokymia and may be hypertrophic.

(3) EMG shows fibrillation, fasciculation, and doublet, triplet, or multiplet single unit discharges that have a high intraburst frequency. This abnormal activity continues during sleep and general anesthesia, and is abolished by curare and sometimes, peripheral nerve block.

(4) The tumor most frequently involved is thymoma. Neuromyotonia is associated with antibodies to voltage-gated potassium channels (VGKC).

Key Signs

- Muscle cramps
- Weakness
- Undulating myokymia
- Excessive sweating

e. Paraneoplastic autonomic dysfunction

(1) Usually develops in association with other PNS, such as PEM or LEMS.

(2) Symptoms often precede the detection of the tumor, usually a SCLC. The autonomic dysfunction may result from adrenergic or cholinergic nerve dysfunction at the pre- or post-ganglionic level.

(3) There are three disorders that can be life-threatening: esophageal and gastrointestinal dysmotility with intestinal pseudo-obstruction, cardiac dysrhythmias, and orthostatic hypotension. Other accompanying symptoms may include dry mouth, erectile dysfunction, anhidrosis, and sphincter dysfunction.

f. Lambert-Eaton myasthenic syndrome

(1) A disorder of the neuromuscular junction characterized by impaired acetylcholine release from the presynaptic motor terminal

(2) Symptoms include fatigue, proximal muscle weakness, muscle aches, and vague parasthesias.

(3) Muscle reflexes are diminished or absent, but after a brief muscle contraction, reflexes may potentiate. Similarly, after brief exercise strength may improve.

(4) Dry mouth and other symptoms of autonomic dysfunction are common.

(5) Neurologic symptoms typically precede or coincide with the diagnosis of the tumor, usually a SCLC.

(6) Nerve conduction studies show small-amplitude compound muscle action potentials (CMAP). At slow rates of repetitive nerve stimulation, a decremental response is seen. At fast rates, facilitation occurs and there is an incremental response of at least 100%. Similar findings are obtained after maximal voluntary contraction of the muscle.

(7) LEMS results from an immunologic attack against the presynaptic voltage-gated calcium channels (VGCC), interfering with the release of acetylcholine vesicles.

(8) The detection of antibodies to P/Q-type VGCC is used as a serologic test for LEMS.

Key Signs

- Fatigue
- Proximal muscle weakness
- Muscle reflexes diminished or absent
- Muscle aches
- Dry mouth

g. Polymyositis and dermatomyositis (PM/DM)

(1) Inflammatory disorders of the muscle that are likely autoimmune in nature

(2) The association of PM/DM with cancer is

rare, and the existence of paraneoplastic PM is controversial.

(3) In women the most common tumors are ovarian and breast cancer; in men, lung and gastrointestinal cancer.

(4) Patients with PM/DM typically present with myalgia and proximal muscle weakness of subacute onset, elevated serum levels of creatine kinase, and EMG evidence of myopathy.

(5) In DM the classic skin manifestations include purplish discoloration of the eyelids (heliotrope rash) with edema, and erythematous, scaly lesions over the knuckles.

(6) Clinical, electromyographic, and pathological findings of PM/DM are similar in patients with and without cancer.

(7) Cutaneous involvement may occur without myopathy (amyopathic dermatomyositis).

(8) The course of PM/DM is independent of the malignant disease.

Key Signs

- Myalgia and proximal muscle weakness (PM/DM)

- Heliotrope rash with edema (DM)

- Erythematous, scaly lesions over the knuckles (DM)

h. Acute necrotizing myopathy

(1) Patients develop muscle pain and proximal weakness, associated with high levels of serum creatine kinase.

(2) Symptoms evolve rapidly to generalized weakness, often leading to death in a few weeks.

(3) Muscle biopsy shows prominent necrosis with minimal or absent inflammation.

(4) Several types of tumors are involved, including SCLC, cancer of the gastrointestinal tract, breast, kidney and prostate.

Key Signs

- Muscle pain and proximal weakness

Laboratory Testing

1. Neuroimaging, in particular MRI studies, are usually normal in the early stages of most PNS,

except for paraneoplastic limbic encephalitis, and the encephalitis associated with antibodies to Ma proteins. Cerebellar atrophy is a common finding in the late stages of paraneoplastic cerebellar degeneration.

2. CSF

a. May reveal pleocytosis, increased proteins, oligoclonal bands, and intrathecal synthesis of IgG.

b. Later in the course of the disease the CSF may contain no cells, but the proteins often remain elevated.

c. If paraneoplastic antibodies are identified, the same antibodies are usually found in the serum.

d. Blood tests

(1) The presence of paraneoplastic antibodies confirms the paraneoplastic origin of the neurologic disorder and focuses the search for the tumor to certain organs, depending on the type of antibody detected (Table 11–2).

(2) If paraneoplastic antibodies are negative, other blood tests, such as analysis for cancer markers (CEA, CA-125, CA-15-3, and PSA, among others) may support the suspicion of cancer.

(3) In patients with peripheral neuropathies, immunoelectrophoresis may disclose M-proteins in serum or urine, suggesting a plasma cell dyscrasia.

e. A skeletal survey to rule out lytic or osteosclerotic lesions suggestive of myeloma should be carried out in all patients with peripheral neuropathy and M protein in serum or urine.

f. If a lung cancer is suspected, the study of choice is CT of the chest.

g. Because of the common association of breast and gynecological cancers with PNS, mammogram and pelvic CT scan or ultrasound should be carried out in all women with a suspected PNS. A stool guaiac examination is useful when the above tests are negative.

h. Men with symptoms of limbic and brainstem encephalitis should be examined with testicular ultrasound.

i. When all tests are negative, a body positron emission tomographic (PET) study may uncover the neoplasm.

Concepts for the Diagnosis of PNS

• Rule out metastatic and nonmetastatic complications.

• Examine serum and CSF for paraneoplastic antibodies.

• PNS can occur without paraneoplastic antibodies.

• If no tumor is found with standard tests, consider body PET scan.

---

j. The discovery of a tumor different from the neoplasm usually associated with a specific antibody (i.e., anti-Hu and prostate cancer rather than SCLC) should raise the suspicion of a second neoplasm. This suspicion is fostered if the tumor does not express the corresponding antigen.

Treatment

1. Effect of antineoplastic therapy
   a. Improvement of neurologic symptoms after treatment of the tumor has been reported for almost all PNS.

b. The significance of antineoplastic therapy on the PNS is difficult to assess because of
   (1) The low incidence of PNS
   (2) The lack of effective treatment for some cancers
   (3) The rapid, irreversible neuronal damage characteristic of many PNS

c. Despite these difficulties, recent studies of large series of patients with anti-Hu associated PEM, which is considered one of the most refractory syndromes to treatment, indicate an association between complete tumor response to therapy and stabilization of the neurologic disorder.

d. Two other disorders that indicate an association between tumor treatment and improvement of PNS are POM and encephalitis associated with antibodies to Ma2. In the latter, improvement or regression of the PNS is common after successful treatment of the tumor, usually a germ-cell neoplasm of the testis. The fact that this type of tumor usually responds to therapy may explain the favorable neurologic outcome.

2. Effect of immunosuppressive treatment
   a. Immunosuppressive treatments are effective in PNS directly mediated by antibodies (i.e.,

---

TABLE 11–3. PARANEOPLASTIC NEUROLOGIC SYNDROMES: RESPONSE TO TREATMENT[a]

Syndromes That *Usually Respond* to Treatment

• LEMS	3,4-diaminopyridine, IVIg, plasma exchange, immunosuppressants[b]
• Myasthenia gravis	Plasma exchange, IVIg, immunosuppressants
• Dermatomyositis	Steroids, immunosuppressants, IVIg
• Opsoclonus-myoclonus (pediatric)	Steroids, ACTH
• Neuropathy (osteosclerotic myeloma)	Radiation therapy, chemotherapy

Syndromes that *May Respond* to Treatment

• Limbic/brainstem encephalitis with antibodies to Ma proteins	IVIg, steroids
• Limbic encephalitis without anti-Hu	Steroids
• Cerebellar degeneration with anti-Tr	Tumor
• Opsoclonus-myoclonus (adults)	Steroids, protein A column, clonazepam, diazepam, baclofen
• Opsoclonus/ ataxia with anti-Ri	Steroids, cyclophosphamide
• Vasculitis of nerve and muscle	Steroids, cyclophosphamide
• Guillain-Barré (Hodgkin's disease)	Plasma exchange, IVIg
• Stiff-man syndrome	Steroids, diazepam, baclofen, IVIg
• Neuromyotonia	Plasma exchange

Syndromes that Usually *Do Not Respond* to Treatment

• Cerebellar degeneration
  Associated with SCLC (irrespective of anti-Hu status)
  Associated with anti-Yo antibodies (cancer of ovary, breast)
• Encephalomyelitis / sensory neuronopathy / autonomic dysfunction (central or peripheral)

Syndromes that *May Improve Spontaneously*

• Lower motor neuropathy and lymphoma
• PCD associated with Hodgkin's disease
• Acute polyradiculopathy associated with Hodgkin's disease
• Opsoclonus / myoclonus (pediatric and adult)

Abbreviations: IVIg: intravenous immunoglobulin; ACTH: adrenocorticotropic hormone; LEMS: Lambert-Eaton myasthenic syndrome; PCD: paraneoplastic cellular degeneration.
[a]For all paraneoplastic syndromes the management should initially focus on detecting and treating the tumor.
[b]Immunosuppressants may include: prednisone, azathioprine

LEMS, myasthenia gravis, neuromyotonia), and some syndromes involving areas of the nervous system that have not been irreversibly damaged (i.e., acute and chronic demyelinating sensorimotor neuropathies, vasculitic neuropathy, DM, POM).

b. The current experience suggests that patients with PNS of the CNS with severe deficits established for several weeks or months (i.e., PEM, PCD, sensory neuronopathy) do not benefit from immunosuppressive therapies.

> **Concepts for the Treatment of PNS**
>
> • Prompt detection and treatment of the tumor
>
> • PNS of the CNS rarely improve after symptom stabilization.
>
> • Individualize for each PNS of the peripheral nervous system.

Prognosis

1. Many PNS have a progressive course that in weeks or months results in severe deficits or death.

2. Progression to severe disability is rarely seen in the neuromuscular disorders that develop after the diagnosis of the tumor, such as some sensorimotor neuropathies or cachectic myopathy.

3. Some patients with PCD (particularly without anti-Yo antibodies), and some patients with anti-Hu associated sensory neuronopathy may have a mild, indolent clinical course and stabilize with moderate neurologic deficits.

4. Spontaneous improvement can be observed in some disorders (Table 11–3).

Bibliography

Dalmau J, Gultekin HS, Posner JB: Paraneoplastic neurologic syndromes: Pathogenesis and physiopathology. Brain Pathol 9:275–284, 1999.

Dalmau J, Posner JB: Paraneoplastic syndromes affecting the nervous system. Semin Oncol 24:318–328, 1997.

Dropcho EJ: Remote neurologic manifestations of cancer. Neurol Clin 20:85–122, 2002.

Rosenfeld MR, Dalmau J: The clinical spectrum and pathogenesis of paraneoplastic disorders of the central nervous system. Hematol Oncol Clin North Am 15:1109–1128, 2001.

Rudnicki SA, Dalmau J: Paraneoplastic syndromes of the spinal cord, nerve, and muscle. Muscle Nerve 23:1800–1818, 2000.

12 Neurologic Complications of Chemotherapy and Radiotherapy

Sudhakar Tummala
Morris D. Groves

Definitions

1. The therapeutic/toxic ratio of cancer therapy is often low.

2. Toxicities from chemotherapy and radiation therapy include acute, subacute, chronic, and late effects.

3. Nervous system complications of radiation may occur when primary neural structures are included in the radiation ports, or secondarily when radiation damages blood vessels supplying the nervous system structures.

Epidemiology and Risk Factors

1. Radiation injury

   a. Brain necrosis develops in 1% to 5% of patients who receive whole-brain irradiation.

   b. Fraction size is the major determinant of brain irradiation toxicity. Keep daily dose of radiation ≤2 Gy if long-term survival expected; ≤3 Gy if intent is palliation.

   c. Factors that increase the likelihood of damage: Higher total radiation dose or fraction size, higher total volume of nervous tissue irradiated, increased time after completion of radiation therapy, and presence of radiosensitizing diseases (diabetes, hypertension).

   d. Complications are less common with stereotactic radiation than with standard external beam radiation.

   e. Neurologic complications from radiation (Table 12–1) are classified according to the time interval between radiation and development of clinical findings.

   f. Radiation-induced cognitive dysfunction and leukoencephalopathy without necrosis is a frequent complication in long-term survivors.

2. Chemotherapy: History of hereditary neuropathy or neuropathy of other causes increases risk of chemotherapy-induced neuropathy.

3. Radiotherapy combined with chemotherapy may increase neurotoxicity.

Etiology and Pathophysiology

1. Radiation toxicity

   a. Acute encephalopathy is due to breakdown of the blood–brain barrier, with resulting edema and increased intracranial pressure. Early delayed toxicity is probably caused by transient oligodendroglial damage and resulting radiation-induced demyelination. Late delayed toxicity is due to damage to both astrocytes and oligodendrocytes, together with vascular necrosis and thrombosis.

   b. Late cognitive dysfunction is due to diffuse white matter spongiosis, miliary foci of necrosis, and demyelination.

   c. Radiation-induced vascular damage is caused by DNA damage to the endothelium, pathology that is similar to severe atherosclerosis and that involves large intracranial and extracranial vessels.

2. Chemotherapy toxicity (each drug with specific mechanisms of injury)

   a. Posterior reversible encephalopathy syndrome (PRES) has pathologic changes of interstitial edema with petechial microhemorrhages and arteriolar fibrinoid necrosis. Predominance of the posterior circulation involvement may be due to less sympathetic innervation of the posterior cerebral arteries, resulting in loss of autoregulation as systemic blood pressure increases.

   b. Cerebral venous thrombosis: Increase in endogenous thrombin generation coupled with an acquired antithrombin III deficiency induced by L-asparaginase predisposes to thrombosis. Other inherited procoagulant polymorphisms may increase the risk for thrombosis in patients receiving L-asparaginase.

   c. Methotrexate (MTX) neurotoxicity: Results from deficiency of S-adenosylmethionine and tetrahydrobiopterin, increased levels of homocysteine or other amino acids that are N-methyl-D-aspartate agonists. Risk factors for MTX neurotoxicity include renal insufficiency (MTX eliminated by kidneys), decreased cen-

TABLE 12–1. RADIATION-INDUCED INJURY TO THE CENTRAL NERVOUS SYSTEM

LOCATION	ACUTE: MINUTES TO 1 WEEK	TIME AFTER RADIATION	
		EARLY DELAYED: 4 TO 16 WEEKS	LATE DELAYED: 4 MONTHS TO YEARS
Brain	Acute encephalopathy	Somnolence syndrome Increased focal signs with worsening MRI Rhombencephalopathy Transient cognitive dysfunction	Radiation necrosis Dementia Endocrinopathy Radiation arteriopathy Radiation-induced tumor
Spinal cord		Lhermitte's sign	Transverse myelopathy Hemorrhagic myelopathy Motor neuron syndrome
Cranial nerves		Anosmia Dysgeusia Hearing loss	Visual loss Hearing loss, hair cell damage Lower cranial nerve paralysis
Peripheral nerves	Paresthesias	Brachial or lumbosacral reversible plexopathy	Brachial or lumbosacral late plexopathy (prominent myokymia on EMG suggests radiation plexopathy) Radiation-induced tumor

tral nervous system/cerebrospinal MTX clearance due to meningeal leukemia or hydrocephalus, high local drug concentrations from MTX given through malpositioned or nonfunctioning ventricular reservoirs, and MTX given concurrently with or after radiotherapy.

Clinical Features

1. Radiation toxicity

   a. Acute encephalopathy: Characterized by mild headache, nausea, drowsiness, fever, or worsening of neurologic signs. Can be severe with clinical picture of brain herniation.

   b. Early delayed radiation toxicity simulates tumor recurrence in 15% of patients and presents with recurrent focal symptoms. Neuroimaging shows increased size and contrast enhancement of the lesion. Imaging changes resolve spontaneously; steroids accelerate resolution. Most patients recover in 6 to 8 weeks.

   c. Late delayed radiation toxicity (radiation necrosis) usually develops 1 to 2 years after radiotherapy and can recapitulate the previous symptoms of brain tumor; new focal neurologic signs can appear.

   d. Myelopathy can appear in two forms

      (1) Progressive myelopathy that begins as Brown-Séquard syndrome and evolves into paraparesis or quadriparesis.

      (2) Degeneration of cauda equina roots with anterior horn cell chromatolysis with clinical findings of asymmetry with atrophy, fasciculation, and areflexia.

   e. Late cognitive decline

      (1) Pattern of deficits in attention, memory, visuospatial skills, executive dysfunction in absence of aphasia, apraxia, or agnosia suggestive of white matter damage.

      (2) Can simulate normal pressure hydrocephalus with gait difficulty and urinary incontinence, and can progress to severe dementia.

   f. Radiation-induced tumors may appear years to decades after irradiation of the nervous system, and include meningiomas, sarcomas, and gliomas; malignant peripheral nerve sheath tumors, and schwannomas.

   e. Radiation-induced hypothalamic-pituitary dysfunction can include growth hormone deficiency (most common), hyperparathyroidism, and hypothyroidism.

2. Chemotherapy-induced neurotoxicity

   a. Produces a variety of clinical pictures (Table 12–2).

   b. PRES can be caused by various immunosuppressants and chemotherapies (cyclosporin, tacrolimus, cisplatin, cytarabine, gemcitabine) and is clinically indistinguishable from the same syndrome in patients with eclamptic, hypertensive, or uremic encephalopathy. Symptoms include headache, altered mental status, seizures, and vision changes (cortical blindness, hemianopia, visual neglect, blurred vision, ocular flutter, oculogyric crisis).

   c. Cerebral venous and sagittal sinus thrombosis seen in patients receiving L-asparaginase.

d. Peripheral neuropathy

(1) Acute or subacute Guillain-Barré–like syndrome can be caused by suramin (15% of patients) or ara-C (cytarabine) as a consequence of selective demyelination.

(2) Vincristine and vinblastine can cause distal sensorimotor axonal neuropathy with foot or wrist drop, vocal cord paresis, or ophthalmoplegia.

(3) Cisplatin can cause pure sensory neuropathy/neuronopathy involving predominantly large fibers with well-preserved pain and temperature sensation.

(4) Autonomic neuropathy and symptoms are common and may precede areflexia with vincristine.

Key Signs: Radiation-Induced Toxicity

- Acute encephalopathy: Headache, nausea, drowsiness, fever, worsening of neurologic signs; can be severe, with clinical picture of brain herniation

- Early delayed toxicity simulates tumor recurrence and presents with recurrent focal symptoms.

- Late delayed toxicity (radiation necrosis) in 1 to 2 years can present with the previous symptoms of brain tumor and new focal neurologic signs.

- Two forms of myelopathy: Progressive begins as Brown-Séquard syndrome and evolves into paraparesis or quadriparesis; degeneration of cauda equina roots, with clinical findings of asymmetry with atrophy, fasciculation, and areflexia

- Late cognitive decline

- Radiation-induced tumors

- Radiation-induced hypothalamic-pituitary dysfunction, including growth hormone deficiency (most common), hyperparathyroidism, and hypothyroidism

Key Signs: Chemotherapy-Induced Neurotoxicity

- Acute and chronic encephalopathy

- Aseptic meningitis

- Headaches without meningitis; seizures

- Cerebellar syndrome

- Visual loss

- Myelopathy

- Peripheral neuropathy

Drugs Causing Peripheral Neuropathy

- Cisplatin
- Taxanes
- Vinca alkaloids
- Procarbazine
- Etoposide
- Cytarabine

TABLE 12–2. NEUROTOXICITY OF CHEMOTHERAPY

CLINICAL SIGNS	AGENTS
Acute encephalopathy	Glucocorticoids, methotrexate, cisplatin, vincristine, asparaginase, procarbazine, 5-fluorouracil, cytarabine, nitrosoureas, tacrolimus, cyclosporin A, interleukin-2, ifosfamide, interferons, tamoxifen, etoposide (VP-16)
Chronic encephalopathy	Methotrexate, carmustine (BCNU), cytarabine, carmofur, fludarabine
Aseptic meningitis	Intravenous immunoglobulin, levamisole, monoclonal antibodies, metrizamide, OKT-3, cytarabine (intrathecal), intrathecal methotrexate
Headaches without meningitis	Retinoic acid, tamoxifen
Seizures	Methotrexate, etoposide, cisplatin, vincristine, asparaginase, nitrogen mustard, carmustine, dacarbazine, m-AMSA (amsacrine), busulphan, cyclosporin
Cerebellar syndrome	5-Fluorouracil, cytarabine, vincristine, cyclosporin A, procarbazine
Visual loss	Tamoxifen, cisplatin
Myelopathy	Intrathecal: methotrexate, cytarabine, thiotepa
Peripheral neuropathy	Vinca alkaloids, cisplatin, hexamethylmelamine, procarbazine, 5-azacitidine, etoposide, teniposide, cytarabine, taxanes, suramin, mitotane, misonidazole

---

Drugs Causing Cerebellar Dysfunction

- Cytarabine
- 5-Fluorouracil
- Ifosfamide
- Procarbazine
- Phenytoin
- Vincristine
- Cyclosporin A

Differential Diagnosis

1. Radiation injury must be differentiated from recurrent or metastatic tumor. If leukoencephalopathy is seen on imaging, conditions that affect white matter should be considered (infection, vitamin B_{12} deficiency, demyelinating diseases).

2. Chemotherapy-induced peripheral neuropathy is usually obvious, but one must also consider direct neural invasion by primary tumors (especially hematologic malignancies) or metastasis, pressure palsies from weight loss and immobility, paraneoplastic neuropathies, radiation-induced plexopathy, and metabolic neuropathies (vitamin B_{12} deficiency, diabetes).

Laboratory Testing

1. Radiation toxicity: Neuroimaging and neurocognitive evaluation required to document the injury. Biopsy occasionally required.

2. Chemotherapy toxicity: Nerve conduction velocities and quantitative sensory testing (QST) establish baseline and early neuropathy changes.

Radiologic Features

1. Radiation necrosis
   a. In the brain, standard magnetic resonance imaging (MRI) cannot distinguish radiation necrosis from tumor recurrence. Specialized imaging with positron emission tomography and MR spectroscopy may help distinguish tumor from radionecrosis (positive predictive value 88% and 86%, respectively).
   b. In radiation-induced myelopathy, MRI shows cord with edema, increased signal, and contrast enhancement.

2. Radiation-induced vascular damage
   Arteriogram often demonstrates unusually long

stenosis, atypical location of stenosis (proximal or distal bifurcation of common carotid) or moyamoya-like changes.

3. In PRES, MRI (FLAIR images most sensitive) shows predominant involvement of subcortical white matter in posterior circulation distribution. Can see simultaneous involvement of cortex, anterior brain, brainstem, and cerebellum.

4. White matter hyperintensity alone can be seen on MRI with toxic leukoencephalopathy from radiotherapy or chemotherapy toxicity.

Treatment

1. Radiation toxicity
   a. Acute encephalopathy is treated with steroids.
   b. Late delayed radiation toxicity is treated with steroids (often ineffective), surgical resection, anticoagulation (heparin and warfarin), hyperbaric oxygen, or pentoxifylline.
   c. Late cognitive decline may improve with ventriculoperitoneal shunt (patients could still improve despite a negative large-volume spinal tap test), and occasionally neurostimulants.
   d. Radiation-induced vascular damage (carotid artery) can be treated with carotid artery stenting (preferred) or surgery.

2. Chemotherapy toxicity
   a. Identify the toxicity early and limit further exposure. Early detection can be achieved by following serial conduction velocities and QST (for small fiber neuropathy).
   b. Steroids, vitamin B_6, and folinic acid benefit some patients, and a few experimental approaches are being explored to try to prevent neuropathy from developing.
   c. Glutamine may reduce severity of paclitaxel-induced neuropathy.
   d. Methotrexate encephalopathy is treated with folinic acid rescue. IV aminophylline (competitive antagonist of adenosine receptors) or thymidine may also benefit some patients with acute MTX toxicity.

Key Treatment

Radiation Injury

- Steroids
- Surgical resection
- Anticoagulation

Chemotherapy Injury

- Limit further exposure
- Steroids, vitamin B$_6$, folinic acid
- Glutamine for paclitaxel-induced neuropathy
- Folinic acid rescue for methotrexate encephalopathy

Prognosis and Complications

1. Radiation toxicity: Acute changes are usually completely reversible. Late central nervous system effects of radiotherapy are very difficult to treat and are often gradually progressive.
2. Chemotherapy toxicity: PRES is usually reversible, although some children can have permanent neurologic sequelae. Neuropathies usually gradually improve over weeks to months after the offending agent is removed, although large-fiber neuropathies can take over a year until improvement is seen.

Prevention

1. Radiation toxicity
   a. In patients with large brain tumors (primary or metastatic), high-dose (8 to 16 mg) dexamethasone prior to the initiation of radiotherapy may curtail toxicity.

b. Routine neurocognitive tests allow for early distinction between direct effect of tumor versus side effects of therapy.

2. Chemotherapy toxicity
   a. Cerebral venous thrombosis
      Enoxaparin has been studied to prevent cerebral venous thrombosis in children who receive L-asparaginase.
   b. Peripheral neuropathy: Patients with hereditary peripheral neuropathies require dose adjustment of neurotoxic agents.

Bibliography

Casey SO, Sampaio RC, Michael E, et al.: Posterior reversible encephalopathy syndrome: Utility of fluid-attenuated inversion recovery MR imaging in the detection of cortical and subcortical lesion. AJNR Am J Neuroradiol 21:1199–1206, 2000.

Glantz MJ, Burger PC, Friedman AH, et al.: Treatment of radiation induced nervous system injury with heparin and warfarin. Neurology 44:2020–2027, 1994.

Guibert FK, Napolitano M, Delattre JY: Neurologic complications of radiotherapy and chemotherapy. J Neurol 245:695–708, 1998.

Shuper A, Stark B, Kornreich L, et al.: Methotrexate treatment protocols and the central nervous system: Significant cure with significant neurotoxicity. J Child Neurol 15:573–580, 2000.

Thiessen B, DeAngelis LM: Hydrocephalus in radiation leukoencephalopathy. Arch Neurol 55:705–710, 1998.

1 | Diagnostic Testing

Michael J. Ruckenstein

BASIC AUDIOMETRIC ASSESSMENT

A basic audiometric assessment includes the following tests:

1. Pure tone assessment of auditory thresholds
2. Speech audiometry (speech reception threshold, speech discrimination testing)
3. Tympanometry
4. Acoustic reflex testing

Pure Tone Audiogram

1. Measures auditory thresholds to pure tone stimuli
2. Stimuli presented via a standard earphone (signal passes through external and middle ears to inner ear = *air conduction*) and via a bone oscillator (provides direct stimulation to the inner ear only = *bone conduction*).
3. Frequencies presented are measured in Hertz (Hz, cycles/second) and include 250, 500, 1000, 2000, 4000, and 8000 Hz (air only)
4. Threshold intensity is measured in decibels hearing level (dB HL). This is a logarithmic scale; hence percentages of hearing loss cannot be calculated from these measures. A measure of 0 dB HL represents the mean pure tone threshold derived from a large number of young adults.
5. Stimuli must be presented in a soundproof booth with equipment that is calibrated regularly.
6. Stimuli are presented to one ear at a time. In certain cases of unilateral hearing loss, the presented signal may actually be perceived by the nontest, better hearing ear, potentially creating a situation in which thresholds appear better than they actually are. In air conduction, if the hearing loss in the test ear is 40 dB or greater than that in the nontest ear, the signal may cross over, and be perceived by the nontest ear. Bone conduction is a very efficient transfer of sound to both ears, and therefore, it is always assumed that any stimulus could be delivered via a bone oscillator and be perceived by both ears. To eliminate the nontest ear from perceiving the pure tone stimulus, a masking white noise is placed in the nontest ear whenever there is potential for crossover of the stimulus to the nontest ear.

Indications

1. Any patient complaining of hearing loss
2. Any patient who may potentially be at risk for hearing loss in the future (e.g., monitoring for noise exposure, ototoxic drug exposure)

Key Indications

- Any complaint of hearing loss
- Patients at risk for hearing loss, e.g., from noise or ototoxic drugs

Contraindications

Children under 5 years old and the mentally challenged will generally need a modified technique using behavioral observation or reinforcement or evoked potential audiometry.

Key Contraindications

- Children under 5 years of age need modified technique
- Patients who are mentally challenged need modified technique

Abnormal Findings

1. Hearing loss is generally defined as
   a. Normal: –10–25 dB HL
   b. Mild hearing loss: 26–40 dB HL
   c. Moderate hearing loss: 41–55 dB HL
   d. Moderate to severe hearing loss: 56–70 dB HL
   e. Severe hearing loss: 71–90 dB HL
   f. Profound hearing loss: 91 dB + HL
2. Hearing loss may be *conductive* (implying a defect in the external or middle ear conductive mechanism), which is defined by abnormalities in air conduction thresholds in the presence of normal bone conduction thresholds.
3. Hearing loss due to pathology in the inner ear or VIII cranial nerve is referred to as *sensorineural*, and is indicated by identical abnormalities recorded using air and bone conduction techniques.
4. A *mixed* hearing loss contains both conductive and sensorineural components.

Key Abnormal Findings

- Conductive hearing loss
- Sensorineural, i.e., hearing loss resulting from pathology of the inner ear or VIII cranial nerve
- Mixed, i.e., both conductive and sensorineural

Complications
None

Speech Reception Threshold (SRT)

The lowest intensity at which a person can correctly repeat 50% of common bisyllabic words (e.g., baseball).

Indications
As per pure tone audiogram

Key Indication

- As per pure tone audiogram

Contraindications
1. Difficulty in language comprehension
2. Age less than 5 years

Key Contraindications

- Difficulty with language comprehension
- Children under 5 years of age

Abnormal Findings
The SRT is generally used as a corroboration of findings on the pure tone audiogram. The SRT should approximate the mean pure tone thresholds obtained at 500, 1000, and 2000 Hz (the pure tone average—PTA). Situations in which the SRT is better than the PTA may indicate the presence of pseudohypoacusis (e.g., malingering).

Key Abnormal Findings

- Used to corroborate findings on pure tone audiogram
- Results better than the pure tone average may indicate pseudohypoacusis (e.g., malingering)

Complications
None

Speech Discrimination Testing

Measures the ability of a patient to repeat a list of monosyllabic, phonetically balanced words. Scores are reported as percent correct.

Indications
As per pure tone audiogram

Key Indication

- As per pure tone audiogram

Contraindications
None

Abnormal Findings
Any degree of hearing loss can cause a decrement in the understanding of speech. However, a discrimination score that is considerably lower than that expected for the level of pure tone hearing loss (e.g., 40% discrimination score with a mild to moderate hearing loss) may be a sign of the presence of a retrocochlear lesion (e.g., an acoustic neuroma).

Key Abnormal Finding

- A score considerably lower than expected for the pure tone hearing loss may indicate an acoustic neuroma.

Tympanometry

The tympanic membrane vibrates most efficiently, and thus transmits sounds most effectively, when the air pressure in the external ear equals that of the middle ear. Conversely, when the air pressure of the external ear exceeds that of the middle ear, the tympanic membrane becomes rigid and more sound is reflected back into the external ear. Tympanometry employs these principles to provide an estimate of air pressure within the middle ear. A probe that contains pressure and sound transducers, as well as a microphone, is sealed into the external ear canal. A probe tone, typically 220 Hz, is emitted while the pressure within the ear canal is varied. The intensity of the reflected sound is measured and used to derive the sound transmitted (*admitted*) into the middle ear. The *admittance* is then plotted against the external canal air pressure (providing a *tympanogram*)

Indications
1. The presence of a conductive hearing loss
2. To support a diagnosis of eustachian tube dysfunction or otitis media

Key Indications

- Conductive hearing loss
- Supports a diagnosis of eustachian tube dysfunction or otitis media

Contraindications
Temporal bone fracture with potential for pneumocephalus

Key Contraindication

- Temporal bone fracture with potential for pneumocephalus

Normal Findings
In the normal middle ear, the maximal sound admittance (to the middle ear) at normal atmospheric pressure (0) as the eustachian tube is equalizing middle ear pressure with that of the external environment.

Key Normal Finding

- Maximal sound admittance (to the middle ear) at the normal atmospheric pressure of 0 as the eustachian tube equalizes middle ear pressure with that of the external environment

Abnormal Findings
1. A tympanogram in which the middle ear pressure is normal but the sound admittance is low indicates a stiff conducting mechanism, such as that seen in otosclerosis (type As tympanogram).
2. Conversely, a normal middle pressure with very high admittance (type Ad tympanogram) indicates the presence of an ossicular discontinuity.
3. A flat tympanogram (type B) has been associated with fluid within the middle ear (e.g., otitis media with effusion).
4. Negative middle ear pressure (type C tympanogram) is characteristic of eustachian tube dysfunction.
5. Presence of a perforation in the tympanic membrane will result in inability to create a seal due to the presence of the eustachian tube.

Key Abnormal Findings

- Normal middle ear pressure and low sound admittance indicate a stiff conducting mechanism, as in otosclerosis.

- Conversely, normal middle ear pressure and very high admittance indicate ossicular discontinuity.
- A flat tympanogram may indicate fluid in the middle ear.
- Negative middle ear pressure is characteristic of eustachian tube dysfunction.
- Perforation in the tympanic membrane results in an inability to create a seal owing to the presence of the eustachian tube.

Complications
None

Acoustic Reflexes

A loud sound (70 to 100 dB above thresholds) presented to one ear will elicit a contraction in the stapedius muscle in both the ipsilateral and the contralateral ear. The stiffening of the ossicular chain resulting from this contraction can be detected by tympanometry. The reflex pathway involves sound being conducted via the VIII cranial nerve to the trapezoid body to the cochlear nucleus. From the ipsilateral cochlear nucleus, fibers pass to the ipsilateral facial motor nucleus and then to the ipsilateral stapedius muscle. Fibers from the ipsilateral trapezoid body also course to the ipsilateral medial superior olive, where they pass to *both* the ipsilateral and contralateral facial motor nucleus.

Indication
Stapedial reflex testing can yield results that may support a variety of clinical diagnoses, but that are not sufficiently sensitive or specific to confirm any of these diagnoses.

Key Indication

- Results of stapedial reflex testing may support various clinical diagnoses, but these results are not sufficiently sensitive or specific to confirm a diagnosis.

Contraindications
None

Normal Findings
A stimulus provided at 70 to 100 dB above threshold should elicit both an ipsilateral and contralateral stapedial reflex.

- Stimulus at 70 to 100 dB above threshold should elicit an ipsilateral and a contralateral stapedial reflex.

Abnormal Findings

1. Acoustic reflexes may be useful in screening patients who are feigning a severe to profound hearing loss.

2. An acoustic neuroma may cause an elevation in reflex thresholds and reflex decay, where the intensity of the reflex weakens by 50% or more within the first 10 seconds of the stimulus.

3. A brainstem lesion may eliminate the contralateral reflexes but not the ipsilateral reflexes.

4. A lesion in the facial nerve proximal to the branch to the stapedius muscle will eliminate the reflex on the side of the tumor.

5. A minor conductive hearing loss will eliminate the reflex on the affected side, whereas a conductive loss greater than 30 dB will eliminate both ipsilateral and contralateral reflexes when the affected side is stimulated.

6. Mild to moderate sensorineural hearing loss may result in reflexes that can be elicited with a stimulus of reduced intensity. Severe to profound hearing loss will generally abolish the ipsilateral and contralateral reflex.

Key Abnormal Findings

- May be used to screen for feigning a severe to profound hearing loss

- Minor conductive hearing loss will eliminate the reflex on the affected side.

- Conductive hearing loss over 30 dB will eliminate both the ipsilateral and contralateral reflexes on stimulation of the affected side.

- Mild to moderate sensorineural hearing loss may result in reflexes that can be elicited with a reduced-intensity stimulus.

- Severe to profound loss generally eliminates both the ipsilateral and contralateral reflexes.

- Acoustic neuroma may cause an increase in reflex thresholds and decay.

- A brainstem lesion may eliminate the contralateral but not the ipsilateral reflex.

- A facial nerve lesion proximal to the branch to the stapedius muscle will eliminate the reflex on the side of the lesion.

Complications
None

Otoacoustic Emissions

Otoacoustic emissions (OAEs) are acoustic signals produced by the outer hair cells of the cochlea and can be recorded by a microphone placed within the external auditory canal. They may occur spontaneously in approximately 45% of the population. They may also be evoked in virtually 100% of the population by a rapid click stimulus (transient evoked OAEs) or by the simultaneous presentation of two tones of different frequencies (distortion product OAEs). OAEs *cannot* be used to estimate audiometric thresholds.

Indications

1. The indications for the performance of OAE measurements have not yet been fully delineated, but they may be useful in the following situations.

2. As part of a neonatal hearing screening protocol

3. As an objective measure in evaluating a patient suspected of presenting with pseudohypoacusis.

4. As part of an ototoxic drug monitoring protocol

Key Indications

- May be useful in screening neonatal hearing, as an objective measure to evaluate patients presenting with pseudohypoacusis, or as part of an ototoxic drug-monitoring protocol

Contraindications
The presence of a known middle ear effusion or other middle ear abnormalities

Key Contraindications

- Known middle ear effusion
- Other known middle ear abnormalities

Normal and Abnormal Findings
As mentioned previously, evoked OAEs should be present in virtually all normal hearing patients. Evoked OAEs will be absent in cases of middle ear and inner ear pathology, and in many cases of retrocochlear pathology.

Complications
None

Auditory Brainstem Response

The auditory brainstem response (ABR) is also known as the *brainstem auditory evoked response* (BAER) or the *brainstem evoked response* (BSER). The ABR is an electroencephalographic (EEG) response evoked by an auditory stimulus. It is recorded using the differential amplification technique, with the active electrode placed on the vertex, the reference electrode placed on the mastoid tip, and the ground electrode placed on the forehead. The auditory stimulus is typically a broadband click, but short, frequency-specific tonepips can be used. Five waves are typically identified in a 10-msec time window. Waves I and II are generated by the proximal and distal aspects of the cochlear nerve, with waves III, IV, V generated primarily by the cochlear nucleus, the superior olivary complex, and the lateral lemniscus, respectively. The patient must be relaxed or sedated during recording to avoid contaminating myogenic potentials.

Indications

1. To estimate the auditory thresholds in patients in whom behavioral audiometry cannot be performed (e.g., a child)

2. As part of the work-up in patients suspected of presenting with pseudohypoacusis (e.g., malingering)

3. As part of a neonatal hearing screening program

4. Intraoperative monitoring (e.g., during resection of an acoustic neuroma)

5. For many years, ABR was the screening test of choice for the evaluation of the presence of a retrocochlear lesion (e.g., an acoustic neuroma). However, recent data do not support its use for this indication, with magnetic resonance imaging (MRI) now being the screening test of choice.

Key Indications

- In estimating auditory thresholds when behavioral audiometry cannot be done, as in children

- As part of a workup for pseudohypoacusis (e.g., malingering)

- As part of a screening neonatal hearing

- In intraoperative monitoring, e.g., for acoustic neuroma

Contraindications
None

Normal Findings
Normal ABR responses should manifest the following characteristics

1. Normal waveform morphology
2. Normal absolute latencies for waves I, III, and V
3. Normal I to III and III to V latencies (2 milliseconds each)
4. Normal I to V latencies (4 milliseconds each)
5. A difference in the absolute wave V latencies for the two ears of less than 3 milliseconds.

Key Normal Findings

- Normal waveform morphology

- Normal absolute latencies for waves I, III, and V

- Normal I to III and III to V latencies

- Normal I to V latencies

- Difference in the absolute wave V latencies for the two ears

Abnormal Findings
Loss of all waveforms may indicate a severe to profound sensorineural loss.

Increased latencies may indicate the presence of a retrocochlear lesion.

Key Abnormal Findings

- Loss of all waveforms may indicate severe to profound sensorineural loss.

- Increased latencies may indicate a retrocochlear lesion.

Complications
None

BALANCE FUNCTION TESTING

Currently available balance function tests include electronystagmography, rotational chair, and dynamic posturography.

Electronystagmography

The electronystagmograph (ENG) is a battery of tests designed to record eye movements in response to visual and vestibular stimuli. Eye movements can be recorded with electrodes or goggles fitted with an infrared camera. Tests performed on ENG include the following.

1. Smooth pursuit: Foveal tracking of a point target,

moving back and forth in a horizontal plane, presented at varying frequencies

2. Saccades: Rapid eye movements to bring objects in the peripheral visual field into focus on the fovea. Saccades are evaluated for accuracy, latency, and velocity.

3. Optokinetic nystagmus: Involves the stimulation of the entire retina (as opposed to just the fovea) with repetitive, continuously moving stimuli. The appropriate stimulus is a rotating stripe that fills the entire visual field. The eye follows the vertical stripe (analogous to a smooth pursuit) and then performs a quick saccade to focus on the next stripe.

4. Spontaneous and gaze-evoked nystagmus: The presence of nystagmus in the absence of visual fixation is recorded with eyes looking straight ahead, and 30 degrees to the right, left, up, and down.

5. Static positional nystagmus: The presence of nystagmus in the absence of visual fixation is recorded in 7 to 11 different head and body positions.

6. Rapid positioning nystagmus: This is equivalent to the Dix-Hallpike or Bárány maneuver, in which the patient is rapidly positioned into the supine position with the head hyperextended and turned to the left or right.

7. Caloric testing: The nystagmus is recorded when the ear is stimulated with water or air equally above (warm) or below (cool) room temperature. Ice water stimulation may be used if the warm or cool stimulations fail to elicit a response. Caloric stimulation excites or inhibits activity within the horizontal semicircular canal of the inner ear, which, in turn, elicits rapid eye movements (nystagmus) via the vestibular ocular reflex.

Indications

Balance tests are not diagnostic of any particular pathological entity. Given this fact, balance tests are indicated when specific information is desired.

1. Site of lesion: Balance testing can help in confirming the side involved in a peripheral vestibular loss. Signs of a central lesion can also be elicited.

2. Extent of lesion: ENG testing can provide a quantitative measure of the extent of a peripheral vestibular lesion

3. Determination of whether the patient is a candidate for vestibular rehabilitation therapy

Key Indications: Balance Tests

- Cannot be used to diagnose a particular pathology

- Can give information about the site and extent of a lesion

- Can determine candidacy for vestibular rehabilitation therapy

Contraindications

1. In the case of a perforated tympanic membrane, an air or closed-loop (balloon) irrigator should be used.

2. Children may have difficulty cooperating with an ENG.

3. Results of oculomotor testing may be inaccurate in patients with visual impairment or abnormalities in function of the extraocular muscles.

Key Contraindications

- An air or closed-loop irrigator should be used when the tympanic membrane is perforated.

- Children may have difficulty cooperating during electronystagmography testing.

- Results of oculomotor testing can be inaccurate in patients with visual impairment or abnormal function of the extraocular muscles.

Normal Findings

1. Saccades and smooth pursuit: Other than elderly patients, all adults should be able to perform smooth pursuit and saccade testing.

2. Spontaneous, gaze-evoked, and positional nystagmus

   a. Normal patients will frequently manifest some degree of spontaneous or positional nystagmus. The criteria for abnormal findings on these exams are listed below.

   b. Dynamic positioning testing (Dix–Hallpike maneuver) should not elicit symptoms or nystagmus.

   c. Physiologic "end-point" nystagmus may be detected on extreme lateral or vertical gaze positions. This normal finding will fatigue within a minute.

3. Caloric testing. The velocities of the slow components of the nystagmus evoked by warm and cool caloric stimulations are used to calculate a unilateral peripheral vestibular weakness. Depending on individual laboratory norms, generally a unilateral

weakness of less than 25% is considered to be within normal limits. Caloric testing may also be evaluated for directional preponderance, a measure designed to reveal if the nystagmus in one direction is stronger in response to bithermal caloric stimuli.

Key Normal Findings

- Adequate performance in testing of saccades and smooth pursuit

- Some degree of spontaneous or positional nystagmus is normal.

- Dynamic positioning test (Dix–Hallpike maneuver) should not elicit symptoms or nystagmus.

- Physiologic "end-point" nystagmus may be detected on extreme lateral or vertical gaze positions, but this normal finding will fatigue within a minute.

- In caloric testing, a unilateral weakness of less than 25% is considered to be in normal limits.

Abnormal Findings

1. Saccades and smooth pursuit: Saccades are evaluated for accuracy, latency, and velocity. Accuracy is controlled by the posterior vermis of the cerebellum. Thus, undershoots (hypometria) or overshoots (hypermetria) of saccades more commonly are associated with cerebellar pathology, and less frequently with pathology within the basal ganglia and brainstem. Latency and velocity of saccades are controlled by the pontine reticular formation. Slow saccades can result from a variety of causes including medications, or pathology within the brainstem, cerebellum, or basal ganglia. Long latencies typically are associated neurodegenerative conditions (e.g., Alzheimer's disease and Parkinson's disease) or from lesions in the brainstem and cerebellum.

2. Inability to maintain smooth pursuit can result from pathology throughout the central nervous system, most commonly in the brainstem or cerebellum.

3. Spontaneous, gaze-evoked, and positional nystagmus: Although somewhat controversial, the following criteria represent a reasonable approach to the definition of pathologic findings on these tests.

   a. Spontaneous nystagmus greater than 5 degrees per second

   b. Persistent nystagmus of less than 6 degrees per second in four or more positions

   c. Sporadic nystagmus of less than 6 degrees per second in all positions tested

d. Direction-changing nystagmus in a given head position

4. Caloric testing: A unilateral weakness of greater than 25% is usually indicative of a peripheral vestibular loss (paresis). A directional preponderance is often associated with a unilateral weakness or spontaneous nystagmus. In the absence of these findings, the presence of a directional preponderance is nonlocalizing and should be correlated with the results of the remainder of the test.

Key Abnormal Findings

- In testing of saccades for accuracy, undershoots (hypometria) or overshoots (hypermetria) are associated with cerebellar pathology.

- Slow saccades can result from various causes, including medications and pathology in the brainstem, cerebellum, or basal ganglia.

- Long latencies in saccades are associated with a neurodegenerative condition (e.g., Alzheimer's disease or Parkinson's disease) or a lesion in the brainstem or cerebellum.

- Inability to maintain smooth pursuit may result from pathology throughout the central nervous system, most commonly in the brainstem or cerebellum.

- In caloric testing, a unilateral weakness of greater than 25% may indicate peripheral vestibular loss (paresis).

- In caloric testing, a directional preponderance is associated with a unilateral weakness or spontaneous nystagmus.

Complications
None

Rotational Chair

Rotational chair testing is performed in the dark, with eye movements recorded with an infrared camera or electrodes. The chair is rotated at frequencies ranging from 0.01 to 1.28 Hz, with the slow component of the nystagmus being the outcome measured. When compared with caloric testing, rotational chair provides a more physiologic stimulus to the inner ear. The frequency of the stimulus can be varied and quantified.

Indications

1. As per ENG

2. The rotational chair is often more easily applied to a child, who can sit on mother's lap during the testing

- As per electronystagmography
- More easily used with children because they can sit on their mother's lap

Contraindications
None

Normal Findings
Comparing head velocity to eye velocity for the derivation of phase, gain, and symmetry. Patient data are compared to established patient norms.

1. Phase: Also known as *phase angle,* it is measured in degrees and provides a measure of the timing relationship between head movement and eye movement.
2. Gain: Measured by dividing the velocity of the slow component of the eye movements by the velocity of the head
3. Symmetry: A comparison of the slow component eye movements to the right compared to the left

Key Normal Findings

- Patient data are compared to established norms for phase, gain, and symmetry.

Abnormal Findings

1. Phase: Increased phase angle (phase lead) is indicative of a peripheral vestibular loss but cannot localize the side of pathology. The significance of a decreased phase angle has not been completely elucidated, but it may indicate the presence of cerebellar pathology.
2. Symmetry: Asymmetries can be noted in central or peripheral disease. However, in the absence of other central findings, an asymmetry to a particular side would be consistent with a peripheral vestibular loss on that side.
3. Gain: A reduction in gain is most commonly seen in bilateral peripheral vestibular loss. A unilateral vestibular loss, particularly if it is acute, may cause a mild reduction in gain.

Key Abnormal Findings

- Increased phase angle (phase lead) indicates peripheral vestibular loss.
- Decreased phase angle may indicate the presence of cerebellar pathology.

- Asymmetries can be seen in central or peripheral disease.
- In the absence of other findings, asymmetry to one side is consistent with a peripheral vestibular loss on that side.
- Reduced gain is seen in bilateral peripheral vestibular loss.
- A mild, acute reduction in gain is seen in unilateral vestibular loss.

Complications
None

Dynamic Posturography

The sensory organization test provides quantitative information pertaining to a patient's functional ability to maintain balance under varying sensory conditions. Force plates on which the patient stands measure the movement of a patient's center of gravity. Six conditions are measured in which the patient's visual and somatosensory (proprioreceptive) inputs are altered. In the first three conditions, the platform is fixed, providing stable proprioceptive inputs. In condition one, the patient stands with eyes open; in the second condition the eyes are closed (Romberg test). In the third condition, the eyes are open and the visual surround moves, attempting to match the patient's visual sway. This creates a sensory conflict, in which the vestibular and proprioreceptive inputs tell the patient that he or she is swaying, while the visual input erroneously indicates that the patient is stable. Conditions four, five, and six replicate conditions one, two, and three, with the exception that the platform is allowed to sway with the patient. This limits the contributions to balance made by the proprioceptive receptors.

Indications
As part of balance function testing protocol, it is the only test that provides information about the patient's functional ability to maintain balance. It is particularly helpful as part of a vestibular rehabilitation protocol.

> **Caveat**
>
> As part of balance function testing, dynamic posturography is the only test that provides information about the patient's functional ability to maintain balance. It is particularly helpful in vestibular rehabilitation.

Contraindications
None

Normal Findings

Normal patients should be able to maintain their balance in all six sensory conditions.

Key Normal Finding

- Maintenance of balance in all six sensory conditions

Abnormal Findings

The pattern of performance may indicate an inability to use certain information (e.g. vestibular, visual) to maintain balance, a preferential reliance on particular cues to maintain balance, or inconsistent results not attributable to physical pathology (e.g. malingering).

Key Abnormal Findings

- Inability to use, for example, vestibular or visual information to maintain balance

- Reliance on cues to maintain balance

- Inconsistent results not attributable to pathology, e.g., in malingering

Complications

None

Bibliography

Campbell K: Essential Audiology for Physicians. San Diego, Singular, 1998.

Jacobson GP, Newman CW, Kartush JM: Handbook of Balance Function Testing. St. Louis, Mosby–Year Book, 1993.

Ruckenstein MJ, Shepard NT: Balance function testing: A rational approach. Otolaryngol Clin North Am 33:507–518, 2000.

Shepard NT, Telian SA: Practical Management of the Balance Disorder Patient. San Diego, Singular, 1996.

2 Hearing Loss

Michael J. Ruckenstein

Definition

A decrease in auditory perceptual sensitivity that can be measured using objective techniques. Hearing loss is defined as *conductive*, secondary to pathology of the external or middle ear, or *sensorineural*, resulting from pathology of the inner ear or the eighth cranial nerve.

Epidemiology and Risk Factors

Hearing loss is a pervasive problem affecting virtually all adults as they age. The major risk factors for hearing loss are the following.

1. Aging
2. Noise exposure
3. Ototoxin exposure
4. Head trauma
5. Chronic infection

Etiology and Pathophysiology

Conductive Hearing Loss

1. Congenital
   a. Congenital aural atresia of the external ear canal with or without middle ear involvement
   b. Congenital ossicular abnormalities
2. Acquired
   a. Trauma to the temporal bone may result in ossicular dislocation (most commonly of the incus), tympanic membrane perforation, or posttraumatic stenosis of the external canal.
   b. Barotrauma (air flight, scuba dive) may cause a ruptured tympanic membrane or a middle ear effusion.
   c. Metabolic: Otosclerosis is a genetic, metabolic disorder that causes disease of the otic capsule of the temporal bone. It occurs more commonly in women and in Caucasians. A conductive hearing loss results from an overgrowth of otic capsule bone, fixing the stapes.
   d. Neoplasms: Benign and malignant neoplasms of the external and middle ear are rare causes of conductive hearing loss. Examples of benign neoplasms include osteomas, adenomas, and glomus tumors. Squamous cell carcinoma and adenocarcinoma can also involve the external and middle ear, either primarily or via secondary spread.
   e. Infections
      (1) Otitis externa is an acute bacterial (*Staphylococcus aureus, Pseudomonas aeruginosa*), or fungal (*Candida, Aspergillus*) infection of the external ear. In addition to hearing loss, it will present pain, itching, and aural discharge.
      (2) Acute otitis media is a suppurative infection of the middle ear most commonly caused by *Streptococcus pneumoniae, Haemophilus influenza,* or *Branhamella catarrhalis.*
      (3) Otitis media with effusion (serous otitis media) represents a persistent effusion of fluid within the middle ear, typically subsequent to acute otitis media or barotrauma. It is much more common, and persistent, in the pediatric population.
      (4) Chronic suppurative otitis media is defined as a chronic or recurrent suppurative infection of the middle ear in the presence of a perforation of the tympanic membrane.
      (5) A cholesteatoma is a benign neoplasm of the middle ear that typically presents with a history of hearing loss and infection. It is an ingrowth of tympanic membrane epithelium into the middle ear. The accumulation of squamous debris within it makes it prone to infection. Conductive hearing loss results from erosion of the ossicles. It can also erode into the inner ear, facial nerve, and posterior and middle cranial fossas.
   e. Immune and Inflammatory: Wegener's granulomatosis can cause chronic otitis media. Although rare, rheumatoid arthritis can affect the ossicular joints.
   f. Iatrogenic: Patients undergoing radiation therapy to the head and neck, particularly to the nasopharyngeal region, can develop eustachian tube dysfunction and otitis media with effusion.

Sensorineural Hearing Loss

1. Congenital
   a. The overall incidence of congenital hearing loss is approximately 1/1000 live births. Approximately 50% of cases of congenital hearing loss

331

are genetic; the remainder are acquired (see below).

b. The most common etiology of acquired neonatal deafness is congenital cytomegalovirus (CMV) infection.

c. Congenital osseo-membranous and membranous inner ear anomalies (e.g., Mondini's dysplasia) are rare entities resulting from defective in utero development. They are not typically genetic in etiology.

2. Acquired

a. Idiopathic: Presbycusis (hearing loss associated with aging) is the most common sensorineural hearing loss. Its etiology is multifactorial, with genetic and environmental factors playing roles. It results from degeneration of sensory hair cells, afferent nerve fibers, and/or the structures of the cochlear lateral wall responsible for metabolic function (stria vascularis, spiral ligament).

b. Trauma

(1) Noise-induced hearing loss remains a common cause of cochlear dysfunction. It most frequently results from a cumulative exposure to industrial and/or recreational noise. An acoustic trauma refers to acute hearing loss suffered from exposure to a short, explosive noise (e.g., gunshot).

(2) Head injury can cause a temporal bone fracture resulting in violation of the inner ear or cochlear nerve. A "labyrinthine concussion" represents a more mild form of hearing loss resulting from head trauma that occurs in the absence of an overt fracture.

(3) Barotrauma (typically from a SCUBA dive) can result in a permanent hearing loss.

(4) Perilymph fistula (PLF) is a rare disorder in which the membranes of the round window or oval window of the cochlea are violated, allowing for leakage of inner ear perilymph fluid into the inner ear. A PLF typically occurs after trauma or ear surgery and presents with fluctuating symptoms of hearing loss and vertigo, often in response to straining.

c. Toxic

(1) Cisplatin is the most common drug to cause hearing loss.

(2) The aminoglycosides can result in hearing loss and vestibular loss, with amikacin being more cochleotoxic than vestibulotoxic.

(3) Furosemide may potentiate the ototoxic effects of the aminoglycosides.

(4) At high doses, erythromycin may cause a reversible sensorineural hearing loss.

(5) Quinine and its derivatives, as well as aspirin, are more commonly associated with tinnitus.

d. Genetic

(1) Genetic hearing loss may be syndromal (25%) or nonsyndromal (75%).

(2) Most cases of genetic hearing loss are autosomal recessive, and tend to present in childhood with more severe hearing loss.

(3) Autosomal dominant forms of hearing loss (20% to 25% of cases) have a more variable presentation. They may present with moderate to profound hearing loss that can progress through adulthood.

(4) Rare forms of genetic hearing loss result from X-linked or mitochondrial mutations.

e. Infectious

(1) The most common cause of virus-mediated hearing loss is CMV. It may present at birth with the full signs of cytomegalovirus inclusion disease. More commonly, it presents with progressive hearing loss in an otherwise asymptomatic patient.

(2) Herpes zoster may present with otalgia hearing loss associated with facial paralysis (Ramsay Hunt syndrome).

(3) A variety of viruses can cause sudden sensorineural hearing loss. Measles, mumps, and rubella are now rare causes of hearing loss.

(4) Syphilis, in its late secondary or tertiary forms, may present with progressive hearing loss with or without vertigo.

(5) While Lyme disease is a common infectious cause of facial paralysis, it has not been shown to mediate inner ear or eighth nerve pathology.

(6) Bacterial meningitis remains the most common cause of acquired deafness in children.

(7) Patients with human immunodeficiency virus (HIV) may suffer hearing loss from a variety of etiologies. The virus can mediate direct pathologic effects on the nerve. Other opportunistic infections (e.g., cryptococcal meningitis) have been associated with hearing loss. These patients also have an increased incidence of syphilis. Malignancies of the central nervous system, which may affect this patient population, particularly CNS lymphoma, may also manifest with hearing loss.

f. Neoplasm

(1) Vestibular schwannomas (acoustic neuromas) arising off the eighth cranial nerve typically present with asymmetric sensorineural hearing loss. The incidence of these tumors is approximately 10 adults per million population per year.

(2) Meningiomas and other benign and, rarely, primary or metastatic malignant neoplasms can affect the eighth cranial nerve.

(3) Benign neoplasms of the petrous apex of the temporal bone, such as epidermoids or cholesterol granulomas, may present with hearing loss and other symptoms, such as vertigo, facial paralysis, and facial pain.

g. Immune: A variety of organ nonspecific autoimmune diseases typically associated with vasculitides can rarely cause hearing loss (e.g., lupus erythematosus, polyarteritis nodosa). Cogan's syndrome is an autoimmune disorder defined by the presence of progressive bilateral hearing loss, vertigo, and nonsyphilitic interstitial keratitis. A rare organ-specific autoimmune inner ear disease has been defined that responds to immunosuppressants.

h. Metabolic: In extreme cases, hypothyroidism may be associated with hearing loss. Associations between diabetes mellitus and hypercholesterolemia and hearing loss have been made, but a cause-and-effect relationship has not been definitively established.

i. Idiopathic: Ménière's disease is an idiopathic disorder characterized by fluctuating, progressive hearing loss, recurrent episodes of vertigo, and tinnitus.

Clinical Features

1. Hearing loss typically manifests as distortion of the perception of speech and sound. Patients with sensorineural hearing loss typically complain of difficulty in discerning speech in a crowded or noisy environment.

2. Otalgia in children most commonly results from an otitis media. In an adult, otalgia is most frequently referred from other nonotologic sites (e.g., cervical spine, temporomandibular joint, dentition, upper aerodigestive tract).

3. Otorrhea is a sign of otitis externa or otitis media.

4. Aural fullness may be a sign of middle ear pathology, but it is also seen in patients with low-frequency sensorineural hearing loss (e.g., Ménière's disease). It may also occur in the absence of otologic pathology, in which case it is thought to be referred from myofacial disorders of the head and neck.

5. Fluctuations in hearing may be caused by conductive or sensorineural hearing loss.

6. Hyperacusis is the perception of normal sounds as being too loud, almost painful. This is seen in inner ear or eighth nerve pathology.

7. Diplacusis occurs when a patient perceives the same sound as having different pitches, depending on which ear is perceiving the sound. This is seen in inner ear or eighth nerve pathology.

8. Tinnitus is typically a manifestation of sensorineural hearing loss and rarely can be seen in patients with conductive loss.

9. Vertigo, when associated with hearing loss, is typically a manifestation of inner ear or eighth nerve pathology.

Key Signs

- Distinguish between conductive and sensorineural causes
- Distinguish between acute (sudden) and chronic hearing loss

Conductive

- Acute: otitis externa, acute otitis media, trauma, cerumen impaction
- Chronic: chronic otitis media, cholesteatoma, and otosclerosis

Sensorineural

- Acute: typically a viral cause
- Chronic: aging, noise exposure, genetic mutations, ototoxicity, trauma, neoplasm

General

- Otorrhea, aural fullness, tinnitus, hyperacusis, diplacusis
- Vertigo in eighth nerve and inner ear pathology

Differential Diagnosis

1. Conductive hearing loss: Differentiating between causes of conductive hearing loss is usually fairly straightforward. History and physical examination will suggest the presence of infection, serous effusion, or neoplasm. A normal examination in the presence of a conductive hearing loss is typically associated with a diagnosis of otosclerosis.

2. Sensorineural hearing loss: The duration and rapidity of symptoms is most helpful in differenti-

ating the cause of sensorineural hearing loss. An acute (sudden) sensorineural hearing loss is typically viral in origin, or may rarely be caused by a neoplasm. A rapidly progressive (over weeks to months) hearing loss implicates an infectious, autoimmune, or neoplastic cause. Slowly progressive hearing loss in a younger patient most commonly results from a genetic or viral (CMV) cause. In an older patient, a slowly progressive hearing loss typically results from presbycusis. Noise-induced hearing loss or ototoxicity are implicated when patients are exposed to these toxins.

Audiometric Testing

1. Any patient with the complaint of hearing loss requires an audiometric assessment performed by a certified audiologist in appropriate facilities.

2. Certain patterns of hearing loss may implicate specific etiologies.
    a. Ménière's disease will typically involve the low frequencies, for example.
    b. Noise-induced hearing loss will cause a maximal hearing loss at 4 kHz.
    c. Congenital hearing losses often manifest a hearing loss at mid-frequencies ("cookie-bite" pattern).

Laboratory Testing

Laboratory testing is indicated in patients with rapidly progressive hearing loss.
1. Complete blood count
2. Sedimentation rate
3. Antinuclear antibodies
4. Antiphospholipid antibodies
5. Rheumatoid factor
6. Complement levels
7. Fluorescent treponemal antibody absorption test (FTA-ABS [MHA-TP])
8. Western blot test for anti–Heat Shock Protein: 70 antibodies (associated with steroid-responsive hearing loss)
9. Thyroid function tests have typically been included in this work-up but are rarely revealing.

Radiologic Studies

1. Magnetic resonance imaging (MRI) scan with a contrast agent is indicated in any patient with asymmetric sensorineural hearing loss, to rule out the presence of a retrocochlear lesion such as acoustic neuroma.

2. Computed tomography (CT) scan of the temporal bone is indicated in cases of suspected congenital anomalies of the inner ear, chronic otitis media with cholesteatoma, and in cases of neoplasms of the external and middle ear.

 Key Tests

- Audiometric testing for all patients presenting with hearing loss

- Blood tests for all patients with rapidly progressing hearing loss

- MRI scan for all patients with asymmetric sensorineural hearing loss to rule out lesion

- CT scan of temporal bone when congenital anomalies of the inner ear, chronic otitis media, and neoplasms are suspected

Treatment

1. Conductive hearing losses are often remedial to surgical intervention (e.g., ventilation tube insertion, tympanoplasty, ossiculoplasty, stapedectomy).

2. Otosyphilis should be treated according to neurosyphilis protocols.

3. Sudden sensorineural hearing loss is treated with prednisone (1–2 mg/kg) for 2 weeks. A taper is only required if symptoms recur after discontinuation of therapy.

4. Autoimmune inner ear disease is treated with immunosuppressants. Prednisone (1–2 mg/kg) is the drug of first choice, typically given for 1 month and then tapered. Methotrexate (15–20 mg/week) can be used as part of a steroid-sparing regimen. Cyclophosphamide, at rheumatologic doses, has been employed when patients fail to be controlled on prednisone and methotrexate.

5. Hearing aids offer remediation for most forms of hearing loss.

6. Cochlear implants offer excellent remediation to patients of all ages who have severe to profound hearing loss and who demonstrate no benefit from hearing aids.

7. Surgical intervention remains the treatment of choice for acoustic neuromas. Focused-beam radiation protocols (gamma knife, linacc [linear accelerator]) are under evaluation.

8. Surgical exploration and repair is indicated when a perilymph fistula is strongly suspected.

Key Treatment

- Hearing aids are the mainstay of treatment for chronic sensorineural hearing loss.

- Cochlear implants offer superb remediation of severe to profound hearing loss in children and adults.

- Conductive hearing losses can generally be addressed with topical or oral antibiotics, or with surgical intervention.

Prognosis and Complications

1. The prognosis for conductive hearing loss is generally much more favorable than for sensorineural loss, with most forms of sensorineural hearing loss being irreversible.

2. Chronic otitis media with cholesteatoma may be complicated by meningitis, extradural or intradural abscesses, sigmoid sinus thrombosis, facial paralysis, labyrinthitis, or abscesses of the head and neck.

3. Approximately 30% to 40% of patients with sudden sensorineural hearing loss will benefit from steroid administration.

4. Surgical intervention can preserve hearing in 60% to 70% of acoustic neuroma tumors that are less than 1.5 cm in diameter.

Prevention

1. Genetic counseling is indicated in families with identified genetic forms of hearing loss.

2. Ototoxicity can be difficult to prevent, as individuals show varying susceptibilities to the ototoxic effects of medications. Thus, following serum levels of potentially ototoxic drugs has not proven reliable. Otoacoustic emission testing or high-frequency audiometry in patients undergoing treatment with ototoxic medications may identify early-onset hearing loss.

3. All work environments that expose their employees to potentially ototoxic levels of noise are required to have a hearing loss monitoring and prevention program in place. Patients exposed to recreational noise exposure (e.g., guns, workshop) should be counseled to wear hearing protectors.

Pregnancy

Hearing loss secondary to otosclerosis may be accelerated during pregnancy.

 Bibliography

Dew LA, Shelton C: Complications of temporal bone infections. In Cummings CW (ed): Otolaryngology, Head and Neck Surgery. St. Louis, Mosby, 1998, pp. 3047–3075.

Harris JP: Immunologic disorders affecting the ear. In Cummings CW (ed): Otolaryngology, Head and Neck Surgery. St. Louis, Mosby, 1998, pp. 3172–3185.

Jennings CR, Jones NS: Presbycusis. J Laryngol Otol 115: 171–178, 2001.

Resendes BL, Williamson RE, Morton CC: At the speed of sound: Gene discovery in the auditory system. Am J Hum Genet 69:923–935, 2001.

Ruckenstein MJ: Vertigo and dysequilibrium with associated hearing loss. Otolaryngol Clin North Am 33:535–562, 2000.

Seidman MD, Ahmad N, Bai U: Molecular mechanisms of age-related hearing loss. Ageing Res Rev 1:331–343, 2002.

3 Tinnitus

Michael J. Ruckenstein

Definition

1. The perception of sound(s) not generated from the external environment.
2. Tinnitus is classified as *pulsatile* or *continuous*.

Epidemiology and Risk Factors

1. Continuous tinnitus accounts for 95% of cases of tinnitus and affects approximately 40 million Americans.
2. Pulsatile tinnitus is a rare disorder.
3. The main risk factor for continuous tinnitus is hearing loss, specifically sensorineural hearing loss.
4. Pulsatile tinnitus usually has a vascular etiology.

Caveat

• Pulsatile tinnitus is a rare disorder.

Etiology and Pathophysiology

Continuous Tinnitus

1. The continuous tinnitus signal is generated by a malfunction in the peripheral auditory system.
2. Peripheral auditory dysfunction typically manifests as hearing loss, although some patients who complain of tinnitus do not manifest audiometric abnormalities.
3. A variety of theories have been proposed to explain the mechanisms involved in the generation of the tinnitus signal; however, none of these theories have been definitively validated.
4. Critical to the understanding of the patient with tinnitus is that while many patients perceive tinnitus, only 5% to 10% of these patients suffer from tinnitus. That is, only a small number of patients with tinnitus actually find the tinnitus distressing.
5. The degree of clinical symptomatology attributed by the patient to the tinnitus cannot be correlated with any unique attribute, such as pitch, intensity, character of the tinnitus tone, duration of the tinnitus, or associated hearing loss.
6. Based on these observations and other data, it is probable that the clinical pathology (distress) associated with tinnitus derives not from the generation of the tinnitus itself, but the failure of central adaptation to the continuous tinnitus signal.
7. Failure of central adaptation to the meaningless tinnitus signal is felt to result from an aversive response of the patient to the signal, which may be promoted by coexistent psychopathology (e.g., anxiety, depression, obsessive compulsive personality disorder).

Pulsatile Tinnitus

1. Pulsatile tinnitus results from a vascular lesion in proximity to the inner ear. Such lesions include
   a. Arteriovenous malformations (AVMs)
   b. Stenotic lesions involving the intracranial carotid artery
   c. Dehiscence of the bone overlying the intratemporal carotid artery
   d. Vascular neoplasms (typically glomus tympanicum or glomus jugulare tumors)
2. Pseudotumor cerebri can be associated with bilateral pulsatile tinnitus.
3. Patients with conductive hearing loss may hear their own blood flow through the intratemporal carotid artery; they do not perceive external masking sounds.

Clinical Features

Continuous Tinnitus

1. Patients with continuous tinnitus may complain of perceiving tones with a variety of characteristics (e.g., whistling, buzzing, ringing, cricket chirping, grinding). The nature of the tone perceived is not clinically significant with regard to treatment or prognosis.
2. Tinnitus is more audible (and distressing) in quiet environments.
3. Any drug (e.g., caffeine) or activity (e.g., exercise) that increases heart rate and cardiovascular tone will temporarily increase the perceived intensity of tinnitus.
4. Anxiety states and painful conditions that increase central nervous system alertness will increase the perceived intensity of the tinnitus.
5. Certain medications, including aspirin, furosemide, and quinine-containing compounds, will

actually increase tinnitus generation. The effects of these drugs are generally reversible.

6. Patients who suffer from tinnitus will complain of decreased ability to concentrate and insomnia.

7. Patients who suffer from tinnitus will often manifest coexistent psychopathology.

8. A sensorineural hearing loss will be detected in most patients with continuous tinnitus.

Pulsatile Tinnitus

1. Patients will present with a pulsing sound in one, and sometimes both, ears.

2. The pulse is more audible in quiet environments or during straining.

3. A patient with pseudotumor cerebri will manifest the typical body habitus.

4. Patients with conductive hearing loss will have decreased auditory acuity.

5. Patients with a dehiscence of the bone overlying the jugular bulb may describe a low-pitched "venous hum."

6. A retinal examination should be performed in patients suspected of suffering from pseudotumor cerebri.

7. Auscultation should be performed for bruits of the neck, the pre- and postauricular regions, the ear canal, and the orbit.

Key Signs

- Continuous: variety of perceived tones

- Pulsatile: pulsing sound more audible in quiet environments

Laboratory Testing

Audiometric assessments are indicated in patients with pulsatile and continuous tinnitus.

Radiologic Testing

1. Magnetic resonance imaging (MRI) scan with paramagnetic enhancement is indicated in patients with asymmetric hearing loss or asymmetric tinnitus.

2. MRI scan with paramagnetic enhancement and MR arteriography of the head and neck are indicated in patients with pulsatile tinnitus.

3. A cerebral angiogram may be indicated to verify (and possibly treat) abnormalities identified on MRA and in patients with severe pulsatile tinnitus in whom the MRA is negative.

4. A computed tomography (CT) scan of the temporal bone is indicated to determine the extent of bony involvement of glomus tumors.

Key Tests

- Audiometric assessment

- MRI scan with paramagnetic enhancement of head and neck (plus MRA for pulsatile)

- CT scan for tumors

Treatment

Continual Tinnitus

1. The patient should be counseled as to the cause of the tinnitus and its benign nature.

2. Modifications to the patient's environment should be made to avoid silent surroundings; leaving a television or radio on to provide background noise is often helpful. Similar results can be achieved by a fan or by commercially available devices that play environmental sounds.

3. Drugs that exacerbate tinnitus (caffeine, aspirin) should be avoided.

4. Hearing aids are effective tinnitus maskers in patients with significant hearing loss.

5. Traditional tinnitus masking, where a masking device is used to completely block out the tinnitus signal, is usually ineffective and has largely been abandoned.

6. Jastreboff's Tinnitus Retraining Therapy incorporates a multimodality approach to treat tinnitus sufferers and has been shown to be effective in a subset of tinnitus patients.

7. Coexistent psychopathology must be addressed.

Pulsatile Tinnitus

1. AVMs and other vascular malformations are addressed by interventional radiology or neurosurgical resection.

2. Glomus tumors are generally resected, with radiation therapy serving as an adjuvant option.

3. Conductive hearing loss is addressed with otologic surgery or hearing aids.

Key Treatments

- Simple environmental measures to ensure ambient sound

- Addressing coexistent psychopathology caused by distress

Prognosis and Complications

1. The vast majority (95%) of tinnitus patients adapt to the tinnitus signal and experience no significant distress.

2. A few tinnitus patients will present with severe symptoms that significantly impact their activities of daily living. These patients present a therapeutic challenge and should be treated with multimodality therapy, typically including psychiatric intervention.

Prevention

As per prevention of hearing loss

Bibliography

Dobie RA: A review of randomized clinical trials in tinnitus. Laryngoscope 109:1202–1211, 1999.

Jastreboff PJ, Jastreboff MM: Tinnitus Retraining Therapy (TRT) as a method for treatment of tinnitus and hyperacusis patients. J Am Acad Audiol 11:162–177, 2000.

Kaltenbach JA: Neurophysiologic mechanisms of tinnitus. J Am Acad Audiol 11:125–137, 2000.

Lockwood AH, Salvi RJ, Burkard RF: Tinnitus. N Engl J Med 347:904–910, 2002.

Weissman JL, Hirsch BE: Imaging of tinnitus: A review. Radiology 216:342–349, 2000.

4 Vertigo

Michael J. Ruckenstein

Definition

1. Vertigo is an illusion of movement of self or surround, typically rotatory in nature.
2. Vertigo may be peripheral in etiology; resulting from pathology within the eighth cranial nerve or the inner ear.
3. Central vertigo results from pathology within the brainstem or cerebellum.

CENTRAL VERTIGO

Epidemiology and Risk Factors

1. History of migraines
2. History of atherosclerotic vascular disease
3. History of cardiac arrhythmias or embolic disease
4. Family history of neurofibromatosis type 2 (NF2)

Etiology and Pathophysiology

1. Central vertigo results from pathology within the brainstem or cerebellum
2. Pathology within these structures leading to vertigo may include vascular (occlusive, hemorrhagic) demyelinative, or rarely neoplastic etiologies.
3. The pathophysiology of migrainous vertigo has not been completely established, but it likely involves transient ischemia of either the peripheral vestibular system or the vestibular nuclei.

Clinical Features of Central Vertigo

1. Migrainous vertigo
   a. May occur in patients with active migraine headaches or with a history of migraine headaches that have resolved
   b. Vertigo duration of minutes to hours
   c. No associated history of unilateral auditory dysfunction
   d. Most commonly occurs in a headache-free interval rather than concurrent with the headache.
   e. May occur as part of a symptom cluster associated with basilar migraines (migraine headache associated with symptoms of posterior fossa pathology, e.g. vertigo, diplopia, parasthesias).

2. Vertebrobasilar insufficiency (VBI)
   a. Recurrent episodes of vertigo typically lasting minutes
   b. Typically associated with other neurologic symptoms (diplopia, dysarthria, dysphagia, drop attacks, loss of motor tone, parasthesias)
   c. VBI may present with symptoms isolated to vertigo in up to 25% of cases.
3. Multiple sclerosis (MS)
   a. A demyelinating disorder such as MS is suspected in young adult patients presenting with vertigo and other neurologic complaints.
   b. Vertigo may be the initial presenting complaint in 5% of patients with MS.
   c. Vertigo may affect up to 50% of patients with MS during their lifetimes.
4. Lateral medullary syndrome (Wallenberg's syndrome)
   a. Results from occlusion of the posterior inferior cerebellar artery
   b. Symptoms include vertigo, ipsilateral ataxia, ipsilateral facial hypesthesia, ipsilateral Horner's syndrome, ipsilateral vocal cord paresis, and contralateral pain and temperature sensory dysfunction.
5. Pontine syndrome
   a. Occurs from occlusion of the anterior inferior cerebellar artery
   b. Symptoms include vertigo and ipsilateral tinnitus, hearing loss, ataxia, facial hemianesthesia, facial paralysis, Horner's syndrome; contralateral hemibody sensory loss may also develop.
6. Cerebellar infarction
   a. May present with isolated vertigo
   b. Significant ataxia may accompany the vertigo.
7. Neoplasm
   a. Acoustic neuroma (vestibular schwannoma): Classically present with unilateral hearing loss and imbalance. 20% to 30% of these patients complain of vertigo
   b. Meningioma: Petroclival meningiomas may present with symptoms similar to those caused by acoustic neuromas
   c. NF2 is defined by the presence of bilateral acoustic neuromas. This genetic disorder may also be diagnosed in a patient with a first-degree relative with NF2 and a single acoustic

neuroma or two of the following: glioma, meningioma, neurofibroma, schwannoma, or premature cataract.

d. Metastases to the cerebellopontine angle may present with symptoms similar to those seen in acoustic neuromas; however, they more frequently cause a facial paralysis.

PERIPHERAL VERTIGO

Epidemiology and Risk Factors of Peripheral Vertigo

1. Most peripheral vestibular disorders are idiopathic in etiology.

2. Head trauma, a history of vestibular neuronitis, or a history of inner ear disease may predispose the patient to develop benign positional vertigo (BPV)

3. BPV is the most common peripheral vestibular disorder.

4. The incidence of Ménière's disease is 10 to 150 cases per 100,000 people

Etiology and Pathophysiology of Peripheral Vertigo

1. Benign positional vertigo

   a. BPV results from calcium-containing crystals that enter the posterior semicircular canal of the labyrinth.

   b. In most cases, the crystals (canaliths) are free-floating within the canal.

   c. When the head is rotated in a specific position, gravity can pull on the crystals, resulting in movement of the perilymph and stimulation of the posterior canal.

   d. These crystals are believed to arise from the otoconial crystals of the otolith organs.

   e. Rarely, canaliths will enter the horizontal or anterior canal.

2. Ménière's disease

   a. Ménière's disease has been thought to result from excess fluid within the endolymphatic compartment of the inner ear (endolymphatic hydrops)

   b. Increases in fluid accumulation would result in rupture of the membranes separating the endolymph and perilymph.

   c. Rupture of the membranes would cause a potassium efflux into the perilymph, resulting in loss of function of sensory hair cells (i.e., the potassium intoxication hypothesis).

   d. Repair of the ruptured membranes would result in a re-establishment of the inner ear fluid and a return to electrolyte balance.

   e. Recent data have brought into question the validity of the potassium intoxication hypothesis and the centrality of endolymphatic hydrops in the pathogenesis of Ménière's disease.

3. Vestibular neuronitis is thought to result from a viral infection of the vestibular nerve.

4. Labyrinthitis may be viral or bacterial (secondary to meningitis or otitis media).

Clinical Features of Peripheral Vestibular Disorders

1. Benign positional vertigo

   a. Vertigo lasting for seconds

   b. Elicited by a rapid change in head position in a nonaxial plane (e.g., rolling over in bed, looking up quickly)

   c. Can be evoked on physical examination by performing a Dix-Hallpike maneuver, in which the patient is rapidly placed in the supine position, with the head turned to the right or left and hanging slightly over the edge of the table.

   d. In the provocative head position, the patient will develop an upbeat and rotatory nystagmus in posterior canal BPV, a downbeat and rotatory nystagmus in anterior canal BPV, and a horizontal nystagmus in horizontal canal BPV.

2. Ménière's disease

   a. Ménière's disease can only be diagnosed when the patient manifests the symptom triad of fluctuating and progressive sensorineural hearing loss, episodic vertigo lasting for hours, and tinnitus. Aural fullness is another common complaint.

   b. This disorder is typically unilateral at the time of onset, but in approximately 45% of cases it will become bilateral.

3. Vestibular neuronitis

   a. Single event of true rotatory vertigo lasting for days

   b. Associated with nausea and vomiting

   c. No associated hearing loss

4. Labyrinthitis

   a. Less common than vestibular neuronitis

   b. Presents with a single episode of vertigo associated with sensorineural hearing loss

   c. More commonly viral in etiology

d. Bacterial labyrinthitis is a rare disorder that presents with vertigo and hearing loss due to local spread of infection from either meningitis or otitis media.

Key Symptoms

- Distinguish between central and peripheral vertigo.

- Determine the cause.

Caveat

- Bacterial labyrinthitis is a rare disorder that presents with vertigo and hearing loss owing to an infection.

Laboratory Testing

1. Auditory testing is indicated in patients reporting auditory deficits associated with their symptoms of vertigo

2. Balance tests are not able to provide a specific diagnosis, but they can help in

   a. Differentiating between central and peripheral vertigo

   b. Determining the side of lesion in peripheral disorders

   c. Determining whether the patient is a candidate for vestibular rehabilitation physical therapy

3. Laboratory testing

   a. In cases of suspected Ménière's disease, a fluorescent treponemal antibody absorption test (FTA-ABS [MHA-TP]) is required to rule out otosyphilis

   b. The reader is referred to appropriate sections of this book for a discussion of the work-up for patients suspected of having a central vascular or degenerative disorder

4. Radiologic testing

   a. Magnetic resonance imaging (MRI) scans with paramagnetic enhancement are indicated in cases of vertigo.

      (1) Associated with other symptoms of central nervous system dysfunction

      (2) Asymmetric hearing loss to rule out a retrocochlear lesion (e.g., acoustic neuroma)

   b. MR arteriography scans of the head and neck are indicated in bad cases of vertigo suspected of resulting from vascular pathology (e.g., vertebrobasilar insufficiency).

TABLE 4–1. KEY SIGNS

Central vertigo
General
 History of migraines, atherosclerotic vascular disease, cardiac arrhythmias or embolic disease, family history of neurofibromatosis type 2
Migrainous vertigo
 Active migraines or history of migraines
 Lasts for minutes to hours
 Not associated with unilateral auditory dysfunction
 May be part of a symptom cluster
Vertebrobasilar insufficiency
 Recurrent episodes
 Lasts for minutes
 May be associated with other neurologic symptoms
Multiple sclerosis
 Young adult patient
 Other neurologic complaints
 Affects up to one half of patients
Lateral medullary syndrome (Wallenberg's syndrome)
 Ipsilateral: ataxia, facial hypesthesia, Horner's syndrome, vocal cord paresis
 Contralateral: pain, temperature sensory dysfunction
Pontine syndrome
 Ipsilateral: tinnitus, facial hemiesthesia, facial paralysis, Horner's syndrome, hearing loss
 Contralateral: hemibody sensory loss
Cerebellar infarction
 Isolated vertigo
 Significant ataxia may accompany vertigo
Neoplasms
 General: unilateral hearing loss and unilateral imbalance
 Meningioma: symptoms similar to acoustic neuroma
 Neurofibromatosis type 2: bilateral acoustic neuroma
 Metastases: facial paralysis
Peripheral vertigo
General: most are idiopathic
Benign positional vertigo (BPV):
 Lasts for seconds
 Elicited by rapid change in head position
 Evoked by Dix-Hallpike maneuver
 In provocative head position,
  Posterior canal BPV: upbeat, rotatory nystagmus
  Anterior canal BPV: downbeat, rotatory nystagmus
  Horizontal canal BPV: horizontal nystagmus
Ménière's disease:
 Triad of fluctuating, progressive sensorineural hearing loss, episodic vertigo lasting for hours; tinnitus
 Aural fullness
 Unilateral at onset
 Almost half become bilateral
Vestibular neuronitis
 Single event of true rotatory vertigo
 Last for days
 Nausea and vomiting
 No hearing loss
Labyrinthitis
 Single event of vertigo with sensorineural hearing loss

Key Tests

- Auditory testing

- Balance testing

- For Ménière's disease, an FTA-ABS or MHA-TP to rule out otosyphilis

• MRI for central pathology

• MRA for vascular pathology

TREATMENT

Central Vestibular Disorders

1. The reader is referred to appropriate sections of this book for discussions pertaining to the treatment of central vascular or demyelinating disorders

2. When infrequent, migrainous vertigo is treated with a vestibular suppressant (e.g., diazepam, 2 to 5 mg, orally 3 times a day, or meclizine, 25 mg orally 3 times a day). Migraine drug prophylaxis (e.g., nortriptyline, 50 mg, QHS) when the migrainous vertigo occurs frequently (e.g., once or twice a month).

Peripheral Vestibular Disorders

1. The Epley canalith repositioning maneuver is the treatment of choice for the treatment of acute BPV (see Part IX, Chapter 5, Benign Positional Vertigo, Figure 5–1).

2. The mainstays of treatment for Ménière's disease include diuretics and a low-salt diet. Whether these treatments address the underlying pathology or reflect the considerable nonspecific (or placebo) response seen in patients with Ménière's disease is unclear.

3. Vestibular suppressants are used for acute vertiginous episodes associated with Ménière's disease.

4. Surgical options for patients with Ménière's disease that is not responsive to conservative regimens include gentamicin inner ear perfusion, endolymphatic shunt surgery, vestibular nerve section, or labyrinthectomy.

5. Viral vestibular neuronitis and labyrinthitis are treated with vestibular suppressants. The addition of corticosteroids (e.g., prednisone 1–2 mg/kg per day for 7 to 14 days) may diminish the degree of vestibular deficit or hearing loss associated with these disorders.

6. Bacterial labyrinthitis is treated with antibiotics and corticosteroids. Surgical intervention is required if the etiology is otitis media

7. Vestibular rehabilitation physical therapy is very useful in treating patients with symptoms of a noncompensated vestibular loss. These residual symptoms of imbalance and lightheadedness can

TABLE 4–2. KEY TREATMENTS

Central vertigo
Vestibular suppressants for migrainous vertigo
See corresponding chapters for treatments of central vascular or demyelinative disorders: vertebrobasilar insufficiency, multiple sclerosis, lateral medullary syndrome (Wallenberg's syndrome), pontine syndrome, cerebellar infarction, neoplasms
Peripheral vertigo
Benign positional vertigo: Epley canalith repositioning maneuver
Ménière's disease: diuretics, and low-salt diet; vestibular suppressants for acute episodes; surgical options
Vestibular neuronitis: vestibular suppressants
Labyrinthitis: vestibular suppressants; surgical intervention if the cause is otitis media
Bacterial labyrinthitis: antibiotics and corticosteriods

be seen subsequent to vertiginous episodes resulting from any of the causes discussed above.

8. Surgical resection remains the treatment of choice for acoustic neuromas. Focused stereotactic radiation therapy may be a therapeutic alternative.

 Key Treatments

• Central vertigo: Migrainous vertigo, vestibular suppressant

• Peripheral vertigo: Benign positional vertigo, Epley canalith repositioning maneuver

• Ménière's disease, vestibular neuronitis, and labyrinthitis, vestibular suppressants

Prognosis and Complications

1. Vertigo resulting from any peripheral cause can be well controlled and carries an excellent prognosis.

2. The resolution of imbalance and ataxia subsequent to a central event carries a more guarded prognosis, particularly for recovery of balance function.

 Bibliography

Baloh RW: Episodic vertigo: central nervous system causes. Curr Opin Neurol 15:17–21, 2002.

El-Kashan HK, Telian SA: Diagnosis and initiating treatment for peripheral system disorders. Otolaryngol Clin North Am 33:563–577, 2000.

Ruckenstein MJ: Vertigo and dysequilibrium with associated hearing loss. Otolaryngol Clin North Am 33:535–562, 2000.

Ruckenstein MJ, Rutka JA, Hawke M: The treatment of Ménière's disease: Torok revisited. Laryngoscope 101:211–218, 1991.

Shepard NT, Telian SA, Smith-Wheelock M, et al.: Vestibular and balance rehabilitation therapy. Ann Otol Rhinol Laryngol 102:198-205, 1993.

Solomon DW: Distinguishing and treating causes of central vertigo. Otolaryngol Clin North Am 33:579–601, 2000.

Definition

1. Benign paroxysmal positional vertigo (BPPV) is characterized by brief bouts of a spinning sensation and nystagmus provoked by changes in head orientation with respect to gravity. The nystagmus is elicited by positional testing and has a specific direction and duration.

2. In the vast majority of cases, BPPV involves the posterior semicircular canal of the labyrinth of one inner ear, resulting in the characteristic upbeating and torsional nystagmus elicited with Dix-Hallpike testing. In less than 10% of cases, it may be present bilaterally or involve other canals.

Epidemiology and Risk Factors

1. Most common etiology for vertigo
2. Predisposing factors
   a. Increasing incidence with age
   b. Head trauma in 10% of cases and 20% of bilateral cases
   c. Following vestibular neuritis, even if caloric response is absent on affected side
   d. Migraine
   e. Ménière's syndrome
   f. Family history
3. Incidence about 64 per 100,000. In elderly patients, the incidence may be as high as 8%.

Etiology and Pathophysiology

1. All of the features of typical BPPV are explained by the abnormal presence of mobile, dense particles in the posterior semicircular canal of the vestibular labyrinth. This material is calcium carbonate crystals (otoconia) dislodged from the otolith organ.

2. When the head is tilted with respect to gravity, particles will move in the canal to the lowest point. Particle movement causes fluid (endolymph) flow within the canal similar to that caused by continuous head rotation or caloric stimulation.

Clinical Features

1. Spinning sensation "like a clock"
   a. When sitting or standing, brought about by pitch-plane head movement, e.g., looking up at a high shelf or rising from a bent-over position
   b. Rolling over in bed, lying down or arising in the morning
2. Nausea and possibly vomiting, diaphoresis, pallor (motion sickness)
3. Imbalance and falls possible
4. The duration of the actual vertigo must be less than 1 minute, typically less than 30 seconds.
   a. Patients often overestimate duration.
   b. Nausea and dysequilibrium may persist.
   c. Several spells may occur in succession if provocative head movements are repeated.
5. Elicited with the Dix-Hallpike maneuver
   a. Patient's head is rotated horizontally 45 degrees while sitting with legs extended on the examination table (Fig. 5–1A).
   b. Keeping the head turned, the patient is then deliberately brought into the supine position (Fig. 1B).
   c. Observe for nystagmus and asks about the onset and duration of vertigo.
      (1) The nystagmus is best observed without fixation, using Fresnel lenses or having the patient look at a blank wall.
      (2) Nystagmus occurs after a latency of several seconds
      (3) Quick phases have upbeating and torsional components, so the upper poles of the eyes beat toward the dependent ear.
      (4) May reverse direction when brought back into the seated position.
      (5) Fatigues with repeated maneuvers, but it is not necessary to establish this.
   d. The patient is brought back upright before repeating the series of movements with the head turned in the opposite direction.

Key Signs

- Vertigo after change in head position (rolling over in bed, looking up)

- Dix-Hallpike maneuver elicits nystagmus and vertigo.

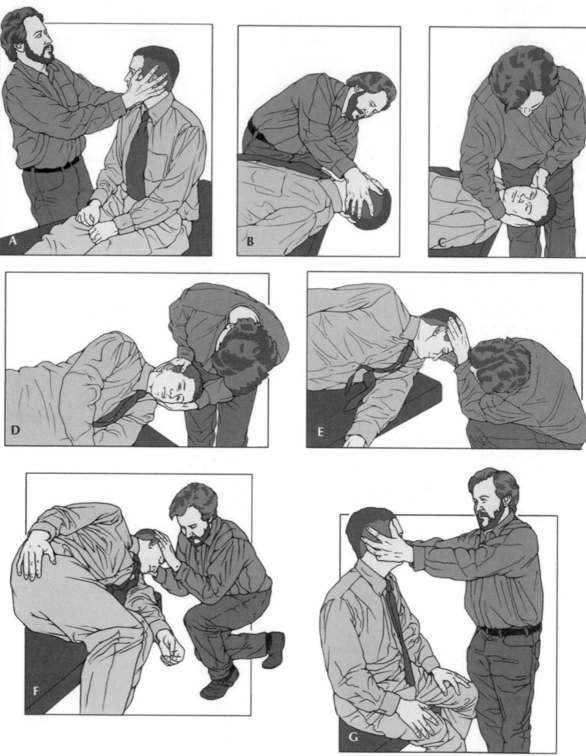

Figure 5–1. Canalith repositioning procedure shown for treatment of benign paroxysmal positional vertigo involving the right posterior semicircular canal. The procedure begins with the Dix-Hall pike maneuver on the affected side (**A** and **B**). **A.** With the patient seated on the examining table, the examiner rotates the head 45 degrees horizontally. **B.** With the head held at the 45 degree position, the patient is eased into the supine position, with the head extending beyond the edge of the examining table. **C.** The head is then rotated 90 degrees away from the affected ear. **D** and **E.** With the head held in position, the patient rolls into the lateral decubitus position (away from the affected ear). **F** and **G.** After a brief interval the patient is brought upright. This is facilitated by keeping the head turned, with the chin close to the chest, and having the patient draw his knees upward, toward the chest while allowing his legs to fall away from the table edge.

- Nystagmus has all of these features: latency, up-beating and torsional direction (toward dependent ear), duration less than 60 seconds.

- Frequently associated with nausea and imbalance

Differential Diagnosis

1. BPPV may be diagnosed with certainty if the nystagmus has *all* of the following characteristics: it begins following a latency of usually 2 to 10 seconds, it has an upbeating and torsional direction, lasts less than 1 minute (generally less than 30 seconds), and is most strongly elicited in the appropriate head position.

2. Lateral (horizontal) semicircular canal variant

   a. Vertigo is elicited in the supine patient by turning the head.

   b. Nystagmus is horizontal, may have little or no latency, and can last more than 1 minute.

   c. Nystagmus will change direction when the head is turned so that the other ear is down.

   d. When due to free-floating debris in the horizontal canal, nystagmus is geotropic—quick phases beat toward the ground.

   e. When due to material adherent to the cupula of the canal, nystagmus is ageotropic—quick phases beat away from the ground.

   f. When nystagmus is geotropic, it is strongest with the affected ear downward.

   g. When nystagmus is ageotropic, it is strongest with the affected ear upward.

2. Brainstem and cerebellar lesions can cause a persistent or transient positional vertigo and nystagmus.

   a. Common in posterior fossa tumors, Chiari malformation, cerebellar degeneration, and multiple sclerosis

   b. Purely vertical or purely torsional positional nystagmus is central in origin.

   c. Gaze-evoked nystagmus or spontaneous downbeat nystagmus are *not* consistent with BPPV.

3. Microvascular compression affecting the eighth cranial nerve may rarely be a cause of positional vertigo.

   a. Nystagmus may be elicited with hyperventilation as well as with certain head positions.

   b. This condition responds well to carbamazepine.

4. Presyncopal dizziness may be positional, but it does not occur with rolling over in bed.

Laboratory Testing

Electronystagmography may document the presence of nystagmus during positional testing,

1. Most laboratories record only horizontal and possibly vertical components of eye rotation; torsional nystagmus is not accurately reflected in the tracings.

2. A description of the nystagmus by the person performing the test can be helpful, especially if symptoms are noted or if a video eye-movement-recording system is used.

3. Caloric and standard rotational chair testing only reflect lateral canal function; because the posterior canal is innervated by a different division of the eighth nerve, BPPV can still occur in an ear with an absent response to ice-water irrigation.

Radiologic Features

There are no radiographic findings in BPPV.

Key Tests

- No findings on radiography for BPPV

- Electronystagmography

Treatment

1. The canalith repositioning procedure (CRP; Epley maneuver) is a safe and effective treatment in most patients with posterior canal BPPV, and is easily performed at the bedside at the time of diagnosis.

2. The affected side must first be determined by the Dix-Hallpike maneuver, as the treatment depends on which ear is involved.

3. In bilateral cases, treat one ear initially, and if necessary treat the second ear several days later.

4. A series of head rotations (Fig. 5–1) moves the responsible material around the posterior canal and into the vestibule, where it does not cause symptoms.

   a. CRP begins by again performing the Dix-Hallpike maneuver on the affected side (Fig. 5–1A and B).

   b. The latency before onset of the nystagmus and the duration of nystagmus are noted.

   c. When symptoms and eye movements abate, without sitting upright, the head is rotated on the supine body 90 degrees away from the affected ear (Fig. 5–1C), so that the nonaffected ear is now toward the ground.

   d. Maintain all positions for the same amount of

time (latency + duration of nystagmus seen initially).

e. Next, the head is kept turned on the body as the patient rolls into the lateral decubitus position (away from the affected ear), so that the nose is now pointed downward (Fig. 5–1D and E).

f. After the appropriate interval, keeping the chin tucked toward the chest and the head turned, the patient is brought into the upright sitting position. This is facilitated by having the knees brought toward the chest and dangling the legs off the side of the examination table (Fig. 5–1F and G).

g. Be certain to hold the patient securely at this point, as he or she may experience a strong sensation of vertigo and imbalance as the debris moves out of the canal.

5. The whole procedure should be repeated at least once to confirm the success of the therapy, and repeated procedures may be necessary before no nystagmus is noted.

6. Patients are advised to keep the head upright for the remainder of the day.

 Key Treatments

- Canalith repositioning maneuver
- Brandt-Daroff exercises

Prognosis and Complications

1. Nausea and vomiting may occur in susceptible individuals during testing. Pretreatment with an antiemetic medication (e.g., promethazine) may be used.

2. When moving material out of the posterior canal, there is a chance that it will relocate into another canal (on the same side). The most frequent conversion is from the posterior to the horizontal semicircular canal.

a. This is more likely to occur if the head is not maintained in the proper position when the patient is brought upright (Fig. 5–1F and G).

b. If particles do enter the horizontal canal, it may be treated by a log-roll maneuver: Beginning with the affected ear downward and the patient lying flat on the table, the head and body are rotated 360 degrees in the direction of the unaffected ear, and the patient is instructed to sleep for several nights with the affected ear upward.

3. BPPV may recur in up to 50% of cases.

4. Patients, spouses or caregivers may be instructed in performing a repositioning procedure if the affected side is known.

5. Occasionally, patients will require physical therapy for gait and balance training with a therapist trained in vestibular rehabilitation.

Prevention

1. Brandt-Daroff exercises were effectively used to treat BPPV prior to development of the CRP, and when performed after treatment can reduce recurrence and continued symptoms.

a. Patient sits on the edge of the bed and turns the head 45 degrees to right.

b. Maintaining the head turn, the patient lies on left side (the legs may be brought up onto the bed if desired) so the head is pointed 45 degrees upward.

c. This position is held until any provoked symptoms resolve.

d. The patient returns to the sitting position, and only then turns the head back to center.

e. The whole sequence is then repeated with a left head turn and lying on the right side.

2. These exercises have an important role in recovery, and should be initiated the day following CRP treatment

a. Often patients are reluctant to assume positions that previously reliably reproduced their symptoms, and may experience anxiety and even nausea as a conditioned response.

b. Repeated exercises can habituate these maladaptive responses.

c. Performance of Brandt-Daroff exercises once each morning may also reduce the risk of recurrence.

d. If the BPPV nevertheless has returned, finding out first thing in the morning while still seated in bed is preferable to discovering it under potentially more hazardous conditions.

e. The affected ear can be determined, since vertigo is generally present only on one side (symptoms with head turned right and lying on the left side = left posterior canal BPPV).

3. Avoiding positions in which the head is partially upside down may be helpful in cases with frequent recurrence of BPPV.

Pregnancy

1. There is no known adverse effect of treatment during pregnancy

2. No increased incidence of BPPV in pregnancy has been reported

Bibliography

Buttner U, Helmchen C, Brandt T: Diagnostic criteria for central versus peripheral positioning nystagmus and vertigo: A review. Acta Oto-Laryngologica 119:1–5, 1999.

Epley JM: Positional vertigo related to semicircular canalithiasis. Otolaryngol Head Neck Surg 112:154–161, 1995.

Furman JM, Cass SP: Benign paroxysmal positional vertigo. N Engl J Med 341:1590–1596, 1999.

Lanska DJ, Remler B: Benign paroxysmal positioning vertigo: Classic descriptions, origins of the provocative positioning technique, and conceptual developments. Neurology 48:1167–1177, 1997.

David Solomon

Definition

1. Facial nerve palsy results from a lesion affecting the seventh cranial nerve distal to its exit from the lateral pons, but shares features with brainstem lesions involving the nucleus.

2. Bell's (idiopathic facial) palsy is the term used for most cases of acute facial palsy for which no immediate cause is apparent, although there is evidence for a viral etiology, specifically herpes simplex type I.

Epidemiology and Risk Factors

1. The incidence is about 25/100,000 per year, with each side of the face having similar incidence.

2. Less than 1% of cases are bilateral.

3. Increased risk in endemic areas for Lyme disease

4. Increasing incidence with age

5. Diabetes causes a fourfold increased risk.

6. Family history is positive in 10% of cases

7. May occur early in human immunodeficiency virus infection, or in later stages of acquired immunodeficiency syndrome

Etiology and Pathophysiology

Likely etiology of Bell's palsy is acute inflammation and edema of the facial nerve, resulting in compression and ischemia or entrapment within the facial canal of the temporal bone.

1. Focal conduction block is the mildest form of injury; no wallerian degeneration occurs, and fibers distal to the lesion and can conduct impulses.

2. Axonal damage results in distal degeneration.

3. Injury to endoneurium and perineurium compromises regrowth of the nerve.

Clinical Features

1. The weakness is in a "peripheral" pattern, involving that half of the face

   a. Cranial nerve VII innervates muscles of facial expression, posterior digastric, and platysma.

   b. Frontalis muscle is involved, unlike "central" lesions.

2. Evolves over hours to 2 days

3. Usually weakness is complete; partial in one third of cases

4. Intraparenchymal ipsilateral brainstem lesions involving the facial nucleus or fascicles will also have a "peripheral pattern," but these lesions usually involve the abducens nerve or are associated with a contralateral hemiparesis and/or ataxia.

5. Hypesthesia of the posterior wall of the external auditory canal (Hitzelberger's sign)

6. Localization of lesion can sometimes be determined from associated features.

   a. Hyperacusis occurs in one third of cases because of paralysis of the stapedius muscle. It indicates lesion in the tympanic segment of nerve or proximally in the labyrinthine segment, the internal auditory canal, or the subarachnoid space.

   b. Loss of taste sensation from the anterior two thirds of the tongue is due to involvement of nervus intermedius, or chorda tympani. This indicates lesion in the mastoid segment at a point prior to exit via stylomastoid foramen or proximally.

   c. Isolated facial motor paralysis occuring distal to the stylomastoid foramen is due to parotid lesions (tumor, sarcoidosis, mononucleosis), trauma, or retromandibular lymphadenopathy.

7. Pain around the ear and facial sensory changes are commonly described.

8. Bell's phenomenon, the normal upward rotation of the eyes during attempted closure, becomes visible because of the inability to close the eyelid.

9. Synkinesis or contracture (see below) indicates subacute onset, chronic nerve compression, or recurrent palsy.

Key Signs

- Unilateral facial weakness involving upper and lower facial muscles

- Onset over less than 48 hours

- Associated with hyperacusis and loss of taste

Differential Diagnosis

1. Central facial palsy occurs in lesions of the contralateral cortex, subcortical white matter, or internal capsule.
   a. Corticobulbar fibers from the lower third of the precentral gyrus pass in the genu of the internal capsule and reach the pons via the medial part of the cerebral peduncle.
   b. Most fibers decussate and innervate the portion of the contralateral facial motor nucleus in the pons that controls the lower face.
   c. Facial expressions elicited by emotional responses or with laughter may be spared.

2. Herpes zoster oticus (Ramsay Hunt syndrome) is acute peripheral facial palsy associated with severe ear pain and a lesion.
   a. Occurs in response to varicella-zoster virus (VZV) reactivation in the geniculate ganglion, with antibody titers often corroborating the diagnosis.
   b. Vesicular lesions are usually found in the external ear or ear canal; sometimes on the soft palate.
   c. Shingles may be absent, but an increase in serum and cerebrospinal fluid (CSF) VZV antibody titer may be found.
   d. Extension to the eighth cranial nerve may cause vertigo and hearing changes, while less often cranial nerves V, IX, X and upper cervical nerves may become involved.
   e. Only 50% of affected patients regain normal facial function.

3. Lyme neuroborreliosis can present with facial palsy alone.
   a. Lyme-induced facial palsies may be as common or more common than idiopathic Bell's palsy in endemic areas.
      (1) Northeast, Midwest, and Western United States and wherever white-tailed deer, white-footed mice, or both are found.
      (2) Most common in summer months, except in the West when it occurs from January to May.
   b. The disease evolves in stages.
      (1) Stage I: pathognomonic "bull's-eye rash" or erythema chronicum migrans, headache, fever, stiff neck, and myalgias
      (2) Stage II (early disseminated): occurs with neurologic manifestations in 15% of patients weeks to months after the rash
   c. Cranial nerve palsies, especially VII, are frequent

   d. CSF examination shows an aseptic meningitis with lymphocytic predominance.
   e. Antibodies directed against *Borrelia burgdorferi* may be present in the CSF, and polymerase chain reaction testing is available.
   f. Lyme infection can cause both an axonal and a demyelinative neuropathy.
   g. Intravenous antibiotic therapy is indicated (ceftriaxone, 2 g/day, for 14 days).

4. Trauma is a leading cause of facial nerve paralysis.
   a. 80% of temporal bone fractures are longitudinal, with facial nerve damage occurring in up to 20% of injuries.
   b. Transverse temporal bone fractures are less common (20%) but carry a 50% risk of facial nerve injury, along with hearing loss and vertigo.
   c. Birth trauma accounts for 80% of facial palsies in the newborn.

5. Acute otitis media is the main cause of facial palsy in children, but it remains rare before 10 years of age. Chronic otitis may develop palsy secondary to cholesteatoma.

6. Tumor accounts for 5% of facial palsies.
   a. One fourth of neoplastic cases present with sudden weakness mimicking Bell's palsy.
   b. Malignancy as a cause of peripheral facial palsy is suggested when
      (1) Weakness progresses over weeks instead of days
      (2) No return of function is seen within 6 weeks of onset or an incomplete paresis does not resolve in 2 months.
      (3) Paralysis is preceded by an adventitious facial movement disorder
      (4) Ear or face pain persists
      (5) Recurrent palsy occurs with involvement of neighboring cranial nerves, and when a mass is present in the ear, neck, or parotid gland.

7. Sarcoidosis is a chronic noncaseating granulomatous inflammatory disease with hilar adenopathy.
   a. VII is most commonly affected cranial nerve, with abrupt onset of weakness following parotitis.
   b. Elevated serum calcium and angiotensin-converting enzyme levels
   c. Confirmed with conjuctival or lip biopsy; gallium scan

8. Möbius' syndrome is a congenital condition causing facial diplegia and abduction deficits.
   a. Facial palsies may be complete or partial and

are generally accompanied by other cranial neuropathies, most commonly VI and XII.

   b. When skeletal and craniofacial abnormalities are also present, there is little risk of familial recurrence (<2%); familial transmission is more common (25% to 30%) when no skeletal defects are found.

9. Melkersson-Rosenthal syndrome is a rare sporadic condition with recurrent, sequential, bilateral facial palsies, facial nonpitting edema, migraine headache, and lingua plicata (fissuring of the tongue).

10. Facial diplegia is a feature of myotonic and facioscapulohumeral muscular dystrophy (Table 6–1).

Laboratory Testing

1. Serum studies: Lyme titer, ACE, treponemal antibodies, thyroid stimulating hormone, glucose. Also consider lead, HIV, Epstein-Barr, PPD (purified protein derivative) for tuberculosis

2. Audiogram is helpful to evaluate the stapedius reflex and eighth nerve involvement.

3. Prognosis for recovery may be predicted by recording the compound motor action potential (CMAP) generated by a supramaximal electrical stimulus (electroneurography).

   a. This test should not be performed within 10 days of onset.

   b. ENOG is most reliable 2 to 3 weeks after onset.

      (1) If the CMAP amplitude is reduced by

TABLE 6–1. DIFFERENTIAL DIAGNOSIS OF PERIPHERAL FACIAL NERVE PALSY

Idiopathic (Bell's palsy)*
Infectious: Herpes simplex, herpes zoster, otitis media, Lyme,* human immunodeficiency virus,* syphilis,* mononucleosis,* mastoiditis, poliomyelitis, meningitis,* malaria, leprosy, rubella, mumps,* osteomyelitis, cat-scratch disease
Inflammatory: Guillain-Barré syndrome,* sarcoidosis,* multiple sclerosis, arteritis, Melkersson-Rosenthal syndrome,* Behçet syndrome, Wegener's granulomatosis, lymphomatoid granulomatosis, Kawasaki disease, angioedema, Tolosa-Hunt syndrome, amyloidosis, idiopathic cranial pachymeningitis*
Neoplastic: Schwannoma, neurofibroma, meningioma, cholesteatoma, parotid gland tumor, metastasis, carcinomatous meningitis,* leukemia
Metabolic: Diabetes mellitus, hypothyroidism, uremia, porphyria
Trauma*: Surgery, temporal bone fracture (transverse > horizontal)
Other: Congenital and familial, Paget's disease,* osteoporosis, hypertension, post vaccination, pontine infarction, myasthenia gravis, external carotid artery aneurysm, lumbar extradural blood patch, vascular malformation, pseudotumor cerebri

*Also commonly found in bilateral facial nerve palsy.
From Stern BJ, Wityk RJ, Lewis RF: Disorders of the cranial nerves and brain stem. In Joynt RJ (eds), Clinical Neurology, revised ed. Philadelphia, Lippincott Co, 1993, pp. 1–90.

greater than 90% compared to the intact side, the prognosis for recovery is poor.

      (2) Though controversial, some evidence suggests that surgical decompression of the meatal foramen might improve outcome in patients with poor prognosis based on electrophysiologic studies (see below).

Radiologic Features

1. VII nerve enhancement within the internal auditory canal may be seen in Bell's palsy, but may also be due to schwannoma, Lyme disease, lymphoma, hemangioma, sarcoidosis, or spread of tumor from the subarachnoid space.

2. Magnetic resonance imaging (MRI) with gadolinium should be performed when there is suspicion of a cerebellopontine angle tumor (hearing loss, gradual onset of weakness), other neurologic deficits, trauma, recurrent palsy, and if no recovery is noted after 1 month.

3. Computed tomography (CT) scan is the study of choice to rule out temporal bone fracture.

Key Tests

• Serum studies

• Audiogram

• Electroneurogram

• MRI with gadolinium for tumor

• CT scan to rule out fracture

Treatment

1. For Bell's palsy, early treatment with oral steroids is *probably* effective to improve facial functional outcome: Oral prednisone, 1 mg/kg per day, for 10 days, followed by a taper to zero over 10 days.

2. Early treatment with antiviral agents in combination with prednisone is recommended as *possibly* effective to improve facial functional outcome: Oral acyclovir, 500 mg, 4 times a day for 10 days.

3. There is not enough evidence to recommend facial nerve decompression to improve recovery.

4. Surgical anastomosis of cranial nerve XII to VII is an option in patients with poor recovery of function.

5. In Ramsay Hunt syndrome, antiviral therapy with valacyclovir, 1 g orally 3 times a day for 2 weeks, should be initiated within 48 hours.

Key Treatments

- Oral steroids
- Antiviral therapy
- Eye protection

Prognosis and Complications

1. More than two thirds of patients have a complete recovery, with 84% achieving near-normal function.

2. Bell's palsy leaves more than 8,000 people in the United States each year with permanent facial weakness.

3. Very few patients with partial weakness have residual long-term deficits.

4. In complete palsies, the reappearance of facial movement within 1 month of onset predicts an excellent recovery.

5. Regrowth of axons occurs at approximately 1 mm/day if surrounding glial elements and connective tissue remains intact

   a. Regenerating motor fibers may be misdirected from their intended target (aberrant regeneration) and motor units often have abnormal activity, resulting in contractures.

   b. Synkinesis is the abnormal concurrent activation of different muscles not usually contracting together.

      (1) Tearing when eating

      (2) Eye closure with mouth opening or contraction around the mouth with blinking

      (3) When severe, botulinum toxin injections may be helpful.

6. Painful neuromas adjacent to the injured nerve may result from growth of axon sprouts outside of the nerve sheath.

7. Corneal damage may occur if the lid does not close completely and the eye is not protected. Lubricants and patching are strongly advised.

8. Approximately 10% of patients with Bell's palsy will have a recurrence (on either side).

Prevention

Recent findings suggest that antibiotic treatment for Lyme disease at the time of exposure may prevent infection.

Pregnancy

Facial palsy is more likely to occur during pregnancy, particularly in the third trimester.

1. Frequency of Bell's palsy in pregnant women is 45/100,000 births.

2. For nonpregnant women the incidence is 17.4/100,000 per year.

Facial Motor Paroxysms

1. Hemifacial spasm consists of frequent, repetitive unilateral involuntary movement of facial nerve innervated muscles.

   a. May be brief, lasting less than 1 second, or prolonged

   b. Usually involves several muscles, often with blinking.

   c. Accompanied by high frequency motor unit discharges on electromyography (EMG).

   d. The mechanism in most cases is likely neurovascular compression by ectatic vessels in the posterior circulation.

      (1) Rule out compressive lesions (arteriovenous malformation, tumor, Paget's disease).

      (2) May follow Bell's palsy or stroke

      (3) Appearance in young adult patients suggests multiple sclerosis.

   e. Treatment with botulinum toxin is often performed, but it requires repeated injections.

   f. Suboccipital craniectomy for microvascular decompression of cranial nerve VII is an effective treatment.

   g. Carbamazepine, baclofen, or clonazepam may be effective.

2. Blepharospasm is a bilateral sustained forceful closure of the eyes. It is an involuntary focal dystonia, although it may be reduced when the patient is distracted

3. Facial myokymia usually occurs in the obicularis oculi, is often benign, and is more likely to occur with anxiety, fatigue, or after exercise.

   a. Involuntary wormlike, writhing, undulating small movements just under the surface of the skin.

   b. EMG showing a pattern of quiet alternating with rhythmic burst discharges

   c. Reported with brainstem lesions (multiple sclerosis, pontine neoplasm)

   d. Can occur after radiation therapy

   e. When generalized throughout the body and

associated with stiffness and hyperreflexia, it is termed Isaacs' syndrome.

4. Tardive dyskinesia (cervicolinguomasticatory syndrome) is involuntary dystonic or dyskinetic movements of the lips, face, jaw, tongue, or limbs. It occurs with the chronic use of neuroleptic medications.

5. Trismus is a spasm of the masseter muscles, and is a classic sign of tetanus from *Clostridium* infection.

   a. Initially occurs in response to sensory stimulation, then becomes spontaneous.

   b. Tetanus also involves spinal extensors; abdominal and laryngeal muscles.

6. Palatal tremor (palatal myoclonus), is brief, rhythmic involuntary movements of the soft palate.

   a. Essential palatal tremor involves the tensor veli palatini, innervated by the third division of the trigeminal nerve.

      (1) Associated with an audible click due to the origin of the muscle near the eustachian tube.

      (2) Benign course, but tinnitus may be disabling

   b. Symptomatic palatal tremor is rhythmic contraction of the levator veli palatini, innervated by cranial nerve VII.

      (1) Associated with pseudohypertrophy of the inferior olive, a hyperintense area on T_2-weighted MRI images in the upper medulla.

      (2) Olivary hypertrophy is contralateral to the tremor when unilateral, and cerebellar signs may be found on the same side as the tremor.

      (3) Occurs with lesions affecting the outflow of the cerebellum from the dentate nucleus via the superior cerebellar peduncle, the red nucleus, or the central tegmental tract (Guillain-Mollaret triangle).

   c. Persists during sleep

Caveat

• Hemifacial spasm in young adult patients suggests multiple sclerosis.

Bibliography

Adler CH, Zimmerman RA, Savino PJ: Hemifacial spasm: Evaluation by magnetic resonance imaging and magnetic resonance tomographic angiography. Ann Neurol 32:502–506, 1992.

Adour KK: Diagnosis and management of facial paralysis. N Engl J Med 307:348, 1982.

Deuschl G, Toro C, Valls-Solé J, et al.: Symptomatic and essential palatal tremor. 1. Clinical, physiological and MRI analysis. Brain 117:775–788, 1994.

Grogan PM, Gronseth GS: Practice parameter: Steroids, acyclovir, and surgery for Bell's palsy (an evidence-based review). Report of the Quality Standards Subcommittee of the American Academy of Neurology. Neurology 56:830–836, 2001.

Illingworth RD, Porter DG, Jakubowski J: Hemifacial spasm: A prospective long-term follow up of 83 cases treated by microvascular decompression at two neurosurgical centres in the United Kingdom. J Neurol Neurosurg Psychiatry 60:72–77, 1996.

Stern BJ, Wityk RJ, Lewis RF: Disorders of the cranial nerves and brain stem. In Joynt RJ (ed): Clinical Neurology, revised ed. Philadelphia, Lippincott, 1993, pp.1–90.

7 Disorders of Smell and Taste
David Solomon

Definition

1. Disorders of smell may involve the olfactory receptors, first cranial nerve, frontal compressive lesions, and limbic structures.

2. Nerve-related disorders of taste are covered in Chapter 6.

Epidemiology and Risk Factors

1. Age: More than three fourths of individuals over 80 years of age have major deficits perceiving and identifying odors.

2. Reduced sensitivity for taste sensation occurs with normal aging.

3. Many medications that otherwise healthy elderly patients use further decrease sensitivity. In one study, average detection thresholds for salt were more than 10 times higher for elderly patients taking an average of 3.4 medications to treat one or more medical conditions.

4. More severe deficits occur in patients with protein malnutrition.

Etiology and Pathophysiology

1. Olfactory receptors in the nasal mucosa are examples of regenerating neural tissue derived from ectodermal stem cells.

   a. Fibers penetrate the cribiform plate of the ethmoid bone, and enter the olfactory bulb.

   b. The olfactory tract runs along the orbital surface of the frontal lobes dorsal to the optic nerves and chiasm and divides into the medial and lateral olfactory stria.

   c. Projections are contralateral (via the anterior commissure) and ipsilateral to the piriform cortex, amygdaloid, and septal nuclei and hypothalamus.

   d. This represents the only sensory system without a thalamic relay.

2. Anosmia may be an early sign of several neurodegenerative disorders (Parkinson's disease, Alzheimer's disease).

3. Histologic changes characteristic of Alzheimer's disease are common in the olfactory bulb and its projection areas, even in the nondemented elderly.

4. Anosmia is most commonly due to nasal or sinus inflammation or upper respiratory infection, and is then bilateral.

5. Head trauma, with or without skull fracture, is a common cause of anosmia. Rhinorrhea should be examined for glucose; if present, a cerebrospinal fluid (CSF) leak is likely, and meningitis may ensue.

6. Unilateral anosmia may precede frontal lobe symptoms if mass lesions in that area are compressing the olfactory nerve; smell should be evaluated in patients with frontal lobe signs.

Clinical Features

1. Patients with anosmia experience decreased taste sensation, as olfaction plays a large role in perception of taste. If taste is lost due to olfactory dysfunction, appreciation of food temperature and spiciness should be maintained.

Key Signs

- Anosmia and rhinorrhea suggest a CSF leak after head trauma

- Decreased taste suggests anosmia

Differential Diagnosis

1. Anosmia is a component of the Foster-Kennedy syndrome (frontal mass lesion), along with ipsilateral optic atrophy and contralateral papilledema.

2. Raised intracranial pressure alone may impair the sense of smell.

3. Kallmann's syndrome is an X-linked disorder with ansomia and hypogonadism.

4. Hallucinations of unpleasant odors are a common aura of temporal lobe epilepsy.

Caveat

- Anosmia may be early sign of Parkinson's disease or Alzheimer's disease.

Laboratory Testing

1. Testing consists of determining if patients can perceive the smell of a non-noxious substance (which can excite trigeminal fibers in the nasal mucosa) in each nostril.
2. Formal evaluation can be performed at the bedside (University of Pennsylvania Smell Identification Test; commercially available from Sensonics, Inc. Haddonfield, NJ).

Radiologic Features

Frontal lobe mass

Key Tests
• Rhinorrhea for glucose
• Smell Identification Test at bedside
• Imaging for fontal lobe lesion

Treatment

Nutritional considerations in elderly to keep food palatable and appetizing.

Key Treatment
• Nutritional consultation for advice about inadvertent noncompliance

Prognosis and Complications

1. Patients with anosmia may not detect dangerous conditions such as a gas leak or smoke from a house fire.
2. Loss of sweet sensation may cause diabetics to unknowingly exceed sugar intake.
3. Sodium-sensitive hypertensive patients may inadvertently be noncompliant in their diet.

Bibliography

Doty RL: Olfactory capacities in aging and Alzheimer's disease: Psychological and anatomic considerations. Ann NY Acad Sci 640:20, 1991.

Mann NM: Management of smell and taste problems. Cleve Clin J Med 69:329–336, 2002.

Nores JM, Biacabe B, Bonfils P: Olfactory disorders due to medications: analysis and review of the literature. Rev Med Interne 21:972–977, 2000.

Schiffman SS: Taste and smell losses in normal aging and disease. JAMA 278:1357–1362, 1997.

8 Facial Numbness

Definition

1. Facial numbness can occur with lesions involving cortex, subcortical white matter, thalamus, brainstem, and fifth (trigeminal) nerve.

2. Fifth nerve lesions causing numbness may be preganglionic, involve the gasserian ganglion, or occur in one or more of the three major divisions (ophthalmic, V1; maxillary, V2; mandibular V3) or their peripheral branches.

Epidemiology and Risk Factors

1. Epidemiology depends on which of the diverse etiologies are being considered.

2. Risk factors include multiple sclerosis, connective tissue disease, malignancy, cerebrovascular disease

Etiology and Pathophysiology

1. The trigeminal nerve is the largest of the cranial nerves.

2. The motor portion innervates the masseter, temporalis, pterygoids, tensor tympani, tensor veli palatini, mylohyoid, and anterior belly of the digastric muscles.

   a. Cortical supranuclear motor pathways are bilateral, but predominantly contralateral.

   b. Upper motor neurons are in the lower third of the precentral gyrus, and project via the corona radiata, internal capsule, and cerebral peduncle, with decussation in the upper pons.

   c. Corticobulbar fibers project onto trigeminal neurons in the motor nucleus of cranial nerve V in the mid-pons, medial to the main sensory nucleus, near the floor of the fourth ventricle.

   d. Lower motor neuron axons exit the anterolateral pons into the subarachnoid space.

   e. The motor nerve enters Meckel's cave (on the medial petrous bone in the middle cranial fossa) and runs beneath the gasserian ganglion, exiting the middle fossa via the foramen ovale as part of mandibular division (V3).

3. The trigeminal sensory system processes pain and temperature sensation, tactile and proprioceptive signals from the face and mucous membranes.

4. The gasserian (or semilunar) ganglion is located in Meckel's cave, and contains cell bodies of the sensory root. Central processes enter the pons and may bifurcate, with ascending branches terminating in the main nucleus and mesencephalic nucleus, and descending branches terminating in the spinal tract and nucleus.

5. The rostral-caudal extent of the brainstem trigeminal nuclei extends from the midbrain to the nucleus of the spinal tract in the upper cervical cord.

6. The mesencephalic nucleus contains the cell bodies of sensory neurons carrying proprioceptive and stretch information from the masticatory muscles.

   a. These are the only cell bodies of primary afferents located within the central nervous system; all other primary sensory neurons are located in ganglia outside the brain or spinal cord.

   b. Collaterals from these sensory afferents synapse on neurons in the motor nucleus, establishing a two-neuron reflex arc constituting the jaw jerk response (masseter reflex).

   c. Jaw jerk is elicited by tapping the chin downward while the mouth is open and relaxed.

   d. This reflex may be seen in hyperexcitable states, but it suggests upper motor neuron dysfunction above the level of the pons.

   e. It is a useful sign deciding if hyperactive limb reflexes are due to a cervical myelopathy (absent jaw jerk) or to a process above the foramen magnum.

7. The main (principal) nucleus is located posterior and lateral to the motor nucleus. Tactile and proprioceptive modalities ascend in the ventral crossed quintothalamic tract with the medial lemniscus and in the dorsal uncrossed trigeminothalamic tract. Second-order neurons in the spinal nucleus carrying pain, temperature, and touch sensation cross at the pontine and medullary levels and ascend in the trigeminothalamic tract to the thalamus.

   a. When sensory findings follow the distribution of a main division or peripheral branch, an extra-axial lesion is suspected. Central lesions, due to the somatotopic organization of the sensory representation in the nucleus, tend to cause an "onion-skin" pattern of facial sensory loss, with caudal lesions affecting lateral aspects of the face, and midline facial sensation representation in the rostral spinal nucleus.

b. Ophthalmic division fibers travel ventrally in the spinal tract and reach the most caudal levels of the spinal nucleus (located medial to the spinal tract), as far as the C3 to C4 level of the cervical cord, continuous with Lissauer's tract. Intraoral and perioral facial sensation is represented in the more dorsal part of the tract and the rostral spinal nucleus in the mid-pons.

c. Corneal reflexes (via V1) depend on the function of the facial nerve, which innervates the obicularis oculi muscles.

(1) When testing the corneal reflex on the side of a facial weakness, the consensual response seen in the fellow-eye can be reliably used to indicate an intact afferent arm of the reflex.

(2) A diminished corneal reflex can also occur with a contralateral parietal lobe lesion. The sternutatory reflex is a sneeze elicited by tickling the nasal mucosa.

d. The nasopalpebral (glabellar tap, obicularis oculi) reflex is a blink response to tapping the bridge of the nose. It normally extinguishes with repeated testing; failure to habituate to this stimulus may be associated with dementia or degenerative conditions.

e. Sensation over the neck up to the angle of the jaw and neck is supplied by the upper cervical roots via the great auricular nerve. Numbness involving both the lower face (V3) and the upper neck is either nonphysiologic or due to an intramedullary lesion.

Clinical Features

1. Depressed corneal reflex
2. Sensory loss over the face and intraoral mucous membranes
3. Bilateral idiopathic trigeminal neuropathy associated with connective tissue disorders
   a. Painless numbness in the V2 and V3 distributions
   b. Loss of taste
   c. Corneal reflexes are usually preserved
4. Weakness in muscles of mastication when V3 is involved

Key Signs

- Depressed corneal reflex
- Sensory loss
- Weakness in muscles of mastication

Differential Diagnosis

1. Trigeminal sensory neuropathy is a slowly progressive condition that may herald the development of connective tissue disease.

2. The most common abnormalities leading to facial numbness are associated with particular locations.
   a. Brainstem: Multiple sclerosis, infarction, glioma
   b. Subarachnoid: Neurovascular compression, schwannomas–acoustic and trigeminal, meningiomas, epidermoid cysts, lipomas, metastatic disease, carcinomatous meningitis
   c. Meckel's cave and cavernous sinus: Meningiomas, trigeminal schwannomas, epidermoid cysts, metastases, pituitary adenomas, aneurysms
   d. Extracranial: Malignant tumors, perineural spread of tumor

3. Examination findings and subjective complaints may not distinguish between lesions at the various portions of the trigeminal system, so magnetic resonance imaging including T_2-weighted images of the whole brain and high-resolution axial and coronal T_1-weighted images of the skull base obtained with and without contrast enhancement should be performed

4. Numb cheek syndrome results from a malignant infiltration of the infraorbital nerve by recurrent squamous cell carcinoma of skin in two thirds of patients.

5. A similar etiology is responsible for numb chin (Roger's sign) syndrome, which may also have pain and swelling associated with a mental neuropathy. It usually occurs in patients with systemic cancer: lymphoreticular neoplasms, breast and lung metastases to the mental canal, or leptomeningeal involvement.

6. Raeder's paratrigeminal neuralgia is described as facial pain or numbness or trigeminal motor weakness with a Horner syndrome. It is associated with lesions in the middle cranial fossa, and should be distinguished from a painful Horner syndrome, which is more vascular in quality.

7. Gradenigo's syndrome involves V1 and the abducens nerve, caused by a lesion at the apex of petrous bone. It was more common as a complication of otitis prior to antibiotic therapy.

8. Lateral lesions in the cavernous sinus affect abducens first, whereas sellar lesions affect III first then V1, sometimes V2 and oculosympathetic nerves, which enter the orbit with V1 (V3 is not present in the cavernous sinus).

9. Herpetic neuralgia (herpes zoster ophthalmicus; shingles) is a severe, burning, aching pain usually in the V1 distribution,

   a. May involve the facial nerve (external ear) with an ipsilateral palsy (Ramsay Hunt syndrome).

   b. Pain may precede the vesicular eruption by up to 1 week, and may persist indefinitely as postherpetic neuralgia.

   c. A contralateral hemiparesis rarely occurs weeks after the onset of herpes zoster ophthalmicus due to a necrotizing arteritis and occlusion of ipsilateral cerebral vessels.

10. Trigeminal schwannomas

    a. 0.4% of brain tumors

    b. Middle cranial fossa location in 50%; posterior fossa, in 30%

    c. Ipsilateral numbness, pain and dysesthesia, diminished corneal reflex, headache

    d. Weakness of the muscles of mastication is found in 30% to 45%.

    e. Abnormal function of other cranial nerves is noted in 75% of patients with trigeminal schwannoma. The cranial nerves most commonly affected, in order of frequency, are VI, VIII, VII, III, II, IX, X, and least often IV.

11. Bilateral, perioral numbness or paresthesia is commonly associated with hyperventilation.

Key Findings

- Numb chin or numb cheek syndrome

- Metastatic involvement of mental or infraorbital nerve

Caveat

- May be initial presenting symptom of breast cancer

Laboratory Testing

1. Appropriate serology to rule out systemic autoimmune diseases

   a. Sjögren's syndrome, scleroderma, systemic lupus erythematosus, rheumatoid arthritis, sarcoidosis, Wegener's granulomatosis, giant cell arteritis

2. Titers or polymerase chain reaction for herpes simplex, zoster, hepatitis A, Whipple's disease, syphilis

3. PPD (purified protein derivative) for tuberculosis

4. Glucose, hemoglobin A1c, sickle cell disease

5. Electromyogram of masseter

Radiologic Features

1. Lesions in the area of the petrous apex of the temporal bone that cause erosion include epidermoid tumor, giant petrous apex cholesterol cyst (granuloma), acoustic schwannoma, trigeminal schwannoma, meningioma, mucocele, chordoma, metastasis, osteochondroma, and chondrosarcoma (Grossman and Yousem, 1994).

2. Cavernous sinus imaging for carotid cavernous fistula

Key Tests

- Blood tests to rule out autoimmune diseases, sickle cell disease, herpes simplex and zoster, hepatitis A, Whipple's disease, syphilis

- Electromyogram of masseter

- Imaging for lesion or fistula

Treatment

Treat underlying condition if identified.

Motor Syndromes

1. Trismus is the inability to open the jaw, with painful spasms of the masseter muscles. It is seen in tetanus, certain myopathies, dystonic reactions, and infection of the pterygomandibular space.

   a. Trismus dolorificus is a painful locking of the jaw thought to result from trigeminal neuralgia. It may frequently occur in psychogenic disease.

2. Ocular masticatory myorhythmia is pathognomonic of central nervous system Whipple's disease. EMG shows rhythmic contraction of muscles of mastication associated with smooth pendular convergent–divergent eye movements with a frequency of about 1 Hz.

3. Gustatory sweating (Frey syndrome) occurs with abnormal regeneration of parasympathetic fibers after damage to the auriculotemporal branch of the mandibular nerve. Flushing and diaphoresis of one side of the face occurs when eating spicy foods.

Pregnancy

Schwannomas tend to increase in size during the third trimester and progress after delivery

Bibliography

Grossman RI, Yousem DM: Neuroradiology. St. Louis, C.V. Mosby, 1994.

Lecky BF, Hughes RC, Murray NF: Trigeminal sensory neuropathy. Brain 110:1463–1485, 1987.

Majoie CB, Verbeeten B, Jr., Dol JA, Peeters FL: Trigeminal neuropathy: Evaluation with MR imaging. Radiographics 15:795–811, 1995.

Williams LS: Advanced concepts in the imaging of perineural spread of tumor to the trigeminal nerve. Top Magn Reson Imaging 10:376–383, 1999.

Disorders of Cranial Nerves IX and X

David Solomon

GLOSSOPHARYNGEAL NERVES

Definition

1. The glossopharyngeal (IX) cranial nerve carries sensation from the ear and pharynx, taste, and autonomic fibers regulating blood pressure.
2. Isolated lesions cause mild dysphagia, decreased ipsilateral gag reflex and palatal droop, loss of taste over the posterior one third of the tongue, and anesthesia of the soft palate, posterior tongue, and pharyngeal wall
3. Glossopharyngeal neuralgia is transient, stabbing severe pain in the ear, base of the tongue, tonsillar fossa or beneath the angle of the jaw, in the distribution of auricular and pharyngeal branches of the vagus and glossopharyngeal nerves. This is considered in Part XI, Headaches.

Epidemiology and Risk Factors

1. Brainstem infarction
2. Cerebellopontine angle lesions
3. Skull base and nasopharyngeal tumors; e.g., jugulotympanic glomus tumor derived from chemorector cells
   a. Reddish-blue mass visible behind the tympanic membrane
   b. Pulsatile bruit and tinnitus; ear pain
   c. Most commonly involves cranial nerves IX and X
   d. Cranial nerves VII, VIII, XI, and XII are affected less frequently
   e. Hypertension, tachycardia, tremor, or vascular headaches accompany functional tumors.
4. Retropharyngeal abscess
5. Surgery and trauma

Etiology and Pathophysiology

1. Autonomic signals include carotid sinus and aortic baroreceptor afferents.
   a. Hering's nerve is the afferent from the carotid sinus, which joins the ninth nerve.
   b. The afferent arm of the carotid sinus reflex is stimulated by high blood pressure or carotid massage, resulting in increased efferent vagal activity.
2. Subarachnoid course is via the rostralmost rootlets, emerging from the lateral aspect of the medulla at the level of the inferior olive and inferior cerebellar peduncle.
3. Exits via the jugular foramen (see Multiple Cranial Nerve Syndrome section in Chapter 10) and travels in the parapharyngeal space in proximity to the internal carotid artery.
4. Main branches carry touch and pain sensation from the tympanic membrane and eustachian tube (Jacobson's nerve), external auditory meatus, skin near the ear and mastoid, mucous membranes of the posterior pharynx, tonsils and posterior soft palate, and join the trigeminal system in the brainstem.
5. Efferent innervation to the stylopharyngeus muscle, which is active (along with tenth nerve innervated muscles) during swallowing
6. Parasympathetic fibers, via the otic ganglion, stimulate parotid and mucosal secretory glands.
7. Taste is carried from pharyngeal mucous membranes and from the posterior third of the tongue.

Clinical Features

1. Bilateral supranuclear lesions cause pseudobulbar palsy, with spastic dysarthria, exaggerated gag reflex, and emotional lability
2. Lesions can cause the gag reflex to be lost after ipsilateral stimulation of the posterior pharynx and loss of taste on the posterior tongue, though no deficit in swallowing or sensation may be appreciated even after surgical section.
3. Rarely, carotid sinus hypersensitivity may be a cause of syncope resulting from hyperactivity of the baroreceptor reflex, by irritation of either the glossopharyngeal nerve or the carotid sinus.
   a. Hypotension leading to syncope occurs in reponse to a reflex bradycardia or asystole from activation of the dorsal motor nucleus of the vagus.
   b. Neck movements, external compression, or cervical masses may trigger hypotension and/or bradycardia.
   c. Demyelination of the ninth nerve can be a

359

cause of blood pressure lability and hypertension in Guillain-Barré syndrome.

Key Signs: Glossopharyngeal Nerve

- Unilateral loss of gag reflex
- Loss of taste over posterior tongue
- Rare cause of syncope

Differential Diagnosis

1. Pain in the distribution of Jacobson's nerve may be mistaken for an otitis media

2. Glossopharyngeal irritation may be a cause of excessive salivation, paroxysmal coughing, hoarseness, or syncope

3. Lateral medullary infarction (Wallenberg's syndrome) usually involves other cranial nerve nuclei as well.

Laboratory Testing

Autonomic testing can quantitate salivary secretion from the parotid gland.

Radiologic Features

Imaging of the jugular foramen and neck soft tissues may reveal adenopathy or malignancy.

Treatment

1. Surgical sectioning of the glossopharyngeal nerve rootlets

2. Chemical block or radiofrequency lesioning of the glossopharyngeal nerve at the jugular foramen

Key Treatments: Glossopharyngeal Nerve Disorders

- Surgical intervention
- Chemical block
- Radiofrequency lesioning

Pregnancy

Glomus jugulare tumors are more common among adult females.

VAGUS NERVE LESIONS

Definition

1. Vagus nerve lesions result in palatal and pharyngeal muscle weakness; vocal cord paralysis.

2. Vocal cord paralysis: Most of the intrinsic muscles of the larynx are innervated by the recurrent laryngeal nerve, which is a branch of cranial nerve X. The paretic vocal cord lies near the midline when viewed with laryngoscopy

Epidemiology and Risk Factors

1. Because of the long course of the vagus nerve, there can be many causes of vocal cord paralysis.

2. Risk factors include malignancy, neck surgery, granulomatous disease, mitral valve disease, and thoracic aortic aneurysm.

3. Idiopathic recurrent laryngeal neuropathy accounts for one quarter to one third of patients with isolated vocal cord paralysis. Men are affected more often than women. The left recurrent laryngeal nerve is more commonly affected than the right.

Etiology and Pathophysiology (Table 9–1)

1. The vagus carries fibers from three nuclei in the medulla.

   a. The nucleus ambiguus is the source of motor fibers to intrinsic laryngeal muscles.

TABLE 9–1.   KEY CAUSES OF NERVE DYSFUNCTION

Recurrent laryngeal nerve dysfunction
  Malignancy is the most common cause of unilateral vocal cord paralysis
  Adenopathy from malignancy, fungal disease, or granulomatous disease
  Thyroid or parathyroid carcinoma or surgery
  Idiopathic cause (25%)
  Bilateral involvement is uncommon, usually is due to thyroid surgery
Vagus Nerve Dysfunction
  Malignancy: Lung (most common), thyroid, breast, esophageal cancer
  Surgery or trauma: Thyroidectomy, pneumonectomy, coronary artery bypass graft, carotid endarterectomy, penetrating neck or chest trauma, postintubation, whiplash injuries, posterior fossa surgery
  Neurologic cause (5%–10%): Wallenberg's syndrome (lateral medullary stroke), syringomyelia, encephalitis, Parkinson's disease, polio, multiple sclerosis, myasthenia gravis, amyotrophic lateral sclerosis, progressive bulbar palsy, Guillain-Barré syndrome, diabetes
  Inflammation: Rheumatoid arthritis can involve the connective tissue of the vocal cord
  Infection: Syphilis, tuberculosis, thyroiditis, viral
  Idiopathic cause (20% to 25%): Sarcoidosis, lupus erythematosus, polyarteritis nodosa, left atrial hypertrophy (Ortner's syndrome)

b. Dorsal nucleus neurons provide parasympathetic innervation to bronchi, heart, and gut.

c. Nucleus of the tract of solitarius fibers carry sensation from the pharynx, larynx, and esophagus.

2. The vagus nerve exits the skull via the jugular foramen, along with glossopharyngeal and accessory nerves, where skull base lesions can result in compression.

3. In the neck, the vagus nerve travels behind the jugular vein and carotid artery.

a. Lymphadenopathy or tumor in the neck at the level of C6 can cause recurrent laryngeal nerve compression, Horner's syndrome, and phrenic nerve dysfunction (Rowland-Payne syndrome)

4. Pharyngeal branches to muscles of the soft palate and pharynx

5. Auricular branch carries sensation from parts of external auditory canal, tympanic membrane, and skin behind the ear.

6. Parasympathetic branches to the carotid artery and heart branch from the vagus in the neck and thorax.

7. Right recurrent laryngeal nerve loops around the subclavian artery and ascends between the esophagus and trachea to the larynx

8. Left recurrent laryngeal nerve traverses the mediastinum, passing under the aorta before ascending into the neck to innervate the intrinsic laryngeal musculature.

9. Thoracic and abdominal vagal branches supply the lungs, esophagus, stomach, and intestines to the descending colon

10. Epilepsy patients with vagal nerve stimulators may have intermittent symptoms related to the device.

11. Other etiologies

a. Thoracic aortic aneurysm or aortic surgery

b. Systemic lupus erythematosus

c. Whiplash injury

d. Mitral valve disease with left atrial enlargement

Clinical Features

1. Vagus nerve paralysis

a. Ipsilateral flattening of palatal arch, failure to elevate arch with phonation, and deviation of uvula toward intact side

b. Dysphagia worse with liquids

c. Nasal quality of articulation

2. Unilateral vocal cord paralysis

a. Hoarse, breathy voice

b. Airway compromise and/or aspiration usually not a problem

3. Bilateral lesions cause respiratory distress, severe dysphagia, absent cough, and weak, nasal voice

Key Signs: Vagus Nerve Paralysis

- Ipsilateral flattening of palatal arch
- Palatal arch not elevated on phonation
- Dysphagia worse with liquids
- Hoarse, breathy voice
- Respiratory distress with bilateral lesions

Differential Diagnosis

1. Extrapyramidal motor disorders (Parkinson's disease, multiple system atrophy) may be a cause of dysarthria, hoarseness, or swallowing difficulty.

2. Neuromuscular junction (myasthenia) causes should be considered.

Laboratory Testing

1. Chest radiograph

2. Computed tomography (CT) or magnetic resonance imaging (MRI) scan of the neck (and thorax if the left side is affected)

3. Barium swallow

4. Thyroid scan

5. Laboratory tests have small yield, but may yield a diagnosis with normal imaging: complete blood count, thyroid function tests, erythrocyte sedimentation rate, rheumatoid factor, parathyroid hormone, calcium and glucose levels, PPD, VDRL, fungal titers, Lyme titers, and lumbar puncture

6. Lower cranial nerve deficits should prompt evaluation of the lateral skull base with CT or MRI

7. Laryngeal electromyography cricothyroid muscle

Key Tests

- Chest radiograph
- CT or MRI of neck and thorax (when left side is affected), of lateral skull base (with lower cranial nerve deficits)
- Barium swallow
- Thyroid scan
- Laryngeal electromyography

Treatment

1. Surgical options
   a. Intracordal injection
   b. Selective reinnervation
   c. Medialization to move the cord into more of an adducted position
2. Indications for early intervention for unilateral vocal cord paresis:
   a. The known etiology leaves no chance of recovery
   b. Intractable aspiration
   c. Psychological or professional factors
3. Otherwise, wait 6 months or use temporary treatments.
4. Speech and swallowing physical therapy

Key Treatments: Vagus Nerve Paralysis

• Surgical intervention

Prognosis and Complications

About 60% of idiopathic unilateral vocal cord paralyses recover or compensate to near normal voices within 1 year.

Bibliography

Rushton JG, Steven JC, Miller RH: Glossopharyngeal (vago-glossopharyngeal) neuralgia: A study of 217 cases. Arch Neurol 38:201–205, 1981.

Stern BJ, Wityk RJ, Lewis RF: Disorders of the cranial nerves and brain stem. In Joynt RJ (eds): Clinical Neurology, revised ed. Philadelphia, Lippincott, 1993, pp. 1–90.

10 Disorders of Cranial Nerves XI and XII and Multiple Cranial Neuropathies

David Solomon

CRANIAL NERVE XI

Definition

1. The spinal accessory nerve (XI) is purely motor and is made up of components originating in the medulla (innervating the pharynx and larynx after joining the vagus nerve) and cervical cord (innervating the ipsilateral sternocleidomastoid and trapezius muscles).

2. The accessory nucleus extends from C1 through C6 in the ventral horn of the cervical cord. Motor roots exit the cord at multiple levels, collect to form the spinal part of XI, and enter the skull through the foramen magnum. The cranial portion of XI arises in the nucleus ambiguus, exits the lateral medulla caudal to the vagus, and joins the spinal part of the nerve before leaving the skull via the jugular foramen.

Epidemiology and Risk Factors

Skull base lesions

Etiology and Pathophysiology

1. Hemispheric strokes affect the contralateral trapezius and result in weakness of shoulder elevation and head tilting away from the lesion.
   a. The rostral accessory nucleus receives bilateral cortical projections.
2. Nuclear lesions are uncommon.
   a. Intraparenchymal lesions of upper cervical cord and lower medulla
   b. Syringomyelia
3. Nerve lesions within the cranium and foramen magnum
   a. Also involve IX, X, and XII
   b. Extramedullary neoplasms
   c. Meningitis
   d. Trauma
4. Retroparotid and retropharyngeal course
   a. Nasopharyngeal carcinoma
   b. Can involve other lower cranial nerves and sympathetic chain (ipsilateral Horner's syndrome)

5. Cervical posterior triangle
   a. Rarely, injured during carotid endarterectomy
   b. Internal jugular vein catheterization
   c. Shoulder dislocation
   d. Radiation therapy

Clinical Features

1. Weakness turning the head away from the side of the nerve lesion
2. Ipsilateral weakness of shoulder shrug and head tilting
3. Bilateral weakness, affecting head flexion
4. No sensory disturbance

Key Signs

- Weakness in head turning away from the affected nerve (with unilateral lesions)
- Neck flexion weakness (with bilateral lesions)
- Absent shoulder shrug and weakness of head tilting (ear to shoulder) on the side of the nerve lesion

Differential Diagnosis

1. Idiopathic neuritis: moderate to severe unilateral shoulder pain at onset, with atrophy and weakness becoming apparent days later as pain subsides
   a. Clinically similar to idiopathic brachial plexopathy/neuralgic amyotrophy (Parsonage-Turner syndrome)
   b. Variable outcome
2. Bilateral neck and shoulder muscle weakness
   a. Amyotrophic lateral sclerosis (ALS)
   b. Myasthenia gravis
   c. Polymyositis
   d. Fascioscapulohumeral muscular dystrophy

Key Findings

- Fasciculations, atrophy, and decreased strength of trapezius and sternocleidomastoid muscles

Laboratory Testing

1. Electromyography (EMG) of sternocleidomastoid (SCM) and trapezius
2. Cranial nerve XI accessible in the neck, so trapezius compound motor action potentials can be measured

Key Tests

• EMG of trapezius and sternocleidomastoid

Radiologic Features

Skull base tumors in the area of the jugular foramen

Treatment

Depends on etiology

Prognosis and Complications

Depends on etiology

Prevention

No data available

Pregnancy

No data available

CRANIAL NERVE XII

Definition

1. Hypoglossal nerve arises from a medial column of motor neurons below the fourth ventricle in the medulla. Fibers pass near the ipsilateral pyramid and medial lemniscus before exiting the lateral aspect of the medulla between the inferior olive and the pyramid.
2. Nerve rootlets join to form cranial nerve XII, which exits the skull via the hypoglossal canal. It then travels near the internal carotid artery and jugular vein to the angle of the mandible, where it divides into branches innervating various muscles of the tongue.

Epidemiology and Risk Factors

1. About half of XII lesions are due to tumor.
2. Unilateral hypoglossal palsies are found in roughly one-fifth of patients with Chiari malformations.

3. Medial medullary infarctions also occur.
   a. They are less common than lateral medullary strokes.
   b. They present with ipsilateral tongue weakness and fasciculations, contralateral hemiplegia sparing the face (pyramid), and loss of contralateral position and vibration sensation (medial lemniscus).
   c. Occlusion of the anterior spinal artery or vertebral artery is responsible.

Etiology and Pathophysiology

See Table 10–1.

Clinical Features

1. Tongue weakness, fasciculations, or atrophy
2. Tongue protruding toward weak side (unilateral lesions)
3. Dysarthria, especially for lingual sounds ("la" and "ta")
4. Dysphagia with difficulty manipulating food in the mouth

Key Signs

• Asymmetrical tongue weakness, atrophy, and fasciculation

• Dysarthria

TABLE 10–1. CAUSES OF XII NERVE PALSY: 100 CASES

Cause	No.
Tumor	49* (18 bilateral)
Metastatic	12
Chordoma	8
Nasopharyngeal	7
Lymphoma	6
Acoustic schwannoma	3
Trauma (gunshot wounds)	12
Stroke	6
Hysteria	6
Surgery	5
Multiple sclerosis	5 (4 bilateral)
Infection (mucor, AIDS, TB)	4
Guillain-Barré	4
Other†	6
Unknown	3

Abbreviations: AIDS, acquired immunodeficiency syndrome; TB, tuberculosis.
*Other tumors: pontine glioma, glomus tumor, meningioma, ependymoma, medulloblastoma, epidermoid, cholesteatoma, hemangiosarcoma, giant-cell tumor, craniopharyngioma, plasmacytoma.
†Other etiologies: syringomyelia, Chiari malformation, cavernous angioma, diabetes, spinocerebellar degeneration, chronic inflammatory demyelinating polyneuropathy.
Adapted from Keane JR: Twelfth-nerve palsy: analysis of 100 cases. Arch Neurol 53:561–566, 1996.

Differential Diagnosis

1. Giant cell (temporal) arteritis can present with headache and infarction of the tongue in patients over 50 years of age.

2. Tongue fasciculations are seen with ALS.

3. Viral infection is associated with ipsilateral headache, which spontaneously reverses over several months.

Laboratory Testing

1. Glossodynia (pain felt in the tongue) occasional symptom of vitamin B_{12} deficiency

2. Erythrocyte sedimentation rate (ESR)

Radiologic Features

1. Skull base or neck tumors or masses

2. Vertebral artery or anterior spinal artery occlusion on angiography

Key Radiologic Findings

- Medullary infarction
- Skull base tumors
- Neck masses

Treatment

1. Depends on underlying etiology

2. Speech therapy

Key Treatment

- Speech therapy for swallowing evaluation and articulation

Prognosis and Complications

Only 15 of the cases reported in Table 10–1 resolved with minimal or no disability.

Prevention

No data are available.

Pregnancy

No data are available.

MULTIPLE CRANIAL NERVE SYNDROMES

1. Tumors of the skull base infiltrating the retroparotid space can affect cranial nerves IX, X, XI, and XII and cause Horner's syndrome (Mackenzie's syndrome).

2. Endolymphatic sac tumors are usually papillary cystadenomas associated with von Hippel-Lindau syndrome that extend into the cerebellopontine angle. They are locally invasive and can cause facial nerve paralysis and lower cranial nerve palsies.

3. Arnold-Chiari malformation, with or without syringobulbia should be considered in patients with unexplained sensorineural hearing loss, headache, vertigo, ataxia, dysequilibrium, dysphagia, or other lower cranial nerve dysfunction, especially if accompanied by cervical pain, spasticity, or weakness.

4. Spontaneous or traumatic internal carotid artery dissection may occur.

   a. Unilateral headache or neck pain (carotidynia), contralateral hemiparesis, and Horner's syndrome are the usual presentation; however, lower cranial nerves may be involved owing to compression by a mural hematoma resulting in dysarthria, dysphagia, depressed gag, or hoarseness.

   b. Dissection in the subadventitial layer may occur without carotid stenosis and therefore not be seen with conventional angiography, but MRI shows a hematoma or thrombosed aneurysm in the absence of luminal narrowing.

5. Swallowing is a coordinated sequence of muscular contractions involving five of the cranial nerves.

   a. Food is kept in the mouth by orbicularis contraction (VII) in the lips.

   b. Muscles of mastication (V3 motor) prepare the consistency of the bolus.

   c. The location of the food or liquid in the mouth is determined from sensory input (V3 sensory).

   d. The tongue (XII) pushes material up against the soft palate (sensed by IX).

   e. The hyoid (XII) and stylopharyngeus (IX) elevate the larynx, pushing the epiglottis over the trachea.

   f. The soft palate elevates (X), closing off the nasopharynx.

   g. Finally, the upper esophageal sphincter is relaxed (X), allowing food to enter the digestive tract and be propulsed by peristalsis.

6. Wilson's disease is a cause of dysarthria and drooling in young patients, associated with a movement disorder or psychiatric symptoms.

7. Mucormycosis infection causes a rapidly evolving cranial neuropathy that must be recognized and treated promptly to avoid a fatal outcome.

   a. Look for the classic eschar or black crusting of the nasal mucosa in a debilitated or diabetic patient with exophthalmos, chemosis, stroke, or cranial nerve deficits.

   b. This demands an urgent otolaryngologic surgical evaluation and antifungal treatment.

8. Infectious mononucleosis caused by the Epstein Barr virus in children

9. Hypertrophic cranial pachymeningitis

   a. Rare inflammatory disorder that typically causes progressive cranial neuropathies, headaches, and cerebellar dysfunction

   b. Usually idiopathic; has appeared as a plaque-like extension of a fibrous orbital pseudotumor

   c. Increased intracranial pressure, lower cranial neuropathy, and cervical radiculopathy occur during the sixth decade and are identified by MRI, which shows diffuse dural thickening and enhancement. Cerebrospinal fluid (CSF) usually shows only mild pleocytosis.

   d. Dural biopsy may show granulomas, which may require surgical excision when a mass effect is present.

   e. Other causes of dural enhancement must be ruled out, including syphilis, tuberculosis, fungal infection, sarcoidosis, rheumatoid arthritis, metstatic cancer, meningioma, fibroma, Wegener's granulomatosis, and intracranial hypotension (CSF leak).

   f. Steroid therapy may help initially, and other immunosuppressive agents may be required.

   g. Diffuse leptomeningeal gliomatosis may be present, originating from occult anaplastic ectopic glia or astrocytoma.

   h. It may present with papilledema and hydrocephalus or multiple cranial neuropathies.

   i. Prognosis is poor, as the disorder is generally unresponsive to radiotherapy and chemotherapy.

   j. Tumors of peripheral nerve sheath origin, sporadic schwannomas, and neurofibromas can originate from cranial nerves or nerve roots.

MOTOR CRANIAL NEUROPATHY

1. When only motor weakness in multiple cranial nerve distributions is noted, localization to the muscle, neuromuscular junction, or motor nerve must be determined.

2. Motor neuropathies such as porphyria (usually in young individuals with abdominal pain), buckthorn berry, thallium, and tick paralysis are rare causes.

3. Polio is associated with pleocytosis in the CSF.

4. Diphtheria can cause a demyelinating motor neuropathy with paralysis of palatal and pharyngeal muscles and internal ophthalmoplegia during the weeks following an upper respiratory infection with *Corynebacterium diphtheriae*.

   a. It may progress to cause a Guillain-Barré-like syndrome.

   b. Treatment with antibiotics and antitoxin can prevent long-term sequalae.

5. Guillain-Barré syndrome (acute inflammatory demyelinating polyneuropathy) commonly affects bulbar motor nerves with facial weakness, ptosis, ophthalmoparesis, and oropharyngeal and lingual weakness progressing rapidly over hours to days, ultimately requiring ventilation in many cases.

6. Botulism in adults may present with ophthalmoparesis, facial weakness, and bulbar palsy, sparing sensory and cognitive function.

   a. Appendicular and diaphragmatic weakness may follow, and reflexes may be depressed or absent.

   b. Usually the result of eating contaminated (home canned) foods but may result from wound infection with *Clostridium botulinum*.

   c. Diagnosis can be confirmed with electrophysiologic testing, showing an increase in compound motor action potential amplitude following maximal exercise or with high-frequency (20–50 Hz) stimulation.

7. Lambert-Eaton syndrome may cause a slowly progressive motor cranial neuropathy that rarely affects respiration.

Bibliography

Brazis PW, Masdeu JC, Biller J: Localization in Clinical Neurology, 4 ed. Philadelphia, Lippincott Williams & Wilkins, 2001.

DeToledo JC, David NJ: Innervation of the sternocleidomastoid and trapezius muscles by the accessory nucleus. J Neuroophthalmol 21: 214–216, 2001.

Keane JR: Twelfth-nerve palsy: analysis of 100 cases. Arch Neurol 53:561–566, 1996.

Mamelak AN, Kelly WM, Davis RL, Rosenblum ML: Idiopathic hypertropic cranial pachymeningitis. Report of three cases. J Neurosurg 79:270–276, 1993.

Patten J: Neurological Differential Diagnosis, 2nd ed. New York, Springer, 1996.

11 Auditory Hallucinations

Christos Ballas
Jeffrey P. Staab

Definition

1. *Hallucinations* are sensory perceptions that occur in the absence of causal stimulation; yet they retain all of the characteristics of normal perceptions.
   a. Hallucinations vary from simple to complex perceptions. The level of complexity is an important clue to etiology (see Clinical Features, below).
   b. Hallucinations are spontaneous, unwilled, and cannot be controlled.
      (1) Some patients learn to identify situations where hallucinations may be exacerbated.
      (2) Patients also may learn to ignore low-level hallucinations.
2. Hallucinations are common in primary psychiatric disorders and some medical and neurologic conditions (e.g., toxic-metabolic states).
   a. In psychotic disorders, *auditory hallucinations* are more prevalent than hallucinations in other sensory modalities.
   b. When *visual hallucinations* predominate, medical and neurologic conditions must be suspected.
3. *Illusions,* in contrast to hallucinations, are altered perceptions of actual stimuli that are modified by an individual's mood or cognitive state. Prominent illusions also suggest medical or neurologic conditions.

Pathophysiology

1. The causes of auditory hallucinations are unknown, though several neurotransmitter systems have been implicated, among them, dopamine serotonin, and NMDA.
   a. Dopamine
      (1) All antipsychotic medications block at least one type of dopamine receptor.
         (a) The clinically effective doses of older generation (so-called typical) antipsychotics (e.g., haloperidol, chlorpromazine) are directly proportional to their D_2 receptor affinity.
         (b) Newer generation (atypical) antipsychotics block other dopamine receptor subtypes. For example, the clozapine D_4 receptor blockade may be partially responsible for its superior efficacy in controlling hallucinations.
      (2) Psychostimulants, which increase dopaminergic activity, are well-known causes of hallucinations, particularly when abused.
   b. Serotonin
      Increasing evidence implicates serotonergic systems in hallucinations, particularly via the 5HT2A receptor subtype.
      (1) D-lysergic acid diethylamide (LSD) and other hallucinogens are potent 5HT2A agonists.
      (2) Atypical antipsychotics are robust 5HT2A antagonists.
      (3) Activation of the 5HT2A receptor may stimulate glutaminergic transmission (see under NMDA).
   c. NMDA
      (1) Recent data suggest that NMDA receptors and glutamate may be involved in hallucinations, although the significance of this is not understood well. Potent hallucinogens such as phencyclidine (PCP) and ketamine activate NMDA receptors.
2. Neuroanatomical correlates of auditory hallucinations have not been established definitively, but neuroimaging studies indicate that abnormalities may exist in the structure and function of the superior temporal (Heschl's) gyrus.

Clinical Features of Auditory Hallucinations (Table 11–1)

1. Symptom characteristics
   a. Sounds, noises, or simple words (e.g., clicks, buzzes, machinery noises)
      (1) Most common with medical or neurological syndromes (e.g., auras)
   b. Musical hallucinations
      (1) A relatively rare phenomenon, most often reported in patients with deafness.
      (2) May be caused by strokes or mass lesions in the area of Heschl's gyrus and associated auditory pathways.
      (3) Patients with primary psychotic disorders

367

TABLE 11-1. KEY DIAGNOSTIC FEATURES OF AUDITORY HALLUCINATIONS

	DIFFERENTIAL DIAGNOSIS	
CLINICAL CHARACTERISTICS	PRIMARY PSYCHIATRIC DISORDER	MEDICAL OR NEUROLOGIC ILLNESS
Simple sounds (buzzes, clicks, machinery noises)	+	+++
Musical hallucinations	+	+++
Distorted hearing (e.g., phonophobia, hearing loss)	+	+++
Voices (single words, name called)	+/−	+/−
Voices (full sentences, commands, commentary)	+++	+
Voices (chronic, mumbled)	+++	+
Auditory >> visual or other hallucinations	+++	+
Visual or other hallucinations >> auditory	+	+++
Multi-modality or cross-modality hallucinations	+	+++
Response to internal stimuli	++	++
Pseudohallucinations	+/−	+/−

may report hearing music, but this occurs with other psychotic symptoms (hallucinations, delusions, thought disorder).

c. Full sentences

(1) Most often experienced as a clear voice; sometimes perceived as a murmuring voice or whisper

(2) May be single or multiple voices, male or female, known or unknown

(3) Commonly spoken to the patient (i.e., the voice speaks in the second person); may direct the patient's behavior (command hallucinations)

(4) Often characterized as coming from outside the head, although this distinction has little clinical utility.

(5) Common in schizophrenia and related disorders

(a) May also occur in mood disorders

(b) Relatively infrequent in medical or neurologic conditions

d. Schneider's "First Rank" symptoms (1959)

(1) Audible thoughts

(2) May echo the patient's own thoughts or say them out loud

(3) Voices carrying on discussions or arguing among themselves (third person)

(4) Voices commenting on the patient or people and situations in the patient's life

(5) Originally defined as pathognomonic for schizophrenia, but also may occur in mood disorders.

e. Multimodal hallucinations

(1) Simultaneous perceptions in two different sensory modalities (e.g., seeing and hearing rats in the corner)

(a) Common in delirium

(b) Also occur in feigned psychosis

(c) Rare in primary psychotic disorders (patients may have separate auditory and visual hallucinations)

(2) Cross-modal perceptions (e.g., "hearing colors")

(a) Usually caused by hallucinogens

Key Symptoms

- Sounds, noises, words, full sentences
- Schneider's "First Rank" symptoms

2. Signs of auditory hallucinations

a. "Responding to internal stimuli"

(1) Talking to or looking at something that is not there

(2) Being distracted by something that others cannot see or hear

b. Plugging ears

c. Radios or other devices used to "drown out the voices"

d. Helmets, hats, or wraps worn to prevent voices from "coming in"

Key Signs

- Responding to internal stimuli
- Plugging ears
- Using devices to drown out voices
- Wearing helmets, hats to prevent voices from coming in

3. Pseudohallucinations

a. Apparent perceptual experiences, but understood to exist only subjectively

b. Often described as metaphors or similes

(1) "It was as if I could hear my thoughts."

(2) "It was like I could hear God's voice in my head."

c. No relationship to mental illness, per se

(1) Hallucinations are pathologic states, while pseudohallucinations are not necessarily so.

Differential Diagnosis

1. No pathology
   a. Isolated or infrequent hallucinations that occur in the absence of other neuropsychiatric symptoms are common.
   More than one-third of the general population has experienced a hallucination in their lifetime.
   b. Prominent, persistent, or recurrent hallucinations strongly suggest a pathological state, particularly hallucinations that occur during daytime, wakeful states.
2. Schizophrenia and related disorders
   a. Schizophrenia: All subtypes
   b. Schizophreniform disorder
   c. Schizoaffective disorder
3. Mood disorders
   a. Major depressive disorder with psychotic features
   b. Bipolar disorder: Hallucinations may occur in mania or depression
   c. In mood disorders, hallucinations are usually mood congruent (i.e., consistent with the mood state).
      (1) Negative or derogatory with depression
      (2) Grand, important, or special in mania
4. Substance-related hallucinations
   a. Acute effects (i.e., intoxication)
      (1) Cocaine
      (2) Amphetamines and other psychostimulants
      (3) Hallucinogens: e.g., LSD, PCP, mescaline
      (4) "Designer" or "club" drugs: e.g., Ecstasy and ketamine
   b. Withdrawal
      (1) Alcohol
      (2) Benzodiazepines
      (3) Barbiturates
   c. Chronic effects
      (1) Persistent or recurrent hallucinations (e.g., "LSD flashbacks")
      (2) Alcoholic hallucinosis
5. Cognitive disorders
   a. Dementia complicated by psychosis
   b. Delirium: Any cause. Includes toxic-metabolic states, infection, intracranial pathology, withdrawal from central nervous system (CNS) depressants, "sundowning," "ICU psychosis"
6. CNS conditions
   a. Tumor
      (1) Especially temporal lobe tumors
      (2) Palinacousis is the persistence or recurrence of sounds
   b. Infections: Encephalitis more likely than meningitis
   c. Stroke: Temporal lobe, auditory cortex
   d. Migraine: Auras
   e. Seizures, particularly complex partial epilepsy
      (1) Auras
      (2) Periictal hallucinations
7. Sleep-related hallucinations: Hypnogogic and hypnopompic hallucinations; sleep paralysis

Laboratory Testing

1. There are no specific laboratory tests for auditory hallucinations.
2. Laboratory evaluation is geared toward ruling out medical illnesses.
   a. For primary psychiatric disorders in patients with unremarkable medical histories and normal physical examinations, few tests are needed.
      (1) Drug screen
      (2) Rapid plasma reagent
      (3) Thyroid stimulating hormone (if mood symptoms are present)
   b. Additional testing is dictated by the medical history and examination.
   c. For suspected delirium, a more extensive investigation is warranted.
      (1) Serum electrolytes, blood urea nitrogen, creatinine, glucose, calcium, transaminases
      (2) Complete blood count
      (3) Pulse oximetry and/or arterial blood gases; possible chest radiograph
      (4) Urinalysis
      (5) Drug screen
      (6) Electrocardiogram
      (7) Head imaging
      (8) Lumbar puncture (if meningitis or encephalitis is suspected)
      (9) Electroencephalogram (for any suspicion of ictal events)

Key Test

- Rule out medical illnesses

Treatment

1. Auditory hallucinations are managed best by treating the underlying illness (e.g., schizophrenia,

depression, delirium). Refer to Part XXV for details.

2. In some cases, patients may benefit from specific treatment of auditory hallucinations, in addition to interventions for the underlying illness.

  a. Mood disorders with psychosis:

    (1) Antipsychotics often needed in combination with antidepressants or mood stabilizers

  b. Conditions in which behavioral disturbances accompany auditory hallucinations.

    (1) Delirium

    (2) Drug withdrawal

    (3) Dementia complicated by psychosis

    (4) Central nervous system illnesses

    (5) There are two therapeutic options in these cases

      (a) Typical neuroleptics

        (i) Considerable clinical experience, few rigorous studies

        (ii) Higher potency agents (e.g., haloperidol, fluphenazine) have fewer anticholinergic side effects that may worsen the cognitive impairments associated with delirium or dementia.

        (iii) Start with relatively low doses (1–2 mg 2 to 4 times a day) and titrate to effect.

          (a) See chapter on schizophrenia for common side effects.

          (b) QTc prolongations and ventricular dysrhythmias, including torsades de pointes, have occurred with typical neuroleptics. These effects are more common in medical settings, where these medications are used to control the behavioral disturbances of delirium.

            • Most likely at doses above 35 mg per 24 hours.

            • More likely with intravenous than intramuscular or enteral routes of administration.

      (b) Atypical neuroleptics

        (i) Rapidly growing clinical experience, emerging treatment studies

        (ii) May be better tolerated

        (iii) Parenteral preparations have not been marketed yet.

        (iv) High cost is a consideration in situations where these drugs may be needed for only a few days (e.g., delirium, drug withdrawal). Typical neuroleptics may be more cost effective in these cases, without substantial risk of tardive dyskinesia from short-term exposure.

 Key Treatment

• Treat underlying illness

 Bibliography

David AS: Auditory hallucinations: Phenomenology, neuropsychology and neuroimaging update. Acta Psychiatrica Scand Suppl 395:395–104, 1999.

Fenelon G, Marie S, Ferrior JP, Guillard A: Musical hallucinations (translation). Rev Neurol (Paris) 151:216–217, 1995.

Ohayon MM: Prevalence of hallucinations and their pathological associations in the general population. Psychiatry Res 97:153–164, 2000.

Tucker GJ: Seizure disorders presenting with psychiatric symptomatology. Psychiatric Clin North Am 21:625–635, 1998.

1 Optic Neuritis

Paul W. Brazis
Andrew G. Lee

Definition

1. *Optic neuritis* (ON) is the general term for idiopathic, inflammatory, infectious, or demyelinating optic neuropathy.

2. If the optic nerve is swollen, it is termed *papillitis* or *anterior* ON

3. If the optic nerve is normal, it is called *retrobulbar* or *posterior* ON

Clinical Features

1. Acute, usually unilateral loss of visual acuity and/or visual field

2. Relative afferent pupillary defect (RAPD) in unilateral or bilateral but asymmetric cases

3. Periocular pain common (90%), especially with eye movement

4. Usually normal (65%) appearing or less commonly swollen (35%) optic nerve head

5. Usually young adult patient (< 40 years) but may occur at any age

6. Eventual visual improvement over several weeks in most patients (90%) to normal or near-normal visual acuity

   a. 88% improve at least one Snellen line by day 15

   b. 96% improve at least one Snellen line by day 30

   c. Visual recovery may continue for months (up to 1 year)

   d. May suffer residual deficits in contrast sensitivity, color vision, stereopsis, light-brightness, visual acuity, or visual field

Key Clinical Features

- Acute, usually unilateral, loss of visual acuity, visual field, or both (acuity may worsen over several days to 2 weeks)

- A RAPD in unilateral or bilateral but asymmetric cases

- Periocular pain, especially with eye movement

- Normal or swollen optic nerve head

- Young adult patient

- Eventual visual improvement

Etiology

1. Most cases are idiopathic or demyelinating in etiology.

2. Occasionally ON may be associated with other disorders.

   a. Polyneuropathies

      (1) Guillain-Barré syndrome (including Miller Fisher syndrome)

      (2) Chronic inflammatory demyelinating polyradiculoneuropathy

   b. Infections

      (1) Bacteria: Syphilis, tuberculosis, Lyme disease, *Bartonella henselae* (cat-scratch disease), mycoplasma, Whipple's disease, brucellosis, beta-hemolytic streptococcus, meningococcus

      (2) Fungi: Aspergillus, histoplasmosis, cryptococcus

      (3) Rickettsiae (e.g., Q fever, epidemic typhus)

      (4) Protozoa: Toxoplasmosis

      (5) Parasites: Toxocariasis, cysticercosis

      (6) Viruses: Adenovirus, hepatitis A, hepatitis B, cytomegalovirus (CMV), coxsackie B, rubella, chickenpox, herpes zoster, herpes simplex virus I, Epstein-Barr virus (infectious mononucleosis), measles, mumps, influenza, HTLV-1, Creutzfeldt-Jakob disease

      (7) Human immunodeficiency virus (HIV) or acquired immunodeficiency syndrome (AIDS)-related

         (a) Primary HIV-related optic neuritis

         (b) Syphilis

         (c) Cat-scratch disease (*Bartonella henselae*)

         (d) Cryptococcus

         (e) Histoplasmosis

         (f) CMV

         (g) Herpes zoster

(h) Hepatitis B

(i) Toxoplasmosis

(8) Postvaccination (e.g., smallpox, tetanus, rabies, influenza, hepatitis B, bacille Calmette-Guérin (bCG), trivalent measles-mumps-rubella vaccine, and Mantoux tuberculin skin test)

(9) Focal infection or inflammation (e.g., paranasal sinusitis or mucocele, postinfectious, malignant otitis externa)

b. Systemic inflammations and diseases

(1) Behçet's disease

(2) Inflammatory bowel disease

(3) Reiter's syndrome

(4) Sarcoidosis

(5) Systemic lupus erythematosus

(6) Sjögren's syndrome

(7) Mixed connective tissue disease

(8) Rheumatoid arthritis

c. Miscellaneous

(1) Birdshot chorioretinopathy

(2) Acute posterior multifocal placoid pigment epitheliopathy

(3) Autoimmune optic neuropathy

(4) Familial Mediterranean fever

(5) Bee or wasp sting

(6) Snakebite

(7) Postpartum optic neuritis

(8) Neuromyelitis optica (Devic's disease)

(9) Recurrent optic neuromyelitis with endocrinopathies

Laboratory Testing

1. The Optic Neuritis Treatment Trial (ONTT)

   a. Randomized, controlled clinical trial

   b. Enrolled 457 patients at 15 U.S. clinical centers between 1988 and 1991

2. All ONTT patients underwent testing for collagen vascular disease including antinuclear antibody (ANA), serologic testing for syphilis (e.g., fluorescein treponema antibody absorption test), and a chest radiograph for sarcoidosis. A lumbar puncture was optional.

   a. ANA positive less than 1:320 in 13% and 1:320 or greater in 3%. Only one patient was eventually diagnosed with a collagen vascular disease.

   b. FTA-ABS positive in six patients (1.3%) but none had syphilis

   c. No chest radiographs revealed sarcoidosis.

3. Neuroimaging

   a. All ONTT patients underwent magnetic resonance imaging (MRI) of the head

   b. MR scans may demonstrate contrast-enhancing optic nerve

   c. Periventricular white matter signal abnormalities consistent with multiple sclerosis (MS) have been reported in 40% to 70% of cases of isolated ON

   d. Computed tomography (CT) scan less sensitive than MRI

Development of MS

1. The 5-year cumulative probability of clinically definite (CD) MS was 30%

2. Brain MR scan performed at study entry was strong predictor of CDMS

   a. 5-year risk of CDMS was 16% (n = 202) with no MR lesions

   b. Risk was 51% (n = 89) with 3 or more MR lesions

Recommendations of ONTT

1. Laboratory testing
   Chest radiograph, laboratory tests (e.g., syphilis serology, collagen vascular disease studies, serum chemistries, complete blood counts, etc.) and lumbar puncture are not necessary for typical ON but should be considered in atypical cases

2. Neuroimaging

   a. Not for diagnosis of optic neuropathy in typical cases

   b. Powerful predictor of MS

 Key Tests

- In atypical cases only: Chest radiograph, blood tests, and lumbar puncture

- Neuroimaging is not necessary for diagnosis, but important for prognosis (i.e., MS risk) and treatment.

Treatment

1. ONTT randomization arms

   a. Intravenous methylprednisolone sodium succinate (250 mg every 6 hours for 3 days) followed by oral prednisone (1 mg/kg per day for 11 days)

   b. Oral prednisone (1mg/kg per day for 14 days)

   c. Oral placebo for 14 days followed by a short oral taper

2. ONTT treatment results

a. Intravenous steroids accelerated visual recovery but provided no long-term benefit to vision

b. "Standard dose" oral prednisone alone did not improve the visual outcome and was associated with an increased rate of new attacks of ON

c. Intravenous followed by oral corticosteroids reduced the rate of development of CDMS during the first 2 years, particularly in patients with MRI abnormalities, but by 3 years the treatment effect had subsided.

d. ONTT recommended that oral prednisone in standard doses be avoided in ON

3. Interferon therapy in ON

a. In a double-blind, randomized trial, 383 patients who had a first acute demyelinating event (optic neuritis, incomplete transverse myelitis, or a brainstem or cerebellar syndrome) and evidence of prior subclinical demyelination on MRI of the brain (two or more silent lesions of at least 3 mm diameter thought characteristic of MS) were randomly assigned to receive weekly intramuscular injections of 30 μg of interferon beta-1a (193 patients) or to receive weekly injections of placebo (190 patients).

b. All received initial treatment with corticosteroids.

c. During 3 years of follow-up, the cumulative probability of the development of CDMS was significantly lower in the interferon beta-1a group than in the placebo group (rate ratio, 0.56). At 3 years, the cumulative probability of CDMS was 35% in the interferon beta-1a group and 50% in the placebo group.

d. As compared with the patients in the placebo group, patients in the interferon beta-1a group had a relative reduction in the volume of brain lesions, fewer new lesions or enlarging lesions, and fewer gadolinium-enhancing lesions at 18 months.

e. Interferon beta-1a at the time of a first demyelinating event may be beneficial for patients with brain lesions on MRI that indicate a high risk of CDMS

Key Treatment: Intravenous Corticosteroids

- Speeds recovery by 2 to 3 weeks
- No effect on visual function at 1 to 3 years
- No effect on recurrence of optic neuritis in affected eye

- Reduces risk of attacks of clinical MS in first 2 years after treatment in patients without clinical MS who have abnormal MRI at onset of visual loss

Prognosis of ON in ONTT

1. Visual recovery generally begins within the first 2 weeks, with much of the recovery occurring by the end of 1 month.

2. If recovery is incomplete at 6 months, some further improvement may continue for up to 1 year.

3. No significant difference in visual acuity comparing the three treatment groups at 6 months

4. After 12 months, visual acuity was 20/40 or greater in 93% of patients, greater than 20/20 in 69%, and 20/200 or lower in 3%. Results were similar in each treatment group.

5. The only predictor of poor visual outcome was poor visual acuity at the time of study entry; even so, of 160 patients starting with a visual acuity of 20/200 or worse, all had at least some improvement, and only 8 (5%) had visual acuities that were still 20/200 or worse at 6 months.

6. At 5-year follow-up for 347 (87%) of 545 patients, the affected eyes had normal or only slightly abnormal visual acuities in most patients, and results did not significantly differ by treatment group. Visual acuity in affected eyes was 20/25 or better in 87%, 20/25 to 20/40 in 7%, 20/50 to 20/190 in 3%, and 20/200 or worse in 3%.

7. Recurrence of ON in either eye occurred in 28% of patients and was more frequent in patients with MS and in patients without MS who were in the prednisone treatment group. Most eyes with a recurrence retained normal or almost normal visual function.

Risk Factors for Developing MS Following ON

1. Increased risk
   a. Abnormal MRI (3 or more lesions)
   b. Prior nonspecific neurologic symptoms
   c. Increased cerebrospinal fluid (CSF) oligoclonal bands
   d. Increased CSF immunoglobulin
   e. Previous optic neuritis
   f. HLA-DR2 and HLA-B7
2. Decreased risk
   a. Normal MRI
   b. Absence of pain*

*We consider these findings in a patient with optic neuritis to be atypical for demyelination and thus likely require further evaluation.

c. Marked disc edema*
d. Retinal exudates or macular star*
e. Bilateral simultaneous onset*
f. Onset in childhood*

---

*We consider these findings in a patient with optic neuritis to be atypical for demyelination and thus likely require further evaluation.

Bibliography

Beck RW, Cleary PA, Trobe JD, et al.: The effect of corticosteroids for acute optic neuritis on the subsequent development of multiple sclerosis. N Engl J Med 329: 1764–1769, 1993.

Beck RW, Trobe J: What we have learned from the Optic Neuritis Treatment Trial. Ophthalmology 102:1504–1508, 1995.

Jacobs LD, Beck RW, Simon JH, et al.: Intramuscular interferon beta-1a therapy initiated during a first demyelinating event in multiple sclerosis. N Engl J Med 343:898–904, 2000.

Lee AG, Brazis PW: Clinical Pathways in Neuro-Ophthalmology. An Evidence-Based Approach. New York, Thieme, 1998.

Optic Neuritis Study Group: The clinical profile of optic neuritis: Experience of the Optic Neuritis Treatment Trial. Arch Ophthalmol 109:1673–1678, 1991.

Optic Neuritis Study Group: The 5-year risk of MS after optic neuritis. Experience of the Optic Neuritis Treatment Trial. Neurology 49:1404–1413, 1997.

Optic Neuritis Study Group: Visual function 5 years after optic neuritis. Experience of the Optic Neuritis Treatment Trial. Arch Ophthalmol 115:1545–1552, 1997.

2 Optic Neuropathy

Paul W. Brazis
Andrew G. Lee

Definition

1. Unilateral or bilateral impairment of optic nerve function. Diagnosis is usually made on clinical grounds alone (see below).

2. Wide differential diagnosis including congenital, hereditary, infectious, inflammatory, infiltrative, ischemic, demyelinating (optic neuritis), and compressive etiologies.

Clinical Features

1. Variable decreased visual acuity

2. Variable decreased color vision

3. Any visual field defect (e.g., central, cecocentral, arcuate, altitudinal)

4. Ipsilateral relative afferent pupillary defect (RAPD) in unilateral or bilateral asymmetric cases.

5. Light-near dissociation of the pupils (react better to near than to light) in bilateral and symmetric cases.

6. Optic disc edema or atrophy (although optic nerve may appear normal in retrobulbar optic neuropathy)

Key Signs

- Decreased visual acuity

- Decreased color vision

- Visual field defect (e.g., central, cecocentral, arcuate, altitudinal)

- Ipsilateral RAPD in unilateral or bilateral asymmetric cases

- Light-near dissociation of the pupils (react better to near than to light) in bilateral and symmetric cases

- Optic disc edema or atrophy (although optic nerve may appear normal in retrobulbar optic neuropathy)

Differential Diagnosis

1. Ischemic optic neuropathy (ION): Clinical syndrome characterized by acute loss of vision, evidence of an optic neuropathy (e.g., dyschromatopsia, RAPD), and usually a swollen optic nerve in elderly patients (anterior ION). Rarely posterior ION (normal-appearing disc) may occur.

   a. Etiology

      (1) Arteritic ION: An inflammatory giant cell arteritis (GCA) affecting medium to large-sized vessels in elderly patients

      (2) Nonarteritic ION: Not due to GCA but due to other vasculopathic risk factors (e.g., diabetes, hypertension)

   b. Clinical features–nonarteritic ION

      (1) Acute onset of usually painless (pain may occur in 8% to 12%) loss of visual acuity and/or visual field (usually altitudinal defect) in a middle-aged or older patient (usually over 50 years of age).

      (2) Usually unilateral (but may be sequential)

      (3) Edema of optic nerve head (anterior ischemic optic neuropathy or AION) with or without peripapillary hemorrhages initially, followed later by sector or diffuse optic nerve pallor

      (4) Most common cause of unilateral optic disc swelling in adults over 50 years of age

      (5) Due to posterior ciliary artery ischemia

      (6) Systemic associations

         (a) Atherosclerotic risk factors including hypertension, diabetes, and increased lipids

         (b) May be caused by nocturnal hypotension.

         (c) Small cup to disc ratio (less than 0.2) is structural optic disc risk factor for AION ("disc at risk")

         (d) Other causes

            (i) Collagen vascular disease

            (ii) Antiphospholipid antibody syndrome

            (iii) Acute blood loss

            (iv) Surgery (hypotension or anemia)

            (v) Post-cataract extraction

            (vi) Migraine

   c. Clinical features–arteritic ION

      (1) Similar clinical features to nonarteritic AION; occasionally normal-appearing disc (posterior ION)

(2) Usually more severe visual loss (but may be any level of visual loss) and markedly pallid disc edema (chalky white)

(3) May be unilateral or bilateral simultaneous ION (as opposed to unilateral nonarteritic AION)

(4) May present with transient visual loss or transient diplopia (not seen in nonarteritic form)

(5) Cup to disc ratio often greater than 0.2 in uninvolved eye (i.e., "disc at risk" often not present)

(6) Constitutional signs of GCA common

   (a) New-onset headache

   (b) Scalp tenderness or temporal artery nodularity

   (c) Jaw claudication

   (d) Anorexia, fatigue, malaise, weight loss

   (e) Polymyalgia rheumatica

Key Clinical Features: Giant Cell Arteritis as Cause of Ischemic Optic Neuropathy

- Bilateral simultaneous or rapidly sequential involvement

- Suspicious eye findings (e.g., simultaneous choroidal or retinal arterial occlusion with ION, pallid disc edema)

- Recent history of transient visual loss (amaurosis fugax) or diplopia

- Cup to disc ratio greater than 0.2 in uninvolved eye (i.e., "disc at risk" not present)

- New-onset headache

- Jaw claudication

- Polymyalgia rheumatica

d. Laboratory testing

   (1) Erythrocyte sedimentation rate (ESR) and C-reactive protein (CRP) test abnormal in approximately 70% to 90% of patients with GCA (NOTE: From 10% to 30% of patients may have a normal ESR despite biopsy proven GCA.)

   (2) If ESR/CRP elevated or if there is a high index of suspicion for GCA, perform temporal artery biopsy.

e. Treatment

   (1) Nonarteritic ION

      (a) Treat underlying vasculopathic risk factors.

   (b) Aspirin therapy may reduce risk in fellow-eye (controversial)

   (c) No known effective treatment of non-arteritic ION

   (d) Avoid nocturnal hypotension.

(2) Arteritic ION

   (a) Oral prednisone (1.0 to 1.5 mg mg/kg per day) with a slow taper over months to years. Begin steroid treatment immediately; check ESR; follow clinical status and constitutional symptoms

   (b) Consider intravenous corticosteroids for severe visual loss, monocular patients, or oral steroid failures.

f. Prognosis

   (1) Nonarteritic

      (a) Often static visual loss

      (b) Vision may deteriorate over first 1 to 2 weeks in approximately 25% of patients

      (c) May spontaneously improve over months in approximately 43% of patients, but improvement is usually mild

      (d) Fellow-eye may be affected by ION in 12% of cases

   (2) Arteritic

      (a) Often severe and bilateral visual loss

      (b) Untreated disease leads to bilateral severe visual loss; 65% of patients develop arteritic ION in fellow-eye if untreated

Key Treatments

Nonarteritic ION

- No known effective treatment

- Treat underlying vasculopathic risk factors.

- Aspirin therapy

- Avoid nocturnal hypotension

Arteritic ION

- Begin oral prednisone treatment immediately

- Consider intravenous corticosteriods for severe visual loss, monocular patients, or those who fail oral steriods

2. Optic neuritis

3. Optic disc edema with macular star (neuroretinitis)

   a. Definition: Descriptive term encompassing a heterogeneous group of disorders characterized by swelling of the optic disc, peripapillary and macular exudates (often deposited in the pattern of a star), and, often, vitreous inflammatory cells

b. Etiology
  (1) Often "idiopathic"
  (2) Infectious etiologies especially consider
    (a) Cat-scratch disease
    (b) Syphilis
    (c) Toxoplasmosis
    (d) Lyme disease
    (e) Tuberculosis
    (f) Toxocara
  (3) Inflammatory etiologies
    (a) Sarcoid
    (b) Lupus erythematosus
    (c) Autoimmune

c. Clinical features
  (1) Age of onset: Usually childhood to young adult
  (2) May affect either gender
  (3) Bilateral involvement in 5 % to 33%
  (4) Pain with eye movement may or may not be present
  (5) Approximately 50% have antecedent viral infection
  (6) Impaired visual acuity, impaired visual field, dyschromatopsia; RAPD in unilateral or asymmetric bilateral cases
  (7) Optic disc swelling with retinal and macular exudates, especially macular star formation (star may take 1 to 2 weeks to develop after onset of disc swelling)
  (8) Vitreous inflammatory cells occur in 90% of cases

d. Differential diagnosis: Other processes that may cause a macular star
  (1) Vascular disease: AION, branch or central retinal artery occlusion, hypertensive retinopathy, diabetic retinopathy, polyarteritis nodosa, Eales disease
  (2) Papilledema
  (3) Optic disc tumor or infiltrate
  (4) Acute neuroretinopathy associated with progressive facial hemiatrophy (Parry-Romberg syndrome)
  (5) Diffuse unilateral subacute neuroretinitis

e. Laboratory testing
  (1) Syphilis serology

  (2) *Bartonella henselae* serology (for cat-scratch disease): may be most common etiology
  (3) Lyme serology (in endemic regions)
  (4) Toxoplasmosis titers (if clinical and fundus picture consistent with toxoplasma lesion)
  (5) Toxocara titers (if clinical and fundus picture suspicious)
  (6) Tests for tuberculosis (e.g., purified protein derivative skin testing)
  (7) Chest radiograph

f. Treatment
  (1) Treat specific infection
  (2) Corticosteroids sometimes used but benefit unknown

g. Prognosis
  (1) Usually benign and resolves spontaneously even without treatment
  (2) Optic atrophy and macular retinal pigment epithelial impairment may result in residual impaired vision
  (3) Not a risk factor for the development of multiple sclerosis (vs. optic neuritis)

Caveat

• Cat-scratch disease may be the most common cause of optic disc edema with macular star.

 Key Signs

• Antecedent viral infection in half of patients, who are children and young adults

• Impaired visual acuity, impaired visual field, dyschromatopsia, RAPD

• Optic disc swelling with retinal and macular exudates, especially macular star formation

• Vitreous inflammatory cells

 Key Tests

• Blood tests: syphilis, *Bartonella henselae,* Lyme disease, toxoplasmosis titer, toxocara titer

• Tuberculosis test

• Chest radiograph

Key Treatment

- Treat specific infection.

4. Toxic or nutritional optic neuropathy

   a. Etiology

      (1) Nutritional deficiencies

         (a) Pernicious anemia

         (b) Dietary deficiency (e.g., vegetarian diet, alcoholism)

         (c) Vitamin B_{12} deficiency

         (d) Folate deficiency

      (2) Toxins

         (a) Ethambutol

         (b) Ethanol and tobacco (tobacco alcohol amblyopia)

         (c) Many drugs (e.g., amantadine, amiodarone, cisplatin)

   b. Clinical features

      (1) Visual field defect: Typically bilateral central or cecocentral scotomas

      (2) Bilateral and symmetric visual loss

      (3) Slowly progressive

      (4) Optic nerve appearance may appear normal until late in course

      (5) Optic atrophy usually develops eventually.

   c. Evaluation of painless progressive bilateral optic neuropathy (presumed toxic or nutritional optic neuropathy)

      (1) Magnetic resonance imaging (MRI) of the optic nerves (exclude bilateral compressive optic neuropathy)

      (2) Vitamin B_{12} level (serum)

      (3) Folate level (serum and erythrocyte)

      (4) Complete blood count with differential

      (5) Urine heavy metal screen (mercury, lead, arsenic) if history suggests exposure

      (6) Syphilis serology

      (7) Leber's hereditary optic neuropathy mutational analysis

      (8) Consider lumbar puncture and other laboratory studies (e.g., chest radiograph, antinuclear antibodies, sedimentation rate, angiotensin-1-converting enzyme, cytoplasmic neutrophil antibodies, paraneoplastic antibody screen) if an inflammatory or infiltrative process is suspected.

Key Signs

- Visual field defect

- Bilateral and symmetric visual loss

- Slowly progressive

- Eventually, optic atrophy develops

Key Tests: Painless Progressive Bilateral Optic Neuropathy

- MRI of optic nerves

- Blood tests: vitamin B_{12} level, folate level (serum and erythrocyte), syphilis screening, CBC with differential, screening for heavy metals if history of exposure

- Leber's hereditary optic neuropathy mutational analysis

- Consider lumbar puncture

- Consider additional blood tests if an inflammatory or infiltrative process is suspected.

5. Radiation optic neuropathy (RON)

   a. Definition: Thought to be an ischemic disorder of the optic nerve that usually results in irreversible severe visual loss months to years after radiation therapy to the brain or orbit.

   b. Clinical features

      (1) Most often a retrobulbar optic neuropathy and, thus, the optic nerve may initially appear normal.

      (2) Approximately three quarters of patients have bilateral involvement.

      (3) The visual loss is characteristically rapid and progressive, with the disc becoming pale over 4 to 6 weeks

      (4) Final vision is often poor. No light perception in 45% and worse than 20/200 in an additional 40% of affected eyes (i.e., 85% of eyes with RON have a final visual acuity of 20/200 or worse)

      (5) Rarely, RON presents as an anterior optic neuropathy with optic disc swelling, usually in the setting of radiation retinopathy after treatment of orbital or intraocular lesions.

      (6) Increased risk of RON

         (a) Concomitant chemotherapy

         (b) Patient with hormone-secreting pituitary adenoma

(c) Diabetes

(d) Increased age

(e) Increased risk with increasing dose of radiation exposure to optic nerve

(7) Diagnosis of RON is suspected from the clinical setting and usually confirmed by MRI.

    (a) Unenhanced T_1- and T_2-weighted images show no abnormalities but, in some cases, enhancement is seen in optic nerves, chiasm, and possibly the optic tracts.

    (b) This enhancement usually resolves over several months.

c. Differential diagnosis

(1) Recurrent tumor (main consideration!)

(2) Empty sella syndrome (arachnoiditis): but generally no MRI optic nerve enhancement in these cases

(3) Secondary new tumor in field of radiation

    (a) Meningioma or glioma

    (b) Dural tumor (e.g., fibrosarcoma)

    (c) Cranial bone tumor (e.g., osteosarcoma)

    (d) Peripheral nerve tumor (e.g., malignant schwannoma)

(4) Adhesive arachnoiditis

(5) Non–radiation-induced ischemic optic neuropathy

(6) Carcinomatous meningitis

(7) Paraneoplastic optic neuropathy or retinopathy

(8) Chemotherapy-related complications or toxicity

    (a) Tamoxifen retinopathy

    (b) Cisplatinum toxicity

    (c) Intra-arterial BCNU (cisplatin), etoposide phosphate, and carboplatin

(9) Unrelated primary optic nerve tumors

(10) Metastatic tumor to optic nerve

(11) Increased intracranial pressure and papilledema (generally no MRI enhancement)

(12) Venous sinus thrombosis with papilledema

d. Treatment

(1) No effective proven treatment

(2) May rarely improve with corticosteroids

(3) Hyperbaric oxygen therapy may be of benefit if given early in the course (e.g., within 72 hours of onset of symptoms), although most patients have only limited improvement.

Key Signs

• Rapid and progressive visual loss

• Disc becomes pale over 4 to 6 weeks

Key Treatments

• No effective proven treatment

• Rarely improves with corticosteriods

• Hyperbaric oxygen therapy within 72 hours of onset of symptoms

6. Compressive optic neuropathy

a. Etiology

(1) Intracranial or intraorbital benign and malignant tumors

    (a) Meningioma

    (b) Glioma

    (c) Craniopharyngioma

    (d) Pituitary adenoma

    (e) Lymphoma and leukemia

    (f) Germinoma

    (g) Sinus histiocytosis with lymphadenopathy

    (h) Nasopharyngeal cancer

    (i) Metastasis

(2) Extramedullary hematopoiesis

(3) Orbital fractures with bone fragment, hematoma, or edema

(4) Pneumatocele

(5) Inflammatory or infectious diseases (e.g., mucoceles)

(6) Idiopathic hypertrophic cranial pachymeningitis

(7) Primary bone diseases (e.g., osteopetrosis, fibrous dysplasia, craniometaphyseal dysplasia, Paget's disease, aneurysmal bone cyst, pneumosinus dilatans)

(8) Vascular etiologies

    (a) Orbital hemorrhage

    (b) Orbital venous anomalies

    (c) Carotid artery and anterior communicating artery aneurysms

    (d) Dolichoectasia of the carotid artery

    (e) Supraclinoid carotid artery compression

    (f) Arteriovenous malformations

(9) Thyroid ophthalmopathy with compres-

sion by enlarged extraocular muscles or stretch from severe proptosis

(10) Hydrocephalus

(11) Iatrogenic (e.g., intracranial catheters, postoperative)

b. Clinical features

(1) Painless, progressive, gradual loss of visual function (visual acuity, visual field, and color vision),

(2) Relative afferent pupillary defect (in unilateral or asymmetric cases)

(3) Optic disc edema or atrophy (but the optic disc may initially appear normal)

(4) Orbital or intracanalicular lesions may produce abnormal blood vessels on the disc head called optociliary *shunt* vessels. These vessels probably represent collateral (versus shunt) circulation between the retinal and choroidal venous circulation that allows venous blood to bypass the compression at the level of the optic nerve.

(5) Orbital signs such as proptosis, chemosis, or conjunctival injection should direct the imaging studies to the orbit.

c. Evaluation

(1) Generally MRI of the head and orbit with gadolinium and fat saturation sequences

(2) CT scan may be helpful in acute trauma, bone lesions, acute hemorrhage or thyroid eye disease.

Key Signs

- Painless, progressive, gradual loss of visual function

- Relative afferent papillary defect

- Optic disc edema or atrophy

- Abnormal blood vessels on the disc head called *shunt* vessels

Key Tests

- MRI of the head and orbit with gadolinium and fat saturation sequences

- Computed tomography (CT) scan for acute trauma, bone lesions, acute hemorrhage, thyroid eye disease

7. Infiltrative or inflammatory optic neuropathy

a. Etiology

(1) Neoplastic

(a) Plasmacytoma and multiple myeloma

(b) Carcinomatous meningitis

(c) Leukemia

(d) Lymphoma

(2) Paraneoplastic disease

(3) Infectious etiologies

(a) Cryptococcal meningitis

(b) Aspergillus

(c) Mucormycosis

(d) Cysticercosis

(e) Lyme disease

(f) Tuberculosis

(g) Syphilis

(h) Cat-scratch disease

(i) Human immunodeficiency virus (acquired immunodeficiency syndrome)

(4) Inflammatory diseases

(a) Churg-Strauss angiitis

(b) Contiguous sinus disease

(c) Behçet's disease

(d) Sarcoidosis

(e) Wegener's granulomatosis

(f) Systemic lupus erythematosus

(g) Sjögren's syndrome

(h) Relapsing polychondritis

(j) Polyarteritis nodosa

(j) Inflammatory bowel disease

b. Clinical features

(1) Infiltrative or inflammatory optic neuropathy may present with the typical features of an optic neuropathy discussed above.

(2) Patients with inflammatory autoimmune optic neuropathy often have a progressive or recurrent steroid-responsive or steroid-dependent clinical course.

c. Evaluation

(1) MRI of head and orbit with gadolinium and fat suppression

(2) Lumbar puncture with cytology

(3) Additional laboratory studies (e.g., complete blood count, syphilis serology, antinuclear antibody, Lyme titer, chest radiograph) should be considered.

Key Tests

- MRI of head and orbit with gadolinium and fat suppression sequences

- Lumbar puncture with cytology

- Consider blood tests: CBC, syphilis screening, antinuclear antibody, Lyme disease

- Consider chest radiograph

8. Traumatic optic neuropathy
   a. Clinical features
      (1) History of direct or indirect impact injury to the head, face, or orbit
      (2) Unilateral or bilateral visual loss
      (3) Variable loss of visual acuity (range 20/20 to no light perception)
      (4) Variable loss of visual field
      (5) Relative afferent pupillary defect (unilateral or bilateral but asymmetric cases)
      (6) Commonly normal or less commonly swollen optic nerve
      (7) Eventual ipsilateral optic atrophy
      (8) Exclusion of other etiologies of visual loss in the setting of trauma (e.g., open globe, traumatic cataract, retinal detachment)
   b. Pathophysiology
      (1) Compressive or direct mechanical injury
         (a) Laceration of nerve
         (b) Optic nerve contusion, edema, and swelling
         (c) Avulsion or transection of nerve
         (d) Bone fragment or fracture
      (2) Hemorrhage
         (a) Retrobulbar bleed with increased intraorbital pressure
         (b) Subperiosteal hematoma
         (c) Optic nerve sheath hematoma
      (3) Vascular injury
         (a) Vasospasm
         (b) Ischemia
         (c) Infarction
   c. Evaluation: Neuroimaging, preferably CT of brain and orbit with axial and coronal views and thin sections
   d. Treatment
      (1) No proven therapy (care must be individualized)
      (2) Corticosteroids (variable doses and regimens reported in literature)
      (3) Consider surgical decompression of optic canal.

Key Signs

- History of direct or indirect impact injury to head, face, or orbit
- Visual loss
- Variable loss of visual acuity
- Variable loss of visual field
- Relative afferent papillary defect
- Normal (common) or swollen (less common) optic nerve

Key Test

- CT of brain and orbit with axial and coronal views and thin sections

Key Treatments

- Care must be individualized because there is no proven therapy.
- Corticosteriods
- Surgery for decompression of optic canal

9. Hereditary optic neuropathy
   a. Three clinical groups:
      (1) Those without associated neurologic signs and symptoms
      (2) Those with neurologic signs and symptoms
      (3) Those in whom the optic neuropathy is secondary to the underlying systemic disease
   b. Kjer optic neuropathy and Leber's hereditary optic neuropathy most common
   c. Clinical features of dominant optic atrophy (Kjer)
      (1) Onset in first decade of life (usually age 4 to 6 years) in 58% of patients
      (2) 12.5% to 22.6% unaware of visual difficulties and discovered to have optic atrophy as a consequence of examination of another affected family member; imperceptible onset
      (3) Impaired visual acuity: Mean initial visual acuity 20/60 and the median final visual acuity 20/80
      (4) Often inability to perceive blue color (tritanopia) or generalized dyschromatopsia
      (5) Central, paracentral, or cecocentral scotomas; may show characteristic inversion of peripheral field with more constriction to blue isopters than red
      (6) Optic atrophy: Occasionally subtle; usually temporal; rarely diffuse
      (7) Visual prognosis is relatively good in Kjer's dominant optic atrophy with stable or slow progression of visual loss.
   d. Clinical features of Leber's hereditary optic neuropathy (LHON)
      (1) Usually occurs in young males (up to 80%

to 90% of cases in the United States), although it may rarely occur in females and develop at any age

(2) Some patients with presumed "tobacco-alcohol amblyopia" or nutritional deficiency amblyopia may actually harbor a LHON; therefore, testing for Leber's mutations may be indicated in patients with presumed toxic or nutritional optic neuropathy.

(3) "Primary" mitochondrial DNA mutations (e.g., 11778, 3460, 14484)

(4) Every son and daughter of a female carrier inherits the LHON trait; only women pass it on.

(5) 20% to 83% of men at risk develop visual loss.

(6) 4% to 32% of women at risk develop visual loss.

(7) Age at onset: 13 to 35 years (range 5 to 80 years)

(8) Visual acuity loss

  (a) Usually acute, rapid, unremitting, and painless

  (b) Ultimately 20/200 to hand motions (20/20 to no light perception range)

  (c) Sequential bilateral involvement (second eye in weeks to months later); interval between onset in two eyes 0 to 15 months

  (d) Simultaneous onset in 42% to 55%

  (e) Progression of visual loss: Mean 3.7 months (range, acute to 2 years)

  (f) Color vision severely affected

  (g) Visual field loss (central or cecocentral scotomas; especially central 25 to 30 degrees)

(9) Fundus findings at the time of visual loss: Triad of the "suspect fundus"

  (a) Telangiectatic microangiopathy

  (b) Apparent swelling of nerve fiber layer around disc (*pseudoedema*)

  (c) Fluorescein angiogram often shows pseudoedema but may rarely reveal true disc leakage.

(10) Prognosis

  (a) Most patients remain unchanged.

  (b) Some patients (especially specific mutations) experience spontaneous improvement (may occur gradually over 6 months to 1 year or may suddenly improve up to 10 years after onset)

(11) Evaluation and associations

  (a) Exclude other etiologies for optic neuropathy (see above)

  (b) Testing for mitochondrial DNA mutations (e.g., 11778, 3460, 14484) available (some patients are negative though for known mutations)

  (c) Occasional cardiac conduction defects

  (d) Dystonia described with 11778 (most common mutation) and 3460 mutation

  (e) Postural tremor occurs with increased frequency in all forms.

  (f) MS-like illness in up to 45% of females with 11778 mutation; rarely described women with 3460 mutation or men with 11778 mutation

  (g) Thoracic kyphosis in some patients with 3460 mutation

(12) Treatment

  (a) Medical therapy remains unproven: Multivitamins; folate; vitamin B_{12}; thiamine, 100 mg/day; coenzyme Q (ubiquinone), 30 mg daily or 40 mg 3 times a day; ibedinone and other coenzyme Q10 analogues

  (b) Avoid alcohol, tobacco, and other environmental toxins

  (c) Consider electrocardiogram in selected cases

  (d) Low vision assessment

Key Signs: Kjer Optic Neuropathy

- Onset in first decade of life

- Impaired visual acuity

- Inability to perceive blue color

- Central, paracentral, or cecocentral scotomas

- Optic atrophy, usually temporal

Key Signs: Leber's Hereditary Optic Neuropathy

- Usually in young males, 13 to 35 years of age

- Visual acuity loss is acute, rapid, unremitting, and painless

- Visual field loss

- Sequential bilateral involvement, with interval between onset in two eyes is 9 to 15 months; simultaneous onset in almost half of patients

- Progression of visual loss

- Color vision severely affected

- Triad of the suspect fundus: Telangiectatic microangiopathy, pseudoedema, fluorescein angiography shows pseudoedema

Key Treatments

- Medical therapy is unproven.

- Avoid alcohol, tobacco and other environmental toxins

Evaluation of an Atypical or Unexplained Optic Neuropathy

1. First line testing
   a. MRI of optic nerve(s)
   b. If MRI negative, consider laboratory testing.
      (1) Erythrocyte sedimentation rate
      (2) Complete blood count with differential
      (3) Syphilis serology (e.g., fluorescein treponema antibody absorption, rapid plasma reagin)
      (4) Antinuclear antibody if signs of systemic lupus erythematosus
      (5) Chest radiograph or CT chest if considering sarcoid or tuberculosis (PPD [purified protein derivative] skin testing)
      (6) Angiotensin-converting enzyme for sarcoid
   b. Lumbar puncture if progression or suspicious of meningeal process

2. Second line testing
   a. Gallium scan if sarcoidosis suspected and CT of chest or chest radiograph negative
   b. PPD skin testing if tuberculosis suspected
   c. Anti-double-stranded DNA, complement levels, etc. if systemic lupus erythematosus or other collagen vascular disease suspected
   d. Leber's hereditary optic neuropathy mutation blood test in select cases
   e. Heavy metal screen if exposure history suggested
   f. Serum vitamin B_{12} and folate levels
   g. Lyme titer if endemic area or exposure history
   h. Paraneoplastic antibody profile
   i. Consider more specific serologic studies if infectious process is suspected (e.g., titers for toxoplasmosis, toxocara, *Bartonella* [cat-scratch disease])

Bibliography

Brazis PW, Lee AG: Focal points: Neuro-ophthalmic problems caused by medications. Am Acad Ophthalmol 15:1–14, 1998.

Chalmers RM, Harding AE: A case-control study of Leber's hereditary optic neuropathy. Brain 119:1481–1486, 1996.

Hayreh SS, Podhajsky PA, Raman R, et al.: Giant cell arteritis: Validity and reliability of various diagnostic criteria. Am J Ophthalmol 123:285–296, 1997.

Ischemic Optic Neuropathy Decompression Trial Research Group: Optic nerve decompression surgery for nonarteritic anterior ischemic optic neuropathy (NAION) is not effective and may be harmful. JAMA 273:625–632, 1995.

Lee AG, Brazis PW: Clinical Pathways in Neuro-Ophthalmology. An Evidence-Based Approach. New York, Thieme, 1998.

Man PY, Tumbull DM, Chinnery PF: Leber hereditary optic neuropathy. J Med Genet 39:162–169, 2002.

3 Pupillary Disorders

Paul W. Brazis
Andrew G. Lee

Anatomy of Pupillomotor Fibers

1. Pupil is formed by the muscles and pigmented stroma of the anterior uveal tract (the iris).
2. There are two types of iris muscles.
   a. Circumferential sphincter found in the margin of the iris, innervated by the parasympathetic nervous system
   b. Radial pupillodilator muscles, innervated by the sympathetic nervous system
3. Afferent pathway of the pupillary reflex
   a. Begins in the retinal nerve fiber layer and retinal ganglion cells
   b. Travels as optic nerve axons into the optic disc head
   c. Travels to the optic chiasm (nasal fibers cross) and optic tract
   d. Just prior to the lateral geniculate body, fibers branch to the brachium of superior colliculus in the dorsal midbrain.
   e. Synapse in the pretectal mesencephalic nuclei
   f. Project to the ipsilateral and contralateral Edinger-Westphal (E-W) nuclei
4. Efferent pathway: Parasympathetic
   a. Parasympathetic pathway travels with the third cranial nerve
      (1) Brainstem fascicle
      (2) Peripheral third nerve
   b. Pupil fibers lie within the superior and medial portion of the nerve in the subarachnoid space.
   c. Enter with the third nerve into the wall of the cavernous sinus
   d. Enter the orbit as the inferior division to the ciliary ganglion
   e. The majority of these fibers synapse within the ciliary ganglion and travel as short ciliary nerves to the iris sphincter.
5. Efferent pathway: Sympathetic–three neuron arc (i.e., central, preganglionic, and postganglionic neuron)
   a. Central neuron (first-order neuron)
      (1) Begins in the posterior hypothalamus
      (2) Descends in reticular formation
      (3) Multiple synapses in the brainstem
      (4) Synapsing in the intermediolateral gray matter of spinal column at the lower cervical and upper thoracic spine (cilio-spinal center of Budge-Waller) level of C8 to T2.
   b. The second-order neuron (preganglionic)
      (1) Exits in the ventral roots via the white rami (mainly T1 level)
      (2) Travels rostrally (without synapse) through the sympathetic paraspinal ganglia
      (3) Synapse in the superior cervical ganglion
   c. Third-order neuron (postganglionic)
      (1) Travels with the carotid artery to the cavernous sinus
      (2) Within the substance of sinus some fibers join briefly with the sixth cranial nerve.
      (3) Then proceed onto the trigeminal nerve (ophthalmic branch) nasociliary branch to the iris dilator via the long posterior ciliary nerves

Relative Afferent Pupillary Defect (RAPD)

1. Testing for the relative afferent pupil defect (Marcus Gunn's pupil)
   a. Should be done under low background illumination
   b. Patient fixating a distant target to relax accommodation
   c. The examiner should use a bright light source such as an indirect head lamp or Fenhoff transilluminator
   d. Move (swing) the light briskly and rhythmically from eye to eye for a fast count of about 3 seconds with equal stimulation time to each eye.
2. The normal pupil response (no RAPD)
   a. Constriction ipsilateral and contralateral to stimulation by direct light
   b. No dilation of the pupil upon swinging the light from the ipsilateral to the contralateral eye
3. An abnormal response
   a. Immediate dilation of the pupil on swinging the light to the involved eye from the normal contralateral eye (4+ RAPD)
   b. Slower but definite dilatation of the involved pupil (3+ RAPD)
   c. Initially no change; then dilatation of the involved eye (1–2+ RAPD)
   d. Initial constriction followed by an ESCAPE to a

larger size compared with the normal fellow-eye (trace RAPD)

4. Clinical correlation of the RAPD

   a. RAPD correlates roughly with the size and density of the visual field defect and is less tightly correlated with visual acuity.

   b. RAPD occurs in patients with retinal (ipsilateral), optic nerve (ipsilateral, may be subtle), or optic tract (contralateral) disease.

   c. No RAPD from media disease alone (e.g., cataract, corneal disease)

   d. No RAPD with retrogeniculate disease in adults

   e. RAPD rarely in vitreous hemorrhage or amblyopia

   f. May not see RAPD if bilateral anterior visual pathway involvement (e.g., bilateral optic neuropathy) that is relatively symmetric

   g. May have contralateral RAPD to pretectal lesion without visual loss

   h. May be useful to quantitate RAPD with neutral density filters

Key Normal Findings: RAPD Absent

- Ipsilateral and contralateral constriction to direct light stimulation

- No dilatation of pupil on quickly moving a light from the ipsilateral to the contralateral eye

Key Abnormal Findings: RAPD Present

- Pupil dilatation is immediate on quickly moving a light from the normal to the involved eye

- Slower but definite dilatation of the involved eye

- No change initially, then dilatation of the involved eye

- Initial constriction, then an ESCAPE to a larger size compared with the normal eye

Anisocoria (Unequal Pupil Size)

1. Determine light reaction (anisocoria greater in the light or dark)

   a. If the light reaction is normal (anisocoria greater in the dark), then differential diagnosis includes

      (1) Physiologic anisocoria

      (2) Horner's syndrome (sympathetic denervation)

      (3) Sympathetic overaction

   b. Pupils do not react equally to light (anisocoria greater in the light)

      (1) Tonic pupil (e.g., Adie's syndrome)

      (2) Third nerve palsy

      (3) Pharmacologic mydriasis

      (4) Iris trauma

2. Physiologic anisocoria (about 20% of normal persons)

   a. Lid position normal (no ptosis)

   b. Pupil size may vary from day to day

   c. Equal anisocoria in light and dark

   d. Usually <1 mm of difference between pupils

   e. Cocaine test (see below) negative for Horner's syndrome

Key Signs: Anisocoria

Anisocoria with Normal Light Reaction (Anisocoria Greater in Dark)

- Physiologic anisocoria

- Horner's syndrome

- Sympathetic overaction

Anisocoria with Pupils That Do Not React Equally to Light (Anisocoria Greater in Light)

- Tonic pupil (e.g., Adie's syndrome)

- Third nerve palsy

- Pharmacologic mydriasis

- Iris trauma

3. Horner's syndrome (oculosympathetic disruption)

   a. Common examination findings

      (1) Ptosis (usually <2 mm) due to weak Müller's muscle of upper lid (may also have lower lid "upside down ptosis")

      (2) Moderate ipsilateral miosis

      (3) Apparent enophthalmos (ptosis and upside-down ptosis)

      (4) Anhidrosis on ipsilateral face

      (5) Dilatation lag (affected pupil dilates slower than unaffected pupil when lights turned off)

   b. Less common examination findings

      (1) Upside-down ptosis (lower lid smooth muscles)

      (2) Increased amplitude of accommodation

(3) Decreased intraocular pressure

(4) Lighter iris (heterochromia iridis) in congenital (or rarely acquired) cases

c. Horner's syndrome: Diagnosis

(1) Horner's syndrome can be confirmed by instilling in both eyes one drop of a 10% cocaine solution. Another drop is instilled 1 minute later, and the result is read in 45 minutes with the patient in the dark. The normal pupil dilates after cocaine instillation, which blocks the presynaptic reuptake of norepinephrine at the neuromuscular junction in the dilator muscle, but in Horner's syndrome the pupil fails to dilate as well. A postcocaine anisocoria of 0.8 mm or greater is significant.

(2) Topical 1% hydroxyamphetamine (Paredrine) releases norepinephrine into the synaptic cleft. It should be instilled at least 48 hours after the cocaine test and dilates a pupil in Horner's syndrome only if the lesion is preganglionic.

(3) No pharmacologic test is available to differentiate a first-order from a second-order neuron Horner's syndrome.

d. Etiologies of Horner's syndrome

(1) A Horner's syndrome may result from a lesion anywhere along the three-neuron pathway.

(2) Patients with a central or first-order Horner's syndrome can usually be identified by the presence of associated hypothalamic, brainstem, or spinal cord signs or symptoms. A central Horner's syndrome may be seen with hypothalamic hemorrhage, or with tumor, but it occurs most commonly after brainstem vascular lesions.

(3) The preganglionic (intermediate or second-order) Horner's syndrome patient may have neck or arm pain, anhidrosis involving the face and neck, brachial plexopathy, vocal cord paralysis, or phrenic nerve palsy. It may occur in isolation, however. The following etiologies may produce a second-order lesion.

(a) Neoplasm located in the neck, head, brachial plexus, or lung (e.g., glomus tumors, breast cancer, sarcomas, lung cancer, lymphoreticular neoplasms, neurofibroma, or thyroid adenoma) may cause a second-order Horner's syndrome.

(b) Cervicothoracic abnormalities causing a Horner's syndrome include a cervical rib, pachymeningitis, hypertrophic spinal arthritis, foraminal osteophyte, ruptured intervertebral disc, thoracic aneurysm, herpes zoster in T3–T4 distribution, and continuous thoracic epidural analgesia.

(c) Neck, brachial plexus or lung trauma or surgery, including birth trauma (Klumpke's paralysis), upper cervical sympathectomy, anterior C3–C6 fusion, and radical thyroid surgery.

(4) The postganglionic (third-order) Horner's syndrome patient may have ipsilateral pain and other symptoms suggestive of cluster or migraine headaches (e.g., tearing, facial flushing, rhinorrhea).

(a) Ipsilateral carotid artery occlusive disease

(b) Dissection of the internal carotid artery (e.g., traumatic, spontaneous). The association of a third-order Horner's syndrome and orbital and/or ipsilateral head pain or neck pain of acute onset is so characteristic that it should be considered diagnostic of internal carotid artery dissection unless proven otherwise.

(c) Postganglionic Horner's syndrome due to cavernous sinus lesions (e.g., thrombosis, infection, neoplasm) usually is associated with other localizing signs such as ipsilateral third, fourth, or sixth nerve palsy or trigeminal nerve dysfunction. Inflammatory, neoplastic, or vascular disease of the cavernous sinus may result in ipsilateral retroorbital pain and a Horner's syndrome (Raeder's paratrigeminal neuralgia). Other causes of a third-order Horner syndrome include infectious or inflammatory lesions (e.g., cervical lymphadenopathy, otitis media, petrositis, sphenoid sinus mucocele, herpetic geniculate neuralgia, meningitis, sinusitis), neoplasms (e.g., cervical node metastasis, cervical sympathetic chain schwannoma or neurolemommas), systemic peripheral or autonomic disorders (e.g., diabetes, amyloidosis, Shy-Drager syndrome, AIDS), trauma (e.g., basilar skull fracture), giant cell arteritis, and Wegener's granulomatosis.

(d) A Horner's syndrome that alternates from one eye to the other ("alternating" Horner's syndrome), usually over days to weeks, has been described with cervical cord lesions, syringomyelia, radiation myelopathy, and Shy-Drager syndrome.

Key Signs: Horner's Syndrome

- General: ptosis, moderate ipsilateral miosis, apparent enophthalmos, anhidrosis on ipsilateral face, dilatation lag

- First-order (central): Associated hypothalamic, brainstem, or spinal cord signs or symptoms

- Second-order (intermediate): Neck or arm pain, anhidrosis involving the face and neck, brachial plexopathy, vocal cord paralysis, phrenic nerve palsy

- Third-order (postganglionic): Ipsilateral pain and symptoms suggestive of cluster or migraine headaches

- Alternating Horner's syndrome: Alternates from one eye to the other

4. Parasympathetic dysfunction

   a. If anisocoria is present and one of the pupils, generally the larger one, reacts poorly to light (anisocoria greater in light), the diagnosis can be narrowed to four possibilities:

   (1) Third nerve palsy

      (a) Acute pupillary dilatation and unresponsiveness is characteristic of compression of the third nerve in the subarachnoid space, usually by the uncus of the temporal lobe or by an internal carotid-posterior communicating artery aneurysm.

      (b) Pupillary sparing is the rule with ischemic (e.g., diabetic) oculomotor neuropathy.

      (c) Although an extra-axial lesion (e.g., unruptured intracranial aneurysm) compressing the third nerve may cause a dilated pupil in isolation (or with minimal ocular motor nerve paresis), in the absence of an extraocular motility deficit and/or ptosis, an isolated dilated pupil is usually not due to third nerve paresis. In addition, although intracranial aneurysms, especially those involving the posterior communicating artery–internal carotid artery junction, often produce a fixed and dilated pupil, this is almost always associated with other signs of a third nerve palsy.

   (2) Damage to the ciliary ganglion or the short ciliary nerves results in a tonic pupil.

      (a) Initially there is an isolated internal ophthalmoplegia (a fixed, dilated pupil with loss of accommodation), but later there is mydriasis with a poor or absent reaction to light but a slow constriction to prolonged near effort (light-near dissociation).

      (b) Redilatation after constriction to near stimuli is slow and tonic.

      (c) Segmental vermiform movements of the iris borders may be evident on slit-lamp examination (due to sector palsy of other areas of the iris sphincter).

      (d) Cholinergic supersensitivity (see below) of the denervated iris sphincter may be demonstrated.

      (e) Tonic pupils are thought to be due to damage of the ciliary ganglion or short ciliary nerves with subsequent collateral sprouting, resulting in the iris sphincter being almost entirely innervated by accommodative elements.

      (f) They occur from local damage to the ciliary ganglion or short ciliary nerves, as part of a widespread peripheral or autonomic neuropathy, or idiopathically in otherwise healthy individuals (Adie's tonic pupil syndrome). A tonic pupil may also be seen with hyporeflexia and progressive segmental hypohidrosis (Ross syndrome).

   (3) Damage to the iris due to ischemia, trauma, or an inflammatory process may cause mydriasis. Clinical characteristics suggesting abnormalities of the iris structure as a cause for mydriasis include

      (a) No associated ptosis or ocular motility disturbance (vs. third nerve palsy)

      (b) The pupil is often irregular with tears in the pupillary margin due to tears in iris sphincter (vs a smooth margin in drug-related pupillary abnormalities).

      (c) Irregular contraction of the pupil to light, the eventual development of iris atrophy may occur, and poor or no response of the pupil to 1% pilocarpine.

   (4) Mydriasis may be induced by the instillation of a parasympathicolytic drug (e.g., atropine, scopolamine). Unilateral mydriasis may follow the use of transdermal scopolamine to prevent motion sickness,

the accidental instillation into the eye of fluids from certain plants (e.g., jimsonweed) that contain belladonna and atropine-like alkaloids, and exposure to certain cosmetics and perfumes.

(a) A careful history is usually all that is required in patients with inadvertent or intentional (e.g., glaucoma medication, treatment with topical cycloplegics for uveitis) exposure to agents that may affect pupil size.

(b) In general, in accidental pharmacologic pupillary abnormalities, a large pupil indicates increased sympathetic tone with dilator stimulation (e.g., ocular decongestants, adrenergic inhalants in the intensive care unit, etc.) or decreased parasympathetic tone with sphincter block (e.g., belladonna alkaloids, scopolamine patch, anticholinergic inhalants, lidocaine injection in orbit). Small pupils indicate decreased sympathetic tone or increased parasympathetic stimulation (e.g., pilocarpine glaucoma drops, anticholinesterases such as from a flea or tick collar or insecticides).

(c) Nurses, physicians, and other health care workers are particularly prone to inadvertent or intentional exposure to pharmacologic mydriatics.

(d) The pupil size of patients with pharmacologic sphincter blockade is often quite large (>8 mm), often on the order of 10 to 12 mm in diameter, which is much greater than the mydriasis usually seen in a typical third nerve palsy or tonic pupil syndromes.

(e) The pupils are evenly affected 360 degrees (vs. a tonic pupil) and smoothly affected around without irregularity (vs iris trauma).

(f) Adrenergic pharmacologic mydriasis (e.g., phenylephrine) may be clinically distinguished by blanched conjunctival vessels, residual light reaction, and a retracted upper lid due to sympastimulation of the upper lid retractor muscle. Many "eye-whitening" drops (e.g., oxymetazoline, phenylephrine) contain sympathomimetics.

(5) Pharmacologic testing of the dilated pupil.

(a) Cholinergic supersensitivity is characteristic of a tonic pupil and causes pupillary constriction when dilute 0.1% pilocarpine is instilled. This drug has little effect on the normal pupil.

(b) A stronger solution of pilocarpine (1%) causes pupil constriction in the case of a third nerve lesion but does not modify pupillary size if the anisocoria is due to an atropinic drug or to iris damage. Constriction after the application of 1% pilocarpine (after failing to constrict with a 0.1% solution) may also occur with prior instillation of a parasympathetic agent that is "wearing off," with the use of a sympathomimetic agent, or with acute Adie's syndrome.

Key Signs: Mydriasis

Related to Iris Structure Abnormalities

- Irregular pupil with tears in papillary margin due to tears in iris sphincter
- Irregular contraction of the pupil to light
- Eventual development of iris atrophy
- Poor or no response to 1% pilocarpine

Related to Exposure to Drugs

- A careful history for exposure to agents that may affect pupil size
- Health care providers are particularly prone to unintentional exposure.
- Pupil is much larger than with mydriasis seen in third nerve palsy or tonic pupil
- Pupils are evenly affected (compared with a tonic pupil) and smoothly affected around without irregularity (compared with iris trauma)

5. Argyll Robertson pupil

a. The Argyll Robertson pupil is characteristically seen in patients with neurosyphilis.

b. Pupils are bilaterally (but may be asymmetric) miotic and irregular, with variable iris atrophy. A decreased or absent pupillary light reaction is noted with an intact near response (light-near dissociation)

6. Light-near dissociation may also be seen with midbrain lesions (e.g., dorsal midbrain syndrome, encephalitis/meningitis, Wernicke's encephalopathy and alcoholism, demyelination, pineal tumors,

vascular disease). Other causes of light-near dissociation include sarcoidosis, diabetes, aberrant regeneration of the oculomotor nerve, Adie's syndrome, familial amyloidosis, paraproteinemic neuropathy, syringomyelia, spinocerebellar ataxia type I, and myotonic dystrophy. Diabetics of long-standing and patients with myotonic dystrophy may have small, poorly reactive pupils.

Key Signs: Argyll Robertson Pupil

- Neurosyphilis

- Pupils are bilaterally (but may be asymmetric) miotic and irregular, with variable iris atrophy.

- Decreased or absent papillary light reaction is noted with an intact near response.

Caveat

- Patients with long-standing diabetes or myotonic dystrophy may have small, poorly reactive pupils.

Bibliography

Keane JR: Oculosympathetic paresis. Arch Neurol 36:13–16, 1979.

Lee AG, Brazis PW: Clinical Pathways in Neuro-Ophthalmology. An Evidence-Based Approach. New York, Thieme, 1998.

Loewenfeld IE, Thompson HS: The tonic pupil: A reevaluation. Am J Ophthalmol 63:46–87, 1967.

Nadeau SE, Trobe JD: Pupil sparing in oculomotor palsy: A brief review. Ann Neurol 13:143–148, 1983.

Thompson HS, Pilley SFJ: Unequal pupils. A flow chart for sorting out the anisocorias. Surv Ophthalmol 21:45–48, 1976.

4 Ptosis, Lid Lag, and Lid Retraction

Paul W. Brazis
Andrew G. Lee

The Normal Eyelid

1. In normal adults, the upper lid just covers the upper cornea, and the lower lid lies slightly below the inferior corneal margin.
2. Eyelid opening occurs with contraction of the levator palpebrae superioris muscle (oculomotor nerve).
3. Accessory muscles for lid elevation
   a. Müller's muscle (sympathetic innervated)
   b. Frontalis muscle (innervated by the temporal branch of the facial nerve) helps
4. Eyelid closure occurs when levator motor neuronal activity ceases.
5. Rapid and firm eye closure is a function of the orbicularis oculi muscles, which are controlled by the facial nerve.
6. Motor neurons for both levator muscles are in the unpaired central caudal nucleus, located at the dorsal caudal pole of the oculomotor complex adjacent to the medial rectus and superior rectus subdivisions.

Ptosis

1. Measurement of ptosis
   a. Ptosis can be measured with the limbus or central light reflex used as reference points.
   b. The usual position of the adult upper eyelid margin is 1.5 mm below the upper limbus or 3 to 4 mm above the light reflex (the margin reflex distance).
   c. If the vertical distance from limbus to limbus is 11 mm, then 4 mm of ptosis would result in bisection of the center of the cornea or pupil by the lid margin.
   d. The palpebral fissure and upper eyelid fold are measured in the primary position of gaze. Normally, the upper lid fold is located 5 to 7 mm above the upper lid margin.
   e. Levator function is the amount of excursion of the upper eyelid from maximal straight down-gaze to maximal upgaze. Levator function is usually 10 to 12 mm or more. The contraction of the frontalis muscle should be neutralized by pressure over the center of the eyebrow. About 2 mm of movement probably is transmitted from contraction of the superior rectus muscle, so that a measurement of 2 mm or less can be considered no levator function. Movement of 4 mm or less is classified as poor levator function; from 5 to 7 mm as fair levator function; and 8 mm or more as good levator function.

2. Etiologies of ptosis
   a. Supranuclear, nuclear (third), and infranuclear lesions include third nerve palsy, oculosympathetic lesions (Horner's syndrome), lesions of the neuromuscular junction (myasthenia gravis), diseases of the muscle, and local mechanical lid abnormalities.
   b. A unilateral (pseudo) ptosis may be associated with eyelid retraction on the opposite side due to Hering's law of equal innervation.
   c. Supranuclear ptosis
      (1) May be unilateral or bilateral
      (2) Unilateral supranuclear ptosis is usually due to a lesion of the opposite cerebral hemisphere, especially ischemic lesions (e.g., middle cerebral artery infarction).
      (3) Bilateral supranuclear ptosis may be seen with unilateral or bilateral hemispheric disease.
      (4) Bilateral supranuclear ptosis associated with supranuclear downward gaze paralysis, but with other oculomotor functions relatively intact, has been described with midbrain lesions (e.g., glioma).
   d. Apraxia of eyelid opening
      (1) Refers to an inability to open the eyes voluntarily in the absence of ptosis or blepharospasm
      (2) Not true ptosis but difficulty in overcoming levator inhibition
      (3) Etiologies
         (a) Right hemisphere or bilateral cerebral hemispheric lesions
         (b) Diseases of the extrapyramidal system: Huntington's disease, Parkinson's disease, progressive supranuclear palsy, amyotrophic lateral sclerosis-parkinsonism-dementia complex, Shy-Drager syndrome, neuroacanthocyto-

sis, adult-onset Hallervordan-Spatz syndrome, Wilson's disease, cortical-basal ganglionic degeneration

   (c) Focal inferior and lateral frontal lobe cortical degeneration

   (d) Motor neuron disease

   (e) Post-bilateral stereotactic subthalamotomy

   (f) Post-implantation of bilateral subthalamic nucleus electrical stimulators for Parkinson's disease

   (g) Unilateral putaminal hemorrhage

   (h) Idiopathic

e. Ptosis may also occur with lesions of the oculomotor nucleus, fascicle, or nerve, and is often associated with other signs of oculomotor dysfunction (e.g., mydriasis, ophthalmoplegia). Lesions of the central caudal nucleus cause bilateral ptosis.

f. A mild ptosis is also evident with oculosympathetic lesions (Horner's syndrome), in which case there is associated miosis.

g. Ptosis may also occur with diseases of the neuromuscular junction (e.g., myasthenia gravis, Lambert–Eaton myasthenic syndrome, and botulism); myopathic processes (e.g., myotonic muscular dystrophy, chronic progressive external ophthalmoplegia, and dermatomyositis); and the Miller Fisher variant of Guillain-Barré syndrome.

h. In myasthenia gravis, Cogan's "eyelid twitch sign" may be observed. When the patient is asked to look up after having kept the eyes directed downward for 20 to 30 seconds, the affected upper eyelid may twitch before setting in a ptotic position.

i. Local mechanical factors may also cause ptosis, including levator tendon damage due to ocular surgery or thyroid eye disease. Mechanical causes of ptosis include tumors or cysts of the conjunctiva, infection (e.g., preseptal or orbital cellulitis), cicatricial scarring (e.g., posttraumatic, postsurgical, or postinflammatory), inflammation, and edema (e.g., Graves' disease), infiltration (e.g., amyloid, sarcoid, neoplastic, Waldenström's macroglobulinemia), primary or metastatic tumors or orbital pseudotumor, contact lenses wear, contact lens migration, foreign body reaction, giant papillary conjunctivitis, and disinsertion of the levator from excessive eyelid manipulation. Prolonged hard contact lens wear may induce a lower position of the upper eyelid and eventually lead to ptosis through levator disinsertion.

j. Disinsertion of the levator tendon may occur with age, resulting in unilateral or bilateral involutional ptosis in the elderly.

   (1) Unlike congenital ptosis, in which the dystrophic levator precludes normal eyelid excursion, the lid continues to move normally in upgaze and downgaze in aponeurotic disinsertion (excursion of the eyelid from downgaze to upgaze is usually 9 mm or more).

   (2) Congenital ptosis usually is the result of abnormal development of the levator and may often coexist with superior rectus muscle paresis (both muscles originate from a common embryologic tissue mass). With congenital ptosis the levator is fibrotic and dystrophic, so that lid elevation in upgaze is poor (lack of levator contraction), and the lid fails to follow the globe in downgaze (inability of the muscle to relax). Levator function (i.e., excursion of the eyelid from downgaze to upgaze) is thus poor (5 mm or less).

k. False ptosis (pseudoptosis) may occur with mechanical impairment of upward eyelid movement (e.g., with orbital tumor); orbital inflammation and eyelid swelling; an anophthalmic socket, with microphthalmia or phthisis bulbi; lid retraction in the opposite eye; and on the side opposite a hypertropic eye (when the hypertropic eye fixes, the opposite eye becomes hypotropic and demonstrates an apparent ptosis).

Etiologies

• Supranuclear lesions

• Lesions of the oculomotor complex

• Oculosympathetic lesions (Horner's syndrome)

• Lesions of the neuromuscular junction

• Diseases of the muscle

• Local mechanical lid abnormalities

Eyelid Retraction and Lid Lag

1. The upper lid position is abnormal if it exposes a white band of sclera between the lid margin and the upper corneal limbus. This may be due to

a. Lid retraction (related to overactivity of the levator muscle, contracture of the levator, hyperactivity of Müller's muscle), which may be noted in the primary position

b. Lid lag, which is noted on attempted down-gaze.

2. Etiologies of lid lag and lid retraction

a. Neurogenic eyelid retraction and lid lag may be due to supranuclear, nuclear or infranuclear lesions affecting the levator or conditions that produce hyperactivity of the sympathetically innervated Müller's muscle.

b. Dorsal mesencephalic supranuclear lesions may result in eyelid retraction, which is seen when the eyes are in the primary position of gaze or on looking upward (Collier's sign, or "posterior fossa stare").

c. Lid lag may occur on a supranuclear basis in progressive supranuclear palsy, likely a result of defective inhibition of the levator nuclei during downgaze.

d. Lid lag may occur in Guillain-Barré syndrome (only observed on downgaze)

e. Lid retraction may also occur with Parkinsonism and Fisher's syndrome

f. Ipsilateral ptosis and contralateral superior eyelid retraction may be due to a nuclear oculomotor nerve syndrome (plus-minus lid syndrome).

g. Paradoxic lid retraction may occur with jaw movement or swallowing (Marcus Gunn's phenomenon). This trigemino-oculomotor synkinesis occurs on a congenital basis.

h. Eyelid retraction may also occur with aberrant regeneration of the oculomotor nerve (when the eye adducts), with congenital or acquired abducens palsies (on abduction), with levator denervation supersensitivity after oculomotor palsies, and with irritative oculosympathetic lesions (Claude Bernard syndrome).

i. Eyelid retraction may also occur if there is ptosis of the opposite eyelid (especially when the ptosis is due to disease at or distal to the neuromuscular junction) when fixating with the eye with the unilateral ptosis (due to Hering's law).

j. Other causes for lid retraction include prolonged steroid use, local application of phenylephrine, an enlarged globe, recession of the superior rectus, or nondysthyroid cicatricial retraction (e.g., due to scar after trauma, herpes zoster).

k. Eyelid retraction and lid lag may also occur with neuromuscular diseases, including myasthenia gravis, familial periodic paralysis, myotonic syndromes, and thyroid eye disease.

l. Thyroid eye disease is one of the most common etiologies for acquired unilateral or bilateral sustained lid retraction; the retraction is due to pathologic shortening of the levator muscle. On looking down, the eyelid pauses and then follows the eye (Graefe's sign) and, in the primary position, there is upper lid retraction with infrequent and incomplete blinking (Stellwag's sign).

m. Volitional lid retraction may occur and is usually bilateral and associated with furrowing of the brows (frontalis contraction).

n. Retraction of the lower eyelid may be the earliest clinical lid sign of a lesion of the facial nerve, and facial nerve lesions are the most common cause of lower lid retraction.

Caveat

Thyroid eye disease is one of the most common causes for acquired sustained lid retraction, which is due to pathologic shortening of the levator muscle.

Bibliography

Bartley GB: The differential diagnosis and classification of eyelid retraction. Ophthalmology 103:168–176, 1996.

Jankovic J: Apraxia of lid opening. Movement Disord 10:5, 1995.

Lee AG, Brazis PW: Clinical Pathways in Neuro-Ophthalmology. An Evidence-Based Approach. New York, Thieme, 1998.

Schmidtke K, Buttner-Ennever JA: Nervous control of eyelid function. A review of clinical, experimental and pathologic data. Brain 115:227–247, 1992.

5 Ocular Motor Palsies

Paul W. Brazis
Andrew G. Lee

Diplopia

Horizontal binocular diplopia is usually due to disease processes affecting the medial and/or lateral rectus muscles, the innervation of these muscles (including ocular motor cranial nerves and neuromuscular junction), or processes affecting fusion or convergence and divergence mechanisms.

1. If the patient complains of vertical diplopia in primary gaze, often one of the vertically acting extraocular muscles is underacting (e.g., right and/or left inferior rectus, superior rectus, inferior oblique, or superior oblique)

2. To identify the muscle or nerve involved, subjective and objective tests should be used.

3. Misalignment (deviation) of the visual axis when only one eye is viewing is referred to as a *phoria*. Misalignment of the visual axis with both eyes viewing is called a *tropia*.

4. When *strabismus* (misalignment of the visual axes) exists, it is named by the direction of deviation (e.g., turned in: esodeviation; turned out: exodeviation; turned down: hypodeviation; turned up: hyperdeviation; intorted: incyclodeviation; extorted: excyclotorsion)

5. Strabismus may be *comitant* (the deviation is stable in nonextremes of gaze) or *incomitant* (the deviation varies in different gaze positions). Eye deviations from childhood strabismus are typically comitant while most of the acquired deviations are incomitant.

6. The alternate cover test is performed by having the patient fixate on a target in each of the nine positions of gaze. The three-step test can be applied with the cover-uncover examination in the evaluation of vertical diplopia due to a single muscle paresis. The deviation can be measured with prisms (in prism diopters).

   a. Determine whether there is a right or left hypertropia or hyperphoria in primary position. For example, if there is a right hypertropia in primary position, there is paresis of the right eye depressors (right inferior rectus or superior oblique) or left eye elevators (left superior rectus or inferior oblique).

   b. Compare the amount of vertical deviation in right and left gaze. For example, if the right hypertropia increases in left gaze, either the

right superior oblique or left superior rectus is underacting.

   c. Compare the vertical deviation in right head tilt and left head tilt (Bielschowsky maneuver). For example, if the vertical deviation increases with right head tilt, the right superior oblique must be weak; if the hyperdeviation increases on left head tilt, the left superior rectus is weak.

Disease of the Ocular Muscles

1. Disease of isolated extraocular muscles, particularly when it affects the lateral rectus or the superior oblique or causes patterns of weakness that resemble central involvement, may be difficult to differentiate from neurogenic weakness.

2. A mechanical restriction of the superior oblique tendon at the pulley may prevent the upward and inward movement of the globe (Brown's superior oblique tendon sheath syndrome). Episodic vertical diplopia results as a consequence of intermittent trapping of the eye on gaze downward and inward or in the field of action of the superior oblique, mimicking paresis of the inferior oblique muscle. This syndrome may be caused by swelling of the superior oblique tendon behind the pulley and may be congenital or acquired.

3. Thyroid (Graves') ophthalmopathy

   a. The myopathy of dysthyroid orbitopathy is attributed to inflammation and fibrosis of the muscles, sparing tendinous insertions.

   b. The inferior recti are usually most severely affected, followed by the medial recti, superior recti, and oblique muscles. The lateral rectus is rarely affected.

   c. Vertical diplopia caused by asymmetric involvement of the inferior or superior rectus muscles is the most common presentation

   d. Other components of dysthyroid orbitopathy include orbital congestion, upper lid retraction, lid lag on looking down, proptosis, conjunctival injection, and optic neuropathy due to compression of the optic nerve by enlarged extraocular muscles in the orbital apex

4. Myasthenia gravis (MG) should be considered in any case of diplopia and may mimic any pattern of neurogenic paresis.

   a. Diplopia may occur in 90% of patients with myasthenia gravis, and 15% will manifest only

393

ocular signs. Of these, 50% to 80% go on to develop generalized MG usually within 2 to 3 years of onset.

b. Any muscle or combination of muscles may be affected, and weakness characteristically increases with sustained effort (i.e., fatigue).

c. May mimic internuclear ophthalmoplegia, gaze palsy, one-and-a-half syndrome, complete external ophthalmoplegia, or other central lesions

d. Unfortunately, certain intracranial mass lesions (e.g., parasellar tumors and aneurysms or midbrain gliomas) may mimic the weakness and fatigability of the lids and extraocular muscles seen with MG.

Caveat

- Diplopia occurs in 90% of patients with MG.

---

5. Botulism, like MG, affects the neuromuscular junction and can cause similar eye findings, usually associated with blurred vision secondary to accommodative paresis.

6. Orbital pseudotumor (idiopathic orbital inflammation)

a. Neuroimaging showing a focal or diffuse usually unilateral orbital inflammatory lesion

b. Histopathology demonstrating a fibro-inflammatory lesion

c. Investigations eliminating identifiable local or systemic causes

d. May be confined to one or multiple extraocular muscles

e. Clinical findings include acute or subacute orbital pain, diplopia, conjunctival chemosis and injection, ptosis, and proptosis.

f. Often monophasic but recurrent episodes may occur

Oculomotor Nerve (Cranial Nerve III) Palsy

1. Localization of Lesions: Lesions can affect the third nerve in the brainstem (nucleus or fascicular portion), subarachnoid space, cavernous sinus, superior orbital fissure, or orbit.

a. Lesions affecting the third nerve nucleus

(1) Oculomotor nucleus: Ipsilateral complete cranial nerve (CN) III palsy; contralateral ptosis and superior rectus paresis

(2) Oculomotor subnucleus: Isolated muscle palsy (e.g., inferior rectus) may occur

(3) Isolated levator subnucleus: Isolated bilateral ptosis

b. Lesions affecting the third nerve fasciculus

(1) Isolated fascicle: Partial or complete isolated CN III palsy with or without pupil involvement

(2) Paramedian mesencephalon: Plus-minus syndrome (ipsilateral ptosis and contralateral eyelid retraction)

(3) Fascicle, red nucleus, superior cerebellar peduncle: Ipsilateral CN III palsy with contralateral ataxia and tremor (Claude's syndrome)

(4) Fascicle and cerebral peduncle: Ipsilateral CN III palsy with contralateral hemiparesis (Weber's syndrome)

(5) Fascicle and red nucleus/substantia nigra: Ipsilateral CN III palsy with contralateral choreiform movements (Benedikt's syndrome)

a. Lesions affecting the third nerve in the subarachnoid space: Complete CN III palsy with or without other cranial nerve involvement; superior or inferior division palsy

b. Lesions affecting the third nerve in the cavernous sinus: Painful or painless CN III palsy; with or without palsies of CN IV, VI, and V1; CN III palsy with small pupil (Horner's syndrome); primary aberrant CN III regeneration may occur

c. Lesions affecting the third nerve in the superior orbital fissure: CN III palsy with or without palsies of CN IV, VI, V1; often with proptosis

d. Lesion affecting the third nerve in the orbit

(1) Oculomotor nerve; superior or inferior branch lesion: CN III palsy; superior or inferior CN III branch palsy

(2) Optic nerve, orbital structures: Visual loss, proptosis, lid swelling, chemosis

2. Etiologies of oculomotor nerve lesions by location

a. Nuclear oculomotor nerve palsy

(1) Infarction or hemorrhage

(2) Tumor

(3) Infection

(4) Trauma

(5) Multiple sclerosis (MS)

b. Fascicular oculomotor nerve palsy

(1) Infarction or hemorrhage

(2) Tumor

(3) MS

(4) Trauma including surgery and radiation therapy

c. Subarachnoid space

(1) Aneurysms of the internal carotid-

posterior communicating, superior cerebellar, basilar, or posterior cerebral arteries

(2) Tumors, especially meningiomas, chordomas, metastases, or primary tumors of the third nerve

(3) Glioblastoma multiforme

(4) Infectious or inflammatory processes of the meninges (e.g., sarcoidosis and Wegener's granulomatosis) and carcinomatous or lymphomatous meningitis

(5) Subarachnoid hemorrhage with leukemia

(6) Pseudotumor cerebri

(7) Spontaneous intracranial hypotension

(8) Trauma, especially during neurosurgical procedures

(9) Nerve infarction from diabetes, atherosclerosis, giant cell arteritis, or systemic lupus erythematosus (nerve infarction may also occur in the cavernous sinus or anywhere along the course of nerve)

(10) Uncal herniation

(11) Hydrocephalus

d. Cavernous sinus/superior orbital fissure lesions

(1) Aneurysm of the internal carotid or posterior communicating artery

(2) Dural carotid cavernous sinus fistula

(3) Cavernous sinus thrombosis or infection (e.g., tuberculoma); superior ophthalmic vein thrombosis

(4) Tumors, including pituitary adenoma, meningioma, esthesioneuroblastoma, arachnoid cyst, neurinoma, nasopharyngeal carcinoma, myeloma, lymphoma, Hodgkin's disease, and metastases

(5) Pituitary infarction or hemorrhage (pituitary apoplexy)

(6) Wegener's granulomatosis

(7) Gammopathy

(8) Mucocele of the sphenoid sinus or sphenoid sinusitis

(9) Tolosa-Hunt syndrome or other granulomatous diseases

e. Orbital lesions

(1) Infections, inflammations, and granulomatous processes (e.g., orbital pseudotumor)

(2) Sphenoid sinus mucocele

(3) Tumors

(4) Dural arteriovenous malformation

(5) Trauma

f. Unknown localization

(1) Congenital

(2) Migraine

(3) Viral infections (including herpes zoster ophthalmicus or Ramsay Hunt syndrome) and immunizations

(4) Lyme disease

(5) Diffuse neuropathic processes (e.g., Fisher's syndrome and chronic inflammatory polyradiculoneuropathy)

(6) Cervical carotid artery dissection, stenosis, or occlusion

(7) Subdural hematomas

(8) Toxic effects of drugs

(9) Dental anesthesia

(10) Radiation therapy

Localization of Oculomotor Nerve Lesions

• Nuclear

• Fascicular

• Subarachnoid space

• Cavernous sinus/superior orbital fissure

• Orbit

• Unknown

---

1. Months to years after the occurrence of an oculomotor lesion, clinical findings of aberrant regeneration of the third nerve may be seen.

a. Findings include elevation of the lid on downgaze (pseudo-von Graefe phenomenon) or on adduction, but lid depression during abduction.

b. The lid-gaze synkinesis is best seen with attempted adduction in downgaze.

c. Other findings with aberrant regeneration include limitation of elevation and depression of the eye with occasional eyeball retraction on attempted vertical gaze, adduction of the eye on attempted elevation or depression, and suppression of the vertical phase of the optico-kinetic response.

d. Aberrant regeneration may be seen after oculomotor damage due to congenital causes, trauma, aneurysm, migraine, and syphilis but is almost never caused by ischemic neuropathy.

e. Long-standing lesions, such as meningiomas of the cavernous sinus, trigeminal neuromas, pituitary tumors, or large aneurysms, may present as a primary aberrant regeneration of the third nerve without a history of a third nerve palsy.

2. Ocular neuromyotonia (ONM) is a rare disorder characterized by episodic (lasting seconds to minutes) horizontal or vertical diplopia, occurring

either spontaneously or after sustained (10 to 20 seconds) eccentric gaze.

   a. OMN may affect the oculomotor, trochlear, or abducens nerve. Most patients have had prior radiation therapy to the sellar or parasellar region (months to years before onset of the ONM) for tumors, although in some cases no responsible structural lesion or history of radiation therapy is noted. Rarely ONM may be due to a compressive lesion.

   b. Thought to reflect impaired muscle relaxation due to inappropriate discharges from oculomotor, trochlear, or abducens neurons or axons with unstable cellular membranes.

   c. Responds well to carbamazepine

Key Signs

Lesions Affecting the Third Nerve Nucleus

- Ipsilateral complete CN III palsy; contralateral ptosis and superior rectus paresis

- Isolated muscle palsy

- Isolated bilateral ptosis

Lesions Affecting the Third Nerve Fasciculus

- Partial or complete isolated CN III palsy with or without pupil involvement

- Plus-minus syndrome

- Claude's syndrome

- Weber's syndrome

- Benedikt's syndrome

Trochlear Nerve (Cranial Nerve IV) Palsy

1. Diagnosis: Patients with a unilateral trochlear nerve palsy demonstrate hypotropia, excyclotropia, or head tilt.

   a. Hypotropia may occur in the normal eye if the affected eye is fixating; if the unaffected eye is fixating, hypertropia occurs in the involved eye. This hypertropia is usually most prominent in the field of gaze of the involved superior oblique muscle (i.e., down and in), especially in cases of acute or recent onset. The hypertropia may also be most prominent in the field of gaze of the ipsilateral overacting inferior oblique muscle in subacute or chronic cases or evident in the entire paretic field (spread of comitance). Duction testing may variably reveal underaction of the ipsilateral superior oblique muscle, overaction of the ipsilateral inferior oblique

muscle, or overaction of the contralateral superior oblique muscle.

   b. Excyclotropia is usually evident on fundus examination and double Maddox rod testing (Maddox rods of different colors over each eye). This cyclotropia is symptomatic only in acquired (vs. congenital) cases.

   c. Head tilt is incorporated to eliminate the hypertropia and, rarely, the cyclotropia. This head tilt is present in approximately 70% of patients and is usually away from the involved side but may be paradoxical (toward the involved side) in about 3%. Paradoxical head tilt presumably results in a greater separation of images, thus allowing one of the images to be ignored.

2. Diagnosis: Bilateral fourth nerve palsies result in an inability to depress either eye fully in adduction. There may be associated bilateral overaction of the inferior oblique muscles. Bilateral fourth nerve palsies are suggested by

   a. A right hypertropia in left gaze and left hypertropia in right gaze.

   b. A positive Bielschowsky test on tilt to either shoulder ("double Bielschowsky test").

   c. A large excyclotropia (>10 degrees).

   d. V-pattern esotropia (15 prism diopters or more difference in esotropia between upgaze and downgaze). The "V" pattern is caused by a decrease of the abducting effect of the superior oblique(s) in depression and overaction of the superior oblique muscle(s).

   e. Underaction of both superior oblique muscles and/or overaction of both inferior oblique muscles.

   f. In general, bilateral fourth nerve palsies tend to have a smaller hypertropia in primary position than do unilateral fourth nerve palsies.

3. Localization of trochlear nerve palsies (structure affected followed by clinical findings)

   a. Lesions affecting the trochlear nucleus and/or fascicles (superior oblique palsy contralateral to lesions)

     (1) Nucleus/fascicles alone: Isolated trochlear palsy (rare)

     (2) Pretectal region: Vertical gaze palsy (dorsal midbrain syndrome)

     (3) Superior cerebellar peduncle: Dysmetria on side of lesion

     (4) Medial longitudinal fasciculus (MLF): Ipsilateral paresis of adduction with nystagmus of contralateral abducting eye

     (5) Descending sympathetic pathways: Ipsilateral Horner's syndrome

(6) Anterior medullary velum: Bilateral trochlear nerve palsies

b. Lesions affecting the trochlear nerve within the subarachnoid space (superior oblique palsy usually ipsilateral to lesion unless mesencephalon is compressed)

(1) Trochlear nerve in isolation: Isolated trochlear nerve palsy

(2) Superior cerebellar peduncle: Ipsilateral dysmetria

(3) Cerebral peduncle: Contralateral hemiparesis

c. Lesions affecting the trochlear nerve within the cavernous sinus and/or superior orbital fissure

(1) Trochlear nerve alone: Isolated trochlear nerve palsy (rare)

(2) Cranial nerves III, VI, sympathetic: Ophthalmoplegia; pupil small, large, or spared; ptosis

(3) Cranial nerve V (ophthalmic branch): Facial or retroorbital pain; sensory loss (forehead)

(4) Increased venous pressure: Proptosis; chemosis

d. Lesions affecting trochlear nerve within orbit

(1) Trochlear nerve, trochlea, superior oblique muscle or tendon: Superior oblique palsy

(2) Mechanical restriction of superior oblique tendon: Brown's superior oblique tendon sheath syndrome

(3) Other ocular motor nerves or extraocular muscles: Ophthalmoplegia, ptosis, restricted ocular movements

(4) Optic nerve: Visual loss, optic disc swelling or atrophy

(5) Mass effect: Proptosis, chemosis, eyelid swelling

4. Etiologies for a fourth nerve palsy based on localization

a. Midbrain (nuclear/fascicular) lesions

(1) Aplasia of the nucleus

(2) Arteriovenous malformation

(3) Demyelination

(4) Hemorrhage

(5) Ischemia/infarction

(6) Tumor (e.g., glioma)

(7) Trauma (including surgical)

(8) Sarcoidosis

(9) Arachnoid cyst of quadrigeminal cistern

b. Lesion in subarachnoid space

(1) Aneurysm (e.g., superior cerebellar artery)

(2) Hydrocephalus

(3) Infections (e.g., mastoiditis, meninigitis)

(4) Wegener's granulomatosis

(5) Superficial siderosis of central nervous system

(6) Post-lumbar puncture or spinal anesthesia

(7) Pseudotumor cerebri

(8) Trauma, including surgery

(9) Neoplasm (e.g., carcinomatous meningitis, cerebellar hemangioblastoma, ependymoma, meningioma, metastasis, neurolemmoma/schwannoma, pineal tumors, trochlear nerve sheath tumors)

(10) Fisher's syndrome

(11) Churg-Strauss syndrome

c. Lesions in cavernous sinus

(1) Neoplasm (e.g., meningioma, pituitary adenoma)

(2) Infectious (e.g., herpes zoster, mucormycosis)

(3) Inflammation

(4) Tolosa-Hunt syndrome

(5) Wegener's granulomatosis

(6) Internal carotid artery aneurysm

(7) Superior ophthalmic vein thrombosis

(8) Foramen ovale electrode placement

(9) Balloon test occlusion of cervical internal carotid artery

d. Orbital lesions

(1) Neoplasm

(2) Infection

(3) Infiltration

(4) Waldenström's macroglobulinemia

(5) Inflammation

(6) Progressive systemic sclerosis

(7) Trauma

(8) Orbital floor fracture

e. Other lesions causing trochlear nerve palsy

(1) Migraine

(2) Congenital

(3) Cephalic tetanus

Localization of Trochlear Nerve Palsies

- Nuclear/fascicular
- Subarachnoid
- Cavernous sinus/superior orbital fissure
- Orbit
- Unknown (e.g., congenital)

5. Myokymia of the superior oblique muscle, a uniocular rotatory microtremor, may cause episodes of vertical oscillopsia, shimmering, or transient diplopia.

   a. This condition is usually benign in isolation.

   b. It may follow a superior oblique palsy.

   c. Natural history of recurrent spontaneous remissions and relapses

   d. May respond to carbamazepine

   e. May be alleviated by strabismus surgery

 Key Signs: Trochlear Lesions

Lesion of the Nucleus or Fascicle

• Dorsal midbrain syndrome

• Dysmetria on the side of the lesion

• Ipsilateral paresis of adduction with nystagmus of contralateral abducting eye

• Ipsilateral Horner's syndrome

• Bilateral trochlear nerve palsies

Lesion of the Nerve within the Subarachnoid Space

• Isolated trochlear nerve palsy

• Ipsilateral dysmetria

• Contralateral hemiparesis

Lesion of the Nerve within the Cavernous Sinus or Superior Orbital Fissure

• Ophthalmoplegia; pupil small, large, or spared; ptosis

• Facial or retroorbital pain; sensory loss in forehead

• Proptosis, chemosis

Lesion of the Nerve within the Orbit

• Superior oblique palsy

• Brown's superior oblique tendon sheath syndrome

• Ophthalmoplegia, ptosis, restricted ocular movements

• Visual loss, optic disc swelling or atrophy

• Proptosis, chemosis, eyelid swelling

Abducens Nerve (Cranial Nerve VI) Palsy

1. Localization

   a. Lesions affecting abducens nucleus

      (1) Abducens nucleus: Ipsilateral horizontal gaze palsy. Etiologies include Möbius syndrome (gaze palsy with facial diplegia), Duane's retraction syndrome (gaze palsy with globe retraction and narrowing of palpebral fissure with adduction)

      (2) Dorsolateral pons may cause other findings including ipsilateral gaze palsy, facial paresis, dysmetria; occasionally with contralateral hemiparesis (Foville's syndrome).

   b. Lesions of the abducens fascicle

      (1) Abducens fascicle: Isolated ipsilateral abduction deficit

      (2) Anterior paramedial pons: Ipsilateral CN VI palsy, ipsilateral CN VII palsy, contralateral hemiparesis (Millard-Gubler syndrome)

      (3) Prepontine cistern: CN VI palsy with or without contralateral hemiparesis (if corticospinal tract involved)

   c. Lesion of abducens nerve in petrous apex (Dorello's canal): CN VI palsy, deafness, facial (especially retroorbital) pain (Gradenigo's syndrome)

   d. Lesion in the cavernous sinus: Isolated CN VI palsy; CN VI palsy plus Horner's syndrome; also may affect CN III, IV, and VI

   e. Superior orbital fissure syndrome: CN VI palsy with variable affect on CN III, IV, and V1; proptosis

   f. Orbital lesion: CN VI palsy; visual loss; variable proptosis, chemosis, lid swelling

2. Etiology of a sixth nerve palsy based on localization

   a. Nuclear (horizontal gaze palsy)

      (1) Congenital (e.g., Möbius syndrome)

      (2) Demyelinating

      (3) Infarction or ischemia

      (4) Neoplasm (pontine and cerebellar)

      (5) Trauma

      (6) Wernicke-Korsakoff syndrome

   b. Fascicular abducens nerve palsy

      (1) Demyelination

      (2) Infarction

      (3) Neoplasm

      (4) Trauma

      (5) Hematoma

   c. Subarachnoid lesions

      (1) Aneurysm or vascular abnormality (e.g., persistent primitive trigeminal artery, posterior inferior cerebellar aneurysm)

      (2) Carcinomatous or leukemic meningitis

      (3) Chiari malformation or basilar impression

(4) Following procedures (e.g., cervical traction, lumbar puncture, myelography, post vaccination, shunting for hydrocephalus, spinal or epidural anesthesia)

(5) Inflammatory (e.g., retropharyngeal space inflammation, necrotizing vasculitis, sarcoidosis, systemic lupus erythematosus, Wegener's granulomatosis)

(6) Fisher's variant (Guillain-Barré syndrome)

(7) Infectious (e.g., Lyme disease, syphilis, tuberculosis, cryptococcal meningitis, cysticercosis, encephalitis)

(8) Neoplasm (e.g., abducens nerve tumor, cerebellopontine angle tumor, clivus tumor, leukemia, metastatic, skull base tumor, nasopharyngeal carcinoma, trigeminal nerve tumor, capillary hemangioma)

(9) Nonlocalizing sign of increased intracranial pressure (e.g., pseudotumor cerebri, meningitis of any type, intracranial tumor, venous sinus thrombosis)

(10) Spontaneous cerebrospinal fluid leak with intracranial hypotension

(11) Trauma (excluding surgical)

(12) Epidural hematoma of clivus (posttraumatic)

d. Petrous apex lesions
  (1) Neoplasm (e.g., nasopharyngeal carcinoma)
  (2) Infection (e.g., complicated otitis media, mastoiditis)
  (3) Thrombosis of inferior petrosal or transverse/sigmoid sinus
  (4) Trauma (e.g., basilar skull fracture)
  (5) Inflammatory

e. Cavernous sinus lesions
  (1) Cavernous sinus thrombosis
  (2) Cavernous sinus fistula
  (3) Superior ophthalmic vein thrombosis
  (4) Neoplasm (e.g., nasopharyngeal carcinoma, pituitary adenoma, plasmacytoma, lymphoma, Hodgkin's disease, hemangioma, hemangioendothelioma, meningioma, sixth nerve tumors, sphenoid sinus tumors, skull base tumors, squamous cell cancer of pterygopalatine fossa, subarachnoid diverticulum)
  (5) Sphenoid sinus mucocele
  (6) Ischemia
  (7) Inflammatory or infectious (e.g., herpes zoster, actinomycoses, Tolosa-Hunt syndrome)

(8) Internal carotid artery diseases (e.g., aneurysm, dissection, dolichoectasia, balloon test occlusion, cisplatin infusion)

(9) Post radiofrequency rhizotomy for trigeminal neuralgia

f. Orbital lesions
  (1) Neoplastic
  (2) Inflammatory
  (3) Infectious
  (4) Traumatic

g. Localization uncertain
  (1) Infectious mononucleosis
  (2) *Mycoplasma pneumoniae* infection
  (3) Lyme disease
  (4) *Campylobacter jejuni* enteritis
  (5) Creutzfeldt-Jakob disease
  (6) Progressive multifocal leukoencephalopathy (PML) in AIDS
  (7) Lymphoma
  (8) Guillain-Barré syndrome
  (9) Fisher's syndrome
  (10) Chronic inflammatory demyelinating polyradiculoneuropathy
  (11) Pregnancy

Localization of Abducens Nerve Palsies

- Nuclear (conjugate gaze palsy)
- Fascicular
- Subarachnoid
- Cavernous sinus/superior orbital fissure
- Unknown

 Key Signs: Abducens Nerve Lesions

- Lesion of the abducens fascicle: Isolated ipsilateral abduction deficit; ipsilateral CN VI and CN VII palsy, Millard-Gubler syndrome: CN VI palsy with or without contralateral hemiparesis

- Lesion of the abducens nerve in Dorello's canal: CN VI palsy, deafness, Gradenigo's syndrome

- Cavernous sinus lesion: Isolated CN VI palsy, CN VI palsy plus Horner's syndrome; also may affect CN III, IV, VI

- Superior orbital fissure syndrome: CN VI palsy with variable affection of CN III, IV, VI; proptosis

- Orbital lesion: CN VI palsy, visual loss, variable proptosis, chemosis, lid swelling

Bibliography

Brazis PW: Subject review: Localization of lesions of the oculomotor nerve: Recent concepts. Mayo Clin Proc 66:1029–1035, 1991.

Brazis PW: Palsies of the trochlear nerve: Diagnosis and localization—recent concepts. Mayo Clin Proc 68:501–509, 1993.

Brazis PW, Lee AG: Binocular vertical diplopia. Mayo Clin Proc 73:55–66, 1998.

Brazis PW, Lee AG: Acquired binocular horizontal diplopia. Mayo Clin Proc 74:907–916, 1999.

Lee AG, Brazis PW: Clinical Pathways in Neuro-Ophthalmology. An Evidence-Based Approach. New York, Thieme, 1998.

Paul W. Brazis
Andrew G. Lee

6 Nystagmus

Definitions

Nystagmus may be defined as a rhythmic biphasic ocular oscillation containing pathologic slow eye movements that are responsible for its genesis and continuation.

1. Jerk nystagmus is generally named according to the direction of the fast, corrective component. Thus, horizontal nystagmus to the left implies that the eyes tend to drift slowly to the right, corrected by quick saccades to the left that bring the eyes back to where the patient wishes to look.

2. It is useful to note whether the oscillations are confined to one eye (monocular), involve mainly one eye (e.g., binocular asymmetric or dissociated), or involve both eyes symmetrically (e.g., conjugate binocular symmetric).

Monocular Eye Oscillations and Asymmetric Binocular Eye Oscillations

1. Spasmus nutans
    a. Often a benign syndrome characterized by a triad of head nodding, nystagmus, and abnormal head posture.
    b. Onset in the first year of life and remits spontaneously within 1 month to several years (up to 8 years) after onset.
    c. Often intermittent, asymmetric or unilateral, and of high frequency and small amplitude with a "shimmering" quality. The nystagmus is usually horizontal but may have a vertical or torsional component.
    d. The irregular head nodding with spasmus nutans has horizontal, vertical, or mixed components.
    e. Patients often also demonstrate a head turn or tilt. Complete triad is not necessary for diagnosis.
    f. Exclude tumor (neuroimaging) of the optic nerve, chiasm, third ventricle, or thalamus (especially if visual loss or optic atrophy present).

2. Monocular nystagmus may occur in adults or children with acquired monocular visual loss and consists of small, slow vertical pendular oscillations in primary position of gaze.
    a. It may develop years after uniocular visual loss (Heimann-Bielschowsky phenomenon) and may improve if vision is corrected.
    b. Monocular, small-amplitude, fast-frequency, and predominantly horizontal nystagmus in children may be caused by unilateral anterior visual pathway disease.

3. Acquired monocular pendular nystagmus may also occur with multiple sclerosis, neurosyphilis, and brainstem infarct (thalamus and upper midbrain) and may be vertical, horizontal, or multivectorial.

4. Monocular rotatory nystagmus may occur with brainstem lesions.

5. Nystagmus is seen only in the abducting eye in internuclear ophthalmoplegia (INO) and in pseudo-INO syndromes. INO is due to a lesion of the medial longitudinal fasciculus (MLF) and consists of puresis of the ipsilateral adducting eye and nystagmus in the contralateral abducting eye on attempted lateral gaze.

6. Superior oblique myokymia may also cause vertical oscillopsia, vertical or torsional diplopia, or both.

Key Signs

- Spasmus nutans and its mimickers
- Monocular visual deprivation or loss
- Monocular pendular nystagmus
- Internuclear ophthalmoplegia (MLF syndrome)
- Superior oblique myokymia

Dysconjugate Bilateral Symmetric Eye Oscillations

1. If the ocular oscillations involve both eyes to a relatively equal degree, the next step in evaluation involves determining whether the eye movements are disconjugate (the eyes moving in opposite directions) or conjugate (both eyes moving in the same direction).

2. When the oscillations are disconjugate, the examiner should determine whether the oscillations are vertical or horizontal. Vertical disconjugate eye oscillations are usually due to see-saw nystagmus. Horizontal disconjugate eye oscillations include

401

convergence-retraction nystagmus (nystagmus retractorius), divergence nystagmus, repetitive divergence, and oculomasticatory myorhythmia.

a. See-saw nystagmus

(1) Refers to a cyclic movement of the eyes with a conjugate torsional component and a disjunctive vertical component: while one eye rises and intorts, the other falls and extorts; the vertical and torsional movements are then reversed, completing the cycle.

(2) This nystagmus is usually pendular. See-saw jerk nystagmus has been described with brainstem lesions affecting the mesodiencephalon or lateral medulla.

(3) Responsible lesions for see-saw nystagmus include large, extrinsic suprasellar lesions that compress the mesodiencephalon bilaterally (e.g., parasellar tumors) or focal mesodiencephalic or lateral medullary brainstem lesions (e.g., infarction).

(4) If a patient with pendular see-saw nystagmus has a focal lesion, then the lesion is usually a large, extensive, suprasellar lesion compressing or invading the brainstem bilaterally at the mesodiencephalic junction.

(5) Pendular see-saw nystagmus may also be congenital.

(6) If the see-saw nystagmus has an underlying jerk waveform, then the patient will have an intrinsic focal brainstem lesion, either in the lateral medulla (usually on the side opposite the torsional quick phases) or in the mesodiencephalon on the same side as the quick phases.

(7) Other disease processes causing see-saw nystagmus include syringomyelia and syringobulbia, brainstem or thalamic vascular disease, multiple sclerosis, trauma, hydrocephalus, albinism, septo-optic dysplasia, Leigh's disease, retinitis pigmentosa, Arnold-Chiari type 1 malformation, and paraneoplastic encephalitis with testicular cancer and anti-Ta antibodies

Key Signs: See-Saw Nystagmus

• Cyclic movement of eyes, with conjugate torsional and distinctive vertical components

• Usually pendular

b. Horizontal dysconjugate eye oscillations

(1) Convergence-retraction nystagmus

(a) Adduction (convergence movement) accompanied by retraction of the eyes into the orbit; occurs spontaneously or on attempted upgaze.

(b) Primarily a saccadic disorder as the convergence movements are not normal vergence movements but asynchronous, adducting saccades.

(c) Mesencephalic lesions affecting the pretectal region are most likely to cause this type of nystagmus. Often associated with abnormalities of vertical gaze.

(2) Divergence nystagmus (with divergent quick phases) may occur with hindbrain abnormalities (e.g., Chiari malformation) and is associated with downbeat nystagmus. These patients have slow phases directed upward and inward.

(3) Repetitive divergence consists of a slow divergent movement followed by a rapid return to the primary position at regular intervals. This rare disorder has been described with coma from hepatic encephalopathy.

(4) Oculomasticatory myorhythmia refers to acquired pendular vergence oscillations of the eyes associated with concurrent contraction of the masticatory muscles.

(a) There is a smooth, rhythmic eye convergence, which cycles at a frequency of approximately 1 Hz, followed by divergence back to the primary position.

(b) Rhythmic elevation and depression of the mandible is synchronous with the ocular oscillations that persist in sleep and are unaltered by stimuli.

(c) A distinct movement disorder recognized only in Whipple's disease.

Key Signs

Convergence-Retraction Nystagmus

• Retraction of eyes into orbit spontaneously or on attempted upgaze

• Eye movements are asynchronous, adducting saccades.

Oculomasticatory Myorhythmia

• Smooth, rhythmic eye convergence followed by divergence back to the primary position

• Rhythmic elevation and depression of the mandible

> **Caveat**
>
> • Oculomasticatory myorhythmia is recognized only in Whipple's disease

Binocular Symmetric Conjugate Nystagmus

Binocular symmetric conjugate eye oscillations may be divided into pendular nystagmus and jerk nystagmus.

1. Binocular symmetric pendular conjugate eye oscillations
   a. Congenital nystagmus
      (1) May be noted at birth or in early infancy, or may emerge or enhance in teenage or adult life, often without apparent provocation.
      (2) Congenital nystagmus may be wholly pendular or have both pendular and jerk components.
      (3) Congenital jerk nystagmus has a slow phase with a velocity that increases exponentially as the eyes move in the direction of the slow phase.
      (4) Although irregular, congenital nystagmus is generally conjugate and horizontal, even on upgaze or downgaze (uniplanar); visual fixation accentuates it and active eyelid closure or convergence attenuates it.
      (5) The nystagmus decreases in an eye position ("null region") specific for each patient.
      (6) When patients are tested with a hand-held optokinetic tape or drum, the quick phase of the elicited nystagmus generally follows the direction of the tape (reversed optokinetic nystagmus).
   b. Latent nystagmus
      (1) It appears when one eye is covered. Both eyes then develop conjugate jerk nystagmus, with the viewing eye having a slow phase directed toward the nose (i.e., the quick phase of both eyes beat toward the side of the fixating eye).
      (2) Although present at birth, latent nystagmus is often not recognized until later in life, when an attempt is made to determine monocular visual acuity during vision screening at school.
      (3) Latent nystagmus is usually associated with strabismus, especially esotropia.
      (4) A marker for congenital ocular motor disturbance and does not indicate progressive structural brain disease

   c. Acquired pendular nystagmus
      (1) May be wholly horizontal, wholly vertical, or have mixed components (circular, elliptical, or windmill pendular nystagmus).
      (2) Pendular nystagmus may be symmetric, dissociated, or even monocular and often causes distressing oscillopsia and decreased visual acuity.
      (3) Damage to the dentatorubroolivary pathways (Guillain-Mollaret triangle) is found in some cases of acquired pendular nystagmus, which is most often caused by multiple sclerosis, stroke, or tumor of the brainstem or other posterior fossa structures.
      (4) Other causes of acquired binocular pendular nystagmus include Pelizaeus-Merzbacher disease, mitochondrial cytopathy, Cockayne's syndrome, neonatal adrenoleukodystrophy, and toluene addiction.
      (5) Pendular nystagmus may also appear with blindness or monocular loss of vision; in the latter case, it may be monocular.
      (6) Palatal myoclonus is a continuous rhythmic involuntary movement of the soft palate that may be accompanied by synchronous movements of other adjacent structures, such as the face, pharynx, larynx, or diaphragm.
         (a) The association of pendular nystagmus with palatal myoclonus is not infrequent, and the condition is then termed *oculopalatal myoclonus*.
         (b) Damage to the dentatorubroolivary pathways (Guillain-Mollaret triangle) is found in cases of oculopalatal myoclonus, which is most often caused by multiple sclerosis or vascular lesions of the brainstem.
         (c) Magnetic resonance imaging often shows enlargement of the inferior olivary nuclei.

 Key Signs

Congenital Nystagmus

• Dampened by convergence or eye closure

• Usually pendular

• Null zone often present

• Uniplanar (usually horizontal in all fields of gaze)

• Inversion of optokinetic nytstagmus

Latent Nystagmus

- Appears when one eye is covered
- The viewing eye has the slow phase directed toward the nose
- Usually associated with strabismus, especially esotropia

Acquired Pendular Nystagmus

- Wholly horizontal, wholly vertical, or mixed
- Symmetric, dissociated, or monocular
- Sometimes associated with palatal myoclonus

2. Binocular symmetric jerk nystagmus: May be divided into those present in primary position and those present predominantly on eccentric gaze. May be predominantly horizontal, torsional, or vertical. Predominantly horizontal forms include congenital nystagmus, latent nystagmus, vestibular nystagmus, periodic alternating nystagmus, drug-induced nystagmus, and epileptic nystagmus. Spontaneous symmetric conjugate jerk nystagmus in primary gaze that is purely torsional is a form of central vestibular nystagmus. Spontaneous symmetric conjugate jerk nystagmus in primary gaze that is predominantly vertical includes upbeat nystagmus and downbeat nystagmus.

   a. Horizontal nystagmus in the primary position is often the result of peripheral vestibular disease.

   (1) Vestibular nystagmus has a linear (constant velocity) slow phase.

   (2) The horizontal component is diminished when the patient lies with the intact ear down and is exacerbated with the affected ear down.

   (3) Peripheral vestibular lesions induce a tendency for the eyes to drift in a direction parallel to the plane of the diseased canal. Horizontal nystagmus with the slow component toward the lesion (the opposite vestibular nuclei drive the eyes toward the diseased side) results from unilateral horizontal canal or total labyrinthine destruction. In the latter case there is a torsional slow component causing the upper part of the globe to rotate toward the side with the lesion.

   (4) Although constant for a particular position of gaze, the slow-phase velocity is greater when the eyes are turned in the direction of the quick component (Alexander's law).

   (5) Nystagmus due to peripheral vestibular disease is most prominent, or only becomes apparent, when fixation is prevented.

   b. Periodic alternating nystagmus (PAN)

   (1) The eyes exhibit primary position nystagmus, which, after 60 to 120 seconds, stops for a few seconds and then starts beating in the opposite direction

   (2) May be congenital, but it is often acquired and caused by disease processes at the craniocervical junction.

   (3) Described with tumors, trauma, encephalitis, spinocerebellar degenerations, cerebellar masses, ataxia telangiectasia, neurosyphilis, multiple sclerosis, vascular disease, craniocervical malformations (e.g., Chiari malformation), hepatic encephalopathy, phenytoin intoxication, and after visual loss.

   (4) Likely caused by lesions of the cerebellar uvula and nodulus or their connections with the brainstem vestibular nuclei.

   (5) Baclofen, a GABA-B agonist, may abolish PAN

   c. Drug-induced (nonspecific) nystagmus

   (1) May be predominantly horizontal, predominantly vertical, predominantly rotatory, or, most commonly, mixed.

   (2) It is most often seen with tranquilizing medications and anticonvulsants.

   d. Nystagmus may occur as an epileptic phenomenon.

   (1) Epileptic nystagmus is usually horizontal, may be seen with epileptiform activity ipsilateral or contralateral to the direction of the slow component of the nystagmus.

   (2) Often is associated with altered states of consciousness, although consciousness may be preserved during the attacks.

   e. Spontaneous jerk nystagmus that is purely torsional is a rare form of central vestibular nystagmus. Purely torsional nystagmus may be seen with brainstem and posterior fossa lesions, such as tumors, syringobulbia, syringomyelia with Chiari malformation, lateral medullary syndrome, multiple sclerosis, trauma, vascular anomalies, postencephalitis, and sarcoidosis, and as part of the stiff-man syndrome.

Key Signs

Horizontal Nystagmus

- Constant-velocity slow phase
- The velocity is greater when the eyes are turned in the direction of the quick component (Alexander's law)

- Horizontal component diminishes when the patient lies down with intact ear down and is exacerbated with the affected ear down.

Periodic Alternating Nystagmus

- The eyes exhibit primary position nystagmus that, after 1 to 2 minutes, stops for a few seconds and then starts beating in the opposite direction

Predominantly Vertical Jerk Nystagmus

1. Downbeat nystagmus
   a. Usually present in primary position, but is greatest when the patient looks down (Alexander's law) and in lateral gaze.
   b. May occur with cervicomedullary junction disease, midline medullary lesions, posterior midline cerebellar lesions, or diffuse cerebellar disease.
   c. Most responsible lesions affect the vestibulocerebellum (flocculus, paraflocculus, nodulus, and uvula) and the underlying medulla. Damage to the nuclei propositus hypoglossi and the medial vestibular nuclei (the neural integrator) in the medulla has also been suggested as the cause of the nystagmus.
   d. Etiologies of downbeat nystagmus
      (1) Craniocervical anomalies, including cerebellar ectopia, Chiari malformation, platybasia, basilar invagination, and Paget's disease
      (2) Familial cerebellar degenerations
      (3) Posterior fossa tumors
      (4) Increased intracranial pressure (e.g., due to supratentorial mass) and hydrocephalus
      (5) Brainstem or cerebellar infarction, anoxia, or hemorrhage
      (6) Dolichoectasia of the vertebrobasilar artery
      (7) Intermittent vertebral artery compression by an osteophyte
      (8) Encephalitis, including herpes simplex encephalitis and HTLV-1 infection
      (9) Heat stroke
      (10) Cephalic tetanus
      (11) Multiple sclerosis and other leukodystrophies
      (12) Syringomyelia/syringobulbia
      (13) Trauma
      (14) Alcohol, including alcohol-induced cerebellar degeneration
      (15) Wernicke's encephalopathy
      (16) Paraneoplastic cerebellar degeneration (including testicular cancer with anti-Ta antibody)
      (17) Superficial siderosis of the central nervous system
      (18) Congenital
      (19) Vitamin B_{12} deficiency
      (20) Thiamine deficiency
      (21) Magnesium deficiency
      (22) Drugs, including lithium, toluene, and anticonvulsants (e.g., phenytoin, carbamazepine, felbamate)
      (23) Transient finding in otherwise normal infants
      (24) Idiopathic

2. Upbeat nystagmus
   a. Damage to the central projections of the anterior semicircular canals, which tend to deviate the eyes superiorly, has been suggested to explain upbeat nystagmus.
   b. Upbeat nystagmus is usually worse in upgaze (Alexander's law) and, unlike downbeat nystagmus, it usually does not increase on lateral gaze.
   c. Damage to the ventral tegmental pathways, which may link the superior vestibular nuclei to the superior rectus and inferior oblique subnuclei of the oculomotor nuclei, may cause the eyes to glide down, resulting in upbeat nystagmus.
   d. Etiologies include medullary disease, lesions of the anterior cerebellar vermis, perihypoglossal and inferior olivary nuclei of the medulla, pontine tegmentum, brachium conjunctivum, midbrain, and brainstem. Medullary lesions invariably involve the perihypoglossal nucleus and adjacent medial vestibular nucleus, nucleus intercalatus, and ventral tegmentum, which contain projections from vestibular nuclei that receive inputs from the anterior semicircular canal.
   e. Etiologies of upbeat nystagmus
      (1) Primary cerebellar degenerations and atrophies
      (2) Chiari malformation
      (3) Posterior fossa tumors
      (4) Brainstem or cerebellum infarction or hemorrhage
      (5) Multiple sclerosis
      (6) Meningitis and brainstem encephalitis
      (7) Thalamic arteriovenous malformation
      (8) Wernicke's encephalopathy
      (9) Behçet's syndrome

(10) Congenital, including cases associated with Leber's congenital amaurosis and other congenital anterior visual pathway disorders

(11) Pelizaeus-Merzbacher disease

(12) Fisher's syndrome (ataxia, areflexia, and ophthalmoplegia)

(13) Middle ear disease

(14) Organophosphate poisoning

(15) Tobacco-induced

(16) Anticonvulsant intoxication

(17) Cyclosporine A

(18) Paraneoplastic syndrome with testicular cancer and anti-Ta antibodies

(19) Transient finding in otherwise healthy neonates

Key Signs

- Downbeat nystagmus is greatest in downgaze (Alexander's law) and in lateral gaze.

- Upbeat nystagmus is worse in upgaze (Alexander's law) and does not increase on lateral gaze.

Binocular Symmetric Jerk Nystagmus Present in Eccentric Gaze

1. Gaze-evoked nystagmus

   a. The eyes fail to remain in an eccentric position of gaze but drift to midposition.

   b. The velocity of the slow component decreases exponentially as the eyes approach midposition.

   c. A "leaky" neural integrator or cerebellar (especially vestibulocerebellar) lesion may result in this type of nystagmus, which is more pronounced when the patient looks toward the lesion.

   d. Cerebellopontine angle tumors may cause Bruns' nystagmus, a combination of ipsilateral large-amplitude, low-frequency nystagmus that is due to impaired gaze holding, and contralateral small-amplitude, high-frequency nystagmus that is due to vestibular impairment

   e. Gaze-evoked nystagmus may be a side effect of medications, including anticonvulsants, sedatives, and alcohol.

   f. Gaze-evoked nystagmus has been described with adult-onset Alexander's disease with involvement of the middle cerebellar peduncles and dentate nuclei, and is also a feature of familial episodic vertigo and ataxia type 2 that is responsive to acetazalomide.

g. Physiologic or endpoint nystagmus is a benign low-amplitude jerk nystagmus with the fast component directed toward the field of gaze. It usually ceases when the eyes are brought to a position somewhat less than the extremes of gaze.

2. Rebound nystagmus

   a. Seen in some patients with brainstem and/or cerebellar disease (e.g., olivocerebellar atrophy, brainstem/cerebellar tumor or stroke, Marinesco-Sjögren syndrome, Dandy-Walker cyst, Gerstmann-Sträussler-Scheinker disease, adult-onset Alexander's disease, etc.).

   b. After keeping the eyes eccentric for some time, the original gaze-evoked nystagmus may wane and actually reverse direction so that the slow component is directed centrifugally (centripital nystagmus); it becomes obvious if the eyes are returned to midposition (rebound nystagmus).

Key Signs

Gaze-Evoked Nystagmus

- Eyes fail to remain in an eccentric position of gaze but drift to midposition

- Velocity of the slow component decreases exponentially as the eyes approach midposition

Rebound Nystagmus

- After keeping the eyes eccentric for some time, the original gaze-evoked nystagmus may wane and actually reverse direction so that the slow component is directed centrifugally; it becomes obvious if the eyes are returned to midposition (rebound nystagmus).

1. Binocular symmetric conjugate jerk nystagmus that is induced includes optokinetic nystagmus, rotational/caloric vestibular nystagmus, positional nystagmus, Valsalva-induced nystagmus, and hyperventilation-induced nystagmus.

2. Positional vertigo of the benign paroxysmal type, also known as *benign paroxysmal positioning vertigo* or *positional nystagmus*, is usually idiopathic

   a. Possibly related to degeneration of the macula of the otolith organ or to lesions of the posterior semicircular canal

   b. Otoconia detached from the otoconial layer (by degeneration or trauma) gravitate and settle on the cupula of the posterior canal causing it to be heavier than the surrounding endolymph and thus sensitive to changes in the direction of gravity (with positional change).

c. After rapid head tilt toward the affected ear or following head extension, when the posterior semicircular canal is moved in the specific plane of stimulation, an ampullofugal deflection of the cupula occurs, with a rotational vertigo and concomitant nystagmus.

d. Some patients show a strong horizontal nystagmus induced by lateral head positioning suggesting lateral (rather than posterior) semicircular canal irritation (lateral canal or horizontal canal variant of benign paroxysmal positional vertigo).

e. Other causes of positional vertigo include trauma, infection, labyrinthine fistula, ischemia, demyelinating disease, Chiari malformation, and, rarely, posterior fossa tumors or vascular malformations.

3. Nystagmus induced by the Valsalva maneuver may occur with Arnold-Chiari malformation or perilymph fistulas.

4. Hyperventilation may induce nystagmus in patients with tumors of the eighth cranial nerve (e.g., acoustic neuroma or epidermoid tumors), after vestibular neuritis, or central demyelinating lesions.

Bibliography

Brazis PW, Masdeu JC, Biller J: Localization in Clinical Neurology, 4th ed. Philadelphia, Lippincott Williams & Wilkins, 2001.

Lee AG, Brazis PW: Clinical Pathways in Neuro-Ophthalmology. An Evidence-Based Approach. New York, Thieme, 1998.

Leigh RJ, Averbuch-Heller L, Tomsak RL, et al.: Treatment of abnormal eye movements that impair vision: Strategies based on current concepts of physiology and pharmacology. Ann Neurol 36:129–141, 1994.

Leigh RJ, Zee DS: The Neurology of Eye Movements, 3rd ed. New York, Oxford University Press, 1999.

7 Orbital Disorders

Paul W. Brazis
Andrew G. Lee

Mass Lesions of the Orbit

1. Tumors of the orbit may or may not be symptomatic.

    a. Optic nerve compression: May show optic disc swelling followed by atrophy. May be visually asymptomatic.

    b. Optociliary shunt vessels. The triad of optociliary veins, disc pallor, and visual loss (the Hoyt-Spencer sign) is characteristic of chronic optic nerve compressive lesions, especially sphenoorbital optic nerve sheath meningiomas.

    c. Limitation of ocular movements and diplopia

    d. Proptosis

    (1) May be seen with disease of the cavernous sinus and may rarely be due to intracranial disease (e.g., a tumor of the middle cranial fossa may cause pressure on the veins of the cavernous sinus leading to secondary intraorbital venous congestion and "false localizing" proptosis).

    (2) Intermittent proptosis may occur with venous angioma within the orbit. Develops when the patient strains, cries, bends the head forward, hyperextends the neck, coughs, or blows the nose against a closed nostril and when the jugular vein is compressed. During these episodes, the eye may become tense and painful, the pupil may enlarge, and occasional bradycardia or syncope may develop (oculocardiac syndrome).

    (3) Pulsation of the globe may occur with congenital sphenoid dysplasia, with orbital-cranial encephalocele with neurofibromatosis, from orbital arteriovenous malformations or venous varices, due to tricuspid regurgitation, with arterial pulsation of the orbital vein, due to arteriovenous fistula, or from transmission of pulsations of intracranial pressure via surgical or traumatic defects in the orbital wall.

    (4) The most common cause of unilateral or bilateral exophthalmos in the adult is Graves' disease.

    (5) Causes of pseudoexophthalmos include an enlarged globe (e.g., due to myopia, buphthalmos, or congenital cystic eye), eyelid or palpebral fissure asymmetry (e.g., due to lid retraction, ptosis, seventh nerve palsy, or postsurgical effect), extraocular muscle abnormality (weakness or paralysis), shallow or asymmetric bony orbits, or contralateral enophthalmos (e.g., metastatic breast cancer, orbital floor fracture, or congenital bone defect).

    (6) Rather than causing proptosis, scirrhous carcinoma of the breast or carcinoma of the lung, gastrointestinal tract, or prostate metastatic to the orbit may cause progressive fibrotic change and enophthalmos.

    (a) This enophthalmos may be caused by posterior traction and tethering on the eyeball or by the tumor mass destroying the orbital wall resulting in "biologic orbital decompression."

    (b) Other causes of enophthalmos include senile orbital fat atrophy, traumatic orbital floor fracture, traumatic orbital fat atrophy, facial hemiatrophy (Parry-Romberg syndrome), facial osteomyelitis, and orbital fat necrosis.

    (c) Spontaneous enophthalmos and ptosis of the globe (hypoglobus), unassociated with orbital trauma, may be associated with ipsilateral chronic maxillary sinusitis or hypoplasia. The apparent dissolution and resorption of the orbital floor causes the loss of inferior support and orbital expansion. Enophthalmos and hypoglobus unassociated with prior trauma, surgery, or other symptoms have been called the "silent sinus syndrome," which is ipsilateral maxillary sinus hypoplasia and orbital floor resorption.

    e. Swelling of the eyelids and chemosis

    f. Gaze-evoked amaurosis

    (1) Loss of vision whenever the eye is placed in an eccentric position of gaze

    (2) Noted most often with cavernous hemangiomas and optic nerve sheath meningiomas

    (3) Has been described with orbital osteoma, glioma, medial rectus granular cell myoblastoma, varix, pseudotumor cerebri, orbital trauma, and metastatic orbital tumor

(4) Thought to be due to decreased blood flow to the retina or optic nerve with eye movement (e.g., the mass compresses the central retinal artery)

(5) Although most often due to intrinsic orbital disease, gaze-evoked monocular obscurations in lateral and upward gaze have also been described with pseudotumor cerebri.

g. Facial pain and paresthesias. Several branches of the trigeminal nerve may be affected by orbital disease, especially those of the ophthalmic division, which has a large number of branches passing through the orbit.

(1) The extent of cutaneous sensory loss is indicative of the position of the orbital disease, with the lacrimal, supraorbital, or supratrochlear nerves being affected by disease along the orbital roof, and the zygomatic and infraorbital nerves being affected by diseases along the orbital floor.

(2) Disease at the orbital apex or the superior orbital fissure may cause hypesthesia affecting several or even all of the periorbital dermatomes.

(3) If a tumor erodes through the floor of the orbit, it may damage the maxillary division of cranial nerve V (the trigeminal nerve), resulting in ipsilateral maxillary pain, anesthesia, or both, over the distribution of the maxillary branch of the trigeminal nerve.

(4) Orbital pain is common with orbital lesions, especially with orbital malignancy or inflammatory disease.

Caveat

- The triad of optociliary veins, disc pallor, and visual loss (Hoyt-Spencer sign) is characteristic of chronic optic nerve compressive lesions, especially sphenoorbital optic nerve sheath meningiomas.

---

2. Common orbital disorders of children

a. Orbital cellulitis: Most common cause of proptosis in children

b. Rhabdomyosarcoma: Most common primary orbital malignancy in children

c. Capillary hemangioma and lymphangioma: Most common benign primary orbital tumors in children

d. Dermoid and epidermoid cysts

e. Leukemia

f. Optic nerve glioma

g. Neurofibroma

h. Orbital pseudotumor

i. Metastatic neuroblastoma: Most common metastatic cancer to orbit in children

j. Retinoblastoma

k. Bilateral proptosis in children: Consider leukemia or metastatic neuroblastoma

---

Common Orbital Disorders of Children

- Orbital cellulitis: Most common cause of proptosis in children

- Rhabdomyosarcoma: Most common primary orbital malignancy in children

- Capillary hemangioma and lymphangioma: Most common benign childhood primary orbital tumors

- Dermoid and epidermoid cysts

- Leukemia

- Optic nerve glioma

- Neurofibroma

- Orbital pseudotumor

- Metastatic neuroblastoma: Most common childhood metastatic cancer to orbit

- Retinoblastoma

- Bilateral proptosis in children: Consider leukemia or metastatic neuroblastoma

---

3. Common orbital disorders of adults

a. Thyroid-related orbitopathy (Graves' disease): Most common cause of unilateral and bilateral exophthalmos

b. Cavernous hemangioma or lymphangioma: Most common benign primary orbital tumor in adults

c. Lymphocytic lesions (e.g., benign reactive lymphoid hyperplasia, atypical lymphoid hyperplasia, malignant lymphoma)

d. Meningioma

e. Lacrimal gland tumors

f. Dermoid and epidermoid tumors

g. Metastatic or secondarily invasive tumors

h. Infections (e.g., mucormycosis, aspergillosis)

Caveat

- The most common cause of exophthalmos in adults is Graves' disease.

Common Orbital Disorders of Adults

- Thyroid-related orbitopathy (Graves' disease): Most common cause of unilateral and bilateral exophthalmous

- Cavernous hemangioma or lymphangioma: Most common benign primary orbital tumor in adults

- Lymphocytic lesions (e.g., benign reactive lymphoid hyperplasia, atypical lymphoid hyperplasia, malignant lymphoma)

- Meningioma

- Lacrimal gland tumors

- Dermoid and epidermoid tumors

- Metastatic or secondarily invasive tumors

- Infections (e.g., mucormycosis, aspergillosis)

---

4. Manifestation of orbital metastatic tumors
   a. Five syndromes
      (1) Infiltrative: Characterized by prominent restriction of motility, a firm orbit, ptosis, and often enophthalmos
      (2) Mass: Characterized by proptosis, displacement of the globe, and often a palpable orbital mass
      (3) Inflammatory: Characterized by pain, chemosis, erythema, and periorbital swelling
      (4) Functional: Characterized by cranial nerve findings (e.g., problems with ocular motility) disproportionate with the degree of orbital involvement
      (5) Silent: Orbital metastatic lesions detected by computed tomography (CT) or magnetic resonance imaging (MRI) but asymptomatic
   b. Infiltrative and mass lesion syndromes are by far the most common manifestations.
   c. Direct metastases to the orbital muscles may occur, especially with carcinoma of the breast and malignant melanoma.
5. Orbital pseudotumor (idiopathic orbital inflammation)
   a. A clinicopathologic entity with the following diagnostic criteria:
      (1) A unilateral orbital mass lesion, clinically presenting with signs of mass effect, inflammation, and/or infiltration
      (2) Neuroimaging showing a focal or diffuse inflammatory lesion
      (3) Histopathology demonstrating a fibroinflammatory lesion

(4) Investigations eliminating identifiable local or systemic causes
   b. When the inflammatory process is confined to one or multiple extraocular muscles, the process is referred to as *orbital myositis*, although some authors feel that orbital pseudotumor and orbital myositis may be distinct clinicotherapeutic entities.
   c. Patients present with acute or subacute orbital pain and diplopia. Findings include conjunctival chemosis and injection, ptosis, and proptosis.
   d. The process may be unilateral or bilateral and usually resolves with corticosteroid therapy or radiation therapy.
   e. The illness is often monophasic but recurrent episodes may occur.
   f. Orbital myositis may be associated with systemic diseases, such as Crohn's disease, celiac disease, systemic lupus erythematosus, Whipple's disease, rheumatoid arthritis, linear scleroderma, and Wegener's granulomatosis.
   g. Orbital myositis may occasionally be paraneoplastic.
   h. Neuroimaging in patients with orbital myositis reveals enlarged, irregular muscles, usually with tendinous insertion involvement. Intracranial extension of the inflammatory process may occur.
   i. Differential diagnosis of orbital pseudotumor
      (1) Thyroid eye disease
      (2) Orbital cellulitis (e.g., orbital apex syndrome) including aspergillosis, mucormycosis, *Bipolaris hawaiiensis*, actinomycosis, cysticercosis, trichinosis.
      (3) Low flow dural-cavernous sinus fistula
      (4) Lymphoid hyperplasia
      (5) Lymphoma
      (6) Hodgkin's disease
      (7) Giant cell arteritis
      (8) Orbital polymyositis and giant cell myocarditis
         (a) A rare, distinct nosologic entity characterized by progressive, often painful bilateral ophthalmoplegia with thickened extraocular muscles and cardiac arrhythmia often leading to death.
         (b) Pathologically, the extraocular and cardiac muscles showed diffuse mononuclear and giant cell inflammation.

(c) Cardiac transplantation may be life-saving.

(9) Sarcoidosis of the extraocular muscles: May cause bilateral painful or painless ophthalmoplegia with enlargement of the extraocular muscles on neuroimaging.

(10) Sinus histiocytosis with massive lymphadenopathy (Rosai-Dorfman disease)

    (a) A benign histoproliferative disease characterized by massive cervical lymphandenopathy, fever, and leukocytosis

    (b) Characterized pathologically by enlarged lymph node sinuses containing large histiocytes with phagocytosed lymphocyte

    (c) May be associated with bilateral or unilateral proptosis with orbital involvement of the extraocular muscles

(11) Erdheim-Chester disease

    (a) An idiopathic condition characterized by infiltration of the heart, lungs, retroperitoneum, bones, and other tissues by a fibrosing xanthogranulomatous process composed of xanthomatous histiocytes and Touton giant cells.

    (b) Often fatal due to cardiomyopathy, severe lung disease, or chronic renal failure.

    (c) Orbital infiltration with this disease may produced proptosis, ophthalmoplegia, xanthelasma, disc swelling, blindness due to optic atrophy, and bilateral enhancing orbital masses on neuroimaging.

(12) Orbital amyloidosis: May be localized to the extraocular muscles, causing ptosis, proptosis, restricted ocular motility, and enlarged extraocular muscles on neuroimaging

(13) Orbital metastases, especially from breast cancer, may present as a bilateral infiltrative process ("orbital pseudotumor" presentation).

(14) Seminoma may rarely present with bilateral nonspecific inflammatory or Graves-like orbitopathy. The etiology of this exophthalmous is not known and not related to direct orbital metastasis. The orbitopathy may regress in response to steroids or excision of primary tumor.

j. Biopsy is required to exclude other diseases, except in pure myositic locations, in which the clinicopathologic picture is rather unique and surgical biopsy may damage the muscle, and in posterior locations, in which the optic nerve may be at risk during surgery.

k. Pathology studies in orbital myositis reveal inflammatory infiltrate composed mainly of small well-differentiated mature lymphocytes, admixed with plasma cells, in a diffuse or multifocal pattern. The muscle fibers are swollen and separated by edema and fibrosis, with loss of normal striations and degeneration of muscle fibers.

l. Other atypical histopathologic patterns such as extensive sclerosis, true vasculitis, granulomatous inflammation, and tissue eosinophilia can be used for subclassification of orbital pseudotumor in general. There is no unequivocal correlation between clinicotherapeutic outcome and these atypical findings.

Key Signs

Orbital Metastatic Tumors

- Infiltrative syndrome: Prominent restriction of motility, a firm orbit, ptosis, and often enophthalmos

- Mass syndrome: Proptosis, displacement of globe, and often palpable orbital mass

- Inflammatory syndrome: Pain, chemosis, erythema, and periorbital swelling

- Functional syndrome: Cranial nerve findings disproportionate to orbital involvement

- Silent syndrome: Asymptomatic orbital metastatic lesions detected on CT or MRI scan

Orbital Pseudotumor

- Mass effect

- Inflammation

- Infiltration

- Orbital myositis

- Systemic diseases (e.g., Crohn's disease, celiac disease, systemic lupus erythematosus, Whipple's disease, rheumatoid arthritis, linear scleroderma, Wegener's granulomatosis

Key Tests

General

- Biopsy required to exclude other diseases

- Pathologic studies

Orbital Pseudotumor

- Neuroimaging

- Histopatholgy

- Investigations to eliminate identifiable local or systemic causes

1. Cavernous sinus and superior orbital fissure syndrome

   a. Painful ophthalmoplegia may be seen with processes affecting the orbit, superior orbital fissure, or cavernous sinus

   b. Cavernous sinus and superior orbital fissure lesions often damage the ocular motor nerves (cranial nerves III, IV, and VI), the ophthalmic branch of the trigeminal nerve, and the oculosympathetic fibers in varying combinations

   c. Medial lesions in the cavernous sinus, such as a carotid artery aneurysm, may affect only the ocular motor nerves but spare the more laterally located ophthalmic branch of the trigeminal nerve, resulting in painless ophthalmoplegia. In contrast, lesions that begin laterally present with retroorbital pain first, and only later does ophthalmoparesis supervene.

   d. Various disorders cause cavernous sinus or superior orbital fissure syndrome.

      (1) Aneurysm of the internal carotid artery or carotid artery occlusion

      (2) Tumors (e.g., meningioma, pituitary adenoma, nasopharyngeal carcinoma, cavernous hemangioma or hemangiopericytoma, lymphoma, myeloma, Waldenström's macroglobulinemia)

      (3) Cavernous sinus thrombosis

      (4) Tolosa-Hunt syndrome (idiopathic granulomatous inflammation of cavernous sinus)

      (5) Infections (e.g., herpes zoster, aspergillosis, mucormycosis)

      (6) Neurosurgical complications

      (7) Carotid-cavernous sinus fistula

Bibliography

Brazis PW, Masdeu JC, Biller J: Localization in Clinical Neurology, 4th ed. Philadelphia, Lippincott Williams & Wilkins, 2001, pp. 163–166.

Goldberg RA, Rootman J: Clinical characteristics of metastatic orbital tumors. Ophthalmology 97:620–624, 1990.

Goldberg RA, Rootman J, Cline RA: Tumors metastatic to the orbit: A changing picture. Surv Ophthalmol 35:1–24, 1990.

Leigh RJ, Zee DS: The Neurology of Eye Movements, 3rd ed. New York, Oxford University Press, 1999.

Mombaerts I, Goldschmeding R, Schlingemann RO, Koornneef L: What is orbital pseudotumor? Surv Ophthalmol 41:66–78, 1996.

Mombaerts I, Koornneef L: Current status of treatment of orbital myositis. Ophthalmology 104:402–408, 1997.

8 Papilledema and Pseudotumor Cerebri

Paul W. Brazis
Andrew G. Lee

Papilledema

1. Definition: The term *papilledema* should be used only to denote disc swelling from increased intracranial pressure
2. Clinical features
   a. Usually bilateral but may be unilateral or asymmetric
   b. Usually preserved visual acuity and color vision early (unlike other optic neuropathies)
   c. May have transient visual obscurations lasting seconds
   d. Visual field defects may occur: Enlarged blind spot, generalized constriction, glaucomatous-like defects, eventual peripheral constriction (especially nasally)
   e. No afferent pupillary defect unless severe and asymmetric or unilateral (uncommon)
   f. Ophthalmoscopic findings
      (1) Early papilledema
         (a) Minimal hyperemia and capillary dilatation
         (b) Early opacification of nerve fiber layer (peripapillary retina loses its superficial linear and curvilinear light reflex and appears red without luster)
         (c) Absence of venous pulsations
         (d) Peripapillary retinal nerve fiber layer hemorrhages
      (2) Fully developed papilledema
         (a) Engorged retinal veins and numerous splinter hemorrhages at or adjacent to disc margin
         (b) Disc surface grossly elevated
         (c) Surface vessels become obscured by opaque nerve fiber layer.
         (d) May have tortuous retinal veins
         (e) Paton's lines (circumferential retinal folds) or choroidal folds
         (f) Exudates (e.g., macular star or hemistar) and hemorrhages in macula may produce decreased vision.
         (g) In acute cases (e.g., subarachnoid hemorrhage), subhyaloid hemor-

rhages may occur that may break into vitreous (Terson's syndrome).
      (3) Chronic papilledema
         (a) Hemorrhages and exudates slowly resolve.
         (b) Central cup, which is initially retained even in severe cases, ultimately becomes obliterated
         (c) Initial disc hyperemia changes to milky gray, small, hard exudates; refractile, drusen-like bodies appear on disc surface
         (d) Nerve fiber layer defects may develop.
         (e) Optociliary "shunt" vessels may develop.
      (4) Atrophic papilledema (pale disc edema)
         (a) Optic disc pallor with nerve fiber bundle visual field defects
         (b) Retinal vessels become narrow and sheathed.
         (c) Occasional pigmentary changes or choroidal folds in macula
         (d) Selective loss of peripheral axons while sparing central axons (i.e., preservation of good central visual acuity) initially but may develop central visual loss over time
3. Syndromes causing increased intracranial pressure
   a. Primary idiopathic pseudotumor cerebri syndrome
   b. Secondary cause
      (1) Hydrocephalus and shunt
      (2) Mass lesions: Tumor, hemorrhage, large infarction, abscess
      (3) Meningitis/encephalitis
      (4) Subarachnoid hemorrhage
      (5) Trauma
      (6) Arteriovenous malformations with high blood flow overloading venous return
      (7) Intracranial or extracranial venous obstruction
      (8) Secondary pseudotumor cerebri syndrome due to certain systemic diseases, drugs, or pregnancy

4. Clinical and laboratory testing
   a. Rule out malignant hypertension.
   b. Consider blood dyscrasias.
   c. Consider other causes of disc edema (see Part X, Chapter 1, Optic Neuritis).

5. Neuroimaging
   a. Required in all patients
   b. Computed tomography (CT) in acute setting, acute vascular processes (e.g., subarachnoid, epidural, subdural, or intracerebral hemorrhage, acute infarction), or head trauma. CT studies are also indicated in patients with contraindications to magnetic resonance imaging (MRI—e.g., pacemakers, metallic clips in head, metallic foreign bodies) or in patients who are too large to fit into the machine or too claustrophobic to obtain an adequate MRI study.
   c. MRI with and without contrast is the modality of choice. In selected cases, consider MR angiography or MR venography for arterial disease or venous obstruction, respectively.

6. Lumbar puncture
   a. If neuroimaging shows no structural lesion or hydrocephalus, then lumbar puncture is warranted.
   b. Studies should include an accurate opening pressure, to evaluate for intracranial hypertension, as well as cell count and differential, glucose, protein, cytology, and appropriate studies for microbial agents.

Key Tests

- Rule out malignant hypertension.
- Consider blood dyscrasias.
- Consider other causes of disc edema.
- Neuroimaging is required in all patients.
- CT in acute setting
- MRI is modality of choice.
- Lumbar puncture if neuroimaging shows no lesion or hydrocephalus

Pseudotumor Cerebri (PTC)

1. Definition
   a. Usually idiopathic
   b. May be due to certain systemic diseases, drugs, pregnancy, and intracranial or extracranial venous obstruction

2. Criteria for the diagnosis of PTC
   a. Increased intracranial pressure (usually greater than 200 mm of water) must be documented in an alert and oriented patient. Spinal fluid pressures between 200 and 250 mm H_2O may occur normally in obese patients and when elevated spinal fluid pressure is suspected, confirmation requires values greater than 250 mm H_2O.
   b. No localizing neurologic findings (except for cranial nerve VI palsy and papilledema)
   c. Cerebrospinal fluid contents normal (including protein and glucose) with no cytologic abnormalities.
   d. Neuroimaging (MRI with and without contrast and, possibly MR venography) should be normal with no evidence of hydrocephalus, mass lesion, meningeal enhancement, or venous occlusive disease.

3. Associated conditions
   a. Drugs: Hypervitaminosis A, steroid withdrawal, anabolic steroids, lithium, nalidixic acid, the insecticide chlordecone (Kepone), isoretinoin, ketaprofen (Orudis) or indomethacin in Bartter's syndrome, thyroid replacement in hypothyroid children, danazol, all-*trans*-retinoic acid (ATRA or tretinoin), cyclosporine, exogenous growth hormone, and probably tetracycline and minocycline.
   b. Systemic diseases: Behçet's syndrome, renal failure, Addison's disease, hypoparathyroidism, systemic lupus erythematosus, sarcoidosis (most of these likely cause pseudotumor cerebri syndrome by venous sinus obstruction or impairment of venous sinus drainage).

4. Epidemiology
   a. Typically obese women in the childbearing years
   b. Approximately 10% to 15% of patients are male, and, when it occurs in children, there is usually no gender preference.
   c. PTC in a man, especially a thin man, should raise the possibility of venous occlusive disease or a secondary pseudotumor cerebri syndrome.

5. Risk factors
   a. Female sex, obesity, and recent weight gain
   b. Iron deficiency anemia, thyroid dysfunction, pregnancy, antibiotic intake, and the use of oral contraceptives were no more common in PTC patients than in a case-controlled study.
   c. Elevated vitamin A levels have been noted in patients with idiopathic PTC. Serum retinol

concentrations were significantly higher in patients with idiopathic PTC compared to controls even after adjusting for age and body mass index.

6. Clinical features of PTC

    a. Headache may often be pulsatile, be of gradually increasing intensity during the day, awaken the patient at night; it may be precipitated by changes in posture, and is often transiently relieved by lumbar puncture.

    b. Pain in a cervical nerve root distribution (possibly from a dilated nerve root sleeve) or retro-ocular pain with eye movement may occur.

    c. Transient visual obscurations last seconds; may be unilateral or bilateral, related to changes in posture; do not correlate with the degree of intracranial hypertension or the extent of disc swelling; and are not considered to be harbingers of permanent visual loss

    d. Intracranial noises (pulse synchronous tinnitus) are common with PTC and are perhaps due to transmission of intensified vascular pulsations via cerebrospinal fluid under high pressure to the walls of the venous sinuses.

    e. Diplopia is often mild and usually due to a sixth cranial nerve palsy (nonlocalizing sign of raised intracranial pressure)

    f. Papilledema in majority. It may be asymmetric, rarely unilateral, and even occasionally absent.

7. Visual loss in PTC

    a. Visual field and, eventually, visual acuity loss are the major causes of morbidity in PTC.

    b. Complete blindness and optic atrophy may occur.

    c. Hypertension and recent weight gain have been reported to be significant risk factors for visual loss.

    d. Blind spot enlargement is common and may be improved with refraction alone (refractive scotoma due to disc swelling and increased peripapillary edema).

    e. Visual field defects in PTC patients are typically "disc-related" defects—most commonly loss of the inferonasal field or general constriction of isopters, followed by arcuate defects, central loss, or altitudinal defects

8. Evaluation of PTC

    a. Thorough history, especially medication use, pregnancy, intercurrent illnesses, and recent weight gain

    b. Consider blood work (sedimentation rate, complete blood count, syphilis serology, calcium, creatinine, and electrolytes)

    c. MRI and lumbar puncture to confirm diagnosis

    d. Complete eye exam including perimetry (Goldmann and/or automated) and optic disc stereo photography.

9. Medical treatment and follow-up

    a. Goals of treatment

        (1) Alleviate symptoms (e.g., headache)

        (2) Preserve visual function

    b. Monthly follow-up for 6 to 12 months: Visual fields, stereo optic disc photos, visual acuity, relative afferent pupillary defect (RAPD) testing, until papilledema has regressed

    c. Medical treatment

        (1) Acetazolamide (e.g., Diamox sequels 500 mg daily at bedtime for 3 days, then 500 mg twice a day – up to 2 to 4 g/day)

        (2) Furosemide (Lasix) of anecdotal benefit

        (3) Consider Topamax (topiramate): may help headache; weak carbonic anhydrase inhibitor, causes decreased appetite (may help with obesity) of anecdotal benefit

    d. Weight reduction beneficial but difficult to achieve

    e. Treat headache symptomatically if no response to acetazolamide

    f. Consider high-dose methylprednisolone and acetazolamide if acute, severe visual loss occurs.

    g. Repeated lumbar punctures have never been systematically studied prospectively and are of questionable benefit.

10. Surgical treatment

    a. Optic nerve sheath fenestration (ONSF)

    b. Lumboperitoneal shunt (LPS)

    c. Surgical indications

        (1) Progressive visual field defect despite medical therapy

        (2) Acute, severe visual loss

        (3) Anticipated hypotension induced by treatment of high blood pressure or renal dialysis

        (4) Headache unresponsive to standard headache medications (LPS)

    d. Surgical therapy—ONSF versus LPS

        (1) Either procedure may improve vision and prevent deterioration of vision

        (2) Approximately one third of patients undergoing ONSF will not experience headache relief and only about 75% of ONSFs

appear to be functioning 6 months after surgery.

(3) LPS failure is common. Most shunt failures occur within 2 to 3 months of the initial LPS (cumulative risk, 37%), and only rarely is the first shunt revision required more than 1 year after initial LPS.

(4) No prospective, randomized study comparing ONSF with LPS

(5) Other neurosurgical procedures, such as subtemporal decompression or stereotactic ventriculoperitoneal shunt, may also alleviate the signs and symptoms of PTC. The use of programmable shunts may decrease side effects of overshunting.

Key Signs

- Headache
- Pain in a cervical nerve root distribution
- Transient visual obscurations lasting seconds
- Intracranial noises (pulse synchronous tinnitus)
- Mild diplopia
- Papilledema in most cases

Key Tests

- Thorough history
- Blood tests
- MRI
- Lumbar puncture
- Complete eye examination, including perimetry and optic disc stereo photography
- Spinal fluid pressure

Key Normal Findings

- Cerebrospinal fluid analysis
- Neuroimaging
- No cause of "secondary" pseudotumor cerebri is evident

Key Treatments

- Closely monitor acuity, visual fields, color vision, disc appearance
- Weight loss
- Acetazolamide
- Consider furosemide; topiramate if acetazolamide intolerant.
- Consider surgical procedures (lumboperitoneal shunt or optic nerve sheath fenestration) if vision decreases or severe headache occurs that fails medical therapy
- LPS may be better than ONSF for headache alone or headache and visual loss
- ONSF may be superior to ONSF for visual loss alone (fewer complications)

Bibliography

Corbett JJ: Problems in the diagnosis and treatment of pseudotumor cerebri. Can J Neurol Sci 10:221–229, 1983.

Corbett JJ, Mehta MP: Cerebrospinal fluid pressure in normal obese subjects and patients with pseudotumor cerebri. Neurology 33:1386–1388, 1983.

Corbett JJ, Thompson HS: The rational management of idiopathic intracranial hypertension. Arch Neurol 46: 1049–1051, 1989.

Giuseffi V, Wall M, Siegel PZ, Roojas PB: Symptoms and disease associations in idiopathic intracranial hypertension (pseudotumor cerebri): A case-control study. Neurology 41:239–244, 1991.

Lee AG, Brazis PW: Clinical Pathways in Neuro-Ophthalmology. An Evidence-Based Approach. New York, Thieme, 1998.

Shin RK, Balcer LJ: Idiopathic Intracranial Hypertension. Curr Treat Options Neurol 4:297–305, 2002.

Wall M, George D: Idiopathic intracranial hypertension. A prospective study of 50 patients. Brain 114:155–180, 1991.

Visual Illusions and Hallucinations

Paul W. Brazis
Andrew G. Lee

Definitions

1. Illusions are misperceptions of external stimuli attributable to disordered processing of visual stimuli (e.g., optical illusions) that disappear with the eyes closed (unlike hallucinations).

2. Hallucinations are not based on incoming stimuli.

Etiology of Illusions—Usually Optical Aberrations

1. Astigmatic lenses (distortion of shape)

2. Lenticular abnormalities (multiple images, altered color)

3. Brunescence (yellow-brown tint): Often due to cataracts

4. Cyanopsia (blue tint): Sometimes noted after cataract removal

5. Erythropsia (red tint): Consider vitreous hemorrhage or hyphema

6. Distortions due to tear film abnormalities, such as dry eyes, or corneal disease

7. Different indexes of refraction

8. Retinal diseases: May cause micropsia, macropsia, metamorphopsia

9. Other visual illusory phenomena

   a. Polyopia (seeing a single target as multiple)

      (1) Unlike binocular diplopia, cerebral polyopia occurs with monocular viewing, both images are perceived with equal clarity, does not resolve with a pinhole, and is unchanged with viewing monocularly with either eye or binocularly.

      (2) Most instances of cerebral polyopia involve only double vision and are due to occipital or parieto-occipital lesions.

      (3) However, the subjective experience of multiple copies of the same image in a gridlike pattern (entomopia or "insect eye") has been described with migraine.

   b. Cerebral macropsia, micropsia, or metamorphopsia, palinopsia (persistence or recurrence of the visual image once the object has been removed) may occur with occipital disease.

      (1) With palinopsia, the image recurs immedi-

ately after diverting the gaze or when the stimulus object is withdrawn.

      (2) The image is frequently achromatic, may be revived by blinking, is not affected by eye closure, and moves in the direction of the eye movements (rarely, opposite to eye movements).

      (3) These illusory phenomena occur on the same side as an impaired but not blind visual field and are associated with occipitotemporal disease, often epileptogenic.

      (4) Also, palinopsia may occur during recovery from cortical blindness in the recovering portion of the visual field.

      (5) Most cases of palinopsia occur with focal, nondominant parietooccipital or occipitotemporal lesions.

      (6) Specific causes of palinopsia include tumor, ischemia, trauma, arteriovenous malformation, abscess, migraine, carbon monoxide poisoning, drugs (e.g., mescaline, LSD, trazodone, "Ecstasy," interleukin 2), multiple sclerosis, and cerebral vasculitis.

      (7) Palinopsia may also be the presenting manifestation of Creutzfeldt-Jakob disease or may follow enucleation.

   c. Visual allesthesia (transposition of an object seen in a visual field to the contralateral visual field) may be noted with occipital disease.

   d. Focal seizures arising in the neocortex of the temporal lobe may give rise to visual illusions ("déjà vu," already seen; "jamais vu," never seen before) or to experiential illusions ("déjà vécu," already lived; "jamais vécu," never experienced before). The patient feels a strong sense of familiarity with scenes or experiential situations that in reality he or she has never seen or experienced before or, on the contrary, a sense of strangeness about visual stimuli such as the face of a close relative or experiential situations that should be familiar.

Visual Hallucinations

1. Visual hallucinations may occur in a number of psychiatric, medical, neurologic, and ocular disorders, as well as in drug-induced states.

   a. Vitreous detachment may cause brief, vertical

flashes of light (Moore's lightning streaks) in the temporal visual fields seen predominantly with eye movement. The flashes of light indicate mechanical stimulation of the retina and are best seen in the dark or with the eyes closed, when the flashes do not compete with ambient light.

b. Optic neuritis may be associated with bright flashes of light induced by eye movement (movement phosphenes) or in response to sudden loud sound.

c. Patients with amaurosis fugax (transient visual loss often due to embolic phenomena) may experience colored bright light flashes or scintillations, as may patients with dissecting carotid aneurysms.

d. Patients with restrictive thyroid ophthalmopathy may occasionally complain of flashing lights in the superior visual field on upgaze, possibly phosphenes as a result of either compression of the globe by a tight inferior rectus muscle or traction on the insertion of the inferior rectus muscle.

2. Simple visual hallucinations

a. Consist of flashes of light (photopsias) or lines of different colors that adopt simple patterns (zig-zagged, circlular, fortification pattern)

b. Often accompany a defective field of vision and indicate inferomedial occipital disease, usually migraine or an epileptogenic lesion

c. Elementary visual hallucinations with occipital epileptic seizures are predominantly multicolored, with circular or spherical patterns as opposed to the predominantly black-and-white zig-zagged linear patterns of migraine.

Key Signs: Simple Visual Hallucinations

- Flashes of light or lines of different colors that adopt a simple pattern, e.g., zig-zagged or circular

- Accompany a defective field of vision and indicate inferomedial occipital disease

- Migraine: Black-and-white zig-zagged linear patterns

- Occipital epileptic seizures: Multicolored with circular or spherical patterns

3. Complex visual hallucinations

a. Include landscapes, animals, etc.

b. May be related to temporal lobe dysfunction.

c. Autoscopic phenomena (hallucinations of the self) and illusory phenomena, such as micropsia

and metamorphopsia, may be seizure manifestations.

d. Among structural lesions, tumors have the greatest tendency to induce hallucinations.

e. Peduncular hallucinations

(1) May be seen with lesions in the upper midbrain that also involve the thalamus, often bilaterally

(2) Usually complex visual hallucinations that have an oneroid (dreamlike) quality.

(3) Often hypnagogic

(4) Usually known to be unreal

(5) May be of normal or lilliputian proportions

(6) May be pleasant to the patient

(7) Destruction of the pars reticulata may be critical for the development of peduncular hallucinosis.

(8) Postulated to be a release phenomenon related to damage to the ascending reticular activating system (ARAS), the rostral projection of which extends from the midbrain to the intralaminar thalamic nuclei.

f. An etiologically nonspecific type of complex visual hallucinations may occur in the elderly with impaired vision (Charles Bonnet syndrome).

(1) These recurrent vivid hallucinations occur in the presence of normal cognition and insight and are usually associated with severe visual deprivation.

(2) Hallucinations usually occur in the evening and are often made up of small, brightly colored people or objects with a cartoonlike appearance.

(3) The patient is usually aware of the unreality of these hallucinations and may note that the hallucinations change size or character when the subject reaches out to touch them.

(4) Thought to be the result of a release phenomenon in ventral temporo-occipital cortex, an area that is poorly activated by visual stimulation in these patients.

g. Other positive visual phenomena experienced by patients with partial visual loss include tessellopsia (regular, repeating patterns), dendropsia (branching patterns), and hiperchromatopsia (hyperintense, brilliant colors).

Key Signs: Complex Visual Hallucinations

- Include landscapes, vehicles, animals, and people

- Have a dreamlike quality

- Often hypnagogic
- Known to be unreal
- Of normal or lilliputian proportions
- May be pleasant
- Charles Bonnet syndrome in the elderly

4. Classification of simple and complex hallucinations:

a. Those due to increased irritability of the cerebral cortex ("ictal"), which are typically stereotyped and more likely to be associated with other seizure manifestations

b. Those due to impaired vision, typically with visual acuity of 20/50 or less ("release hallucinations"), which are less stereotyped, longer in duration or continuous, likely to occur in the blind portion of the visual field, and perceived as unreal by the patient

   (1) They may range in complexity from simple phosphenes to well-formed visions, such as people, vehicles, or furniture.

   (2) Release hallucinations are thought to represent the liberation of endogenous cerebral visual activity from "control" by higher visual inhibitory centers and may result from lesions anywhere in the visual pathways (retina to occipital cortex), regardless of the complexity of the hallucination.

5. Migraine

a. The presence of a small area of visual loss or a mild disturbance of vision that progressively increases over 15 minutes or more is highly characteristic of migraine.

b. This visual abnormality is usually bilateral and homonymous. The patient need not have headache for this diagnosis to be made.

c. Most patients have some abnormal positive visual symptoms associated with the episodes, most commonly fortification spectra around an area of scotoma, scintillations, or distortions within the area of visual disturbance resembling "heat waves" or "water running down a glass"

d. The typical visual aura starts as a flickering, uncolored, zig-zagged line in the center of visual field that gradually progresses and expands toward the periphery of one hemifield and often leaves a temporary scotoma.

e. Migrainous visual accompaniment often occur in individuals over age 50 years and often occur in the absence of headache in this age group.

   (1) These episodes probably are not associated with an increased stroke risk.

   (2) The spells are usually stereotyped, begin gradually and progress, last several minutes to one hour, usually include positive visual phenomena (bright images, colors, movement of images), and affect both eyes.

   (3) Migrainous visual accompaniments are usually benign may occur with amyloid angiopathy of the central nervous system.

f. Patients may experience a large number of consecutive (mostly) visual auras, very often without headache (migraine aura status). Between the auras, the patient is without symptoms. Episodes can last for weeks, and within this period several migraine auras can occur on one day.

g. Abnormal visual disturbances similar to those with migraine, often associated with headache, may rarely occur with cerebral structural lesions, such as arteriovenous malformations of the occipital lobe or brain tumors, but these usually do not have the characteristic build-up and resolution of visual symptoms. Instead these lesions usually produce symptoms that steadily increase in frequency and duration until they are present daily.

h. Differential diagnosis of migraine-like hallucinations

   (1) Occipital lobe tumors may rarely produce scintillating scotomas that mimic migraine. In most of these cases, the tumors were diagnosed only after the patients eventually developed papilledema or when a homonymous visual field defect was documented.

   (2) Arteriovenous malformations (AVMs) of the occipital lobes may also produce visual symptoms and headache that may simulate migraine.

      (a) Visual symptoms with occipital AVMs are usually brief, episodic, unformed, and not associated with the angular, scintillating figures that occur with migraine.

      (b) They also tend to occur consistently in the same visual field.

      (c) However, the clinical symptoms classically noted with migraine may occasionally occur with occipital AVMs.

   (3) Idiopathic occipital epilepsy and visual seizures.

      (a) The ictal elementary visual hallucinations are stereotyped for each patient, usually lasting seconds.

      (b) They consist of mainly multiple, bright colored, small circular spots, circles, or balls.

(c) Mostly, they appear in a temporal hemifield often moving contralaterally or in the center, where they may be flashing.

(d) They may be multiple and increase in size in the course of a seizure and may progress to extra-occipital manifestations and convulsions.

(e) Blindness occurs usually from the beginning, and postictal headache, often indistinguishable from migraine, is common

(f) Elementary visual hallucinations in occipital seizures are entirely different from the visual aura of migraine in that they are mainly colored, have a circular pattern, have the same onset regarding localization, are often brief (lasting seconds, occasionally minutes). They develop fast and then individual components may multiply or move together to the contralateral side, they often occur daily, and they may be associated with other seizure manifestations. Conversely, the visual aura of migraine starts with predominantly flickering achromatic or black-and-white (rarely colored) linear and zig-zagged patterns in the center of vision which gradually expanding over minutes toward the periphery of one hemifield and often leave a scotoma. Migraine rarely occurs daily.

(4) Symptoms similar to the scintillating scotomas of migraine may also occur with acute vitreous or retinal detachment. In these patients, the visual symptoms are clearly monocular, last longer than typical migrainous visual aura, and occur without any associated headache.

(5) Scintillating scotomas have also been described associated with internal carotid artery dissection.

6. Evaluation of patients with visual hallucinations

a. Patients with typical expanding migraine scintillations and positive phenomena lasting 20 to 30 minutes that have been noted to occur on different sides at different times, and headaches that have been documented to occur on different sides at different times usually do not require further work-up.

b. However, any patient with abnormalities on visual field examination suggesting a retrochiasmal lesion or any patient with atypical migraine-like phenomena, especially patients with visual symptoms that are brief, episodic, unformed, and not associated with the angular, scintillating figures that occur with migraine, requires magnetic resonance imaging (MRI) and MR angiography to investigate the possibility of occipital AVM, venous sinus thrombosis, or tumor.

c. When either "migraine" headache or visual symptoms are restricted to one side of the head (even if the visual field exam is normal), a neuroimaging study should be performed to investigate the possibility of an occipital AVM.

d. Patients with migraine and symptoms or signs of collagen vascular disease require a collagen vascular disease profile.

e. Electroencephalography or a trial of anticonvulsant medications is warranted if occipital epilepsy is likely.

Key Tests

- Often no work-up is necessary if symptoms are characteristic and examination is normal.

- Any patient with abnormalities on visual field examination suggesting a retrochiasmal lesion or with atypical migraine-like phenomena—especially with visual symptoms that are brief, episodic, unformed, and not associated with the angular, scintillating figures that occur with migraine—requires MR imaging and MR angiography.

- When either "migraine" headache or visual symptoms are restricted to one side of the head (even if the visual field examination is normal), a neuroimaging study should be performed.

- Patients with migraine and symptoms or signs of collagen vascular disease require a collagen vascular disease profile.

- Electroencephalography or a trial of anticonvulsant medications is warranted if occipital epilepsy is likely.

Bibliography

Brazis PW, Masdeu JC, Biller J: Localization in Clinical Neurology, 4th ed. Philadelphia, Lippincott Williams & Wilkins, 2001, pp. 475–477.

Lee AG, Brazis PW: Clinical Pathways in Neuro-Ophthalmology. An Evidence-Based Approach. New York, Thieme, 1998.

Norton JW, Corbett JJ: Visual perceptual abnormalities: hallucinations and illusions. Semin Neurol 20:111–121, 2000.

Panayiotopoulos CP: Visual phenomena and headache in occipital epilepsy: a review, a systematic study and differentiation from migraine. Epileptic Disord 1:205–216, 1999.

1 **Migraine**

Randolph W. Evans

Epidemiology and Risk Factors

1. One year prevalence: 18% women, 6% men. In the United States, 28 million persons have migraine per year.

2. Lifetime prevalence: 25% women, 8% men

3. Migraine begins before the age of 20 in 50% and over the age of 50 in 2%.

4. Prevalence is highest from the ages of 25 years to 50 years.

5. About 70% of migraineurs have a positive family history in a first-degree relative.

   a. First-degree relatives of those with migraine with aura have a fourfold greater risk of migraine with aura, and those with migraine without aura have a 1.9-fold increased risk of migraine without aura.

   b. Family histories are often inaccurate because many migraineurs do not know they have migraine.

   c. Mode of transmission is unclear; genetic heterogeneity is present.

6. In the United States, prevalence is highest among Caucasians, intermediate among African Americans, and lowest among Asian Americans.

7. Prevalence is highest in low-income and low-education groups in the United States.

8. High prevalence among neurologists (lifetime of 47% in males and 63% in females).

9. Frequency can range from once in a lifetime to daily.

   a. 1–12 per year, 38%

   b. 1–3 per month, 37%

   c. 1 per week, 11%

   d. 2–6 per week, 14%

10. About 50% of migraineurs have medically diagnosed migraine. Many patients and some doctors misdiagnose migraine as "sinus."

11. Co-morbidity (greater than coincidental association of two disorders in the same individual). Migraineurs have an increased prevalence of many disorders.

    a. Mitral valve prolapse, patent foramen ovale, and hypertension

    b. Stroke and epilepsy

    c. Atopic allergies, asthma, and irritable bowel syndrome

    d. Depression, bipolar disease, anxiety disorders, and panic attacks

---

Facts About Migraine

- 28 million persons in the United States suffer migraines each year.

- Prevalence (lifetime): 25% women, 8% men

- Prevalence highest in those between the ages of 25 years to 50 years

- In the United States, prevalence highest among Caucasians, intermediate among African Americans, and lowest among Asian Americans

- Low-income and low-education groups have the highest rate of migraine in the United States.

- High prevalence among neurologists (lifetime of 47% in males and 63% in females)

- Frequency of migraine can range from once in a lifetime to daily.

Etiology and Pathophysiology

1. Incompletely understood. Migraine is a neurovascular headache.

2. Migraine aura is a slow march of visual or other neurologic symptoms associated with changes in neuronal activity that result in spreading depression from the occipital cortex. Excitatory changes produce increased blood flow followed by reduced blood flow from neuronal inhibition.

3. The trigeminovascular system may constitute the anatomic substrate for migraine pain.

   a. The pain-producing cranial nerves and dura

      (1) Input passes through the ophthalmic division of the trigeminal ganglion to the trigeminocervical complex (the trigeminal nucleus caudalis and dorsal horns of C_1 and C_2), which produces pain in the head (especially the ophthalmic division) and upper posterior neck.

b. The peripheral branches of the trigeminal nerve which are activated during migraine

(1) The pain results from neurogenic inflammation produced by the antidromic release of calcitonin gene-related peptide by trigeminal nerve endings and associated with the release of other pain substances from plasma, platelets, and mast cells (e.g., histamine, prostaglandin, serotonin).

(2) This release induces the vasodilatation and extravasation of plasma proteins and the sensitization of trigeminal nociceptive nerve endings.

(a) Throbbing pain and exacerbation by activities such as bending over, head movement, coughing, and walking may be due to mechanical hypersensitivity of meningeal C-fiber nociceptors.

(3) Nitric oxide released from blood vessels, perivascular nerve endings, or brain tissue can trigger migraine pain.

c. Central processing of pain signals in the trigeminocervical complex

(1) Second-order neurons receive input and project rostrally to the contralateral thalamus (ventrobasal complex and medial nuclei) and then activate cortex (anterior cingulate, insular, and frontal), periaqueductal gray matter (dorsal raphe nuclei), and locus coeruleus.

(2) Aminergic areas in the periaqueductal gray matter and locus coeruleus influence the incoming pain and cortical blood flow.

(3) A continuous discharge in this pain-control system might result from stimulation from the cortex or the hypothalamus owing to stress or to excessive afferent input from the special senses or from cerebral or extracranial vessels.

(a) Migraine prodrome may originate in the hypothalamus.

d. Ergot derivatives and triptans are 5-hydroxytriptamine (5-HT)$_{1B/1D}$ agonists.

(1) They active the 5-HT receptors present in cranial vessels and second-order trigeminal neurons, which leads to inhibition of cyclic aminomonophosphate production.

(2) Cranial vasoconstriction, peripheral neuronal inhibition, and central trigeminal nucleus inhibition result.

Clinical Features

1. General features

a. Unilateral in 60%, bilateral in 40%

(1) Often more intense in the frontotemporal and ocular regions before spreading to the parietal and occipital area.

(2) Any region of the head or face may be affected, including the parietal region, the upper or lower jaw or teeth, the malar eminence, or the upper anterior neck. Unilateral or bilateral posterior neck pain occurs in up to 75% of migraines and can lead to diagnostic confusion with tension-type headaches.

(3) 15% report side-locked headaches, migraine always occurring on the same side.

b. Throbbing pain is reported in 85%, although up to 50% of migraneurs describe nonthrobbing pain during some attacks.

c. Headache lasts 4 to 72 hours untreated or unsuccessfully treated.

(1) Median untreated attack duration is 24 hours

(2) Migraine persisting for more than 72 hours is termed "status migrainosus."

d. Untreated, 80% have moderate-severe intensity of pain; 20% mild pain.

e. Pain is usually increased by physical activity or movement.

f. Nausea occurs in about 80%; vomiting, in about 30%.

g. Photophobia (light sensitivity) is present in about 90%; phonophobia (noise sensitivity), in about 80%.

h. Migraine without aura (common) 80% of migraineurs; with aura (classic), in 20%

i. 45% of migraineurs have at least one autonomic symptom due to parasympathetic activation (lacrimation, eye redness, ptosis, eyelid edema, nasal congestion, and rhinorrhea). Of these, 45% have both nasal and ocular symptoms, 21% have only nasal symptoms, and 34% have only ocular symptoms. These symptoms result in diagnostic confusion with "sinus" and allergies.

j. Prodromal symptoms (premonitory phenomena) may be present in about 10% and precede the migraine attack by hours or up to 1 or 2 days.

(1) Changes in mental state may be reflected by depressed, hyperactive, euphoric, talk-

ative, irritable, drowsy, or restless behaviors.

(2) Neurologic symptoms may include photophobia, difficulty concentrating, phonophobia, dysphasia, hyperosmia, and yawning.

(3) General symptoms may include stiff neck, food cravings, cold feeling, anorexia, sluggishness, diarrhea or constipation, thirst, and fluid retention.

k. Triggers or precipitating factors are present in about 85% of migraineurs who report an average of three triggers. There are numerous triggers

(1) Stress is reported by about 50%. Other persons may report migraines triggered by let down after stress, vacations, or crying.

(2) Missing a meal (40%), lack of sleep, oversleeping, and fatigue

(3) Environmental triggers: changes in weather, heat, high humidity, high altitude

(4) Sensory triggers: bright lights, glare, flickering lights, loud noise, strong smells such as perfume or cigarette smoke

(5) Menses is a trigger for about 50% of female migraineurs.

(6) Up to 50% report alcohol as a trigger (can be all forms of alcohol or only one type such as red wine or beer).

(7) 10% to 45% report food triggers such as chocolate, dairy foods (particularly cheese), citrus fruit, fried fatty foods, and nitrates and nitrites in cured meats or fish (e.g., frankfurters, bacon, and lox).

(8) Other triggers include head trauma, exertion, and nitroglycerin.

Key Precipitating Factors or Triggers

Triggers or precipitating factors present in about 85% of those affected; an average of three triggers are usually reported:

• Stress (approximately 50%)

• Missing a meal (40%), lack of sleep, oversleeping, fatigue

• Environmental: changes in weather, heat, high humidity, high altitude

• Sensory: bright lights, glare, flickering lights, loud noise, strong smells such as perfume or cigarette smoke

• Menses (about 50% of female patients)

• Alcohol (up to 50%)

• Food (10%–45%) such as chocolate, dairy foods (particularly cheese), citrus fruit, fried fatty foods, and nitrates and nitrites in cured meats or fish (e.g., frankfurters, bacon, and lox)

• Head trauma, exertion, and nitroglycerin

l. Resolution phase or postdrome

(1) Frequent symptoms include changes in mood, weakness, tiredness, and reduced appetite.

(2) May report feeling tired and washed out, irritable, or experiencing poor concentration ("mashed potato brain"). Less often, unusually refreshed or euphoric.

m. Sleep

(1) Sleep may relieve migraine, especially in children.

(2) Migraine can also begin during sleep and cause awakening or can be present upon awakening at the usual time.

2. Migraine without aura: about 80%

a. International Headache Society (IHS) criteria

(1) At least five attacks fulfilling criteria (2)–(4)

(2) Headache lasting 4 to 72 hours (untreated or unsuccessfully treated)

(3) Headache has at least two of the following characteristics:

(a) Unilateral location

(b) Pulsating quality

(c) Moderate or severe intensity (inhibits or prohibits daily activities)

(d) Aggravation by walking stairs or similar routine physical activity

(4) During headache at least one of the following

(a) Nausea and/or vomiting

(b) Photophobia and phonophobia

(5) History, physical, and neurologic examinations do not suggest another disorder.

3. Migraine with aura: 20%

a. IHS criteria

(1) At least two attacks fulfilling criterion (2)

(2) At least three of the following four characteristics:

(a) One or more fully reversible aura symptoms indicating brain dysfunction.

(b) At least one aura symptom develops gradually over more than 4 minutes or 2 or more symptoms occur in succession.

(c) No single aura symptom lasts more than 60 minutes.

(d) Headache follows aura with a free interval of less than 60 minutes (it may also begin before or with the aura).

(3) History, physical examination and, when appropriate, diagnostic tests exclude a secondary cause.

b. Most migraineurs with aura also have migraine without aura.

c. Total duration of the aura is usually less than 1 hour. If the aura lasts more than 1 hour but less than 1 week, then it is "migraine with prolonged aura" (also termed "complicated migraine").

d. Aura symptoms

(1) Visual aura: the most common aura; present in 99% of cases

(a) Two types: positive visual phenomena with hallucinations and negative visual phenomona or scotomas with either incomplete or complete loss of vision in a portion or the whole of the visual field

(b) Most visual auras have a hemianoptic distribution.

(c) Photopsias consist of small spots, dots, stars, unformed flashes or steaks of light, or simple geometric forms and patterns that typically flicker or sparkle.

(d) Scintillating scotomas

(i) Also called "fortification spectra" (looks like a medieval fortified town as viewed from above) or *teichopsia* ("seeing fortifications"). Fortification spectra present in about 10%.

(ii) A scotomatous arc or band with a shimmering or glittering, bright, zigzag border.

(iii) The visual alteration usually commences in the center of the visual field and slowly extends laterally.

(iv) The scotoma frequently is semicircular or horseshoe-shaped.

(e) Occasionally, objects may appear to change in size and shape (metamorphopsia). Includes macropsia, micropsia, telescopic vision (objects larger than normal), teleopsia (objects too far away), mosaic vision, and Alice in Wonderland syndrome (episodes of distorted body image). Multiple images can also be present.

(f) Most consist of flickering, colored or uncolored, unilateral or bilateral zig-zag lines or patterns, semicircular or arcuate patterns, wavy lines, or irregular patterns.

(g) Headaches are usually contralateral but can occasionally be unilateral, on the side of the visual symptoms.

(2) Sensory aura: present in about 30% of migraine with aura.

(a) Numbness, tingling, or pins and needles sensations which are usually unilateral.

(b) Cheiro-oral (hand-mouth) distribution is common.

(c) Sensory symptoms often slowly spread in distribution, e.g., from hand to mouth.

(d) The hand and then the face, alone or in combination, are the parts of the body most commonly affected. Paresthesia of one side of the tongue is typical. Less often, the leg and trunk may be involved.

(3) Motor aura is rare: Often sensory ataxia or a heavy feeling is misinterpreted as "weakness."

(4) Speech and language disturbances may occur in up to 20% of cases.

(a) Patients often report speech disturbance occurring as the spreading paresthesias reach the face or tongue.

(b) Slurred speech and, with involvement of the dominant hemisphere, paraphasic errors and other types of impaired language production, and impaired comprehension may occur.

(c) Duration is usually less than 30 minutes.

(5) Other aura symptoms: Rarely, other symptoms include dejà vu and olfactory and gustatory hallucinations

(6) Combinations of aura symptoms

(a) Visual symptoms frequently occur alone.

(b) Sensory, speech, and motor symptoms are usually associated with visual symptoms or with one or more of the other symptoms.

(c) When two or more aura symptoms are present, they almost always occur in succession and not simultaneously.

4. Migraine aura without headache (acephalgic migraine).

   a. Migraine aura can occur without headache, often in those with migraine with or without aura. Visual aura is the most common.

   b. Episodic vertigo without headache or auditory or other neurologic symptoms lasting minutes to days can also be an aura.

   c. In older persons, can be confused with transient ischemic attacks and are termed "late-life migraine accompaniments" (see Part XI, Chapter 8, Headaches in Patients Over the Age of 50).

   d. Rarely, migraineurs have persistent visual aura.

      (1) Usually simple, unformed hallucinations in the entire visual field of both eyes may be described as a million dots, television static, clouds, dots, heat waves, flashing or flickering lights, lines of ants, rainlike pattern, snow, squiggles, bubbles, and grainy vision.

      (2) Occasionally, palinopsia (the persistence of visual images), micropsia, or formed hallucinations.

      (3) Might respond to preventive treatment with divalproex sodium.

5. Pediatric migraine and variants including familial hemiplegic, basilar, ophthalmoplegic, benign paroxymal vertigo of childhood, abdominal, confusional, and "footballer's" are discussed in Part XI, Chapter 6, Headaches during Childhood and Adolescence. Posttraumatic migraine is also discussed in Part XIII, Chapter 1, Mild Head Injury and the Postconcussion Syndrome.

6. Part XI, Chapter 7, Headaches in Women, reviews other migraine topics including menstrual, menopause, oral contraceptive use, and headaches during pregnancy and postpartum.

7. Benign episodic mydriasis

   a. Transient isolated mydriasis with normal vision and pupillary reactivity to light may occasionally accompany migraine headaches, typically in young adults or children.

      (1) Duration of episodes 15 minutes to 24 hours often associated with blurred vision.

      (2) Episodes average 2 to 3 per month

   b. Eyelid or motility abnormalities are absent

   c. Dilation of the pupil is from either parasympathetic insufficiency of the iris sphincter or sympathetic hyperactivity of the iris dilator.

   d. Angle-closure glaucoma should be excluded

Key Clinical Features

- Unilateral headache, 60%; bilateral headache, 40%
- Thobbing pain 80%, nausea 80%, vomiting 30%
- Photophobia 90%, phonophobia 80%
- At least one autonomic symptom in 45%
- Without aura, 80%; with aura, 20%

Differential Diagnosis

1. Although most migraines can be diagnosed on the basis of clinical criteria, some may have features of tension and migraine ("migrainous" especially when occurring in persons with definite migraine) or cluster and migraine ("cluster-migraine").

2. First severe migraine attacks, the worst migraine attacks, or migraine with a thunderclap onset ("crash" migraine) may raise concerns about possible other causes such as subarachnoid hemorrhage or meningitis (see Part XI, Chapter 5, First or Worst Headaches).

3. With the first attack, 7% of patients with multiple sclerosis present with significant headaches that may be confused with migraine. In addition, migraine may be as much as twice as common in those with multiple sclerosis as in controls.

Laboratory Testing

1. Electroencephalograms are not indicated except when there is a question of a seizure disorder or in the case of migraine with altered consciousness—e.g., confusional or basilar migraine.

2. Blood tests are generally not helpful except as a baseline when monitoring for side effects of medications.

3. Lumbar puncture is not indicated except in some special cases (e.g., first or worst migraine, crash migraine, persistent or unusual auras, or to rule out pseudomigraine (see Part II, Chapter 1, Lumbar Puncture and Cerebrospinal Fluid Evaluation).

Radiologic Features

1. The routine use of neuroimaging for migraine is not indicated when there is no recent change in headache pattern, no history of seizures, and no other focal neurologic signs or symptoms.

2. Indications for neuroimaging (usually magnetic resonance imaging—MRI) in migraineurs include

the following: unusual, prolonged, or persistent aura; increasing frequency, severity, or change in clinical features; migraine status; first or worst migraine; migraine with a sudden onset and severe intensity ("crash" migraine); new onset over the age of 50 years; variants including basilar confusional, hemiplegic, and aura without headache; late-life migraine accompaniments; and posttraumatic migraine.

3. White matter abnormalities (WMA) are present on MRI scans more often in migraineurs (variably reported in 12% to 46%) than in controls (2% to 14%).

   a. WMA, foci of hyperintensity on both proton-density and T_2-weighted images in the deep and periventricular white matter, are due to either interstitial edema or periventricular demyelination.

   b. Although the cause is not certain, various hypotheses have been proposed, including increased platelet aggregration with microemboli, abnormal cerebrovascular regulation, and repeated attacks of hypoperfusion during the aura.

   c. Although antiphospholipid antibody syndrome can cause WMAs, this disorder is no more common in people with migraine than in controls.

   d. In some cases, nonspecific WMA present on MRI scans of migraineurs can be incorrectly diagnosed as signifying multiple sclerosis.

      (1) There are several features of WMA that are more typical of multiple sclerosis than migraine as visualized on T_2-weighted and FLAIR scans, including primarily periventricular rather than peripheral location, oval rather than round or punctate shape, irregular or fuzzy margins rather than sharply defined edges, and oriented perpendicular to the ventricles.

      (2) Corpus callosum or infratentorial lesions are more likely due to multiple sclerosis, as are lesions greater than 6 mm in diameter.

   e. WMA may also be present in systemic lupus erythematosus (SLE) but are not specific for central nervous system (CNS) involvement. Migraine is more common in patients with SLE than in controls.

Indications for Considering Neuroimaging

- Unusual, prolonged, or persistent aura
- Increasing frequency, severity, or change in clinical features
- Migraine status
- First or worst headache
- Crash migraine
- Onset over the age of 50 years
- Posttraumatic migraine

Treatment

1. Acute (symptomatic)

   a. General principles

      (1) Early treatment when the headache is mild is much more effective than later treatment when the migraine is moderate-severe in intensity.

      (2) Frequent use of acute medications can lead to rebound (recurring headache induced by repetitive and chronic overuse of acute headache medications.)

         (a) Generally, the use of acute therapy should be restricted to a maximum of 2 to 3 days per week.

      (3) Different patients may respond to different medications at different times.

      (4) There are numerous options which are briefly summarized here. Refer to standard pharmacology textbooks and references for more information.

      (5) Patients benefit from stratified care.

         (a) Treatment based on attack characteristics including peak intensity, time to peak intensity, associated symptoms, and disability

         (b) Individually tailored to specific patient needs

         (c) Use nasal, parenteral, or rectal forms of medication in patients with significant nausea or vomiting or gastroparesis. Antinausea medications such as promethazine or prochlorperazine may help.

> PEARL
>
> - Early treatment—when the headache is mild—is much more effective than when the migraine is moderate–severe in intensity.
>
> - Medications for acute headaches should be used only 2 to 3 days per week; their frequent use may lead to rebound.
>
> - Treatment should be based on attack characteristics such as peak intensity, time to peak intensity, associated symptoms, and disability.

b. Over-the-counter medications including aspirin, acetaminophen, aspirin plus caffeine, and nonsteroidal anti-inflammatory drugs (NSAIDs)

c. Opioid combinations and butalbital combinations and butorphanol nasal spray; use should be restricted because of the potential for rebound headaches and habituation.

d. Prescription NSAIDs (oral such as naproxen and intramuscular ketorolac) and isomeheptene combinations.

e. Ergotamine ± caffeine. Used extensively before triptans became available but much less now. Overuse can result in rebound and dependence. Contraindications are the same as for dihydroergotamine (see below).

f. Dihydroergotamine (DHE). Can be administered as nasal spray (NS) or by subcutaneous (SC), intramuscular (IM), or intravenous (IV) injection.

(1) Does not result in dependence.

(2) NS provides relief in 65%; parenteral administration, in about 90%

(3) May cause nausea. Can be administered with metoclopromide, promethazine, or prochlorperazine.

(4) Contraindications

(a) Concurrent use of a triptan. Use of the two drugs should be separated by at least 24 hours because of the potential for additive vasoconstriction.

(b) Coronary artery disease, cerebral, and peripheral vascular disease, and uncontrolled hypertension. In patients with risk factors including older age, consider the possibility of undiagnosed

coronary artery or peripheral vascular disease. (CAD or PVD).

(c) Pregnancy and breast-feeding

(5) For acute migraine, can administer NS or as IM or SC dose of 1 mg.

(6) For an attack that has climaxed, can administer prochlorperazine 5 mg IV or metoclopramide 5–10 mg IV followed immediately by 0.5–0.75 mg DHE given slowly over 2 to 3 minutes. If the patient is not improving in 30 to 60 minutes, another 0.5 mg DHE can be given IV without prochlorperazine or metoclopramide.

g. Triptans ($5\text{-HT}_{1B/1D}$ agonists)

(1) 2-hour efficacy (reduction of moderate to severe pain to mild or no pain) 80% with sumatriptan SC; 65% to 70% with sumatriptan, rizatriptan, and zolmitriptan, and almotriptan PO, and less with naratriptan and frovatriptan succinate.

(2) Triptans are more effective and more likely to result in pain freedom with treatment of migraine when pain is mild.

(3) Options

(a) Sumatriptan tablet (25 mg, 50 mg, 100 mg), nasal spray (5 and 20 mg), and subcutaneous injectable (6 mg)

(b) Zolmitriptan tablet (2.5 mg and 5 mg) and orally disintegrating tablet (2.5 and 5 mg)

(c) Naratriptan tablet (1 mg and 2.5 mg)

(d) Rizatriptan tablet (5 and 10 mg) and orally dissolvable wafer (10 mg)

(e) Almotriptan 12.5 mg tablet

(f) Frovatriptan succinate 2.5 mg tablet

(4) Contraindications include

(a) Coronary artery disease, cerebral and peripheral vascular disease, and uncontrolled hypertension

(b) In those with risk factors including older age, consider the possibility of undiagnosed CAD and PVD.

(5) Side effects are usually mild and transient and include chest pressure/heaviness, jaw tightness, dizziness, somnolence, asthenia/fatigue, nausea, and paresthesias. Recurrence (return of episodic headache during the same attack after acute treatment) is common with triptans, occurring in 20% to 40% of patients, depending on the triptan, about 11 hours later. A second dose will usually relieve the recurrent headache.

Key Treatment

Acute Headaches

- Over-the-counter medications such as aspirin, acetaminophen, aspirin plus caffeine, and NSAIDs

- Opioid and butalbital combinations and butorphanol nasal spray

- Prescription NSAIDs and isometheptene combinations

- Ergotamine ± caffeine

- Dihydroergotamine

- Triptans

h. Intractable migraine and migraine status: options

(1) Intravenous fluids and electrolyte replacement as indicated

(2) Sumatriptan 6 mg SC

(3) Intractable migraine may respond to metoclopramide 10 mg IV and DHE 0.5 to 1.0 mg (depending upon response) IV every 8 hours for 2 to 3 days as indicated. DHE and triptans should not be used within 24 hours of each other.

(4) Prochlorperazine 5 to 10 mg IV

(5) Ketorolac 30 to 60 mg IM

(6) Corticosteroids (single or rapidly tapering dose of prednisone starting at 80 mg a day or dexamethasone 6 mg PO or IV)

(7) Parenteral narcotics such as meperidine with promethazine

(8) Valproate sodium 500 mg diluted in 50 ml of saline administered IV over 5 to 10 minutes: can be repeated every 8 hours for 2 days

(9) Droperidol (2.5 mg IM or IV)

(10) Magnesium sulfate 1 g IV over 15 minutes.

2. Preventive (prophylactic)

a. Guidelines for use of prophylactic treatment

(1) Migraine significantly interferes with patient's daily routine despite acute treatment

(2) Acute medications contraindicated, ineffective, have interolerable side effects, or are overused

(3) Frequent headache (2 or more attacks per week)

(4) Uncommon migraine type (hemiplegic, basilar, prolonged aura, or migrainous infarction)

(5) Cost of both acute and preventive treatments

(6) Patient preference

b. General principles for administering prophylactic treatment

(1) Start low and increase dose slowly

(2) Perform an adequate trial of 2 to 3 months at an adequate dose

(3) Discontinue or taper off (depending on the drug) overused medications that may be causing rebound and that may decrease the efficacy of preventive treatment

(4) Monitor with a headache diary

(5) Educate the patient about the rationale for treatment and possible side effects; address the patient's expectons for treatment.

(6) Consider co-existent or co-morbid disease

(a) Some medications may treat two disorders such as migraine and epilepsy, hypertension, depression, bipolar disorder, and insomnia.

(b) Co-existent diseases (e.g., depression or asthma may be relative contraindications in the use of beta-blockers)

(c) In women who are pregnant or might become pregnant, the potential for teratogenicity should be considered (see Section XI, Chapter 8, Headaches in Women)

(7) Withdraw some medications especially at moderate-high doses slowly (e.g. tricyclic antidepressants and beta-blockers)

(8) Those with mild responses to one preventative may benefit from the addition of a second.

(9) First line preventatives reduce the frequency more than 50% in about 50–60% of migraineurs.

c. Antidepressants

(1) Tricyclic antidepressants such as amitriptyline and nortriptyline starting at 10 to 25 mg at bedtime slowly increasing the dose as appropriate. Efficacy typically at a dose range up to 150 mg. Protriptyline, which is nonsedating, may also be effective.

(a) Side effects include drowsiness, weight gain, dry mouth, and constipation. May lower the seizure threshold in those with frequent seizures (amitriptyline more so than nortriptyline).

(b) Amitriptyline and nortriptyline may treat more than one disorder for patients with sleep disturbance and/or depression.

(2) Fluoxetine, a second-line drug: Has questionable efficacy in migraine. Venlafaxine might be effective.

d. Beta-blockers (starting dose and upper range)

(1) Propranolol (40-240 mg in divided doses), propanolol long-acting (60–160 mg once daily)

(2) Atenolol (50–100 mg)

(3) Metoprolol (50–200 mg)

(4) Nadolol (40–160 mg)

(5) Timolol (10–30 mg in divided doses)

(6) Contraindications

(a) Asthma, congestive heart failure, sinus bradycardia, second- and third-degree heart block

(b) May exacerbate depression

(c) In diabetics, may block the symptoms and signs of hypoglycemia

(d) Some authorities urge caution in the use of beta-blockers in migraine with prolonged aura and basilar migraine because of the potential for limiting compensatory vasodilator capacitance.

(7) Side effects include tiredness, fatigue, dizziness. Need to monitor for symptomatic bradycardia and hypotension.

(8) The failure to respond to one beta-blocker does not generally predict the failure to respond to another.

(9) May treat more than one disorder if the patient also has hypertension, essential tremor, or anxiety/panic attacks.

e. Anticonvulsants

(1) Divalproex sodium

(a) Starting dose of 500 mg day (administered twice daily or, with extended-release tablet, once a day). May dose up to 1500 mg/day for migraine (for epilepsy, need to monitor serum levels; in migraine, serum levels may be helpful for monitoring toxicity but not predicting efficacy)

(b) Contraindicated in patients with hepatic disease or significant hepatic dysfunction

(c) Side effects include nausea, asthenia, somnolence, weight gain, hair loss, tremor, dizziness, and teratogenic potential (neural tube defects in 1% to 2%). Can also cause thrombocytopenia and abnormal coagulation. Very rare side effects, which can be fatal: liver failure (usually during the first 6 months of treatment) and pancreatitis

(d) Obtain baseline hematologic and liver function studies and then at periodic intervals. Platelet counts and coagulation profile prior to planned surgery

(e) Consider for migraineurs with prolonged or atypical migraine aura.

(f) May be useful as monotherapy in those with migraine and epilepsy or bipolar disease

(2) Topirimate

(a) Start at 25 mg daily (bedtime dosing may be preferable) and increase by 25 mg weekly. Can be given in a single daily dose if not on a hepatic enzyme inducer. If bothersome side effects, wait before increasing dose or decrease dose. Effective dose for migraine may be up to 300 mg; efficacy often at 100 mg daily.

(b) Side effects include somnolence, fatigue, decreased appetite, weight loss, dizziness, paresthesias of hands and feet (persistent paresthesias may improve by taking potassium chloride 20 to 40 mEq per day or vitamin C), psychomotor slowing, and difficulty with speech, language, concentration, and memory (cognitive side effects less at lower doses used for migraine than for epilepsy). Kidney stones, which usually pass without surgery in 1.5% or less. Very rare reports of secondary angle-closure glaucoma occurring during the first month of treatment.

(c) No need for baseline or periodic blood work.

(d) May be useful for patients with migraine who are overweight or who also have epilepsy, bipolar disease, or essential tremor.

(3) Gabapentin

(a) Start at 300 mg given three times daily. May increase up to 2400 mg daily in three divided doses.

(b) Side effects include somnolence, dizziness, asthenia, and ataxia.

(c) No need for baseline or periodic blood work.

(d) May be useful for those with migraine and essential tremor or epilepsy.

f. Other preventatives

(1) Verapamil

(a) Start at 120 to 240 mg per day in three divided doses or once daily with the extended-release preparation, going up to 240 mg daily.

(b) Contraindications: severe left ventricular dysfunction, hypotension, sick sinus syndrome, or second- or third-degree atrioventricular block, atrial flutter or fibrillation with an accessory bypass tract. Combination use with beta-blockers may produce excessive bradycardia and atrioventricular block.

(c) Side effects include constipation, hypotension, atrioventricular block, edema, headache, and nausea.

(d) Efficacy for migraine prevention is poorly established. Flunarizine, a calcium channel blocker not available in the United States, has well-demonstrated efficacy. Consider use as a second-line treatment or in migraineurs with coexistent stroke, prolonged or atypical migraine aura, or basilar migraine.

(2) NSAIDs such as naproxen 500 mg per day and ketoprofen 150 mg per day may be modestly effective.

(3) Methysergide

(a) Highly effective but use restricted to refractory severe migraine due to side effects

(b) Start at 1 mg daily and increase, as indicated by 1 mg every third day to a daily dose of 3 to 6 mg in three divided doses.

(c) Contraindications include cardiovascular diseases, severe hypertension, history of thrombophlebitis, peptic ulcers, pregnancy, familial fibrotic disorders, lung diseases, collagenoses, and liver and kidney diseases.

(d) Side effects include nausea and vomiting, diarrhea, leg pain, edema, dizziness, sedation, and lassitude. Use triptans and ergotamine with caution because of additional vasoconstrictor effect of methysergide.

(e) Long-term use may rarely lead to retroperitoneal, heart valve, and pleural fibrosis (1/2500).

(i) Manufacturer's labeling recommends use for 6 months followed by 3 to 4 weeks off the drug before starting again.

(ii) With long-term use, period laboratory testing for fibrotic reactions is recommended.

(4) Magnesium
Daily oral magnesium (e.g., trimagnesium dicitrate 300 mg twice daily) has been reported both as effective and as ineffective.

(5) Riboflavin
400 mg daily may be effective based upon one randomized controlled trial.

(6) Feverfew (the herb *Tanacetum parthenium*) 50 to 82 mg per day may be modestly effective.

(7) Coenzyme Q10 150 mg a day may be effective.

(8) Botulinum toxin injections may be effective.

Key Preventive Treatments

- Antidepressants
- Beta-blockers
- Anticonvulsants

g. Behavioral and physical treatments

(1) Relaxation training (including progressive muscle relaxation, autogenic training, and meditation or passive relaxation), thermal biofeedback combined with relaxation training, electromyographic biofeedback, and cognitive-behavioral therapy are all somewhat effective in preventing migraine.

(2) Acupuncture might be effective but further study is needed.

Bibliography

Evans RW, Mathew NT: Handbook of Headache. Philadelphia, Lippincott Williams & Wilkins, 2000.

Goadsby PJ, Lipton RB, Ferrari MD: Drug therapy: Migraine—current understanding and treatment. N Engl J Med 346:257–270, 2002.

Olesen J, Tfelt-Hansen P, Welch KMA: The Headaches, 2nd ed. Philadelphia, Lippincott Williams & Wilkins, 2000.

Silberstein SD, Lipton RB, Dalessio DJ: Wolff's Headache and Other Head Pain, 7th ed. New York, Oxford University Press, 2001.

US Headache Consortium: Evidence-based guidelines for migraine headache. *www.aan.com*, 2000.

2 Tension-type, Chronic Daily Headache, and Drug-induced Headache

Randolph W. Evans

TENSION-TYPE HEADACHE

Epidemiology and Risk Factors

1. The one year prevalence has been variably reported from 30% to 90%.
2. The lifetime prevalence is 78%, 63% men and 86% women.
3. Male to female ratio about 1:1.3
4. Prevalence peaks in the fourth decade.

Etiology and Pathophysiology

1. Multifactorial and poorly understood
2. Can arise from sustained contraction of pericranial muscles (muscle contraction headache)
   a. There is no correlation between muscle contraction, tenderness, and the presence of headache.
   b. There may be as much or more muscle contraction in those with migraine as in those with tension-type headache.
3. May be referred from upper cervical structures (joints, ligaments, and muscles)
4. May be due to abnormal neuronal sensitivity and pain facilitation
   a. Prolonged pain input from the periphery may cause central sensitization in the trigeminal nucleus caudalis neurons.
5. May be triggered by physical or psychological stress, lack of sleep, anxiety, and depression.
6. Tension-type headache in migraineurs may be different than in non-migraineurs.
   a. May respond to triptans in migraineurs.
   b. May have typical migraine triggers.
   c. Light or noise sensitivity more likely to accompany

Clinical Features

1. Episodic tension-type headache
   a. International Headache Society (IHS) Criteria
      (1) At least ten previous headache episodes fulfilling the criteria. Number of days with the headache less than 180/year or 15/month.
      (2) Headache lasting from 30 minutes to 7 days
      (3) At least two of the following pain characteristics:
         (a) Pressing/tightening (non-pulsating quality)
         (b) Mild or moderate severity
         (c) Bilateral location
         (d) No aggravation by walking stairs or similar routine physical activity
      (4) Both of the following:
         (i) No nausea or vomiting (anorexia may occur)
         (ii) Photophobia and phonophobia are absent; one but not the other is present
   b. Character of pain
      (1) Variably described as pressure, soreness, tightness, a band or cap on the head, or weight on the head
      (2) Occasionally pulsating during severe pain episodes
   c. Location
      (1) 90% bilateral
      (2) Can be unilateral in the presence of trigger points or oromandibular dysfunction
2. Chronic tension-type headache
   a. IHS criteria
      (1) Average headache frequency is at least 15 days/month or 180 days/year for 6 months.
      (2) The same pain characteristics as for episodic tension-type headache
      (3) Both of the following:
         (a) No vomiting
         (b) No more than one of the following: nausea, photophobia, or phonophobia
   b. Some patients may have continuous headaches for years.

431

Key Clinical Findings: Tension-Type Headache

- Usually non-throbbing
- 90% bilateral
- Mild-moderate severity
- No nausea or vomiting

Differential Diagnosis

1. Secondary causes of headache should be excluded as appropriate (see Part I, Chapter 6, Headaches)
2. Medication rebound can cause frequent headaches.

Treatment

1. Acute headaches may respond to aspirin, acetaminophen, or combinations with caffeine; nonsteroidal anti-inflammatory drugs (NSAIDs); isometheptene combinations; butalbital combinations; and muscle relaxants.
   a. Overuse may lead to rebound headaches.
   b. Frequent butalbital use can also result in dependency.
2. Frequent headache may require preventive medications.
   a. Tricyclic medications are generally more effective than selective serotonin reuptake inhibitors (SSRIs).
   b. Other migraine preventives (see Part XI, Chapter 1, Migraine) may be helpful, especially when tension-type and migraine are both present.
   c. Tizanidine
      (1) An α_2-adrenergic agonist that inhibits the release and effectiveness of norepinephrine at both central sites (e.g., the locus coeruleus) and the spinal cord. It acts as a central muscle relaxant and has antinociceptive effects.
      (2) The most commonly reported adverse events include dry mouth, drowsiness, and dizziness. Less common side effects include asthenia, hypotension, elevated liver enzymes (reversible on drug discontinuation), nausea, speech difficulties, and dyskinesia.
         (a) Baseline and periodic aminotransferase monitoring is recommended.
      (3) Can start with 2 mg at bedtime and titrate upward to the maximum tolerated dose or a maximum daily dose of 18 mg, divided over three dose intervals per day, depending upon response.
      (4) May be beneficial for chronic tension-type and chronic daily headaches.

Key Treatment: Tension-Type Headache

- Acute headaches: aspirin, acetaminophen, or combinations with caffeine; NSAIDs; isometheptene combinations; butalbital combinations; muscle relaxants
- Frequent headaches may require preventative medications (see text under "Treatment")

CHRONIC DAILY HEADACHE

Definition

1. Headache 15 or more days per month
2. Includes different headache types
   a. Transformed migraine (chronic migraine) with or without medication overuse
      (1) Previous history of intermittent migraine usually by age 20 to 30 years
      (2) In 80%, gradual transformation from episodic to chronic daily headache (CDH), which may be associated with analgesic overuse and psychological factors (depression, anxiety, abnormal personality profile, and home or work stress).
      (3) In 20%, sudden transformation, which may be triggered by head or neck trauma, flulike illness, aseptic meningitis, operations, and medical illnesses.
      (4) Migraine characteristics to a significant degree intermittently or continuously
   b. Chronic tension-type headache with or without medication overuse
   c. Hemicrania continua with or without medication overuse
      (1) Rare entity with constant, unilateral pain of variable intensity
      (2) Painful exacerbations associated with ptosis, lacrimation, and nasal stuffiness
      (3) Responds dramatically to indomethacin
   d. New daily persistent headache with or without medication overuse
      (1) Fairly rapid onset of a daily persistent headache without a prior history of increasingly frequent migraine or tension-type headache
      (2) Probably heterogeneous disorder of uncer-

tain cause. Some cases may be triggered by a viral infection.

Key Types of Chronic Daily Headache

- Transformed migraine
- Chronic tension-type with or without medication overuse
- Hemicrania continua
- New daily persistent headache

Epidemiology

1. In adults, about 3% of men and 5% of women. About 1% of adolescents.
2. More than 50% with chronic tension-type headache and about 35% with transformed migraine
3. 0.5% of the population has chronic severe daily headache.

Differential Diagnosis

1. Rule out secondary causes of headache as appropriate (see Part I, Chapter 6, Headaches).
2. Consider contribution of medication rebound.
3. Occasionally, pseudotumor cerebri can present with headaches without papilledema.

Treatment

1. Taper medications that may be causing rebound (see below).
   a. The headaches may get worse before improving, which may not occur before 3 to 6 weeks.
   b. For outpatients, headaches may lessen with the transitional use of a tapering dose of prednisone (60 mg for 2 days, 40 mg for 2 days, and 20 mg for 2 days) for 6 days or the combination of tizanidine and a long-acting NSAID.
2. Acute medications
   a. Longer-acting NSAID (e.g. naproxen sodium), baclofen, tizanidine, and hydroxyzine 50 mg orally three times a day as needed which are not associated with rebound.
   b. May use acute migraine agents as appropriate but limit to 2 to 3 days per week. Dihydroergotamine has little potential for causing rebound but frequent use of triptans can.
3. Preventive medications
   a. Same as with chronic tension-type headaches (above). Consider use of tricyclics, SSRI, dival-

proex sodium, topiramate, beta-blockers, etc. (see Part XI, Chapter 1, Migraine).
   b. Start at a low dose and gradually increase until the drug is effective or until side effects occur or the ceiling dose for the medication has been reached.
   c. Have the patient keep a headache diary so efficacy can be monitored.
   d. Combination therapy may be helpful in some cases.
   e. The effect of treatment may not be apparent for weeks.
   f. Treatment may not be effective until rebound is eliminated.
4. Inpatient treatment
   a. May be indicated if outpatient therapy fails, for detoxification, or if there is significant medical or psychiatric co-morbidity.
   b. Medication detoxification
      (1) Tapering of narcotics is preferable, but abrupt withdrawal can be done with close supervision. Clonidine patch or 0.1 to 0.3 mg orally two or three times daily may reduce symptoms of opioid withdrawal.
      (2) Abruptly stopping butalbital, a short acting barbiturate, may trigger withdrawal, which can include apprehension, muscle weakness, tremors, dizziness, twitches, seizures, psychosis, and delirium.
         (a) Seizures usually occur on the second or third day of withdrawal but can occur up to the eighth day
         (b) To avoid withdrawal reaction, can taper by one tablet q3-5 days or substitute a long-acting barbiturate, phenobarbital at 30 mg three times daily for the first 2 days and then 30 mg daily for the next 2 days.
   c. Intravenous dihydroergotamine (DHE) regimen (as described in Part XI, Chapter 1, Migraine)
   d. DHE regimen may be combined as appropriate with other medications such as NSAIDs, oral or intravenous corticosteroids, intravenous prochlorperazine, and intravenous valproate sodium (as described in Part XI, Chapter 1, Migraine). One or more of these other treatments can be used in those who can not tolerate DHE or have a contraindication to it.
5. Behavioral therapy and psychological and psychiatric referral, as appropriate, may be beneficial.
6. Physical therapy may be useful if there is a myofascial contribution to the headaches.

7. Trigger point injections, occipital nerve blocks, and botulinum toxin injections may be effective in some cases.

8. Patient education

Key Treatment: Chronic Daily Headache

General

• Taper medications that may cause rebound

Medications for Acute Headache

• Nonrebound medications such as longer-acting NSAID (e.g. naproxen sodium), baclofen, tizanidine, and hydroxyzine

• Migraine agents can be used 2 to 3 three times a week

Preventative Medications

• Tricyclics, SSRI, divalproex, topirimate, beta-blockers

Inpatient Treatment

• May be indicated if outpatient therapy fails; for detoxification; or if there is significant medical or psychiatric co-morbidity

Other

• Behavioral therapy and psychologic and psychiatric referral as appropriate

• Trigger point injections, occipital nerve blocks, and botulinum toxin injections may be effective in some cases.

• Patient education

Prognosis

1. Even with optimal therapy, about one third of those who improve will have return of their daily headache and medication overuse pattern.

2. Regular follow-up is important.

3. There is a minority of patients with intractable CDH resistant to current treatments.

DRUG-INDUCED HEADACHE

Acute Drug-Induced Headache

1. Many drugs can cause this condition, including
   a. Nitroglycerin, antihypertensives (beta-blockers, calcium channel blockers, angiotensin converting enzyme inhibitors, and methyldopa), dipyridamole, hydralazine, sildenafil
   b. Histamine receptor antagonists (such as cimetidine and ranitidine)

c. NSAIDs, especially indomethacin
   d. Cyclosporine, amphotericin, griseofulvin, tetracycline, and sulfonamides

Drug-Induced Aseptic Meningitis

1. Numerous causes
   a. NSAIDs
   b. Antibiotics (trimethoprim/sulfamethoxazole, sulfasalazine, cephalosporins, ciprofloxacin, isoniazid, and penicillin)
   c. Intrathecal drugs and diagnostics (antineoplastics such as methotrexate and cytarabine; gentamicin; corticosteroids; spinal anesthesia; baclofen; repeated iophendylate for myelography; and radiolabeled albumin)
   d. Intraventricular chemotherapy
   e. Intravenous immunoglobulin
   f. Vaccines (polio; measles, mumps, and rubella; and hepatitis B)
   g. Other drugs such as carbamazepine, muromonab CD-3, and ranitidine

2. Clinical presentation is the same as that of viral meningitis.

3. Cerebrospinal fluid (CSF) findings are similar to viral meningitis except for neutrophil predominance in most cases. Intravenous immunoglobulin is an exception, with eosinophils in the CSF.

4. The prognosis is generally good with discontinuation of the causative agent.

Key Types of Drug-Induced Headache

• Acute drug-induced

• Drug-induced aseptic meningitis

• Medication rebound

Chronic Drug-Induced Headache

1. Definition

   a. Also called analgesic, drug, medication abuse, medication misuse, or rebound headache

   b. Rebound headache

   (1) Frequent use of some immediate-relief medications can result in recurring or persistent headache in those with preexisting headache and an individual susceptibility.

   (2) The actual dose limits and time needed to develop rebound headaches have not been defined in rigorous studies.

(3) The best evidence is from a study of short-term caffeine withdrawal.

    (a) Adults with a low-moderate daily caffeine intake of an equivalent of about 2.5 cups of coffee (mean of 235 mg) per day

    (b) Upon withdrawal of caffeine, 50% had a headache by day 2

    (c) Nausea, depression, and flulike symptoms are common with withdrawal

(4) In patients with frequent headaches, routinely obtain a history of caffeine use in over-the-counter and prescription medications as well as beverages and ice cream. Some examples:

    (a) 12 ounces of Coca-Cola contains 45 mg

    (b) 8 ounces of brewed coffee contains 135 mg

    (c) A Fiorinal tablet contains 40 mg, and 2 Excedrin Migraine tablets contain 130 mg

(5) Overuse is related to the frequency of use and total consumption such as the following:

    (a) Three or more simple analgesics (aspirin and/or acetaminophen) a day (more than 1000 mg) more often than 5 days a week. Frequent use of short-acting NSAIDs such as ibuprofen can also be a cause.

    (b) Combination analgesics containing barbiturates (more than 3 tablets per day) or benzodiazepines more often than three times a week

    (c) Narcotics (more than one tablet per day) or ergotamine (1 mg orally or 0.5 mg rectally) more often than twice a week

    (d) Triptans may also induce rebound.

2. Epidemiology and risk factors

  a. Prevalence perhaps 1% of migraineurs and 0.5% of those with chronic tension-type headache

  b. Persons with migraine and tension-type headache are especially susceptible to drug-induced headache.

  c. Most patients with chronic headache overuse symptomatic medications.

3. Pathophysiology

  a. Not known

  b. Some hypotheses:

    (1) Central sensitization

    (2) Peripheral sensitization with alternation of nerve terminal sensitivity

    (3) Increased activity of the on-cells in the brainstem's pain-modulation system

    (4) Kindling

    (5) Depletion of 5-HT and upregulation of its postsynaptic receptors

4. Clinical features

  a. The headaches are refractory, daily, or near daily.

  b. The headaches occur in those with a primary headache disorder who use immediate-relief medications frequently, often in excessive quantities.

  c. The headache can vary in severity, type, and location.

  d. The threshold for headache is low.

  e. Headaches may be accompanied by asthenia, nausea, restlessness, anxiety, irritability, memory problems, difficulty with concentration, and depression.

  f. A drug-dependent rhythmicity may be present with frequent early morning headaches (e.g., 2 A.M. to 5 A.M.)

  g. Tolerance may develop over time, so that increasing doses are taken.

  h. Habituation and dependence (the psychological and physical need to repeatedly use drugs) may develop especially with butalbital, opiates, and caffeine. Beware of the warning behaviors of substance abuse and misuse (I)

    (1) Unauthorized dose escalations

    (2) Frequent phone calls, especially on weekends and after hours, for more medication

    (3) Doctor shopping or obtaining medications from multiple physicians and emergency rooms

    (4) Reporting medications as lost, ruined, stolen, or left behind when out of town (e.g., stolen purses and ingestion by household pets)

    (5) Frequent office visits for medications

    (6) Resistance or unwillingness to reduce medications or use alternative symptomatic and preventative medications (e.g., "This is the only drug that works," or "I am allergic or experience side effects with those other drugs.")

    (7) Refusal to sign release to obtain information from other physicians or failure to disclose the names of prior or current physicians

i. Withdrawal symptoms occur when the medications are abruptly stopped.

j. Spontaneous improvement of headache occurs on discontinuing the medications.

k. Preventive headache medications may not be effective until the symptomatic medications are tapered off.

5. Treatment (see above under CDH)

6. Prognosis and complications

a. Withdrawal therapy can result in a 50% or greater improvement in headache frequency in about 70%.

b. The relapse rate is about 40%.

c. Frequent drug use can lead to a variety of complications including peptic ulcer disease (with NSAIDs and aspirin) and analgesic nephropathy, and hepatic failure.

7. Prevention

a. Try to limit symptomatic medication use that can cause headaches to 10 events or 24 tablets or capsules per month and limit use to 2 days/week. Individual susceptibility to rebound is variable.

b. Limit or avoid caffeine ingestion in those susceptible to caffeine withdrawal headaches.

Bibliography

Evans RW, Mathew NT: Handbook of Headache. Philadelphia, Lippincott Williams & Wilkins, 2000.

Olesen J, Tfelt-Hansen P, Welch KMA: The Headaches, 2nd ed. Philadelphia, Lippincott Williams & Wilkins, 2000.

Silberstein SD, Lipton RB, Dalessio DJ: Wolff's Headache and Other Head Pain, 7th ed. New York, Oxford University Press, 2001.

Silberstein SD, Liu D: Drug overuse and rebound headache. Curr Pain Headache Rep 2000. 6:240–247, 2002.

Silberstein SD, Welch KM: Painkiller headache. Neurology. 59:972–974, 2002.

3 Cluster Headache

Randolph W. Evans

Epidemiology and Risk Factors

1. About 0.4% of the general population

2. Male:female ratio of 5:1

3. Can occur at any age including childhood and adolescence (rare before the age of 10) but usually begins in the third or fourth decade of life

4. 90% have episodic cluster and 10% chronic (cluster period lasts for more than 1 year without remission, or remission lasts less than 14 days).

Etiology and Pathophysiology

1. Incompletely understood

2. Genetic factors in some cases

   a. Positive family history in 7%.

   b. First-degree relatives have a 14-fold increased risk of cluster headache.

3. Activation of the trigeminovascular system as in migraine may explain the pain.

4. Autonomic features due to activation of the cranial parasympathetic fibers

   a. Fibers originate from first-order neurons within the superior salivatory nucleus which has a functional brainstem connection to the trigeminal nucleus caudalis

   b. These fibers travel with the seventh cranial nerve and synapse in the pterygopalatine ganglia.

   c. Postganglionic fibers provide vasomotor and secretomotor innervation to the cerebral blood vessels and the lacrimal and nasal mucosal glands, respectively.

5. A postganglionic Horner's syndrome during attacks is indicative of involvement of the carotid sympathetic plexus. The cavernous carotid artery, where the parasympathetic, sympathetic, and trigeminal fibers converge, is a likely location.

6. The circadian, circannual, and seasonal rhythmicity of cluster suggests a periodic disturbance of the suprachiasmatic nucleus of the hypothalamus. Hypothalamic abnormalities have been demonstrated in positron emission tomography scan and morphometric magnetic resonance imaging studies

Clinical Features

1. Periodicity

   a. Individual cluster attacks occur during attack phases or cluster periods.

   b. Most patients have one to two annual cluster periods with each lasting between 1 and 3 months.

   c. Some patients have a seasonal propensity.

   d. Remission usually lasts between 6 months and 2 years.

   e. Circadian periodicity

      (1) Usually one to two attacks per day although some patients will have up to eight attacks per day

      (2) In individuals, the attacks usually occur at the same time each day.

         (a) The most common times of onset are 1–2 A.M., 1–3 P.M., and 9 P.M.

         (b) The nocturnal attacks may correlate with the onset of the first period of rapid eye movement sleep.

2. Symptoms and signs

   a. Unilateral severe pain with the most common sites, in order of decreasing frequency, retroorbital, temporal, and infraorbital. But can occur in other locations including the neck.

      (1) The headache may alternate sides between cluster periods or, rarely, within the same period.

      (2) Pain is described as constant, boring, pressing, burning, or stabbing, and about 30% describe throbbing or pulsating.

   b. There is a rapid onset of 5 to 15 minutes and usually short duration of 30 to 45 minutes, although a minority may have pain persisting up to 3 hours (and rarely longer).

   c. During attacks, most patients prefer to walk, sit, kneel, stand, or jog in place. Many find it difficult to lie down and feel restless and agitated.

   d. Autonomic symptoms are present in over 97%.

      (1) Lacrimation and conjunctival injection are each present in 80%.

      (2) Ipsilateral congestion or clear drainage of the nares is present in 75%.

(3) A partial Horner's syndrome with a slight ipsilateral ptosis or miosis or a combination of both is present in about 65% of cases and may persist between attacks in later stages of the disorder in some patients.

(4) Increased forehead sweating may occur in a minority of patients during attacks.

(5) Erythema of the eyelid or a circumscribed area of the face or forehead may be present.

e. Nausea, light sensitivity, and noise sensitivity present in some patients. Occasionally, a visual aura may precede the headache.

3. Precipitating factors

a. Small quantities of alcohol can trigger attacks during cluster periods but not during remission.

b. Nitroglycerin and histamine can trigger attacks during cluster periods.

Key Clinical Findings

• Periodicity

• Unilateral severe pain

• Duration usually 30 to 45 minutes but may last up to 3 hours

• Ipsilateral lacrimation and conjunctival injection in 80%

• Ipsilateral congestion or clear nares drainage in 75%

• Partial Horner's syndrome during headache in 65%

Differential Diagnosis

1. Symptomatic or secondary cluster headache

a. Can be due to head trauma or iatrogenic trauma (orbital enucleation and dental extraction)

b. A variety of pathologies have been associated with cluster-like headaches which are usually atypical because of the lack of periodicity, lack of response to medications, or the presence of abnormal neurologic signs. Include arteriovenous malformations, aneurysms, sphenoid sinusitis, parasellar tumors, upper cervical cord meningioma and infarction, subdural hematoma, cerebral metastases, and temporal arteritis.

2. Cluster headaches can usually be diagnosed based upon the clinical criteria without the need for neuroimaging

3. Neuroimaging, preferably MRI, may be considered for patients with the following:

a. A pattern of clusterlike headache that does not conform to the clinical criteria

b. Onset of cluster headache after age 40

c. A progressive pattern of headaches

d. Chronic cluster headache

e. Any focal neurologic deficit other than Horner's syndrome

Indications for Neuroimaging

• Clusterlike headache that does not conform to the clinical criteria

• Onset of cluster headache after age 40

• Progressive pattern of headaches

• Chronic cluster headache

• Any focal neurologic deficit other than Horner's syndrome

4. Cluster-migraine and cluster-tic

a. Migraine can occur with cluster features such as recurring cluster periods and diurnal periodicity and shorter duration than migraine but without autonomic features or Horner's syndrome associated with cluster.

b. Cluster-tic

(1) Cluster and trigeminal neuralgia may be present at the same time in a patient.

(2) Some patients may have three types of pain attacks: trigeminal neuralgia-like, cluster-like, and neuralgic pain immediately followed by a cluster-like headache.

5. Chronic paroxysmal hemicrania and short-lasting unilateral neuralgiform headache with conjunctival injection and tearing (SUNCT) (see Part XI, Chapter 4, Brief Head and Facial Pains)

Treatment

1. Acute (see Part XI, Chapter 1, Migraine, for side effects and contraindications)

a. Inhalation of 100% oxygen at a rate of 7 to 10 liters/minute for 15 to 20 minutes with a loosely applied face mask is effective in about 70%. Oxygen has a cerebral vasoconstrictive effect and reduces calcitonin gene-related peptide release during attacks.

b. Sumatriptan 6 mg subcutaneously

(1) Effective in 90% of patients for 90% of their attacks

(2) Efficacy within 15 minutes in up to 75%

(3) There is no tachyphylaxis or rebound effect.

(4) Intranasal sumatriptan or oral triptans are less efficacious.

c. Intravenous dihydroergotamine (DHE) 1 mg may provide relief in less than 10 minutes. With intramuscular and intranasal administration, the same dose takes longer to work.

> **WARNING**
>
> Triptans and DHE should not be used within 24 hours of each other.

d. Topical 4% lidocaine administered as nose drops may be effective

(1) Patients lie supine with the head tilted toward the floor at 30 degrees and turned to the side of the headache.

(2) A nasal dropper may be used and the dose (1 mL of 4% lidocaine) may be repeated once after 15 minutes.

e. Butorphanol nasal spray might be tried if other treatments are not effective or are contraindicated. There is a significant potential for habituation and addiction.

Key Treatment: Acute Cases

- Inhalation of 100% oxygen
- Triptans
- DHE
- Topical 4% lidocaine given as nose drops
- Butorphanol nasal spray (addiction potential)

2. Transitional treatments

a. Medications that may induce rapid suppression of attacks during the time interval before a preventive becomes effective.

b. Prednisone 60 mg daily for 3 days then 10 mg decrements every 3 days given in the morning to prevent interference with sleep

c. Ergotamine tartrate 1 mg orally twice a day including a bedtime day if nocturnal attacks occur. Contraindicated in peripheral and cardiovascular disease. Ergotamine and triptans should not be used within 24 hours of each other.

d. DHE 0.5 to 1.0 mg subcutaneously or intramuscularly every 8 to 12 hours

e. A greater occipital nerve block on the side

ipsilateral to the attacks with corticosteroid (120 mg of methylprednisolone or 40 mg of triamcinolone) and 3 ml. of 1% lidocaine may produce a temporary remission.

3. Preventive medications (see Part XI, Chapter 1, Migraine, for information on side effects and contraindications)

a. Verapamil is the drug of choice for episodic and chronic types.

(1) Total daily dose starting at 120 to 240 mg in three divided doses, slowly increasing up to 480 mg. Doses up to 1200 mg per day have been used in chronic cluster headache.

(2) Baseline and serial electrocardiograms are indicated to monitor for the development of heart block when using a dose of 240 mg per day or higher.

b. Methysergide for younger patients without contraindications for episodic cluster (2 mg three times per day up to 12 mg daily). May be best to avoid combining with ergotamine, DHE, or triptans because of potential for additive vasoconstrictor effect.

c. Divalproex sodium (500 to 2000 mg daily)

d. Lithium carbonate (150 to 300 mg tid)

(1) Used more for chronic than for episodic cluster

(2) Need to closely monitor for side effects

e. Topiramate (50 to 125 mg per day)

f. Baclofen 10 mg three times per day

g. Melatonin 10 mg at bedtime

h. Topical capsaicin 0.025% cream applied via a cotton-tipped applicator 0.5 inch up the nostril ipsilateral to the side of the headache three times daily for 7 days might be effective.

i. For chronic or intractable cases, can use combination therapy.

Key Treatment: Preventive Medications

- Verapamil
- Methysergide
- Divalproex sodium
- Lithium carbonate
- Topiramate
- Baclofen

4. Surgical treatment

a. Indications

(1) Total resistance to medical treatment

(2) Strictly unilateral pain

(3) Stable psychological and personality profiles with low addiction potential.

b. Percutaneous radiofrequency retrogasserian rhizotomy

(1) Good to excellent results in 70%

(2) Loss of facial sensation and corneal reflex required

(3) V1 and V2 lesions adequate for orbital pain

(4) A repeat radiofrequency lesion can be made for recurrence, which occurs in 20% of patients.

(5) Transient complications include hyperacusis, tinnitus, jaw deviation, chewing, and ice-pick pain

(6) Persistent complications include facial anesthesia/hypesthesia, corneal anesthesia, and occasionally anesthesia dolorosa.

b. Gamma knife radiosurgery to lesion the trigeminal nerve root may be an effective treatment.

c. Percutaneous retrogasserian glycerol rhizolysis may also be an effective treatment with much less risk for corneal anesthesia or facial anesthesia compared to radiofrequency surgery. The recurrence rate is about 40%.

Prognosis

1. About 20% of patients with episodic cluster can develop a chronic pattern.
2. About 30% of patients with the chronic type can develop episodic cluster with remission periods.
3. Most patients will develop longer remission periods with increasing age.

 ## Bibliography

Bahra A, May A, Goadsby PJ: Cluster headache: A prospective clinical study with diagnostic implications. Neurology 58:354–361, 2002.

Evans RW, Mathew NT: Handbook of Headache. Philadelphia, Lippincott Williams & Wilkins, 2000.

Olesen J, Tfelt-Hansen P, Welch KMA: The Headaches, 2nd ed. Philadelphia, Lippincott Williams & Wilkins, 2000.

Peres MF, Stiles MA, Siow HC, et al.: Greater occipital nerve blockade for cluster headache. Cephalalgia 22:520–522, 2002.

Silberstein SD, Lipton RB, Dalessio DJ: Wolff's Headache and Other Head Pain, 7th ed. New York, Oxford University Press, 2001.

TRIGEMINAL NEURALGIA

Epidemiology and Risk Factors

1. About 15,000 new cases per year in the United States
2. 90% of cases begin after the age of 40
3. 3:2 female:male prevalence

Etiology and Pathophysiology

1. About 80% due to vascular compression of the trigeminal nerve at the root entry zone, most commonly by a branch of the superior cerebellar artery
   a. May result in focal demyelination, which leads to increased firing rates in trigeminal primary afferents (antidromic discharges) and impairment of segmental inhibition in the trigeminal nucleus
   b. Produces a hyperactive sensory circuit with painful paroxysmal bursts of activity in the wide dynamic range neurons of the nucleus caudalis
   c. Hypersensitivity of low-threshhold mechanoreceptors in the trigeminal nucleus oralis may also occur, leading to rapid firing rates typically associated with noxious stimuli but now occurring in response to non-noxious stimuli or sensory triggers.
2. A multiple sclerosis plaque in about 4% of cases. Especially consider as the cause in new onset under the age of 40 years.
3. Perhaps 5% are due to tumors: trigeminal schwannomas, meningiomas, lymphomas, lipomas, epidermoid tumors, acoustic schwannomas, metastases, tumors of the skull base, and pituitary tumor with cavernous sinus invasion.
4. Other causes include basilar artery aneurysm, venous compression, synringobulbia, brainstem infarction, chronic oral or dental disease, and sinusitis.

Clinical Features

1. Severe sharp, shooting, or electric shock-like sensation lasting seconds to 2 minutes

2. Usually in unilateral maxillary and mandibular trigeminal distributions either in one or both. Uncommonly in the ophthalmic division.
3. 4% of cases are bilateral with asynchonous pain usually due to multiple sclerosis.
4. In about 90% of cases, trigger zones are present.
   a. Non-painful stimuli usually in the central part of the face around the nose and lips trigger pain.
   b. Stimuli can include talking, chewing, washing the face, brushing the teeth, shaving, facial movement, and cold air.
   c. After a paroxysm of pain, there is a refractory period lasting up to several minutes where stimulation of the trigger zone will not trigger pain.
5. Facial grimacing or spasm may accompany the pain (tic douloureux)
6. Between painful paroxyms, the patient is usually pain-free, although dull aching may persist for a few minutes after attacks of long duration or multiple clustered attacks.
7. Multiple attacks may occur for weeks or months.
8. About 50% will have spontaneous remissions for at least 6 months.
9. Physical examination is usually normal except for trigger zones. Up to 25% of patients will have sensory loss.
10. Pretrigeminal neuralgia—a rare disorder
    a. A dull continuous toothache in the upper or lower jaw which evolves into typical trigeminal neuralgia after a period of months to years.
    b. A diagnosis of exclusion
    c. May respond to medical treatments used for trigeminal neuralgia

Key Clinical Features: Trigeminal Neuralgia

- Paroxysmal attacks of severe facial pain
- Attacks occur usually in a maxillary and/or mandibular trigeminal distribution.
- Attacks last seconds to 2 minutes.
- Trigger zones are usually present.

Radiologic Features

1. Magnetic resonance imaging preferred
2. Helps to exclude multiple sclerosis and neoplasms as the cause
   a. Present in about 9% of cases
   b. Often present in those with atypical features (sensory loss, constant ache), less than 40 years of age, and with pain in more than one trigeminal division.
3. Magnetic resonance angiography may demonstrate microvascular compression.

Treatment

1. Medications
   a. General principles
      (1) Start with a low dose and slowly increase depending upon efficacy and side effects.
      (2) Monotherapy preferable but polypharmacy may be necessary (e.g., carbamazepine and baclofen)
         (a) Medications may become less effective over time; e.g., carbamazepine provides pain relief in up to 80% initially and in the short term but decreases to 56% in the long term
      (3) If the patient is pain free for 6 to 8 weeks, can try tapering the medication and assess whether a remission is present.
   b. Options (usual maintenance total daily dose range in parentheses)
      (1) Carbamazepine (400–800 mg in two or three divided doses)
      (2) Oxcarbazepine (600–1800 mg in two divided doses)
      (3) Baclofen (40–80 mg in three to six divided doses)
      (4) Phenytoin (300–500 mg in a single dose or in three divided doses)
      (5) Clonazepam (1.5–8 mg in three divided doses)
      (6) Divalproex sodium (500–1500 mg in two divided doses)
      (7) Topiramate (25–400 mg in a single dose or two divided doses)
      (8) Lamotrigine (150–400 mg in two divided doses)
      (9) Gabapentin (900–2400 mg in three divided doses)
      (10) Pimozide (4–12 mg in a single dose or two divided doses)

Key Treatment: Medications

- Carbamazepine
- Oxcarbazepine
- Baclofen
- Phenytoin
- Clonazepam
- Divalproex sodium
- Topiramate
- Lamotrigine
- Gabapentin
- Pimozide

2. Surgical options
   a. About 30% of patients fail medical therapy
   b. Extracranial peripheral denervation of trigeminal branches
      (1) Useful for the elderly with a short life expectancy or for those who are medically unfit for a more invasive procedure
      (2) Lidocaine relieves pain for hours to days, alcohol for 6 to 18 months, freezing for 4 to 14 months, and neurectomy for 20 to 30 months.
   c. Radiofrequency thermocoagulation of the gasserian ganglion
      (1) Greater than 90% initial effectiveness with about a 15% 2-year recurrence rate
      (2) Side effects include dysesthesias in up to 25% (corneal anesthesia in 20% if ophthalmic division is involved).
   d. Glycerol trigeminal rhizotomy
      (1) Injection of glycerol into the gasserian ganglion. General anesthesia is not needed.
      (2) Effective in up to 90%, but a 50% recurrence by 2 years
      (3) Mild sensory loss is common.
   e. Percutaneous balloon compression of the gasserian ganglion
      (1) Effective in over 80% with a 28% recurrence rate
      (2) Risk of intracranial hemorrhage and autonomic dysfunction
   f. Microvascular decompression
      (1) Suboccipital retromastoid craniectomy for vascular decompression of the trigeminal nerve at the root entry zone
      (2) Vascular loops: 85% arterial, usually from

the superior cerebellar artery, and 15% venous

   (3) 80% have complete pain relief and about 8% partial relief; at 10 years, 70% have pain relief and 4% partial relief.

   (4) Risks include death (0 to 1%), intracranial hemorrhage or stroke (1% to 2%), permanent hearing loss in up to 5%, and mild sensory loss in about 10%.

g. Gamma knife radiosurgery

   (1) Radiation (70–80 Gy) delivered to the trigeminal nerve root entry zone

   (2) About 80% pain free after a mean follow-up of 16 months

   (3) Time to initial relief varies from 1 to 120 days with a mean of 14 days

   (4) Long-term follow-up is not available, and there is uncertainty concerning the possibility of delayed radiation complications.

GLOSSOPHARYNGEAL NEURALGIA

Epidemiology

1. Rare disorder. Perhaps 1500 new cases per year in the United States.
2. Glossopharyngeal neuralgia is present along with trigeminal neuralgia in about 10% of cases.

Etiology

1. Usually due to microvascular compression.
2. Uncommon causes include oropharyngeal malignancy, peritonsillar infection, and multiple sclerosis.

Clinical Features

1. Paroxysms of severe stabbing or burning unilateral pain lasting a few seconds to less than 2 minutes.
2. Distribution within the posterior part of the tongue, tonsillar fossa, pharynx, or beneath the angle of the lower jaw, or in the ear
3. Pain may be triggered by swallowing (especially cold liquids), talking, coughing, yawning, or sneezing.
4. Occasionally a trigger zone is present within the pre-auricular or post-auricular area, the neck, or the external auditory canal.
5. Up to 2% of patients can lose consciousness during paroxysms do to bradycardia or asystole.
6. Neurologic examination is normal.
7. Remissions may occur.

Treatment

1. May respond to the medications used in trigeminal neuralgia (see above)
2. Surgical options
   a. Intracranial sectioning of the glossopharyngeal nerve and the upper rootlets of the vagus nerve.
   b. Microvascular decompression of the glossopharyngeal nerve is also effective.

ICEPICK HEADACHE OR IDIOPATHIC STABBING HEADACHE

1. Sharp stabbing pain anywhere in the head occurring either as single episodes lasting from a fraction of a second to 1 to 2 seconds or as brief repeated volleys of pain.
2. Usually unilateral but may be bilateral.
3. Usually occur around the orbit or the temple and less frequently in the occipital and parietal areas. Attacks usually recur in the same area. Icepick pain occurring in the eye has also been termed *ophthalmodynia periodica*.
4. There are no associated symptoms or signs.
5. Frequency may vary from one attack in a year to 50 attacks per day.
6. Etiology not known. Perhaps due to spontaneous discharges of trigeminal afferent fibers.
7. Occurs in about 40% of migraineurs and about 2% of adults. May also occur in patients with cluster headaches and rarely in temporal arteritis. Can occur at any age including childhood.
8. Often, reassurance is the only treatment. For frequent attacks, can try indomethacin 25 to 50 mg three times a day.

COLD STIMULUS HEADACHE (ICE CREAM HEADACHE OR BRAIN FREEZE)

1. Holding ice or ice cream or frozen yogurt in the mouth or swallowing a cold food or drink as a bolus may cause moderate-severe pain in the palate and throat or less often referred to the forehead, temple, or ears. Usually bilateral but may be unilateral pain. Lasts less than 5 minutes, usually less than one minute.
2. Common in the general population.
3. Probably due to a direct effect of cold receptors in the oropharynx.

OCCIPITAL NEURALGIA

1. Common disorder. Pain may be in the distribution of the lesser or greater occipital nerve and referred

anteriorly to the fronto-temporal area or retro-orbital with greater occipital neuralgia.

2. Occasionally brief paroxyms of stabbing pain but more often longer duration aching or throbbing. Can be unilateral or bilateral.

3. Can occur without any apparent reason in any age group or posttraumatically (see Part XIII, Chapter 7, Whiplash Injuries for more information including treatment).

NECK-TONGUE SYNDROME

1. Uncommon disorder characterized by acute unilateral occipital pain and numbness of the ipsilateral tongue precipitated by sudden movement, usually rotation of the head.

2. Can occur without any obvious abnormalities or be associated with degenerative spondylosis, ankylosing spondylitis, psoriatic arthritis, and genetically determined laxity of ligaments of joint capsules.

3. Due to transient subluxation of the atlantoaxial joint that stretches the joint capsule and the C2 ventral ramus (which contains proprioceptive fibers from the tongue originating from the lingual nerve to the hypoglossal nerve to the C2 root).

EAGLE'S SYNDROME

1. An uncommon disorder due to an elongated styloid process alone or the combined lengths of the process and stylohyoid or stylomandibular ligaments exceed 40 mm.

2. Symptoms include dysphagia and unilateral pharyngeal aching radiating to the ear worse with swallowing. Pain may be intermittent or continuous.

3. Digital palpation of an elongated styloid process can precipitate or increase pain.

4. May respond to transpharyngeal injection of steroid and local anesthetic or surgical excision.

EXPLODING HEAD SYNDROME

1. A sensation of a loud bang in the head like an explosion can awaken people from sleep.

2. Ten percent of cases are associated with the sensation of a flash of light.

3. Etiology is not known.

SHORT-LASTING UNILATERAL NEURALGIFORM HEADACHE WITH CONJUNCTIVAL INJECTION AND TEARING (SUNCT SYNDROME)

1. Extremely rare

2. Attacks of unilateral moderately severe orbital or temporal stabbing or throbbing pain lasting 5 to 250 seconds typically associated with ipsilateral conjunctival injection and lacrimation.

3. Attack frequency is 3 to 100 per day. Trigger zones may be present.

4. Usually idiopathic. Rarely due to posterior fossa vascular malformations.

5. Usually resistant to therapy. Might respond to carbamazepine, topiramate, gabapentin, lamotrigine or retrogasserian glycerol rhizolysis.

PAROXYSMAL HEMICRANIAS

1. Chronic paroxysmal hemicrania (CPH)
   a. Uncommon. 2:1 female predominance. Age of onset from 3 to 81 years with a mean of 33 years.
   b. Almost always unilateral throbbing, boring, pulsatile, or stabbing pain of moderate-severe intensity. Attacks can occur while awake or awaken from sleep.
   c. Maximal pain usually in the ocular, temporal, maxilllary, and frontal regions.
   d. During attacks, one or more ipsilateral autonomic symptom is usually present: lacrimation, ptosis, conjunctival injection, nasal congestion, and rhinorrhea.
   e. Attacks occur one to 40 times per day, lasting 2 to 120 minutes.
   f. About 10% of patients can trigger attacks by bending or rotating their head.
   g. Secondary causes include intracranial neoplasms and vascular abnormalities, collagen vascular disease, and Pancoast's tumor.
   h. Always responds to indomethacin 25 to 50 mg three times a day. May also respond to aspirin, verapamil, steroids, naproxen, and acetazolamide.

Key Clinical Findings: CPH

- Almost always unilateral

- Can occur while awake or awaken from sleep

- One or more ipsilateral autonomic symptoms are usually present during attacks.

- Attacks occur 1 to 40 times per day, lasting 2 to 120 minutes
- Always responds to indomethacin

2. Episodic paroxysmal hemicrania
   a. Rare. No gender preference
   b. Same headache and associated autonomic symptoms as CPH.
   c. Daily attack frequency from 2 to 30 with attacks lasting 3 to 30 minutes each.
   d. Unlike CPH which has no remissions, remissions range from 1 to 36 months. The headache phase lasts 2 weeks to 4.5 months.
   e. Always responds to indomethacin
3. Paroxysmal hemicranias versus cluster headache
   a. Similar location, pain, and associated autonomic symptoms
   b. Compared to cluster headache, paroxysmal hemicranias are generally shorter lasting, more frequent, and respond absolutely to indomethacin.

Bibliography

Evans RW, Mathew NT: Handbook of Headache. Philadelphia, Lippincott Williams & Wilkins, 2000.

Evans RW, Pearce JM: Exploding head syndrome. Headache 41:602–603, 2001.

Olesen J, Tfelt-Hansen P, Welch KMA: The Headaches, 2nd ed. Philadelphia, Lippincott Williams & Wilkins, 2000.

Pareja JA, Antonaci F, Vincent M: The hemicrania continua diagnosis. Cephalalgia 21:940–946, 2001.

Silberstein SD, Lipton RB, Dalessio DJ: Wolff's Headache and Other Head Pain, 7th ed. New York, Oxford University Press, 2001.

5 First or Worst Headaches

Randolph W. Evans

Definition

A new type of headache that may be a first primary headache (e.g. migraine or cluster) or worst headache including those with sudden onset can be of primary or secondary origin.

Epidemiology

In the emergency department: 1% of patients have the chief complaint of acute headache and about 20% of those with the worst headache of their life have a subarachnoid hemorrhage.

Differential Diagnosis

1. Table 5–1 lists possible causes.
2. Meningitis, encephalitis, sinusitis, periorbital cellulitis, cerebral venous thrombosis, optic neuritis, migraine, ischemic cerebrovascular disease, and cerebral vasculitis usually have a subacute onset but may have a sudden onset.
3. An acute severe headache associated with neck rigidity raises concern about subarachnoid hemorrhage, meningitis, and systemic infections.

> PEARLS
>
> Many first or worst headaches are due to migraine.
>
> Beware: migraine is a diagnosis of exclusion.
>
> Many secondary headaches mimic migraine.

SUBARACHNOID HEMORRHAGE (SAH)

(also see Part III, Chapter 5, Subarachnoid Hemorrhage and Saccular Aneurysm)

Epidemiology

1. About 32,500 cases of nontraumatic SAH occur each year in the United States.
2. 80% are due to ruptured intracranial aneurysms, resulting in 18,000 deaths; 5% are due to a rupture of an intracranial arteriovenous malformation (AVM).
3. The prevalence of intracranial saccular aneurysms is about 2%, with 93% of aneurysms ≤10 mm. The mean age of rupture of aneurysms is around 50 years.

Clinical Features

1. Headache is present in 90% of those with SAH.
2. The classic headache is sudden, severe, and continuous, often with nausea, vomiting, meningismus, focal neurologic findings, and loss of consciousness. Typically described as "worst headache of my life."
3. 12% report a feeling of a "burst."
4. Mild gradually increasing headache in 8%; sudden severe headache in 92%.
5. Headache can be present in any location, unilateral or bilateral.
6. Presentations: 33% headache only; 75% headache, nausea, and vomiting; 66% sudden severe headache with loss of consciousness or focal deficits; 50% with none or minimal headache and slight nuchal rigidity or moderate to severe headache with no neurologic deficit or a cranial nerve deficit.; and 50% similar to meningitis: headache, stiff neck, nausea and vomiting, photophobia, and low-grade fever.
7. Stiff neck present in 75% during the first 24 hours.
8. Transient loss of consciousness in up to 33%.
9. A sentinel headache (retrospective diagnosis of a minor leak) or warning leak occurs in 50% patients before a major rupture of a saccular aneurysm.
   a. Accurate diagnosis can be lifesaving.
      (1) Major SAH has a morbidity and mortality of 30% to 70% and occurs in 30% to 50% of patients in the days or weeks after the sentinel headache.
      (2) 50% of major SAHs occur within 1 week of the sentinel headache.
   b. About 50% of those with sentinel headache do not seek medical attention. Sentinel headaches are commonly misdiagnosed by physicians as migraine, sinusitis, hypertension, and flu. Beware of new-onset "migraine."
   c. Usually sudden onset. Duration usually 1 to 2 days but can last several minutes to several hours to 2 weeks.

TABLE 5–1. DIFFERENTIAL DIAGNOSIS OF THE ACUTE SEVERE NEW ONSET HEADACHE—"FIRST OR WORST"

Primary headache disorders
  Migraine
  Cluster
  Benign exertional or cough headache
  Benign orgasmic cephalgia
Posttraumatic
Associated with vascular disorders
  Acute ischemic cerebrovascular disease
  Subdural and epidural hematomas
  Parenchymal hemorrhage
  Unruptured saccular aneurysm
  Subarachnoid hemorrhage
  Systemic lupus erythematosus
  Temporal arteritis
  Internal carotid and vertebral artery dissection
  Cerebral venous thrombosis
  Acute hypertension
  Pressor response
  Pheochromocytoma
  Pre-eclampsia
Associated with nonvascular intracranial disorders
  Intermittent hydrocephalus
  Pseudotumor cerebri
  Post–lumbar puncture
  Related to intrathecal injections
  Intracranial neoplasm
  Pituitary apoplexy
Acute intoxications
Associated with noncephalic infection
  Acute febrile illness
  Acute pyelonephritis
Cephalic infection
  Meningoencephalitis
  Acute sinusitis
Spontaneous intracranial hypotension
Acute mountain sickness
Disorders of eyes
  Acute optic neuritis
  Acute glaucoma
Cervicogenic
  Greater occipital neuralgia
  Cervical myositis
Trigeminal neuralgia

From Evans RW: First or worst headaches. In Evans RW, Mathew NT, Handbook of Headache. Philadelphia, Lippincott Williams & Wilkins, 2000, p 107, with permission.

  d. Associated symptoms or signs in 70%.
  e. The diagnosis of sentinel headache should be considered in **every** patient with sudden severe and unusual headache or face pain.

Key Clinical Features: Sentinal Headache

Headache can be in any location, unilateral or bilateral 70% have associated symptoms or signs:

- 30% nausea and vomiting
- 30% neck pain and stiffness
- 15% blurred or double vision
- 20% motor or sensory abnormalities
- 20% drowsiness
- 20% dizziness
- 20% transient loss of consciousness

Laboratory Testing

1. Computed tomography (CT) of the brain is the initial imaging study of choice to detect SAH
   a. After the initial event, the probability of detecting aneurysmal hemorrhage on CT: first 24 hours, 95%; day 3, 74%; 1 week, 50%; 2 weeks, 30%; and 3 weeks, almost 0%.
2. From more than 3 to 14 days after the hemorrhage, magnetic resonance imaging (MRI; using the fluid-attenuated inversion recovery or FLAIR sequence) is more sensitive than CT.
3. **A lumbar puncture should be performed on all patients with a new- onset headache suspicious for SAH who have normal CT or MRI scans.**
4. In cases of suspected SAH, a CT or MRI study should be performed first because lumbar puncture can result in clinical deterioration and death after SAH.
5. Red blood cells are present in virtually all cases of SAH and variably clear from about 6 to 30 days.
6. When the cerebrospinal fluid obtained from the first lumbar puncture is bloody, the only certain way to distinguish SAH from a traumatic tap is the presence of xanthochromia (see Part II, Chapter 1, Lumbar Puncture and Cerebrospinal Fluid Evaluation).
7. Xanthochromia is variably present from 2 to 12 hours after SAH.
8. If the CT or MRI and/or lumbar puncture studies demonstrate SAH, a four-vessel cerebral arteriogram should be performed to try to identify the source of the bleed. Multiple aneurysms may be present in 20% to 30% of cases.
9. Magnetic resonance angiography can detect up to 90% of saccular aneurysms with a size of ≥5 mm. False-positive studies can occur. Confirmation with a cerebral arteriogram is necessary.

THUNDERCLAP HEADACHE

1. A sudden severe headache with maximal onset within 1 minute without evidence of SAH2.
2. Most cases are due to primary disorders but a small percentage are due to secondary causes (Table 5–2).
3. Aneurysmal mechanisms of thunderclap headache include aneurysmal expansion, thrombosis, and intramural hemorrhage.

TABLE 5–2. SOME CAUSES OF THUNDERCLAP HEADACHE

Primary causes
  "Crash" migraine
  Benign thunderclap headache
  Benign orgasmic, cough, and exertional headache
Secondary causes
  Ruptured and unruptured intracranial saccular aneurysm
  Cerebral vasospasm
  Ischemic and hemorrhagic stroke
  Acute hypertension (e.g., pheochromocytoma)
  Posttraumatic headache
  Cerebral venous thrombosis
  Carotid artery or vertebral artery dissection
  Spontaneous intracranial hypotension
  Pituitary apoplexy
  Occipital neuralgia
  Erve virus

4. A normal CT scan does not mean the absence of pathology.

5. A MRI scan (in some cases with MR angiography) can detect unruptured aneurysms, cerebral venous sinus thrombosis (a MR venogram may also be indicated), carotid or vertebral artery dissections, spontaneous intracranial hypotension, and pituitary hemorrhage.

Bibliography

Becker K: Epidemiology and clinical presentation of aneurysmal subarachnoid hemorrhage. Neurosurg Clin N Am 9:435–444, 1998.

Edlow JA, Caplan LR: Primary care: avoiding pitfalls in the diagnosis of subarachnoid hemorrhage. N Engl J Med 342:29–36, 2000.

Evans RW: First or worst headaches. In Evans RW, Mathew NT (eds): Handbook of Headache. Philadelphia, Lippincott Williams & Wilkins, 2000.

Khajavi K, Chyatte D: Subarachnoid hemorrhage. In Gilman S (ed): MedLink Neurology. San Diego, MedLink, 2003.

Linn FHH, Rinkel GJE, Algra A, van Gijn J: Headache characteristics in subarachnoid haemorrhage and benign thunderclap headache. J Neurol Neurosurg Psychiatry 65:791–793, 1998.

Van Gijn J, Rinkel GJ: Subarachnoid haemorrhage: Diagnosis, causes, and management. Brain 124:249–278, 2001.

Weir B: Headaches from aneurysms. Cephalalgia 14:79–87, 1994.

6 Headaches During Childhood and Adolescence

Randolph W. Evans

Epidemiology

1. By the age of 7 years, 40% of children have had headaches.
   a. 2.5% have frequent nonmigraine types
   b. 1.4% with migraine
2. By age 15, 75% have had headaches
   a. 15.7% with frequent tension type
   b. 5.3% with migraine, 1.5% migraine with aura
   c. 54% with infrequent nonmigraine types

MIGRAINE

Epidemiology

1. 20% of migraineurs have the onset before 10 years of age and 45% before 20 years of age.
2. Before puberty, prevalence is the same for boys and girls; after puberty, the female to male ratio is 3:1.
3. The risk of a child developing migraine is 70% when both parents have migraine and 45% when one parent is affected.
4. Motion sickness and sleepwalking both occur much more often in children with migraine.

Clinical Features

1. Migraine without aura
   a. The most common type
   b. Duration often less than adults and can be as little as 1 hour
   c. More often bilateral distribution (65%, typically frontal and temporal) than unilateral
2. Migraine with aura
   a. 20% have the gradual onset of a visual aura before or during the onset of headache usually lasting less than 30 minutes.
   b. May describe spots, colors, dots, or lights in both eyes. Rarely, visual distortions and hallucinations ("Alice in Wonderland" syndrome) including metamorphopsia, micropsia, macropsia, zoom vision, or mosaic vision (fracture of image into facets).

Key Clinical Findings: Childhood Migraine

- Without aura: 80%
- Duration can be as little as 1 hour
- 65% bilateral, 35% unilateral
- Visual aura usually lasts less than 30 minutes.

---

3. Familial hemiplegic migraine
   a. Rare variant: migraine with aura that includes hemiplegia or hemiparesis
   b. At least one first-degree relative has migraine and has had at least one hemiparetic attack.
   c. Autosomal dominant on chromosome 19 due to a mutation in a brain-specific P/Q calcium channel subunit.
   d. Attacks may occur on the same or different sides from episodes to episode.
   e. The face, arm, and leg typically become paretic with a slow, spreading progression.
   f. May be an associated alteration of consciousness ranging from confusion to coma. Aphasia may be present if the dominant hemisphere is involved.
   g. Diagnosis of exclusion: Consider partial seizures, congenital and acquired heart disease, infectious/inflammatory causes (e.g., varicella encephalitis), vascular and hematologic disorders, cerebrovascular malformations, and head trauma.
4. Basilar migraine
   a. Migraine with aura symptoms originating from the brainstem or both occipital lobes.
   b. Two or more aura symptoms of the following types: visual, dysarthria, vertigo, tinnitus, decreased hearing, double vision, ataxia, bilateral paresthesias, bilateral paresis, and decreased level of consciousness.
   c. Rare disorder. Frequently occurs in children. More than a third have their first attack in the second decade of life and two thirds have the first attack in their second or third decade of life. Rarely presents over the age of 50.
   d. Those with basilar migraine may have other types of migraine as well.

449

e. Aura usually lasts from 5 to 60 minutes but can last up to 3 days.

f. Visual symptoms including blurred vision, teichopsia (shimmering colored lights accompanied by blank spots in the visual field), scintillating scotoma, graying of vision. May start in one visual field and then spread to become bilateral.

g. Diplopia may be present in up to 16% of cases.

h. Vertigo (which can be present with tinnitus), dysarthria, gait ataxia, and paresthesias (usually bilateral but may alternate sides with a hemidistribution) may be present alone or in various combinations.

i. In 50% of cases, bilateral motor weakness occurs.

j. Impairment of consciousness often occurs including obtundation, amnesia, syncope, and, rarely, prolonged coma.

k. A severe throbbing headache, typically with a bilateral occipital location, is present in 96%.

l. Nausea and vomiting typically occur, and light and noise sensitivity occur in up to 50%.

m. Diagnosis of exclusion with differential similar to hemiplegic migraine.

n. Treatment

(1) Avoid triggers

(2) Analgesics or nonsteroidal antiinflammatory drugs (NSAIDs) for acute pain. Many authorities recommend not using ergotamine, triptans, and dihydroergotamine because of the potential for vasoconstriction and stroke (although there are reports of effective use of triptans without significant side effects).

(3) Preventive medication often not necessary but can try verapamil, valproic acid, and Topamax. Some experts recommend avoiding use of beta-blockers, which may limit any compensatory vasodilator capacitance.

o. Prognosis and complications

(1) Frequency decreases as patients enter their 20s and 30s.

(2) Stroke is a rare complication.

(3) Occasionally, focal or generalized seizures may follow the aura.

5. Ophthalmoplegic migraine

a. Rare condition that may occur at any age but typically occurs in infants and children under the age of 12.

b. As the intensity of an ipsilateral severe headache subsides after a day or more, paresis of one or more of cranial nerves III, IV, and VI occurs. Patients typically have multiple recurrent episodes.

c. The third nerve is involved in 80% of cases, initially with ptosis and then with oculomotor paresis. Mydriasis is present in more than 50% of cases.

d. Early high dose corticosteroids may be beneficial. Recovery usually occurs in a week to 4 to 6 weeks. After multiple attacks, recovery may be incomplete.

e. Diagnosis of exclusion especially after initial episode. Consider Tolosa-Hunt syndrome (granulomatous inflammation in the cavernous sinus), parasellar lesions, diabetic cranial neuropathy, collagen vascular disease, and orbital pseudotumor (an idiopathic infiltration of orbital structures).

6. Benign paroxysmal vertigo of childhood

a. Onset usually between 2 and 5 years of age but can be before 1 year of age or as late as 12 years.

b. Unprovoked stereotypical episodes of true vertigo (with a sensation of movement as described by verbal children) usually lasts for seconds or minutes but may last for hours. The child becomes pale, cannot maintain an upright position, and wishes to remain still.

c. No complaint of headache or alteration of consciousness, although nausea or other abdominal discomfort may follow the vertigo.

d. Treatment is usually not necessary.

e. As the child becomes older, the episodes of vertigo may be associated with migraine headaches or become less severe and disappear. Other types of migraine may then occur in 21%.

f. Diagnosis of exclusion. Partial seizures can produce true vertigo.

7. Abdominal migraine (cyclical vomiting)

a. Criteria

(1) Family history of migraine

(2) A history of migraine with or without aura

(3) Recurrent identical attacks of abdominal pain

(4) No abdominal symptoms between attacks

(5) Onset of attacks of abdominal pain in early childhood or early adult life (before age 40), mainly in females

(6) Episodes lasting from 1 to several hours

(7) Pain usually located in the upper abdomen

b. Episodes may be associated with nausea and vomiting and pallor or flushing.

c. Prevalence peaks at ages 5 to 9 years.

d. Diagnosis of exclusion. If there is alteration of consciousness, consider a seizure disorder.

e. Drugs used for migraine prevention and symptomatic treatment may be helpful.

8. Confusional migraine

a. Migraine with a headache, which can be minimal, associated with a confusional state that can last from 10 minutes to 2 days.

b. Agitation and impaired memory may be present. May be inattention, distractibility, and difficulty maintaining coherent speech or action.

c. Diagnosis of exclusion.

9. "Footballer's" migraine

a. Acute minor head trauma can trigger migraine in children and adolescents.

10. MELAS syndrome

a. Mitochondrial encephalomyopathy, lactic acidosis, and strokelike episodes (MELAS): a rare disorder

b. Can present as episodic migraine early in the course of the disease.

c. Features

(1) Strokelike episodes before age 40

(2) Encephalopathy with seizures, dementia, or both

(3) Evidence of a mitochondrial myopathy with lactic acidosis, ragged-red fibers, or both.

(4) At least two of the following present:

(a) Normal early development

(b) Recurrent headache

(c) Recurrent vomiting

(5) Most patients have exercise intolerance, limb weakness, short stature, hearing loss, and elevated cerebrospinal fluid protein.

d. 90% of cases are due to an A-to-G point mutation in the mitochondrial geneencoding for tRNA at nucleotide position 223243. The other 10% are due to seven other mitochondrial DNA point mutations. All children of mothers with MELAS are affected through maternal transmission of mitochondrial DNA.

Treatment

1. Non-medication

a. Identify and avoid migraine triggers.

b. Biofeedback, stress management, and progressive relaxation training may be beneficial.

c. Education about migraine for the patient and parents or caretakers

d. Acute headaches

(1) Aspirin should be avoided before the age of 15 years because of the potential for Reye's syndrome

(2) Headaches in children 6 years of age and younger are typically brief and resolve with acetaminophen and/or sleep

2. There are numerous symptomatic and preventive medications that may be helpful in appropriate cases. The contraindications and the many potential side effects are reviewed in pharmacology references.

3. Table 6–1 lists symptomatic medications that may be of benefit. Children with significant nausea or vomiting may benefit from the use of metoclopramide 0.2 mg/kg orally (up to 10 mg) or promethazine 0.5 mg/kg orally or in suppository form.

a. In those with frequent headaches, total weekly doses of symptomatic medications and caffeine should be carefully monitored because of the potential for rebound headaches

b. Prolonged migraine may respond to an inpatient intravenous protocol of an antiemetic, metoclopramide, and dihydroergotamine (DHE).

TABLE 6–1. SYMPTOMATIC TREATMENT FOR MIGRAINE IN CHILDREN AND ADOLESCENTS (INITIAL DOSES)

MEDICATION	DOSAGE
Acetaminophen	10–15 mg/kg PO
Pseudoephedrine HCL	30 mg PO
Ibuprofen	10 mg/kg PO
Naproxen sodium	5 mg/kg PO
Butalbital 50 mg, acetaminophen 325 mg, caffeine 40 mg	6–9 yr, 1/2 tablet; 9–12 yr, 3/4 tablet; >12 yr, 1 tablet
Isometheptene mucate, dichloralphenazone 100 mg, and acetaminophen 325 mg	6–12 yr, 1 capsule; >12 yr, 1–2 capsules
Sumatriptan	0.06 mg/kg SC (6 mg maximum); 25–50 mg PO; 5 or 20 mg NS
Zolmitriptan	6–8 yr, 1.25 mg; >9 yr, 2.5 mg
Rizatriptan	6–8 yr, 2.5 mg; 9–11 yr, 5 mg; >12 years, 5-10 mg
Dihydroergotamine	6–9 yr, 0.1 mg/dose; 9–12 yr, 0.15 mg/dose; 12–16 yr, 0.2 mg/dose

Triptans and DHE should not be given within less than 24 hours of each other.

(1) Metoclopramide 0.2 mg/kg (up to 10 mg) can be given orally or intravenously 30 minutes prior to DHE.

(2) DHE (see Table 6–1 for initial doses) can be given intravenously every 6 hours for a maximum of 12 doses.

(3) The DHE may be increased by 0.05 mg/dose the the point where the patient develops mild abdominal discomfort. The protocol should be continued at the dose prior to the onset of abdominal discomfort.

(4) If metoclopramide causes an extrapyramidal syndrome, diphenhydramine can be given (1 mg/kg, maximum dose of 50 mg) orally, intramuscularly, or intravenously.

(5) For persistent cases or in the case of a significant myofascial component, may use intravenous ketorolac 7.5 to 15 mg every 6 hours alternating with DHE.

4. Preventive medications should be considered for children and adolescents with frequent migraines that are not responsive to symptomatic medications or that significantly interfere with school, home, or other activities.

a. Table 6–2 provides information on specific medications.

b. Because of the rare complication of fatal hepatotoxicity, which rarely occurs in children older than 10 years of age, divalproex sodium should be avoided in children under 10 years of age unless other medications have failed, in which case it should be used as monotherapy.

Prognosis

1. By age 22 years, 50% of males and 60% of females still have migraine.

2. In those with severe migraine beginning between the ages of 7 and 15, 20% are migraine free by 25 years of age, but 50% continue to have migraines into later life.

EPISODIC TENSION-TYPE HEADACHES

1. The most common recurrent headache

2. Features

a. Duration of 30 minutes to many days

b. Bilateral with a pressing or tightening quality

c. Mild to moderate intensity

d. Not worsened by routine physical activity

e. Light or noise sensitivity may be present but nausea is absent.

TABLE 6–2. PREVENTIVE MEDICATIONS FOR MIGRAINE IN CHILDREN AND ADOLESCENTS

MEDICATION	DOSAGE
Propranolol	<14 yr, initial dose10 mg PO bid; may increase by 10 mg/day each week to 20 mg tid maximum >14 yr, initial dose 20 mg PO bid; may increase by 20 mg/day each week up to 240 mg/day. Equivalent long-acting doses may be used.
Nadolol	0.25–1 mg/kg, initial dose
Cyproheptadine HCl	≥6 years, 4 mg PO hs. May be slowly increased to 12 mg PO hs or 8 mg PO hs and 4 mg PO q.am
Amitriptyline or nortriptline	10 mg PO hs. May be increased every 2 weeks to 50 mg PO hs <12 yr and 100 mg PO hs >12 yr
Divalproex sodium	>10 yrs, 125–250 mg PO hs; slowly increase to 500–1000 mg in 2 divided doses. Equivalent extended–release doses may be used.
Topiramate	Initial dose 0.25–1 mg/kg or 15 mg or 25 mg. Can be given once daily for headaches. Increase by initial dose once weekly to 50–100 mg total daily dose given bid in children or qd in adolescents.

Key Clinical Findings: Episodic Tension-Type Headaches

- Duration of 30 minutes to days
- Bilateral with pressing quality
- Mild to moderate intensity
- Light or noise sensitivity may be present but no nausea

3. Treatment

a. Symptomatic treatment with acetaminophen or a NSAID may be effective.

b. Frequent use of symptomatic medications or caffeine can lead to rebound headaches.

c. Non-medication approaches for frequent headaches

(1) Adequate sleep, regular exercise, and avoidance of caffeine may help.

(2) Biofeedback, stress management, and progressive relaxation training may also be worthwhile.

(3) If school or family problems, stress, depression, or anxiety are prominent, psychological or psychiatric evaluation may be indicated.

d. If there is a significant muscle contraction component, muscle relaxants, NSAIDs, physical therapy, and a trial of a transcutaneous electrical nerve stimulator may be warranted.

e. Frequent headaches may improve with preventives such as amitriptyline, nortriptyline, and paroxetine.

CHRONIC NONPROGRESSIVE HEADACHES

1. Most commonly chronic tension type, mixed (both distinct migraine and tension headaches or headaches with features of both), transformed migraine (episodic migraine transforming into daily or near daily headaches usually from medication rebound), and medication rebound.

2. Medication rebound

   a. Medications that can cause rebound include acetaminophen, ibuprofen, and other NSAIDs, combination drugs with agents such as butalbital, acetaminophen, aspirin, caffeine, and codeine, propoxyphene, ergotamine, and triptans.

   b. The number of doses of analgesics taken per week can range from as few as 8 to more than 80.

   c. Discontinuing the analgesics alone or in some cases starting a preventive can dramatically reduce the frequency of headaches in many cases. Other treatments listed above for frequent tension-type headaches may also be helpful. Divalproex sodium may be useful in some cases. Intractable headaches may respond to the intravenous DHE regimen.

3. New daily persistent headaches

   a. Develops for the first time over less than 3 days

   b. Etiology often unknown

   c. Can be due to a postviral syndrome

4. Acute infectious mononucleosis

   a. Typical picture of a 7-day prodromal illness followed by a 4-day to 3-week acute illness with fever, headache, malaise, pharyngitis, cervical lymphadenopathy, and mononuclear leukocytosis with atypical lymphocytes

   b. Transient hepatic dysfunction and splenomegaly and hepatomegaly may be present.

   c. The monospot or heterophile antibody test is positive.

   d. Persistent Epstein-Barr infection can cause longer duration chronic headaches.

ACUTE SEVERE HEADACHES

1. Frequency of causes different than in adults

   a. Aneurysmal subarachnoid hemorrhage is uncommon–fewer than 2% of cases occur in those under 18 years of age.

   b. Subarachnoid hemorrhage is more likely due to ruptured arteriovenous malformations, which outnumber aneurysms by nearly 10 to 1 in childhood.

2. Most commonly due to infection (e.g., viral upper respiratory infections, sinusitis, streptococcal pharyngitis, and viral meningitis) and migraine.

3. Brain abscess a rare cause

   a. Usually present with symptoms of less than 2 weeks duration

   b. Symptoms variably present include headaches, nausea and vomiting, fever, seizures, nuchal rigidity, and papilledema.

Chronic Progressive Headaches

1. Primary brain tumors.

   a. Rare cause of headaches. The annual incidence of pediatric primary brain tumors is about 2–3/100,000; 60% are posterior fossa, 40% are supratentorial.

   b. Headache present in about 65%, vomiting in 65%, and changes in personality in about 50%. About one third of headaches always associated with vomiting.

2. Hydrocephalus

   a. Obstructive or noncommunicating is due to a blockage of cerebrospinal fluid (CSF) pathways at or proximal to the outlet foramina of the fourth ventricle, the foraminas of Luschka and Megendie (e.g., aqueductal stenosis, Chiari malformation, neoplasms, inflammatory ventriculitis)

   b. Communicating due to blockage of CSF in the basal subarachnoid cisterns, in the subarachnoid spaces over the brain surface, or within the arachnoid granulations (e.g., leptomeningeal inflammation).

   c. Small children may present with symptoms and signs of raised intracranial pressure including headaches, vomiting, irritability, lethargy, and poor feeding.

   d. Older children may present with headaches, often worse in the morning, vomiting, cranial nerve VI palsies, papilledema, and altered levels of consciousness.

e. The headaches are often bilateral and are made worse by coughing, sneezing, straining, or bowel movement.

3. Other causes

a. Chronic subdural and epidural hematomas, pseudotumor cerebri, malformations (Chiari and Dandy-Walker), hypertension, and medication rebound.

Bibliography

Carlow TJ: Oculomotor ophthalmoplegic migraine: is it really migraine? J Neuroophthalmol 22:215–221, 2002.

Evans RW: Headaches during childhood and adolescence. In Evans RW, Mathew NT (eds): Handbook of Headache. Philadelphia, Lippincott Williams & Wilkins, 2000.

Linder SL, Winner P: Pediatric headache. Med Clin North Am 85:1037–1053, 2001.

Peatfield RC, Welch KMA: Basilar artery migraine. In Olesen J, Tfelt-Hansen P, Welch KMA (eds): The Headaches, 2nd ed. Philadelphia, Lippincott Williams & Wilkins, 2000.

Winner P, Gladstein J: Chronic daily headache in pediatric practice. Curr Opin Neurol 15:297–301, 2002.

7 Headaches in Women

Randolph W. Evans

Epidemiology and Risk Factors

1. Women have headaches more than men
   a. The lifetime prevalence of headaches is 99% in women and 93% in men.
   b. The lifetime prevalence for migraine is 25% for females and 8% for males. The one-year prevalence is 18% for females and 6% for males.
   c. The lifetime prevalence for tension-type headaches is 88% for women and 69% for men.
2. The gender ratio increases from menarche, peaks at 42 years of age, and then declines.
   a. The female incidence of migraine with aura peaks between the ages of 12 and 13, and migraine without aura peaks between the ages of 14 and 17.

Pathophysiology

1. Estrogen levels are a key factor in the increased prevalence of migraine in women.
   a. Migraine prevalence increases at menarche.
   b. Estrogen withdrawal during menstruation is a common trigger.
   c. Estrogen administration in oral contraceptives and hormone replacement therapy can trigger migraines.
   d. Migraines typically decrease during the second and third trimesters of pregnancy.
   e. Migraines are common immediately postpartum with the precipitous drop in estrogen levels.
   f. Migraines generally improve with physiologic menopause.
2. Exactly how changes in estrogen levels influence migraine is not understood.
   a. Fluctuations in estrogen levels can result in changes in prostaglandins (which sensitize pain receptors and increase neurogenic inflammation), prolactin release, opioid regulation, and melatonin secretion.
   b. These fluctuations can also cause changes in neurotransmitters including the catecholamines, noradrenaline, serotonin, dopamine, and endorphins.

MENSTRUAL MIGRAINE

Epidemiology

1. Menstruation is a trigger for about 50% of migraineurs.
2. 14% of women with migraines have headaches only with menstruation and at no other time of the month.
3. The duration, severity, and response to treatment of menstrual migraine is similar to migraine occurring at other times.

Treatment

1. Symptomatic treatment is the same as for other migraines (see Part XI, Chapter 1, Migraine).
2. Interval or short-term preventive treatment of menstrual migraine starting 2 to 3 days before and continuing during the menses may be helpful for some women with regular menses and migraines poorly responsive to symptomatic medications. There are many potentially effective medications.
   a. Amitriptyline or nortriptyline 25 mg orally at bedtime
   b. Long-acting propranolol 60–80 mg daily or nadolol 40 mg daily
   c. Nonsteroidal anti-inflammatory drugs such as naproxen sodium, 550 mg twice daily
   d. Ergotamine 1 mg daily or twice daily or dihydroergotamine 1 mg subcutaneously or intramuscularly
   e. Sumatriptan 50 mg daily or naratriptan 1 mg orally twice daily for 5 days perimenstrually
   f. Transdermal estradiol 100 μg on menstrual day −3 and replaced on days −1 and +2
3. Continuous combined oral contraceptive use
   a. Rather than skipping the pill-free week, a lower estrogen dose is administered (e.g., Mircette)

Key Treatment: Menstrual Migraine

- Usual migraine symptomatic drugs (triptans, etc.)
- Interval preventive medications
- Continuous combined oral contraceptive use

MENOPAUSE AND MIGRAINE

1. Two thirds of women with prior migraine improve with physiologic menopause

2. Surgical menopause results in worsening of migraine in two-thirds of cases.

3. Estrogen replacement therapy has a variable effect on migraine.

   a. 45% improve, 46% worsen, and 9% are unchanged.

   b. When migraines increase on estrogen replacement, the following strategies may be beneficial:

      (1) Reduce estrogen dose

      (2) Change estrogen type from conjugated estrogen (Premarin) to pure estradiol (Estrace) to synthetic estrogen (Estinyl) to pure estrogen (Ogen)

      (3) Convert from interrupted to continous dosing in the case of estrogen withdrawal migraine.

      (4) Convert from oral to parenteral administration (e.g., Alora, Climara, Estraderm, or Vivelle-Dot)

      (5) Add androgens.

ORAL CONTRACEPTIVE (OC) USE AND MIGRAINE

1. Onset and frequency

   a. Migraines may occur for the first time on OCs.

   b. The effect of OC use is variable on preexisting migraine: may increase, decrease, or stay the same. Low-estrogen-dose OCs usually have no effect or may improve migraine.

   c. When new-onset migraine occurs or the frequency increases, 30% to 40% may improve when OCs are discontinued. Improvement may not occur for up to 1 year.

2. Risk of stroke

   a. There is an increased risk of stroke in women with migraine, although the absolute risk is still small.

      (1) In women ages 35 to 44 years, the approximate incidence of ischemic strokes per 100,000 women/year is 3.6 in those without migraine, 11 in migraine without aura, and 22 in migraine with aura.

      (2) In women ages 25 to 34 years, the respective incidence is 1.3, 4, and 8 per 100,000 women/year.

   b. Controversial topic. Depending on the study, low-estrogen-dose OCs may not increase the risk of stroke. High-estrogen-dose OCs used in the past do increase the risk of stroke.

   c. Progestin-only oral contraception does not increase the risk of stroke.

3. OC use in migraineurs

   a. Most women with migraine without aura can safely take low-estrogen-dose OCs when there are no other contraindications.

   b. Those with migraine with aura such as visual symptoms lasting less than 1 hour can also take the medication.

   c. Women with aura symptoms such as hemiparesis or aphasia or prolonged focal neurologic symptoms and signs lasting more than 1 hour might best avoid starting low-estrogen-dose OCs and stop the medication if already taking.

   d. In prescribing OCs, other risk factors should be considered, including older age, cigarette smoking, diabetes, uncontrolled hypertension, and coronary artery disease.

   e. Progestin-only OCs and the many other contraceptive options can be considered as appropriate.

HEADACHES DURING PREGNANCY AND POSTPARTUM

Neuroimaging

1. With appropriate indications (see Chapter 6, Headaches), neuroimaging should be performed.

2. With the use of lead shielding, a standard computed tomography (CT) scan of the head exposes the uterus to less than 1 mrad (a dose of >15 rads is necessary to result in deformities that might justify pregnancy termination).

   a. CT is the study of choice for the evaluation of acute head trauma acute subarachnoid hemorrhage.

   b. There is no known risk associated with intravenous contrast for CT but avoid if possible.

3. There is no known risk of magnetic resonance imaging (MRI) without or with gadolinium contrast during pregnancy. Contrast should be avoided if possible.

4. There are potential medico-legal considerations in performing imaging during pregnancy.

Differential Diagnosis

1. Includes pre-eclampsia, eclampsia, and cerebrovascular disease including an increased risk of cerebral venous thrombosis (see Part III, Chapter 9, Stroke in Pregnancy and the Postpartum Period)

2. Pseudotumor cerebri can develop or worsen during pregnancy.

   a. Pregnancy is not a risk factor.

   b. Visual outcome is the same for the pregnant and nonpregnant patient.

3. Brain tumors

   a. Pregnancy does not increase the risk of a primary brain tumor.

   b. Meningiomas may increase in size during pregnancy and then regress postpartum.

   c. 25% of macroprolactinomas will expand enough to cause problems during pregnancy.

   d. Choriocarcinomas usually follow a molar pregnancy but can rarely follow term delivery, abortion, and ectopic pregancy. Brain metastases occur in 20% of cases.

4. Infection

   a. Pregnancy is a state of relative immunosuppression.

   b. Coccidioidomycosis, tuberculosis, listeriosis, and malaria have an increased risk of spread to the central nervous system when acquired during pregancy.

Migraine

1. Depending on the study, 1% to 10% of migraine has the new onset during pregnancy, usually during the first trimester. About 5% of women will have the new onset of migraine during the postpartum period.

2. Course during pregnancy

   a. Preexisting migraine improves or disappears in 60%, is unchanged in 20%, and is more frequent in 20%.

   b. Strictly menstrual migraine improves in 85% of pregnancies.

   c. The improvement often occurs during the second and third trimesters.

   d. When improvement occurs with the first pregnancy, improvement occurs in about 50% of subsequent pregnancies.

   e. About 40% of women have headaches during the first postpartum week, especially between days 3 and 6.

      (1) Often a mild to moderately severe bifrontal pain associated with photophobia and nausea

      (2) More frequent in women with a personal or family history of migraine

      (3) May be triggered by rapidly falling estrogen levels

Key Clinical Findings: Migraine During Pregnancy

- New onset of migraine in 1% to 10% of pregnancies

- Preexisting migraine improves or disappears in 60%

- More frequent in 20%

- Improvement often occurs during the second and third trimesters

3. Treatment

   a. Non-mediation approaches include avoidance of triggers, ice, sleep, and biofeedback.

   b. Symptomatic medications

      (1) Need to consider the potential of risk for the fetus and the potential for medication rebound and habituation with some drugs.

      (2) Acetaminophen, a U.S. Food and Drug Administration (FDA) Class B drug (no evidence of risk in humans, but there are no controlled human studies), is the drug of choice.

      (3) Aspirin is rated as FDA Class C (risk to humans has not been ruled out) during the first and second trimesters and Class D (positive evidence of risk to humans from human or animal studies) during the third trimester.

         (a) There are multiple possible adverse effects.

         (b) Low-dose aspirin is generally safe when used to prevent pre-eclampsia or for the treatment of antiphospholipid antibody syndrome. There may be an increased risk of abruptio placentae.

      (4) Caffeine in small doses of less than 300 mg a day is FDA Class B and probably safe. However, several studies have raised concern over an increased risk of miscarriage with moderate to high caffeine intake. The most prudent recommendation would be to ingest 100 mg or less per day.

      (5) Butalbital is FDA Class C but there has been no evidence of an association with malformations. Overuse can result in rebound headaches, habituation in the mother, and fetal dependence and neonatal withdrawal.

      (6) If acetaminophen alone is ineffective, some patients will benefit from the addi-

tion of butalbital or butalbital and caffeine, which can also be combined with codeine.

(7) Codeine, FDA Class C, is probably safe in reasonable amounts.

(8) Meperidine, methadone, and butorphanol (all FDA Class C) are probably not teratogenic.

(9) Nonsteroidal anti-inflammatory drugs are FDA Class B during the first two trimesters but should be avoided during the third trimester because of the potential for adverse events.

(10) Ergotamine and dihydroergotamine are both FDA Class X, contraindicated in pregnancy. (The actual risk is not clear, however.)

(11) Triptans are FDA Class C. Although there is no evidence of teratogenicity at this time, the use of triptans during pregnancy should be avoided.

(12) Antiemetics may be necessary if prominent nausea or vomiting is present. The following are generally considered reasonably safe during pregnancy, especially with occasional use.

   (a) Prochlorperazine, promethazine, and chlorpromazine are all FDA Class C.

   (b) Metoclopramide is FDA Class B.

c. Prolonged migraine

(1) May be treated with 10 mg of prochlorperazine intravenously and intravenous fluids. The addition of parenteral narcotics may also be helpful.

(2) Magnesium sulfate 1 g in D5W or normal saline administered intravenously over 15 minutes

(3) Migraine status may respond to the administration of intravenous corticosteroids such as dexamethasone 4 mg intravenously.

d. Preventive medications

(1) Frequent severe migraines especially associated with nausea and vomiting may justify the use of preventive medication.

(2) Valproic acid (FDA Class D) should be avoided because of the 1% to 2% risk of neural tube defects when taken between day 17 and day 30 after fertilization.

(3) Beta-blockers are the preventive of choice if contraindications are not present.

   (a) Atenolol, nadolol, propranolol, metoprolol, and timolol are all FDA Class C.

   (b) There may be an increased incidence of small for gestational age infants.

   (c) Propranol may cause fetal and neonatal toxicity.

(4) Tricyclic antidepressants

   (a) Amitriptyline and nortriptyline are FDA Class D.

   (b) Doxepin and protriptyline are FDA Class C.

   (c) These drugs are associated with a low risk of harm to the fetus.

   (d) Tricyclics should be stopped at least 2 weeks before the due date because there have been reports of infants with respiratory distress and feeding difficulties when a tricyclic is continued through delivery.

(5) Fluoxetine (FDA Class C) is questionably effective for migraine but might be beneficial for chronic daily headache.

(6) Verapamil (FDA Class C) is probably safe during pregnancy.

e. Breast-feeding and migraine medications

(1) Maternal medications usually compatible with breast-feeding include acetaminophen, barbiturates (which may cause infant sedation), caffeine (which may cause irritability or poor infant sleep pattern in higher maternal doses), nonsteroidal anti-inflammatory drugs, beta-blockers, narcotics, valproic acid, and verapamil.

(2) The effect on the nursing infant of antidepressants such as amitriptyline and fluoxetine is not known but may be of concern.

(3) Caution is advised when using a triptan during lactation. Expressing and discarding all milk for 8 hours after the dose would largely avoid the baby's exposure.

B Bibliography

The American Academy of Pediatrics Committee on Drugs: The transfer of drugs and other chemicals into human milk. Pediatrics 93:137–150, 1994.

Boyle CA: Management of menstrual migraine. Neurology 53 (4 Suppl I):S14–18, 1999.

Evans RW: Headaches in women. In Evans RW, Mathew NT (eds): Handbook of Headache. Philadelphia, Lippincott Williams & Wilkins, 2000.

Marcus DA: Pregnancy and chronic headache. Expert Opin Pharmacother 3:389–393, 2002.

Silberstein SD: Headache and female hormones: what you need to know. Curr Opin Neurol 14:323–333, 2001.

8 Headaches in Patients Over the Age of 50

Randolph W. Evans

Epidemiology

1. The prevalence of headache decreases with advancing age (Table 8–1).

2. 66% of headaches in the elderly are primary compared to 90% in younger persons.

3. Many of the numerous causes of headaches are listed in the box below.

New-Onset Headaches Occurring Over the Age of 50

Primary headaches
  Migraine
  Tension
  Cluster
  Hypnic
Secondary headaches
  Neoplasms
  Subdural and epidural hematomas
  Head trauma
  Cerebrovascular disease
  Temporal arteritis
  Trigeminal neuralgia
  Postherpetic neuralgia
  Medication-induced and rebound
  Systemic disease
  Diseases of the cranium, neck, eyes, ears, and
    nose
  Parkinson's disease
Exertional headache due to angina

MIGRAINE

Epidemiology

1. New onset over the age of 50 represents only 2% of all migraineurs.

2. Migraine prevalence decreases with older age: Over the age of 70 year, 5% in women and 2% in men.

Clinical Features

1. Migraine with aura is less common than in younger persons.

2. In contrast, those with a history of migraine with aura when younger may develop migraine aura without headache.

3. Late-life migrainous accompaniments: transient visual, sensory, motor, or behavioral neurologic manifestations that are similar or identical to the auras of migraine with aura.

   a. Headache is associated with only 50% of cases and may be mild.

   b. Headaches occur more often in men than women.

   c. Complaints from most to least common: visual symptoms (blindness, homonymous hemianopsia, and blurring of vision), paresthesias (numbness, tingling, pins-and-needles sensation, or a heavy feeling of an extremity), brainstem and cerebellar dysfunction (ataxia, clumsiness, hearing loss, tinnitus, vertigo, and syncope), and disturbances of speech (dysarthria or dysphasia).

   d. Some features help to distinguish migraine from transient ischemic attacks (TIA).

      (1) Gradual build-up of sensory symptoms; a march of sensory paresthesias

      (2) Serial progression from one accompaniment to another—e.g., from flashing lights to paresthesias, paresis, or dysphasia.

      (3) Often a duration of 15 to 25 minutes; 90% of TIAs last for less than 15 minutes

      (4) The progression of scintillating scotomas over approximately 20 to 30 minutes is unique and is considered to be pathognomonic for migraine.

      (5) Multiple stereotypical episodes: may be a "flurry" of episodes

      (6) Usually benign natural history without permanent sequelae

      (7) Evaluation for other causes of TIA should be considered, especially when the patient is seen after the first attack or there are unusual aspects.

      (8) If episodes are frequent, can consider preventive treatment with medications such as verapamil, antiplatelet medications (e.g., aspirin, dipyridamole, clopidigrel), divalproex sodium, and topiramate. Beta-blockers should be avoided because of the potential for worsening vasospasm.

459

TABLE 8–1. PREVALENCE OF HEADACHES AT VARIOUS AGES

Age (years)	Women (%)	Men (%)
21–34	92	74
55–74	66	53
75+	55	22

(9) For acute treatment, there is a potential risk of increasing cerebral vasospasm with ergotamine, dihydroergotamine, and triptans.

Key Clinical Features: Late-Life Migraine Accompaniments

- Headache in only 50% of cases
- More common in men than in women
- Visual and sensory auras the most common
- Serial progression of one accompaniment to another
- Duration usually 15 to 25 minutes

Treatment

1. Ergotamine, dihydroergotamine, and triptans should not be used in patients with coronary artery disease, cerebrovascular disease, peripheral vascular disease, or uncontrolled hypertension.

2. Before using a triptan in patients without these contraindications, a screening cardiac evaluation might be considered, especially if they have risk factors.

3. Preventive treatment with tricyclic antidepressants may be contraindicated in some patients with prostatism, glaucoma, or cardiac dysrhythmias.

4. Beta-blockers may be contraindicated in some patients with diabetes mellitus, congestive heart failure, or bronchial asthma.

5. Drugs used for other indications such as estrogen replacement therapy (also see Part XI, Chapter 7, Headache in Women) or nitrates may trigger migraines.

TENSION-TYPE HEADACHE

1. 10% have onset after 50 years of age.

2. The prevalence over the age of 65 years is 27%.

3. The diagnosis of new-onset tension-type headaches is one of exclusion.

CLUSTER HEADACHES

1. Age of onset is typically between 20 and 50 years, but occasionally can occur in the 70s.

HYPNIC HEADACHE

1. Rare disorder that occurs in people over the age of 40

2. Only occurs during sleep when the headache causes awakening at a consistent time.

3. Headache is bilateral more often than unilateral, throbbing or non-throbbing, and mild to severe in intensity.

4. Duration can range from 15 minutes to 6 hours and can occur frequently, as often as nightly for many years.

5. Diagnosis of exclusion because other types of headache can awaken from sleep including:
   a. Other primary headaches: migraine, cluster, and chronic paroxysmal hemicrania
   b. Secondary causes include drug withdrawal, temporal arteritis, sleep apnea, oxygen desaturation, pheochromocytoma, neoplasms, communicating hydrocephalus, subdural hematomas, and vascular lesions.

6. Medications that may be effective include caffeine (1 or 2 cups of caffeinated beverage or a 50 to 60 mg caffeine tablet before bedtime), lithium carbonate (300 mg at bedtime), indomethacin, atenolol, cyclobenzaprine, melatonin, prednisone, and flunarizine (not available in the United States).

Key Clinical Features: Hypnic Headache

- Rare disorder only in those older than 40 years
- Headache awakens from sleep at a consistent time
- Bilateral more often than unilateral, mild to severe
- Duration from 15 minutes to 6 hours
- Can be frequent as often as nightly for years

TEMPORAL ARTERITIS
(also see Part XX, Chapter 9, Temporal Arteritis and Polymyalgia Rheumatica)

lmost always occur over the age of 50, with a mean age of onset of about 70. Ratio of women to men is 3:1.

Clinical Features

1. Headache is the most common feature reported by 60% to 90% of patients.

2. Pain is usually throbbing but may be sharp, dull, burning, or lancinating.

3. Pain may be intermittent or continuous and is more often severe than moderate or mild.

4. Pain may be worse at night when lying on a pillow, when combing the hair, or when washing the face.

5. The location is variable, bilateral or unilateral. In 25% of cases the headache is only in the temple and does not involve the temple at all in 29%. Can mimic occipital neuralgia with unilateral nuchal-occipital pain and marked tenderness over the greater occipital due to inflammation of the occipital artery.

6. About half of the patients with temporal arteritis have tenderness or decreased pulsation of the superficial temporal arteries.

Laboratory Testing

1. According to the American College of Rheumatology 1990 criteria, three out of the following five criteria should be satisfied:
   a. Age at least 50 years
   b. New onset of localized headache
   c. Temporal artery tenderness or decreased pulse
   d. Erythrocyte sedimentation rate (ESR) of at least 50 mm/hour
   e. Positive histology

2. The ESR varies with older age. A formula for the upper limits of normal that includes 98% of healthy persons: age in years divided by 2 for men and age in years plus 10 divided by 2 for women. The ESR is not specific for temporal arteritis and can be elevated in any infectious, inflammatory, or rheumatic disease.

3. The ESR has been reported as normal in 10% to 36% of those with temporal arteritis. When abnormal, the ESR averages 70 to 80 mm/L.

4. In one study, the C-reactive protein was more sensitive (100%) than ESR (92%) for detection of temporal arteritis. The combination of C-reactive protein and ESR above the cutoff values gave the best specificity (97%).

5. The superficial temporal artery biopsy makes the diagnosis with certainty but has a false-negative rate ranging from 5% to 44% in various series.

Treatment

1. In the absence of contraindications, treatment is typically started with prednisone at a dosage of 40 to 80 mg/day. The headache will typically improve within 24 hours.

2. The initial dose is maintained for about 4 weeks and then slowly reduced over many months, depending on the clinical effect, the ESR, and occurrence of side effects.

3. Long-term treatment is usually required because the disease is active for at least 1 year and an average of 3 to 4 years.

POSTHERPETIC NEURALGIA

The persistence of pain after the initial outbreak of herpes zoster for more than 1 to 6 months (there are different definitions in the literature)

Epidemiology and Risk Factors

1. Annual incidence of acute herpes zoster is about 400/100,000 people

2. The incidence greatly increases with older age. Different studies variably report the annual incidence as 40 to 160/100,000 for those under 20 years of age to 450 to 1100/100,000 for those 80 years or older.

3. The lifetime risk of developing acute herpes zoster for those who live into their 70s and 80s is as high as 40%. The lifetime risk of a second or third attack in healthy people is about 5%.

4. Postherpetic neuralgia (PHN), the most common neurologic complication of varicella zoster infection, occurs in about 10% to 15% of those with acute zoster.

5. PHN develops in 50% of those older than 50 years of age and in 80% of those older than age 80.

6. Zoster involving the face nearly doubles the risk of developing PHN, which lasts longer than PHN in other locations.

7. Zoster is more common in immunocompromised patients who are also at greater risk of developing generalized zoster with diffuse cutaneous lesions and internal organ development.

Key Risk Factors: Postherpetic Neuralgia

- Most common neurologic complication of varicella zoster infection

- Occurs in about 10% to 15% of those with acute zoster

- Develops in 50% of those older than 50 years of age and in 80% of those older than age 80

- Zoster involving the face nearly doubles the risk of developing PHN, which lasts longer than PHN in other locations.

Etiology and Pathophysiology

1. Acute herpes zoster occurs when the dormant varicella zoster virus (from a previous chickenpox infection) is reactivated in the trigeminal, geniculate, or dorsal root ganglion, replicates, and travels down the sensory nerve to infect the skin in the corresponding dermatome.

2. A hemorrhagic inflammation involving the dorsal root ganglia and nerve is present.

3. In patients with PHN, fibrosis and cell loss in the dorsal root ganglion with loss of myelin occurs.

Clinical Features

1. Herpes zoster most commonly occurs in the thoracic region. The next most commonly involved area is a trigeminal distribution, usually in the ophthalmic division (herpes zoster ophthalmicus), in 23% of cases. There is almost always unilateral involvement.

2. Involvement of the geniculate ganglion can result in vesicles in the external auditory canal with severe ear pain and an ipsilateral facial palsy, Ramsay Hunt syndrome (see Part I, Chapter 15, Neurologic Eponyms).

3. Uncommonly, an extraocular muscle paresis may be associated as a result of involvement of the third, fourth, or sixth cranial nerves. Optic neuritis is a rare complication and may occur preceding and after the viral exanthem.

4. Radicular pain occurs with zoster and may precede the eruption of grouped vesicles (shingles) by days to weeks. The pain is usually sharp or stabbing.

5. Occasionally, pain occurs with a rash, zoster sine herpete.

6. Typically, the vesicles crust, the skin heals, and the pain resolves within 3 to 4 weeks of the onset of the rash.

7. Three types of pain may be present in PHN, varying from person to person.

    a. A constant burning or deep aching

    b. An intermittent spontaneous pain with a jabbing or lancinating quality

    c. A superficial, sharp, or radiating pain or itching provoked by light touch, allodynia, which is present in 90% of those with PHN and often interferes with sleep.

Key Clinical Findings: Postherpetic Neuralgia

- A constant burning or deep aching

- An intermittent spontaneous pain with a jabbing or lancinating quality

- Allodynia (present in 90% of those with PHN and often interferes with sleep)

Laboratory Testing

1. The diagnosis of herpes zoster is primarily a clinical one.

2. Tzanck cell test smears of the skin lesions may demonstrate intranuclear inclusions. Virus from vesicles can be isolated in cell culture.

3. Antibody titers rise after primary varicella-zoster virus infection and can be used to confirm diagnosis retrospectively. Patients with zoster or immune deficiency may not demonstrate a rise in antibody.

4. During acute zoster, varicella-zoster virus DNA can be demonstrated in white blood cells by polymerase chain reaction.

Treatment

1. For the treatment of acute zoster, oral corticosteroids (prednisone starting at 60 mg/day and tapering off over 2 weeks) may reduce acute pain but not the risk of PHN.

2. Famciclovir (500 mg every 8 hours for 1 week) and valacyclovir (1 g every 12 hours for 1 week) reduce the risk and duration of PHN. (The doses of both drugs are reduced in renal insufficiency.)

3. Nerve blocks can be effective treatment for acute pain of zoster.

4. For high-risk patients over the age of 55 years, epidural bupivacaine (0.25% 6–12 ml every 6 to 8 or 12 hours) and methylprednisolone (40 mg every 3 to 4 days) for 1 to 3 weeks as needed has been reported as decreasing the prevalence of PHN to 1.6%.

5. Numerous treatments are available for PHN with varying efficacies.

    a. Up to 61% of patients may have pain relief with use of tricyclic antidepressants including amitriptyline, nortriptyline, and desipramine. Start with a low dose and then slowly increase to an optimal dose with the most pain relief and tolerable side effects. Anecdotally, other antidepressants such as fluoxetine may be effective.

b. Gabapentin is effective in the treatment of pain and sleep disturbance.

c. Topical agents including capsaicin, lidocaine, aspirin, and nonsteroidal anti-inflammatory drugs may also be useful.

d. Opioids such as sustained release oxycodone (10 mg every 12 hours slowly increasing as necessary to 30 mg every 12 hours) and oral levorphanol may be effective when other drugs fail or cannot be tolerated.

e. Transcutaneous electrical nerve stimulation with the electrodes placed above and below the involved area may help about one third of patients.

f. For extracranial PHN, administration of 60 mg of intrathecal methylprednisolone and 3 ml of 3% lidocaine weekly for 4 weeks results in a good to excellent pain response in 91%. However, there is the long-term potential side effect with this treatment of adhesive arachnoiditis.

Key Treatment: Postherpetic Neuralgia

- Tricyclic antidepressants including amitriptyline, nortriptyline, and desipramine

- Gabapentin

- Topical agents such as capsaicin, lidocaine, aspirin, and nonsteroidal anti-inflammatory drugs

- Opioids such as sustained-release oxycodone and oral levorphanol

- Transcutaneous electrical nerve stimulation

- Intrathecal methylprednisolone and lidocaine

Prognosis and Complications

1. PHN can last for years.

2. Complications of herpes-zoster

   a. Rarely, herpes-zoster can cause arteritis and ischemic and hemorrhagic stroke from the spread of the virus to the vessels both hematogenously and through the sensory nerves (especially with herpes-zoster ophthalmicus).

b. Zoster encephalitis
   (1) Develops in immunocompromised persons with the rash or weeks to months later
   (2) Mental status changes and multifocal neurologic deficits

c. Zoster myelitis may occur in immune competent and incompetent patients.
   (1) Typically presents with motor deficits ipsilateral to the rash, which can spread to the contralateral cord

d. Cranial and peripheral nerve palsies can occur in 5% of those with zoster.

Prevention

Hopefully, the varicella vaccine will prevent chickenpox and these late complications. Although not certain, the varicella vaccine may only provide immunity for perhaps 6 years and revaccination may be necessary to provide lifetime immunity.

OTHER MEDICAL CONDITIONS

1. Headache associated with muscle contraction may occur more often in Parkinson's disease. Amantidine and levodopa can cause headaches in some cases.

2. Chronic obstructive lung disease, severe anemia, chronic renal failure, hypercalcemia, and hyponatremia can cause headaches.

Bibliography

Amlie-Lefond C, Jubelt B: Varicella-zoster virus infections of the nervous system. In Gilman S (ed): MedLink Neurology. San Diego, MedLink, 2003.

Dodick DW, Mosek A, Campbell JK: The hypnic ("alarm clock") headache syndrome. Cephalalgia 18:152–156, 1998.

Evans RW: Headaches over the age of 50. Evans RW, Mathew NT (eds): Handbook of Headache. Philadelphia, Lippincott Williams & Wilkins, 2000.

Fisher CM: Late-life migraine accompaniments: further experience. Stroke 17:1033–1042, 1986.

Lee AG, Brazis PW: Temporal arteritis: A clinical approach. J Am Geriatr Soc 47:1364–1370, 1999.

Salvarani C, Cantini F, Boiardi L, Hunder GG: Polymyalgia rheumatica and giant-cell arteritis. N Engl J Med 347:261–271, 2002.

Watson CPN: A new treatment for postherpetic neuralgia. N Engl J Med 343:1563, 2000.

9 Other Headaches

Randolph W. Evans

COUGH, EXERTIONAL, AND SEXUAL HEADACHES

Epidemiology

1. The lifetime prevalence of benign, cough, exertional, and sexual headaches is 1% for each.
2. All three types occur more often in men.

Benign Cough Headache

1. Bilateral headache of sudden onset lasting less than 1 minute and precipitated by coughing. The term also includes headache brought on by sneezing, blowing the nose, laughing, crying, weightlifting, bending, stooping, or straining with a bowel movement.
   a. Weightlifting can also produce a benign acute bilateral nuchal-occipital or nuchal-occipital parietal headache than can persist as a residual ache for days or weeks.
   b. About 25% have the onset after a respiratory infection with cough.
2. Infrequent type of headache with a mean age of onset of 55 years
3. Diagnosis made after neuroimaging excludes pathology such as Chiari malformation, platybasia, basilar impression, brain tumors, cerebral aneurysm, carotid stenosis, and vertebrobasilar disease.
4. Treatments that may be effective include indomethacin, a single lumbar puncture, and methysergide. Some patients may have an abrupt recovery after extraction of an abscessed tooth.

Benign Exertional Headache

1. Bilateral usually throbbing headache brought on by physical activity lasting from 5 minutes to 24 hours. Activities include running, rowing, tennis, and swimming. In some persons, one activity may precipitate the headache but not others.
2. Exercise can trigger a migraine in migraineurs.
3. Depending on the clinical scenario and number of headaches, it may be necessary to exclude secondary causes including subarachnoid hemorrhage, sinusitis, brain tumors, pheochromocytoma, cardiac ischemia (anginal headache), and intracranial arterial dissection.
4. May be prevented by a warm-up period or avoiding the particular activity. Indomethacin may be preventive. Migraineurs with exertional headache may respond to migraine preventive medications.

Key Clinical Findings: Benign Exertional Headache

- Bilateral usually throbbing headache
- Brought on by a variety of physical activities
- Typically lasts 5 minutes to 24 hours
- Secondary causes should be excluded in some cases.

Headache Associated with Sexual Activity

1. Three types of benign headache are precipitated by sexual excitement. All are bilateral and may be prevented or eased by stopping sexual activity before orgasm.
   a. The dull type is a dull ache in the head or neck that intensifies as sexual excitement increases. Probably due to muscle contraction.
   b. The explosive type is a sudden severe headache occurring at orgasm. The headache may be severe for minutes to 4 hours, followed by a milder headache lasting up to 48 hours.
   (1) 40% of those with the explosive type also have exertional headache.
   (2) Occurs more often when a persons tries to have more than one orgasm after a brief interval.
   (3) A personal or family history of migraine is common.
   (4) Especially when diagnosing the first sex headache, need to exclude subarachnoid hemorrhage (sexual activity a precipitant for up to 12% of ruptured saccular aneurysms). Rarely, pheochromocytoma is a cause. Sildenafil can cause headache in about 10% of users.
   (5) In some patients, this headache can be prevented by weight loss, an exercise program, a more passive role during intercourse, variation in posture, and limita-

tion of additional sexual activity on the same day.

(6) In some patients, the headache may be prevented by a taking medication 30 to 60 minutes before sex such as indomethacin, ergotamine, or a triptan. Those with frequent sex headaches may respond to migraine preventive medications such as beta-blockers or verapamil.

c. A postural headache similar to a post–lumbar puncture headache can occur, presumably due to a dural tear and cerebrospinal fluid (CSF) leak triggered by sex.

Key Clinical Findings: Explosive Sex Headache

- Precipitated by sexual activity

- Bilateral with a duration of minutes to hours

- May be prevented or eased by ceasing sexual activity before orgasm

- Not associated with any intracranial pathology such as a ruptured aneurysm

CHIARI TYPE I MALFORMATION AND HEADACHE

1. Hernation of the cerebellar tonsils below the level of the foramen magnum

2. Usually congenital but can be acquired with reversible descent due to lumbar puncture, overdraining CSF shunts, and spontaneous intracranial hypertension.

3. Female to male ratio 3:2.

4. Associated with syringomyelia in 40% (most commonly between the levels of C4 and C6).

5. All patients with tonsillar herniations greater than 12 mm and 70% of those with herniations of 5 to 10 mm are symptomatic.

6. Presentations include foramen magnum compression, central cord syndrome, cerebellar dysfunction, bulbar palsy, and paroxysmal intracranial hypertension. Syncope can occasionally occur with headache similar to basilar migraine or with Valsalva-like maneuvers or exercise.

7. Headaches may be similar to migraine and tension types. Can last from seconds to hours or may be continuous. Can be unilateral or bilateral in various locations including suboccipital-occipital, vertex, temporal, frontal, or orbital.

8. If the tonsillar herniation is less than 5 mm, consider other causes of the headaches.

LOW CEREBROSPINAL FLUID PRESSURE HEADACHES

Etiology and Pathophysiology

1. CSF shunt overdrainage

2. CSF leak due to trauma including lumbar puncture, cranial or spine trauma both from injury and from surgery

3. Associated with other medical conditions such as severe dehydration, diabetic coma, uremia, hypernea, meningoencephalitis, and severe systemic infection.

4. Spontaneous where the cause is often uncertain but may be due to meningeal diverticulae, spondyltic dura tear, weak and attenuated dura, connective tissue disorders, and trivial trauma.

5. Pathophysiology the same as post–lumbar puncture (see Part II, Chapter 1, Lumbar Puncture and Cerebrospinal Fluid Evaluation)

Clinical Features

(also see Part II, Chapter 1, Lumbar Puncture and Cerebrospinal Fluid Evaluation)

1. Orthostatic throbbing or nonthrobbing headache

2. A chronic daily headache can worsen when upright and improve when recumbent.

3. Other manifestations may include stiff neck, interscapular pain, nausea/vomiting, diplopia most often due to a cranial nerve VI palsy, dizziness, hearing complaints, blurred vision, light sensitivity, face numbness, radicular upper limb symptoms. Rare manifestations include stupor, coma, cerebellar ataxia, Parkinson's disease, and increased prolactin with galactorrhea.

Laboratory Testing

1. Lumbar puncture usually demonstrates a reduced opening pressure of 0 to 7 cm H_2O, although the pressure can be in the normal range especially if the procedure is performed after a period of bed rest.

2. CSF analysis may be normal or can demonstrate a moderate, primarily lymphocytic pleocytosis, the presence of red blood cells, and elevated protein that can even exceed 500 mg/dl.

3. Magnetic resonance imaging (MRI) scan of the brain may reveal diffuse pachymeningeal enhancement with gadolinium, and in some cases, subdural fluid collections. Reversible descent of the cerebellar tonsils may be present.

4. Spine MRI may reveal extra-arachnoid or extra-dural fluid, the diverticula, and the location of the

leak. Myelography followed by a computed to-mography (CT) scan may also help to identify the location of the CSF leak.

5. Color Doppler imaging of the superior ophthalmic vein may show an increased diameter of the vein and higher mean maximum flow velocity.

6. Meningeal biopsy (which is usually not necessary for the diagnosis) may show a thin zone of fibroblasts and thin-walled blood vessels in an amorphous matrix in the subdural aspect of the dura.

Treatment

1. Many patients improve spontaneously with bed rest. Oral or intravenous caffeine may help (see Part II, Chapter 1, Lumbar Puncture and Cerebro-spinal Fluid Evaluation).

2. Lumbar epidural blood patch usually helps. Re-peated patches may be necessary in the spontane-ous type.

3. Surgery is occasionally indicated when the loca-tion of the dural tear is found and is not responsive to other treatments.

NEOPLASMS

1. The prevalence of adults with primary and meta-static brain tumors who complain of headache at the time of diagnosis has been variably reported as 31% to 71%.

2. The neurologic examination can be normal. Papilledema is present in about 40% of patients. Headache is usually associated with other prob-lems such as a new-onset seizure, confusion, prolonged nausea, hemiparesis, or other focal findings.

3. Headache is most often bifrontal but may be in other locations of the head and neck and unilat-eral.

4. Headache quality usually is similar to tension type, but occasional patients have headaches similar to migraine without aura and rarely, migraine with aura and cluster headaches

5. Most headaches are intermittent with a moderate to severe intensity but a significant minority report only mild headaches relieved by simplege analge-sics. The classic brain tumor headache (severe, worse in the morning, and associated with nausea and vomiting) occurs in a minority of patients with brain tumors.

6. Pituitary adenomas
   a. Headache may be present in up to 72%. May be intermittent or continuous, is usually bilat-

eral, and more frequently occurs in the anterior half of the head.
   b. Pituitary macroadenomas can cause trigeminal neuralgia and clusterlike headaches.
   c. Acute pituitary apoplexy (hemorrhage of a pituitary macroadenoma with compression of neighboring neural and vascular structures) produces headache in 83% of cases, which may be variably associated with visual disturbance, ocular palsies, nausea/vomiting, altered menta-tion, meningismus, and fever.

7. Headache is present in up to 62% of patients with meningeal carcinomatosis (see Part VIII, Chapter 10, Meningeal and Spinal Metastases)

8. Colloid cysts of the third ventricle can present with paroxysmal severe headache or episodic positional headaches.

VASCULAR DISORDERS

1. Stroke
   a. Headache present in 29% with bland infarcts, 57% with parenchymal hemorrhage, 36% with transient ischemic attacks, and 17% with lacu-nar infarcts.
   b. The headache may be prior to the clinical deficit, at, or after the onset.
   c. Unilateral (to the side of the cerebral ischemia) headache of mild to moderate severity usually reported but many be severe and incapacitat-ing. Nausea, vomiting, and light and noise sensitivity are variably present.

2. Carotid endarterectomy
   a. A benign ipsilateral frontotemporal intense headache may follow carotid endarterectomy with a latency of 36 to 72 hours.
   b. Headache can also be due to postoperative intracerebral hemorrhage, which is a complica-tion of 0.75% of endarterectomies. May occur with a range of 0 to 18 days with a mean of 3 days after surgery.

3. Unruptured arteriovenous malformation (AVM)
   a. Migrainelike headaches with and without vi-sual symptoms can be associated with AVMs, especially those in the occipital lobe which is the predominant location of about 20% of parenchymal lesions.
   b. 95% of patients with AVMs have headaches always occurring on the same side, but about 15% of those with migraine also have side-locked headaches.
   c. Typical migraine due to an AVM is the excep-tion, as there are usually associated problems with headache from an AVM, which may

include papilledema, a visual field cut, a cranial bruit, short duration of headache or scotoma, and seizures.

4. Carotid and vertebral artery dissections
  a. Epidemiology
    (1) 2.5% of all patients with a first stroke have an internal carotid artery (ICA) dissection, with 90% involving the cervical carotid artery and 10% the intracranial carotid artery. The frequency of vertebral artery (VA) dissections is about 1/3 that of carotid.
    (2) 20% of spontaneous ICA and almost half of VA dissections are bilateral. Occasionally, combined ICA and VA dissections occur.
    (3) More than 70% of the patients are younger than 50 years of age.
  b. Etiology and pathophysiology
    (1) Due to penetration of circulating blood through an intimal tear into the subintimal, medial, and less commonly, adventitial layers of the vascular wall that extends for varying distances along the vessel
    (2) Risk and predisposing factors for spontaneous dissections include migraine, hypertension, oral contraceptives, fibromuscular dysplasia, temporal arteritis, polyarteritis nodosa, meningovascular syphillis, Ehlers-Danlos syndrome, Marfan syndrome, cystic medial necrosis, and moyamoya disease.
    (3) Trauma dissections due to penetrating or nonpenetrating injuries have derived from minor or trivial trauma such as coughing, blowing the nose, turning the head, sleeping in the wrong position, sports activities, chiropractic manipulation, yoga exercises, sexual activity, and whiplash neck injuries.
  c. Clinical features
    (1) Extracranial ICA dissection
      (a) Head, face, orbital, or neck pain, usually ipsilateral to the side of the dissection is the initial manifestation in 80%.
        (i) The onset of the headache is usually gradual, but about 10% have a thunderclap headache or sudden severe headache.
        (ii) The headache is usually a constant steady aching or sharp pain and less often, throbbing.
        (iii) Facial pain, including ear pain, is reported by about 33%, and orbital and eye pain in about 40%

of patients. Usually anterolateral neck pain is present in 25%.
      (b) An incomplete ipsilateral Horner's syndrome with ptosis and miosis but not anhydrosis is present in about 50% of cases due to damage of the sympathetic fibers.
      (c) Focal cerebral ischemic symptoms may precede the headache or follow the headache by up to 4 weeks.
      (d) Neurologically normal, 50%; mild deficits only, 21%, moderate to severe deficits, 25%; and death, 4%.
      (e) Subjective or objective bruits or both are present in about 45%.
      (f) Uncommon accompaniments include syncope, amaurosis fugax, scalp tenderness, neck swelling, visual scintillations, CN VI palsy, CN XII palsy, and involvement of the chorda tympani.
    (2) Intracranial ICA dissection typically presents with a severe ipsilateral headache and a major stroke.
    (3) VA dissection
      (a) Headache and posterolateral neck pain, unilateral or bilateral, present in 88%. Headache, usually aching or sharp; less often, throbbing. Can present with thunderclap headache in 20%.
      (b) Deficits can be due to vertebrobasilar distribution stroke or transient ischemic attacks, especially lateral medullary syndrome.
      (c) Neurologically normal or mild deficits, 83%; moderate to severe deficits, 11%, and death, 6%.
  d. Radiologic features
    (1) Arteriograms are the standard study. May reveal stenosis, often irregular and tapered; dissecting aneurysms; intimal flaps, and occlusion of distal branches. Irregular narrowing may give a "wavy ribbon" appearance, and severe narrowing may produce a "string sign."
    (2) Axial MRI may demonstrate the abnormal lumen and intramural clot.
    (3) MRA is 95% sensitive for ICA and 20% sensitive for VA dissections (much less due to technical artifacts). Spiral CT may have similar sensitivities.
    (4) Carotid duplex ultrasound may show a tapering luminal stenosis and a double lumen with reduced or absent distal carotid artery flow. VA ultrasound is less sensitive.

e. Treatment

(1) In the absence of subarachnoid hemorrhage, intracranial hemorrhage, a massive stroke, or other contraindications, heparin followed by warfarin is standard to prevent thrombus propagation and embolic stroke.

(2) Because most arteries will heal within 3 months, a follow-up study such as a MRA or arteriogram is typically done. Then a decision is made about whether to continue warfarin.

f. Prognosis

(1) With or without anticoagulation, a complete or excellent recovery occurs in about 85% of those with ICA and VA dissections.

(2) The recurrence rate for second dissections is 2% for the first month and then about 1% per year.

5. Cerebral venous thrombosis

a. Headache present in 80% and is often the first manifestation.

b. Variable headache, diffuse or unilateral, ranging from mild to severe intensity. Usually constant but can be intermittent. Usually subacute onset but can have a thunderclap presentation.

c. Headache is almost always associated with the following signs: papilledema in up to 80% of cases; at some time during the course of the disease, focal deficits in 50% and partial and/or generalized seizures in 40%.

6. Anginal headache (see Part XI, Chapter 8, Headaches in Patients Over the Age of 50)

HYPERTENSION

1. Mild or moderate hypertension does not usually cause headache.

2. Headaches due to severe hypertension are usually a bioccipital throbbing but can be generalized or a frontal throbbing. The headache is often present in the morning.

3. Hypertensive encephalopathy can present with headache, nausea, and vomiting, which may be associated with visual symptoms. Papilledema, focal neurologic deficits, seizures, and decreased levels of consciousness may be present.

4. A sudden severe headache can occur due to an acute pressor response due to the ingestion of wine or foods with a high tyramine level in people taking monoamine oxidase inhibitors. Illicit drugs with sympathomimetic actions such as cocaine, methamphetamine, and methylenedioxymethamphetamine ("ecstasy") can also cause acute hypertension and stroke.

5. Pheochromocytoma

a. Up to 92% of patients report a rapid-onset bilateral, severe, throbbing headache which lasts less than one hour in 70%. Nausea is present in 50% of cases.

b. Symptoms and signs of adrenergic stimulation are common, with sweating, palpitations, and tachycardia each reported by about 70% of patients.

c. Anxiety, dizziness, abdominal pain, chest pain, weight loss, heat intolerance, nausea/vomiting, pallor (less often flushing), syncope, and orthostatic hypotension may also occur.

d. Many patients have spells lasting between 15 and 60 minutes occurring from several times per day to once or twice a year.

e. Paroxysms can be triggered by physical exertion, certain medications, emotional stress, changes in posture, and increases in intraabdominal pressure.

CAROTIDYNIA

1. Neck pain associated with carotid artery tenderness especially near the bifurcation. Facial pain may also occur alone or with the neck pain.

2. Need to exclude carotid artery disease (dissection, occlusion or stenosis, aneurysm, fibromuscular dysplasia, and temporal arteritis) with appropriate testing such as carotid ultrasound, MRA, angiography, and a erythocyte sedimentation rate and C-reactive protein.

3. Acute monophasic carotidynia

a. May have a viral basis

b. Typically occurs in young or middle-aged adults and persists for an average of 11 days

c. Analgesics, nonsteroidal anti-inflammatory drugs such as indomethacin, or a short course of corticosteroids may relieve the pain.

Key Clinical Findings: Acute Monophasic Carotidynia

- Anterior neck and/or facial pain
- Carotid artery tenderness near the bifurcation
- Diagnosis of exclusion
- May have a viral basis
- Occurs in young or middle-aged adults
- Persists for an average of 11 days

4. Chronic or recurrent carotidynia

   a. Recurring pain lasting minutes to hours with episodes occurring daily or weekly in adults

   b. Diagnosis of exclusion. Should exclude carotid disease as noted above. Evaluation by an ENT physician to exclude nonvascular abnormalities such as thyroiditis and Eagle's syndrome (see Part XI, Chapter 4, Brief Head and Facial Pains) may be useful.

   c. May be related to migraine.

   d. May respond to treatment with indomethacin, a short course of corticosteroids, and migraine preventive medications.

PARANASAL SINUSITIS

1. Acute sinusitis

   a. Lasts from 1 day to 4 weeks. Subacute sinusitis from 4 to 12 weeks.

   b. Nasal congestion, purulent nasal drainage, and facial tenderness and pain are commonly present.

   c. Fever is present in 50%.

   d. Ansosmia, pain on mastication, and halitosis may also be present.

   e. Maxillary sinusitis

      (1) Pain is usually in the cheek, the gums, and the maxillary teeth; less often in the periorbital, supraorbital, or temporal areas.

      (2) Pain is improved when the patient lies supine and worse when the head is upright.

      (3) The maxillary sinus is tender to palpation.

   f. Frontal sinusitis

      (1) Severe frontal headaches with tenderness over the frontal sinus on percussion or palpation

      (2) The pain is less when the head is upright and worse when the patient lies supine.

      (3) Complications include brain abscess, meningitis, subdural or epidural abscess, osteomyelitis, subperiosteal abscess, orbital edema, orbital cellulitis, and orbital abscess.

   g. Sphenoid sinusitis

      (1) 3% of all cases of acute sinusitis; usually associated with pansinusitis

      (2) Headache may be frontal, occipital, temporal, or a combination and periorbital.

      (3) The pain is less when upright and worse when the patient is supine and with standing, walking, bending, or coughing. Frequently associated with nausea and vomit-

ing. Photophobia and eye tearing may be present.

      (4) Nasal discharge and drainage are present in 30% and fever in more than 50%.

      (5) May be misdiagnosed as migraine, meningitis, trigeminal neuralgia, or brain tumor.

      (6) Complications include bacterial meningitis, cavernous sinus thrombosis, subdural abscess, cortical vein thrombosis, ophthalmoplegia, and pituitary insufficiency. A parameningeal focus may cause an aseptic meningitis.

Key Clinical Findings: Sphenoid Sinusitis

- Headache may be in various locations.
- Nausea and vomiting often present
- Pain less when upright
- Pain worse when supine and with standing, walking, bending, or coughing
- Nasal discharge and drainage in 30% and fever in 50%
- Often misdiagnosed

   h. Ethmoid sinusitis

      (1) Produces pain in the periorbital, retroorbital, temporal, inner canthal area, or between the eyes. Usually associated with rhinitis.

      (2) Coughing, straining, or lying supine can worsen the pain, whereas keeping the head upright lessens it.

      (3) Complications include meningitis, orbital cellulitis, cavernous sinus thrombosis, and cortical vein thrombosis.

2. Chronic sinusitis. Present for more than 12 weeks.

   a. Usually low-grade and diffuse headache often accompanied by nasal obstruction, congestion, and fullness

   b. Symptoms often increase during the day.

3. Radiologic features

   a. Plain sinus radiographs can diagnose acute maxillary or frontal sinusitis but are often inadequate for ethmoid or sphenoid disease.

   b. CT of the sinuses in the coronal plain is highly sensitive for the detection of nasal and paranasal sinus disease. However, a routine CT scan of the head may inadequately cover these areas.

   c. MRI scan of the brain routinely visualizes the paranasal sinuses.

   d. Radiographic evidence of sinusitis is present in

40% of adults without symptoms as an incidental finding.

TEMPOROMANDIBULAR DISORDERS (TMD)

1. TMD are common in the general population, with at least one sign present in 75% and at least one symptom in 33%. Bruxism (grinding or clenching of teeth) occurs during sleep in up to 20% of the population.

2. Only 5% of patients with signs of TMD require treatment, and fewer than 5% have associated headache.

3. Pain, which is usually localized in the muscles of mastication, the preauricular area, or the temporomandibular joint (TMJ), is the most common presenting symptom. The pain is usually aggravated by jaw function.

4. Because both the ear and the TMJ have sensory innervation from the auriculotemporal nerve, otalgia is a common initial symptom.

5. Signs include limited or asymmetric jaw movements, joint noise on movement, and locking on opening.

6. Joint noises are caused by poor lubrication in the joint, associated with inflammation, arthritis, or a slipped fibrous disc. Joint noises and joint displacement are common in asymptomatic persons.

7. Examination

   a. The extraoral exam includes palpation of the TMJ both laterally (the lateral capsule of the TMJ) and endaurally (the posterior recess and capsule) for tenderness.

   b. Mandibular range of motion can be measured vertically and laterally. The maximum vertical opening (measured with a ruler from the incisal edge of the upper and lower central incisors) normally measures 35 to 55 mm.

   c. Deviation of the mandible midline to one side is usually due to a failure of the condyle to slide forward on the side to which the chin is deviating.

   d. Lateral excursion distance to the right and left (measured from the midline of the maxillary central incisors to the midline of the mandibular central incisor teeth) usually ranges from 8 to 15 mm. Protrusive or forward mandibular movements can also be measured.

8. Etiology

   a. Myofascial pain is the most common cause of pain arising from the TMJ. Can be associated with stress, grinding the teeth, and bruxism.

   b. Other causes include synovitis, trauma, osteoarthritis, anterior disc displacement, adhesions, bony ankylosis, systemic arthropathies, and tumors.

9. Treatment

   a. Usually responds to conservative reversible therapies. Referral to a dentist may be necessary.

   b. An oral appliance or bite plate that fits between the upper and lower teeth is worn at night and sometimes during the day. This device relieves pressure or unloads the TMJ by creating a space between the upper and lower teeth and distributing forces throughout the dental arch.

   c. A soft diet and the application of moist heat help to relieve exacerbations

   d. Physical therapy including home programs can be helpful.

   e. Patient education may help to reduce clenching or grinding habits.

   f. Some patients may benefit from stress-reduction techniques such as biofeedback.

   g. Medications may be helpful such as nonsteroidal anti-inflammatory drugs, muscle relaxers, tricyclic antidepressants, and the judicious use of narcotics.

   h. Surgery is occasionally indicated.

SEIZURE DISORDERS

1. Benign occipital epilepsy, benign rolandic epilepsy, and temporal and occipital lobe epilepsy can cause seizures that mimic some features of migraine.

   a. A seizure is more likely if the aura lasts less than 5 minutes and is associated with alteration of consciousness, automatisms, and abnormal motor activity such as tonic-clonic movements.

   b. Migraine is more likely if the aura lasts more than 5 minutes and has positive (e.g., tingling, scintillations) and negative features (e.g., visual loss, numbness).

2. Unilateral or bilateral headaches can occur during a temporal lobe seizure.

3. Hemicrania epileptica or synchronous ipsilateral ictal headache with migraine features is a cause of headaches associated with a seizure.

   a. Most patients have both ictal headache and some other seizure manifestation, although ictal headaches may be the only manifestation.

   b. The seizure discharges, usually on the same side as the ipsilateral headache, begin and end simultaneously with the headache.

   c. The headaches usually last a few seconds to minutes.

4. About 50% of patients have postictal headaches after partial complex and generalized tonic-clonic

seizures. The headaches can resemble those of the migraine and tension type.

CENTRAL PAIN SYNDROME

1. Central lesions of the second-order trigeminal neurons, the quintothalamic tract, the ventrobasal nuclei of the thalamus, the parietal lobe, and the cerebellum can cause diminished pain and burning sensations in the face and scalp. This was originally termed *thalamic pain syndrome.*

2. The ipsilateral extremities and trunk are usually also involved. Diminished pinprick and temperature sensation are usually present.

3. Patients also report mechanical and thermal, especially cold, hyperalgesia (allodynia).

4. Etiology
   a. Complication of 8% of strokes; onset of pain may be delayed for 1 to 2 months after the stroke
   b. Other causes include multiple sclerosis, tumors, and abscesses.

5. Treatment
   a. Often difficult
   b. Some patients may respond to tricyclics (e.g., amitriptyline), antiseizure drugs (including carbamazepine, valproic acid, gabapentin, and lamotrigine), narcotics, clonidine, neuroleptics, and intravenous lidocaine.

Bibliography

Evans RW, Mathew NT: Handbook of Headache. Philadelphia, Lippincott Williams & Wilkins, 2000.

Evans RW, Pascual J: Orgasmic headaches: clinical features, diagnosis, and management. Headache 40:491–494, 2000.

Förderreuther S, Henkel A, Noachtar S, Straube A: Headache associated with epileptic seizures: epidemiology and clinical characteristics. Headache 42:649–655, 2002.

Moki B: Headaches in cervical artery dissections. Curr Pain Headache Rep 6:209–216, 2002.

Olesen J, Tfelt-Hansen P, Welch KMA: The Headaches, 2nd ed. Philadelphia, Lippincott Williams & Wilkins, 2000.

Silberstein SD, Lipton RB, Dalessio DJ: Wolff's Headache and Other Head Pain, 7th ed. New York, Oxford University Press, 2001.

1   Sleep and Testing

Carl E. Rosenberg

Normal Sleep

1. All mammals sleep, including *Homo sapiens*.
2. The average human sleep need is 8 hours (range, 4–10 hours)
3. Sleep is divided into REM and non-REM sleep.
   a. REM (rapid eye movement)
      (1) Active sleep in premature infants and neonates
      (2) Paradoxical sleep in animals
      (3) Tonic REM occurs when the eyes are quiet.
      (4) Phasic REM occurs when the eyes are moving.
      (5) Automonic variability is highest during phasic REM.
      (6) Muscle atonia is occurs with REM sleep.
      (7) The electroencephalogram (EEG) shows a mixture of beta, alpha, and theta waves
      (8) Brain metabolism is almost as high as in waking.
      (9) Most dreams, certainly emotionally laced dreams, happen in REM sleep.
      (10) Current theory links REM sleep with the storing of memory.
   b. Non-REM sleep
   (1) Light sleep
      (a) Stage 1
         (i) The transition between waking and sleep
         (ii) The alpha rhythm disappears.
         (iii) The EEG background is a mixture of alpha, theta, and occasional delta waves.
      (b) Stage 2
         (i) The EEG background is similar to stage 1 sleep.
         (ii) Sleep spindles and/or K-complexes appear.
         (iii) A sleep spindle is an EEG spindle, usually 11 to 14 Hz, lasting 0.5 to 1.5 seconds
         (iv) The K-complex consists of a negative EEG wave followed by a posi-

tive component lasting 0.5 seconds or more
   (2) Deep sleep
      (a) 20% or more of the epoch, 30 seconds, is dominated by delta waves of 2 Hz or less, with a peak to trough amplitude of 75 μV or more ("sleep delta").
      (b) Sleep spindles can be seen in deep sleep.
      (c) Deep sleep has been divided into stage 3 and stage 4.
         (i) Stage 3: 20% to 50% of the epoch is sleep delta.
         (ii) Stage 4: over 50% of the epoch shows sleep delta.
         (iii) Current practice is to combine stages 3 and 4 into *deep sleep*.
         (iv) Brain metabolism is least in deep sleep.
      (3) The EEG background shows a gradual slowing as non-REM sleep progresses from light sleep into deep sleep.
4. Sleep cycle
   a. Classic sleep cycle
      (1) Lasts 90 to 120 minutes
      (2) Stage1 → stage 2 → deep sleep → stage 2 → REM
   b. Deep sleep dominates the sleep cycle in the early part of sleep.
   c. The first sleep cycle need not have REM sleep.
   d. Sleep cycles in the latter part of sleep may have little or no deep sleep.

Polysomnography (PSG)

1. Multichannel and modality measurement of physiologic parameters during sleep
2. An epoch of sleep is a 30-second page of sleep
3. Minimal requirements
   a. EEG: C3-A2 & O1-A2 (C4-A1 & O2-A1)
   b. EOG: LOC-A2 & ROC-A1
   c. Electromyography (EMG): Chin, left leg, right leg
   d. Electrocardiogram (ECG)

472

e. Airflow via thermistor or pressure monitor

f. Chest wall and abdomen motion via induction coil or piezoelectric monitor

g. Sao_2

h. Video monitor

i. A technician to monitor the patient

4. Possible additional channels

   a. Any number or combination of EEG channels

   b. Left and right arm EMG channels

   c. Chest wall EMG

   d. Snoring microphones

   e. Esophageal intrathoracic pressure monitors

   f. End tidal Co_2, used primarily with children

   g. Reflux

   h. Penile tumescence

   i. Treatment measures

      (1) Continuous positive airway pressure (CPAP)

      (2) CPAP airflow

   j. Any other physiologic monitor that does not cause multiple arousals

5. Traditional measures

   a. Sleep staging

      (1) Each epoch is staged as to wake or stage of sleep

      (2) Sleep latency

         (a) Time to first three epochs of stage 1 or first epoch of any other stage of sleep

         (b) Normal (90% confidence limits): 5 to 38 minutes

      (3) Sleep efficiency

         (a) Percentage of time in bed when the subject is asleep

         (b) Total sleep time/Time in bed

         (c) Normal: 74% to 94%

      (4) REM latency

         (a) Time to first epoch staged as REM

         (b) 43 to 137 minutes

      (5) Normal distribution of sleep stages

         (a) Stage 1: 1% to 8%

         (b) Stage 2: 39% to 68%

         (c) Deep sleep: 5% to 37%

         (d) REM: 14% to 28%

      (6) Arousals index

         (a) Number of arousals/Hours of sleep

         (b) Often arousals and awakenings are combined

      (7) Epileptic events

   b. Respiratory measures

      (1) Respiratory rate and rhythm

      (2) Apnea-hypopnea index: Number of apneas and hypopneas/Hours of sleep

      (3) Baseline Sao_2

      (4) Lowest Sao_2

      (5) Mean Sao_2

   c. ECG rate, rhythm, and variability

   d. Technician comments and activity seen on the video monitor

6. Risks and contraindications

   a. Polysomnography (PSG) is essentially a noninvasive study, with no more risk than traditional EEG.

   b. Trained personnel must place more invasive monitors; esophageal pressure and reflux monitors.

   c. Sleep laboratories usually have minimal medical support and cannot handle inpatients.

Polysomnography

Measures of Sleep

- Sleep latency, REM latency, sleep efficiency
- Stage 1: 4%
- Stage 2: 54%
- Stage 3: 21%
- REM: 21%

Respiratory Measures

- Apnea-hypopnea index
- Sao_2
- Rate and rhythm

Multiple Sleep Latency Test (MSLT)

1. A measure of daytime sleepiness

2. PSG is performed the night before the MSLT

3. MSLT consists of four to five scheduled naps at 2-hour intervals

   a. The subject is not allowed to sleep between naps

   b. For each nap the subject is put in a dark quiet room and encouraged to go to sleep

   c. The subject is given up to 20 minutes to fall asleep

   d. Once the subject is asleep, the examiner allows 15 minutes to elapse to see if any REM sleep occurs

e. Two measures come from each nap
   (1) The sleep latency (time to first epoch scored as sleep)
   (2) The sleep latency is set at 20 minutes, if the patient does not fall asleep within 20 minutes
   (3) Whether or not REM sleep is seen
   (4) The time to REM sleep is irrelevant
   (5) If REM sleep is seen within the 15-minute window it is called a *sleep-onset REM (SOREM)* Note that this definition does not require that the first epoch of sleep be REM.
   f. If only one SOREM is seen in the first four naps, a fifth nap becomes necessary
4. The final report yields two measures
   a. The mean sleep latency (average of the sleep latencies from each nap)
      (1) Normal: ≥ 10 minutes
      (2) Pathologic: ≤ 5 minutes
      (3) Sleepy is between
   b. The number of SOREMs (naps with REM sleep)
      (1) Zero or one SOREM is normal
      (2) Two or more SOREMs are abnormal

Multiple Sleep Latency Test

Perform a PSG the night before

Mean Sleep Latency

- Average of the sleep latencies from all the naps
- Normal: ≥10 minutes
- Sleepiness: 5–10 minutes
- Pathological sleepiness: ≤5 minutes

Number of Naps with REM

- Normal: none or 1
- Abnormal: ≥2

Narcolepsy

- Mean sleep latency: < 5 minutes
- Two or more SOREMs

Controversial or Experimental Testing

1. Unattended pulse oximetry
   a. Sensor and position dependent
   b. Cannot distinguish the type of respiratory event
   c. Oximetry alone misses apnea in 33% of patients
2. Unattended snoring monitors
   a. Snoring volume need not correlate with the degree of apnea
   b. Often misses apneas
3. Home/unattended PSG
   a. Complicated systems, often confusing patients
   b. Very expensive to send a technician into the home for set-up
   c. Higher rate of failed studies due to technical problems in the unattended environment
   d. Risk of losing equipment
4. Split-night studies
   a. Used in obstructive sleep apnea
   b. The first half of the study is used to confirm obstructive sleep apnea
   c. CPAP is titrated during the second half of the study
   d. Most useful in the presence of severe obstructive sleep apnea
   e. The reported acceptance of CPAP varies.
   f. The degree of REM sleep apnea may be missed or underestimated.
   g. Highly dependent on the time asleep

 ## Bibliography

Carskadon MA, Dement WC, Mitler MM, et al.: Guidelines for the multiple latency sleep test (MSLT): A standard measure of sleepiness. Sleep 9:519–524, 1986.

Chesson AL, Feber RA, Fry JM, et al.: The indications for polysomnography and related procedures. An American Sleep Disorders Association review. Sleep 20:423–487, 1997.

Iber C, O'Brien C, Schluter J, Davies S, et al.: Single night studies in obstructive sleep apnea. Sleep 15:221–227, 1991.

Kryger MH, Roth T, Dement WC (eds): Principles and Practice of Sleep Medicine, 3rd ed. Philadelphia, W.B. Saunders, 2000.

Rechtschaffen A, Kales A (eds): A Manual of Standardized Terminology: Techniques and Scoring System for Sleep Stages of Human Subjects. Los Angles, UCLA Brain Information Service/Brain Research Institute, 1968.

Walseben JA, Kapur VK, Newman A, et al.: Sleep and reported daytime sleepiness in normal subjects: The Sleep Heart Health Study. In preparation, 2001.

2 Insomnia and Circadian Rhythm Disorders

Carl E. Rosenberg

Definition

1. *Insomnia* is simply a difficulty in sleeping.
2. *Sleep onset insomnia* is a difficulty falling asleep.
3. *Sleep maintenance insomnia* is a difficulty staying asleep.
4. *Early morning insomnia* is early morning awakening.
5. It is important to realize that these are clinical descriptions and not diagnoses.
6. Circadian rhythm disorders represent a problem in the "scheduling" of sleep
   a. This may be a problem only in relation to the demands imposed by a person's work or school schedule.
   b. This may be a problem intrinsic to the timing of sleep.

Epidemiology

1. Transient insomnia, days to weeks, affects about 50% of adults during their lifetime.
2. Chronic insomnia, over 6 weeks, is thought to afflict 25% of the adult population.
3. Women are 1.3 times more likely than men to complain of insomnia.
4. There is a strong association between insomnia and psychiatric conditions, especially depression. Often the severity of the insomnia corresponds to the severity of the psychiatric condition.

Clinical Features and Differential Diagnoses

1. Sleep onset insomnia
   a. Primary or psychophysiologic insomnia
      (1) Difficulty falling asleep
      (2) Anxiety about falling asleep
      (3) Performing inhibiting activities of sleep in bed such as arguments, watching television, or excessive reading
      (4) Often these patients sleep better in a novel environment.
      (5) These patients will complain bitterly as to feeling listless or fatigued during the day, but never sleepy.
   b. Delayed sleep phase
      (1) Very common in teenagers and professionals
      (2) Basically a persistent jet lag where the patient goes to bed late and is forced to awaken early.
      (3) Sleep is normal and refreshing when these patients can sleep until they awaken normally.
      (4) These patients complain of both sleep onset insomnia and daytime sleepiness.
   c. Shift-work syndrome
      (1) This is similar to delayed sleep phase in that there are often simultaneous complaints of insomnia and sleepiness.
      (2) The problem is that the change of shifts never allows the patient to attain a stable sleep/wake cycle.
   d. Secondary sleep onset insomnia associated with drugs
      (1) Withdrawal from sedative-hypnotics, including alcohol
      (2) Use of stimulants, including caffeine, nicotine, cocaine, and amphetamines
2. Sleep maintenance insomnia
   a. Two patterns
      (1) Awakening during the night for an hour or more
      (2) Prolonged repetitive awakenings
   a. This can be due to sleep/wake cycle disorders
      (1) Irregular sleep pattern
      (2) Shift-work syndrome
      (3) Aging with deterioration of the circadian pacemaker
   c. Sleep disrupters
      (1) Obstructive sleep apnea
         (a) The patient with obstructive sleep apneas: Sleep disrupted with awakening due to respiratory events.
         (b) The patient's bed-partner: Sleep disrupted with arousals due to the patient's snoring.

475

(2) Reflux

(3) Asthma

(4) Use of sedative-hypnotics with awakening when they "wear off." This includes alcohol.

(5) Note that nocturnal seizures do not usually present with insomnia.

3. Early morning awakening

a. Most often associated with depression

b. Can be seen in a short sleeper who retires at a "normal" time.

c. REM-related obstructive sleep apnea

4. Secondary insomnia in association with a psychiatric illness.

a. This can mimic any of the clinical pictures of insomnia.

b. Early morning awakening is a hallmark of depression.

c. Note that severely depressed patients can complain of hypersomnolence as well.

d. A careful history and insight on the part of the practitioner is needed to distinguish between primary and secondary insomnias and the role of psychiatric illness.

5. Disruption of the sleep/wake cycle in Alzheimer's disease

a. Sleeping patterns become almost random

b. This is the second most common reason for these patients to be institutionalized.

c. There is an accelerated degeneration of the superchaismatic nucleus.

6. Medications can cause insomnia.

a. Antihypertensives, including clonidine, beta-blockers, methyldopa, reserpine

b. Anticholinergics (ipratropium bromide)

c. Central nervous system stimulants such as methylphenidate

d. Hormones: oral contraceptives, thyroid preparations, cortisone, and progesterone

e. Sympathomimetics including bronchodilators (e.g., terbutaline, albuterol), theophylline, pseudoephedrine

f. Antineoplastics such as medroxyprogesterone and interferon alpha

 Key Signs

Sleep Onset Insomnia

- Primary or psychophysiologic insomnia: Difficulty falling asleep, anxiety about falling asleep, inhibiting activities of sleep in bed, fatigue during the day but are not sleepy; sleep better in a novel environment

- Delayed sleep phase: Common in teenagers and professionals; a persistent jet lag where the patient goes to bed late and is forced to awaken early; sleep is normal and refreshing when the patient can sleep until awakening normally; complaints of both sleep onset insomnia and daytime sleepiness.

Sleep Maintenance Insomnia

- Awakening during the night for an hour or more

- Prolonged repetitive awakenings

Early Morning Awakening

- Most often related to depression

- REM-related obstructive sleep apnea

Secondary Insomnia in Association with a Psychiatric Illness

- A careful history is required to distinguish between primary and secondary insomnias and the role of psychiatric illness

- Severely depressed patients may complain of hypersomnolence

Medications that Cause Insomnia

- Antihypertensives

- Anticholinergics (ipratropium bromide)

- CNS stimulants

- Hormones, sympathomimetics, antineoplastics

Use of Sedative-Hypnotics for Sleep

- Short term, maximum 2 weeks

- Acute stressful situations, such as the loss of a loved one

- Short half-life medications for sleep onset insomnias; longer for sleep maintenance insomnias

- May be useful in shift-work syndrome

Laboratory Testing

1. Basically there are no specific laboratory tests needed for the diagnosis of insomnias.

2. Polysomnography

a. Used to rule out other possibilities such as obstructive sleep apnea.

b. To "prove" to the patient that the patient sleeps.

c. Only about one third of the patients who complain about insomnia will actually show an abnormal delay to sleep onset or waking on a polysomnogram.

3. Sleep diary
   a. A record kept by the patient of bedtime, sleep times, time out of bed, and any naps
   b. Two typical weeks usually provides sufficient sleep diary data.
4. Actigraphy
   a. This computerized test is not a standard clinical tool.
   b. The system counts the movements of a limb and then the software estimates whether the patient is awake or asleep on the basis of these counts over time.
   c. It is about 80% accurate.
   d. These devices can measure for 3 to 7 days, depending on the sampling rate and the model.
   e. Can be used to document the presence or degree of insomnia.

 Key Tests

- No laboratory tests needed for the diagnosis of insomnias
- Polysomnography
- Sleep diary
- Actigraphy

Treatment

1. Psychophysiologic
   a. The treatment for this condition is relearning how to go to sleep.
   b. Cognitive treatment
      (1) Principles of sleep hygiene
      (2) Relaxation therapy
      (3) Hypnosis
   c. Sleep restriction
      (1) Limits the time in bed to increase sleep efficiency
      (2) Patient instructions
         (a) The patient's sleep time is estimated.
         (b) The patient time to retire is based on the required time to rise.
         (c) The patient may retire progressively earlier as long as sleep remains uninterrupted
2. Use of sedative-hypnotics for sleep (Table 2–1)
   a. Short term, maximum 2 weeks
   b. Useful in acute stressful situations, such as the loss of a loved one
   c. Short half-life medications for sleep onset insomnias; longer for sleep maintenance insomnias
   d. May be useful in shift-work syndrome

TABLE 2–1. SEDATIVE-HYPNOTIC MEDICATIONS

Medication	Dose (mg)	Onset of Action (min)	Duration of Action (hrs)
Triazolam	0.125–0.25	15–30	1.5–5
Zaleplon	15–30	30	4
Zolpidem	5–10	30	1.5–4
Lorazepam	1–4	30–60	8–24
Flurazepam	15–30	20	7–10
Temazepam	15–30	45–60	3–25
Clonazepam	0.5–2	20–60	19–60

3. Delayed sleep phase
   a. Chronotherapy
      (1) The patient retires 3 to 4 hours later every day until the desired schedule is achieved.
      (2) The patient stays awake for 24 hours then continues until the desired bedtime.
   b. Chronotherapy can be supplemented by the techniques used for psychophysiologic insomnia.
4. Shift-work syndrome
   a. Very difficult to treat
   b. Current modalities include
      (1) Light therapy
      (2) Scheduling only with phase delays, no advances
      (3) Short-term sedative use
      (4) Change of employment
   c. The ability to tolerate this condition varies widely among individuals.
5. Insomnias in the context of psychiatric disease
   a. Treatment is directed at the underlying disease.
   b. Can be supplemented by the treatments for psychophysiologic insomnia
6. Sleep disruption with Alzheimer's disease
   a. Very difficult to treat
   b. Behavioral intervention by keeping the patient awake and active during the day
   c. Keep the patient clean and dry at night

 Key Treatment

- Psychophysiologic: Relearning how to go to sleep, cognitive treatment, and sleep restriction
- Use of sedative-hypnotics for sleep
- Delayed sleep phase: Chronotherapy, plus the techniques for psychophysiologic insomnia
- Insomnias in the context of psychiatric disease: Treat underlying condition, plus the techniques for psychophysiologic insomnia
- Both shift-work syndrome and sleep disruption with Alzheimer's disease are difficult to treat.

Sleep Hygiene

- Avoid naps

- Maintain a regular schedule

- Avoid bright light before retiring

- Keep clock face away from view at night

- Avoid heavy exercise and meals before sleep

- Develop a bedtime ritual, including a time to "unwind" before sleeping

- Observe that the bed is for only two activities, one of which is sleep.

Bibliography

Czeilser CA, Richardson GS, Coleman RM, et al.: Chronotherapy: Resetting the circadian clocks of patients with delayed sleep phase insomnia. Sleep 4:1–12, 1981.

Edinger JD, Wohlgemuth WK, Radtke RA, et al.: Does cognitive-behavioral insomnia therapy alter dysfunctional beliefs about sleep? Sleep 24:591–599, 2001.

The International Classification of Sleep Disorders, Revised. Rochester, MN, American Sleep Disorders Association, 1997.

Janson C, Lindberg E, Gislason T, et al.: Insomnia in men: A 10-year prospective population based study. Sleep 24:425–430, 2001.

Morin CM, Hauri PJ, Espie CA, et al.: Nonpharmacologic treatment of chronic insomnia. Sleep 22:1134–1156, 1999.

3 Periodic Limb Movements and Restless Legs

Carl E. Rosenberg

Definitions

1. Periodic limb movements (PLMs)
   a. Also known as *nocturnal myoclonus, periodic leg movements*
   b. In the legs: Rhythmic motions consisting of dorsiflexion of the great toe and ankle possibly associated with flexion of the knee and hip
   c. Note the curious similarity to the "triple flexion reflex"
   d. The arms can also be involved
   e. The activity can be unilateral, bilateral, or may switch from side to side
   f. A single movement lasts 0.5 to 5.0 seconds
   g. The movements come in clusters with a frequency of one every 20 to 40 seconds
   h. A cluster can last minutes to hours
   i. More common in non-REM sleep
2. Restless legs syndrome (RLS)
   a. Four clinical criteria are necessary
      (1) A desire to move the limbs associated with paresthesias or dysesthesias
      (2) Motor restlessness
      (3) Symptoms only occur or are worst at rest and are partially or completely relieved by activity
      (4) Symptoms are worse in the evening or at night
   b. A common mistake is to call periodic limb movements restless legs

Epidemiology

1. Periodic limb movement syndrome
   a. Increases as patients age
      (1) Rarely, under 30 years of age
      (2) 5% of those between 30 and 50
      (3) 29% of those over 50
      (4) 44% of those over 65
   b. Present in 11% of asymptomatic healthy adults
2. Restless legs syndrome
   a. Patients present in middle age
   b. Symptoms have started in their 20s
   c. Prevalence is between 5% and 15% but often does not result in a visit to a physician

Etiology and Pathophysiology

1. Both the etiology and pathophysiology of PLMS and RLS are unknown.
2. It is likely that these conditions are mediated by the spinal cord.
3. The periodicity suggests some form of neural pacemaker.
4. The influence of cortical influences is unknown.

Clinical Features and Differential Diagnoses

1. PLMS
   a. Most patients are asymptomatic
   b. Frequently the complaints come from the bed partner
   c. Complaints of insomnia
   d. Complaints of daytime sleepiness
   e. Patients are older
   f. Differential diagnosis
      (1) Sleep starts
      (2) Epilepsy
      (3) Nocturnal leg cramps
2. RLS
   a. Four essential features (see above)
   b. Complaints of both sleep onset and sleep maintenance insomnia
   c. Periodic leg movements
   d. There can be a family history of RLS
   e. Patients are older
   f. Differential diagnosis
      (1) Akathisia
      (2) Peripheral neuropathy
      (3) Chronic pain
3. Associated conditions
   a. Polyneuropathy
   b. Uremia
   c. Iron deficiency
   d. Rheumatoid arthritis

479

Minimal Criteria for Restless Legs Syndrome

- Desire to move associated with paresthesias or dysesthesias

- Motor restlessness

- Worse or only present at rest with relief in activity

- Worse in the evening or at night

Testing

1. Neurologic examination is normal
2. Limb movements are confirmed by polysomnography
    a. PLM Index: Number of movements/Hours of sleep
    b. PLM Arousal Index: Number of movements with arousals/Hours of sleep
    c. Norms have not been determined.
    d. These indices may help in determining whether to treat PLMs.
3. Metabolic studies
    a. Serum iron
    b. Ferritin
    c. Serum magnesium
    d. Serum vitamin B_{12} and folate

Treatments

1. Clonazepam, 0.5 to 2.0 mg
2. Dopamine agonists
    a. Pergolide, 0.1 to 0.5 mg
    b. Pramipexole, 0.125 to 1.0 mg
3. Caridopa/levodopa
    a. 10/100 to 25/250 mg
    b. Long-acting, 50/100 mg

4. Anti-epileptic
    a. Gabapentin, 200 to 400 mg
    b. Carbamazepine, 100 to 400 mg
5. Opiates: Codeine is begun with 15 mg and titrated
6. Numerous and varied medications have been reported to be effective in small numbers of patients

Key Treatment Sequence

- Clonazepam

- Dopamine agonist

- Carbidopa/levodopa

- Anti-epileptics

- Opiates

- Other

Bibliography

Bucher SF, Seelos KC, Oertel WH, et al.: Cerebral generators involved in the pathogenesis of the restless legs syndrome. Ann Neurol 41:639–645, 1997.

Chesson AL, Wise M, Davila D, et al.: Practice parameters for the treatment of restless legs syndrome and periodic limb movement disorder. An American Academy of Sleep Medicine Report, Standards of Practice Committee of the American Academy of Sleep Medicine. Sleep 22:961–968, 1999.

Henning WA: Restless legs syndrome: a sensorimotor disorder of sleep/wake motor regulation. Curr Neurol Neurosci Rep 2:186–196, 2002.

Walters AS: Toward a better definition of the restless legs syndrome. The International Restless Legs Syndrome Study Group. Mov Disord 10;634–642, 1995.

Winkleman J, Wetter TC, Collado-Seidel V, et al.: Clinical characteristics and frequency of the hereditary restless legs syndrome in a population of 300 patients. Sleep 23:597–602, 2000.

4 Obstructive Sleep Apnea
Carl E. Rosenberg

Definition

1. In obstructive sleep apnea the posterior pharynx narrows or closes with inspiration. The respiratory block persists until an increased inspiratory pressure overcomes the mechanical block. *Obstructive sleep apnea* is defined as repetitive blockages during sleep.
2. The respiratory block causes respiratory events.
   a. *Apnea:* A complete cessation of airflow. The standard definition requires that it be longer than 10 seconds for clinical significance.
   b. An *obstructive apnea* is an apnea showing continued respiratory effort from the chest or abdomen.
   c. A *mixed apnea* is an apnea showing respiratory effort but that effort disappears during the respiratory event.
   d. A *central apnea* is an apnea without respiratory effort throughout its duration.
   e. *Hypopnea:* A partial cessation of airflow. The standardized American Academy of Sleep Medicine definition requires a 10-second duration, 30% loss of amplitude of airflow, and 4% decrease in Sao_2. The evolving standard is to consider all hypopneas meeting the standard definition as obstructive.

Epidemiology and Risk Factors

1. Obstructive sleep apnea occurs in 3% to 5% of the adult population.
   a. It occurs more often in men. Like other conditions, female risk increases after menopause.
   b. Obstructive sleep apnea is more likely to occur in people of African descent.
2. The risk of obstructive sleep apnea increases with obesity. However, excess weight is not a prerequisite.
3. Obstructive sleep apnea shows a strong association with heart disease and hypertension.

Caveat

• Obstructive sleep apnea shows a strong association with heart disease and hypertension.

Etiology and Pathophysiology

1. The pathophysiology is a complex interaction of skeletal and soft tissue anatomy, neuromuscular tone, and pulmonary function.
2. The muscles of the tongue and posterior pharynx decrease in tone during sleep.
3. This "floppy" tube collapses with the decreased pressure associated with inspiration.
4. The Venturi effect due to this narrowing results in vibration of the uvula and soft palate, namely, snoring. The volume of snoring is not well correlated with the severity of the apnea.
5. Any condition increasing "floppiness," narrowing the size of the size of the airway, or decreasing the ability to exchange air can exacerbate this condition.

Clinical Features

1. Excessive daytime sleepiness
   a. Passive sleepiness is sleepiness or falling asleep when engaged in activities not requiring motor activity or involving personal safety. These include reading, watching television, and going to movies.
   b. Active sleepiness is sleepiness or falling asleep when engaged in activities requiring motor activity or involve personal safety. These include driving, working with machinery, and conversations.
   c. Women will often refer more to fatigue than true sleepiness.
   d. Patients' reports of their sleepiness vary greatly and need not correlate with the degree of obstructive sleep apnea.
2. Loud disruptive snoring often resulting in partners sleeping separately.
3. Respiratory pauses manifested in breaks in snoring, awakenings with gasping, or reports that the patient stops breathing.
4. Hypertension often accompanies obstructive sleep apnea. Frequently there is a history of this hypertension being difficult to control.
5. Patients often complain of difficulty maintaining concentration, attention, or memory.
6. Patients will describe decreased libido or other difficulty with sexual function.

Key Signs

- Excessive daytime sleepiness
- Loud, disruptive snoring
- Respiratory pauses
- Hypertension
- Difficulty in concentration, attention, or memory
- Decreased libido

Differential Diagnosis

1. Depression: Patients with obstructive sleep apnea often have complaints similar to patients with depression. This can occur with or without daytime sleepiness.
2. Conditions with excessive daytime sleepiness
   a. Sleep-wake cycle disorders
   b. Narcolepsy
   c. Idiopathic and secondary hypersomnolence
   d. Long sleeper
3. Primary snoring

Laboratory Testing

1. Polysomnography
   a. All-night sleep testing (see Part XII, Chapter 1, Sleep and Testing)
   b. RDI (respiratory distress index)
      (1) Normal: RDI ≤ 5.
      (2) Mild: $5 \leq RDI \leq 15$
      (3) Moderate: $15 \leq RDI \leq 30$
      (4) Severe: RDI < 30
   c. Lowest Sao_2
   d. Cardiac arrhymias
2. Substitutes (all less than adequate)
   a. Nocturnal oximetry
   b. Recording of snoring
   c. Automated continuous positive airway pressure (CPAP) with recording of airflow limitations
   d. Actigraphy

Key Test

- Polysomnography

Treatment

1. Maintain continuous positive airway pressure
   a. This creates an air splint, keeping the posterior pharynx open.
   b. The patient needs to wear a mask (usually over the nose only) all night every night. The condition returns whenever the CPAP device is not used.
   c. The CPAP pressure is adjusted during a polysomnogram. The pressure is raised until both the respiratory events and snoring are eliminated.
2. Uvulopalatopharyngoplasty (UPPP)
   a. Removal of the uvula and much of the soft palate as possible
   b. Eliminates obstructive sleep apnea in 50% of patients.
3. Jaw advance
   a. The mandible of the jaw is separated and advanced. The base of the tongue is tethered down and may be de-bulked. The jaw is wired shut for up to 2 weeks.
   b. There are several variations on this theme.
   c. This procedure eliminates obstructive sleep apnea in 70% of patients.
4. Weight loss
   a. Usually a substantial loss of 50 pounds or more is required.
   b. It is difficult to lose weight without an accompanying treatment for the obstructive sleep apnea.
5. Ineffective treatments for moderate or worse obstructive sleep apnea. These treatments may be effective in correcting snoring alone.
   a. Somnoplasty
   b. Laser-assisted uvuloplasty
   c. Dental devices

Key Treatment

- Continuous positive airway pressure
- Uvulopalatopharyngoplasty
- Jaw advance
- Weight loss

Prognosis

1. Untreated obstructive sleep apnea
   a. Increased risk of heart disease and stroke

b. Exacerbation of hypertension; it is not clear if obstructive sleep apnea can cause hypertension

c. Worsening daytime sleepiness with attendant risk of accident

d. Decreased cognitive function (as measured on the Wechsler Adult Intelligence Scale, etc.) in severe cases. This deficit reverses with treatment.

2. Reversal of symptoms and risks with successful treatment.

Bibliography

American Academy of Sleep Medicine: Sleep related breathing disorders in adults: Recommendations for syndrome definition and measurement techniques in clinical research. Sleep 22:667–689, 1999.

Baldwin C, Griffith KA, Nieto J, et al.: The association of sleep-disordered breathing and sleep symptoms with the quality of life in the sleep heart health study. Sleep 24:96–105, 2001.

Flemons WW: Clinical practice. Obstructive sleep apnea. N Engl J Med 347:498–504, 2002.

Loube DI, Gray PC, Strohl KP, et al.: Indications for positive airway pressure treatment of adult obstructive sleep apnea patients: A consensus statement. Chest 115:863–866, 1999.

5 Parasomnias

Carl E. Rosenberg

Definitions

1. A parasomnia is an episodic event occurring in association with an individual's sleep.
2. Parasomnias are divided according to sleep cycle.
   a. Non-REM (rapid eye movement) sleep
   b. REM sleep
   c. Not definitely associated with one state or the other
3. Neurologists are usually asked to determine whether the event is epileptic.

Epidemiology

1. There is little known about the epidemiology of these disorders.
2. The non-REM disorders of arousal can begin as early as the age of 2 years and usually disappear by adolescence.
3. The prevalence of REM behavioral disorder is estimated at 0.5%.
   a. 90% in men
   b. Increased incidence with narcolepsy

Pathophysiology

1. Non-REM parasomnias, disorders of arousal, have a strong hereditary component.
2. REM parasomnias
   a. REM behavioral disorder is characterized by a failure of the system controlling atonia during REM sleep.
   b. It has been seen in the presence of
      (1) Acute withdrawal
      (2) Use of antidepressants
      (3) Cerebral insults: Trauma, vascular, infectious, and degenerative.
      (4) Idiopathic

Clinical Features

1. Non-REM disorders of arousal
   a. Sleepwalking
      (1) Can appear as merely sitting up in bed, extend to actual walking, or even attempts to escape
      (2) It is unusual for this to begin in adulthood
      (3) The patient is difficult to awaken and is amnesic of the event
      (4) It is not dangerous to awaken sleepwalkers, but they will be confused on awakening.
      (5) Sleepwalkers can hurt themselves.
   b. Sleep terrors (a.k.a. night terrors)
      (1) Abrupt arousal from sleep
      (2) Children show behaviors suggesting intense fear
      (3) Children do not recall the event in the morning.
      (4) This condition is not associated with a psychiatric condition, nor is it a response to a traumatic waking event.
   c. In adults these two forms often merge their behaviors.
   d. These events occur in the first half of sleep.
2. REM parasomnias
   a. REM behavioral disorder
      (1) Motor behavior occurring after 90 minutes of sleep, usually late in sleep.
      (2) These patients frequently injure themselves, usually by falling out of bed.
      (3) The patient may remember a dream or dream fragments, usually frightening.
      (4) Differential diagnosis
         (a) Epilepsy
         (b) Posttraumatic stress syndrome
         (c) Arousals with nightmares
   b. REM sleep–related sinus arrest
      (1) Episodes of asystole lasting up to 9 seconds and occurring in REM sleep only
      (2) Discovered in young healthy adults, most asymptomatic.
      (3) Waking electrocardiogram is entirely normal.
3. Other parasomnias
   a. Sleep starts
      (1) A myoclonic-like contraction of legs, and possibly other limbs, occurring at sleep onset.
      (2) These can be repetitive.
      (3) They usually do not indicate any pathology.
      (4) They can be seen in association with uremia.

484

b. Sleep enuresis
  (1) Bed-wetting that persists beyond 5 years of age.
  (2) There is a strong hereditary pattern.
  (3) It can persist into early adulthood.
  (4) Differential diagnosis
      (a) Nocturnal seizures
      (b) Enuresis returning after a patient has been dry can indicate a urologic problem.
      (c) Can be seen with obstructive sleep apnea

Distinguishing Arousal Disorders from REM Behavioral Disorder

Arousal Disorders
- Occur in the early part of sleep
- Strong family history
- Most adults have a history of childhood events

REM Behavioral Disorder
- Occurs in the latter part of sleep
- Appears later in life

Laboratory Testing—Polysomnography

1. Extra electroencephalogram (EEG) channels are often vital in distinguishing epileptic events from nonepileptic events.
2. Video monitoring is imperative.
3. Limb electromyelographic (EMG) electrodes may be of value.
4. Most of these paramonias are episodic, and a single polysomnogram is frequently normal.
5. Non-REM disorders of arousal
   a. Prior to the event the EEG shows deep sleep dominated by high-voltage slow delta waves.
   b. The event begins
      (1) There is an acute arousal, possibly heralded by hypersynchrony.
      (2) Muscle activity can obscure the record.
      (3) The EEG shows a pattern consistent with light sleep.
6. REM behavioral disorder
   a. Prior to the event
      (1) The EEG shows REM sleep.
      (2) The EMG while suppressed, often shows an increased number of muscle twitches.
   b. The event begins
      (1) The EEG continues to show REM sleep until an arousal or the event subsides
      (2) Prominent muscle activity is noted on the EMG.

Treatment

1. Non-REM disorders of arousal
   a. In children the primary treatment is to reassure the parents.
   b. In adults
      (1) Benzodiazpines
      (2) Tricyclic antidepressants
      (3) Carbamazepine
      (4) Hypnosis
2. REM behavioral disorder
   a. Clonazepam, 0.5 to 1.0 mg
   b. Environmental safety
3. REM-related sinus arrest
   a. Unknown
   b. No treatment?
   c. Pacemaker?
4. Enuresis
   a. Reassurance
   b. Alarm
   c. Tricyclic antidepressants
   d. Desmopressin (DDAVP)
   e. Urologic evaluation
   f. Look for an underlying sleep disorder or epilepsy in adults.

Bibliography

Hublin C, Kaprio J, Partinen M, Koskenvuo M: Nocturnal enuresis in a nationwide twin cohort. Sleep 21:579–585, 1998.

Kryger MH, Roth T, Dement WC (eds): Principles and Practice of Sleep Medicine. Philadelphia, W.B. Saunders, 2000.

Rattenborg NC, Linblom S, Best J, et al.: Sinus arrest during REM sleep in young adults. N Engl J Med 311:1106–1110, 1984.

Schenck CH, Mahowald MW: REM sleep behavior disorder: clinical, developmental, and neuroscience perspectives 16 years after its formal identification in SLEEP. Sleep 25:120–138, 2002.

Schenck CH, Pareja JA, Patterson AL, et al.: Analysis of polysomnographic events surrounding 252 slow-wave sleep arousals in thirty-eight adults with injurious sleep walking and sleep terrors. J Clin Neurophysiol 15:159–166, 1998.

6 Narcolepsy and Hypersomnias   *Carl E. Rosenberg*

Definition

1. Hypersomnias are conditions with increased need for sleep during the day (normal waking time) independent of the amount of sleep gained during the night (normal sleeping time).
2. Narcolepsy is a condition in which the increased sleep need is for REM sleep. Elements of REM sleep can appear without sleep.

Epidemiology and Risk Factors

1. Narcolepsy
   a. Narcolepsy requires a hereditary propensity combined with an unknown environmental inciting factor or event.
   b. Secondary narcolepsy is rare but has been reported, i.e., in multiple sclerosis.
   c. The prevalence is 0.05%.
   d. Males and females are equally affected.
   e. Onset is typically during the second or third decade of life.
2. Hypersomnias
   a. *Idiopathic hypersomnolence* is an unexpected increased need for sleep. It is usually a diagnosis of exclusion.
   b. *Secondary hypersomnolence* is an increased need for sleep usually seen in the context of diffuse cerebral injury, i.e., head trauma, progressive multifocal leukodystrophy, and so on.

Etiology and Pathophysiology

1. Narcolepsy
   a. There is a genetic predisposition acted on by environmental factors.
   b. Of narcoleptics, 85% share the HLA type DQB1*0602 (however, 12% to 38% of the population share this HLA allele).
   c. May be caused by damage to the hypocretin system.
      (1) Hypocretin I and II are synthesized in the posterior and lateral hypothalamus.
      (2) These neurons project to monoaminergic and cholinergic centers of the ascending reticular activating system.
      (3) Hypocretin in the cerebrospinal fluid may

be entirely absent or present at a reduced level.
      (4) A neuropathologic study in humans revealed a great reduction in hypocretin-producing cells.
2. Hypersomnolence: Little is known about the pathophysiology or epidemiology of this condition.

Clinical Features

1. Narcolepsy
   a. Excessive daytime sleepiness
      (1) Classically these are *sleep attacks*, unexpected bouts of severe sleepiness. The patient feels much better after a brief nap. The sleepiness persists if a nap is postponed or omitted.
      (2) Sleep attacks often occur in a boring or monotonous situation.
      (3) The patient need not go into REM in every nap.
      (4) Sleepiness is the first symptom of narcolepsy, often beginning around 15 years of age.
   b. Cataplexy
      (1) This is an acute loss of tone in some or all muscles during waking.
      (2) Cataplexy is most often elicited by laughter, but it can occur with other intense emotions.
      (3) Usually occurs with or after the onset of excessive daytime sleeping. The delay may be from 1 to 30 years.
      (4) Frequency can vary from daily to once a year.
   c. *Sleep paralysis* is a persistence of REM sleep atonia into waking. It occurs on awakening.
   d. Hypnogogic hallucinations
      (1) A "dream" that persists into waking. Often such dreams are frightening.
      (2) Often associated with sleep paralysis making them even more frightening.
   e. Complaints of poor or nonrestorative sleep. This occurs late in the course of the disease.
   f. Of patients with narcolepsy, 80% have sleepiness with at least one of the other symptoms;

20% have sleepiness, cataplexy, sleep paralysis, and hypnogogic hallucinations.

2. Hypersomnia
   a. Daytime sleepiness despite "sufficient" sleep.
   b. The degree of daytime sleepiness should be confirmed with polysomnography (PSG) and a multiple sleep latency test (MSLT).
   c. Diagnosis of exclusion
   d. Look for possible causes of the hypersomnia such as head trauma or encephalopathy.

Key Signs: Narcolepsy

- Excessive sleep during the day
- Cataplexy
- Sleep paralysis
- Hypnogogic halluncinations

Differential Diagnosis

1. Obstructive sleep apnea: Patients are very sleepy during the day. They can be mistaken for narcoleptics if they are thin with a weak history of snoring.
2. It may be difficult to distinguish between narcolepsy and hypersomnia on the basis of history alone. The MSLT may distinguish between the two.
3. Sleep–wake cycle disorders including delayed sleep phase: Patients complain of daytime sleepiness and insomnia. A careful sleep history and sleep diary should answer the question.
4. Isolated sleep paralysis can be seen in normal individuals.
5. Severe sleep deprivation can cause sleep paralysis or even cataplexy.
6. Depression: Patients with depression often complain of daytime sleepiness.
7. Hypothyroidism: Patients have daytime fatigue, other signs of hypothyroidism, and often snore.

Laboratory Testing

1. PSG
   a. Most often the polysomnogram is normal.
   b. It may show extra REM cycles.
2. MSLT
   a. Narcolepsy
      (1) Two or more sleep onset REMs (SOREMs)
      (2) A mean sleep latency shorter than 5 minutes

   (3) HLA testing can be used as evidence against a diagnosis of narcolepsy; it is not useful in confirming the diagnosis (see above).
   b. Hypersomnia
      (1) One or fewer sleep onset REMs.
      (2) The mean sleep latency is 6.5 minutes or less

Multiple Sleep Latency Test in Narcolepsy

- Mean sleep latency <5 minutes
- Two or more sleep onset REMs (SOREMs)

Treatment

1. For excessive daytime sleepiness
   a. Modafinil, 100 to 400 mg/day
   b. Methylphenidate, 10 to 60 mg/day
   c. Dextroamphetamine, 5 to 60 mg/day
   d. Strategic naps: 15- to 30-minute naps scattered throughout the day.
2. For cataplexy
   a. Fluoxetine, 20 to 60 mg/day
   b. Imipramine, 25 to 200 mg/day
   c. Cloripramine, 25 to 200 mg/day

Prognosis

1. The mean time for the diagnosis of narcolepsy from the onset of symptoms is 15 years.
2. Narcolepsy is a lifelong condition. However, as the demands of maintaining a schedule decrease, the ability to function without medications increases.

 Bibliography

Dement WC, Carskadon MA, Ley R: The prevalence of narcolepsy. Sleep Res 2:147, 1973.

International Classification of Sleep Disorders: Diagnostic and Coding Manual, Revised. Rochester, MN, American Sleep Disorders, 1997.

Mignot E, Lin X, Arrigoni J, et al.: DQB1*0602 and DQA1*0102 are better markers for narcolepsy in Caucasian and black Americans. Sleep 17:S60–S67, 1994.

Overeem S, Mignot E, Gert van Dijk J, Lammers GJ: Narcolepsy: Clinical features, new pathologic insights, and future perspectives. J Clin Neurophysiol 2:78–105, 2001.

Taheri S, Zeitzer JM, Mignot E: The role of hypocretins (orexins) in sleep regulation and narcolepsy. Annu Rev Neurosci 25:283–313, 2002.

1 Mild Head Injury and the Postconcussion Syndrome

Randolph W. Evans

Definition

1. Mild head injury is typically defined by the following criteria: a duration of loss of consciousness of 30 minutes or less or occurrence of being dazed without loss of consciousness, an initial Glasgow Coma Scale (GCS) score of 13 to 15 without subsequent deterioration, and absence of focal neurologic deficits without evidence of depressed skull fractures, intracranial hematoma, or other neurosurgical pathology.

2. The GCS is widely used as a rapid neurologic assessment for baseline and follow-up examinations (see Part XIII, Chapter 2, Moderate and Severe Head Injury, Table 2–1). Moderate head injury is defined by a score of 8 to 12; severe by a score of less than 8.

3. Concussion is a trauma-induced alteration in mental status that may or may not involve loss of consciousness.

4. The postconcussion syndrome (PCS) is a constellation of symptoms and signs that may occur alone or in combination following a usually mild head injury. Loss of consciousness does not have to occur for the PCS to develop.

5. PCS may be subdivided into an early phase and a late or persistent phase in which symptoms and signs persist for more than 6 months.

Epidemiology and Risk Factors

1. Mild head injury accounts for 75% or more of all head injuries.

2. The annual incidence of mild head injury in the United States is about 150 per 100,000 population or about 500,000 persons per year.

3. Estimates of the relative causes of mild head injury in the United States are as follows: motor vehicle accidents, 45%; falls, 30%; occupational accidents, 10%; recreational accidents, 10%; assaults, 5%.

4. About 50% of all patients with mild head injury are between the ages of 15 and 34 years.

5. Motor vehicle accidents are the cause more often in the young, and falls are more common in the elderly.

6. Men are more frequently injured than women with a 2:1 ratio.

7. Between 20% and 40% of people with mild head injuries in the United States do not seek treatment.

8. PCS develops in over 50% of people with mild head injuries.

Etiology and Pathophysiology

1. Can result in cortical contusions due to coup and contrecoup injuries and diffuse axonal injury from shear and tensile strain damage

2. Release of excitatory neurotransmitters including acetylcholine, glutamate, and aspartate may form a neurochemical substrate.

3. Impairment in cerebrovascular autoregulation may occur.

4. Structural and functional deficits have been demonstrated on magnetic resonance imaging (MRI), single photon emission computed tomography (SPECT), positron emission tomography (PET), and magnetic source imaging studies, as well as with neuropathology examination.

Clinical Findings

- Headaches

- Cranial nerve symptoms and signs

- Psychological and somatic complaints

- Cognitive impairment

- Rare sequelae

Clinical Findings

1. Headaches

   a. Epidemiology

      (1) Variably estimated to occur in 30% to 90% of patients who are symptomatic after mild head injury

      (2) Headache prevalence and lifetime duration are greater in people with mild head injury than in those with more severe trauma.

(3) According to International Headache Society (IHS) criteria, the onset of the headache should be within 2 weeks, although some experts suggest 3 months.

(4) Many patients have more than one headache type or headaches with migraine and tension features.

(5) Neck injuries commonly accompany head injuries and can cause headaches.

b. Tension type (see Part XI, Chapter 2, Tension-Type, Chronic Daily Headache, and Drug-Induced Headaches)

   (1) Account for perhaps 85% of PCS headaches

   (2) Can be associated with temporomandibular joint injury (see Part XI, Chapter 9, Other Headaches)

c. Occipital neuralgia (see Part XIII, Chapter 7, Whiplash Injuries)

d. Migraine

   (1) Recurring attacks of migraine with and without aura can result from mild head injury.

   (2) Footballer's migraine

      (a) Original description of young men playing soccer who had multiple migraines with auras triggered only by impact

      (b) Other types of minor head injury in other sports can trigger migraine, often in adolescents with a family history of migraine.

      (c) After minor head trauma, children, adolescents, and young adults can develop a variety of transient neurologic sequelae that are not always associated with headache and that are perhaps due to vasospasm. Five types: hemiparesis; somnolence, irritability, and vomiting; a confusional state; transient blindness, often precipitated by occipital impacts; and brainstem signs

e. Cluster type—a rare consequence

f. Supraorbital and infraorbital neuralgia

   (1) Shooting, tingling, aching, or burning pain that may be associated with decreased or altered sensation and sometimes decreased sweating in the appropriate nerve distribution.

   (2) Pain can be paroxysmal or fairly constant.

   (3) A dull aching or throbbing pain may also occur around the area of injury.

g. Scalp lacerations and local trauma

   (1) In the presence or absence of a laceration, an aching soreness, tingling, or shooting pain over the site of the original trauma can develop.

   (2) Symptoms may persist for weeks or months but rarely for more than 1 year.

h. Subdural and epidural hematomas

   (1) Can result from even minor trauma without loss of consciousness (see Part XIII, Chapter 3, Subdural and Epidural Hematomas)

   (2) Headaches caused by subdural hematomas are nonspecific, ranging from mild to severe and paroxysmal to constant, unilateral or bilateral. They are usually associated with at least one of the following: sudden onset; severe pain; exacerbation with coughing, straining, or exercise; and vomiting or nausea.

   (3) Headaches from epidural hematomas are also nonspecific and may be associated with nausea, vomiting, and memory impairment. They can be unilateral or bilateral.

Key Clinical Findings: Subdural Hematomas and Headaches

- Subdural hematomas can result from even minor trauma without loss of consciousness.

- Headaches are nonspecific, unilateral or bilateral, and associated with vomiting or nausea.

- Headaches may have sudden onset.

- Headaches may worsen with coughing, straining, or exercise.

i. Low cerebrospinal fluid pressure (CSF) headaches arising from a dural root sleeve tear or a cribiform plate fracture (see Part XI, Chapter 9, Other Headaches)

j. Dysautonomic cephalalgia

   (1) Rare headache due to injury of the anterior triangle of the neck or carotid shealth

   (2) Local pain may be followed weeks later by severe unilateral frontotemporal headache, ipsilateral increased sweating of the face, dilation of the ipsilateral pupil, blurred vision, ipsilateral photophobia, and nausea, which can occur a few times per month and last for hours or days.

k. Other types

   (1) Hemorrhagic cortical contusions can cause headache from subarachnoid hemorrhage.

(2) Headache arising from carotid and vertebral artery dissections (see Part XI, Chapter 9, Other Headaches)

(3) Rarely, hemicrania continua can be posttraumatic.

2. Cranial nerve symptoms and signs (also see Part XIII, Chapter 4, Cranial Neuropathy)

a. Dizziness is reported by 53% within 1 week of injury. Can have a central origin or be due to labyrinthine concussion, perilymph fistula, and benign positional vertigo

b. Blurred vision reported by 14%

(1) Usually due to convergence insufficiency

(a) Exact anatomic basis unknown

(b) Horizontal diplopia often after a period of reading

(c) Characterized by failure to maintain the esodeviation required for near tasks

(2) Optic nerve contusions may result in decreased visual acuity and hue discrimination (see Part X, Chapter 2, Optic Neuropathy).

(a) Can occur with indirect injuries, often without orbital or optic canal fracture from forces transmitted to the optic nerve from the globe and orbits; can occur without loss of consciousness after relatively minor head trauma

(b) Sites of injury include anterior or posterior optic nerve.

(c) Mild head injury can also cause diplopia caused by cranial nerve III, IV, and VI palsies.

c. After mild head injury, more than 5% of patients report decreased smell and taste resulting from olfactory nerve damage: the filaments may be torn from the cribiform plate, or the olfactory bulb may be contused or lacerated.

(1) Need to exclude ethmoid fractures, CSF rhinorrhea, and injury to the orbital surface of the frontal lobes

(2) More common with occipital trauma than frontal trauma

(3) Resolves in up to 50% of cases, usually during the first 3 months

d. Light and noise sensitivity reported by about 10%

3. Psychological and somatic complaints

a. Within 3 months of mild headache injury, 51% to 84% of patients have symptoms.

b. At least 35% are depressed; irritability is a symptom in 25%.

c. Posttraumatic stress disorder is common, especially after motor vehicle accidents and assaults.

d. Fatigue reported by 23% at 6 months

e. Sleep disturbance is common.

4. Cognitive deficits

a. Reported by up to 18% at 1 month

b. Common deficits include a reduction in information-processing speed, attention, reaction time, and memory for new information.

5. Rare sequelae

a. The incidence of subdural and epidural hematomas is 1% or less in adults after mild head injury.

b. Diffuse cerebral swelling is a rare potentially fatal complication usually occurring in children and adolescents and caused by impaired cerebral autoregulation.

c. Second impact syndrome

(1) Rare

(2) Diffuse cerebral swelling occurring after a second concussion in someone still symptomatic from an earlier one

(3) Concern over this rare entity is a major reason for guidelines for return to play after sports injuries.

d. Seizures may occasionally result.

e. Nonepileptiform seizures (pseudoseizures) usually follow mild head injury but not more severe head injury.

f. Transient global amnesia. In children, this entity may be due to confusional migraine.

g. Others—cerebral venous thrombosis and postural tremor

Differential Diagnosis

1. In patients with progressive clinical symptoms or an abnormal neurologic examination even after an initially negative computed tomography (CT) scan of the head, consider a delayed or chronic subdural or epidural hematoma.

2. If headaches are becoming more frequent, consider the possibility of medication rebound.

3. With time, other symptoms such as memory complaints of PCS will generally not worsen. In cases in which structural pathology has been excluded by neuroimaging, consider possibilities such as depression, anxiety, hysteria, somatiform disorder, compensation neurosis, and malingering.

Laboratory and Radiologic Testing

1. Electroencephalograms (EEG) are usually not indicated unless there is a suspicion of a seizure disorder.

   a. An abnormal EEG can not be attributed unequivocally to mild head injury in the absence of a preinjury study for comparison.

   b. EEG power spectral analyses or brain mapping are not indicated for routine clinical purposes because of issues of sensitivity and specificity.

2. Although auditory brainstem evoked potentials are sometimes abnormal, there is no correlation between abnormal results and PCS.

3. CT is the procedure of choice for the evaluation of acute head injury.

   a. Although a scan is usually negative, neurosurgical complications are present in up to 3% of mild head injuries.

   b. Skull radiographs are not usually indicated because of the greater sensitivity of CT.

4. Magnetic resonance imaging (MRI) scans

   a. More sensitive than CT in detecting brain contusions and diffuse axonal injury, especially in the frontal and temporal regions and brainstem.

   b. Occasionally MRI will detect an isodense subdural or vertex epidural hematoma not evident on CT.

5. SPECT may detect lesions not found on CT or MRI. However, the findings may not have prognostic significance and may be nonspecific. For example, depression and multi-drug abuse can produce deficits similar to those seen after mild head injury.

6. Neuropsychological testing

   a. Very helpful to evaluate persisting cognitive complaints

   b. Numerous problems associated with test sensitivity, specificity, reliability, and confounding subject characteristics

   c. Patients can be misdiagnosed as brain injured. The psychologist should be familiar with the findings in malingering and exaggerated memory deficits.

7. Neuro-otological evaluation which may include an electronystagmogram, audiogram, and ENT consultation may be indicated for the evaluation of vertigo.

8. Ophthalmologic evaluation, including visual fields, is helpful for patients with nonroutine or persistent visual complaints.

Treatment

1. Treatment is individualized after each of the problems is properly diagnosed.

2. Standard treatments as outlined in other chapters for posttraumatic tension-type headache, occipital neuralgia, migraine, and other. Beware of the potential for medication rebound and habituation from the use of various symptomatic medications.

3. The efficacy of cognitive rehabilitation is controversial.

4. Patients with prominent psychological symptoms may benefit from supportive psychotherapy and the use of antidepressant and antianxiety medications.

5. Benign position vertigo usually resolves with positional exercises.

6. Convergence insufficiency may respond to "pencil pushups" (focusing on the pencil eraser as it is repeatedly brought close to the eyes) or base-out prisms.

7. Education of the patient and family members, other physicians, and when appropriate, employers, attorneys, and representatives of insurance companies about PCS can be very helpful. There is widespread ignorance about the potential effects of mild closed head injury.

8. Return to play in sports

   a. The American Academy of Neurology has published a practice parameter on the management of concussion in sports. The report defines three grades of concussion (Table 1–1) and makes recommendations for initial management after the first event (Table 1–2) and when to return to play after removal from the contest (Table 1–3).

TABLE 1–1. AMERICAN ACADEMY OF NEUROLOGY GRADING SCALE OF CONCUSSION SUSTAINED IN SPORTING EVENTS

GRADE 1

1. Transient confusion
2. No loss of consciousness
3. Concussion symptoms or mental status abnormalities on examination resolve in less than 15 minutes

GRADE 2

1. Transient confusion
2. No loss of consciousness
3. Concussion symptoms or mental status abnormalities on examination last more than 15 minutes

GRADE 3

1. Any loss of consciousness, either brief (seconds) or prolonged (minutes)

TABLE 1–2. INITIAL MANAGEMENT FOLLOWING FIRST EVENT

GRADE	ON-SITE EVALUATION	NEUROLOGIC EVALUATION	SAME DAY RETURN TO PARTICIPATION
Grade 1	Yes	Not required but may be pursued, depending on clinical evaluation	Yes, if normal sideline assessment at rest and with exertion, including detailed mental status examination
Grade 2	Yes	Yes	No
Grade 3	Yes	Yes	No

From Report of the Quality Standards Subcommittee of the American Academy of Neurology: Practice parameter: the management of concussion in sports (summary statement). Neurology 48:581, 1997, with permission.

b. These parameters are practice options because they are based on literature review and expert opinion.

Key Treatment

- Treatment is individualized.
- Standard treatments for posttraumatic tension-type headache, occipital neuralgia, and migraine
- Efficacy of cognitive rehabilitation controversial
- Patients with prominent psychological symptoms may benefit from supportive psychotherapy and antidepressant and antianxiety medications.
- Benign position vertigo usually resolves with positional exercises.
- Convergence insufficiency may respond to "pencil pushups" or base-out prisms.
- Education of the patient and, when appropriate, others about the effects of postconcussion syndrome

Prognosis

1. Risk factors
   a. Persistence and severity of symptoms and neu-

TABLE 1–3. WHEN TO RETURN TO PLAY AFTER REMOVAL FROM CONTEST

GRADE OF CONCUSSION	TIME UNTIL RETURN TO PLAY*
Multiple grade 1 concussions	1 week
Grade 2 concussion	1 week
Multiple grade 2 concussions	2 weeks
Grade 3—brief loss of consciousness (seconds)	1 week
Grade 3—prolonged loss of consciousness (minutes)	2 weeks
Multiple grade 3 concussions	1 month or longer, based on clinical decision of evaluating physician

*Only after being asymptomatic with normal neurologic assessment at rest and with exercise.
From Report of the Quality Standards Subcommittee of the American Academy of Neurology: Practice parameter: the management of concussion in sports (summary statement). Neurology 48:581, 1997, with permission.

ropsychological deficits are not predicted by a loss of consciousness of less than 1 hour compared with a patient just being dazed.

b. Significant predictors for return to work by 3 months after the injury include older age; higher level of education, employment, and socioeconomic status; and greater income.

c. Those with a higher IQ recover faster than those with a lower IQ.

d. Persistent symptoms are more likely with age older than 40 years, female gender, and prior head injury.

2. Symptoms

a. Most patients will recover within a few months.

b. Headaches may persist: one year, 8% to 35%; 2 years, 24%; 4 years, 24%.

c. Dizziness is still reported by 18% at 2 years; subjective memory complaints, by 19% at 4 years.

d. Cognitive deficits usually resolve within 3 to 6 months, although a minority of patients have persistent problems.

3. Effect of litigation

a. Those with litigation are quite similar to those without with regard to improvement of symptoms with time, types of headaches, cognitive test results, and response to antimigraine medications.

b. Symptoms usually do not resolve with the settlement of litigation.

c. Pending litigation may increase the level of stress for some claimants.

d. Some claimants have persisting complaints due to secondary gain, malingering, and psychological disorders.

e. Potential indicators of malingering

(1) Premorbid factors: antisocial and borderline personality traits, poor work record, prior claims for injury

(2) Behavioral characteristics: uncooperative, evasive, or suspicious

(3) Neuropsychological test performance: missing random items, giving up easily, inconsistent test profile, frequently saying "I don't know"

(4) Postmorbid complaints: describing events surrounding the injury in great detail or reporting an unusually large number of symptoms

(5) Others: engaging in general activities not consistent with reported deficits; having significant financial stressors; resistance, and exhibiting a lack of reasonable follow-through on treatments

Bibliography

Evans RW: Postconcussion syndrome. In Evans RW, Baskin DS, Yatsu FM (eds): Prognosis of Neurological Disorders. New York, Oxford University Press, pp. 366–380, 2001.

Evans RW: Posttraumatic headaches. In Evans RW, Mathew NT (eds): Handbook of Headache. Philadelphia, Lippincott Williams & Wilkins, 2000, pp. 117–138.

McCrea M, Kelly JP, Randolph C, et al.: Immediate neurocognitive effects of concussion. Neurosurgery 50: 1032–1040, 2002.

Report of the Quality Standards Subcommittee of the American Academy of Neurology: Practice parameter: the management of concussion in sports (summary statement). Neurology 48:581–585, 1997.

Young WB, Packard RC, Ramadan N: Headaches associated with head trauma. In Silberstein SD, Lipton RB, Dalessio DJ (eds): Wolff's Headache and Other Head Pain, 7th ed. New York, Oxford University Press, 2001, pp. 325–348.

Ajay Jawahar
Anil Nanda

2 Moderate and Severe Head Injury

Definition

A patient with head trauma presenting with an initial Glasgow Coma Scale score (GCS; Table 2–1) of 8 to 12 is categorized as moderate; less than 8, as severe.

Epidemiology and Risk Factors

1. Head injuries in the United States, as in all industrialized countries, are frequent. According to a recent study, an estimated 8.1 million Americans have suffered some form of head injury, of which 1.9 million (23%) were associated with the danger of brain damage. In general, 20% of head injuries were classified as major and potentially life-threatening. Data reveals that of all people injured in traffic accidents in the United States, 70% had head injuries; 66% of these were classified as mild, 24% as moderately severe, and 5% as severe, with 5% mortality.

2. These head injuries resulted in 9.6 million lost days from work and 6.6 million days of hospitalization. Out of all these head injuries, 21% involve contusion of the scalp and face; 62%, laceration of the scalp; and 16%, cerebral contusion or intracerebral hematomas.

Etiology and Biomechanics

1. It is estimated that 75% of all head injuries are the result of traffic accidents, while 25% are of industrial or other origin.

2. Among men under 35, accidents are the chief causes of death and are responsible for more than 50% of deaths in men between 15 and 24 years of age. Among women, accidents are the leading cause of death in those under 25 years of age; they account for 40% of deaths from women 15 to 19 years of age.

3. In trauma to the skull, the hair and scalp have some dampening effect on the impact. However, the brunt of the blow is delivered to the skull, which is elastic enough to be flattened or indented when struck with a blunt object. The maximum indentation occurs instantly and is followed within a few milliseconds by several oscillations. When the skull is bent beyond its elastic tolerance, it breaks. This may result in a simple linear fracture extending from the center of the impact toward the base.

4. A more severe blow results in a stellate fracture, and an even more forceful blow can lead to a depressed fracture. The type of fracture depends not only on the velocity of the blow but also, and more important, on the size and surface of the object striking the skull.

5. A pointed object may perforate the skull, whereas an object with a large, blunt end impacting on the skull at the same velocity may cause a depression.

6. The skull travels faster than the brain under the same impact. Although the brain is frequently contused by the in-bending skull at the site of the impact, severe surface injuries occur in the brain when it is hurled by inertial pressure against the inner table, particularly against its rough, bony prominences. Deeper contusions in the substance of the brain are due to inertial stress from relative movements of the brain and pressure gradients.

7. While so-called coup lesions of the brain occur at or close to the point of impact, the contrecoup lesions develop at approximately the opposite end of impact. The characterization of the biomechanics of the "coup contrecoup" contusions is as follows:

   a. Coup contusions are caused by the slapping effect of the in-bending bone during impact.

   b. The movement of the brain against irregular and rough bony surfaces causes contrecoup contusions.

8. When the head is relatively fixed, a blunt impact causes a coup lesion with no contrecoup effect.

9. When the head is free to move, a blunt impact will cause contrecoup lesion but little or no coup effect.

Pathophysiology

In addition to linear or translational acceleration, rotational acceleration also plays an important role in injuring the brain. It has been shown that the brain oscillates in a rotational axis after any significant blow and that cerebral concussion, gross contusions, and even hemorrhages over the brain surface can be produced by rotational displacement of the head upon extreme motion of the neck. During impact, the

494

TABLE 2–1. GLASGOW COMA SCALE

Eye Opening		
	Spontaneous	4
	To speech	3
	To pain	2
	None	1
Verbal Response		
	Oriented	5
	Confused conversation	4
	Inappropriate words	3
	Inappropriate sounds	2
	No response	1
Motor Response		
	Obeys	6
	Localizes pain	5
	Withdraws from pain	4
	Flexor response	3
	Extensor response	2
	No response	1

cerebrospinal fluid (CSF) contained in the major basal cisterns offers some protection to the brain. However, this protective layer is insufficient in the shallow subarachnoid space around the frontal and temporal lobes. Dural tears, extracerebral and intracerebral hematoma, and contusions can occur at the coup or contrecoup sites in the brain. Such contusions are much more common on the impacted side in depressed fractures. Epidural hematomas arising from a torn meningeal artery are almost invariably on the impact side, but contralateral subdural hematomas develop in about one-third of all patients. The pathophysiology of brain injury can be best understood by studying the changes in cerebral metabolism, cerebral blood flow, the blood–brain barrier, and cerebral edema.

1. Cerebral metabolism
   a. Energy is normally produced in the brain by an oxidative mechanism, but the brain does not have the capacity to store oxygen.
   b. Under normal conditions, cerebral metabolism consumes 25% of total body glucose. When plasma glucose level drops to 70 mg/100 ml, the first signs of cerebral dysfunction start appearing; and at levels below 20 mg/100 ml, coma ensues.
   c. In the case of traumatic or hypoxic damage to the normal aerobic pathways, anaerobic glucose metabolism occurs in the brain as a compensatory mechanism. This results in the formation of lactate as a by-product that dilates cerebral blood vessels and temporarily increases the oxygen supply to the brain.
   d. Severe concussion results in greatly increased lactate production.

2. Cerebral blood flow
   a. Normally, the rate of cerebral blood flow is between 50 and 60 ml/min for each 100 gm of brain tissue.
   b. This constant flow is maintained by an autoregulatory mechanism that is based on active vascular responses.
   c. The arterioles constrict when the perfusion pressure rises, and they dilate when the pressure is low.
   d. Changes in cerebral arterial O_2 and CO_2 concentration also influence cerebral blood flow.
   e. When PO_2 is low, the flow increases markedly, while a decrease of PCO_2 results in alkalosis, constriction of small arteries, and reduction of cerebral blood flow.
   f. Elevated PCO_2 causes acidosis, vasodilatation, and increased flow.
   g. A relatively normal range of arterial blood pressure is required for autoregulation of cerebral blood flow (CBF). The system does not work properly when perfusion pressure falls below 60 mm Hg. When the pressure rises above 150 mm Hg in a normotensive subject, the arterioles become dilated beyond their autoregulatory constrictive capacity.
   h. Autoregulation is easily abolished by trauma. This results in widespread hypoxia with lactic acid accumulation, which in turn causes vasodilatation.
   i. Paradoxical reactions may also develop. A vasodilator stimulus, such as increased arterial PCO_2, may result in a total or regional decreased cerebral blood flow in a traumatized brain.
   j. Cerebral blood flow undergoes considerable change in severe head injuries. Significant reduction in arterial blood perfusion of the entire brain or large portions interferes with normal metabolism and generally has a poor prognosis and outcome.
   k. In the final stages of cerebrovascular decompensation, intracranial and arterial pressures are inseparable, and cerebral blood flow ceases completely. The patient passes into shock and respiratory arrest occurs.

3. Blood–brain barrier
   a. The blood–brain barrier system consists of a series of membranes regulating the passage of fluid and molecules from the intravascular to the extravascular compartments within the brain.
   b. In severe injuries to the brain, the barrier is virtually wiped out by the destruction of anatomic substrates in the contused tissue. The restitution of the barriers depends on the process of tissue healing.
   c. Cerebral healing occurs through the formation of glial scar, which, in itself, is a slow process.

The blood–brain barrier, therefore, may remain leaky for several months, even after complete clinical recovery of a head-injured person. This is demonstrated by a positive radioactive brain scan over the area of injury.

4. Brain edema

   a. Brain edema is caused by accumulation of excess water in the brain tissue.

   b. Traumatic edema is considered vasogenic because the source of the excess water is the bloodstream.

   c. The arteries, veins, and capillaries are all torn in the contused brain. This leads to multiple small hemorrhages within the area.

   d. The red blood corpuscles are soon caught in the mesh of tissue while plasma propagates much further. The site for the development of edema is usually white matter, even in cortical injuries. This is believed to be due to the structural compactness of the gray matter.

   e. The fluid in traumatic edema is like proteinaceous plasma that contains albumin.

   f. The edematous tissue has excess sodium and chloride, but it is low in potassium content.

   g. It is commonly believed that posttraumatic edema is maximal after 24 hours of injury and then begins to subside; however, clinical experience indicates that it can develop within a few hours and can persist for weeks.

Clinical Features

Moderate and severe head injury usually results in the development of intracranial hematomas or cerebral contusions, or both. The various clinical aspects of epidural hematoma and subdural hematoma are discussed in Part XIII, Chapter 3 (Subdural and Epidural Hematomas), so here we will only discuss a few general principles of clinical assessment.

1. State of consciousness

   a. From a purely practical point of view, the state of a patient's consciousness can be described according to the patient's spontaneous activity, response to painful stimulus, and reaction to a set of various verbal commands.

   b. The state of consciousness is usually altered in moderate and severe injuries to the brain. This is caused by a sudden rise of pressure in the region of neurons critical to consciousness.

   c. Cerebral ischemia, diffuse cerebral edema, depolarization of neurons by changes in the neurotransmitter release, and possible physical damage to the neurons also play an important role in altering the patient's consciousness.

   d. Various coma scales are used to evaluate and document the state of consciousness. They are all based on the original Glasgow Coma Scale with different modifications (see Table 2–1).

2. Pupils and ocular movements

   a. The size of the pupils, their equality, and their reaction to light can provide a valuable diagnostic aide in head-injured patients.

   b. The movements of the eyes can also give considerable information about the type and severity of the brain injury.

   c. When the patient is in a stupor or comatose state, it is necessary to depend on the position of the eyes at rest or on reflex eye movements.

   d. Reflex movements include the oculocephalic (doll's-eye) reflex and the oculovestibular reflex. Unconscious patients with diffuse or bilateral hemispheric damage frequently reveal a lack of conjugation between the eyes, resulting in a divergent strabismus.

3. Focal neurologic signs

   a. A variety of neurologic dysfunctions may result from contusions or penetrating injuries to the brain.

   b. In a discrete circumscribed injury, the resulting deficit may also be quite discrete, yet brain dysfunction may be widespread and hardly distinguishable from injury to the total brain mass or generalized brain compression.

4. Decerebrate rigidity

   a. The body, particularly the limbs, of many patients with lethal brain injury are rigid. This extensor hypertonicity of the skeletal muscles is generally considered a sign of mid-brain damage and carries a very grave prognosis.

   b. In full decerebrate rigidity, all four limbs are extended, with the upper limbs being more extended than the lower. The arms are adducted and rotated inwards. The feet are in plantar flexion. All of these patients, with very rare exceptions, are in deep coma.

Key Clinical Features: Examining a Patient with Head Injury

- Consciousness

- Pupils and eye movements

- Focal neurologic deficits

- Posture and rigidity

Intracerebral Hematoma

1. Posttraumatic intracerebral hematomas are related to the contusion of the brain and are caused by rotational acceleration.

2. Most occur in the low frontal or temporal regions. They may be found (1) directly beneath a depressed fracture, (2) adjacent to an area of cortical laceration or contusion, or (3) within the centrum of the lobe without evidence of an overlying contusion.

3. The size of a clinically significant hematoma varies considerably, ranging between 30 and 160 ml.

4. Early hematomas are solid, but they begin liquefying after a few days.

5. Eventually they consist of dark, thick fluid that can be aspirated. Surgical aspiration leaves behind a large cavity filled with CSF that occasionally gets connected to the ventricular system.

Diagnostic Methods

1. Technical diagnostic methods are essential for establishing an accurate diagnosis and have a direct bearing on the management strategies for head-injured patients.

2. A number of diagnostic imaging procedures are available that, when properly selected, lead to a quick and accurate diagnosis of the magnitude of brain injury. Some of the more commonly used imaging modalities are discussed below.

   a. Plain roentgenogram: Radiographic examination of the skull must be a part of the evaluation of any head-injured patient. This should include, posteroanterior (Caldwell), half-axial (Towne), facial (Water), and both lateral views of the skull with the patient lying in a supine position. These radiographs are evaluated for skull fractures, foreign bodies, displacement of the calcified choroids plexus, air-fluid levels in the sinuses, and other objective evidence of significant brain injury.

   b. Computed tomography (CT scanning) consists of determination of density to x-rays of structures within a slice of tissue and presentation of data as a two-dimensional image. This is the single most informative modality in the evaluation of head injured patients. Two main attributes of CT that make it ideally suited to the patient with head injury are (1) the ability to differentiate blood from brain and (2) the ability to depict the effect of trauma on the brain. A routine examination consists of 8 or 10 slices from the base of the skull to the vertex without using any contrast. Blood is visible as a uniformly hyperdense area, while contusions consist of poorly defined areas of mottled density and punctate high-density structures mixed with areas of normal brain density, surrounded by low-density edema.

   c. Cerebral angiography: It is seldom indicated in an acute situation if a CT scanner is available. However, if the CT scan is not available, cerebral angiography is a useful alternative for detecting injury to the cranial contents. It is also useful if the accident is suspected due to the rupture of a pre-existing cerebral aneurysm or arteriovenous malformation. Angiography depicts extracerebral hematomas as well as a CT scan does, but it is unable to differentiate an intracerebral hematoma from a contusion or other avascular mass lesions.

Key Radiologic Features: Head Trauma

- Skull fractures
- Epidural hematoma
- Subdural hematoma
- Contusions
- Intracerebral hematoma
- Blood in the ventricles

Key Tests

- Roentgenogram
- Computed tomography
- Cerebral angiography (if CT not available)

Emergency Treatment

Patients with severe head injuries should be assessed immediately. A proper diagnosis must be established and supportive and/or aggressive treatment instituted without delay. Rapid attention should be paid to the following to serve as a guide to further treatment:

1. Provision for adequate airway and ventilation

2. Observation of vital signs and a search for associated injuries

3. Assessment of the state of consciousness

4. Quick, but thorough, neurologic examination

5. Detailed history of the accident/trauma, if possible

Medical Treatment

1. In all cases of moderate or severe head injury, a catheter should be inserted into a vein of the upper limb and kept open for fluid administration and blood transfusions if necessary.

2. Blood should be drawn for all biochemical tests, hematocrit, and grouping. Central venous pressure monitoring is useful when severe blood loss is suspected.

3. Intravenous fluids should be administered in a restricted fashion during the first two days. The preferred fluid is glucose and N/2 saline.

4. An indwelling catheter in the bladder is helpful in maintaining an accurate intake-output balance chart.

5. Because a rise in intracranial pressure (ICP) either already exists or is anticipated, appropriate measures may be taken early by administering hyperosmotic solutions, corticosteroids, and/or diuretics.

6. Simultaneous administration of corticosteroids and hyperosmolar solutions is generally recommended.

7. Status epilepticus, a potentially life-threatening complication leading to severe cerebral hypoxia, must be stopped immediately.

8. Intravenous infusion of phenytoin sodium at a rate of less than 100 mg per minute in a dosage of 10–17 mg/kg is a safe and effective means of rapidly terminating the status epilepticus. Diazepam is another effective drug for controlling seizures. It should be given as an intravenous injection in adults (5–10 mg). If need arises, the injection can be repeated at 10 to 15 minute intervals up to a maximum dose of 30 mg. The drug should be injected in a large vein, allowing at least 1 minute for delivery of every 5 mg.

Intensive Care

1. Patients with severe head injury should be kept in an intensive care unit as long as necessary.

2. There is evidence to suggest that mortality and morbidity in severe head injury can be reduced by as much as 20% with modern-day intensive care. This decrease results from the avoidance of secondary complications such as cerebral herniation, raised ICP, hypoxia, and other medical complications.

Surgical Treatment

1. Continuous intracranial pressure monitoring is now a routine matter in most neurosurgical centers with head-injury units. It provides immediate information that leads to early detection and correction of increased ICP before herniation develops. It also provides information about the efficacy of the treatment, the extent of injury and, potentially, the final outcome.

2. A variety of subdural, intracortical, and intraventricular catheters and devices are available these days that can be positioned in the cranium to monitor ICP. The placement does not require the patient to be wheeled into the operating room or to be anesthetized.

3. Depressed skull fractures should be elevated and repaired on an emergency basis to prevent infection if the scalp over the fracture is lacerated. Depression under an intact scalp, frequently seen in infants, but occasionally in adults, can be repaired on an elective basis.

4. Missile wounds caused by high-velocity projectiles and resulting in massive brain lacerations should be immediately explored and widely debrided. Small and low-velocity bullets cause many civilian injuries from projectiles with relatively little destruction. These are best treated conservatively unless a major intracranial hematoma is present. The entrance and exit wounds must, of course, be debrided and closed, including the dura.

5. The management of acute epidural and subdural hematomas is discussed in greater details in Part XIII Chapter 3, Subdural and Epidural Hematomas.

Key Treatment

- Perform thorough assessment
- Maintain airway, breathing, and circulation
- Maintain CSF pressure
- Anti-edema drugs
- Anti-convulsants
- Radiology
- Surgery

Assessment and Prognosis in Severe Head Injury

1. In many cases of head injury, it is difficult in the acute stage to establish a prognosis. It has been estimated that 60% of deaths in patients with significant head injury occur before admission to the hospital.

2. The consensus derived from several statistical evaluations indicates that the mortality in primary

brain injury is about 30% except in children below 10 years, in whom it is around 20%.

3. Studies have shown that final restitution of mental functions takes place in about 80% of patients who regain consciousness within a day of the injury.

4. Despite all the advances in treatment and the establishment of intensive care units, the influence of treatment on recovery is still somewhat disputed; some physicians believe that the extent of brain injury in large measure determines the final outcome.

5. It is clear that aggressive treatment, aimed at avoiding secondary damage to the brain due to hypoxic or ischemic events and raised ICP, can salvage patients who otherwise would succumb to the injuries. However, even with early diagnosis and intensive management, the mortality in severe head injuries continues to be high.

Bibliography

Bakay L, Glasauer FE, Alker GJ Jr: Head injury. Boston, Little, Brown, 1980.

Barrow DL (ed): Complications and sequelae of head injury; Neurosurgical topics American Association of Neurosurgeons Park Ridge, IL, 1992.

Cooper PR, Golfinos JG (eds): Head injury, 4th ed. New York, McGraw-Hill, 2000.

Evans RW (ed): Neurology and Trauma. Philadelphia, W.B. Saunders, 1996.

3 Subdural and Epidural Hematomas

Amitabha Chanda
Anil Nanda

Definition

Epidural and subdural hematomas are examples of focal intracranial injury. They differ from each other with regard to their mechanism, presentations, treatment, and outcome. Additionally, the pathogenesis, presentations, treatment, and outcome of acute subdural hematoma are different from those of chronic subdural hematoma. Although, in this chapter, we will primarily discuss traumatic hematomas, it should be remembered that hematomas can occur without trauma.

Epidemiology

1. Epidural hematoma (EDH)
   a. Epidural hematoma, an accumulation of blood between the inner table of the skull and the dura, occurs in less than 2% of patients admitted with head injury.
   b. It is more common in young adults, and less common in children younger than 2 years of age and in adults older than 60 years of age. This may be due to increased adherence of the dura to the inner table of the skull in the elderly. Posterior fossa EDH and bilateral EDH (typically bifrontal) are more common in infants and children.
   c. Epidural hematomas can occur as a result of falls, vehicular accidents, or assaults, among other traumatic events.
2. Subdural hematoma (SDH)
   a. Hemorrhages occurring at the dura–arachnoid interface produce SDH.
   b. Subdural hematomas may be acute, subacute, or chronic. Those that develop immediately after injury are called *acute*, those developing from 3 days to 3 weeks after injury are termed *subacute*, and those appearing later are called *chronic*. However, the subacute variety may present either like an acute SDH or like a chronic SDH. For practical purposes, subdural hematoma is classified into acute and chronic.
   c. Acute subdural hematoma occurs in 5% to 22% of patients admitted to the hospital with severe head injury, and is more likely to occur in elderly people.
   d. Chronic subdural hematoma occurs in 1 to 2

per 100,000 people per year. It commonly occurs in elderly subjects due to shrinking of the brain as a result of atrophy. In a significant proportion there may be no history of overt injury.
   e. Chronic subdural hematomas can occur in younger subjects who have chronic alcoholism or coagulopathies.

Mechanism, Pathogenesis, and Pathology

1. Epidural hematoma
   a. Epidural hematoma occurs solely as a result of the contact effects of trauma. During impact, there is tensile strain on the inner table of the skull and compressive strain on the outer table of the skull. Because bone is less resistant to tensile strain than to compressive strain, the inner table breaks and follows the path of least resistance, leading to torn dural vessels. Although in most EDH (90%) there is an associated skull fracture, it can occur without a skull fracture. Local bending of the bone can cause a tear in a blood vessel without breaking the bone, especially when the bone is compliant. This explains the reduced incidence of fracture with EDH in children.
   b. Epidural hematoma can result from injury to the middle meningeal artery (the most common cause) or vein, diploic veins, and dural venous sinuses. The hematoma enlarges as the dura mater is stripped from the bone by the direct trauma and by the hydrostatic forces of the blood.
   c. Although mostly acute, delayed-onset and chronic epidural hematomas can occur (9% to 10% of all EDH). The risk factors for development of delayed EDH are (a) sudden reduction of intracranial pressure, (b) rapid correction of hypovolemic shock in a polytrauma patient, and (c) a patient with coagulopathy.
   d. In adults, EDH are typically located in the temporal or frontal region. The size of the hematoma depends on the degree of adherence of the dura mater to the skull, depth of incorporation of the vessel into the inner table of the skull, and size of the injured vessel.

e. The hematoma in a typical EDH is clotted. True encapsulation can occur in chronic forms.

2. Acute subdural hematoma (ASDH)

   a. Acute subdural hematoma can occur both by contact effects and by inertial effects.

   b. In uncomplicated subdural hematoma (without cortical contusions/lacerations), there is tearing of the parasagittal bridging veins. In quick succession, accelerations from the strain propagate along the brain surface and through the veins. When the strain tolerance is exceeded, the vein ruptures and a hematoma develops. This typically occurs after a fall or an assault.

   c. The complicated form of subdural hematoma (associated with cortical contusion/laceration) may result either from contact loading or inertial loading.

      (1) During contact loading, coup contusions or lacerations can occur when the brain surface and vessels lying beneath the area of the skull deformation are traumatized. This can occur directly, by compressive strain, or indirectly, by tensile strain caused by high negative pressure.

      (2) The inertial injury is usually associated with diffuse parenchymal injury, and the severity depends on the duration of the acceleration. This diffuse injury is manifested by brain shifting and obliteration of basal cistern and usually has a greater influence on the patient's outcome.

   d. Infantile acute SDH is a special type of ASDH occurring in an infant as a result of minor head trauma without initial loss of consciousness or cerebral contusion. It occurs in children less than 2 years of age and commonly results from a fall backward from a sitting or standing position. It may also be seen in association with child abuse or the "shaken baby syndrome." Additionally, there may be associated retinal or preretinal hemorrhages.

   e. The clotted blood in ASDH is mixed with cerebrospinal fluid (CSF), as there is some tearing of the arachnoid membrane and escape of CSF into the subdural space.

3. Chronic subdural hematoma (CSDH)

   a. Chronic subdural hematoma occurs by the same mechanism as uncomplicated subdural hematoma.

   b. If the amount of blood collected is small or if there is a sizable hematoma in a patient with brain atrophy, there may not be any symptoms. In a week or so, a membrane beneath the dura mater covers the hematoma, and in about 3 weeks a membrane forms between the hematoma and the arachnoid membrane. Eventually, the hematoma liquifies and then enlarges. In some instances, there may be resorption of the hematoma.

   c. To date, it is not known unequivocally why the hematoma enlarges or reduces in size. It is possible that albumin diffuses across the membrane and causes absorption of CSF. Moreover, the hematoma will enlarge with recurrent hemorrhages.

Clinical Features

1. Epidural hematoma: The clinical presentation of EDH depends mainly on the size of the hematoma, its location, the rapidity of collection of blood, and associated brain injury. Depending on these factors, several presentations may occur singly or in combination.

   a. Altered sensorium: The patient may be unconscious from the onset of the injury. This implies diffuse brain injury of some degree apart from the epidural hematoma. If the diffuse injury is mild enough and the hematoma is not too large or too rapidly collected, the patient usually regains consciousness. However, prolonged unconsciousness is expected if the diffuse injury is severe. If there is no diffuse injury, the loss of consciousness may appear late because of raised intracranial pressure or brain shift caused by enlargement of the clot. Thus a patient may be (1) conscious throughout, (2) unconscious throughout, (3) initially conscious and subsequently unconscious, or (4) initially unconscious and subsequently conscious, and that period of consciousness may or may not be followed by unconsciousness. The concept of "lucid interval" [unconsciousness → consciousness (lucid interval) → unconsciousness] has been associated with EDH. However, lucid interval is, in no way, pathognomonic for EDH.

   b. Features of raised intracranial pressure may include headache, vomiting, abducens palsy, papilledema, bradycardia, and hypertension. If the rise in intracranial pressure is progressive or rapid, it may cause loss of consciousness. The features of uncal herniation may appear in the form of ipsilateral pupillary dilatation (from compression of ipsilateral oculomotor nerve) or contralateral hemiparesis (from compression of the ipsilateral cerebral peduncle). In late herniation, bilateral pupillary dilatation (from compression of contralateral oculomotor nerve) and flaccid paralysis (from progressive compression of contralateral cerebral peduncle) appears. The respiratory pattern also changes progressively. Patients with posterior fossa epidural hematoma may have unconsciousness, neck pain/rigidity, vomiting, and cerebellar signs. Additionally, they may suddenly slip into the disastrous consequences of apnea resulting from tonsillar herniation.

c. Focal neurologic deficits (e.g., hemiparesis, monoparesis, or paraparesis) may occur, depending on the location of the hematoma.

d. Seizure may be generalized or focal. However, seizure is more common with subdural hematomas.

Key Signs: Epidural Hematoma*

- Patient may be conscious or unconscious
- Raised intracranial pressure
  - Headache
  - Vomiting
  - Abducens palsy
  - Papilledema
  - Bradycardia
  - Hypertension
- Focal neurologic deficits
  - Hemiparesis
  - Monoparesis
  - Paraparesis
- Seizure

*Signs depend mainly on the size of the hematoma, the rapidity of collection of blood, and associated brain injury.

2. Acute subdural hematoma

a. As with EDH, the clinical features of acute subdural hematoma are related to the size of the hematoma, rapidity of its growth, and severity of diffuse injury to the brain.

b. If diffuse injury is very severe with severe brain swelling, the patient will be unconscious from the very onset, with decerebrate posturing or flaccidity. In such cases, the prognosis remains very poor. In patients who have less severe injuries, the presentation and the level of consciousness depend on the magnitude of the impact injury and rapidity of the hematoma accumulation.

c. Patients may become unconscious later or may have lucid interval. As with EDH, as the intracranial pressure rises, features of coning start. During uncal herniation, sometimes the tentorial edge notches the contralateral cerebral

peduncle quite early, and the patient may have ipsilateral pupillary dilatation and ipsilateral hemiparesis. This is known as Kernohan-Woltman's notch or Kernohan-Woltman's phenomenon.

e. The classical clinical picture of infantile ASDH is an immediate cry followed by a generalized seizure.

Key Signs: Acute Subdural Hematoma*

- Unconsciousness with decerebrate posturing or flaccidity
- Ipsilateral pupillary dilatation
- Ipsilateral hemiparesis
- Immediate cry followed by a generalized seizure (infantile ASDH)

*Signs depend on size of hematoma, rapidity of its growth, and severity of diffuse injury to the brain.

3. Chronic subdural hematoma

Most commonly, the patient has a history of trauma, which may be trivial or even forgotten. After a few weeks, the problems start.

a. Features of raised intracranial tension such as headache, vomiting, and abducens palsy. However, because the collection is slow, the symptoms are not dramatic. In some extreme cases, there may be altered sensorium or unconsciousness.

b. Features of dementia

c. Focal neurologic signs, like hemiparesis and monoparesis

d. Seizure

Key Signs: Chronic Subdural Hematoma

- Raised intracranial tension
  - Headache
  - Vomiting
  - Abducens palsy
- Dementia
- Focal neurologic signs
- Seizure

Diagnostic Radiology

1. Computed tomographic (CT) scan is the "gold standard" of radiologic investigations in head trauma. Plain x-ray films are of only academic interest and are done in a few selected cases.

Usually, non-contrast-enhanced CT scan with bone window is sufficient.

2. The blood seen in EDH and acute SDH usually appears hyperdense in CT scan. In some cases of EDH, the collection may not be hyperdense (in cases of hyperacute collection; if the hematocrit of the patient is very low, in the case of chronic EDH). If the collection is isodense, contrast injection or magnetic resonance imaging (MRI) may be required. Similarly, in CSDH, when the collection is isodense, contrast-enhanced CT scan or MRI may be needed to delineate the collection.

3. Extra-axial hematomas may increase in size for 3 hours. It may be prudent to do CT scans 3 hours after injury, if the situation permits (that is, if patient is stable and not deteriorating).

4. The value of MRI is significant in predicting the age of the clot, which becomes important in chronic subdural hematoma. Sometimes it is very useful in showing the clot of EDH and SDH in vertex or in the floor of the middle cranial fossa. Moreover, its value has already been mentioned in the case of hypodense collections. Postcontrast MRI can also predict, to some degree, the progression of extra-axial hematomas in the acute stage (in a patient who is undergoing conservative treatment or who is under observation). Contrast enhancement indicates extravasation from broken vessels that continue to bleed and will be enlarged.

CT Scan Features of Epidural Hematoma

- Hyperdense, biconvex lesion between the skull and the brain

- Subfalcine/uncal herniation may be seen.

- Hematomas at vertex and floor of the middle cranial fossa may be difficult to see.

CT Scan Features of Acute Subdural Hematoma

- Hyperdense, crescentic area between the skull and the brain

- Usually not as hyperdense as epidural hematoma, as blood is diluted by CSF, which will leak through the torn arachnoid

- Usually widespread

- Features of brain shift; viz. uncal, subfalcine herniation may be seen

- Associated brain swelling evidenced by obliteration of the basal cisterns may be present.

CT Scan Features of Chronic Subdural Hematoma

- First week: Hyperdense, crescentic

- Subsequent 2 weeks: Isodense crescentic

- Beyond 3 weeks: Hypodense, crescentic/lenticular

- Recurrent bleeding causes some mixture of hyperdensity as well.

- Features of brain shift may be evident.

Treatment

The general management of head injury is discussed in Part XIII, Chapter 2, Moderate and Severe Head Injury. After general management, the specific management of the hematoma is necessary.

1. Epidural hematoma: For all practical purposes, the treatment of EDH is surgical. However, in a few selected circumstances, medical management may be undertaken.

    a. Medical management

    (1) With the increased use of CT scan, more and more small EDH are being detected, where nonsurgical management is a treatment option. A transient increase in the size of a hematoma may occur between days 5 and 16 in 50% cases and may require emergency craniotomy.

    (2) The management includes: (a) admission, (b) observation, and (c) serial CT scans to monitor any change in the size of the hematoma until there is resolution or medical treatment is abandoned. However, prompt surgical intervention should be done if there is any sign of deterioration or increase in the size of the hematoma.

Indications for Medical Management of Epidural Hematoma

- Subacute or chronic epidural hematoma

- Minimal neurologic signs/symptoms

- No evidence of any mass effect on CT scan

---

    b. Surgical management
    Most EDH patients require surgical treatment according to established principles.

    (1) A suitable size craniotomy is made, which is at least equal to the extent of the hematoma.

    (2) Hematoma is quickly evacuated, followed

by hemostasis either with bipolar cautery (bleeding from arteries and veins) and/or bone wax (bleeding from diploic veins).

(3) Dural tack up sutures are placed, and if the craniotomy is large, a central tenting suture is also placed.

Indications for Surgery in Epidural Hematoma

• Symptomatic epidural hematoma

• Epidural hematoma larger than 1 cm

• Epidural hematoma increasing in size

• Delayed epidural hematoma

• In pediatric patients, the threshold for surgery should be low, as there is very little room for the clot.

---

2. Acute subdural hematoma

a. Small ASDH are managed nonsurgically with observation, bed rest, diuretics, and other measures in order to reduce intracranial pressure.

b. Minimally symptomatic cases of infantile ASDH may be treated by subdural tap. Chronic persistent cases may need a subduroperitoneal shunt. Large hyperdense collection requires craniotomy and evacuation. However, during craniotomy and evacuation, the child may go into hypovolemic shock.

c. Large ASDH (>1 cm in adults, >5 mm in children) should be promptly evacuated. Smaller ASDH do not need surgical evacuation and surgery may be more injurious in those patients where there is massive brain swelling.

Key Treatment: Acute Subdural Hematoma

Small

• Measures to reduce intracranial pressure (e.g., best rest, diuretics)

Large (>1 cm adults; >5 mm children)

• Prompt surgical evacuation of the hematoma

Infantile ASDH

• Subdural tap (minimally symptomatic cases)

• Subduroperitoneal shunt (chronic persistent cases)

• Craniotomy and evacuation (large hyperdense collection)

d. Principles of surgery

(1) A large craniotomy flap is made.

(2) The dura is opened, and the coagulum is evacuated. Hemostasis is achieved. In most cases, the bleeding source cannot be identified.

(3) The dura is closed with duraplasty. The bone flap may or may not be replaced. Although in face of brain swelling, it is advised to discard bone flap, some authorities argue that this may be more injurious as it may cause strangulation of the vessels on the surface of the brain against the craniotomy edge, thus causing severe venous congestion and swelling of the brain.

3. Chronic subdural hematoma
The surgical treatment of CSDH is controversial. However, the following approaches should be kept in mind:

a. Medical management

(1) Identify and treat coagulopathies, if any.

(2) Start prophylactic anticonvulsants.

(3) Recognize that in selected cases, nonsurgical management can be achieved.

(4) Consider surgical evacuation if the lesion is symptomatic and/or more than 1 cm in thickness, and/or increasing in size.

Key Treatment

• Identify and treat any coagulopathies.

• Start prophylactic anticonvulsants.

• Elect surgical evacuation if lesion is symptomatic and/or more than 1 cm in thickness and/or increasing in size.

b. Surgical treatment

(1) The goal of surgery is to evacuate the hematoma and to minimize or prevent recollection. Usually the surgical results are extremely satisfactory.

(2) Hematoma can be evacuated through a twist drill hole or a burr hole (Table 3–1). Studies failed to show any significant difference in outcome after these two modalities of treatment.

(3) After surgery, measures can be taken to promote continuous drainage (placement of a subdural drain) and prevent reaccumulation (keeping the patient flat). However, these approaches are controversial.

(4) Subdural drain
A ventricular catheter is inserted in the subdural space and connected to a ventricu-

TABLE 3–1. TWIST DRILL AND BURR HOLE SURGERY FOR CHRONIC SUBDURAL HEMATOMA

	TWIST DRILL	BURR HOLE
Incision	Small; around 0.5 cm	Larger to make a burr hole of at least 2.5 cm in diameter
Location of bony opening	Rostral portion of hematoma	Thickest portion of the hematoma and/or temporal region
Dural opening	Done with the twist drill itself or with a 16 to 18 G spinal needle	Dura is opened by a cruciate incision and margins are coagulated with bipolar cautery
Evacuation of hematoma	Allowed to drain via a ventricular catheter	Allowed to drain freely and then the space is irrigated gently with saline
Subdural drain	Preferable	Optional

lostomy drainage bag maintained about 50 to 80 cm below the level of the head. Serial CT scans are done to assess the size of the collection. Most commonly, the drain is removed after 48 to 72 hours. Antibiotic coverage is recommended.

(5) In cases that persistently recur after the above-mentioned procedures, formal craniotomy with excision of the subdural membrane is desirable. It is advisable to not remove the deep membranes adhered to the brain surface.

(6) Complications of surgery

(a) Seizure

(b) Intracerebral hemorrhage

(c) Reaccumulation

(d) Epidural hematoma

Outcome and Mortality

In general, the outcome for patients with these hematomas depends on the general condition of the patient (age, associated medical illness, other injuries), duration of the symptoms, and neurologic status. Size of the hematoma does not have a significant impact on outcome.

1. Epidural hematomas

a. The mortality associated with epidural hematoma varies from 5% to 20% in different series. Mortality is lower in patients who have lucid interval than those who do not (unconscious throughout).

b. Associated intracranial injury implicates worse outcome.

2. Acute subdural hematoma

a. The mortality with acute subdural hematoma is 50% to 90% in different series. A major cause of death is the underlying brain injury. The mortality is higher in older patients and patients receiving anticoagulants.

b. The traditional "Four Hour Rule"

(1) Patients operated on within 4 hours of injury had 30% mortality, and those operated on beyond 4 hours had 90% mortality. Additionally, a functional recovery (Glasgow Outcome Scale of >4) rate of 65% can be achieved if surgery is done within 4 hours.

(2) Other prognostic factors:

(a) Postoperative intracranial pressure: Less than 20 mm Hg had a recovery rate of 79%.

(b) Initial neurologic examination

c. Recently, the magnitude of the importance of the above-mentioned factors has been disputed: delay of surgery affects the outcome significantly, but perhaps not drastically. Also the mode of injury is found to be a significant prognosticator.

3. Chronic subdural hematoma

a. Overall, the prognosis is much better for chronic subdural hematoma than for acute subdural hematoma.

b. Patients with high subdural fluid pressure tend to improve more rapidly. A residual collection after treatment is common, and clinical improvement is not synonymous with complete resolution, especially before 20 days postoperatively. This residual collection does not need any treatment unless it is increasing in size or the patient is showing signs of deterioration.

Bibliography

Ammirati M, Tomita: Posterior fossa epidural hematoma during childhood. Neurosurgery 14:541–544, 1984.

Aoki N, Masuzawa H: Infantile acute subdural hematoma. J Neurosurg 61:273–280, 1984.

Domenicucci M, Signorini P, Strzelecki J, Delfini R: Delayed post-traumatic epidural hematoma. A review. Neurosurg Rev 18:109–122, 1995.

Gennarelli TA, Meaney DF: Mechanisms of primary head injury. In Wilkins RH, Rengachary SS (eds): Neurosurgery, 3rd ed., vol. 2. New York, McGraw-Hill, 1996, pp. 2611–2621.

Markwalder TM, Steinsiepe KF, Rohner M, et al.: The course of chronic subdural hematomas after burr-hole craniotomy and closed-system drainage. J Neurosurg 55:390–393, 1981.

Ramamurthi B: Acute subdural hematoma. In Vinken PJ, Bruyn GW (eds): Handbook of Clinical Neurology, vol 24. Amsterdam, North-Holland, 1976, pp. 275–296.

Rivas JJ, Lobato RD, Sarabia R, et al.: Extradural hematoma: Analysis of factors influencing the course of 161 patients. Neurosurgery 23:44–51, 1988.

Seelig JM, Becker DP, Miller JD, et al.: Traumatic acute subdural hematoma: Major mortality reduction in comatose patients treated within four hours. N Engl J Med 304:1511–1518, 1981.

Wilberger JE Jr, Harris M, Diamond DL: Acute subdural hematoma: Morbidity, mortality, and operative timing. J Neurosurg 74:212–218, 1991.

4 Cranial Neuropathy

*Prasad Vannemreddy
Anil Nanda*

Definition

1. Involvement of cranial nerves by any disease or trauma either directly or indirectly producing clinically relevant symptomatology
2. The most common causes are trauma, tumors, infection, and metabolic diseases such as diabetes and metal poisoning.

Epidemiology

1. The incidence of cranial nerve injury differs by age groups and demographics.
   a. Keane and Baloh provide a comparative tabulation of incidence.
   b. Almost all olfactory grove meningiomas or nasal encephaloceles lead to loss of olfaction.
   c. A 3% incidence of ocular palsy in closed-head injury is recorded by Russell, with a 4.5% incidence of fifth nerve injury in his series of 1,000 cases, whereas facial and eighth nerve injuries closely follow temporal bone fractures.
2. Vestibular schwannomas produce hearing loss in 98% of patients; vestibular nerve dysfunction, in 70%; facial nerve paralysis, in 10%, trigeminal nerve involvement in 30%, and sixth nerve dysfunction in 10%. Hypoglossal neuropathy is reported in 10% of patients after carotid endarterectomy.
3. In pediatric head trauma, oculomotor nerves are most commonly affected, followed by the optic nerve, trigeminal nerve, and facial nerve. Vestibulocochlear and olfactory injuries are rare.
4. Third nerve palsy may be produced by aneurysms of the posterior communicating artery or, less commonly, by basilar artery aneurysms.
5. Intracavernous or supraclinoid aneurysms may present with facial pain syndromes due to compression of the first and second divisions of the trigeminal nerve.

Etiology

1. Blunt head trauma in motor vehicle accidents and gunshot wounds are responsible for most lesions.
   a. Other causes include tumor, infection, metabolic disorders, and operative trauma.
2. Symmetric middle cranial neuropathies result from crushing injuries of the skull.
3. Blunt head trauma is accompanied by basilar fractures and involves the cranial nerves near the fractures.
4. Gunshot wounds take trajectories—horizontal in suicide attempts and anteroposterior in homicidal injuries.
5. Avulsion and stretching of the nerve roots can occur with acceleration and deceleration trauma and in blunt injuries.
   a. These forces damage the nerves at their points of fixation or angulation.
   b. Olfactory esthesioblastomas; optic nerve or chiasmatic gliomas; and schwannomas of trigeminal, facial, and hypoglossal nerves injure the nerves directly, with preservation of function depending on the extent of loss and the size of the tumors.
6. Multiple sclerosis and other demyelinating diseases can present with mononeuropathy or polyneuropathy and usually have remissions and relapses.
   a. Diabetes mellitus is another cause of mononeuropathy that has a fluctuating course.

Clinical Manifestations

1. The 12 pairs of cranial nerves are involved in different orders of preference depending on the patient's age and the mechanism of insult. In general, the olfactory, facial, and vestibulocochlear nerves are damaged most frequently by blunt head trauma, with the lower cranial nerves (IX, X, XI, and XII) being the least commonly injured. In children younger than 10 years of age, abducent and facial nerves are commonly injured.
2. Middle and lower cranial neuropathies are closely associated with basal skull fractures in blunt head trauma. Tumors arising from the skull base injure the cranial nerves in almost the same way as trauma damages the various cranial fossae. Anterior cranial fossa tumors tend to involve the first five cranial nerves, and middle cranial fossa tumors damage the fifth and seventh; the posterior cranial fossa lesions damage the lower cranial nerves.
3. With the exception of oculomotor, abducent, and

facial nerves, altered consciousness obscures examination of cranial nerve injuries, and diagnosis may be delayed significantly.

4. Olfactory nerve

   a. Injury is difficult to establish in an acute trauma phase where nasal bleed and swelling confound the examination.

   b. Summer suggests the overall incidence of olfactory nerve dysfunction to be 7%, increasing to 30 percent with severe head injuries or anterior cranial fossa fractures.

   c. In more than one third of cases, recovery occurs within 3 months.

   d. Irreversible damage usually occurs with tumors of the anterior cranial fossa involving the olfactory grove (e.g., meningiomas, nasopharyngeal carcinoma).

Key Signs: Olfactory Nerve Injury

- Injury is difficult to establish in an acute trauma phase where nasal bleed and swelling confound the examination.

5. Optic nerve

   a. The optic nerve is tethered in the optic canal and is subject to stretch, causing injury during brain shifts.

   b. Most traumatic optic neuropathies result from severe head trauma, and altered consciousness in the patient delays the diagnosis. An afferent pupillary defect in an unconscious patient is useful in the detection of optic nerve injury, whereas in conscious patients, testing for visual fields and acuity usually establishes the diagnosis.

   c. The most common tumor to injure the anterior visual pathways is a pituitary adenoma. The classic description of bilateral temporal hemianopsia results from these tumors as well from the other sellar lesions such as craniopharyngioma, meningioma, and Rathke's cleft cyst.

   d. Unilateral involvement is more common with orbital tumors and lesions of the anterior clinoid process (e.g., medial sphenoid wing meningiomas). Severe papilledema can cause blindness from long-standing, slow growing tumors.

Key Signs: Optic Nerve Injury

- Bilateral temporal hemianopsia (pituitary adenoma)

- Blindness caused by severe papilledema (long-standing, slow-growing tumors)

6. Oculomotor nerve

   a. Trauma is the most common cause of oculomotor neuropathy, and associated facial and orbital injuries compound the diagnosis.
      (1) Ptosis with lateral deviation of the eyeball is the presenting feature, with or without swelling.
      (2) Intraorbital tumors and aneurysms of the posterior communicating artery or basilar artery are the other causes.

   b. Lesions of the cavernous sinus (aneurysms of internal carotid artery, meningiomas, and angiomas) typically involve all of the oculomotor nerves (III, IV, and VI).

   c. Superior orbital fissure syndrome and cavernous sinus thrombosis are more painful conditions that require emergency intervention.

Key Signs: Olfactory Nerve Injury

- Ptosis with lateral deviation of the eyeball with or without swelling

7. Trochlear nerve

   a. Injury to the trochlear nerve is rarely diagnosed. Often a complaint of diplopia after recovery from a severe head injury leads to this diagnosis.

   b. Typically, the double vision is vertical, especially when the patient walks down a flight of stairs.

   c. A lesser distortion of the opposite trochlear nerve may be established by using a red glass to demonstrate reversal of hypertropia on downgaze.

Key Signs: Trochlear Nerve Injury

- Diplopia following recovery from a severe head injury

- Vertical double vision, especially when walking down a flight of stairs

8. Abducent nerve

   a. Lateral rectus palsy in its minor form may not correlate well with abducent nerve injury, and conjugate movements that are controlled by the brainstem sometimes make clinical examination and diagnosis of abducent nerve palsy difficult to establish.

b. Common causes include cerebellopontine angle lesions, chordomas, and brainstem tumors.

9. Trigeminal nerve

a. It is rare to have an injury to the trigeminal ganglion or main trunk within the cranial cavity, but the peripheral branches are often involved in facial lacerations and orbit fractures.

b. Basal skull fractures may involve the trigeminal nerve and are usually combined with injury to abducent and facial nerve palsy.

(1) Injury to the maxillary and ophthalmic divisions results in facial numbness, and involvement of the mandibular branch causes the mastication muscles to become weak.

(2) Transient trigeminal nerve symptoms occur in 22% of cases and are permanent in 11% after microsurgery or stereotactic radiosurgery for vestibular schwannomas.

c. Trigeminal neuralgia (TN, tic douloroux) is probably the most common disease involving the fifth nerve, with an annual incidence of 4 out of 100,000.

(1) It affects women more than men, the right side of the face more than the left; and the second division more often than the first.

(2) 2% of patients with MS have trigeminal neuralgia, whereas 18% of patients with bilateral trigeminal neuralgia have MS.

d. This severe disabling condition is probably caused by ephaptic transmission in the nerve from large-diameter myelinated A fibers to poorly myelinated A-delta and C (nociceptive) fibers.

e. Causes of TN include abnormal vascular loops (most commonly by the superior cerebellar artery) producing compression at the root entry zone or posterior fossa tumors (<0.8% of TN) and multiple sclerosis.

f. Most cases do not require imaging for diagnosis, but it is used for atypical presentation. Tumors producing TN also present with associated neurologic deficits, and pain is almost constant.

Key Signs: Trigeminal Nerve Injury

- Maxillary and ophthalmic injury: Facial numbness; mandibular branch involvement causes weak mastication muscles

- Trigeminal neuralgia: Affects women more than men; the right side of face more often than the left.

- When tumor related, neurologic deficits and almost constant pain result.

10. Facial nerve

a. The long, tortuous, intraosseous course of the facial nerve in the temporal bone makes it highly susceptible to injury in temporal bone fractures. In about 50 percent of cases of transverse temporal bone fractures, the facial nerve within the internal auditory canal is damaged.

b. With longitudinal fractures, the nerve is not directly involved, but a delayed paralysis may ensue secondary to edema.

c. Trauma involving the internal auditory canal injures both facial and vestibulocochlear nerves; facial nerve symptoms, loss of hearing, and vertigo are present.

d. Facial nerve dysfunction

(1) House and Brackmann proposed the clinical grading for facial nerve function (Table 4–1).

(2) Natural tears and Lacrilube are applied if eye closure is impaired.

(3) In the case of complete facial nerve palsy with fifth nerve impairment, early tarsorrhaphy is performed.

(4) Facial reanimation is performed (e.g., hypoglossal-facial anastamosis) after 1 to 2 months if the facial nerve is divided or after 1 year if no function has returned.

TABLE 4–1. HOUSE AND BRACKMANN CLINICAL GRADING FOR FACIAL NERVE FUNCTION

Grade 1	Normal
Grade 2	Mild dysfunction
Grade 3	Moderate dysfunction
Grade 4	Moderate to severe dysfunction
Grade 5	Severe dysfunction
Grade 6	Complete paralysis

Note: Grades 1–3 are associated with acceptable function.

Key Signs: Facial Nerve Injury

- Longitudinal fractures: Delayed paralysis secondary to edema

- Trauma involving the internal auditory canal: Facial nerve symptoms, loss of hearing, and vertigo

11. Vestibulocochlear nerve

    a. The less common transverse fractures of the petrous pyramid damage both facial and vestibulocochlear nerves.

       (1) Cerebrospinal fluid (CSF) leakage is common, and meningitis is a late complication.

       (2) Sudden deafness after a blow to the head is often partially or completely reversible and is usually related to intense acoustic stimulation from pressure waves.

       (3) Vertigo is the most common neuro-otologic sequel to head injury and is positional.

       (4) Vestibular schwannomas produce dysfunction of the vestibulocochlear nerve with varying degrees of hearing loss.

    b. Hearing dysfunction has five classifications according to Gardener and Robertson's modification of the Silverstein and Norrell system.

       (1) Class I is good to excellent, IV is poor, and class V is no function.

       (2) Hearing preservation is possible with vestibular schwannomas of less than 1.5 cm.

       (3) Hearing loss rarely improves postoperatively.

Key Signs: Vestibulocochlear Nerve Injury

- CSF leakage

- Meningitis

- Vertigo

12. Vagus and glossopharyngeal nerves

    a. Injury to these nerves is uncommon. Only a few cases of penetrating trauma as a cause of cranial nerve palsy and (recently) of fractured occipital condyle in closed-head injury have been reported.

    b. Glossopharyngeal neuralgia presents with severe, lancinating pain in the distribution of the ninth and tenth nerves (involving the throat and the base of the tongue and radiating to the ear and the neck).

       (1) These patients rarely present with syn-cope, hypotension, convulsions, and cardiac arrest; the incidence of glossopharyngeal neuralgia to TN is 1:70.

       (2) Trigger zones are rare, and microvascular decompression (MVD) or intracranial nerve divisions provide lasting relief.

Key Signs: Glossopharyngeal Nerve Injury

- Severe, lancinating pain involving the throat and the base of the tongue radiating to the ear and neck

13. Spinal accessory nerve: Injury to the accessory nerve is rare.

    a. Avulsions may be associated with cervical spine trauma.

    b. A more common cause is surgical trauma, which may result from surgery to the deep cervical lymph nodes and the posterior cervical triangle.

    c. Hyperextension neck injuries may occasionally involve the spinal accessory nerve and produce paralysis of the sternomastoid and trapezius.

Key Signs: Spinal Accessory Nerve Injury

- Injury to the accessory nerve is rare.

14. Hypoglossal nerve

    a. The most frequent cause of hypoglossal nerve injury is iatrogenic and is almost always a result of carotid endarterectomy, gunshot wounds, or penetrating injuries.

    b. Hyperextension neck injuries can produce a blunt trauma to the nerve, with or without fracture of the hypoglossal tubercle or occipital condyle.

    c. Tongue weakness ipsilateral to the nerve injury results from this type of injury, and bullet wounds may produce bilateral tongue paralysis.

    d. Lower cranial nerve dysfunction is possible after surgery for cerebellopontine (CP) angle tumors and creates difficulty in swallowing and associated risk of aspiration.

       (1) Various combinations of lower cranial nerve palsies occur with glomus jugulare tumors (jugular foramen syndrome) and are occasionally combined with facial nerve palsy.

       (2) The most common cranial nerve involved is the eighth nerve.

       (3) Other tumors producing multiple cranial

neuropathies are epidermoids, chordomas, and those involving cavernous sinus.

Key Signs: Hypoglossal Nerve Injury

- Lower cranial nerve dysfunction
- Tongue weakness

Radiologic Features

1. Clinical suspicion is the best diagnostic method.
2. Magnetic resonance imaging (MRI) is used to visualize the cranial nerves.
3. Work-up for functional evaluation varies according to the nerve.
   a. Olfactory nerve injuries are evaluated electively by clinical examination.
   b. Compression by ethmoid air cells in the optic canal and fractures across the optic canal can be demonstrated by high-resolution computed tomography (CT) scan, and in nearly half of the cases with optic nerve injury.
4. Diplopia fields are useful for diagnosis and follow-up of oculomotor function.
   a. High-resolution CT and MRI are useful in differentiating the causes for delayed diplopia, including impending tentorial herniation and midbrain contusions associated with trochlear nerve palsy.
5. A good correlation exists between facial nerve injury, or eighth nerve injury, and the type of temporal bone fracture. For both of these nerves, electrophysiologic monitoring is useful in diagnosis and prognostication.
6. Injury to the lower cranial nerves is uncommon, and clinical diagnosis helps in the case of accessory and hypoglossal nerves and is sometimes combined with electromyography.
7. Vagus and glossopharyngeal nerves are rarely injured, and the lesions might not be easily diagnosed.

Key Tests

- MRI (cranial nerves, oculomotor function)
- CT (optic nerve, oculomotor function)
- Electromyography (accessory and hypoglossal nerves)
- Clinical suspicion/diagnosis

Treatment

1. Olfactory nerve
   a. Two objective tests of olfaction are olfactory respiratory reflex and olfactory electroencephalography (EEG).
   b. The former helps in ruling out malingering, while EEG provides a nonspecific alpha response to an odoriferous substance.
   c. A high-resolution CT of ethmoids and frontal fossa is essential in the work-up of anosmia, especially with CSF rhinorrhoea, which frequently accompanies trauma to the anterior cranial fossa and nasal sinuses or surgery for tumors of the anterior cranial fossa.
   d. MRI can demonstrate injury to the basofrontal lobes and the olfactory bulbs.
   e. There is no specific treatment for posttraumatic anosmia other than counseling the patient and providing reassurance.

Key Treatment: Olfactory Nerve

- Posttraumatic anosmia: No treatment besides counseling and reassurance

2. Optic nerve
   a. Clinical evaluation and investigations such as electroretinography and visual evoked potentials must be combined when evaluating visual impairment.
      (1) Prolonged p100 may be indicative of impaired conduction along the optic nerve secondary to compression.
      (2) High-dose steroids (similar to a dosage for acute spinal cord injury) are used in the acute phase.
      (3) Intravenous methylprednisolone 30 mg/kg as a loading dose followed by 5.5 mg/hour for 36 to 48 hours was used by the Graz group.
   b. In patients with delayed-onset loss of vision from compression of the optic nerve and failed steroid treatment, operative approaches in the transcranial, transethmoidal, transmaxillary, and transorbital routes have been described for optic nerve decompression.
   c. Sudden vision loss secondary to pituitary apoplexy is also considered an indication for emergency decompressive surgery.
      (1) Cook and colleagues provide the details of outcome in operative and nonoperative groups. In their meta-analysis, nontreatment was reported to be as effective as

medical or surgical treatment of traumatic optic neuropathy.

Key Treatment: Optic Nerve

- Steroids (acute phase)

- Methylprednisolone, 30 mg/kg intravenously, followed by 5.5 mg/hour for 36 to 48 hours

- Compression causing delayed vision loss: Surgery involving transcranial, transethmoidal, transmaxillary, and transorbital routes

3. Oculomotor nerves

   a. Diplopia fields, CT, and MRI are helpful in establishing a diagnosis.

   b. However, there is no effective treatment for injury to these nerves.

      (1) A therapeutic eye patch controls diplopia, and recovery can be expected to follow in 4 to 6 months.

      (2) Surgery for extraocular muscles in cases of failed recovery should be delayed for 9 months to 12 months or until diplopia is stabilized, and it is especially beneficial in cases of fourth to sixth nerve palsy.

Key Treatment: Oculomotor Nerves

- No effective treatment

- Diplopia can be treated with a therapeutic eye patch.

4. Trigeminal nerve

   a. Disabling neuralgia sometimes accompanies partial injuries to the sensory divisions.

   b. Medical management includes carbamazepine, baclofen, pimozide, phenytoin, capsaicin, clonazepam, and amitriptylin.

      (1) Carbamazepine is most commonly used starting at a low dose that is increased by 200 mg every day up to a maximum of 1200 mg per day.

      (2) Complete or acceptable relief is achieved in up to 69% of cases. Baclofen may be more effective as an adjunct to carbamazepine.

   c. Surgical options include peripheral nerve blocks by phenol or alcohol or neurectomy, percutaneous rhizotomy, Spiller-Frazier retrogasserian rhizotomy, MVD, and stereotactic radiosurgery.

   d. Percutaneous trigeminal rhizotomy is preferred in patients who are a high risk for major

surgery, unresectable tumors, multiple sclerosis, and low life expectancy (<5 years). Rhizotomy is performed using radiofrequency or balloon compression, and results are comparable.

   e. MVD provides long-lasting relief and a low incidence of facial anesthesia.

   f. Failures following a given treatment may be treated using the other options.

   g. Up to 90% of recurrences are in the distribution of the previously involved nerve divisions; 10% involve a new one.

Key Treatment: Trigeminal Nerve

Drugs

- Carbamazepine

- Baclofen (as an adjunct to carbamazepine)

- Pimozide

- Phenytoin

- Capsaicin

- Clonazepam

- Amitriptylin

Surgery

- Peripheral nerve blocks by phenol or alcohol

- Neurectomy

- Percutaneous rhizotomy

- Spiller-Frazier retrogasserian rhizotomy

- Microvascular decompression

- Stereotactic radiosurgery

5. Abducens nerve

   a. Recovery of function to a certain degree is always the rule.

   b. Botulinum toxin, injected into the ipsilateral medial rectus muscle, has also been proposed as a treatment option for a faster recovery.

   c. A prospective multicenter trial recently conducted by the North American Neuro-ophthalmology Society, however, revealed that patients with traumatic abducens palsy treated with either botulinum toxin or conservative measures had similar high recovery rates.

Key Treatment: Abducens Nerve

- Botulinum toxin injected into the ipsilateral medial rectus muscle

6. Facial nerve

   a. Monitoring is preferred, because an excellent spontaneous recovery can be expected with delayed-onset paralysis.

   b. With nonsurgical management, 90% of patients experience good recovery within 6 months.

   c. Absent facial nerve stimulation after 4 days may indicate surgical exploration, especially with transverse fractures of the temporal bone and a discontinuous fallopian canal.

   d. A mastoidectomy and decompression of the nerve under microsurgical techniques with or without graft repair may be beneficial.

Key Treatment: Facial Nerve

- Spontaneous recovery with delayed-onset paralysis is common.

- 90% of patients have good recovery within 6 months without surgery.

- Absent facial nerve stimulation after 4 days may require surgical exploration.

7. Vestibulocochlear nerve

   a. Conductive deafness can be treated surgically by correcting the middle ear, and it has a good prognosis.

   b. There is no specific treatment for sensorineural deafness. Some improvement ensues with partial injuries.

   c. Conversely, perilymph fistula with loss of eighth nerve function indicates surgical exploration. In refractory posttraumatic vertigo, a labyrinthectomy or translabyrinthine VIII nerve section or selective vestibular nerve section (in cases with preserved hearing) may provide relief.

   d. Cochlear implants are undergoing clinical trials and hold promise in the treatment of sensorineural deafness.

   e. Lower cranial nerve palsy

   f. Unilateral paralysis of nerves IX through XII, also known as Collet-Sicard syndrome, requires investigation for underlying causes.

   g. In vascular injuries such as vertebral artery fistulae, and in fractures of the occipital condyle, treatment may be directed to rectify them.

   h. Otherwise, the treatment for cranial nerve palsy is expectant and symptomatic.

Key Treatment: Vestibulocochlear Nerve

- Surgery for conductive deafness

- No specific treatment for sensorineural deafness

- Surgical exploration for perilymph fistula with loss of eighth nerve function

- Lower cranial nerve palsy:

  - Treatment is expectant and symptomatic

  - Surgical exploration for unilateral paralysis of nerves IX through XII

Prognosis and Complications

1. Anosmia following trauma improves in one third of cases, usually during the first 3 months, although recovery may continue for 5 years. Delayed visual loss is potentially reversible.

2. Indirect injury (vascular insult secondary to raised intracranial pressure or tumor compression) results in immediate and almost permanent visual loss. Gjerris reported that 40% to 50% of patients remained blind, and nearly 75% of patients showed no improvement in their deficit.

3. With retained pupillary reflex, the prognosis is more favorable. Recovery of the third nerve usually occurs in 2 to 3 months, with aberrant regeneration that exhibits in the form of disproportionate improvement in adduction and highly variable ptosis.

4. The slender trochlear nerve is usually avulsed from the midbrain and the prognosis is not favorable.

5. The abducent nerve usually shows axonal regeneration in 4 months with functional recovery.

6. Some recovery is expected in partial injuries to the trigeminal nerve.

7. A positive percutaneous stimulation after 4 days of facial nerve trauma indicates excellent prognosis for recovery. In most series, facial palsy makes a good spontaneous recovery.

8. Sensorineural deafness has a poor prognosis, and tinnitus is disabling.

   a. With small tumor size, most patients with vestibular schwannomas can have preserved hearing.

   b. Vestibular symptoms take 6 to 12 weeks to subside, and an intractable postural vertigo with sensorineural deafness may be indicative of perilymph fistula.

Prevention

1. General guidelines for prevention of trauma apply to prevention of cranial nerve injury.
2. In particular, prompt early diagnosis is emphasized to minimize neuronal damage.
3. Iatrogenic injury may be avoided by following accepted surgical principles during operative procedures.

Pregnancy

Medical and surgical treatment of cranial neuropathy should observe standard precautions for pregnancy and lactation.

Anesthesia

Surgical treatment is required in selective situations, and anesthesia follows routine protocol, except for an allowance for intraoperative neuroelectrophysiologic monitoring where short-acting muscle relaxants and inhalation anesthetics are favored.

Bibliography

Cannon CR, Jahrsdoerfer RA: Temporal bone fractures. Review of 90 cases. Arch Otolaryngol Head Neck Surg 109:285–288, 1983.

Cook MW, Levin LA, Joseph MP, Pinczower EF: Traumatic optic neuropathy. A meta-analysis. Arch Otolaryngol Head Neck Surg 122:389–392, 1996.

House WF, Brackman DE: Facial nerve grading system. Otolaryngol Head Neck Surg 93:184–193, 1985.

Jacobi G, Ritz A, Emrich R: Cranial nerve damage after paediatric head trauma: A long-term follow-up study of 741 cases. Acta Paediatr Hung 27:173–187, 1986.

Keane JR, Baloh RW: Posttraumatic cranial neuropathies. Neurol Clin 10:849–867, 1992.

Luxenberger W, Stammberger H, Jebeles JA, Walch C: Endoscopic optic nerve decompression: The Graz experience. Laryngoscope 108:873–882, 1998.

Russel WR: In Brock S (ed): Injuries of the Brain and Spinal Cord and Their Coverings, 4th ed. New York, Springer-Verlag, 1960.

5 Neurorehabilitation of Brain Injuries

David S. Kushner

Definition and Epidemiology

1. Definition: The neurorehabilitation of a traumatic brain injury is a process that involves medical, physical, social, educational, and vocational interventions that can be provided in a variety of institutional and community settings to facilitate functional recovery after brain damage resulting from external mechanical forces.

2. Epidemiology

   a. It is estimated that 8 million traumatic head injuries occur in the United States annually, of which approximately 1 million are initially treated in hospitals.

   b. Most traumatic brain injuries, 75% to 80%, are classified as "mild traumatic brain injuries," also known as concussions (see Classification and Assessment below).

   c. An estimated 300,000 sports-related brain injuries occur each year.

   d. Traumatic brain injuries result in significant economic burden to society annually in terms of direct and indirect costs (estimated at 56 billion dollars by the Centers for Disease Control (CDL) in 2002); individual lifetime costs may exceed 6 million dollars.

Facts about Traumatic Head Injuries

- 8 million traumatic head injuries occur in the United States annually.

- Approximately 1 million of the patients with such injuries are initially treated in hospitals.

- 75% to 80% are classified as mild traumatic brain injuries ("concussions").

- Approximately 300,000 sports-related brain injuries occur each year.

- Direct and indirect costs of traumatic brain injuries were estimated at 56 billion dollars in 2002

---

3. Incidence

   a. The usual causes of traumatic brain injuries are accidents involving motor vehicles, bicycles, pedestrians, construction, and sports, as well as physical violence (both weapon and non-weapon related).

   b. The most common cause of head trauma is motor vehicle accidents.

   c. Falls are a leading cause of head injury in individuals older than 65 years of age.

   d. Adolescents, young adults (15 to 24 years old), and people older than 65 years are at the greatest risk for traumatic brain injury; and men of all ages are at twice the risk of women.

4. Pathophysiology

   a. Primary brain injury may result from penetrating trauma (such as gunshot wounds); from direct impact forces to the head that cause injury beneath the point of contact (coup injury) or opposite the point of contact due to rebound of the brain within the skull (contracoup injury); and from acceleration-deceleration or rotational forces, known as shear forces, generated by the mechanical process and velocity of the traumatic event, that injure axons and small blood vessels within the substance of the brain.

   b. Secondary brain injury may result from any factor that leads to an abnormal increase in the intracranial pressure, an abnormal decrease in the cerebral perfusion pressure, or an abnormal increase in cerebral metabolic demand. (Central factors may include expanding hematomas, acute hydrocephalus, progressive cerebral edema, and protracted seizures. Systemic factors may include hypoglycemia, hypotension, infection, blood loss, and impairment of cardiopulmonary function).

5. Pathologic features

   a. Brain contusions are areas of focal cortical injury involving localized ischemia, edema, and mass effect; they result from direct impact forces or from acceleration-deceleration trauma. Signs and symptoms vary with cortical location and may include focal weakness, numbness, imbalance, incoordination, visual impairments, and neuropsychological impairments.

   b. Intracranial hemorrhages including epidural, subdural, subarachnoid, and intracerebral hemorrhages may complicate any traumatic brain injury. The risk increases with worsening severity of brain injury, though anticoagulant therapy or coagulopathies also increase the risk. Signs may include worsening headache and progressive neurologic deterioration.

c. Cerebral edema may occur secondary to the swelling of injured brain cells (cytotoxic edema), the leakage of proteins and fluid from damaged blood vessels (vasogenic edema) and the expansion in size of the brain ventricles and cisterns (hydrocephalus) resulting in the transependymal flow of cerebrospinal fluid into the brain (hydrostatic edema).

d. Axonal shear injury is the primary pathologic feature common to traumatic brain injury of all classifications (mild, moderate, and severe). Trauma-generated shear forces produce nonuniform strains and distortions within the brain that disrupt axons and small blood vessels, causing physiologic or structural axonal injury roughly proportional to the direction and magnitude of the applied traumatic force.

6. A multitude of somatic, affective, and cognitive symptoms and signs can follow a traumatic brain injury (see Key Symptoms and Signs).

a. The symptoms and signs of brain injury contribute to reversible or irreversible impairments of physical and neuropsychological capacity resulting in functional disabilities affecting mobility, self-care, and the ability to perform the more complex tasks of independent living (such as banking, shopping, homemaking, working, and driving).

b. Functional disabilities contribute to handicaps, which are social disadvantages that may prevent a person from fulfilling his or her expected role in a society (including vocational, educational, and interpersonal relationship roles). Handicaps may be affected by physical or cultural barriers.

c. To facilitate neurorehabilitation interventions and maximize functional recovery, clinicians must determine the various impairments responsible for the disabilities observed after brain injury.

Key Symptoms and Signs: Possible Sequelae of Traumatic Brain Injury

Somatic Disorders

- Headaches
- Dizziness/Vertigo
- Hearing loss
- Tinnitus
- Loss of taste
- Anosmia
- Pain
- Weakness
- Numbness
- Neuroendocrine dysfunction
- Sleep impairment
- Fatigue
- Loss of appetite
- Loss of libido
- Impaired vision
- Diplopia
- Seizures
- Spasticity
- Imbalance/Incoordination
- Tremor/Dystonia

Affective Disorders (Behavior, Mood, Personality)

- Apathy
- Irritability/Lability
- Anxiety/Depression
- Denial
- Bizarre ideation
- Impulsivity/Disinhibition
- Aggression
- Silliness
- Somatization
- Psychosis

Disorders of Cognition

Impairments of Attentional/Arousal

- Coma
- Vegetative state
- Lethargy/Fatigue
- Minimally conscious state
- Psychomotor delay
- Inattention/Hyperarousal

Impairments of Memory

- Anterograde/Retrograde amnesia
- Impaired orientation
- Impaired short/long-term or immediate recall

Continued

Key Symptoms and Signs: Possible Sequelae of Traumatic Brain Injury
(Continued)

Impairments of Perception

• Impaired visual/spatial perception

• Impairment of complex sensory integration (apraxia)

Impairments of Language/Communication

• Aphasias (receptive/expressive)

• Disorders of language pragmatics

Impairments of Intellect/Executive Function

• Concrete reasoning/cognitive rigidity

• Disorders of initiation/sequencing

• Poor insight/planning/problem solving

7. Goals and objectives

a. Goals of traumatic brain injury neurorehabilitation include the prevention of secondary complications (such as seizures, pneumonia, contractures, heterotopic ossification or deep venous thrombosis); treatment to reduce neurologic impairments when possible; compensatory strategies for permanent residual disabilities; patient/caretaker education; and interventions to promote the long-term maintenance of function as well as the promotion of successful community reintegration (including the return to school or to the workplace if possible).

b. Objectives include the reduction of functional disabilities via medical, physical, restorative, adaptive, environmental, and social interventions through a multidisciplinary team of specialists that may variably include physicians, nurses, therapists, psychologists, dieticians, social workers, and orthotists.

Classification and Assessment

1. Definitive signs must be present at the time of head trauma for a traumatic brain injury to be diagnosed. Signs of brain injury may include confusion, amnesia, loss of consciousness, and focal neurologic deficits such as weakness, numbness, imbalance, incoordination, or visual impairment.

2. Patient evaluation after traumatic brain injury and during the neurorehabilitation process involves physical examination, neuroimaging procedures when necessary, and the use of well-validated standardized measurement instruments and scales that complement the physical examination in evaluating functional recovery; facilitate reliable documentation of functional disability severity; help to increase the consistency of treatment decisions; facilitate communication between specialists; and provide a reliable basis for monitoring progress.

3. Traumatic brain injury severity is initially classified as "mild," "moderate," or "severe" at the time of injury based on certain measures including the duration of posttraumatic amnesia (the period during which a patient is unable to form new memories), the duration of loss of consciousness, if any, and the Glasgow Coma Scale score (Tables 5–1 and 5–2). Subdividing patients with a brain injury into these classifications facilitates the determination of appropriate medical treatment and the prognosis for recovery.

a. *Mild traumatic brain injury* has been classified by the American Congress of Rehabilitation Medicine as head trauma with loss of consciousness, if any, lasting less than 30 minutes, Glasgow Coma Scale score of 13 or more, and posttraumatic amnesia of less than 24 hours. The term "concussion" is often used in the medical literature as a synonym for a mild traumatic brain injury.

b. *Moderate traumatic brain injury* has generally been classified to involve a Glasgow Coma Scale Score of 9 to 12, loss of consciousness of 30 minutes to 6 hours, and a posttraumatic amnesia duration of 24 hours to 1 week.

c. *Severe traumatic brain injury* has been generally classified with a Glasgow Coma Scale Score of 8 or less, a loss of consciousness of more than 6 hours, and a posttraumatic amnesia duration of more than one week.

4. Brain injuries of all classifications (mild, moderate, or severe) may be complicated by cortical contusions, intracranial hemorrhages, physiologic or structural axonal shear injury, skull fractures, cranial adnexal injuries (associated injury of head or neck structures, such as cervical spine injury, facial bone fractures, and cranial nerve injuries), and seizures. These complications become more likely with a worsening spectrum of traumatic

TABLE 5–1. MEASURES OF INJURY SEVERITY

• Glasgow Coma Scale
(A quantitative measure of the depth of unconsciousness)
• The Galveston Orientation and Amnesia Test
(A prospective measure of posttraumatic amnesia duration)
• Westmead Posttraumatic Amnesia Scale
(A measure of posttraumatic amnesia duration)

TABLE 5–2. GLASCOW COMA SCALE

Scoring of Eye Opening
4 – opens eyes spontaneously
3 – opens eyes to command
2 – opens eyes to painful stimuli
1 – no eye opening

Scoring of Motor Responsiveness
6 – can follow simple motor commands
5 – localizes painful stimuli
4 – generalized response to pain
3 – decorticate posturing to pain
2 – decerebrate posturing to pain
1 – no motor responsiveness to pain

Scoring of Verbal Responsiveness
5 – appropriate speech
4 – converses though confused/disoriented
3 – minimal confused speech, words/phrases
2 – incomprehensible sounds
1 – no verbal responsiveness

brain injury severity. Special studies including neuroimaging procedures may help to document these abnormalities.

  a. Skull fractures may constitute open or closed head trauma. Open head trauma involves a communication between the intracranial compartment and the air which may occur with linear skull fractures having overlying scalp lacerations, depressed skull fractures, frontal bone fractures, and basilar skull fractures. There is a significant risk for the development of an intracranial infection with open head trauma.

  b. Seizures may result from physiologic or structural neuronal injury. Seizures that occur within or after the first week following trauma, intracerebral hematomas, cortical contusions, and depressed skull fractures may increase the risk for posttraumatic epilepsy.

5. Outcomes measurement instruments: The measurement and prediction of outcomes may help to guide treatment decisions, be useful in research protocols, and assist service providers or policy makers in the allotment of resources. Some of the popular outcomes measurement scales are listed below.

  a. The Glasgow Outcome Scale is not a sensitive measure of individual progress during neurorehabilitation but is useful to provide quantitative population outcomes data (Table 5–3).

  b. The Ranchos Los Amigos Levels of Cognitive Function Scale is widely used as a descriptive measure of an individual's progress, including level of awareness and capacity to interact appropriately, during the neurorehabilitation process (Table 5–4). This scale is not useful in describing deficits of high-level cognition.

  c. The Functional Independence Measure is widely used in rehabilitation to document admission and discharge levels of physical ability including levels of independence in ambulation and self-care activities. This scale is relatively insensitive to cognitive and behavioral deficits.

  d. The neuropsychological testing battery performed by skilled neuropsychologists is useful in assessing specific areas of deficits involved in high-level cognition, as well as neurobehavioral abnormalities and disorders (including deficits related to organic brain injury and deficits that may be related to nonorganic disorders such as anxiety, depression, or malingering).

Neurorehabilitation During Acute Care

1. Neurorehabilitation interventions should begin during an acute hospitalization once the brain injury patient's condition has been stabilized. Interventions include the prevention of secondary complications, the maintenance of homeostasis, the promotion of early mobilization, and the promotion of early return to self-care. Interventions may begin in the intensive care unit or after transfer to a regular hospital ward.

2. The typical acute care brain trauma patient will have multiple medical and physical problems and will display confusion, agitation, and posttraumatic amnesia.

3. Prevention measures include active interventions and regular patient monitoring for secondary complications of traumatic brain injury (including those complications that may occur secondary to the loss of mobility and the impairment of cognition). Possible complications include deep vein thrombosis and pulmonary embolism; skin breakdown; spasticity, joint contractures and heterotropic ossification; pneumonia; falls, fractures

TABLE 5–3. GLASCOW OUTCOME SCALE

Score	Category	Definition
1	Death	
2	Coma/Vegetative state	Unresponsiveness to internal or external stimuli
3	Severe disability	Dependent for daily care by reason of mental/physical impairments
4	Moderate disability	Independent with self-care, but requires sheltered environment
5	Good recovery	Functional independence though minor deficits may persist

Adapted from Jennett B, Bond MR: Assessment of Outcome in Severe Brain Damage: A practical scale. Lancet 1:480–484, 1975.

TABLE 5–4. RANCHOS LOS AMIGOS LEVELS OF COGNITIVE FUNCTION SCALE

I. No response
II. Generalized response to stimuli
III. Localized response to stimuli
IV. Confused agitated behavior
V. Confused non-agitated but inappropriate behavior
VI. Automatic and appropriate behavior
VII. Purposeful and appropriate behavior

and joint dislocations; seizures; posttraumatic hydrocephalus; neuroendocrine disorders (such as syndrome of inappropriate secretion of antidiuretic hormone—SIADH—or diabetes insipidus); occult traumatic injuries (such as spinal cord injury); hypertension, tachycardia and increased cardiac output often due to hypothalamic dysfunction and the increased release of circulating catecholamines).

4. The routine monitoring of basic health functions and health indicators including vital signs, nutrition and hydration status, bladder and bowel function, skin integrity, respiratory status, sleep adequacy, and pain help to assure the maintenance of homeostasis.

5. Early physical and occupational therapeutic interventions include passive or active patient mobilization and the encouragement of early participation in self-care activities. The speech therapist assists in the early assessment and treatment of disorders of cognition, communication, and swallowing. The psychologist participates in the assessment and treatment of disorders of cognition and behavior, and assists with family education and adjustment issues.

6. Early rehabilitation interventions continue during the acute hospitalization while the brain trauma patient is monitored or treated for various medical or surgical conditions.

The Rehabilitation Process

1. Brain trauma rehabilitation may continue in a variety of settings depending on the extent of functional disabilities, medical comorbidities, and the patient's ability to tolerate physical activity following discharge from the acute care hospital.

2. Comprehensive rehabilitation involves an active inpatient multidisciplinary therapeutic team approach to improve as needed an individual's strength, endurance, balance, mobility, transfers, ambulation, the performance of self-care activities, cognition, communication, swallowing, behavior, community re-entry skills; and to assist with patient–family adjustment issues and education.

3. Subacute brain trauma rehabilitation may involve

less active therapies that are provide in a skilled nursing facility for those patients who may be unable to tolerate an active rehabilitation program such as those who may be in a vegetative state or slow to recover.

4. Post-acute rehabilitation may involve the continuation of therapies at home, in an outpatient facility, in a transitional living facility, or in a vocational or school re-entry program. In some cases, where there may be prominent disinhibited or aggressive behavior, further treatment may be necessary in a residential behavioral management program.

5. Medications may be prescribed during the rehabilitation process for a host of reasons including seizure prevention; control of unstable behaviors including agitation/aggression; to increase arousal; to reduce anxiety or depression; to treat pain or to aid sleep. In general, medications that may impair daytime concentration or attention are avoided.

Special Situations

1. Coma intervention
   a. 50% of individuals who are vegetative at 1 month postinjury regain some degree of consciousness within a year; and more than 25% improve to a level of independence. However, emergence from coma complicated by hypoxic injury is far less likely.
   b. Good prognostic indicators for coma recovery include early spontaneous eye opening, conjugate eye movements, reactive pupils, decorticate posturing, and the absence of hydrocephalus or ventilator dependence.
   c. Multidisciplinary therapeutic interventions include multisensory stimulation; treatment of spasticity; interventions to improve joint mobility and orthostatic tolerance; encouragement of protective reflexes; vestibular stimulation; screening for adverse medical events such as undiagnosed seizures, hydrocephalus, or neuroendrocine disorders; avoidance of sedating medications; and trials of medications that may enhance arousal.

2. Mild traumatic brain injury/concussion
   a. 50% of patients with mild head injury develop symptoms, and of those 10% to 15% may develop persistent or disabling problems. Headache and vertigo are the most common postconcussion symptoms. Behavioral or cognitive dysfunction may occur in patients with unilateral or multi-focal abnormalities on neuroimaging.
   b. Treatment is individualized based on a thor-

ough evaluation of each symptomatic complaint. Management should be practical; it should always include patient–family education and, when necessary, somatic medical treatments, psychological-psychiatric therapies, and pragmatic occupational interventions.

3. Pediatric rehabilitation: Children require a specialized rehabilitation environment where they can recover from their injury, regain skills, and learn at age-appropriate levels. Programs emphasize three basic components of a child's life: family, school, and recreation. Individualized educational programs are developed to assist with the eventual transition back into the community school system.

Neurorehabilitation Follow-up

1. Gaps in medical follow-up increase risks for institutionalization of patients having traumatic brain injury and related disabilities. Therefore routine medical follow-up is encouraged by the neurorehabilitation specialist.

2. Responsibility for coordination of outpatient medical care, rehabilitation services, and determination of further rehabilitation needs rests with the neurorehabilitation specialist.

3. Goals of follow-up include assessment of health status, safety, maintenance of function, and adequacy of family or caregiver interventions. Areas of concern include medical, physical, cognitive, emotional, and social function.

4. Sexual function issues are another area of follow-up concern. Adaptive strategies, devices, and counseling can enhance sexual function in patients with disabilities.

5. Functional capacity evaluations are available for patients who are making the transition back to the community to help determine their ability to safely drive a car, operate machinery, or return to work at a particular vocation.

Bibliography

Bajo A, Fleminger S: Brain injury rehabilitation: what works for whom and when: Brain Inj 16:385–395, 2002.

Horn LJ: Systems of care for the person with traumatic brain injury. In Berrol S (ed): Physical Medicine and Rehabilitation Clinics of North America: Traumatic Brain Injury. Philadelphia, W.B. Saunders, 1992; pp. 475–492.

Kushner D: Principles of neurorehabilitation. In Weiner WJ, Gortz CG (eds): Neurology for the Non-neurologist, 4th ed. Philadelphia, Lippincott Williams & Wilkins, 1999; pp. 453–466.

Kushner D: Mild traumatic brain injury: Toward understanding manifestations and treatment. Arch Intern Med 158: 1617–1624, 1998.

Rosenthal M, Griffith ER, Bond MR, Miller JD (eds): Rehabilitation of the Adult and Child with Traumatic Brain Injury. Philadelphia, F.A. Davis, 1990.

Whyte J, Hart T, Laborde A, Rosenthal M: Rehabilitation of the patient with traumatic brain injury. In Delisa JA, Gans BM (eds), Rehabilitation Medicine Principles and Practice, 3rd ed. Philadelphia, Lippincott-Raven, 1998; pp. 1191–1231.

6 Spinal Cord Injury

Aclan Dogan
Anil Nanda

Definition

Spinal cord injury may be defined as an insult to the spinal cord resulting in partial or complete compromise of the functions of the cord such as motor, sensory, autonomic, and reflex functions. Although the most common cause is trauma, a significant number occur as a result of infections, tumors, vascular compromise, or a degenerative disease. Approximately 50% of the trauma cases result in quadriplegia and the other half in paraplegia. The management of spinal cord injuries is continuously evolving.

Epidemiology and Etiology

1. Nationally, nearly 48% of all injuries are the result of motor vehicle accidents. The next most frequent causes are falls, acts of violence (including gunshot and other penetrating wounds), and athletic injuries, which account for 21%, 15%, and 14%, respectively.

2. Approximately 85% of the injured patients are male and 15% female. This male preponderance decreases beyond age 65, when falls become the most common mechanism of spinal cord injury.

3. The most common injuries are to the middle and low cervical levels, which are the most mobile and flexible regions of the spine. The second most common level of injury is at the thoracolumbar junction, which biomechanically is the second most mobile spinal column region.

4. It has been estimated that 8000 to 10,000 traumatic spinal cord injuries occur each year in the United States. Currently in the United States estimates of the prevalence of individuals with chronic paralysis due to spinal cord injury vary between 250,000 and 500,000.

Clinical Findings

1. Detailed neurologic assessment of a cervical spinal cord injury begins with a standard motor and sensory evaluation. Motor function is scored on a scale of 0 to 5 for each muscle tested.

2. Sensory examination should be multimodality and include an assessment of the lateral and dorsal columns. The lateral columns carry pain and temperature sense and can be tested with pinprick or an ice cube. The dorsal columns carry touch, vibration, and position sense and are usually tested acutely with a tuning fork.

3. An important part of the initial neurologic screening is the rectal examination because of the clinical significance of the concept of sacral sparing. Pain or temperature sparing in the sacral area is more significant than retention of touch or vibration perception. Patients with lateral column sacral sparing, who are otherwise totally without motor and sensory function below the injury, may improve significantly, even to the point of walking.

4. Reflex testing is the least reliable part of a neurologic examination with regard to diagnosis and prognosis. Patients with high-velocity injuries may never experience spinal shock and may be hyperreflexive and spastic immediately after injury. They may even have rectal tone.

5. Spinal shock is physiologic transection of the cord associated with flaccid areflexia and no sensation below the level/zone of the injury. The patient should be told initially that because he or she is in spinal shock and has complete lesions, there is only a 3% to 5% chance of significant spontaneous recovery.

6. Approximately 1% of the spinal cord injury population develops what is called an ascending cord necrosis syndrome. It occurs more commonly in young patients of the pediatric and adolescent age group and in patients presenting with a Brown-Séquard syndrome. It most often presents during the first couple of weeks after injury. A swollen cord is often noted on magnetic resonance imaging (MRI) or after computed tomography (CT) myelography. It is not certain whether it represents a problem of ischemia or progressive infarction, but it is thought by most clinicians to be a vascular phenomenon.

7. A physician may "clear" the cervical spine (i.e., decide that significant spinal injury does not exist) simply by examining a patient. It is considered "clear" if the patient has no neck pain and meets the following criteria.
   a. No altered mental status
   b. No neurologic deficits
   c. No intoxication from alcohol or other drugs or medications
   d. No other painful injuries that may divert his or her attention from a neck injury

8. In other cases, such as when patients complain of

521

neck pain, are not fully awake, or have obvious weakness or other signs of neurologic injury, the cervical spine is kept in a rigid collar until appropriate radiologic studies are completed.

Types of Spinal Injury

1. *Bony or ligamentous injury.* Fortunately, most injuries to the spine are not associated with injury to the spinal cord itself. Some of these fractures require only immobilization, such as a rigid collar for cervical spine fractures or some type of brace or body jacket for fractures lower in the spine. Even if the bones and ligaments are not damaged, the muscles and other soft tissues of the neck may sustain an injury that can be painful but is usually not serious. However, other bony or ligamentous injuries may require surgery to stabilize the spine. If left untreated, some bony and ligamentous injuries eventually cause chronic pain or result in progressive deformity of the spine.

2. *Complete spinal cord injury.* Completeness of the injury is based on the presence of detectable function below the level of the injury. Individuals with no detectable sensory or motor function more than three segments below the level of injury should be classified as having a "complete" injury. Almost one half of all spinal cord injuries are complete.

Key Point: Complete Spinal Cord Injury

- No detectable sensory or motor function more than three segments below the level of injury indicates a "complete" injury.

---

3. *Incomplete spinal cord injury.* The term "incomplete" describes an individual's preservation of sensory or motor function (or both) more than three segments below the level of the lesion. Patients with incomplete injuries have a greater probability of experiencing some degree of return of function. Incomplete spinal cord injuries often fall into one of several patterns.

Key Point: Incomplete Spinal Cord Injury

- Preservation of sensory or motor function (or both) more than three segments below the level of the lesion is an "incomplete" injury

---

   a. Central cord syndrome

     (1) Most common in male patients of middle and older age groups who have preexisting cervical spondylosis and stenosis. The spi-

nal cord is compressed anteriorly and posteriorly.

     (2) These patients present with a clinical picture of weakness of the upper extremities (due to injury to the medial segments of the corticospinal tracts) that is greater than that of the lower extremities.

     (3) Most significant deficit is in the distal upper extremities, where they not only have motor and sensory loss but also frequently associated dysesthetic or hyperesthetic sensory abnormalities.

     (4) These patients may also have bowel, bladder, and sexual dysfunction.

Key Signs: Central Cord Syndrome

- Upper extremity weakness
- Motor and sensory loss in the distal upper extremities
  —Dysesthetic or hyperesthetic sensory abnormalities frequently associated with motor and sensory loss
- Bowel, bladder, and sexual dysfunction

---

   b. Anterior cord syndrome

     (1) It is the second most common syndrome.

     (2) This syndrome is often associated with a vertebral fracture or dislocation (or both) and disc herniation that compresses the anterior aspect of the cord and damages the anterior and lateral white matters tracts and the gray matter.

     (3) CT myelograms or MRI scans usually reveal anterior canal compromise and cord compression.

     (4) These individuals present with total loss of motor and lateral column sensory function (pain and temperature) below the level of injury, but dorsal column function (i.e., proprioception, touch, position sense) is spared.

Key Signs: Anterior Cord Syndrome

- Total loss of motor and lateral column sensory function (pain and temperature) below the level of the injury
- Dorsal column function remains

---

   c. Brown-Sequard syndrome

     (1) This pattern of injury classically occurs as a result of a penetrating or stab wound that

produces anatomic severance of the left or right side of the cord.

(2) These patients have ipsilateral loss of dorsal column function (i.e., proprioception, touch, vibration deficit) and motor function as well as contralateral pain and temperature loss that usually begins two levels below the level of injury.

Key Signs: Brown-Sequard Syndrome

- Ipsilateral loss of dorsal column function (i.e., proprioception, touch, vibration deficit) and motor function

- Contralateral pain and temperature loss usually two levels below the injury

d. Conus medullaris syndrome

(1) These cases are unique owing to a combination of spinal cord and nerve root involvement (i.e., conus medullaris and cauda equina injury).

(2) Whereas patients with conus syndrome usually have injuries from T11 to L1, cauda equina syndrome is seen in injuries from L1 down through the sacral levels.

(3) These patients have pure lower motor neuron (peripheral nerve) injuries and flaccid areflexia of not only the lower extremities but also the bowel and bladder.

(4) These patients often present with incomplete, asymmetrical deficits and have good potential for recovery.

(5) Patients with complete conus and cauda equina syndromes are often worse off functionally than their counterparts with complete cord injury, who enjoy the relative benefits of innervation, although they are centrally disconnected from their lower extremities.

(6) They also most often have reflex sphincter and sexual activity.

(7) Their spastic and innervated lower extremities undergo less severe atrophy than is experienced by victims of complete conus or cauda equina injury.

(8) Chronic intractable pain also seems to be more prevalent in patients with severe conus and cauda equina injury than in those with higher-level injuries.

Key Signs: Conus Medullaris Syndrome

- Incomplete, asymmetrical deficits

- Chronic intractable pain

Radiologic Features

1. The radiologic diagnosis of spinal injury begins with x-ray films. In many cases the entire spine is radiographed. Anteroposterior and lateral plain radiographs of the entire spinal column should be obtained immediately after arrival at the trauma center.

2. High-resolution CT with sagittal reconstruction is helpful for visualizing the bony anatomy, including any fractures.

3. Multiplanar high-resolution MRI with T_1-weighted and gradient-echo or T_2-weighted images is most helpful for looking at the spinal cord itself as well as any blood clots, herniated disks, or other masses that may be compressing the spinal cord.

Key Tests: Conus Medullaris Syndrome

- Computed tomography with sagittal reconstruction

- Magnetic resonance imaging scan (T_1-weighted and gradient-echo or T_2-weighted)

Treatment

1. Treatment of spinal cord injury begins in the prehospital setting, with paramedics or other emergency medical services personnel carefully immobilizing the entire spine. In the emergency department, this immobilization is continued while more immediate life-threatening problems are identified and addressed.

2. Standard intensive care unit (ICU) care—maintaining a stable blood pressure, monitoring cardiovascular function, ensuring adequate ventilation and lung function, preventing and promptly treating infection and other complications—is essential if patients with spinal cord injury are to achieve the best possible outcome.

3. In addition to high-quality ICU care, most patients with spinal cord injuries receive high doses of methylprednisolone (bolus of 30 mg/kg over 15 minutes and then maintenance of 5.4 mg/kg for 23 hours). This drug has been shown to improve the outcome slightly after spinal cord injury. To be effective, administration of this drug must begin

within 8 hours after injury; therefore patients often begin receiving it in the emergency room. If the drug was begun within 3 hours of injury, it is generally continued for 24 hours. If the patient did not receive the drug until 3 to 8 hours after injury, it may be best to continue the drug for 48 hours.

4. After the baseline assessments, including the history, physical examination, neurologic examination, and imaging, patients with spinal cord injury are placed in one of several categories.

a. For many injuries of the cervical spine, traction may be indicated to help "reduce" the spine (i.e., bring the spine into proper alignment).

b. Patients without compression on the spinal cord (i.e., patent canal) or spinal fractures or instability are transferred immediately to the ICU and are subjected to a standard acute-care protocol, which includes corticosteroids, if indicated, with no indication for decompression or surgical stabilization.

c. Patients without pressure on the spinal cord but with spinal column instability are taken to the operating room for surgical fusion when systemically stable. In some cases, primary placement in a halo apparatus, Miami-Jackson collar, or a thoracolumbar support with a brace may replace or supplement the need for surgery.

d. Patients with extrinsic spinal cord compression in whom traction is inappropriate (thoracic or lumbar) or it failed to relieve the pressure (cervical) are taken to the operating room, where surgery is performed to reestablish the patency of the spinal canal and the integrity of the spinal column. This includes realigning the spinal column, decompressing the spinal cord or its nerve roots, and stabilizing the spinal column with fusion and possibly instrumentation. The issue of the timing of surgical decompression of an acutely injured spinal cord is currently under intense debate. Traditionally, surgeons have thought that waiting several days was the safest course of action, as there was some evidence that operating immediately might worsen the outcome.

e. Acute surgical decompression is only rarely necessary for cervical injuries. Exceptions to this rule include cervical burst fractures, herniated discs, epidural hematoma, and such severe cervical spine disruption that the patients cannot be managed in a halo collar or without immediate surgical fixation. For example, patients with severe disruption associated with ankylosing spondylitis do best with early surgery.

f. For patients with penetrating wounds of the neck, chest, or abdomen, the life-threatening visceral injuries take priority over their neurologic lesions. Once it is determined that the patient with a spinal cord injury is physiologically stable after the life-saving procedure, he or she is considered for surgical or nonsurgical treatment.

g. Some patients have penetrating wounds of the spinal column and surrounding soft tissues but do not have major visceral injuries that are life-threatening or require surgical exploration. Patients in this category with complete neurologic lesions do not undergo surgical exploration when there are thoracic level injuries. Cervical level injuries are explored only if the bullet is in the canal and impinging on the cord or its roots. In these cases, the goal is to regain a nerve root level or relieve intractable local or radicular pain. Patients with incomplete thoracic and cervical gunshot wounds with neural element compression are all considered surgical candidates.

Key Treatment: Spinal Cord Injuries

- Immobilization
- Standard ICU care
  - Stabilize blood pressure
  - Monitor cardiovascular function
  - Ensure adequate ventilation
- Methylprednisolone administered within 8 hours after injury
- Surgical decompression and stability

Rehabilitation

1. The inpatient rehabilitation phase of care is provided by a multispecialty team of physicians, nurses, and allied health care personnel including rehabilitation nurses and nurse-clinicians; physical, occupational, recreational, and educational therapists; rehabilitation technicians; rehabilitation psychologists; social service specialists; vocational rehabilitation counselors; sexuality and reproduction counselors; dietitians; peer counselors; driver education specialists; and administrative personnel.

2. The overall goal of the rehabilitative phase is to return each patient to society with the greatest possible skills relating to independence and mobil-

ity. It is the consensus that most of the recovery occurs during the first year after injury.

3. The patients should return at least twice annually to a multidisciplinary-staffed spinal cord injury clinic where all body systems as well as the spine and spinal cord function are monitored and reevaluated. It has been shown that such frequent follow-up visits dramatically decrease the number of readmissions historically necessary to treat systemic complications.

Prognosis

Neurologic Improvement

1. Recovery of function depends on the severity of the initial injury. Unfortunately, those who sustain a complete spinal cord injury are unlikely to regain function below the level of the injury.

2. Incomplete injuries usually show some degree of improvement over time, but it varies with the type of injury. Although full recovery is unlikely in most cases, many patients can improve at least enough to ambulate and to control bowel and bladder function.

3. Patients with an anterior cord syndrome tend to do poorly, but most of those with a Brown-Sequard syndrome can expect to reach some of their goals.

4. Patients with a central cord syndrome often recover to the point of being ambulatory and controlling bowel and bladder, but often they are unable to perform detailed or intricate work with their hands.

5. Not surprisingly, young patients and those with incomplete injuries do better than older patients and those with complete injuries.

Mortality

1. Death from spinal cord injury is influenced by several factors. Perhaps the most important is the severity of associated injuries to the chest and abdomen. Many of these associated injuries are fatal.

2. For isolated spinal cord injuries, the mortality rate after 1 year is roughly 5% to 7%.

3. If a patient survives the first 24 hours after injury, the probability of surviving for 10 years is approximately 75% to 80%.

4. The 10-year survival rate for patients who survived the first year after injury is 87%.

Bibliography

Atkinson PP, Atkinson JLD: Spinal shock. Mayo Clin Proc 71:384–389, 1996.

Bracken MB: Steroids for acute spinal cord injury. Cochrane Database Syst Rev 3:CD001046, 2002.

Bracken MB, Shepard MJ, Collins WF, et al.: A randomized, controlled trial of methylprednisolone or naloxone in the treatment of acute spinal cord injury. N Engl J Med 322:1405–1411, 1990.

Green BA, David C, Falcone S, et al.: Spinal cord injuries in adults. In Youmans JR (ed): Neurological Surgery, Philadelphia, W.B. Saunders, 1996; pp 1969–1990.

Schneider RC: The syndrome of acute anterior spinal cord injury. J Neurosurg 12: 95–122, 1955.

Schneider RC, Cherry G, Pantek H: The syndrome of acute central cervical spinal cord injury. J Neurosurg 11: 546–577, 1954.

Waters RL, Adkins RH, Yakura J, et al.: Profiles of spinal cord injury and recovery after gunshot injury. Clin Orthop 267: 14–21, 1991.

7 Whiplash Injuries

Randolph W. Evans

Definition

1. An acceleration/deceleration mechanism of energy transfer to the neck that may result from a rear-end or side-impact motor vehicle collision
2. The term "whiplash," first used in 1928, is best used only as a description of the mechanism of injury and not as a description of the sequelae.

Epidemiology and Risk Factors

1. In 1999, there were 11.9 million motor vehicle accidents in the United States including 3.5 million rear-end collisions.
2. More than 1 million people per year have whiplash injuries in the United States.
3. Women experience persistent neck pain more frequently than men, especially in the 20- to 40-year age group, by a ratio of 7:3
   a. This greater susceptibility may be due either to a woman's narrower neck with less muscle mass supporting a head of roughly the same volume as a man's or to a narrower spinal canal than a man's.

Etiology and Pathophysiology

1. Animal and human studies have demonstrated damage to multiple structures, including intervertebral discs, facet joints, ligaments, and muscle.
2. When symptoms persist for more than 3 months, some physicians advance a variety of nonorganic explanations: emotional problems, a culturally conditioned and legally sanctioned illness, social and peer copying, secondary gain, and malingering.

Clinical Findings

1. Neck pain
   a. Onset within 6 hours in 65%, within 24 hours in an additional 28%, and within 72 hours in the remaining 7%
   b. Most neck pain is due to myofascial and facet (zygapophyseal) joint injury.
      (1) Myofascial trigger points can produce paresthesias in the limbs.
      (2) Facet joints can refer pain in characteristic patterns, depending on level, over various parts of the occipital, posterior cervical, shoulder girdle, and scapular regions.
      (3) Chronic neck pain arises from one or more facet joints in 54% of cases.
2. Headaches
   a. As many as 82% of patients complain of headache in the first weeks 4 weeks after whiplash injury, with an occipital location in 46%, generalized headache in 34%, and other locations in 20%. Headache is present more than half the time in 50% of patients.
   b. Headaches are usually of the muscle-contraction type, often associated with occipital neuralgia.
      (1) The term *occipital neuralgia* is in some ways a misnomer. The pain is not necessarily from the occipital nerve, and usually it does not have a neuralgic quality (paroxysmal, shooting pain), although such pain is present in some cases.
      (2) Greater occipital neuralgia can occur following trauma, but it also occurs without any injury.
      (3) The aching, pressure, stabbing, or throbbing pain may be in a nuchal-occipital and/or parietal, temporal, frontal or periorbital or retro-orbital location only, or in more than one location. The headache can last from minutes to hours to days and can be unilateral or bilateral.
      (4) Lesser occipital neuralgia has similar qualities, but the pain is generally referred more laterally over the head.
      (5) The headache can be due to an entrapment of the greater occipital nerve in the aponeurosis of the superior trapezius or semispinalis capitis muscle, or it can be referred without nerve compression from trigger points in these or other suboccipital muscles.
      (6) Digital pressure over the greater occipital nerve at the mid-superior nuchal line (halfway between the posterior mastoid and the occipital protuberance) reproduces the headache.
      (7) Pain referred from the C2–C3 facet joint or other upper cervical spine pathology and

posterior fossa pathology may produce a similar headache.

(8) Trigger points in other muscles such as the splenius cervicis, upper trapezius, sternocleidomastoid, masseter, temporalis, and occipitofrontalis can also produce referred pain in the head.

(9) Jaw pain associated with headache can be due to temporomandibular joint injury.

c. Can also be referred from the C2–C3 facet joint innervated by the third occipital nerve ("third occipital headache")

(1) Pain in upper cervical region and extending at least onto the occiput and at times toward the ear, vertex, forehead, or eye

(2) Accounts for 50% of persistent headaches

d. Occasionally can precipitate new-onset migraine.

3. Dizziness: Can be due to posttraumatic dysfunction of the vestibular apparatus, brainstem, and cervical proprioceptive system

4. About one third of patients complain of upper limb paresthesias

a. Can be referred from trigger points, facet joints, cervical roots, the brachial plexus, spinal cord compression, and entrapment neuropathies

b. Non-neurogenic thoracic outlet syndrome

(1) Paresthesias radiating down the limb often into the fourth and fifth fingers may be accompanied by subjective complaints of arm heaviness or weakness.

(2) Symptoms may worsen with overhead work, repetitive use, including computer use, and at night.

(3) No objective findings on examination or electromyogram (EMG)

(4) May be due to referred pain and paresthesias from a myofascial injury of the anterior neck muscles, such as the anterior scalene, or from the shoulder area, involving the pectoralis minor and not due to neural or vascular compression

c. Carpal tunnel syndrome can result from acute hyperextension of the wrist on the steering wheel.

5. Subjective complaints of upper limb heaviness, weakness, or fatigue: Can be due to non-neurogenic thoracic outlet syndrome or to reflex inhibition of muscle because of pain; the latter can be overcome by more central effort

6. Some patients also report nervousness and irritability, cognitive disturbances, disrupted sleep, fatigue, and blurred vision. Blurred vision is often due to convergence insufficiency, although oculomotor palsies can occasionally occur.

7. One third of patients complain of interscapular pain and low back pain.

8. Rare sequelae include torticollis, tremor, transient global amnesia, esophageal perforation and descending mediastinitis, hypoglossal nerve palsy, superior laryngeal paralysis, cervical epidural hematoma, and extracranial internal carotid and vertebral artery dissections.

Key Clinical Findings

- Neck pain
- Headaches
- Upper limb paresthesias
- Dizziness

Laboratory and Radiologic Testing

1. A cervical spine x-ray series is often obtained to exclude the occasional fracture or subluxation.

2. In patients with abnormal neurologic examinations or persistent complaints suggesting radiculopathy or myelopathy, a cervical spine magnetic resonance imaging (MRI) study may be indicated.

3. A cervical myelogram followed by computed tomography (CT) scan may be useful if the MRI study demonstrates equivocal findings or if an MRI study cannot be done. Myelography/CT may be more sensitive than MRI in some cases for nerve root compression and for surgical planning.

4. Nerve conduction velocity and EMG studies can provide evidence of radiculopathy, brachial plexopathy, carpal tunnel syndrome, or ulnar neuropathy at the elbow.

5. Because asymptomatic radiographic findings are common, it is often difficult to determine which findings are new and which are preexisting.

a. Cervical spondylosis and degenerative disc disease occur with increasing frequency with older age and often are asymptomatic.

b. Asymptomatic cervical disc protrusions are also common in the general population, occurring in 20% of people 45 to 54 years of age and 57% of those older than 64 years.

Treatment

1. Neck pain

a. Often treated initially with ice then with heat, nonsteroidal anti-inflammatory drugs

(NSAIDs), muscle relaxants, pain medications, and antidepressants such as the tricyclic antidepressants

b. Soft cervical collars can be used during the first 2 to 3 weeks but should then be avoided.

c. Range-of-motion exercises, physical therapy and transcutaneous electrical nerve stimulators may be helpful for patients with persistent complaints.

d. Trigger points

(1) Pain may be reduced or eliminated by trigger point injections with local anesthesia (e.g., 3 cc of 1% lidocaine), dry needling without any injection, sterile water, or sterile saline. An injectable corticosteroid produces no more improvement than a local anesthetic alone.

(2) Physical therapy using myofascial release techniques (e.g., stretch and spray) may also be beneficial.

e. Facet joints

(1) Symptomatic facet joints are identified by anesthetic blocks.

(2) Percutaneous radiofrequency neurotomy with multiple lesions of target nerves can provide at least 50% relief for a median duration of about 9 months.

f. Some patients report benefit from acupuncture or chiropractic treatment. Controlled efficacy studies would be worthwhile.

Key Treatment: Neck Pain

- NSAIDs and muscle relaxants

- Soft cervical collars as needed for first 2 to 3 weeks only

- Range-of-motion exercises, physical therapy

- Trigger point injections

- Facet joint identification and radiofrequency neurotomy as indicated

2. Headaches

a. Those of myofascial origin or caused by occipital neuralgia may be relieved by tricylic antidepressants, muscle relaxants, and NSAIDs. Chronic frequent use of opiates, benzodiazepines, butalbital, and carisoprodol should be avoided because of the potential for habituation and rebound headaches.

b. Those caused by occipital neuralgia may respond to local anesthetic nerve blocks with or without an injectable corticosteroid.

Key Treatment: Headaches

- Tricylic antidepressants

- Muscle relaxants

- NSAIDs

- Local anesthetic nerve blocks with or without an injectable corticosteroid

3. Non-neurogenic thoracic outlet syndrome: May benefit from an exercise program (Peet's exercises)

4. Patient education and a sympathetic approach may increase patient satisfaction with treatment and reduce treatment shopping.

Prognosis

1. Risk factors for persistent symptoms

a. Accident mechanisms: inclined or rotated head position, unprepared for impact, and car stationary when hit

b. Occupant's characteristics: older age, female gender, and stressful life events unrelated to the accident

c. Symptoms: intensity of initial neck pain or headache, occipital headache, interscapular or upper back pain, and multiple symptoms or paresthesias at presentation

d. Signs: reduced range of motion of the cervical spine and objective neurologic deficit

e. Radiographic findings: preexisting degenerative osteoarthritic changes, abnormal cervical spine curves, and narrow diameter of the cervical spinal canal

2. Duration of symptoms (Table 7–1): Most patients recover within 3 months, but a significant minority have persistent symptoms for 1 to 2 years or even longer.

3. Effect of litigation

a. Most patients who are symptomatic when litigation is settled continue to be symptomatic.

b. Litigants and nonlitigants have similar recovery rates and similar response rates to treatment for facet joint pain.

TABLE 7–1. PERCENTAGES OF PATIENTS WITH PERSISTENCE OF NECK PAIN AND HEADACHES FOLLOWING A WHIPLASH INJURY

SYMPTOM	1 WEEK	3 MONTHS	6 MONTHS	1 YEAR	2 YEARS
Neck pain	92	38	25	19	16
Headache	57	35	26	21	15

c. However, there are patients with pain complaints due to secondary gain, exaggeration, malingering, and psychosocial factors.

d. Clinicians should evaluate the merits of each case individually.

Prevention

1. General measures directed at driving safety such as reducing the number of drunk drivers, improving the driving habits of youngsters, and encouraging vigilance and discouraging multi-tasking while driving such as eating, putting on make-up, or talking on a cell phone.

2. Proper use of head restraints can reduce the incidence of neck pain in rear-end collisions by 24%. Adjustable head restraints should be in a position to prevent neck extension. Many drivers maintain the restraint at a position too low to rest their heads.

3. Even though wearing a seat belt and shoulder restraint should be encouraged, 73% of occupants wearing a seat belt develop neck pain as compared to 53% not wearing a seat belt. Rather than a whiplash injury, failure to wear a seatbelt could cause a more serious head injury.

Bibliography

Bogduk N, Tessell R: Whiplash: the evidence for an organic etiology. Arch Neurol 57:590–591, 2000.

Evans RW: Whiplash injuries. In Gilman S (ed): MedLink Neurology. San Diego, CA, MedLink, 2003.

Evans RW: Whiplash injuries. In Evans RW, Baskin DS, Yatsu FM (eds): Prognosis of Neurological Disorders, 2nd ed. New York, Oxford University Press, 2000, pp. 152–167.

Lord SM, Barnsley L, Wallis BJ, et al.: Percutaneous radio-frequency neurotomy for chronic cervical zygapophyseal joint pain. N Engl J Med 335:1721–1726, 1996.

Radanov BP, Sturznegger M, Di Stefano G: Long-term outcome after whiplash injury: a 2-year follow-up considering features of injury mechanism and somatic, radiologic, and psychosocial findings. Medicine 74:281–297, 1995.

8 Reflex Sympathetic Dystrophy and Causalgia

Thomas C. Chelimsky

Definition

1. The International Association for the Study of Pain arrived at a consensus definition in 1996. They used the terms complex regional pain syndromes I and II for reflex sympathetic dystrophy and causalgia, respectively.

2. "CRPS I is a syndrome that usually develops after initiating noxious event, is not limited to the distribution of a single nerve, and is apparently disproportionate to the inciting event. It is associated at some point with evidence of edema, changes in skin blood flow, abnormal sudomotor activity in the region of the pain, or allodynia or hyperalgesia."

3. CRPS II requires a well identified nerve injury.

Epidemiology

1. Neither the incidence nor the prevalence can be determined with any certainty for several reasons.

   a. It is probably underdiagnosed in the primary care community where the disorder is rarely seen.

   b. It is likely overdiagnosed by specialists who have no other real diagnosis to apply to chronic limb pain without a structural underpinning.

   c. There is no patient registry.

2. Preliminary evidence from an ongoing population-based study suggests a prevalence of around 20 per 100,000. This would amount to a prevalence higher than that for trigeminal neuralgia, or 70,000 cases in a country of 350 million people such as the United States. This number may still be small, as a busy pain specialist easily sees 100 new cases per year.

3. Precipitating events include, in order of frequency, immobilization (e.g., casting), fracture, nerve injury, nonspecific tissue trauma, and no clear event in quite a few. When produced by a well defined nerve lesion, the disorder is termed causalgia or complex regional pain syndrome II (CRPS II), in contrast to CRPS I or reflex sympathetic dystrophy (RSD) when this is not the case. The association of RSD with stroke is likely due to an undetected nerve injury in the anesthetic region.

4. Prognosis is varied depending on the stage of the illness, its responsiveness to blocks and pharmacologic manipulation, and the patient's motivation to work toward function in the face of pain. Probably 75% of patients with a disease duration of less than 6 months return to normal function, with quite a few cured; for longer durations of illness, when the probability of cure is small, fewer than 50% achieve these results.

Neuropathology

1. Neither the mechanisms that trigger an RSD nor those that maintain it are understood. RSD is perhaps best conceived as prolongation and exaggeration of the normal neural response to injury.

2. Animal models utilizing nerve injury have produced a similar clinical picture. Inferences drawn from these data suggest roles for several disparate pathophysiologic processes.

   a. Reorganization of the dorsal horn with disturbance of sensory, motor and autonomic functions.

   b. Abnormal central processing at thalamic and cortical (especially right anterior cingulate gyrus) levels amplifying pain signals.

   c. Aberrant sympathetic-somatic connections, with α-adrenergic receptors present on vessels, sweat nerves, and sensory nerve endings and within the dorsal root ganglion itself. Overexpression of nerve growth factor in genetically altered mice has similar consequences.

   d. Neurogenic inflammation occurs at the tissue level.

3. Sympathetically maintained pain refers to pain relieved by a sympathetic block. This term has relatively little pathophysiologic meaning, as sympathetic block in a particular individual is usually not placebo-controlled, and entities other than RSD have clearly been shown to respond to sympathetic block (e.g., shingles).

Symptoms

1. Symptoms fall into four categories: sensory, including pain; motor; autonomic; trophic.

   a. Sensory symptoms are most prominent, as they

include the chief complaint of pain. Hyperalgesia (comprising the first 3 items below) is the rule.

(1) Spontaneous pain

(2) Pain with a nonnoxious stimulus such as a cool breeze or light stroking, termed allodynia

(3) Exaggerated pain with a noxious stimulus

(4) Sensory loss in a stocking or glove distribution may be present.

b. Motor complaints include spasm, dystonic posturing, tremor, weakness, and reduced range of motion (ROM). In some cases, particularly after total knee arthroplasty, reduced passive and active ROM constitutes the only complaint and finding. This presentation seems exquisitely sensitive to an oral course of corticosteroid.

c. Autonomic complaints comprise the cornerstone of the clinical presentation and include vasomotor disturbances, with swelling, protrusion of skin veins, and labile skin color and temperature to extremes, as well as sudomotor abnormalities, with absent (early in the disease course) or excessive (later) sweating.

d. Trophic changes include thickening of the hair and nails, shiny thin skin, and abnormal bones, with periarticular osteoporosis.

2. In addition to symptom categories, the disorder appears to have stages of progression, with a warm, dry limb in the earliest stage; a cool, wet limb in the middle stage; and a severely atrophic but less painful in the last stage.

 Key Symptoms

Sensory

- Hyperalgesia
- Allodynia
- Distal sensory loss
- Paresthesias

Motor

- Spasm
- Reduced range of motion
- Dystonia
- Tremor

Autonomic

- Swelling
- Sweating
- Discoloration
- Labile skin temperature

Trophic

- Thin skin
- Thick hair
- Ridged nails
- Periarticular osteoporosis

Clinical Findings

1. Confirmatory findings parallel the criteria for diagnosis and include sensory, motor, autonomic, and trophic abnormalities. The most typical findings are hypesthesia in a stocking or glove distribution, allodynia to cold or to light stroking, limited ROM or mild dystonic posturing of the extremity, asymmetrical skin temperature, palpably increased sweat production, coarse nails and hair, and taught, shiny skin. Such findings confirm the diagnosis.

2. Because a nerve injury is likely to underlie an RSD, it is important to seek it out on examination through assessment of Tinel's sign and sensory loss in the distribution of the nerve. The finding of a major nerve injury alters the diagnosis from CRPS I to CRPS II and provides additional avenues for treatment.

Laboratory Tests

The diagnosis is primarily clinical. No test can establish the diagnosis, although some tests are helpful for supporting the diagnosis: a bone scan and tests of autonomic function.

1. A three-phase technetium pyrophosphate bone scan yields diffuse uptake in a good proportion of the limbs involved with RSD. The scan can also be helpful for excluding other competing diagnoses, such as stress fractures, metastatic lesions, or underlying osteoporosis. Note that in children the scan shows just the opposite: reduced uptake on the affected side.

2. Autonomic testing can support the diagnosis when resting sweat rates are increased on the affected side compared to the uninvolved side. In addition, the resting skin temperature is predictive for response to a sympathetic block.

3. Plain radiographs show periarticular osteoporosis (Sudek's atrophy) in more advanced cases.

4. Magnetic resonance imaging of the limb may reveal interstitial edema and can exclude other soft tissue causes of pain, if clinically warranted.

5. EMG can diagnose injury to a major nerve underlying the RSD (in a diagnosis of CRPSII) resulting.

 Key Tests

- Tests are supportive only, not diagnostic.
- Plain radiography
- Autonomic testing
- Bone scan
- Electromyography (to diagnose a nerve injury)
- MRI of soft tissue

Differential Diagnosis

1. Differential diagnosis for RSD has two meanings, as RSD is intrinsically associated with some other provocative process. One must therefore, in all cases, attempt to ascertain the cause and in so doing simultaneously evaluate for some of these causative diagnoses as competing diagnoses. They include thrombosis of a vein or artery, compartment syndromes, occult fractures (stress, osteoporotic, malignant), osteomyelitis or cellulitis, and disruption of a nerve. Physical examination should in large part be sufficient to exclude these diagnoses.

2. Phenobarbital and isoniazid can cause RSD and must be stopped before an RSD will resolve.

3. If pain progresses in the same limb or into another limb, RSD progression should be a diagnosis of exclusion; it should never be assumed. In most such cases, the added pain is due to overuse of the second limb or joint, with consequent bursitis or ensethitis, among others.

Treatment

1. The complexity of the RSD syndrome requires an interdisciplinary approach. The disciplines involved in management depend on the specific symptoms exhibited by the patient. If motor involvement is major, both physical therapy and occupational therapy are required. In most cases the syndrome has had major debilitating consequences on the patient's life, and the help of a psychologist is nearly always critical. The administration of sympathetic blocks, if appropriate, necessitates participation of an anesthesiologist. Finally, a physician (a neurologist in our center) must prescribe and modify medications as needed.

2. Management is complex and requires extensive education, particularly emphasizing functional gains over pain relief. Ideal management provides an environment in which the patient learns strategies for continued functional improvement, initially through training (behavioral therapy) and eventually through reconceptualizing the entire problem (cognitive-behavioral therapy) into one that is limited and manageable (rather than a

TABLE 8–1. APPROACHES TO TREATMENT

PROBLEM	INTERVENTION	MEDICATION
Consequences of pain		
Sleeplessness	Relaxation strategies by psychologist	Sedative pain-relieving tricyclic such as amitriptyline or doxepin. (Benzodiazepines should never be used.)
Depression	Counseling (psychiatric)	SSRI
Fear–avoidance	Pacing strategies; control issues	
Sensory		
Shooting pain	Desensitization (OT)	Anticonvulsant such as gabapentin, oxcarbazepine
Burning pain	Desensitization (OT)	Daytime tricyclic such as imipramine
Aching	Mobilization	Nonsteroidal or scheduled opiate (never "as needed")
Allodynia	Contrast baths (OT)	Ketamine or other analgesic ointments prepared at compound pharmacy
Tinel's sign	Strengthening neighboring muscles	Clonidine patch over site of Tinel's
Refractory pain		Spinal cord stimulation
Motor		
Reduced weight-bearing	Stress loading of joints	Moderate to high dose oral corticosteroid for 1–3 weeks
Reduced range of motion	Continuous passive motion machine	Corticosteroid
Spasm	Specific exercises of involved muscles (PT)	Antispastics such as baclofen, tizanidine, or clonazepam
Dystonia	Muscle training reeducation training	Dopaminergic or anticholinergic agents
Autonomic, prominent	Sympathetic block or radiofrequency lesion	Phenoxybenzamine
Trophic: osteopenia	Stress loading	IV or IN calcitonin

Abbreviations: IN, intranasal; OT, occupational therapy; PT, physical therapy; SSRI, selectic serotonin reuptake inhibitors.

process that controls the patient). A specific functional goal should be set by the patient and team together at each stage of progress.

3. For specific issues, optimal approaches are outlined in Table 8–1. Most patients should receive at least one of high-dose corticosteroid (e.g., prednisone 60–80 mg/day for 1–3 weeks). Only steroids and calcitonin emerge as effective treatment for RSD from meta-analyses.

Key Treatment

Interdisciplinary approach addressing

• Behavioral issues

• Psychological obstacles to progress

• Physical deconditioning and other motor dysfunction

• Cutaneous hypersensitivity

• Anesthesiology procedures

Clear goal orientation

Medications selected based on specific issues

Bibliography

Birklein F, Schmelz M, Schifter S, Weber M: The important role of neuropeptides in complex regional pain syndrome. Neurology 57:2179–2184, 2001.

Chemali KR, Gorodeski R, Chelimsky TC: Alpha-adrenergic supersensitivity of the sudomotor nerve in complex regional pain syndrome. Ann Neurol 49:453–459, 2001.

Forouzanfar T, Koke AJ, van Kleef M, Weber WE: Treatment of complex regional pain syndrome type I. Eur J Pain 6:105–122, 2002.

Fukumoto M, Ushida T, Zinchuk VS, et al.: Contralateral thalamic perfusion in patients with reflex sympathetic dystrophy syndrome. Lancet 20:1790–1791, 1999.

Kemler MA, Barendse GA, van Kleef M, et al.: Spinal cord stimulation in patients with chronic reflex sympathetic dystrophy. N Engl J Med 343:618–624, 2000.

Kingery WS: Critical review of controlled clinical trials for peripheral neuropathic pain and complex regional pain syndromes. Pain 79:317–319, 1999.

Perez RS, Kwakkel G, Zuurmond WW, de Lange JJ: Treatment of reflex sympathetic dystrophy (CRPS type 1): a research synthesis of 21 randomized clinical trials. J Pain Symptom Manage 21:511–526, 2001.

Anatomy and Physiology

1. Peripheral nerves are composed of unmyelinated and myelinated axons surrounded by Schwann cells and a supporting tissue.

    a. Unmyelinated axons are surrounded by the plasma membrane of a Schwann cell.

    b. Myelinated axons are surrounded by a Schwann cell that wraps around the axon multiple times, insulating the axon by multiple layers of its cell membrane, which is rich in lipid sphingomyelin.

    c. Nerve fibers are surrounded by three supportive layers that are highly elastic and serve as shields to protect the myelin and axon from external pressure and tension (Fig. 9–1). These layers include

    (1) Endoneurium

    (2) Perineurium

    (3) Epineurium

2. The myelinated axon is completely surrounded by myelin and Schwann cells except at certain gaps, called the nodes of Ranvier, where sodium channels are highly concentrated. In adults the length of myelinated segments, called the internodal segments, is approximately 1 mm, and the nodes of Ranvier measure approximately 1 μm. Saltatory conduction occurs at the nodes of Ranvier owing to their high sodium channel concentration and the low capacitance and high resistance of the internodal myelin.

Classification

1. Compression, traction, laceration, and thermal and chemical injuries may damage peripheral nerves. The pathologic reactions and the pathophysiologic correlates of these focal injuries are limited.

2. In myelinated nerves, peripheral nerve injuries results in axonal loss, demyelination, or both. The nerve injury may or may not destroy the supporting structures partially or completely.

3. Peripheral nerve injuries are classified based on the functional status of the nerve and histologic findings. Seddon's initial classification continues to be popular among surgeons, but Sunderland's revision is more detailed and has better clinical and prognostic implications (Table 9–1).

    a. *Neurapraxia or first-degree nerve injury.* This usually results from brief or mild pressure on the nerve, which may distort the myelin producing segmental demyelination and conduction block without wallerian degeneration.

    b. *Axonotmesis or second-degree nerve injury.* This type of injury occurs with longer or increasing pressure on the nerve and with ischemia or traction. It results in axonal damage with secondary wallerian degeneration distal to the site of injury. However, all the supporting structures (endoneurium, perineurium, epineurium) remain intact.

    c. *Neurotmesis.* This injury follows prolonged or extreme pressure on a nerve, or accompanies lacerations or gunshot wounds. The peripheral nerve injury is severe, resulting in complete disruption of the nerve with all the supporting structures. Because the nerve injury may affect one or more levels of the supporting structures, resulting in different prognoses, this class is often subdivided, as advocated by Sunderland, into three further types.

    (1) *Third-degree nerve injury,* in which the endoneurium is disrupted with intact perineurium and epineurium

    (2) *Fourth-degree nerve injury,* where the endoneurium and perineurium are disrupted, but the epineurium is intact

    (3) *Fifth-degree nerve injury,* where the nerve is transected, resulting in complete discontinuity of the nerve

Diagnosis

1. The diagnosis of peripheral nerve injury often requires a detailed history and neurologic examination, with electrodiagnostic (EDX) studies and surgical findings playing significant roles. The history of the type of injury is extremely important; for example, a history of a stab wound injury is often associated with axonal interruptions and grade 3 to 5 nerve injuries, whereas interoperative compression may be due to grade 1 or 2 nerve injuries.

2. EDX studies, which evaluate the integrity of the myelin sheath and axon exclusively, can only

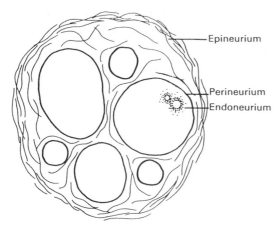

Figure 9–1. Anatomy of a peripheral nerve. (From Sunderland S: Nerve Injuries and Their Repair: A Critical Appraisal. Edinburgh, Churchill Livingstone, 1991; with permission.)

distinguish a neurapraxic injury (first degree or myelin injury) from all other degrees of injury in which there is axonal damage and degeneration. Hence, assessing the extent of the damage to the supporting nerve structures requires anatomic assessment of the nerve during surgery.

3. There are three electrophysiologic consequences of peripheral nerve injury: (1) focal slowing of conduction; (2) conduction block; and (3) axonal loss (conduction failure). The first two are due to disruption of myelin and are relatively benign and often reversible. The third, due to axonal damage, is more severe and may be irreversible. Combined patterns may also occur.

  a. *Focal slowing* of conduction, when isolated, is not associated with weakness or sensory loss but is a convenient method for localizing peripheral nerve lesions. Focal slowing is often the result of widening of the nodes of Ranvier *(paranodal demyelination)*. This may present on EDX studies in one of two ways.

   (1) When all the large myelinated fibers are slowed to essentially the same degree, focal slowing (synchronized slowing) of conduction across the nerve segment is evident on nerve conduction studies. This is shown by either prolongation of distal latencies or slowing of conduction velocities. In contrast, the compound muscle action potentials' (CMAPs) amplitude and duration are not affected and do not change when the nerve is stimulated proximal to the lesion.

   (2) When the speed of impulse transmission is reduced at the lesion site along a variable number of medium or small nerve fibers (average or slower conducting axons), differential (desynchronized) slowing of conduction across the nerve segment is evident. In this situation, the CMAPs are dispersed on stimulations proximal to the lesion and have prolonged duration, with normal (nondispersed) responses on distal stimulation. If this finding is isolated, the speed of conduction along the injury site (latency or conduction velocity) is normal, as at least some of the fastest conducting axons are spared. However, when the latter fibers are also involved, differential slowing is accompanied by slowing of the latency or conduction velocity.

  b. *Conduction block* is caused by blockage of transmission of action potentials across the injured nerve segment. Normally, the action potential travels in a saltatory fashion passing nodes of Ranvier without failure. Conduction block is usually the result of a loss of one or more myelin segments *(segmental or internodal demyelination)*. It may also follow axonal loss before the completion of wallerian degeneration ("axonal" conduction block; see Axonal loss, below). Conduction block is defined as a significant decrease in CMAP amplitude, the area with stimulation proximal to the injury site, or both when compared with

TABLE 9–1. CLASSIFICATION AND DEGREES OF PERIPHERAL NERVE INJURY

Sunderland	First degree	Second degree	Third degree	Fourth degree	Fifth degree
Seddon	Neurapraxia	Axonotmesis	Neurotmesis		
Electrophysiology	Conduction block	Axonal loss			
Pathology	Segmental demyelination	Loss of axons with intact supporting structures	Loss of axons with disrupted endoneurium	Loss of axons with disrupted endoneurium and perineurium	Loss of axons, with disruption of all supporting structures (discontinuous)
Prognosis	Excellent; recovery usually complete in 2–3 months	Slow recovery that is dependent on sprouting and reinnervation	Protracted and can fail due to misdirected axonal sprouts	Unlikely without surgical repair	Impossible without surgical repair

From Katirji B: Electromyography in Clinical Practice: A Case Study Approach. St. Louis, Mosby, 1998; with permission.

the CMAP distal to it, with no evidence of significant temporal dispersion (i.e., prolongation of CMAP duration). Conduction block may involve all the myelinated axons (complete block) or only some of them, leaving the others normal (partial block). A nerve lesion manifesting with conduction block is best localized when it can be bracketed by two stimulation points: one distal to the site of injury (resulting in a normal CMAP) and one proximal to it (resulting in a partial or complete decrease in CMAP).

c. *Axonal loss.* In cases where there has been axonal degeneration, the nerve conduction studies characteristically result in an unelicitable or uniformly low CMAP amplitude, which is not dispersed, at all stimulation points. There are two caveats related to the above findings that may cause diagnostic confusion.

    (1) Although unelicitable or uniformly low CMAP amplitudes are typically seen in cases of axonal degeneration, they are encountered occasionally when there is conduction block (due to segmental demyelination) situated distally along the nerve, between the most distal stimulating point and the recording site.

    (2) Following axonal damage, the distal axon undergoes degeneration (wallerian degeneration), that is completed in 7 to 11 days. However, even soon after axonal transection the distal axon remains excitable. Electrophysiologically, the distal CMAP decreases and reaches its nadir within 5 to 6 days, but the distal sensory nerve action potential lags slightly behind, reaching its nadir at 10 to 11 days (Fig. 9–2). Hence, early after an axon-loss peripheral nerve injury (grades 2–5), a conduction block pattern is common. This is similar to the

conduction block pattern seen with segmental demyelination (first degree injury or neurapraxia), except that repeat studies after completion of wallerian degeneration reveal a decrease in the distal CMAPs, with values similar to those of the proximal CMAPs. This type of conduction block has been referred to as axonal noncontinuity, early axon loss, or axon discontinuity conduction block. It should be noted that identifying a conduction block during the early days of axonal loss is extremely helpful for localizing a peripheral nerve injury, particularly when it is of the closed type, where the exact site of trauma is not apparent. Hence it is important to perform nerve conduction studies as soon as the patient seeks medical attention. Waiting for the completion of wallerian degeneration results in diffusely low CMAPs (regardless of the stimulation site), which does not allow localization of the injury site. Needle electromyography (EMG) is useful, but localization by this method is suboptimal because peripheral nerves may not have motor branches from long segments (e.g., the median and ulnar nerves in the arms).

4. Needle EMG is useful for evaluating and managing peripheral nerve injuries in one of three situations.

a. For axonal loss lesions examined after the completion of wallerian degeneration, where nerve conduction studies are not associated with localizing focal slowing or conduction block, needle EMG helps localize the lesion to a nerve segment.

b. For severe axonal lesions associated with absent sensory and motor nerve conduction studies suggesting a grade 5 injury (neurotmesis), needle EMG may prove that the nerve is in

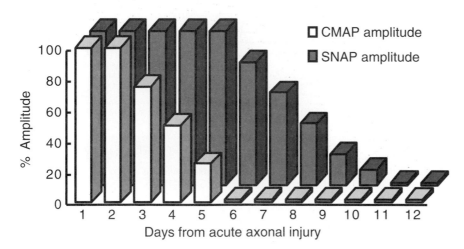

Figure 9–2. Distal compound muscle action potential (CMAP) and sensory nerve action potential (SNAP) after acute axonal nerve injuries. (From Katirji B: Electromyography in Clinical Practice: A Case Study Approach. St. Louis, Mosby, 1998; with permission.)

TABLE 9–2. THERAPY OF PERIPHERAL NERVE INJURIES

NERVE LESION	EMG	OPERATIVE CNAP	THERAPY

Nerve transection	Not done acutely	Not done acutely	Early operation (72 hrs)
			   Sharp laceration: repair by end-to-end suture
			   Blunt laceration: repair 2–4 weeks later
			   Nerve intact: conservative

Nerve incontinuity (focal lesion)	Serial EMG: 2–4 months
	   Axonal integrity /regeneration = conservative treatment
	   No axonal integrity = surgery with operative CNAP
		Surgery
		   CNAP present
		   CNAP absent
			
			Simple neurolysis
			Resection and repair (graft)

Nerve incontinuity (long lesion)	Serial EMG: 4–6 months
	   Axonal integrity /regeneration = conservative treatment
	   No axonal integrity = surgery with operative CNAP
		Surgery
		   CNAP present
		   CNAP absent
			
			Simple neurolysis
			Resection and repair (graft)

Abbreviations: EMG, electromyography; CNAP, compound nerve action potential.
From Gutierrez A, England JD: Peripheral nerve injuries. In Katirji B, Kaminski HJ, Preston DC, et al (eds). Neuromuscular Disorders in Clinical Practice, Boston, Butterworth-Heinemann, 2002; with permission.

continuity by recording from few residual motor unit action potentials (MUAPs).

c. With axonal lesions, needle EMG is extremely useful for following the progress of reinnervation. A progressive proximal-to-distal increase in the number of voluntary MUAPs and the presence of new MUAPs (nascent units) is strong evidence of reinnervation, which may occur spontaneously or after surgical repair.

Treatment

1. The management of peripheral nerve injuries may be conservative or surgical, depending on the extent of the injury (Table 9–2). Often there is associated pain (causalgia) that requires treatment with anticonvulsants, tricyclic antidepressants, or both.

2. In acute nerve lesions associated with neurapraxia and segmental demyelination (first-degree injuries), recovery is often rapid and is completed in 6 to 8 weeks, so long as the offending factor (usually compression) is eliminated.

3. In conditions where there is sharp nerve transection (e.g., injuries caused by glass, knives, or sharp metal edges), immediate repair is indicated and should be done at the same time as the soft tissue repair.

4. For injuries caused by blunt nerve transection (e.g., injuries due to propeller blades, power saws, or compound fractures), the anatomy of the nerve is often distorted, and a certain amount of tissue may have to be trimmed from each stump. Therefore the nerve repair is best accomplished after a delay of several weeks, when the amount of neuroma and scar tissue to be trimmed is more evident.

5. For nerve lesions in continuity, the decision to operate is delayed and based on whether reinnervation has occurred, which requires serial clinical and EDX examinations. In humans, nerves regenerate at an average rate of 1 to 2 mm/day (about 1 inch/month). In general, surgical intervention is warranted if no clinical or EMG evidence of functional reinnervation is evident 3 to 6 months after injury.

6. With surgical intervention, intraoperative electrophysiologic monitoring is extremely important for the decision-making. The presence or absence of the compound nerve action potential across the lesion is the single most important determinant of the type of surgical intervention to be used. An absent potential indicates the need for resection and repair of the nerve, whereas the presence of a response usually indicates that a better result may be achieved by observation, neurolysis, or fascicular repair.

7. Surgical techniques used for nerve repair are end-to-end suturing, neurolysis, split repair, and graft repair. Nerve gaps are best managed by autogenous nerve grafting using an interfascicular grouped fascicular approach. Common donor nerves include the sural and antebrachial cutaneous nerves.

Bibiliography

Chaudhry V, Cornblath DR: Wallerian degeneration in human nerves: serial electrophysiologic studies. Muscle Nerve 15:687–693, 1992.

Dorfman LJ: Quantitative clinical electrophysiology in the evaluation of nerve injury and regeneration. Muscle Nerve 13:822–828, 1990.

Gutierrez A, England JD: Peripheral nerve injuries. In Katirji B, Kaminski HJ, Preston DC, et al (eds): Neuromuscular Disorders in Clinical Practice. Boston, Butterworth-Heinemann, 2002.

Kline DG: Surgical repair of peripheral nerve injury. Muscle Nerve 13:843–852, 1990.

Seddon HJ: Surgical Disorders of the Peripheral Nerves, 2nd ed. New York, Churchill Livingstone, 1975.

Sunderland S: Nerve Injuries and Their Repair: A Critical Appraisal. Edinburgh, Churchill Livingstone, 1991.

Sunderland S: Nerves and Nerve Injuries, 2nd ed. New York, Churchill Livingstone, 1978.

Watchmaker GP, Mackinnon SE: Advances in peripheral nerve repair. Clin Plast Surg 24:63–73, 1997.

10 Mountain Sickness

Randolph W. Evans

Epidemiology and Risk Factors

1. Acute mountain sickness (AMS) develops in about 25% of visitors to altitudes of 6300 to 9700 feet, usually above 8200 feet. About 100 million tourists visit altitudes above 6300 feet worldwide per year.

2. Risk factors include age younger than 60 years, less physically fit, live at sea level, a history of AMS, female gender, obesity, and underlying cardiopulmonary problems. Alcohol inhibits acute ventilatory adaptation to mild hypoxia at moderate altitude.

3. AMS leads to high-altitude cerebral edema (HACE) in 1.5% of cases. HACE usually occurs above 12,000 feet.

Etiology and Pathophysiology

1. As the partial pressure of oxygen decreases with increasing altitude, ventilation increases, resulting in respiratory alkalosis.

2. Hypocapnia alone results in cerebral vasoconstriction, and hypoxia produces a net decline in cerebral vascular resistance and decreased cerebral blood flow.

3. Hypoxia can result in cerebral edema, which may be due to cerebral vasodilatation and elevated cerebral capillary hydrostatic pressure. An increase in sympathetic activity follows, causing an elevated heart rate, pulmonary vasoconstriction, an initial increase in cerebral blood flow followed by a decrease.

Clinical Findings

1. AMS is characterized by headache and at least one of the following: a gastrointestinal disorder (anorexia, nausea, or vomiting), fatigue or weakness, dizziness or lightheadedness, and difficulty sleeping.

2. The headache, which is often pounding, is usually bilateral but may be unilateral.

3. Onset is usually within 12 hours of arrival at altitude but may be delayed by several days.

4. HACE is signaled by a change in mental status and/or ataxia in a person with AMS or high-altitude pulmonary edema.

   a. Urinary incontinence, papilledema, cranial nerve palsies, tremor, and abnormalities in limb tone may also be present. Seizures are rare.

   b. Can result in death from cerebral herniation

5. High-altitude pulmonary edema (HAPE), which can occur along with HACE, usually occurs above 9840 feet.

6. High-altitude retinal hemorrhage is common above 15,000 feet.

Key Clinical Findings

- Headache and at least one of the following:
  - anorexia, nausea, or vomiting
  - fatigue or weakness
  - dizziness
  - difficulty sleeping

Treatment

1. AMS may be treated symptomatically with rest, mild analgesics (nonsteroidal anti-inflammatory drugs—NSAIDs—are quite effective), alcohol avoidance, and adequate hydration.

2. Depending on the severity of symptoms, avoiding going any higher or slowing the rate of ascent or descent may be necessary.

3. Acetazolamide (250 mg orally twice a day) may ameliorate acute symptoms.

4. HACE: initiate immediate descent or evacuation. If descent is not possible, use a portable hyperbaric bag (2 to 4 psi for a minimum of 2 hours), administer oxygen (2 to 4 liters/minute), and dexamethasone (initially 8 mg orally, intramuscularly or intravenously and 4 mg every 6 hours thereafter). If descent is delayed, give acetazolamide.

Prognosis

1. AMS usually resolves after 16 to 72 hours at altitude.

2. When descent is impossible and treatment is unavailable, HACE and HAPE have a mortality up to 50%.

Prevention

1. May be prevented in those planning higher ascents by starting below 8000 feet, resting the first day, and then ascending approximately 1000 feet per day

2. Sleeping at a lower altitude at night may be helpful because hypoxia worsens with sleep.

3. Avoiding alcohol and staying well hydrated may also be helpful.

4. Acetazolamide 125 to 250 mg twice daily starting 24 hours before ascent and continuing for 2 days at high altitude may prevent AMS and improve sleep.

5. Aspirin 320 mg 1 hour before arrival at high altitude and again every 4 hours for two doses (for a total of three doses).

6. Dexamethasone (2 mg every 6 hours or 4 mg every 12 hours orally) starting 24 to 48 hours before arrival at high altitude and continuing for several days may be effective.

7. Ginkgo biloba 120 mg a day orally may also be effective.

 Bibliography

Brundrett G: Sickness at high altitude: a literature review. J R Soc Health 122:14–20, 2002.

Burtscher M, Likar R, Nachbauer W, Philadelphy M: Aspirin for prophylaxis against headache at high altitudes: randomised, double blind, placebo controlled trial. *BMJ* 316:1057–1058, 1998.

Hackett PH, Roach RC: High-altitude illness. N Engl J Med 345:107–114, 2001.

Honigman B, Theis MK, Koziol-McLain J, et al.: Acute mountain sickness in a general tourist population at moderate altitudes Ann Intern Med 118:587–592, 1993.

11 Decompression Sickness

Randolph W. Evans

Epidemiology and Risk Factors

1. Decompression sickness (DCS), also referred to as the *bends* or *caisson disease,* usually affects divers or caisson workers but can also occur in airline pilots during rapid ascent in a nonpressurized cabin.

2. About 900 cases of DCS are reported annually in the United States among recreational SCUBA divers.

3. Most accidents occur in inexperienced divers.

4. The incidence of DCS for recreational divers is 1/5000 to 1/10,000 dives and for commercial divers, 1/500 to 1/1000 dives.

5. Up to 50% of cases occur in people who claim to have been diving within the limits set by a standard table or decompression computer.

6. Divers with a patent foramen ovale are five times more likely to sustain serious sequelae because the gas bubbles that form in the blood can pass directly from the right to the left atrium without being filtered by the lungs. Right-to-left shunts are more common in persons with migraine with aura.

Etiology and Pathophysiology

1. With descent, the partial pressure of the gases breathed by the dive increases proportionately according to Dalton's law. Although oxygen is metabolized, tissues soak up inert nitrogen and become saturated.

2. With ascent, the nitrogen moves from the tissues to the blood and is exhaled by the lungs, a process termed decompression.

3. When ascent is too rapid and the tissues are supersaturated, dissolved gas changes to free gas which creates bubbles.

4. When the filtering capacity of the pulmonary capillaries is exceeded, the bubbles enter the arterial circulation.

5. Manifestations are specific for the tissues in which the bubbles accumulate.

   a. Bubbles in the paravertebral veins, Batson's plexus, can result in stasis and venous infarction in the spinal cord.

   b. Cerebral injury can develop from bubbles occluding vessels or directly disrupting tissue.

   c. Secondary effects such as activation of complement, platelet aggregation, and release of vasoactive mediators can also lead to sequelae.

Clinical Features

1. DCS, which can occur after diving to a depth of more than 25 feet, appears within a few minutes to a few hours after the end of a dive; 85% become symptomatic within an hour and 95% develop symptoms within 24 hours.

2. Mild DCS (type I) is defined by pain, usually in the joints (bends) and/or itching of the skin.

3. Serious DCS (type II) is characterized by neurologic problems.

   a. Involvement of the thoracic spinal cord, the most commonly affected area, leads to low back or pelvic pain and dysesthesias, which may be accompanied by sensory loss, weakness, and incontinence. Divers use the term "hits" to signify spinal cord involvement.

   b. Less often, the brain may be affected, resulting in various symptoms and signs such as headache, confusion, lethargy, vertigo, speech disturbance, hemiparesis, visual impairment, and seizures, depending upon the site of involvement.

4. Rupture of alveoli, which may occur when a diver ascends without venting air from the lungs or from blockage of part of the bronchial tree, can result in additional gas embolism.

   a. During ascent or shortly after surfacing, divers may develop a variety of problems such as acute respiratory distress, headache, cardiorespiratory arrest, and seizures.

   b. Depending on the site of embolism to the brain, cortical blindness, aphasia, and hemiplegia may occur.

   c. Arterial gas embolism and DCS may co-exist.

 Key Clinical Findings

- Mild DCS (type I) is defined by pain in the joints (bends) and/or itching of the skin.

- Serious DCS (type II) is characterized by involvement of the spinal cord or the brain.

Radiologic Features

1. DCS is typically diagnosed based on the history and physical examination.
2. Magnetic resonance imaging studies of the brain and spinal cord may be normal or show only nonspecific abnormalities.

Treatment

1. High concentrations of oxygen should be administered by face mask to increase resorption of gas bubbles.
2. Fluid administration (ideally a hyperosmolar drink such as a juice, rehydration solution or sports drink, or intravenous isotonic fluids without glucose) may result in more rapid elimination of gases while treating dehydration.
3. As soon as possible, the patient should be recompressed in a hyperbaric chamber while breathing oxygen.

Key Treatment

- Administration of high concentrations of oxygen
- Fluid administration
- Recompression in a hyperbaric chamber

Prognosis

1. Prompt treatment usually results in complete recovery.
2. Neurologic deficits may persist in cases where recompression is delayed or not done.

Bibliography

Broome JR: Aspects of neurological decompression illness: a view from Bethesda. J R Nav Med Serv 1995;81:120–126.

Moon RE: Treatment of diving emergencies. Crit Care Clin 1999;15:429–455.

Newton HB: Neurologic complications of scuba diving. Am Fam Physician 63:2211–2218, 2001.

Wilmshurst PT: Brain damage in divers. BMJ 1997;314:689–690.

Wilmshurst PT, Nightingale S, Walsh KP, Morrison WL: Effect of migraine of closure of cardiac right-to-left shunts to prevent recurrence of decompression illness or stroke or for haemodynamic reasons. Lancet 2000;356:1648–1651.

12 Lightning and Electrical Injuries

Randolph W. Evans

Epidemiology and Risk Factors

1. About 100 lightning and 1500 technical electricity-related deaths occur annually in the United States.

2. Routes of lightning injury

   a. A direct strike is the most damaging; more likely if the person is carrying a metal conductor such as an umbrella or golf club above shoulder level.

   b. A side flash or splash injury occurs when lightning first strikes a tall object such as a nearby tree and then arcs to the person standing next to the object or when lightning first strikes another person or an animal and then arcs to the victim.

   c. A ground or side current occurs when lightning strikes the ground first and then travels along the surface before reaching the person.

   d. Occasionally, people can sustain injury indoors while on the telephone, from current conducted through the lines, or in the bath or shower from ground current travelling along the water pipes.

3. Technical electrical injuries can occur from exposure to high-voltage electricity (1000 V or more) and low-voltage electricity.

   a. High-voltage electricity injuries account for about 70% of electrical injuries and deaths and are almost always work-related.

   b. Low-voltage injuries typically occur in the home and are associated with the use of electrical appliances while standing on a wet floor or while in the bathtub, children playing with outlets or wires, or use of faulty electrical equipment.

   c. When the energized conductor is held in the hand, alternating current exposure in the range of 8 to 22 mA at 60 Hz may result in long exposure because of a state of tetanic contraction of flexor muscles of the forearm and hand, which is paradoxically termed "let go current."

Etiology and Pathophysiology

The two major causes of tissue damage are thermal injury and electroporation, which is the production and expansion of transient aqueous pores in the lipid bilayer component of the cell membrane.

Clinical Features

1. Lightning and electrical injuries may result in sudden death or cerebral hypoxia from ventricular fibrillation.

2. Transient loss of consciousness, confusion, and amnesia may also occur.

3. Lightning injury may result in keraunoparalysis, a transient paralysis, usually of the lower limbs, in association with sensory loss and pale skin.

4. Lightning and electrical injuries may also cause acute spinal cord, focal brain, and peripheral nerve damange and rhabdomyolysis.

5. Deep burns are more common with electrical injuries than with lightning injuries.

6. Secondary trauma can occur from falls.

7. Delayed neurologic disorders associated with lightning and electrical injuries include cognitive deficits, motor neuron disease, parkinsonism, choreoathetosis, dystonia, myoclonus, basilar artery thrombosis, seizures, myelopathy, generalized polyneuropathy, and reflex sympathetic dystrophy.

Key Findings

- Sudden death or cerebral hypoxia from ventricular fibrillation

- Transient loss of consciousness, confusion, and amnesia

- Keraunoparalysis

- Acute spinal cord, focal brain, peripheral nerve, and muscle injury

- Deep burns

- Delayed neurologic disorders

Treatment

Evaluation and management depend on the sites, types, and extent of injury.

543

Key Treatment

- Treatment depends on location, type, and extent of injury.

Prognosis

1. About one third of lightning strikes are fatal.

2. The symptoms and signs of keraunoparalysis typically resolve within a few hours.

3. Those with hypoxic encephalopathy as a result of cardiac arrest usually have a poor prognosis.

4. Most patients with spinal cord injuries due to lightning and electrical injuries have permanent disability.

Bibliography

Cherington M: Central nervous system complications of lightning and electrical injuries. Semin Neurol 15:233–240, 1995.

Cherington M: Lightning injuries in sports: Situations to avoid. Sports Med 31:301–308, 2001.

Duff K, McCaffrey RJ: Electrical injury and lightning injury: a review of their mechanisms and neuropsychological, psychiatric, and neurological sequelae. Neuropsychol Rev 11:101–116, 2001.

Jafari H, Couratier P, Camu W: Motor neuron disease after electrical injury. J Neurol Neurosurg Psychiatry 71:265–267, 2001.

Jain S, Bandi V: Electrical and lightning injuries. Crit Care Clin 15:319–331, 1999.

Wilbourn AJ: Peripheral nerve disorders in electrical and lightning injuries. Semin Neurol 15:241–255, 1995.

1   Myasthenia Gravis and Myasthenic Syndromes

David S. Younger

Definition

Myasthenia gravis (MG) is a postsynaptic disorder of the neuromuscular junction that results in weakness and fatigue owing to autoimmune loss of acetylcholine receptors (AChR). It is an important disease for students of neurology because it is the best understood autoimmune disorder, and the historical achievements that have contributed to its understanding span the decades of modern neuroscience.

The term *myasthenia* has traditionally been used interchangeably for acquired autoimmune MG, and the term *myasthenic*, for other syndromes of the neuromuscular junction. A classification of neuromuscular disorders is presented in Table 1–1.

Historical Background

1. The clinical syndrome of MG was identified by Wilks in 1877, but it was named by Jolly in 1985, and the test of repetitive nerve stimulation was later named for him.

2. Even before the mechanism of MG was appreciated, the efficacy of physostigmine was shown by Walker. Dale and colleagues described the chemical nature of transmission at motor end plates, and Harvey and Masland summarized the salient electrophysiologic features of MG in 1941. In that same year, Blalock and later Keynes, described transsternal thymectomy in MG that included as complete a removal of the gland as possible, whether or not a tumor was suspected preoperatively.

3. In 1960, the autoimmune basis of MG was suggested by Simpson, however the immunologic basis of MG awaited the basic understanding of ACh release at motor end plates, as described by Katz and Miledi.

4. Nature provided two gifts that facilitated characterization of the nicotinic AChR in animal and human investigation: first, the neuromuscular toxin, α-bungarotoxin (BuTx) that blocked the AChR; and second, the electric organ of Torpedo, which served as a rich reservoir of AChR.

5. In 1973, Patrick and Lindstrom injected rabbits with AChR from the electric organ of eels intending to make anti-receptor antibodies and to see if they blocked the function of intact receptors. Instead, the immunized rabbits became paralyzed and died; and so-called experimental autoimmune MG was recognized.

6. Fambrough and Drachman later applied BuTx to motor point biopsies in intact muscle from patients with MG and found a marked reduction in the number of AChR, averaging 20% of controls.

7. By 1980, Engel and Lennon reproduced the essential clinical and morphologic correlates of human MG in animals by passive transfer of human myasthenic serum, also with AChR specific monoclonal antibodies.

8. The past two decades have witnessed a spectacular progress in the microstructure, physiology, and molecular composition of the nicotinic AChR; and this has in turn been applied to the clinical problem of MG. Distinct but related genes encode the individual AChR subunits, termed $\alpha,\beta,\delta,\gamma,\epsilon$, and cDNA for each has been cloned showing remarkable homology.

Pathogenesis

The fatigue and weakness of MG is due to the loss of a functioning AchR, resulting in a state of impaired neuromuscular transmission.

1. In response to an incoming nerve action potential, quanta packets of Ach are released into the synaptic cleft where they eventually come in contact with AChR located on the postsynaptic membrane.

2. The reversible binding of a molecule of Ach at the receptor site leads to the transient opening of an ion channel with a net influx of Na^+ producing a depolarizing end plate potential (EPP).

3. EPP normally summate above threshold for the activation of a muscle action potential because of the abundance of AChR and free Ach molecules in the synaptic cleft, the so-called safety factor for neuromuscular transmission.

4. In MG this safety factor is disturbed by the critical reduction in the number of functioning receptors due to circulating blocking, binding, or modulating AChR antibodies, alone or in association with

545

TABLE 1–1. CLASSIFICATION OF NEUROMUSCULAR JUNCTION DISEASES

Autoimmune
Myasthenia gravis
Lambert-Eaton myasthenic syndrome (LEMS) (presynaptic)

Toxic (presynaptic)
Botulism
Snake venom

Congenital
Presynaptic
Ach resynthesis or packaging
Paucity of vesicles

Synaptic
End plate acetylcholinesterase deficiency

Postsynaptic
Slow channel syndrome
AChR deficiency
Mutations of AChR subunit
Low-affinity fast-channel syndrome
High conductance fast-channel syndrome
Severe AChR deficiency

Partially Characterized Defects
Congenital myasthenic syndrome resembling LEMS
AChR deficiency with paucity of secondary synaptic clefts
Familial limb girdle myasthenia

Modified from Bromberg (1999) and Engel (1992).

receptor lysis by activated T and B cells, and membranolytic complement.

5. Not surprisingly, it is possible to partially restore neuromuscular transmission, in the short term by the administration of anticholinesterase medication to increase the amount of available ACh in the synaptic cleft, and in the long term by the use of various types of immunotherapy, and by thymectomy to impede immune-mediated attack on AChR.

Clinical Presentation and Diagnosis

The clinical diagnosis of autoimmune MG is made first by recognizing a pattern of weakness that has the features of fluctuation and variability over the course of a day or over months, leading to perceptible exacerbations and remissions; and then confirmed by the edrophonium test (see below) and by electrodiagnostic and serologic studies.

1. The distribution of weakness is characteristic, affecting ocular, facial, oropharyngeal, and limb muscles.

Key Symptom

• Weakness of the ocular, facial, oropharyngeal, and limb muscles

2. When the injection of up to 10 mg of edrophonium, a fast-acting anticholinesterase drug, slowly over 3 minutes leads to dramatic improvement, the diagnosis is strongly suggested because there are few false-positive results. Formal diagnosis is bolstered, however, by electrodiagnostic testing and the measurement of circulating AChR antibody titers.

3. Electrophysiologic evaluation includes repetitive motor nerve stimulation and single-fiber electromyography (SFEMG). With repetitive nerve stimulation, up to 85% of patients with generalized MG and 10% of those with ocular MG show abnormal decremental responses; with SFEMG, 86% of patients with generalized MG and 63% of those with ocular MG show such a response.

4. A decremental response of 12% to 15% or more, of successive compound muscle action potentials (CMAP) after 3 Hz of repetitive stimulation and aggravation of the block for several minutes after brief exercise is indicative of MG.

5. SFEMG quantitates transmission at individual end plates while the patient voluntarily activates the muscle under examination. This requires intense cooperation by the patient and advanced training on the part of the examiner to be assured of valid results especially when the findings are borderline. Twenty motor unit potentials (MUP) are studied for variability in the time between potentials, which varies among consecutive discharges— termed *jitter;* and calculated as the mean difference between consecutive interpotential intervals. *Blocking* occurs when consecutive impulses do not follow. A typical finding in MG on SFEMG is normal jitter in some potential pairs and increased jitter in others.

6. Three AChR assays are available for the serological evaluation of MG, including binding, blocking, and modulating AChR assays. The binding assay is positive in up to 90% of patients with generalized MG and should be the first line of testing with a specificity of more than 99%. Anti-striational antibodies are useful in the screening of thymoma. Patients with high titers of blocking and modulating antibodies, mediastinal mass on chest computed tomography (CT), and very high titers of anti-striational antibodies may harbor malignant thymoma.

7. Approximately 12% to 17% of patients with generalized MG lack demonstrable serum AChR antibodies, and are classified as seronegative MG. However these patients do not differ clinically from those with elevated titers, and they exhibit favorable responses to anticholinesterase or immunosuppressant drugs, plasmapheresis, intravenous immunoglobulin g (IVIg), and thymectomy. Simi-

larly, significantly reduced numbers of AChR have been noted in motor end-plate biopsies of patients with seronegative generalized MG and ocular MG. In addition, passive transfer of sera from seronegative patients to laboratory animals results in a disorder clinically similar to that induced by seropositive sera.

8. All patients with MG should undergo CT imaging of the chest to exclude a thymoma and at the least to examine for glandular enlargement. There is no role for needle biopsy of a thymomatous mass on chest imaging because of the risk of crisis and spread of a malignant tumor throughout the chest. Rather, all thymic tumors should be removed surgically and promptly by sternal splitting thymectomy. Notwithstanding the fact that nonmalignant thymoma is more common in seronegative and ocular MG, malignant thymoma should be suspected in patients with a rapidly progressive generalized course.

9. The investigation of congenital or genetic forms of myasthenia requires sophisticated morphologic and electrophysiologic studies of the intact neuromuscular junction. These include cytochemical localization of acetylcholinesterase and immune deposits at end plates by intercostal motor point biopsy; electron microscopic and cytochemical evaluation for the size and density of synaptic vesicles and the morphology of nerve terminals and postsynaptic membranes; quantitative assessment of AChR binding sites, in vitro microelectrode studies including noise analysis and patch-clamp recordings for the kinetic properties of AChR ion channels; and the application of molecular genetic analysis to detect mutations in AChR subunits.

Key Tests

- Edrophonium (10 mg)
- Electrophysiological testing
  - Repetitive motor nerve stimulation
  - Single-fiber electromyography (SFEMG)
- Serologic evaluation
  - AChR assays
  - Computed tomography

Treatment

Neurologists must choose the sequence and combination of available anticholinesterase medications, immu-nosuppressant and immunomodulating medications, and thymectomy procedures.

1. Virtually all patients use pyridostigmine bromide (Mestinon), an anticholinesterase inhibitor given in doses of 1 to 3 (60 mg) tablets at 3 to 4 hour intervals while awake, titrated to the severity of symptoms, with increases in the dose until undesirable side effects (abdominal cramping, diarrhea, excessive secretions, and sweating) predominate. However pyridostigmine bromide does not appreciably change the natural history of the disease, and ultimately other modalities must be used to prevent disease progression.

2. Prednisone has been the most widely used immunosuppressant agent in MG since the first reports of its efficacy in 1949. Corticosteroids exert nonspecific immunosuppression at virtually all levels of the immune system from the presentation of antigen-presenting cells (APC) in the thymus, to the activation of B and T cells, the secretion of AChR antibodies, and stabilization of the immune attack upon nicotinic AChR end plates. Up to one-half of patients experience initial exacerbation of MG after commencement of therapy, and roughly two-thirds of patients have an undesirable or life-threatening side effect shortly after commencement of therapy. The unwanted side effects are lessened with gradual increments of the dose beginning at 20 mg on alternate days, and slowly increasing by 5 mg every week until stabilization occurs.

3. Azathioprine (Imuran) has been used in the treatment of MG since the first report of its efficacy in 1969. It exerts a favorable action in MG by the inhibition of T cell activation and T cell–dependent antibody-mediated responses. It is appropriate therapy, as an alternative to prednisone, for patients with generalized disease, especially those with frequent relapses; in those who are not candidates for thymectomy because of age or cormorbid disease; and in MG patients with thymoma before or after thymectomy. There are three drawbacks to its use: First, idiosyncratic side effects occur in about 10% of patients, most often gastrointestinal or flu-like syndromes that necessitate permanent withdrawal of the medication. Second, bone marrow suppression occurs in virtually all patients. Third, there is a delay in onset of the therapeutic effect of 3 months or longer. Slow advancement of the medication is advised, with increments of 25 mg every week upon careful monitoring of chemistries and blood counts until a maintenance dose of 2 to 3 mg/kg per day is

achieved with periodic monitoring of chemistries and blood count thereafter.

4. In 1987 the beneficial effect of cyclosporine was reported, showing an efficacy equal to prednisone and azathioprine in a placebo-controlled trial. It inhibits T cell–dependent antibody responses by reversibly suppressing the clonal expansion of activated helper T cells. However, its cumulative and dose-dependent renovascular side effects limits its practical long-term use.

5. Mycophenolate mofitil (CellCept) has recently been introduced as an adjunctive agent in the treatment of patients with generalized disease refractory to prednisone and azathioprine; however, only a few centers have used it extensively.

6. The hypothesis that MG originated in the thymus gland was first suggested by Weigert in 1901. The earliest transsternal thymectomy in a patient with MG was performed decades later. The benefit of thymectomy in MG without thymoma was subsequently recognized, and it is now known that the thymus contains all of the elements needed for the activation of AChR-specific T cells, and thymectomy suppresses experimental autoimmune MG. The success of transcervical and transsternal thymectomy procedures in promoting sustained remission and improvement; and the often observed fall in antibody titers, especially in those with noninvoluted hyperplastic glands, further strengthens the role of the thymus gland in the pathogenesis and, possibly, perpetuation of the disease. There is general agreement that patients with generalized MG should undergo thymectomy to remove as much of the gland as possible. Nevertheless, there is a need for prospective clinical trials to compare the effectiveness of available thymectomy procedures.

7. Plasmapheresis and IVIg have been widely used in the treatment of MG to effect rapid improvement. One is not a substitute for the other, because they act through different mechanisms, and combining the two may be advisable. The salutary action of plasmapheresis is believed to result from the removal of AChR antibodies from the serum, whereas the benefits of IVIg, although potentially more hypothetical, include the inhibition and downregulation of AChR antibodies, activated T and B cells; and inhibition of membrane attack complex component C5b-9 of complement. The major drawbacks to both therapies are the high relative cost and need for specialized staff and equipment, including a large-bore central catheter for plasmapheresis, and the miniscule but finite risk of transmissible disease and anaphylactic reaction with IVIg.

8. Myasthenic crisis remains a formidable challenge for effective management. Approximately 16% of all patients experience a crisis, defined as the need for mechanical ventilation. Progressive weakness, oropharyngeal involvement, refractoriness to anticholinesterase medication, intercurrent infection, and invasive procedures have all been implicated in the development of crisis. It is now standard practice to treat crisis in an intensive care unit. Crisis is a temporary exacerbation, regardless of the proximate cause, and the goal is to keep the patient alive until it subsides, usually in 2 weeks. The underlying immunologic derangement in crisis in not known. However there is justification for aggressive management with plasmapheresis and IVIg therapy to hasten recovery.

9. The ultimate goal in MG is a cure, or at least effective prevention or inhibition of the immune response to AChR without engendering systemic immunosuppression and unwanted side effects. A number of therapies that would selectively or specifically interfere with the immune pathogenesis of MG are on the horizon. One such therapy employs a genetically engineered "guided missile" of APC to kill AChR-specific T cells.

Key Treatment

Initial Therapy: Ocular or Mild Generalized Disease

First Line

• Pyridostigmine

Second Line

• Prednisone (brief course)

• IVIg

• Plasmapheresis

Chronic Therapy: Moderate-to-Severe Generalized Disease

First Line

• Azathioprine

Second Line

• Prednisone

Third Line

• Cyclosporine

• Mycophenolate mofitil (CellCept)

For more information about MG and related disorder, log on to *www.mgnyc.org*.

Bibliography

Bromberg MB: Myasthenia gravis and myasthenic syndromes. In DS Younger (ed): Motor Disorders. Lippincott Williams & Wilkins. Philadelphia, 1999, pp.163–178.

Ciafaloni E, Sanders DB: Advances in myasthenia gravis. Curr Neurol Neurosci Rep 2:89–95, 2002.

Cohen MS, Younger DS: Aspects of the natural history of myasthenia gravis: Crisis and death. Ann NY Acad Sci 377:670–677, 1981.

Engel AG: Myasthenia gravis and myasthenic syndromes. In LP Rowland and S DiMauro (eds): Handbook of Clinical Neurology, vol. 18. New York, Elsevier 1992, pp. 391–455.

Jaretzki A III, Barohn RJ, Ernstoff RM, et al.: Myasthenia gravis: Recommendations for clinical research standards. Neurology 55:16–23, 2000.

Younger DS, Raksadawan N: Medical therapies in myasthenia gravis. Chest Surg Clin North Am 11:329–336, 2001.

Younger DS, Worrall BB, Penn AS: Myasthenia gravis: Historical perspective and overview. Neurology 48:S1–S7, 1997.

2 Amyotrophic Lateral Sclerosis

David S. Younger
Samrina Hanif

Definitions

1. Amyotrophic lateral sclerosis (ALS) was recocognized as a distinct clinical and neuropathological entity by Charcot more than a century ago.

2. Clinical lower motor neuron (LMN) signs of ALS relate to anterior horn cell degeneration and include weakness, wasting, and fasciculation.

3. Clinical upper motor neuron (UMN) manifestations of ALS relate to corticospinal tract degeneration and include hyperreflexia, spasticity, clonus, and Hoffmann's and Babinski's signs.

4. The clinical spectrum of ALS includes acquired and genetic forms (see Classification of Amyotrophic Lateral Sclerosis). In clinical practice, the diagnosis is made when LMN signs are found in three limbs (or in case of bulbar-onset cases, in lingual and oropharyngeal muscles) in combination with widespread UMN signs. Primary lateral sclerosis (PLS) is a pure clinical UMN syndrome that is sometimes a either a forme fruste of ALS, or a paraneoplastic syndrome related to cancer of the breast or lung. Progressive bulbar palsy (PBP) relates to LMN or motor neuron degeneration in brainstem nuclei, leading to early dysarthria and dysphagia. Motor neuron disease localized to a single limb is termed *monomelic amyotrophy*.

Classification of Amyotrophic Lateral Sclerosis

- Sporadic adult ALS
- Dominant ALS, adult onset
- Dominant ALS, juvenile
- Recessive ALS, juvenile
- Guamanian ALS-PD-dementia
- ALS with other forms of dementia (see text)
- Paraneoplastic ALS (lymphoproliferative disease, small cell lung cancer).

Epidemiology

1. The annual incidence of ALS is approximately 1 to 2 per 100,000 in developed countries (range, 0.5 to 2.4 per 100,000).

2. The mean age of onset is 56 years, with a more common occurrence in men than women (1.3:1).

3. ALS is less common below the age of 40 years, and rare below age 30. The average duration of illness is 3 to 5 years with a large variation in the duration of disease course, with most patients living 5 years after diagnosis, and others surviving for decades.

4. Epidemiologic studies have shown no worldwide or general tendencies, but there are areas of unusually high prevalence that elude interpretation such as clusters of cases in the same football team or small town, that may hide an essential clue to pathogenesis or neurotoxic event.

5. One area of high prevalence was Guam, where the syndrome of ALS-parkinsonism-dementia (ALS-PD-dementia) was described. When genetic causation was deemed unlikely, attention was directed to the possibility of an environmental toxin. Investigators showed that ingestion of the local cycad nut contained an excitatory amino acid and neurotoxin, β-N-methylamino-L-alanine.

Diagnosis

1. The first step in diagnosis of ALS is recognizing the cardinal symptoms and signs as noted above. Most patients complain of some functional impairment that results from weakness, such as difficulty writing, buttoning, holding onto objects, frequent tripping, and, occasionally, falls.

2. Hoarseness, slurred speech, and drooling occur in patients with bulbar-onset ALS.

3. Focal weakness, wasting, fasciculation, and night cramps are perceived by the patient. By the time relentless progression ensues, tendon reflexes are pathologically overactive or clonic, and the diagnosis is clinically inescapable.

4. In the presence of the classical syndrome, most experts agree that confidence in the clinical diagnosis of ALS is probably close to 90% or more, even before extensive testing.

5. When portions of the classical syndrome are missing or there are unusual findings such as ophthalmoparesis, sensory loss, bowel or bladder incontinence, or cerebellar involvement, that confidence decreases and an alternative disease is more likely.

6. Dementia, a common occurrence in older people, can be an associated feature of ALS in more than a dozen different syndromes including Alzheimer, Pick, Lewy body, and Creutzfeldt-Jakob disease; subcortical gliosis, spongy vacuolar angiopathy, Huntington's disease, Guamanian ALS-PD-dementia, familial ALS (FALS), corticobasal degeneration, non-Pick lobar atrophy, progressive supranuclear palsy, and Luysopallidonigral degeneration.

7. The recommended evaluation for suspected ALS is summarized under Key Tests. The role of testing in ALS is twofold. First, to confirm the diagnosis while confidently eliminating other disorders that may bear clinical resemblance to it. Second, to identify a systemic disorder toward which strong therapy might be directed, with the hope of slowing the progression of ALS.

Key Tests

All Patients

- Electromyographic (EMG) and nerve conduction studies (NCS) (all patients)

- Pedigree

- SOD1 gene mutation analysis in blood; if positive, no further testing is necessary in a patient with FALS

Sporadic ALS

- Blood tests: complete blood count, differential, erythrocyte sedimentation rate, chemistries, creatine phosphokinase, quantitative immunoglobulins, immunofixation electrophoresis, T cell subsets, acetylneuraminic acid, Lyme antibody, thyroid and parathyroid function tests, GM1, asialoGM1 and GD1b ganglisoside antibodies, and SOD1 gene analysis

- Lumbar cerebrospinal fluid (CSF) analysis for protein, glucose, cell count, immunoglobulin G, oligoclonal bands, and cytology

- Magnetic resonance imaging (MRI) of the brain and cervical spinal cord

- Muscle biopsy to confirm neurogenic involvement in a clinically involved or unaffected limb

- Chest, abdomen, pelvis computed tomography (CT), and bone marrow studies to exclude occult lymphoproliferative cancer and other malignancies

Familial ALS

1. About 10% of ALS cases are familial with autosomal dominant (AD) inheritance, so called,

FALS-AD, and are clinically indistinguishable from sporadic cases, with an invariably fatal outcome, suggesting that they might share important pathogenic mechanisms.

2. Pathological findings in FALS include degeneration and loss of large motor neurons in the cerebral cortex, brainstem, cervical and lumbar spinal cord, as well as selected nonmotor cells and tracts in the central nervous system (CNS) including the dorsal columns, Clarke's column, and spinocerebellar tracts.

3. Several pathogenic mutations in the gene for Cu/Zn superoxide dismutase occur in FALS-AD on chromosome 21q. CuZn superoxide dismutase 1 (SOD1) is a protein of 153 amino acids encoded by 5 exons within the SOD1 locus whose primary function is to detoxify the superoxide free radical O_2-, converting I to H_2O_2, and in turn to H_2O through the action of catalase or glutathione peroxidase. The mechanisms whereby mutations in the SOD1 gene trigger ALS are not clearly understood; however, several lines of investigation suggest that one or more apoptotic cell death pathways may be activated.

4. Recessive juvenile-onset ALS is characterized instead by chronic slow progression, often into decades, with findings often resembling denervating polyneuropathy. Some affected individuals are markedly spastic or pseudobulbar. The gene locus for FALS resides on chromosome 2q33.

5. One form of juvenile ALS has AD inheritance and resides on chroomosome 9q.

Differential Diagnosis

Various disorders may sometimes be confused with motor neuron disease but are obvious after appropriate evaluation.

1. The spastic paraparesis of multiple sclerosis mimics PLS clinically, but is easily separable by the finding of widespread plaques on brain MRI.

2. Pseudobulbar palsy resembles PBP but is more often due to multiple strokes easily seen on brain MRI.

3. Cervical spondylotic myelopathy is suggested by neck and radicular pain, numbness in the hands, and gait imbalance; but it can also be due to compression by metastatic carcinoma, plasmacytoma, and lymphoma ascertained by cervical spine MRI.

4. Syringomyelia is suggested by cape-like distribution of pain and temperature sensory loss, as well as by LMN signs in the hands, with or without UMN signs.

5. Paraneoplastic enecephalomyelitis usually pre-

cedes or follows diagnosis of small cell cancer of the lung, often in association with sensory neuronopathy.

6. Post-polio muscular atrophy occurs decades after known poliomyelitis, whereas spinal atrophy and myelitis promptly follow irradiation atrophy or myelitis after spinal irradiation.

7. Multifocal motor neuropathy occurs in association with multifocal conduction block on nerve conduction studies (NCS) with or without elevated titers of serum GM1, asialo-GM1, or GD1b autoantibodies.

8. Charcot-Marie-Tooth disease type 2 presents with syndromes of spinal muscular atrophy and with vocal cord paralysis.

9. Myelomatosis mimics motor neuron disease resulting from infiltration of ventral spinal roots by plasma cells, detectable by MRI and cerebrospinal fluid analysis.

10. Pure motor chronic inflammatory demyelinating polyneuropathy is detected by slow velocities on NCS without active denervation on needle EMG.

11. Polyglucosan body disease may mimic ALS, but differs in early dementia and absent tendon reflexes.

12. Myasthenia gravis may be mistaken for PBP but is later recognized by a decremental response on repetitive motor nerve stimulation at 3 Hz, serum AChR antibody titers, and an edrophonium test.

13. Inclusion body myositis, which may present with weakness, wasting, fasciculation, overactive tendon reflexes, and a normal creatine kinase level, is separable by muscle biopsy.

14. Amyloid myopathy is suggested by typical LMN signs, areflexia, monoclonal IgA or IgG monoclonal paraproteinemia, and Bence Jones proteinuria. Diagnosis is established by the finding of extracellular congo-red birefringence and detailed cytochemical stains on a nerve or muscle biopsy.

Overview of Multidisciplinary Integrated Care Approach

1. Over the past several years it has become clear that optimal care of patients with ALS includes attention to both medical and psychosocial needs.

2. The ideal care of a patient with ALS, especially in the later stages, requires a multidisciplinary team composed of neurologist; physiatrist; internist; physical, occupational, and respiratory therapists; speech, swallowing, and communication experts; social worker; and nutritionist.

3. A multidisciplinary integrated medical, palliative, and psychosocial care approach accomplishes

three essential goals: First, the identification of medical problems at an early stage, including the selection of naturopathic, experimental, or other potentially effective medical therapies. Second, effective utilization of medical resources, particularly in the current managed health care environment. Third, maintenance of the highest quality of life by keeping the disruptive features of the disease to a minimum, while encouraging useful coping strategies and treatment options and actively identifying and modifying maladaptive behavior.

Key Treatment: Overview

- An integrated medical, palliative, and psychosocial care approach is essential for managing ALS.

- A multidisciplinary team of specialists—especially in the later stages of disease—is required for optimal care.

Medical Therapies

Although there is no known cure for ALS, medical therapy is given in the hope of slowing progression. There are four classes of agents with a rational basis for their use.

1. Anti-excitotoxic agents such as riluzole block receptors for glutamate, an excitotoxic amino acid, and significantly prolonged survival in patients with predominant bulbar-onset disease in double-blind placebo controlled trials at a dose of 50 mg by mouth twice daily.

2. Neurotrophic factors or nerve growth factors are critical for neuronal functioning and for promoting the propagation of collateral axon sprouting necessary to sustain muscle innervation once the degeneration of neurons begins. Several available neurotrophic factors include ciliary and brain-derived neurotrophic factor, insulin-like growth factor (IGF), that have shown a trend, but not significant effect in ALS.

3. The evidence of impaired oxidative processes in patients with FALS has led to the widespread adoption of high-dose vitamins for their antioxidative properties, especially vitamin E (2,000 U/day), vitamin C (2,000 mg/day), and beta-carotene (25,000 U/day).

4. There is circumstantial evidence for the role of immunologic processes in ALS such as the inordinately more frequent occurrence of concomitant monoclonal paraproteinemia and lymphoproliferative diseases; and the pathological findings of IgG, activated lymphocytes, and macrophages in

human ALS motor neurons at autopsy. IgG from patients with ALS interacted with calcium channels that may promote entry of calcium into motor neurons, thereby contributing to the process of cellular destruction. There has been no observed benefit after treatment with cyclophosphamide, intravenous gamma globulin, prednisone, cyclosporine, total body irradiation, or calcium channel blocking agents in ALS.

Key Treatment: Medical Therapy

- Anti-excitotoxic agents

- Neurotrophic factors

- Vitamins, especially vitamin E (2,000 U/day), vitamin C (2,000 mg/day), and beta-carotene (25,000 U/day)

Palliative Treatment

Palliative therapy should be offered at all stages of the disease to promote the highest level of health and to stimulate confidence, encourage independence, reduce the burden of physical handicaps, and sustain relationships with family, friends, and colleagues.

1. The gradual loss of ambulation due to weakness and spasticity is inevitable. The patient should be guided by a physiatrist and physical and occupational therapists for assistance devices to maintain independence including a cane, walker, ankle foot orthosis, and other bracing maneuvers, lightweight wheelchairs, and self-propelled larger units as needed.

2. Spasticity is treated with physiotherapy and anti-spasticity agents such as tizanidine and oral or intrathecal baclofen.

3. Cramps, often the earliest symptom, can be managed effectively with quinine sulfate, tonic water and bitter lemon beverages, verapamil hydrochloride, gabapentin, and roloxifene.

4. Fasciculations, frequently annoying but never disabling, are generally responsive to clonazepam.

5. Communication impairments resulting from dysarthria lead to isolation and may even limit the ability of patients to communicate such basic needs as suctioning or repositioning. Consultation with a speech therapist is useful to educate patients in oromotor exercises for mild impairments, and to encourage early intervention for evaluation of computer-assisted and electronic communication systems. Verbal communication can be prolonged in tracheotomized patients, as long as speech is intelligible, by cuffless tubes or intermittent positive pressure breathing (IPPB).

6. The evaluation of swallowing difficulty generally includes inspection of the nasopharynx, larynx, and esophageal paths by fiberoptic and barium video fluoroscopic studies. The treatment of mild dysphagia includes dietary counseling and positioning devices for the head and trunk. Management of aspiration is improved by anti-cholinergic agents such as atropine and amytriptyline; assisted coughing or chest physical therapy, oropharyngeal suctioning, and percutaneous endoscopic gastrostomy placement. The routine use of gastrostomy runs counter to the view that death due to starvation or malnutrition is ALS is a painless, final, merciful act and is one of the many options to be considered for prolongation of life.

7. Insomnia resulting from disrupted sleep, intermittment airway obstruction, and frequent daytime naps in patients with ALS is treatable with triazolam.

8. Excessive crying or tearfulness, especially common with ALS, sometimes responds to antidepressant medication.

9. Respiratory symptoms invariably occur in all patients with ALS. The decision to proceed to IPPB and eventually endotracheal intubation or indwelling tracheostomy should be discussed openly with patient and family in advance of impending emergencies, and in association with health care proxy or durable power of attorney to assure implementation of patient wishes.

Key Treatment: Palliative Treatment

- Assistance devices such as a cane, walker, ankle foot orthosis

- Physiotherapy for spasticity

- Clonazepam for fasciculation

- Oromotor excercises for speech impairments

- Anti-cholinergic agents for aspiration

- Triazolam for insomnia

Psychosocial Care

The psychosocial aspects of ALS are most important as the disease progresses relentlessly. With the increasing trend to manage the care of ALS patients in academic medical centers, many patients feel isolated from their local neurologists and primary health care providers who may have a longstanding relationship with the patient and caregivers. Three principles of psychosocial care can optimize the relationship of the treating neurologist and the patient with ALS and caregivers:

1. Empower the patient, and make every effort to foster a balanced team care model that conveys dignity and mutual respect.

2. Try not to force acceptance of the diagnosis of ALS or confront denial directly; rather, try to convey the diagnosis as a challenge, encouraging the patient and caregivers to reflect upon all aspects of their psychological, spiritual, cognitive, and cultural background to facilitate acceptance of the diagnosis and ultimately fatal prognosis.

3. As the care of ALS takes a toll on health care professionals, the treating neurologist and other physicians should be aware of their own coping strategies to ensure optimal communication among interdisciplinary team members, and with the patient and caregivers.

Key Treatment: Psychosocial Care

• Empower the patient.

• Foster a balanced team care model that conveys dignity and mutual respect.

Key Website

• There is an excellent Web site devoted to ALS for patients, family members, caregivers, and health care professionals:
  www.als-nyc.org.

Bibliography

Brown RH Jr.: Recent progress in understanding the inherited motor neuron diseases. In Younger DS (ed): Motor Disorders. Philadelphia, Lippincott Williams & Wilkins, 1999, pp. 357–361.

Lange DJ: Amyotrophic lateral sclerosis. In Younger DS (ed): Motor Disorders. Philadelphia, Lippincott Williams & Wilkins, 1999, pp. 363–367.

Murphy PL, Del Bene M, Albert SM: Multidisciplinary integrated psychosocial and palliative care. In Younger DS (ed): Motor Disorders. Philadelphia, Lippincott Williams & Wilkins, 1999, pp. 523–527.

Pascuzzi RM: ALS, motor neuron disease, and related disorders: a personal approach to diagnosis and management. Semin Neurol 22:75–87, 2002.

Younger DS: Motor neuron disease and malignancy. Muscle Nerve 23:658–660, 2000.

Younger DS, Rowland LP, Latov N, et al.: Lymphoma, motor neuron disease, and amyotrophic lateral sclerosis. Ann Neurol 29:78–86, 1991.

3 Spinal Muscular Atrophy

Natte Raksadawan
David S. Younger

Definition

Late in the nineteenth century, Werndig and Hoffmann described the clinical findings of infantile spinal muscular atrophy. They noted infantile paralysis usually by the third month of life, occurrence in siblings with normal parents, progressive hypotonia and weakness, hand tremor, and death from pneumonia in early childhood. At autopsy there was atrophy of ventral roots of the spinal cord, a decrease in the number of spinal cord motor neurons, and a pattern of atrophy in muscle fibers consistent with loss of innervation. It is now known that the spinal muscular atrophies (SMA) are inherited disorders of spinal motor neurons with a variable clinical expression depending upon age of onset, severity, and allelic genetic localization.

Epidemiology

1. The incidence of infantile SMA (type 1) is 4 to 10/100,000 live births, suggesting a carrier frequency of 1/80 to 1/50.
2. The incidence of childhood and adult SMA (types 2, 3) is 1/19,420 live births, with a prevalence of 1.6/100,000.

Genetic Basis

1. 96% of cases of SMA demonstrate autosomal recessive inheritance. The responsible genetic lesion is a deletion or point mutation in the survival motor neuron (SMN) gene located at the 5q11-q13 chromosome locus. Affected patients receive one abnormal mutant gene from each carrier parent.
2. The SMN gene occurs in two forms, telemetric (SMNt) or SMN1, and centromeric (SMNc) or SMN2. SMN1 and SMN2 each contain nine exons but differ in 8 nucleotides.
3. 95% of affected patients with SMN1 demonstrate homozygous deletion of exons 7 and 8.

Clinical Syndromes

1. The classification of SMA (Table 3–1) is based on overall age at onset and severity, with type 1 (I; Werdnig-Hoffmann) onset by 6 months of age; type 2 (II, Dubowitz disease), between 6 and 18 months; and type 3 (III; (Kugelberg-Welander disease), after 18 months.

2. Molecular genetics has added further precision to classification as well as the recognition of disorders alleleic to SMA1, such as congenital axonal neuropathy and arthrogryposis multiplex congenita.

SMA1

1. SMA1 presents with infantile hypotonia, lingual fasciculation, progressive limb and intercostal muscle weakness, joint contracture, poor sucking reflex, swallowing difficulty, areflexia, and poor motor milestone development, but without disturbance of cognition, sensation, or sphincter tone.

2. Children with SMA1 almost never sit without support when placed. They typically lie in the frog-leg position with a fine tremor of the fingers called *polyminimyoclonus*. There may be no spontaneous movements except in the hands and feet, in striking contrast with the infant's level of social interaction, which is unimpaired.

3. The highest mortality (90%) occurs among infants with onset before 3 months of age owing to the overall severity of the disorder complicated by eventual malnutrition and pulmonary insufficiency.

4. Such severely affected infants tire during feeding, and if breast-fed, they lose weight before it is evident that they are not taking in sufficient calories. Pulmonary insufficiency results from intercostal muscle weakness, leading to pectus excavatum and flaring of the lower ribs, the so-called bell-shaped deformity; bilateral eventration or paralysis of the diaphragm occurs, with an abdominal breathing pattern.

5. Malnutrition and respiratory insufficiency exacerbate fatigue and cause susceptibility to infection, which becomes a life-threatening crisis that forces the decision of whether to embark on endotracheal intubation and parenteral tube feeding.

6. Congenital axonal neuropathy presents with neonatal hypotonia, congenital joint contractures, facial diplegia, ophthalmoplegia, severe weakness, and respiratory failure at delivery that requires mechanical ventilatory support. An antenatal history of decreased fetal movement and polyhydramnios is common.

7. Arthrogryposis multiplex congenita presents with

TABLE 3–1. SPECTRUM OF SMA PHENOTYPES

SMA Type	Onset of Weakness	Life Span	Motor Milestones	Clinical Presentation
CAN	Prenatal	Days	None	Neonatal hypotonia Joint contractures No movement Facial diplegia Ophthalmoplegia Severe weakness and respiratory failure at delivery that requires ventilatory support
AMC-SMA	Prenatal	1 month or less	None	Joint contractures Paralysis Normal facial/extraocular movement
SMA1	Before 6 months	2 years or less	No independent sitting	Infantile hypotonia Joint contractures Normal facial/extraocular movement Variable suck/swallow problems Prognosis depends on respiratory function Areflexia Poor motor development, without disturbance of cognition or sensation Postural tremor of fingers
SMA2	Usually 6 months to 18 months	70% alive at 25 years	Independent sitting or independent ambulation	Prognosis depends on maximum motor and respiratory function achieved
SMA3	After age 18 months	Normal	Independent ambulation	Gradual loss of function over time
SMA4	After age 30 years	Normal	Normal	Very slowly progressive

Abbreviations: CAN: congenital axonal neuropathy; AMC-SMA: arthrogryposis multiplex congenita-SMA.

congenital joint contracture and paralysis that spares extraocular and facial muscles.

SMA2

1. Patients usually achieve normal milestones up to 6 to 8 months of age, although they are hypotonic.

2. The legs tend to be more involved than the arms, leading to failure to walk as a chief complaint. Many patients with SMA2 are able to sit without support if placed in position.

3. Some affected children will occasionally stand or walk with assistance; however, the age for sitting, standing, and walking is always delayed. Walking, if it does occur, is always temporary.

4. Many patients survive to the third or fourth decade, with the difference between survivors and nonsurvivours being good pulmonary function.

SMA3

1. Onset in SMA3 is usually any time after age 18 months, most often signaled by onset of weakness between 1½ and 3 years of age, and referred to as SMA3a; in some cases, onset of weakness occurs after the age of 3 years (SMA3b).

2. Affected children have a history of normal motor milestones and walking until they begin to fall or have difficulty walking up or down stairs.

3. At a later age, onset may be mistaken for limb girdle muscular dystrophy owing to proximal muscular atrophy, waddling gait, lumbar lordosis, genu recurvatum, and a protuberant abdomen; some children may appear very thin, like a "stick man."

4. Some authors have identified adult-onset SMA, which occurs after the age of 21, type 4. This designation, however, is not consistently used in the literature.

Differential Diagnosis

1. SMA1 should be differentiated from other syndromes such as neonatal and infantile hypotonia, or the so-called floppy infant syndrome, as well as from hypoxic-ischemic cerebral injury, brain malformation, peroxisomal disorders, amino and organic aciduria, congenital myopathy, neonatal myasthenia gravis, and mitochondrial encephalomyopathy.

2. The differential diagnosis of SMA2 and SMA3, in addition, includes juvenile amyotrophic lateral sclerosis, X-linked spinobulbar muscular atrophy (Kennedy and Fazio-Londe syndromes); adult Tay-Sach disease, neuronal forms of Charcot-Marie Tooth disease, chronic inflammatory demyelinating polyneuropathy, hereditary neuropathy with propensity to pressure palsies, limb-girdle muscular dystrophy, and dermatomyositis.

Laboratory Testing

1. The diagnostic work-up for SMA has changed since the discovery of the *SMN* gene. The sensitiv-

ity of genetic testing is 96%, 94%, and 82% in SMA1, SMA2, and SMA3, respectively.

2. For infants who have deletions of exons 7 and 9, no further work-up is necessary.

3. If DNA analysis is normal, then a more traditional approach is necessary for diagnosis that includes measurement of serum creatine kinase, nerve conduction studies (NCS) and needle electromyography, and muscle biopsy.

4. The serum CK is often normal in SMA1 and 2, but it may be elevated in SMA3, adding to the confusion with limb girdle muscular dystrophy in children with an uninformative *SMN* gene testing.

5. Motor NCS abnormalities, when present, show mildly reduced compound muscle action potential amplitudes and velocities, with normal distal latencies, in motor nerves innervating weak, wasted, twitching muscles, all of which is indicative of the progressive loss of functioning motor axons.

6. Needle EMG shows variabale acute and chronic denervation potentials including fibrillation, positive sharp waves, and fasciculation potentials with reduced recruitment of large-amplitude and long-duration motor unit potentials.

7. Muscle biopsy shows neurogenic large group atrophy with evidence of type grouping, indicating collateral reinnervation, and variably increased connective tissue that parallels the duration of illness.

Key Tests

- Genetic testing
- Measurement of serum creatine kinase
- Nerve conduction studies
- Needle electromyography
- Muscle biopsy

Management

1. Because there is no cure or known means of slowing the progression of SMA, effective management should focus on prevention and treatment of the complications of the disease, as well as to sustain health and prolonged survival without compromising quality of life (Table 3–2).

2. Up to 80% of SMA1 children die by 1 year of age; the remainder, by age 2. In contrast, 68.5% of SMA2 children survive to 25 years. The outcome of SMA3 is more favorable, with 70% of children still walking by 10 years of age and the possibility of an essentially normal life expectancy.

3. For those patients that survive, and their families, supportive therapy consists of managing the consequences of progressive weakness, restrictive lung disease, impaired nutrition, orthopedic deformities, immobility, psychosocial problems, and family genetic counseling, which may all vary with the age of onset and the severity of illness.

4. The risk of pneumonia increases as pulmonary volumes decrease. Particularly sensitive measures of declining pulmonary reserve are the forced vital capacity, inspiratory and expiratory muscle pressures (P_I and P_E max), and arterial blood gas measurement used by pulmonologists and respiratory therapists to ascertain the need for noninvasive ventilation, which unfortunately does not alter the inevitably poor prognosis in SMA1.

5. Poor nutrition with failure to thrive complicates a weak sucking reflex, aspiration, and easy fatiguability, particularly in infants. A feeding evaluation should be performed by a team of occupational, speech, and swallowing therapists and dietitians to adjust the feeding schedule, positioning, and food textures to maximize caloric intake. Barium swallow radiography using a modified approach or video fluoroscopy is useful in ascertaining the need for gastrostomy feeding.

6. Scoliosis is the most serious orthopedic problem in SMA and occurs primarily among nonwalkers. Spinal orthotics do not prevent or retard scoliosis, but they may help patients to sit comfortably in a wheelchair, and require monitoring of pulmonary function. Corrective scoliosis surgery should be considered after wheelchair dependence com-

TABLE 3–2. KEY COMPLICATIONS OF SPINAL MUSCULAR ATROPHY

COMPLICATION	CHARACTERISTICS
Respiratory insufficiency	Proportional to general weakness
	May occur during sleep before clinically apparent
	Patient responds well to noninvasive ventilation
Failure to thrive	Particularly infants
	Exacerbates weakness and fatigue
	Reduces reserves
Constipation	Very common
	Patient responds to dietary management
Orthopedic deformities	Clubfoot
	Scoliosis, kyphosis
	Flexion contractures
Psychosocial dysfunction	Inadequate intellectual challenge
	Depression rare in patients, in siblings; marital discord

mences because it can improve disabling postures, improve respiratory muscle dynamics, and prolong survival. Clubfoot deformity may also need corrective surgery. Other common deformities include those of flexion contracture secondary to immbolity in the hips, knees, and ankles, all of which may be prevented or ameliorated by daily range of motion exercises.

7. Children with SMA2 and SMA3 should be encouraged to stand and walk with orthoses for as long as possible, and afterward to maintain as normal a posture as possible in the wheelchair to avert disabling scoliosis. However, for some children with SMA2, a power chair is appropriate as close to the second birthday as possible, as children learn to maneuver a joy stick and can achieve a degree of independent mobility. School-age children will benefit from a range of psychosocial and educational services.

8. Once the diagnosis of SMA is made by genetic testing, genetic counseling is the next step in prevention. 98% of parents of an affected SMA child will be obligate carriers of the SMN gene; with a 25% chance that the next child will be symptomatic, and a 50% chance of the carrier state. Genetic counseling, and prenatal diagnosis of high-risk couples reduce the chance of a new symptomatic case.

Key Treatment

- No known cure or means of slowing progression of the disease
- Management should focus on prevention and treatment of disease complications.

For more information about SMA and related motor neuron diseases, patients and families should contact *www.als-nyc.org.*

Bibliography

Dubowitz V: 38th ENMC International Workshop on Spinal Muscular Atrophy Trial Group. Neuromusc Disord 6:293–294, 1966.

Dubowitz V: Infantile muscular atrophy. A prospective study with particular reference to a slowly progressive variety. Brain 87:707–718, 1964.

Eng GD, Binder H, Koch B: Spinal muscular atrophy: Experience in diagnosis and rehabilitation management of 60 patients. Arch Phys Med Rehabil 65:549–553, 1984.

Iannaccone ST: Childhood spinal muscular atrophy. In DS Younger (ed): Motor Disorders. Philadelphia, Lippincott Williams & Wilkins, 1999, pp. 349–356.

Lefebvre S, Burglen, Reboullet S, et al.: Identification and characterization of a spinal muscular atrophy-determining gene. Cell 80:155–165, 1995.

Nicole S, Diaz CC, Frugier T, Melki J: Spinal muscular atrophy: recent advances and future prospects. Muscle Nerve 26:4–13, 2002.

4 Hereditary Spastic Paraplegia

Natte Raksadawan
David S. Younger

Definitions

1. Hereditary spastic paraplegia (HSP) denotes syndrome of familial spastic paraparesis and paraplegia that are heterogeneous in mode of inheritance, gene localization, gene defects, pattern of neurologic presentation, and severity.

2. HSP is clinically classified into "pure" (pHSP) or only progressive spasticity alone; and rarer "complicated" forms in which spasticity is combined with additional neurologic or non-neurologic features. The genetic classification of HSP (Table 4–1) further specifies spastic paraplegia genotypes (SPG).

3. Suggested criteria for HSP include family history, progressive spastic paraparesis, hyperreflexia of the legs, and Babinski signs, in association with sphincter and dorsal column disturbance.

Epidemiology

1. The prevalence of pHSP is 9.6 per 100,000 population.

2. 70% to 80% of cases display autosomal dominant (AD) inheritance, with the remainder autosomal recessive (AR) and X-linked recessive.

pHSP

1. Type 1 AD-pHSP has an onset before age 35, with spasticity as the predominant handicap. Type 2 commences after age 35, typically with muscle weakness, urinary involvement, impaired vibratory and joint position sense.

2. Progression is generally slow, with most patients requiring a cane or wheelchair over a span of 6 decades.

3. The main pathologic findings are degeneration of corticospinal tracts beginning at the medullary pyramids and increasing caudally, with variable degeneration of posterior column nuclei and tracts and with some spinocerebellar tract involvement.

4. With advances in the molecular genetics of HSP, several genes have been cloned and mapped (Table 4–1).

5. Linkage studies reveal 12 SPG mapped to date (SPG 2–4, 5A, 5B, 6–8, 10–13).

6. Gene products for three types of pHSP have been identified: proteolipid protein in SGP2; spastin in SPG4; and paraplegin in SPG7.

7. X-linked pHSP is allelic to another disorder, Pelizaeus-Merzbacher disease, which in its classic form presents in early childhood with slowly progressive spastic paraparesis, dystonia, and cerebellar signs, psychomotor retardation, and nystagmoid eye movements.

Complicated HSP

Three syndromes of complicated HSP have been well studied (Table 4–1).

1. The first is the syndrome of mental retardation, aphasia, shuffling gait, and adducted thumbs (MASA syndrome).

2. The second is the syndrome of X-linked hydrocephalus and aqueduct stenosis (HSAS syndrome).

3. The third is Sjögren-Larsson syndrome, which leads to congenital ichthyosis, mental retardation, spastic diplegia or tetraplegia, glistening white dots on the retina, short stature, seizure disorder, and speech defects.

4. HSP occurs in association with Charcot-Marie

TABLE 4–1. HSP OF KNOWN GENETIC TRANSMISSION

DESIGNATION	MIM#	INHERITANCE	GENE LOCATION/ PRODUCT
pHSP Form			
SGP2	312920	XR	Xq21/PLP
SGP3	182600	AD	14q11.2-q24.3
SGP4	182601	AD	2q22-p21/spastin
SPG5A	270800	AR	8q12-q13
SPG5B	600146	AR	
SPG6	600363	AD	15q11.1
SGP7	602783	AR	16q24.3/paraplegin
SPG8	603563	AD	8q23-24
SPG10	604187	AD	12q13
SPG11	604360	AR	15q13-q15
SPG12	604805	AD	19q13
SPG13	605280	AD	2q24
Complicated HSP Form/Syndrome			
SPG1	312900	XR	Xq28/LICAM
SPG9	601162	AD	10q23.3-24.1
SPG14	605229	AR	3q27-q28
ARSACS		AR	13q12/sacsin
Sjögren-Larsson		AR	17p11.2

Abbreviations: Other Complicated HSP Forms: HSP with: CMT; Silver syndrome; Troyer syndrome; sensory neuropathy; pigmentary skin changes; Kjellin syndrome; epilepsy; thinning of the corpus callosum; MAST syndrome; Kallmann's syndrome; MIM#: Mendelian Inheritance in Man classification number.

Tooth disease; Silver syndrome of associated distal amyotrophy; Troyer syndromes of associated distal (hand) amyotrophy and mild cerebellar signs; with sensory neuropathy; with abnormal skin and hair pigmentation; Kjellin syndrome of associated mental retardation and pigmentary macular degeneration; complex partial, myoclonic, and simple partial epilepsy; thinning of the corpus callosum; MAST syndrome of associated extrapyramidal features; and Kallmann's syndrome of associated hypogonadotrophic hypogonadism and anosmia.

Differential Diagnosis

The differential diagnosis and laboratory evaluation of HSP is summarized in Table 4–2.

1. Obvious AD-pHSP should be distinguished from AD spinocerebellar ataxia through genetic testing of abnormal expansion of CAG trinucleotide repeats.

2. Index cases of pHSP should be tested first and foremost for multiple sclerosis and structural disorders of the brain and spinal cord owing to arteriovenous malformations, brain and spinal cord neoplasms, cervical spondylotic myelopathy, and Arnold Chiari malformation by magnetic resonance imaging (MRI) of the brain and spine. Other readily identifiable causes of HSP include amyotrophic lateral sclerosis (by electrodiagnostic testing); tropical spastic paraparesis, acquired immunodeficiency syndrome, and neurosyphilis (through the addition of retroviral and spirochetal testing in the blood and cerebrospinal fluid); and

subacute combined degeneration of the spinal cord from vitamin B_{12} deficiency. The cause of HSP may lie in a definable metabolic disorder traceable to (1) deficiency of galactocerebrosidase in adult-onset and juvenile-onset of Krabbe leukodystrophy (spastic hemiparesis, visual loss, cerebellar ataxia, and dementia-psychosis); (2) deficiency of sufatidase in metachromatic leukodystrophy (spastic quadriparesis, dementia); (3) deficiency of phytanic acid accumulation owing to Refsum's disease (visual loss, hypertrophic sensorimotor neuropathy, cranial nerve and cerebellar involvement); (4) impaired bile acid synthesis indicative of cerebrotendinous xanthomatosis (dementia, psychiatric disturbances, cerebellar dysfunction, peripheral neuropathy); or (5) increased urine and lysosomal storage of sialic acid owing to Salla disease (mental retardation, psychomotor delay, coarsened facies, spasticity).

3. The differential diagnosis of HSP with retinal disease should lead to consideration of Kjellin syndrome (early adulthood dementia, spastic paraplegia, and yellow retinal flecks of the macula); Laurence-Moon-Bardet-Biedl syndrome (childhood mental retardation, hypogenitalism, ataxia, nystagmus, and retinitis pigmentosa); Cockayne syndrome (mental retardation, normal pressure hydrocephalus, ataxia, sensorineural hearing loss, intention tremor, nystagmus, muscle rigidity, and incontinence); Hallevorden-Spatz disease (dementia, speech problems, choreoathetosis, tremor, wasting, and spasticity); and secondary hereditary dystonia with dopamine sensitivity.

TABLE 4–2. DIFFERENTIAL DIAGNOSIS AND LABORATORY EVALUATION OF pHSP

Diagnosis	Laboratory Tests
Friedrich's ataxia	Genetic test for GAA trinucleotide repeats
Krabbe leukodystrophy	Brain MRI, galactocerebrosidase
Metachromatic leukodystrophy	MRI, arylsulfatase
Refsum's disease	Phytanic acid
Vitamin B_{12} deficiency	B_{12}, methylmalonic acid, homocysteine
Cerebrotendinous xanthomatosis	Bile acid synthesis
Salla disease	Urine and lysosomal sialic acid
Cervical spondylotic myelopathy	Spine MRI
Arnold-Chiari malformation	Brain/spine MRI
Neoplasm	Brain/spine MRI
Cerebral palsy	Birth history
Arteriovenous malfomation	Brain and spine MRI
Multiple sclerosis	Brain/spine MRI, cerebrospinal fluid, trimodal evoked responses
Amyotrophic lateral sclerosis	Electromyographic and nerve conduction studies
Arginase deficiency	Serum arginine, aminoaciduria
Lathyrism	Exposure to *Lathyrus sativus*
Abetalipoproteinemia	Lipoprotein electrophoresis
Dopa-responsive dystonia	L-dopa trial
Tropical spastic paraparesis	Blood/CSF HTLV-1 antibodies
Acquired immunodeficiency syndrome	CD4 count, HIV RNA
Adrenoleukodystrophy/ Adrenomyeloneuropathy	Saturated very long-chain fatty acids

4. X-linked forms of pHSP should be distinguished from adrenomyeloneuropathy, which has been mapped to chromosome Xq28 and encodes peroxisomal membrane protein and is associated with detectably high levels of plasma saturated very long-chain fatty acids.

Therapy and Genetic Counseling

1. There is no effective treatment to slow or halt the progression of HSP.

2. Spasticity may be reduced with oral or intrathecal baclofen.

3. Physical therapy and occupational therapy play important roles in maintaining strength, safe ambulation, and continuing to work as long as possible.

4. Genetic counseling defines the inheritance pattern through an extensive pedigree and can be useful to future generations of childbearing age. The application of prenatal diagnosis has been recently described in AD-pHSP.

Key Treatment

- No known effective treatment for slowing or halting progression of the disease

- Oral or intrathecal baclofen for spasticity

- Physical and occupational therapy for maintaining strength and ambulation

Bibliography

Harding AE: Hereditary spastic paraplegias. Semin Neurol 13:333–336, 1993.

McDermott CJ, White K, Bushby K, Shaw PJ: Hereditary spastic paraparesis: A review of new developments. J Neurol Neurosurg Psychiatry 69:150–160, 2000.

Moser HW: Hereditary spastic paraplegia. In DS Younger (ed): Motor Disorders, Philadelphia, Lippincott Williams & Wilkins, 1999, pp. 269–274.

Tallaksen CME, Durr A, Brice A: Recent advances in hereditary spastic paraplegia. Current Opin Neurol 14:457–463, 2001.

Younger DS: Differential diagnosis of progressive spastic paraparesis. Semin Neurol 13:319–321, 1993.

5 Muscle Cramps

Maria E. Alexianu
David S. Younger

Definition

Cramps are transient, painful, involuntary contractions of a muscle or group of muscles. They ordinarily last a few seconds to several minutes and are provoked by contracting an already shortened muscle. They occur during vigorous exercise and after exercise ceases. Nocturnal cramps typically cause forceful flexion of the ankles and toes. They occur in any muscle, typically the calves.

Epidemiology

1. Most people experience cramps at some time in their lives and at all ages. The overall incidence of cramps in children is 7.3%. They are generally unilateral, with an occurrence of 1 to 4 times per year.

2. The incidence of cramps in patients 65 years or older is greater than 50% and more likely to be seen in association with peripheral vascular disease, arthritis, and female gender.

3. Pregnancy increases the incidence of cramps to 81% in adults, and occurs most often after the 25th week of gestation.

Diseases Associated with Cramps

1. Cramps accompany benign fasciculation in the Denny-Brown, Foley syndrome of cramps and benign fasciculation.

2. Cramps occur in neuromyotonia or Isaacs' syndrome accompanied by myokymia, abnormal postures, pseudomyotonia, and hyperhydrosis.

3. Cramps may be the first sign of a metabolic myopathy, occurring with myalgia on exertion in myoadenylate deaminase deficiency; phosphofructokinase deficiency, phosphoglycerate kinase deficiency, dystrophinopathies, and myotonia congenital; in association with cramp-like rigid contraction in McArdle's disease (phosphorylase deficiency); and in the Brody syndrome of deficient calcium ATPase reuptake in the sarcoplasmic reticulum of type II myofibers.

4. Nocturnal leg cramps accompany restless legs syndrome, sleep-induced myoclonus, sleep paralysis, and bruxism.

5. Cramps are statistically more common in pregnancy, dehydration, excessive sweating, thyrotoxicosis, hypothyroidism, uremia, hypomagnesemia, hypokalemia, hypocalcemia, uremia, gout, liver cirrhosis, stingray injury, and excessive ingestion of licorice.

6. Frequent cramping may be a clue to underlying neurogenic disease such as peripheral neuropathy, ventral root compression, human T-cell lymphotrophic virus type 1–associated spastic paraparesis and tropical ataxic neuropathy, poliomyelitis, post-polio syndrome, spinal muscular atrophy, and amyotrophic lateral sclerosis.

7. Central nervous system disorders that may include cramps include dystonia and Parkinson disease; the stiff-man syndrome, characterized by painful muscle spasm and stiffness; poliomyelitis; and the post-polio syndrome.

8. Drug ingestion may lead to muscle cramps (Table 5–1).

Mechanisms of Cramping

The exact mechanism of cramps remains obscure. They likely derive from a common expression of several mechanisms in many diverse clinical settings.

1. The experimental application of local anesthetic along a perpipheral nerve blocks the electrical discharge of cramp potentials and the severe pain of marked cramping, more effectively than spinal anesthesia, general anesthesia, and intravenous diazepam.

2. The electromyographic (EMG) findings of a cramp consist of high-frequency (200–300 Hz) repetitive motor unit potentials (MUPs), usually beginning with single potentials and followed by doublets. The activity gradually spreads synchronously to adjacent areas of muscle or display more than a single discharge at sites that activate sequentially. The activity waxes and wanes and can continue for several minutes. Muscle stretching first interrupts the discharge, then renders it asynchronous, and eventually stops it altogether. A similar benefit is seen by nerve stimulation at 10 to 40 Hz for several seconds. Afterward the muscle may be irritable, exhibiting spontaneous motor unit potential discharges for several minutes.

2. Nocturnal leg cramps occur mainly during rapid eye movement (REM) sleep and in stages 1 through 3 of non-REM sleep. Nocturnal leg cramps with a known genetic predisposition are

TABLE 5–1. CLINICAL CLASSIFICATION OF CRAMPS

Idiopathic
Nocturnal leg cramps
Sleep disorders
Pregnancy

Association with Systemic Conditions
Dehydration
Electrolyte disturbances
Arthritis
Peripheral vascular disease
Endocrinopathy

Association with Central and Peripheral Nervous System Disorders
Motor neuron disease
Tropical spastic paraparesis
Stiff-man syndrome
Neuromyotonia (Isaacs' syndrome)
Poliomyelitis, post-polio syndrome
Radiculopathy
Peripheral neuropathy

Primary Muscle Disorders
Metabolic myopathy
Dystrophinopathy
Myotonia congenita

Drug-Induced Disorders
Albuterol, anticholinesterases, beta-blockers, DHE (dihydroergotamine), caffeine, cholesterol-lowering agents (statins), cimetidine, chemotherapy agents, diuretics, lithium, hexacarbons, nifedipine, phenothiazines, terbutaline, theophylline, misoprostol, alcohol

usually accompanied by myoclonic jerks and frequent painful awakenings. They are most commonly associated with autosomal dominant inheritance.

3. The pain the accompanies cramps is also multifactorial. Cramps may be due to excitation of pain-sensitive nerve terminals in response to mechanical stimulation; local production of lactic acid; excess accumulation of potassium, creatine, or adenine nucleotides; and inflammatory cell infiltration associated with myalgia, swelling, and local injury following a marked sustained episode of cramping.

Evaluation

1. Infrequent muscle cramps, generally in the calves, in an otherwise normal individual generally do not warrant evaluation.

2. The evaluation of frequent cramps commences with a general medical and neurologic history and examination, and simple blood studies for possible underlying systemic diseases.

3. Nerve conduction studies are performed to ascertain associated peripheral neuropathy and to investigate radiculopathy that may show prolonged distal latency, reduced compound muscle and sensory nerve action potential amplitudes, and reduced velocities in the involved nerves, as well as prolonged F response latencies in affected root myotomes. Concentric needle EMG and quantitative MUP analysis are useful to discern underlying myopathy, to investigate the electrophysiologic appearance of a cramp discharge, and to differentiate a cramp discharge from other abnormal spontaneous discharges.

4. Noctural cramps that fragment sleep warrant further investigation with polysomnography and concomitant EMG needle recording.

5. Muscle biopsy is performed for the diagnosis of metabolic myopathy.

Management and Prognosis

1. Acute management of a painful calf cramp follows passive lengthening of the muscle by forceful dorsal flexion of the foot, and standing or walking on the affected leg.

2. Prevention of further episodes of cramping may follow withdrawal of a potential offending medication or treatment of systemic illness.

3. When cramps recur and disrupt quality of life and sleep, drug treatment to reduce the excitability and contractility of muscle tissue is indicated, including consideration of nighttime quinine salts, tonic water and bitter lemon beverages, verapamil hydrochloride, gabapentin, aspirin, roloxifene, B vitamin supplementation, intramuscular injection of trigger points with 0.5% to 1% xylocaine hydrochloride, and even botulinum injection into calf muscles.

Key Treatment

- Passive lengthening of the muscle followed by forceful dorsal flexion of the foot

- Various medications (e.g., quinine salts, tonic water and bitter lemon beverages, verapamil hydrochloride, gabapentin, aspirin)

Bibliography

Ferrante MA, Wilbourn AJ: Basic principles and practice of electromyography. In Younger DS (ed): Motor Disorders. Philadelphia, Lippincott Williams & Wilkins, 1999, pp. 19–44.
Leung AK, Wong BE, Chan PY, Cho HY: Noctural leg cramps in children: incidence and clinical characteristics. J Natl Med Assoc 91:329–332, 1999.
Riley JD, Antony SJ: Leg cramps: differential diagnosis and management. Am Fam Physician 52:1794–1798, 1995.
Sawaya R, Kanaan N: Nocturnal leg cramps. Clinically mysterious and painful—but manageable. Geriatrics 56:34–42, 2001.

6 Fasciculation

Maria E. Alexianu
David S. Younger

Definition

1. Clinically, fasciculation are visible involuntary twitches of muscle. Electrophysiologically, they correspond to a spontaneous discharge of the motor unit with activation of some or all of the myofibers. A single fasciculation may be as small as a flicker of the surface of the muscle, or large enough to move a small part of the body, such as a finger.

2. Fasciculations occur in various progressive and nonprogressive neuromuscular disorders wherein they may be a clue to a categorical diagnosis of the motor unit.

3. Fasciculation occurs in 70% of normal individuals, exacerbated by extreme exercise, cold temperature, hyperventilation, stress, excessive caffeine and alcohol intake, metabolic derangements, and prescription medication.

4. The exact origin of fasciculation in any one disorder in not well understood, and it is generally assumed that the predominant pathologic process rests with the most likely localization; as for example, in the peripheral nerve process in multifocal motor neuropathy, the ventral root in compressive radiculopathy, and the anterior horn cell in motor neuron disease (Table 6–1).

5. Fasciculation in amyotrophic lateral sclerosis (ALS) could conceivably result from secondary pathological processes extending to other sites capable of initiating spontaneous activity, as for example the distal motor fiber, the axon terminal, and supraspinal segments.

Associated Disorders

1. Two benign fasciculation disorders are benign fasciculation syndrome, and the syndrome of cramps and fasciculation.

2. When localized to myotomal segments, fasciculation may be the signature of poliomyelitis, compressive root disease, or involvement of ventral roots by nonspecific inflammation, as may occur in acute or chronic inflammatory demyelinating polyradiculopathy, myelomatosis, or neurolymphomatosis. Focal weakness, wasting, and fasciculation are the hallmarks of anterior horn cell involvement; when present in three limbs in combination with hyperactive reflexes, this combination makes the diagnosis of ALS virtually inescapable.

3. The ingestion of ciguatera toxin present in infected tropical reef fish leads to systemic illness, toxic neuropathy, and widespread fasciculation.

4. Hyperthyroidism and hyperparathyroidism both lead to systemic manifestations that include widespread fasciculation and hyperreflexia, that may resemble ALS.

5. Anticholinesterase drug overdose and cholinomimetic drugs induce fasciculation in normal individuals. In children, inhalation of isoflurane gas depresses end-plate depolarization and inhibits fasciculations caused by succinylcholine.

6. In the syndrome of multifocal motor neuropathy, with or without conduction block or elevated serum titers of GM1 ganglioside antibodies, fasciculation is limited to muscles innervated by the affected nerves in congruence with a peripheral nerve localization.

7. Radiation therapy can lead to focal motor neuron disease when portions of the spinal cord are incompletely shielded from a contiguous intramedullary glioma or Schwannoma.

8. Brachial plexopathy and lumbosacral plexopathy similarly occur when these structures are inadvertently or purposely included in the field of radiation, as for example in treating apical tumor of the lung and malignant tumors of the plexus.

9. Paget disease of the high cervical cord can lead to basilar invagination and cervical cord compression, resulting in a syndrome of segmental weakness, wasting, and fasciculation, and hyperreflexia reminiscent of ALS.

10. Fasciculation occurs in diverse progressive neurogenetic disorders, among them Machado-Joseph disease (Azorean disease), pallido-luysio-nigral atrophy, myelofibrosis, multisystem atrophy, some gangliosidoses, and olivopontocerebellar atrophy.

Electrophysiology

1. When recorded with a needle electrode, fasciculation potentials fire irregularly with the configuration of motor unit action potentials (MUP). They signify irritability rather than denervation. Their firing frequency varies from a few per minute to one per second.

TABLE 6–1. KEY FEATURES ASSOCIATED WITH FASCICULATIONS

Diseases	Distinguishable Associated Features
Benign fasciculation syndrome	Intermittent, long periods without fasciculations
Cramp-fasciculation syndrome	Legs mainly; cramping more prominent
Electrolyte disturbance Parathyroid disorders	Improves with treatment of underlying disease
Radiculopathy	Limited to one or rarely two myotomes
Motor neuropathy with or without conduction block and elevated titers to GM1 gangliosides	Limited to muscles innervated by involved nerves; lack of atrophy in weak, areflexic muscles; conduction block
Ciguatera infection	Time relationship to food poisoning
Post-radiation motor neuron disease and plexopathy	Focal weakness, atrophy of involved muscles, decreased deep tendon reflexes in the field of radiation
Spinal cord or brainstem tumors	Territorial distribution of fasciculations
Paget's disease of the bone	Brainstem compression symptoms because of basilar invagination
Amyotrophic lateral sclerosis	Widespread fasciculation, with focal weakness, wasting, hyperreflexia; associated with fibrillations and positive sharp waves on EMG.

2. It is possible to differentiate fasciculation potentials from abnormal spontaneous discharges of other causes that lead to focal movement of the surface of muscle by careful electrodiagnostic testing. This is accomplished by concentric needle electromyography (EMG) in which the examiner studies the configuration, firing rate, and synchronicity of the abnormal MUP. Myotonic discharges, myokymic potentials, and cramp potentials may present diagnostic challenges in their differentiation from fasciculation potentials clinically and electrophysiologically.

3. Myotonic discharges are action potentials of single muscle fibers that frequently occur in trains. Their firing frequency and amplitude continuously change, a feature that produces the characteristic EMG pitch variation of a "dive bomber airplane." These potentials are a frequent associated finding of the muscle membrane disorders or channelopathies that result from disturbances of muscle ion channel function and membrane excitability, such as seen in myotonic muscular dystrophy, periodic paralysis, neuromyotonia or Isaacs' syndrome, malignant hyperthermia, episodic ataxia type 1, and hereditary "rippling muscle" disease.

4. Grouped repetitive discharges are the repeated firing of groups of several potentials that display a simple waveform. They can vary in the number of

potentials composing a group and in their firing frequency. When two or more grouped repetitive discharges fire concurrently and asynchronously, it is termed *myokymia,* and can accompany facial myokymia with multiple sclerosis and pontine gliomas; and limb myokymia in conjunction with radiation induced plexopathy, multifocal motor neuropathy, chronic inflammatory demyelinating polyradiculoneuropathy (CIDP), and gold intoxication.

5. Fasciculation potentials in ALS are distinguished by their tendency for more complex and varied EMG appearance, especially in areas of subtle and minor clinically wasting; and the frequent association with fibrillation and positive sharp waves.

Evaluation and Management

1. The management of a patient with fasciculation should be directed toward identifying the underlying disorder and the initiation of effective treatment.

2. Initial evaluation should include a general medical and neurologic history and examination to uncover coexisting motor neuron, nerve root, peripheral nerve, or muscle disease.

3. If indicated, blood studies are useful to ascertain serum parathyroid and calcium level, thyroid function, lymphocyte cell markers for neoplastic disease, as well as routine chemistries, complete blood count, and erythrocyte sedimentation rate (ESR).

4. Electrodiagnostic studies should include a sampling of nerve conductions in the arms and leg, and concentric needle EMG studies of involved muscles to identify benign or symptomatic fasciculation, and to identify a specific neuromuscular disorder.

5. Neuroimaging studies with gadolinium should be obtained if there is suspicion of inflammatory, degenerative, or compressive plexopathy; radiculopathy; or spinal cord disease.

6. There is no effective therapy of benign fasciculation; however, attention to potential provocative factors may be useful.

Key Treatment

- Identify the underlying disorder and initiate effective treatment.

- No effective therapy exists for benign fasciculation.

B Bibliography

Desai J and Swash M: Fasciculations: What do we know of their significance? J Neurol Sci 152:S43–S48, 1997.

Eisen A: Clinical electrophysiology of the upper and lower motor neuron in amyotrophic lateral sclerosis. Semin Neurol 2:141–155, 2001.

Ferrante MA, Wilbourne AJ: Basic principles and practice of electromyography. In DS Younger (ed): Motor Disorders. Philadelphia, Lippincott Williams & Wilkins, 1999, pp. 19–44.

Reed DM, Kurland LT: Muscle fasciculation in a healthy population. Arch Neurol 9:363–367, 1963.

Younger DS: Overview of motor disorders. In DS Younger (ed): Motor Disorders. Philadelphia, Lippincott Williams & Wilkins, 1999, pp. 3–17.

1 Clinical Evaluation of Peripheral Neuropathies

Hazem Machkhas

Evaluating the patient with peripheral neuropathy is challenging and, in a significant number of cases, frustrating for both the diagnostician and patient. The most important hurdle, obviously, is to establish that the symptoms are due to a peripheral neuropathy. The next challenge is to establish a rational differential diagnosis that leads to a systematic diagnostic approach, which should combine cost-effectiveness and minimal discomfort for the patient from excessive testing. Keep the patient well informed throughout this process and emphasize from the onset of the evaluation that the cause remains unidentified in up to 30% of patients with peripheral neuropathy. The last step is to develop a treatment plan, which may be disease-specific (immunomodulation) or symptomatic and supportive.

Etiology

The mnemonic "*dang the rapist*" is helpful for remembering the most common etiologies of peripheral neuropathy.

1. Diabetes: most common cause
2. Alcohol: may be secondary to a direct toxic effect of alcohol on the peripheral nerves, alcohol-related nutritional deficiency, or both
3. Nutritional: deficiency of vitamin B_{12}, vitamin E, or thiamine
4. Guillain-Barré syndrome
5. Trauma: mostly associated with mononeuropathies and plexopathies
6. Hereditary: in addition to the classic hereditary motor sensory neuropathies (HMSN): hereditary sensory and autonomic neuropathies (HSAN), neuropathies associated with peroxisomal disorders (adrenomyeloneuropathy, Refsum's disease), lysosomal disorders (Fabry's disease), disorders of lipoprotein metabolism (Tangier disease), and disorders of porphyrin metabolism
7. Environmental toxins and drugs: major causative agents: lead, arsenic, nitrous oxide, organophosphates, chemotherapeutic agents (cisplatin, vinca alkaloids), phenytoin, colchicine, isoniazid
8. Rheumatic: neuropathies associated with collagen vascular disorders
9. Amyloid: typically painful neuropathy, with signs and symptoms of autonomic failure

10. Paraneoplastic: includes anti-Hu associated sensory neuropathy, paraneoplastic autonomic neuropathy, and paraneoplastic demyelinating polyradiculoneuropathy
11. I: stands for
    a. Other Immune-related neuropathies, such as chronic inflammatory demyelinating polyradiculoneuropathy (CIDP), sarcoid neuropathy, multifocal motor neuropathy (MMN)
    b. Infections: leprosy, Lyme disease, HIV-associated neuropathy
12. Systemic disease: paraproteinemia-related neuropathies, neuropathies associated with thyroid disease, organ failure (renal, hepatic, pulmonary), organ transplantation, critical illness neuropathy
13. Tumors: direct infiltration of peripheral nerves, roots, or plexuses

Symptoms

1. The patient may have the following complaints.
    a. Sensory symptoms
       (1) Loss of feeling: variously described as numbness, deadness, or "like my jaw feels as if I've been to the dentist and received Novocain." Some patients are aware of the loss of feeling only and report an increased threshold to pain (not feeling cuts, bruises, injuries) or are unable to discriminate hot and cold water. These symptoms may be in the hands and feet. Typically, the earliest symptoms are in the feet.
       (2) Abnormal feelings are reported, such as tingling, prickling, or pins and needles. Some patients report the sensation of walking on sand or ground glass. Pressure on the hands or feet may produce uncomfortable, but nonpainful, electrical sensations.
       (3) Pain is the most distressing sensory symptom. It can be a burning sensation (superficial feeling of skin being burned), a deep bony ache (crushing feeling deep in the bone), or jabbing (sharp jolts or short-duration pulses of pain). These symptoms have the uncanny feature of worsening as

the patient is retiring to go to sleep. Some patients describe excessive sensitivity even to light touch (such as a bed sheet touching their feet at night).

(4) There may be poor balance due to loss of proprioceptive signaling in the feet that results in sensory ataxia. Patients describe an inability to walk in the dark, inability to close their eyes in the shower (some patients stop using the shower altogether and resort to baths), and constant use of visual cues to maintain proper gait and stance.

b. Motor symptoms

(1) Weakness: Distal weakness in the lower limbs is described as tripping on the toes, slapping the feet while walking, or difficulty climbing up or down the stairs. Proximal weakness in the lower limbs leads to difficulty when arising from a seated position (especially a low-lying chair, the commode, or getting out of a car) and when going up stairs. Distal weakness in the hands results in a weak grip (dropping things), difficulty buttoning, zipping, or turning a key in a lock.

(2) Atrophy: This normally starts in the feet but goes unnoticed by most patients, who report atrophy only once it reaches the hands.

c. Autonomic symptoms: mostly seen with diabetic neuropathy, amyloid neuropathy, and hereditary sensory and autonomic neuropathies. Symptoms may include

(1) Orthostasis ("I feel faint when I get up")

(2) Gastroparesis: repeated nausea with vomiting, persistent diarrhea, alternating diarrhea and constipation

(3) Incontinence: loss of bladder or bowel control

(4) Impotence (men), ranging from difficulty maintaining an erection to total inability to have one

(5) Dry mucous membranes: dryness of the eyes or mouth

2. What to ask the patient

a. Duration of symptoms

b. Tempo of illness

c. Exacerbating and relieving factors

d. The single most bothersome symptom (which may affect the therapeutic approach)

e. Any medications that had been started within the previous year before the onset of symptoms

f. Developmental history during childhood and adolescence: Was the patient clumsy? Was participation in sports or normal child play precluded by weakness or inability to keep up with same-age peers? These features may indicate a hereditary neuropathy.

g. Is there a history (personal or familial) of spontaneously remitting mononeuropathies? If so, it suggests hereditary neuropathy with liability to pressure palsies or familial amyloid neuropathy.

h. Carefully ask about past medical history. The presence of previously diagnosed diabetes or lupus pinpoints the likely culprit.

i. Is there a family history of such symptoms? Have any family members been diagnosed? Is there a family history of conditions that may predispose to peripheral neuropathy (e.g., diabetes)?

j. Has any previous work-up been done for this condition?

k. Have any treatments been attempted? Have any helped?

l. What are the patient's expectations? This information provides the treating physician with an opportunity to review the detailed steps required to diagnose a peripheral neuropathy. It is important at this juncture to set realistic goals for diagnosis and therapy. Such goals can be revised and reassessed as the diagnostic process evolves.

Key Symptoms

- Distal numbness and tingling (feet more than hands)
- Burning dysesthetic pain that is worse at night
- Distal weakness and atrophy
- Gait difficulty, imbalance
- Orthostasis
- Impotence

Signs

1. Sensory

a. Stocking and glove pattern sensory loss to various modalities in polyneuropathies

b. Sensory loss in individual nerve distribution in mononeuropathy or multiple mononeuropathies

c. Selective loss of pain sensation in small-fiber neuropathies (diabetes, amyloidosis)

d. Selective or preferential loss of proprioception and vibration in neuropathies that predominantly affect posterior columns (vitamin B_{12} neuropathy)

2. Motor

   a. Atrophy, when present, is usually distal, more prominent in the feet.

   b. Tone may be normal or reduced.

   c. Weakness may assume several patterns.

      (1) Symmetrical, predominantly distal weakness is featured in most polyneuropathies.

      (2) Symmetrical, proximal more than distal weakness is characteristic of polyradiculoneuropathies, with chronic inflammatory demyelinating polyradiculoneuropathy (CIDP) the prototype.

      (3) Asymmetrical weakness is seen in mononeuropathy or multiple mononeuropathies (compressive, vasculitic, diabetic).

3. Reflexes

   a. Typically absent or reduced, at least at the ankles, in most neuropathies

   b. May be normal, such as in small-fiber neuropathies

4. Autonomic examination

   a. Orthostatic blood pressure decrease with no change in pulse rate

   b. Absence of heart rate variability in response to Valsalva maneuver

   c. Absence of the normal skin axon-reflex vasodilatation (flare) response

5. Cranial nerves

   a. Examination is typically normal in most peripheral neuropathies.

   b. Facial sensory loss suggests connective tissue disorder (Sjögren's syndrome or scleroderma).

6. Other abnormalities

   a. Skeletal abnormalities: pes cavus, pes planus, hammer toes, joint deformities (Charcot's joints)

   b. Skin changes: distal loss of hair in the lower limbs, dry and thin skin, presence of painless ulcers in the feet

   c. Oral abnormalities: macroglossia in primary amyloidosis, aphthous ulcers in Behçet's disease, sicca complex in Sjögren's syndrome

   d. Organomegaly: seen with amyloidosis, sarcoidosis, and POEMS syndrome (multisystem syndrome combining polyneuropathy organomegaly, endocrinopathy, M protein, and skin changes)

Key Signs

- Glove and stocking pattern sensory loss
- Distal weakness and atrophy
- Fasciculations
- Absent or diminished reflexes, especially ankles
- Absence of skin-axon (flare) reflex
- Neuropathic orthopedic deformities

Tests

1. Blood tests

   a. Routine chemistries, including fasting blood sugar

   b. Complete blood count: anemia or macrocytosis suggests vitamin B_{12} deficiency

   c. Thyroid function studies

   d. Serum protein electrophoresis (SPEP)

   e. Vitamin B_{12} levels

   f. Serologies: rheumatoid factor (RF), antinuclear antibody (ANA), and erythrocyte sedimentation rate (ESR). Usually of low yield as routine screening tests. More advanced serologic testing, including anti-neutrophil cytoplasmic antibody (ANCA), hepatitis serology (to include hepatitis C), cytomegalovirus serology, and Lyme disease serology should be performed in the clinical setting of mononeuritis multiplex (multiple mononeuropathies of vasculitic etiology). Serum cryoglobulins should also be assayed in that setting.

   g. Human immunodeficiency virus (HIV) testing: to be done as indicated.

   h. Autoantibodies: The use of antibody "panels" as a routine part of working up peripheral neuropathy is discouraged, as they lack specificity and sensitivity in that setting. Some important antibodies are associated with peripheral neuropathy, however.

      (1) Anti-ganglioside antibodies: anti-GM1 (multifocal motor neuropathy and Guillain-Barré syndrome) and anti-GQ1b (Miller Fisher syndrome)

      (2) Anti-myelin-associated glycoprotein (anti-MAG) antibodies: not associated with any specific neuropathy but indicate an immune-mediated process that may respond to immunomodulating therapy

      (3) Anti-Hu antibodies: present in up to 90%

of patients with paraneoplastic sensory neuronopathy. Their presence should prompt evaluation of underlying malignancy, frequently found to be small cell lung cancer

  (4) Antisulfatide antibodies: not associated with any specific neuropathy

2. Lumbar puncture: useful in the work-up of suspected inflammatory neuropathies, including Guillain-Barré syndrome and CIDP. Typically shows elevated protein with normal leukocyte count (cytoalbuminogenic dissociation).

3. Electrophysiology: Once the diagnosis of peripheral neuropathy has been suspected on history and examination, nerve conduction studies help confirm the diagnosis; thus they constitute the first step in the work-up. The pattern of abnormalities helps narrow the suspected etiologies of the neuropathy and thus guides the treating physician when selecting a targeted battery of tests.

4. Quantitative sensory testing: measures sensory thresholds to various modalities. It is rarely used in routine clinical settings but is an important tool in clinical trials.

5. Autonomic testing: requires highly specialized laboratories with expertise in the performance and interpretation of autonomic tests.

  a. Quantitative sudomotor axon-reflex test (QSART)

  b. Thermoregulatory sweat test (TST)

  c. Heart rate response to Valsalva maneuver and deep breathing

  d. Tilt-table test

6. Nerve biopsy: Most common site for biopsy is the sural nerve. The yield is highest when biopsy is used judiciously. It may be helpful for diagnosing inflammatory and vasculitic neuropathies, amyloidosis, hereditary neuropathies (especially when DNA testing is negative), and other rare processes (leprosy, tumor infiltration).

7. Skin biopsies: for evaluating intraepidermal nerve fiber density. They are typically used for diagnosing small fiber neuropathies and have a potential role in following the neuropathic process serially.

Key Tests

• Blood tests: fasting blood glucose, serum protein electrophoresis (SPEP), vitamin B$_{12}$, appropriate serologies

• Autoantibodies (use judiciously)

• Lumbar puncture

• Electromyography and nerve conduction studies

• Nerve biopsy

• Punch skin biopsy

Caveat

• The presence of anti-Hu antibodies in patients with paraneoplastic sensory neuronopathy should prompt evaluation of the underlying malignancy (frequently small cell lung cancer).

Treatment

1. Specific therapies: various immunosuppressive and immunomodulatory agents

  a. Prednisone: used primarily for CIDP

  b. Intravenous immunoglobulin (IVIG): used for Guillain-Barré syndrome and CIDP. It may be helpful for multifocal motor neuropathy (MMN) and neuropathies associated with monoclonal gammopathies. There is a possible role in a select group of patients with diabetic amyotrophy.

  c. Plasmapheresis: used for Guillain-Barré syndrome, CIDP, and neuropathies associated with monoclonal gammopathies.

  d. Cyclophosphamide: may be used as first-line treatment in vasculitic neuropathies and MMN.

  e. Other immunosuppressants: Azathioprine, methotrexate, and cyclosporine may be tried in refractory cases, although they have a low chance of succeeding where other modes failed and carry a high potential of toxicity.

2. Symptomatic therapies: mostly agents that help control the potentially debilitating symptoms of painful neuropathies

  a. Anticonvulsants

    (1) Gabapentin: first-line agent in many practices

    (2) Carbamazepine: effective treatment for lancinating pain

    (3) Other seizure medications such as topiramate and lamotrigine may be effective. The limited data available so far is confusing.

  b. Antidepressants

    (1) Tricyclic antidepressants: Amitriptyline has been extensively studied and has proven effectiveness. Nortriptyline may be as effective and has fewer anticholinergic side effects.

(2) Selective serotonin reuptake inhibitors (SSRIs): Clinical experience with their effectiveness is limited.

c. Antiarrhythmics: Limited experience with mexiletine has produced mixed results.

d. Others

    (1) Tramadol: opioid agonist with low potential for addiction and demonstrated effectiveness in diabetic neuropathy patients

    (2) Lidocaine: given intravenously or as a topical patch; suggested to have beneficial effects in diabetic neuropathy patients

    (3) Clonidine: limited experience; trials ongoing for effectiveness in diabetic neuropathy patients.

    (4) Capsaicin: mixed results in previous trials. Most patients report worsening pain associated with its application and discontinue it.

3. Supportive therapies: Orthotic devices are critical for maintaining the ambulatory status of patients and preventing the development of contractures in the latter stages of weakness. This aspect of management should never be overlooked. An integrated approach in conjunction with physical medicine and rehabilitation is essential for optimal results.

Key Treatment

Immunomodulation

- Prednisone
- IVIG
- Plasma exchange
- Cytotoxic drugs

Symptomatic

- Gabapentin
- Amitriptyline
- Tramadol
- Tegretol

Bibliography

Amato AA, Dumitru D: Approach to peripheral neuropathy. In Dumitru D, Amato AA, Zwarts M (eds): Electrodiagnostic Medicine. Philadelphia, Hanley & Belfus, 2002, pp. 885–897.

Cornblath DR, Glass JD: Approach to painful peripheral neuropathies. In Mendell JR, Kissel JT, Cornblath DR (eds): Diagnosis and Management of Peripheral Nerve Disorders. New York, Oxford University Press, 2001, pp. 129–141.

Kissel JT: The role of antibody testing. In Mendell JR, Kissel JT, Cornblath DR (eds): Diagnosis and Management of Peripheral Nerve Disorders. New York, Oxford University Press, 2001, pp. 67–89.

Mendell JR, Kissel JT, Cornblath DR. Clues to the diagnosis of peripheral neuropathy: history and examination of the patient. In Mendell JR, Kissel JT, Cornblath DR (eds): Diagnosis and Management of Peripheral Nerve Disorders. New York, Oxford University Press, 2001, pp. 10–29.

Guillain-Barré Syndrome

Steven Lovitt
Yadollah Harati

Acute Inflammatory Demyelinating Polyneuropathy

1. Definition: The classic form of Guillain-Barré syndrome (GBS) is also known as acute inflammatory demyelinating polyradiculoneuropathy (AIDP) and produces rapidly progressive weakness. By definition, patients should reach their maximal deficit within 4 weeks.

2. Epidemiology
   a. AIDP is the most common cause of acute generalized weakness. The annual incidence is 1 to 2 cases per 100,000, or approximately 3,500 cases.
   b. AIDP has been reported in patients of all ages and races, with a mean age of occurrence of 40 years.
   c. Over 60% of cases are preceded by an infection, most commonly diarrheal illnesses (such as *Campylobacter jejuni*) and upper respiratory tract infections (such as mycoplasma).
   d. AIDP can be associated with systemic conditions such as human immunodeficiency virus (especially during seroconversion), sarcoidosis, lymphoma, and systemic lupus erythematosus, as well as pregnancy and surgical procedures.

3. Neuropathology: Demyelination may occur in any portion of the nerve from the root distally, although most of the damage occurs proximally. Complement is deposited on the outer surface of the myelinated nerve fiber, followed by inflammatory cell infiltration and myelin degeneration. Macrophages invade the Schwann cells and destroy myelin, after which new Schwann cells remyelinate the nerve.

Symptoms and Clinical Findings

1. The most significant symptom in AIDP is weakness. Although it classically starts in the legs and then ascends, weakness may start in the arms, or less commonly, the face or pharyngeal muscles. The weakness reaches its maximal severity within 4 weeks.

2. Up to about one third of patients require ventilatory support. Close monitoring of the forced vital capacity is important and can assist in planning for intubation.

3. Although AIDP is commonly considered to be a pure motor neuropathy, sensory complaints and paresthesias are quite common, especially at the onset of symptoms. Patients may complain of symptoms such as arthralgias, back pain, cramping, or aching.

4. Hyporeflexia or areflexia is nearly universal, although its absence should not delay treatment because it may not be present at the onset of symptoms.

5. Up to 15% of patients develop ophthalmoparesis; ptosis or mydriasis may occur.

6. Autonomic dysfunction occurs in up to 65% of patients, commonly manifesting as orthostatic hypotension, labile blood pressure, anhidrosis, arrhythmia, urinary retention, abdominal distention, facial flushing, and acral vasoconstriction.

7. Despite the advent of intensive care units and immunomodulatory therapy, the mortality rate remains 3% to 5%, most commonly due to autonomic dysfunction (especially arrhythmia), respiratory failure, and sepsis. Although the prognosis is not as grave as it was before the advent of the above factors, recovery may be incomplete, and permanent disability may occur in up to 10% of patients.

Key Signs

- The most significant symptom is weakness, usually starting in the legs.

- Sensory complaints at onset: Arthralgias, back pain, cramping, aching

- Hyporeflexia or areflexia is nearly universal; its absence should not delay treatment because it may not be present at onset of symptoms.

- Autonomic dysfunction: Orthostatic hypotension, labile blood pressure, anhidrosis, arrhythmia, urinary retention, abdominal distention, facial flushing, acral vasoconstriction

Laboratory and Electrophysiologic Studies

1. An elevated cerebrospinal fluid (CSF) protein level occurs in 90% of patients during the course of their illness. Although lumbar puncture will yield normal results in up to 30% of patients during the first week, this number falls to less than 20%

during the second week, and to 10% after 1 month. The CSF protein level rarely exceeds 1.0 gm/dL, and a markedly elevated level should prompt consideration of another diagnosis.

2. Although the CSF is usually acellular, up to 20 cells/mm^3 are seen in up to 5% of patients. A more significantly elevated cell count is commonly seen in the face of HIV infection.

3. Nerve conduction velocity (NCV) studies classically show features of demyelination of motor nerves such as prolonged distal latencies, markedly slow conduction velocity, conduction block, and temporal dispersion. However, early in the clinical course, no such features may be present because of the proximal nature of the demyelination. It is therefore important to perform F-wave studies, as the presence of these responses is dependent on the integrity of the nerve roots. A significant number of patients will have prolonged or absent F waves when first studied, and then develop features of demyelination when restudied. Electromyography (EMG) early in the clinical course may show decreased recruitment, although fibrillations and positive sharp waves develop after 1 to 2 weeks.

Diagnostic Points

- Electrodiagnostic studies including F waves should be performed to confirm demyelination, although a normal study does not rule out early Guillain-Barré syndrome.

- Lumbar puncture: However, normal results do not exclude Guillain-Barré syndrome.

- The threshold for initiating treatment should be low because of the possibility of normal results early in the disease course and the potential for significant morbidity and mortality in untreated illness.

Differential Diagnosis

1. Other rapidly progressive neuropathies such as lead toxicity, tick paralysis, acute intermittent porphyria, diphtheria, neurotoxic shellfish poisoning, and buckthorn neuropathy may mimic AIDP and are discussed later in this section (see Chapter 3, Other Acute Neruopathies).

2. Myasthenia gravis (MG) may be confused with AIDP, especially when patients present in myasthenic crisis. However, MG is more likely to present with diplopia and ptosis due to preferential involvement of the extraocular and levator muscles. MG does not cause autonomic dysfunction and tends to worsen during the day, improving with rest. The muscle stretch reflexes are preserved in MG, and sensory symptoms are absent. As well, in AIDP, respiratory failure occurs only in the setting of severe limb weakness, whereas MG may cause dyspnea at any stage.

3. When polymyositis progresses rapidly, it may easily mimic AIDP. Polymyositis causes predominantly proximal weakness with involvement of the neck flexors; while the proximal musculature is affected in AIDP, the distal muscles are equally involved. Polymyositis may cause dysphagia, but it does not cause other bulbar symptoms or autonomic dysfunction. As well, the elevated creatine phosphokinase level, myopathic features on EMG, normal NCV, and normal CSF help distinguish this condition from AIDP.

4. Botulism also produces rapidly progressive weakness with respiratory failure. Other similar cases occurring in the community may suggest the diagnosis of botulism. Botulism classically begins with bulbar dysfunction followed by descending weakness, as opposed to the classic ascending pattern of AIDP. The early autonomic dysfunction of botulism, manifested by dilated pupils, constipation, and dry mouth, are a key diagnostic clue. As well, the NCV studies are normal in botulism, while repetitive nerve stimulation reveals a decremental response at low rates and an incremental response at high rates.

Caveats

- Myasthenia gravis may be confused with AIDP.

- When polymyositis progresses rapidly, it may mimic AIDP.

- Botulism also produces rapidly progressive weakness with respiratory failure.

Treatment

1. Plasma exchange has been shown in randomized trials to shorten time to independent ambulation and initial improvement, as well as time spent on a ventilator. Although selection bias in those trials resulted in only patients with moderate and severe weakness being included, patients with mild weakness are often treated as well. The optimal number of exchanges necessary remains unclear; patients who received six exchanges during trials did no better than patients receiving four. However, plasma exchange is not available in many institutions, and it can have significant adverse affects in patients with autonomic involvement due to rapid changes in blood pressure and intravascular volume.

2. Intravenous gammaglobulin, 400 mg/kg, for 5 days has also been shown to be efficacious and probably has equal efficacy to plasma exchange. Although it has many side effects, such as aseptic meningitis, renal failure, fluid overload, and thrombogenicity, its availability makes it a good alternative to plasma exchange, especially in patients with autonomic dysfunction.

3. No additional benefit has been shown when combining these two modalities.

4. Supportive care such as respiratory therapy, monitoring of autonomic function (cardiac monitor, frequent vital signs), and prompt treatment of any infections helps prevent additional morbidity and mortality.

Key Treatment

- Prevention and prompt recognition of respiratory insufficiency and autonomic involvement are of utmost importance, because as these are the most common causes of mortality.

- Intravenous gammaglobulin and plasma exchange can hasten recovery

- Selection of treatment should be guided by the availability of prompt treatment and the ability to minimize side effects.

Variants of Guillain-Barré Syndrome

Several other acute autoimmune disorders involving the peripheral nerves may mimic AIDP. Some of these conditions have weakness as the predominant feature, and some lack weakness as the predominant feature. All are frequently preceded by an infectious illness (often diarrheal or respiratory) and have the peak of symptoms within 4 weeks.

1. Acute motor axonal neuropathy (AMAN): Occurs primarily in Northern China, although occasional cases do occur elsewhere. A diarrheal illness, most commonly due to *C. jejuni*, often precedes the onset of symptoms. The rapid onset of weakness with areflexia is similar to that of AIDP, but NCVs show reduced compound muscle action potentials without absent F waves (unless due to low amplitudes of the compound motor action potential [CMAP]) or demyelinating features. CSF shows an elevated protein with normal cell count. Although controlled trials have not been performed on this variant, patients receive the same treatment as in AIDP, with a similar or slightly less favorable prognosis.

2. Acute motor sensory axonal neuropathy

(AMSAN): Although the classic preceding diarrheal illness and rapid onset of symptoms are similar to both AIDP and AMAN, weakness in this disorder is more fulminant and patients rapidly develop quadriplegia, often requiring respiratory support. Ophthalmoparesis, facial weakness, and autonomic dysfunction are also more common. Although patients tend to improve with treatment, recovery is more protracted, and patients have more significant residual deficits than in AIDP.

3. Miller Fisher syndrome: Commonly occurs after a preceding infection, but the symptoms are quite different from AIDP, AMSAN, or AMAN. The classic triad of symptoms is ophthalmoparesis, areflexia, and cerebellar ataxia. Diplopia is usually the first complaint, followed by gait difficulty. Soon, complete ophthalmoparesis, usually with some ptosis, occurs. Pupillary dilitation is uncommon but can occur. Although mild weakness and sensory loss can be present, they are minor and may not be appreciated due to the other obvious deficits. The diagnosis is made on clinical grounds; however, obtaining an antiGQ1B titer provides support as it is elevated in over 95% of cases. Recovery is spontaneous; in a study of 28 untreated patients, the median period between recovery from ataxia and from ophthalmoparesis was 12 days (range 3 to 41 days) and 15 days (range 3 to 46), respectively. At 6 months, all patients were nearly free of ataxia and ophthalmoparesis and had returned to their normal activities. Despite the good prognosis, intravenous immunoglobulin (IVIG) and plasma exchange are often used to hasten recovery despite the lack of clinical trials.

Caveat

- The classic triad of symptoms in Miller Fisher syndrome is ophthalmoparesis, areflexia, and cerebellar ataxia.

4. Acute panautonomic neuropathy: A rare condition that generally presents with onset over 2 weeks, although subacute onset can also occur. Patients commonly present with episodes of orthostatic hypotension and near-syncope, as well as gastrointestinal disturbance manifested as diarrhea, nausea, vomiting, and constipation. Patients may complain of dry mouth and eyes, urinary retention, and blurry vision. Recovery is gradual and patients may be left with significant residual autonomic dysfunction.

5. Pure sensory neuropathy: A few patients have been reported who presented with an acute large fiber

neuropathy without motor involvement. Sensory ataxia, when present, may be severe. Tremor and autonomic dysfunction may be present.

Bibliography

Asbury AK: New concepts of Guillain-Barré syndrome. J Child Neurol 15:183–191, 2000.

Bernsen R, de Jager AE, Schmitz PI, van der Meche FG: Residual physical outcome and daily living 3 to 6 years after Guillain-Barré syndrome. Neurology 53:409-410, 1999.

French Cooperative Group on Plasma Exchange in Guillain-Barré Syndrome: Plasma exchange in Guillain-Barré syndrome: One-year follow up. Ann Neurol 32:94–97, 1992.

The Guillain-Barré Syndrome Study Group: Plasmapheresis and acute Guillain-Barré syndrome. Neurology 35:1096–1104, 1985.

Hahn AF: Guillain-Barré syndrome. Lancet 22:635–641, 1998.

Mori M, Kuwabara S, Fukutake T, et al.: Clinical features and prognosis of Miller Fisher syndrome. Neurology 56:1104–1106, 2001.

Van der Meche FGA, Schmitz PIM: The Dutch Guillain-Barré Study Group. A randomized trial comparing intravenous immune globulin and plasma exchange in Guillain-Barré syndrome. Muscle Nerve 16:1267–1268, 1992.

Visser LH, Schmitz PI, Meulstee J, et al.: Prognostic factors of Guillain-Barré syndrome after intravenous immunoglobulin or plasma exchange. Neurology 53:598–604, 1999.

Steven Lovitt
Yadollah Harati

3 Other Acute Neuropathies

Heavy Metal Toxicity

Although heavy metal toxicity was once not uncommon because of occupational exposure, as the clinical presentation was increasingly recognized efforts were made to minimize exposure. The prevalence of these disorders is therefore now quite low. Although serum and urine heavy metals levels are frequently performed by some physicians in cases of neuropathy in which other testing has not revealed a diagnosis, the diagnostic yield of such testing is very low. Furthermore, these conditions are expected to cause not only a peripheral neuropathy but also numerous systemic manifestations. Table 3–1 gives the causes, signs and symptoms, and treatments for all the neuropathies listed in this chapter. Understanding the clinical presentation for each of the heavy metal toxicity syndromes may help to minimize unnecessary testing.

1. Lead toxicity
   a. Clinical presentation: exposure may occur through ingestion of lead-based paint chips (generally by children) or as a byproduct of distillation of "moonshine" through lead pipes. Occupational exposure may occur in people who manufacture batteries or work with lead extensively, especially in manufacturing pipes or using lead solder. Systemic manifestations include anemia, renal failure, constipation, and abdominal pain. In children, encephalopathy is usually the feature prompting neurologic consultation. In adults, patients develop primarily distal weakness, with wrist drop a classic feature. Foot drop may be seen as well. The weakness is commonly but not necessarily asymmetrical. Sensory changes are absent or minimal, and prominent sensory abnormalities should raise the possibility of another etiology. As well, the absence of systemic abnormalities, especially hematologic manifestations, should raise questions about the diagnosis.
   b. Pathophysiology: Symptoms of lead poisoning are caused by inhibition of δ-aminolevulinic acid dehydratase, an enzyme used in heme biosynthesis.
   c. Treatment: The source of lead poisoning should be identified and eliminated. Ethylene diamine tetraacetic acid (EDTA), penicillamine, and BAL (dimercaprol) have all been used and shown to be effective. No controlled studies

comparing these different treatment modalities have been performed.

2. Thallium toxicity
   a. Clinical presentation: Patients are exposed to thallium either accidentally, via insecticides or rodenticides, or via attempted homicide. The symptom that generally alerts the treating physician to this possibility is alopecia, which occurs in nearly all cases of thallium poisoning. However, alopecia may not develop for several weeks after exposure. Acutely after ingestion, gastrointestinal symptoms such as vomiting, diarrhea, and abdominal pain dominate the clinical presentation. In cases of severe overdose, death occurs from cardiogenic shock. Otherwise, distal paresthesias and pain develop, more prominently in the legs. Distal weakness and numbness ensue, although the muscle stretch reflexes may be preserved. The progression of weakness is often rapid, and muscle atrophy may occur within weeks.
   b. Pathophysiology: Thallium appears to induce an axonal neuropathy. Although it is suspected that thallium somehow competes with potassium at a cellular level, the exact mechanism of action remains unknown.
   c. Treatment: The source of thallium poisoning should be identified and eliminated. Potassium supplements are often administered, although evidence of their efficacy is scant. Oral administration of Prussian blue immediately after ingestion of thallium may lessen thallium absorption, but is not effective if thallium has already been absorbed from the gastrointestinal tract.

3. Arsenic toxicity
   a. Clinical presentation: Nearly all cases of arsenic toxicity result from intentional overdose, either from homicide or suicide attempts. In mild cases, only distal reduction in sensation may be present. With more significant ingestion, gastrointestinal symptoms such as vomiting, diarrhea, and abdominal pain dominate the clinical presentation in the hours after ingestion. Psychosis may occur, and death may occur within a day if cardiovascular collapse ensues. Days later, distal paresthesias and pain begin and spread proximally. Weakness commonly occurs; although the distal musculature is primarily affected, total quadriparesis and

TABLE 3–1. CAUSES, SIGNS AND SYMPTOMS, AND TREATMENT FOR NEUROPATHIES

	EXPOSURE	SIGNS AND SYMPTOMS	TREATMENT
Heavy metal toxicity Lead	Ingestion of lead-based paint chips Moonshine Persons who work with lead	Children: encephalopathy Adults: primarily distal weakness, with wrist drop being a classic feature	Identify and eliminate source Ethylenediaminetetraacetic acid (EDTA), penicillamine, and dimercaprol (BAL)
Thallium	Accidental exposure via insecticides or rodenticides Attempted homicide	Alopecia, but several weeks after poisoning Acute: gastrointestinal symptoms: vomiting, diarrhea, abdominal pain Distal paresthesias and pain, mostly in legs Then rapid distal weakness and numbness Large overdose: death from cardiogenic shock	Prussian blue immediately after ingestion Potassium supplements
Arsenic	Intentional overdose from homicide or suicide attempts	Vomiting, diarrhea, abdominal pain Days later, distal paresthesias and pain begin and spread proximally; weakness Large doses, total quadriparesis and respiratory compromise Chronic exposure, anemia and sloughing of skin of the distal limbs	Identify and eliminate source
Mercury	Inhalation, usually in an industrial setting	Fatigue, tremor, personality change, insomnia Gastrointestinal disturbance and nephrotoxicity may occur	Penicillamine and dimercaprol
Tick paralysis	Neurotoxin secreted in the saliva of a female gravid tick. The toxin has not yet been identified	Children are more commonly affected May be misdiagnosed as Guillain-Barré syndrome Weakness is generally ascending and causes respiratory failure and bulbar weakness Sensory loss is rare Hyporeflexia is always present Has a fulminant course as opposed to Guillain-Barré, which may be progressive over weeks CSF is normal in tick paralysis as opposed to Guillain-Barré	Removal of the tick, including the mouth parts, is curative
Diphtheritic polyneuropathy	Exotoxin secreted by *Corynebacterium diphtheriae*. Rare in US due to mass vaccination, but adults vaccinated in childhood who travel abroad may contract diphtheria	First a tonsillar, pharyngeal, or nasal infection Severe cervical lymphadenopathy and soft tissue swelling, i.e., "bull neck" appearance Life-threatening airway obstruction possible, especially from bleeding if membrane is disturbed Loss of papillary accommodation is common The neuropathy generally occurs after onset of bulbar symptoms	Diphtheria antitoxin Antibiotics
Critical illness polyneuropathy	Underlying cause remains unknown	Occurs in critically ill patients with multiple organ failure, often with sepsis, in the ICU Severe weakness, usually of distal musculature Hyporeflexia or areflexia	If patient survives the critical illness, prognosis is good, and strength is regained spontaneously
Buckthorn neuropathy	Ingestion of buckthorn fruit; neurotoxins in the stone, seeds, and roots of *Karwinskia humboldtiana*	Onset in 5 to 20 days Flaccid paralysis that begins in legs and spreads to arms in days Dyspnea, dysarthria, dysphagia in 1 to 3 days after arm weakness Muscle stretch reflexes limited	Recovery is spontaneous but may take up to 1 year Daily thiamine may hasten recovery
Pyridoxine intoxication	Extremely high doses of pyridoxine, over 200 g/day Lower doses, up to 10 g/day	Acute sensory neuronopathy Severe vibratory and proprioceptive loss Diffuse paresthesias Indolent distal sensory neuropathy	Some patients recover spontaneously after drug is discontinued, but severe residual deficits are common Good recovery after discontinuation of pyridoxine

Table continued on following page

TABLE 3–1. CAUSES, SIGNS AND SYMPTOMS, AND TREATMENT FOR NEUROPATHIES *Continued*

	EXPOSURE	SIGNS AND SYMPTOMS	TREATMENT
Glue-sniffer neuropathy	Exposure to hexacarbons, especially n-hexane; toluene exposure	Rapidly progressive weakness over weeks in patients who sniff glue for its euphoric effects Onset is chronic in patients with severe occupational exposure to organic solvents Severe weakness Hyperhidrosis and blue discoloration of distal limbs Significant acid-base and electrolyte disorders	Prognosis is good with medical management of superimposed medical issues Symptoms may worsen for up to 2 months after exposure—more common in chronic onset
Ciguatera poisoning	Several different toxins produced by dinoflagellates and passed up the food chain to certain species of fish Most cases in the US occur in Florida and Hawaii	Symptoms begin within hours of ingestion of affected fish: diarrhea, vomiting, abdominal cramping Electrolyte disturbance with dehydration Bradycardia and hypotension Paresthesias and pruritis within a few days Reversal of temperature: cold objects produce a burning sensation; hot ones feel cold Feeling of looseness of teeth Myalgias, fatigue, and weakness	Patients may be misdiagnosed or labeled as having a psychiatric illness Most patients fully recover but some have chronic paresthesias and myalgias Treatment is mostly supportive; mannitol may be helpful but only within 2 days of onset of symptoms
Puffer (Fugu) fish intoxication	Tetrodotoxin produced by endocrine glands and concentrated in liver, skin, and reproductive organs of the puffer fish	Rapidly progressive paresthesias that may occur in minutes. Quadriparesis with bulbar and respiratory impairment soon after Coma, hypotension, and cardiac arrhythmia	With supportive care, the prognosis for full recovery is good after the first 24 hours
Paralytic shellfish poisoning	Ingestion of shellfish contaminated by toxin-producing dinoflagellates	Symptoms within minutes, usually with oral or perioral paresthesias Rapidly progressive weakness, with involvement of the respiratory musculature Bulbar and extraocular musculature frequently affected	With supportive care, the prognosis is excellent and occurs within a week

respiratory compromise may occur in larger doses. In cases of chronic exposure, anemia and sloughing of the skin of the distal limbs may occur.

b. Pathophysiology: Arsenic appears to have two major effects on the molecular level: it interacts with sulfhydryl groups in proteins, and it uncouples oxidative phosphorylation. The former is suspected of causing the neurotoxic effects, resulting in axonal degeneration. The mechanism leading to the neuropathy, however, remains unknown.

c. Treatment: The source of arsenic poisoning should be identified and eliminated. BAL is sometimes used to attempt to reverse toxic effects, but the evidence supporting its efficacy is scanty. Penicillamine may be used to attempt to increase arsenic excretion; however, as symptoms generally continue to worsen after ingestion of even a single dose, the efficacy of this treatment is also uncertain.

4. Mercury toxicity

a. Inorganic form: The major source of exposure to inorganic mercury is through inhalation, usually in an industrial setting. Children may be exposed while playing with broken thermometers. The nervous system is preferentially affected due to the metal's lipophilic nature. Fatigue, tremor, personality change, and insomnia are common. Rarely, a predominantly motor neuropathy occurs which mimics Guillain-Barré syndrome (GBS). Gastrointestinal disturbance and nephrotoxicity may occur. Penicillamine and dimercaprol are used as treatment; gradual toxic exposure is common, although acute and severe toxicity may leave significant residual deficits.

b. Organic form: The clinical presentation of organic mercury toxicity has been reviewed extensively due to the Minimata Bay (Japan) epidemic, which occurred as a result of industrial water contamination and ingestion of the fish living in those waters. Patients developed prominent paresthesias, starting distally and spreading proximally, as well as tremor, dysarthria, constriction of the visual fields, speech and hearing impairment, and ataxia.

Tick Paralysis

1. Clinical presentation: Tick paralysis may easily be misdiagnosed as GBS. In both conditions, the

weakness is generally ascending and frequently causes respiratory failure and bulbar weakness. Sensory loss is rare; hyporeflexia is universally present. Nerve conduction velocity studies may show prolonged distal latencies and slowed motor conduction velocities. Several key factors may help to distinguish between the two conditions. Tick paralysis always has a fulminant course, whereas GBS may be progressive over weeks. The cerebrospinal fluid is normal in tick paralysis, whereas albumino-cytological disassociation is seen in GBS. As the tick is often hidden in scalp, axillary, or pubic hair, the diagnosis is easily overlooked unless the patient is thoroughly examined for ticks. An alert electroencephalography technician may make the correct diagnosis while applying the leads. Once the tick is fully engorged, it falls off; therefore, patients may appear to improve spontaneously or in response to plasma exchange or intravenous gammaglobulin. Spontaneous improvement does not occur in GBS. Removal of the tick, including the mouth parts, is curative.

2. Pathophysiology: Symptoms are caused by a neurotoxin secreted in the saliva of a female gravid tick of the genus *Ixodid, Dermacentor,* or *Argasid.* The toxin has not yet been identified, and heterogeneity of neurotoxins may exist between different species of ticks implicated in this disorder. Studies have implicated both a presynaptic and postsynaptic mechanism. Children are more commonly affected, perhaps because their smaller body mass leads to increased susceptibility to the neurotoxin.

Diphtheritic Polyneuropathy

1. Clinical presentation: Patients are first affected by a tonsillar, pharyngeal, or nasal infection. An intrapharyngeal membrane is often described but is not necessarily present. Severe cervical lymphadenopathy and soft tissue swelling may occur, resulting in a "bull neck" appearance. Life-threatening upper airway obstruction can occur, especially due to bleeding if the membrane is disturbed. Bulbar palsy occurs within 2 months from direct spread of exotoxin and results in palatal weakness, manifested as nasal speech and regurgitation. Dysarthria and dysphagia may also occur but are less frequent. Loss of pupillary accommodation is common. A diffuse polyneuropathy from the hematogenous spread of exotoxin may occur up to 2 months after primary infection. Generally, the neuropathy occurs after the onset of bulbar symptoms. Diffuse weakness and hyporeflexia may occur, along with phrenic nerve palsy and ophthalmoparesis. Impairment of vibratory and proprioceptive sensation is common. Interest-

ingly, the facial nerves are relatively spared. As facial weakness is ubiquitous in Guillain-Barré syndrome when associated with respiratory insufficiency, facial sparing may serve as a critical clue in the differential diagnosis of Guillain-Barré syndrome. Lumbar puncture may be normal or may show albumino-cytological disassociation. Electrodiagnostic studies reveal changes consistent with demyelination. Treatment is with diphtheria antitoxin; a test dose should be administered because anaphylactic reactions may occur. Antibiotic therapy is important to ensure that a carrier state does not ensue.

2. Pathophysiology: Symptoms are caused by an exotoxin secreted by *Corynebacterium diphtheriae.* This toxin results in inactivation of ribosomal guanosine triphosphatase and inhibition of protein synthesis, causing a demyelinating neuropathy. Diphtheritic neuropathy is quite rare in the United States because of mass vaccination. However, it has become more common in Eastern European countries. Because adults who were vaccinated in childhood do not have sufficient immunity to prevent diphtheria once exposed, adults may contract diphtheria while traveling abroad; it is an important diagnostic consideration in adults with Guillain-Barré syndrome with a recent travel history.

Critical Illness Polyneuropathy (CIP)

1. Clinical presentation: Several distinct disorders of the peripheral nervous system occur in the ICU setting. Motor neuron, peripheral nerve, myoneural junction, and muscle may all be affected. However, all cause flaccid weakness, and distinguishing between them clinically can be extremely difficult. Complicating the overlapping features is that such patients are critically ill, often encephalopathic and often unable to cooperate with the history and physical examination. Electrodiagnostic studies in this setting are fraught with technical and electrical artifact, making performance and interpretation difficult. The exact incidence of CIP is unknown, but up to 81% of critically ill patients may develop clinical, electrodiagnostic, or histopathologic evidence of neuropathy. CIP occurs in the setting of multiple organ failure, often with superimposed sepsis. A neurologist is often consulted when the patient cannot be weaned from the ventilator. Patients may have severe weakness, usually affecting the distal musculature more severely than the proximal musculature. Decreased sensation may be present in a stocking distribution, but may be impossible to appreciate in the encephalopathic patient. Hyporeflexia or

areflexia is common. Although mild facial weakness may be present, the remainder of the cranial musculature is relatively spared. Electrodiagnostic studies, when correctly interpreted in light of the numerous technical difficulties, are key in localizing the disorder to the peripheral nerve. Repetitive nerve stimulation should be performed to ensure that a decremental response suggestive of neuromuscular junction pathology is not present. Electromyography reveals abnormal spontaneous activity; motor units, when good effort can be obtained, are often of low amplitude. These findings, also seen in severe myopathy, are insufficient to establish a diagnosis. Nerve conduction studies should also be performed, which reveal decreased or absent sensory nerve responses. The creatine phosphokinase level is normal. Nerve biopsy reveals changes consistent with axonopathy. If the patient survives the critical illness, the prognosis for the polyneuropathy appears to be good, and patients regain their strength spontaneously.

2. Pathophysiology: The underlying cause of CIP remains unknown. As the different syndromes of neuromuscular weakness in the ICU setting often overlap, finding the underlying cause in critically ill patients with multiple organ failure is difficult. A systemic inflammatory response syndrome may play a role via cytokines, hypoxia, and ischemia. Insulin resistance causing hyperglycemia and further nerve ischemia may also play a role.

Buckthorn Neuropathy

1. Clinical presentation: Patients may die from toxic effects on the heart, liver, or kidney if a large amount of the buckthorn fruit is ingested. More characteristically, the onset of weakness occurs 5 to 20 days after ingestion. A flaccid paralysis begins in the legs and spreads to the arms within days. Dyspnea, dysarthria, and dysphagia occur 1 to 3 days after arm weakness. Muscle stretch reflexes are diminished; sensory deficits are unusual. Autonomic involvement does not occur; mentation is not affected. Recovery is spontaneous yet protracted and may take up to a year. Daily administration of thiamine may hasten recovery. The plant is native to Mexico and the United States, and essentially all cases occur in these locations.

2. Pathophysiology: Symptoms occur due to neurotoxins in the stone, seeds, and roots of *Karwinskia humboldtiana*. The mechanism of action is unknown. Electrodiagnostic studies in animals suggest a demyelinating process; however, both axonal degeneration and segmental demyelination have been reported in pathologic studies.

Pyridoxine Intoxication

1. Clinical presentation: Patients taking extremely high doses of pyridoxine (over 200 g/day) develop an acute sensory neuronopathy, with severe vibratory and proprioceptive loss. Diffuse paresthesias are common; weakness does not occur, although gait ataxia may mimic lower limb weakness. Some recovery occurs spontaneously after cessation of the drug, but patients commonly have severe residual deficits. With lower doses (up to 10 g/day), an indolent distal sensory neuropathy may occur, with good recovery after drug withdrawal.

2. Pathophysiology: Pyridoxine toxicity causes degeneration of the dorsal root and gasserian ganglion, with involvement of both proximal and distal segments of the nerve.

Glue-Sniffer Neuropathy

1. Clinical presentation: Patients may present with rapidly progressive weakness after sniffing glue for its euphoric effects. The onset is more chronic in patients with severe and chronic occupational exposure to organic solvents. The weakness may be severe enough to cause complete quadriparesis with respiratory failure, and bulbar weakness may also occur. Hyperhidrosis and blue discoloration of the distal limbs can develop from autonomic involvement. Patient care may be complicated by significant acid-base and electrolyte disorders. Prognosis for recovery is good with appropriate medical management of superimposed medical issues. However, symptoms may continue to worsen for up to 2 months ("coasting") after cessation of exposure, although this is more common in cases with more chronic onset.

2. Pathophysiology: Toxicity is due to exposure to hexacarbons, especially n-hexane. Toluene exposure also appears to play a role. The underlying cause is not yet known, but it may involve inhibition of axonal transport or direct toxicity to neurofilaments.

Ciguatera Poisoning

1. Clinical presentation: Symptoms start within hours of ingestion of affected fish. The initial symptoms are gastrointestinal, most commonly diarrhea, vomiting, and abdominal cramping. Electrolyte disturbance with dehydration can ensue. Bradycardia and hypotension may occur, and

in rare cases shock and respiratory failure can develop. Within the next few days, paresthesias and pruritus begin, most severely in the limbs, although the entire body may be affected. A "reversal" of temperature sensation is common, with cold objects producing a burning sensation and warm objects feeling unpleasantly cold. A feeling of looseness of the teeth is also characteristic. Myalgias, fatigue, and weakness may occur. Although most patients eventually make a full recovery, paresthesias and myalgias may become chronic. Patients may not be correctly diagnosed, and often are labeled as suffering from psychiatric illness. Recurrence of symptoms may occur after ingestion of unaffected fish, even months after the initial ingestion. The diagnosis generally rests upon finding a cluster of patients who all ingested fish, although a mouse bioassay test is available. Treatment is mostly supportive, although infusion of mannitol may be helpful if initiated within 2 days of the onset of symptoms.

2. Pathophysiology: Symptoms are caused by ingestion of several different toxins produced by dinoflagellates and passed up the food chain to certain species of fish. The fish are not clinically affected and the toxin, once present, is not affected by heat or cold. Symptoms occur in tropical regions such as the Caribbean and Indo-Pacific. Most cases in the United States occur in Florida and Hawaii. The toxin acts via voltage-gated sodium channels.

Puffer Fish Intoxication

1. Clinical presentation: Puffer fish (Fugu) is considered a delicacy in Japan. Tetrodotoxin is produced by exocrine glands and concentrated in the liver, skin, and reproductive organs. Because of its potential toxicity, chefs must be licensed to prepare Fugu. When prepared in its customary fashion, Fugu ingestion produces tingling of the lips and mouth. In toxic quantities, ingestion of the toxin results in rapidly progressive paresthesias that may occur in minutes. Quadriparesis with bulbar and respiratory impairment soon ensue. Coma, hypotension, and cardiac arrhythmia may occur. A more rapid onset of symptoms implies a worse prognosis; the mortality rate within the first day may approach 60%. However, with supportive care, the prognosis for full recovery is good after the first 24 hours.

2. Pathophysiology: Tetrodotoxin selectively binds to sodium channels, blocking propagation of action potentials through the nerve.

Paralytic Shellfish Poisoning

1. Clinical presentation: Symptoms occur after ingestion of shellfish contaminated by toxin-producing dinoflagellates. The shellfish are not clinically affected. Symptoms start within minutes of ingestion, usually with oral or perioral paresthesias. Rapidly progressive weakness occurs, with preferential involvement of the respiratory musculature. The bulbar and extraocular musculature is also frequently affected. With supportive care, prognosis is excellent and improvement occurs within a week.

2. Pathophysiology: Symptoms are caused by saxitoxin, which selectively binds to sodium channels.

Bibliography

Campellone J: Clinical approach to neuromuscular weakness in the critically ill patient. J Clin Neuromusc Dis 1:151–158, 2000.

Felz MW, Smith CD, Swift TR: A six-year old girl with tick paralysis. N Engl J Med 342:90–94, 2000.

Kane SL, Dasta JF: Clinical outcomes of critical illness polyneuropathy. Pharmacotherapy 22:373–379, 2002.

Kishi Y, Sasaki H, Yamasaki H, et al.: An epidemic of arsenic neuropathy from a spiked curry. Neurology 56:1417–1418, 2001.

Logina I, Donaghy M: Diphtheritic polyneuropathy: A clinical study and comparison with Guillain-Barré syndrome. J Neurol Neurosurg Psychiatry 67:433–438, 1999.

4 Diabetic Neuropathies

Hazem Machkhas
Yadollah Harati

As the prevalence of diabetes has continued to increase in the United States and worldwide (mostly in younger individuals owing to the higher prevalence of obesity), diabetic peripheral neuropathy has displaced leprosy as the most common worldwide etiology of peripheral neuropathy. Although the term *diabetic neuropathy* continues to denote the most commonly occurring distal symmetrical sensorimotor neuropathy, it is important to realize that the neuropathic complications of diabetes span a wide spectrum of cranial and peripheral nerve disorders (Table 4–1).

Epidemiology

1. Current prevalence of diabetes in the United States is approximately 6.5%.

2. At the time of diagnosis of diabetes, 8% of patients have neuropathy.

3. At 25 years after diagnosis of diabetes, up to 50% have neuropathy.

4. The economic impact of diabetes and its complications is staggering and is destined to keep rising. The estimated cost for 1997 was $98 billion. Roughly 1.5% of that ($1.5 billion) was spent on the care of foot ulcers in the Medicare population (more than 65 years of age).

Pathophysiology

Multiple pathogenic mechanisms have been proposed in the origin of diabetic neuropathy. The major theories revolve around metabolic and vascular etiologies. It is likely that multiple mechanisms play a role.

1. Metabolic pathogenesis

    a. Persistent hyperglycemia creates a disturbance in the microenvironment of the nerve by increasing the polyol pathway activity, leading to accumulation of sorbitol and fructose in the nerve. Sorbitol accumulation leads to focal edema.

    b. Polyol accumulation is suspected to lead to *myo*-inositol depletion, which is suspected to result in axonal degeneration and demyelination.

    c. Hyperglycemia is thought to lead to alterations in essential fatty acid metabolism, including the precursors of prostaglandins, more importantly prostaglandin E_1 (PGE_1), which has among its functions a potent vasodilator effect and antiplatelet activity.

    d. Hyperglycemia also leads to accumulation of glycosylation end products, which may cause microvascular disease by depositing in endothelial cells and may increase oxidative stress by releasing reactive oxygen radicals.

2. Vascular pathogenesis

    a. Histopathologic studies in diabetics have demonstrated the presence of vasculopathy in endoneurial and epineurial blood vessels, including thickening or occlusion of the blood vessel wall.

    b. Hemodynamic alterations have been observed at the microvascular level in diabetics, including decreased neural blood flow, increased vascular resistance, reduced oxygen tension, and disturbed vascular permeability.

3. Immune pathogenesis

    a. Perivascular inflammatory cells and microscopic vasculitis have been seen in endoneurial and epineurial blood vessels of a number of patients, predominantly those with proximal asymmetrical neuropathy.

    b. Circulating anti-neuronal autoantibodies have been detected in the sera of some patients, and antibody and complement deposits have been shown in the sural nerve.

4. Nerve growth factor (NGF) deficiency

    a. Animal studies have demonstrated that retrograde transport of endogenous NGF is impaired in diabetic rats.

    b. Serum levels of NGF are reduced in diabetic patients.

5. Oxidative stress

    a. Sustained hyperglycemia, in experimental diabetes, reduces the levels of free radical scavengers in plasma and other organs, including the liver and kidneys. The same effect is suspected in the peripheral nerves.

    b. The reduction in free radical scavengers is compounded by the observation that several of the metabolic consequences of hyperglycemia promote the production of highly reactive oxidants.

582

TABLE 4–1. CLASSIFICATION OF DIABETIC PERIPHERAL NEUROPATHIES

Distal symmetrical sensorimotor polyneuropathy
Proximal diabetic neuropathy(ies)
Diabetic cranial mononeuropathies
Diabetic thoracoabdominal neuropathy
Diabetic autonomic neuropathy
Diabetic limb mononeuropathies (upper or lower limbs)
Diabetic mononeuropathy multiplex

DISTAL SYMMETRICAL SENSORIMOTOR POLYNEUROPATHY

Distal symmetrical sensorimotor polyneuropathy is by far the most common of the diabetic neuropathies. It is predominantly sensory and develops insidiously several years after diabetes is diagnosed. In some patients, however, it is the presenting symptom that leads to the diagnosis of diabetes.

1. Clinical features
   a. Numbness and painless tingling (so-called negative symptoms) are more common than positive symptoms, which include pain, cramping, spasms, prickling, tightness, and a crawling sensation.
   b. Pain is the most prominent feature in about 10% of patients.
   c. Pain and other sensory symptoms usually begin at the toes and typically extend to the feet and mid-calves before involving the fingers.
   d. Most patients exhibit evidence of small and large fiber involvement. In some patients, selective loss of pain (small) fibers predominates, leading to complications such as foot ulcers and arthropathy. When untreated, foot ulcers often lead to osteomyelitis.
   e. Mild distal muscle weakness and atrophy can be seen, usually in patients with long-standing diabetic neuropathy.
   f. Deep tendon reflexes are typically depressed, and absent at the ankles.
   g. Most patients have a degree of clinical or subclinical autonomic dysfunction. Manifestations include orthostatic hypotension, erectile dysfunction, micturition and bladder emptying difficulties, gastroparesis, and diminished sweating of the distal limbs leading to dry skin.

Key Signs: Distal Symmetrical Sensorimotor Polyneuropathy

- Numbness and tingling (feet more than hands)
- Dysesthetic pain (worse at night)
- Distal weakness and atrophy (rare, in severe cases)

- Distal sensory loss (multimodality)
- Depressed deep tendon reflexes

2. Laboratory features
   a. Abnormalities on electrophysiologic studies do not correlate with the severity of the symptoms.
   b. Sensory nerve action potential reduction is one of the earliest, most sensitive changes.
   c. Motor conductions may be normal but in most cases display some mild slowing, especially in the lower limbs, even in individuals without motor symptoms.
   d. Nerve biopsy is not indicated for the routine evaluation of diabetic neuropathy. Typical changes include loss of myelinated and unmyelinated nerve fibers, axonal degeneration and regeneration, and secondary remyelination.

Key Tests: Distal Symmetrical Sensorimotor Polyneuropathy

- Reduction of sensory nerve action potentials
- Motor conduction studies mildly slowed in the lower limbs
- Nerve biopsy is not indicated

1. Treatment
   a. As yet, there are no pharmacologic agents that can slow, prevent, or reverse the nerve fiber damage of diabetic neuropathy.
   b. The most important and so far only measure to slow or prevent the course of diabetic neuropathy (and other diabetic complications) is rigorous blood glucose control.
   c. Experimental trials with aldose reductase inhibitors, recombinant human NGF, and α-lipoic acid (a potent free radical scavenger) are ongoing. *Myo*-inositol supplementation has not been beneficial.
   d. The cornerstone of treatment remains pain control. This is a difficult and frustrating experience and, in many patients, disappointing. Various classes of drugs can be used, and patients in general do not show a uniform response to these drugs. Some agents have shown beneficial results.
      (1) Tricyclic antidepressants: Double-blind trials of amitriptyline have demonstrated significant benefits in reducing burning, aching, sharp, throbbing, and stinging pain. The drug is contraindicated in patients with heart block, recent myocardial infarction, urinary obstruction, and narrow angle

glaucoma. The most bothersome side effects are anticholinergic; if they develop, nortriptyline, which gives similar results, may be substituted.

(2) Anticonvulsants

(a) Phenytoin is usually not effective.

(b) Carbamazepine is useful for treating painful symptoms, but potential toxicity precludes its use unless many other agents have failed.

(c) Gabapentin is now being used for a variety of painful neuropathic syndromes, including diabetic polyneuropathy. It has been shown in double-blind trials to be effective.

(d) Clonazepam has been reported to be quite effective in the treatment of sharp, brief, lancinating pain.

(3) Tramadol, an opioid receptor agonist and inhibitor of norepinephrine and serotonin reuptake, has proven effectiveness in the treatment of painful diabetic neuropathy. It is usually well tolerated and has a low potential for abuse. It should not, however, be used in patients with a history of substance abuse.

(4) Others include baclofen, clonidine, lidocaine, and mexiletine.

Key Treatment: Distal Symmetrical Sensorimotor Polyneuropathy

- No drug can slow, prevent, or reverse nerve fiber damage.
- Rigorous blood glucose control is the only measure to prevent or slow the course of the disease.
- Pain control is the cornerstone of treatment.

PROXIMAL DIABETIC NEUROPATHY

Proximal diabetic neuropathy is variously known as diabetic polyradiculoplexopathy, diabetic amyotrophy, or diabetic femoral neuropathy. It primarily affects the lower limbs; is typically unilateral (but bilateral involvement is not uncommon), and despite the name involves some degree of distal muscle weakness.

1. Clinical features

a. Typically occurs later in life, after age 50

b. Usually preceded or accompanied by substantial unprovoked weight loss (> 30 lb)

c. Onset of illness heralded by pain in the low back area, buttock, or hip

d. Several days to a few weeks later, weakness appears and progresses rapidly. Proximal muscles are prominently involved, but it is not unusual to find a mild degree of distal weakness.

e. Involvement of the upper limbs is rare and, if seen concomitantly with lower limb weakness, suggests other diagnoses (e.g., chronic inflammatory demyelinating polyradiculoneuropathy).

Key Signs: Proximal Diabetic Neuropathy

- Rapid onset of proximal weakness (usually unilateral)
- Pain at onset
- Weight loss

2. Laboratory features

a. Electrophysiologic testing reveals denervation potentials in multiple proximal and paraspinous muscles, predominantly those innervated by the L2-4 nerve roots. There may also be findings of a superimposed polyneuropathy.

b. Pathologically, several observations have suggested a vascular (ischemic)-mediated process, with a possible inflammatory component. Infarcts in the lumbar plexus have been documented at autopsy, and small mononuclear cell infiltrates may be seen in proximal and distal sensory nerves. Sural nerve biopsy is not routinely recommended for this condition.

c. ESR is often significantly elevated.

Key Tests: Proximal Diabetic Neuropathy

- Electrophysiologic testing reveals denervation potentials in multiple proximal and paraspinous muscles
- ESR is often significantly elevated
- Sural nerve biopsy is not routinely recommended

3. Treatment

a. The natural history of the illness suggests a self-limiting condition with total or partial recovery within 9 to 18 months of the onset of symptoms.

b. The observation of inflammation in nerve biopsies of patients with the illness has prompted the suggestion that immunomodulatory therapy may be beneficial. Intravenous immunoglobulin (IVIG) has been proposed as the agent of choice but must be used with extreme caution in this patient population with probable subclinical nephropathy, especially when spontaneous recovery is the norm.

Key Treatment: Proximal Diabetic Neuropathy

• No specific treatment is indicated.

DIABETIC CRANIAL THIRD NERVE PALSY

Although the third cranial nerve is most commonly affected in diabetic cranial neuropathies, diabetic fourth and sixth cranial nerve palsies may occur. The association between diabetes and other cranial palsies, including seventh nerve palsy, is less well established. The following discussion of diabetic third nerve palsy applies also to fourth and sixth nerve palsies.

1. Clinical features
    a. The first symptom in approximately 50% of cases is usually an abrupt onset of sharp, intense retro-orbital, periorbital, or hemicranial pain. Ophthalmoplegia follows within 1 to 2 days. The other 50% are painless.
    b. Sudden diplopia and occasionally severe ptosis are the manifestations of diabetic third nerve palsy. The hallmark of the condition is sparing of the pupil, which helps differentiate this condition from the more serious compressive oculomotor syndromes.
    c. Prognosis is good, with most patients making full recovery within 3 to 6 months.

Key Signs: Diabetic Cranial Third Nerve Palsy

• Orbital pain at onset (in 50% of cases)

• Diplopia and ptosis

• Pupillary sparing

2. Laboratory features
    a. There are no specific laboratory features.
    b. Cerebrospinal fluid (CSF) analysis, if done to exclude other conditions, may show a nonspecifically elevated protein level, common to most diabetic patients.
    c. Brain imaging may be performed to exclude masses, aneurysms, or subarachnoid hemorrhage. It is expected to be normal.

3. Treatment
    a. As the prognosis is quite good, no specific treatment is indicated.
    b. Eye patches are helpful for suppressing diplopia.
    c. Simple analgesics can be given for pain.

Key Treatment: Diabetic Cranial Third Nerve Palsy

• No specific treatment is indicated.

THORACOABDOMINAL NEUROPATHY

Thoracoabdominal neuropathy, variously referred to as diabetic truncal mononeuropathy, diabetic thoracic polyradiculoneuropathy, or diabetic radiculopathy, is a disconcerting entity that is often misdiagnosed as postherpetic neuralgia, even in the absence of any preceding vesicular rash.

1. Clinical features
    a. It is typically seen in patients older than 45 years of age.
    b. It usually occurs in known diabetics but occasionally is the presenting manifestation of undiagnosed diabetes.
    c. Predominant symptom is abrupt or gradual onset of burning dysesthetic pain in the lateral chest or abdominal wall. Pain may intensify at night.
    d. Distribution of the affected areas varies, with some patients displaying well defined dermatomal involvement and others having pain in small ill-defined patches throughout the trunk.
    e. Weakness of the abdominal wall muscles may be seen.
    f. In most cases, significant weight loss precedes or accompanies the onset of pain.
    g. Prognosis is quite good, with gradual resolution of symptoms over 6 to 9 months.

Key Signs: Thoracoabdominal Neuropathy

• Abdominal wall muscle weakness (rare)

• Abrupt or gradual onset of burning dysesthetic pain in the lateral chest or abdominal wall

• Significant weight loss

2. Laboratory features
    a. Electromyography reveals, in some patients, denervation potentials in the abdominal wall, intercostal, and paraspinous muscles.
    b. Nerve pathology is not well defined.

3. Treatment
   a. Pain may be treated with the common agents for neuropathic pain.
   b. If this fails, a lidocaine 5% patch applied locally may substantially reduce the pain.

Key Treatment: Thoracoabdominal Neuropathy

• No specific treatment is indicated

DIABETIC NEUROPATHIC CACHEXIA

Diabetic neuropathic cachexia is an uncommon entity, but awareness of its clinical features is important. Some have argued that it should not be recognized as a separate entity but included in the continuum of features of distal symmetrical sensorimotor polyneuropathy.

1. Clinical features
   a. It occurs almost exclusively in older men with poorly controlled diabetes.
   b. It is heralded by precipitous weight loss, soon followed by debilitating dysesthetic burning pain in the distal limbs and occasionally over the trunk. Typically, there is no associated weakness. Cachexia is so impressive that an underlying malignancy is often suspected.
   c. Once optimal blood glucose control is restored, the prognosis for recovery, including incremental weight gain, is good.

2. Laboratory features
   a. Diagnosis is clinical, and no specific test confirms the initial suspicion.
   b. Electrodiagnostic studies reveal the expected changes seen in the distal symmetrical sensorimotor polyneuropathy.
   c. Nerve pathology is nonspecific, and a nerve biopsy is not recommended as part of the work-up.

3. Treatment
   a. Instituting strict diabetic control is of paramount importance and is the first step toward recovery.
   b. Common drugs used to treat neuropathic pain may help. In some cases the use of narcotics is indicated.

 ## Bibliography

Feldman EL, Russell JW, Sullivan KA, Golovoy D: New insights into the pathogenesis of diabetic neuropathy. Curr Opin Neurol 12:553–563, 1999.

Greene DA, Stevens MJ, Feldman EL: Diabetic neuropathy: scope of the syndrome. Am J Med 107:2S–8S, 1999.

Harati Y: Treatment of diabetic peripheral neuropathies. In Johnson RT, Griffin JW, McArthur JC (eds): Current Therapy in Neurologic Disease. St. Louis, Mosby, 2002; pp. 380–384.

Kelkar P, Masood M, Parry GJ: Distinctive pathologic findings in proximal diabetic neuropathy (diabetic amyotrophy). Neurology 55:83–88, 2000.

Younger DS, Rosoklija G, Hays AP: Diabetic peripheral neuropathy. Semin Neurol 18:95–104, 1998.

5 Chronic Inflammatory Demyelinating Polyradiculoneuropathy

Hazem Machkhas
Yadollah Harati

The earliest descriptions of chronic inflammatory demyelinating polyradiculoneuropathy (CIDP) appeared during the middle of the twentieth century, with reports of a steroid-responsive neuropathy. Over the next two to three decades, the term CIDP was coined, and diagnostic criteria were established. The incidence of CIDP is not known, but it is one of the most commonly acquired neuropathies encountered in tertiary care settings.

Symptoms

1. Although the cardinal disability caused by CIDP is secondary to weakness, sensory symptoms are usually the first to appear and can be quite prominent. Patients complain of subacute onset of numbness and tingling, initially in the feet and subsequently in the hands.

2. About 10% to 20% of patients have painful dysesthetic pain.

3. In a small number of patients, sensory loss is severe enough to produce sensory ataxia.

4. Be aware that a "pure sensory CIDP" may occur, although most of these patients develop some weakness with prolonged follow-up.

5. Various degrees of weakness are reported. The weakness is typically symmetrical. It is more prominent in the lower extremities, although a certain level of upper extremity weakness is almost always present. The complaints of weakness are attributable to proximal and distal muscle involvement.

6. Prominent cranial nerve involvement is uncommon, although a mild degree of clinical or subclinical facial diplegia is seen in up to 15% of patients.

7. Autonomic manifestations are unusual.

8. Some patients present with prominent symptoms of lumbar spinal stenosis or even myelopathy secondary to significant swelling of the nerve roots, leading to compromise of the structures in the central spinal canal.

9. At some point during their illness, up to 5% of patients with CIDP have concomitant central nervous system (CNS) demyelination. Symptoms may include diplopia, vertigo, cerebellar ataxia, and spasticity.

10. The evolution of symptoms is usually slowly progressive. The diagnosis of CIDP requires progression of symptoms for more than 2 months.

Key Symptoms

- Numbness and tingling (feet more than hands)
- Lower limb weakness (almost always)
- Upper limb weakness (not always)

Caveats

- The diagnosis of CIDP requires progression of symptoms for more than 2 months.
- Proximal weakness with no distal involvement suggests a different diagnosis.

Clinical Findings

1. Multimodality symmetrical distal sensory loss occurs in the lower limbs and possibly in the upper limbs.

2. Distal and proximal weakness appears, definitely in the lower limbs and sometimes in the upper limbs. In most cases the same extent of involvement is seen proximally and distally. In some cases proximal weakness is more severe. Proximal weakness with no distal involvement suggests a different diagnosis.

3. Neck flexor weakness is common.

4. Varying degrees of facial diplegia may be seen.

5. Deep tendon reflexes are usually depressed in the affected limbs. Typically, ankle reflexes are absent.

6. Atrophy and fasciculations are not seen in typical cases but may be seen in chronic cases.

7. The presence of upper motor neuron signs (hyperreflexia, spasticity, extensor plantar response) sug-

gests either concurrent CNS demyelination or cord compression due to root hypertrophy.

8. Vertigo and ataxia may be seen with CNS involvement.

 Key Signs

- Proximal and distal weakness (lower limbs more than upper limbs)
- Distal sensory loss (feet more than hands)
- Neck flexor weakness
- Depressed deep tendon reflexes in weak limbs

CIDP as a Manifestation of Concurrent Illness

1. CIDP can be seen in the setting of several conditions whose clinical and electrophysiologic presentations may be similar to that of idiopathic CIDP.
   a. Monoclonal gammopathy: In most cases work-up of the monoclonal gammopathy does not reveal a malignancy, making it a monoclonal gammopathy of unknown significance (MGUS). With prolonged follow-up, 25% of these cases undergo malignant transformation (mostly multiple myeloma).
   b. Inflammatory bowel disease
   c. Connective tissue disease
   d. Human immunodeficiency virus (HIV) infection
   e. Chronic hepatitis
   f. Bone marrow and organ transplantation: frequently in the setting of graft-versus-host disease
2. The response to immunotherapy in these cases is similar to that of idiopathic CIDP. The long-term prognosis depends on the underlying illness.

Pathogenesis

1. An immune-mediated etiology is strongly suspected in CIDP but has never been satisfactorily proven.
2. Certain findings support an immune etiology.
   a. Favorable response to plasma exchange and other immunomodulatory therapies
   b. Presence of mononuclear inflammatory cells in the spinal roots, ganglia, and peripheral nerves in autopsy specimens
   c. Demonstration of immunoglobulins M (IgM)

and G (IgG) deposits at the Schwann cell plasma membrane in the sural nerve
   d. Demonstration of complement membrane attack complex (MAC) deposits in the myelin sheath of some nerve fibers in the sural nerve

Laboratory Tests

1. Routine laboratory tests typically are normal. It is important, especially if suggested by the history and examination, to obtain certain specific tests to exclude concurrent illnesses. Such tests include those for HIV antibody, thyroid function, and antinuclear antibody (ANA); a hepatitis screen; erythrocyte sedimentation rate (ESR); and serum protein electrophoresis.
2. Electrophysiologic testing is paramount for the diagnosis of CIDP and hinges on the demonstration of acquired demyelination.
3. The electrophysiologic criteria set by the American Academy of Neurology are specific but may be too stringent and, accordingly, may miss a significant number of cases. Three of the following criteria must be present.
   a. Slowing of nerve conduction velocities in two or more motor nerves
   b. Partial conduction block or abnormal temporal dispersion in one or more motor nerves
   c. Prolonged distal motor latencies in two or more nerves
   d. Prolonged or absent F-wave latencies in two or more motor nerves
4. Cerebrospinal fluid (CSF) examination: The presence of elevated CSF protein is extremely helpful for supporting the diagnosis of CIDP, but it is not specific. Keep in mind that up to 5% of patients with CIDP may have normal CSF protein. The presence of a leukocyte count of more than 10 cells/mm^3 casts doubt on the diagnosis of idiopathic CIDP. Cell counts up to 50 cells/mm^3 are allowed in HIV positive patients. Other CSF abnormalities sometimes seen but nonspecific are oligoclonal bands and, more rarely, an elevated IgG synthesis rate.
5. Nerve biopsy: The value of a peripheral nerve biopsy (classically the sural nerve) to the diagnosis of CIDP continues to be hotly debated. Some argue that it has no added diagnostic value, and others highlight its importance in difficult cases (e.g., when dealing with concurrent illnesses) and for excluding other etiologies (e.g., vasculitis). The classic histopathologic feature is demyelination and remyelination as seen on teased nerve preparations, semi-thin sections, or both; it is encountered in up to 70% of cases. Axonal degeneration

or a mixed picture of demyelination and axonal degeneration is seen in the remaining 30%. Rarely, the nerve biopsy is normal. Significant inflammation is seen in only 15% to 20% of specimens.

Key Tests

- Electrophysiologic testing: electromyography and nerve conduction studies

- Cerebrospinal fluid analysis

- Sural nerve biopsy

Treatment

1. Prednisone, which gave the disease its early name (steroid-responsive neuropathy), had been the mainstay of therapy for years. The success of oral prednisone therapy was so impressive that only two small controlled trials are found in the literature. Treatment starts at a high dose (80–100 mg/day), with a slow taper over many months. The prohibitive side effects of such therapy have led to the search for other modalities. Pulse intravenous (IV) methylprednisolone therapy has been used as an alternative with good results, but the evidence remains anecdotal.

2. During the past decade, several trials have demonstrated that IV immunoglobulin (IVIG) and plasma exchange are equally effective therapies for CIDP. Because of its ease of administration, IVIG has become the first line treatment in most practices. There have been no studies comparing IVIG and plasma exchange to oral prednisone.

3. In cases resistant to the above modalities, an array of immunosuppressant agents can be used. The data for their effectiveness are scarce. Agents that may be used include azathioprine, cyclophosphamide, and cyclosporine.

Key Treatment

- Prednisone

- Intravenous immunoglobulin

- Plasma exchange

Prognosis

1. The initial treatment of CIDP is quite rewarding. Up to 90% of patients show initial improvement with immunotherapy.

2. Relapse rate with various therapies remains high (50%–60%).

3. In some series, up to 30% of patients achieve a treatment-free remission.

4. Poor prognosis is associated with delay of treatment beyond 1 year from the onset of symptoms, as well as severe weakness at the start of therapy. A less impressive response to therapy is also usually seen in CIDP patients with a concomitant illness.

Caveat

- Poor prognosis is associated with treatment delay, severe weakness at the start of treatment, and concomitant illness.

Bibliography

Dyck PJ, O'Brien PC, Oviatt KF, et al.: Prednisone improves chronic inflammatory demyelinating polyradiculoneuropathy more than no treatment. Ann Neurol 11:136–141, 1982.

Hahn AF, Bolton CF, Pillay N, et al.: Plasma exchange therapy in chronic inflammatory demyelinating polyneuropathy: a double-blind, sham-controlled, cross-over study. Brain 119:1055–1066, 1996.

Hahn AF, Bolton CF, Zochodne D, Feasby TE: Intravenous immunoglobulin treatment in chronic inflammatory demyelinating polyneuropathy: a double-blind, placebo-controlled, cross-over study. Brain 119:1067–1077, 1996.

Kissel JT, Mendell JR: Chronic inflammatory demyelinating polyradiculoneuropathy. In Mendell JR, Kissel JT, Cornblath DR (eds): Diagnosis and Management of Peripheral Nerve Disorders. New York, Oxford University Press, 2001, pp. 173–191.

Pollard JD: Chronic inflammatory demyelinating polyradiculoneuropathy. Curr Opin Neurol 15:279–283, 2002.

Definition

Porphyrias are inherited disorders in which enzymes of the heme biosynthesis pathway have partial activity. Eight enzymes are involved in the synthesis of heme; with the exception of the first, an enzymatic deficit at each step of heme synthesis causes a different form of porphyria. The porphyrias are classified based on the principal site of the deficient enzyme: erythroid, presenting with dermatologic findings; and hepatic, presenting primarily with neurologic sequelae. The common forms presenting with neurologic findings are transmitted via autosomal dominant inheritance with variable penetrance.

Epidemiology

1. Because of the variable penetrance, true figures are not known.
2. The incidence of the genetic defect of the most common form, acute intermittent porphyria (AIP), is estimated to be 5 to 10 per 100,000 in the United States.
3. Variegate porphyria (VP) affects about 3 per 1000 whites in South Africa due to a founder effect.
4. Hereditary coproporphyria (HCP) is much less common, estimated as affecting two per million in Denmark.
5. Only six cases of δ-aminolevulinic acid (ALA) dehydratase porphyria, which is transmitted via autosomal recessive inheritance, have been reported.

Pathogenesis

Symptoms are postulated to be due either to accumulation of heme biosynthetic pathway intermediates or decreased heme production. Both theories have significant flaws, however, so the underlying mechanism is still uncertain.

Symptoms

1. Symptoms are paroxysmal and may occur in the setting of infection, starvation or low-calorie diets, alcohol, or offending medications. Drugs commonly used by neurologists that are generally contraindicated include barbiturates, carbamazepine, valproic acid, phenytoin, ergots, primidone, estrogens, metoclopramide, clonidine, ketamine, and nortriptyline.

2. Autonomic neuropathy. Abdominal pain is nearly always present and can even mimic an acute surgical abdomen, leading to unnecessary surgery, which can further exacerbate attacks. Vomiting, constipation, tachycardia, hypertension, fever, and diarrhea can occur.

3. Weakness. It is usually symmetrical but can be asymmetrical or even focal. It can also progress rapidly and can easily be confused with Guillain-Barré syndrome. Ankle reflexes may be spared even when other muscle stretch reflexes are absent, a key diagnostic clue. Rarely, respiratory failure occurs. Involvement of motor cranial nerves, most commonly VII and X, can occur.

4. Psychiatric symptoms. Depression, anxiety, paranoia, and agitation may occur during acute attacks. Depression and anxiety may become chronic, and distinguishing whether these symptoms are reactive or affective can be difficult. Psychiatric populations screened for porphyria show a significantly higher incidence of the disorder (0.21% of patients in one study) than the general population.

5. Sensory symptoms. Although porphyric neuropathy is commonly thought of as a purely motor and autonomic neuropathy, sensory involvement can occur, manifesting as numbness or paresthesias. However, the sensory involvement is part of the generalized proxysmal neuropathy and is not seen in isolation.

6. Seizures. These may occur during acute attacks, especially in patients with hyponatremia due to the syndrome of inappropriate antidiuretic hormone (SIADH), vomiting, or fluid therapy. When present, they introduce a therapeutic dilemma because many of the drugs used to treat seizures exacerbate porphyria.

 Key Symptoms

- Rapidly progressive weakness

- Abdominal pain

- Tachycardia

- Constipation
- Hypertension
- Seizures

Precipitating Factors

- Porphyrinogenic drugs
- Infection
- Starvation
- Alcohol use
- Surgery

Laboratory Tests

1. Measurement of 24-hour urinary porphyrins is often used as a screening test but does not distinguish between the various forms of porphyria and can be normal between attacks.

2. A definitive diagnosis requires demonstration of reduced enzyme activity. Abnormal values are approximately 50% of normal. Enzyme activity assays of family members may be helpful in ambiguous cases.

 Key Tests

- Screening test for 24-hour urinary porphyrins is used but does not distinguish between the various forms of porphyria and can be normal between attacks.

- Demonstration of reduced enzyme activity (about half the normal values) provides a definitive diagnosis; for ambiguous cases, testing family members may be helpful.

Differential Diagnosis

1. Guillain-Barré syndrome (GBS). Although both diseases can present with rapidly progressive weakness and autonomic dysfunction, severe abdominal pain is not expected with GBS. Diffuse hyporeflexia is the rule, whereas porphyria frequently spares the ankle reflexes. Lumbar puncture is normal during porphyria attacks, whereas albuminocytologic disassociation occurs in GBS. Nerve conduction velocity studies most commonly reveal axonopathy in porphyria, whereas with GBS demyelination is expected.

2. Lead poisoning. Because lead also affects the heme biosynthetic pathway, lead poisoning can cause weakness and abdominal pain. However, lead poisoning is more likely to cause mononeuropathies (especially wrist drop), causes hematologic abnormalities, and is less likely to produce multiple attacks.

3. Multiple sclerosis. Because of the pattern of discrete attacks of weakness, porphyria can be confused with demyelinating disease. The lesions seen on magnetic resonance imaging (MRI) scans and cerebrospinal fluid (CSF) abnormalities in MS help distinguish these conditions.

4. Hereditary tyrosinemia. Patients with this rare condition also present with episodes of pain and weakness. However, such cases are generally seen in the pediatric population, whereas porphyric attacks usually occur after puberty, probably owing to higher levels of endogenous steroids. Tyrosinemia also is associated with Fanconi syndrome and hepatic dysfunction.

Treatment

1. The most important treatment is educating the patient about avoiding factors that may precipitate an attack, such as low-calorie diets or starvation, excessive alcohol, and porphyrinogenic drugs.

2. Some attacks can be aborted by increased carbohydrate intake, orally or intravenously.

3. Intravenous hematin inhibits the first enzyme of the heme biosynthetic pathway and therefore reduces the flow of substrates through the cascade, relieving the enzymatic block. Hematin is the treatment of choice for acute exacerbations and should be given in dosages of up to 4 mg/kg over at least 30 minutes every 12 hours.

4. During acute attacks the pain should be treated with narcotic analgesics. Because attacks are infrequent, the risk of addiction is low. If significant constipation is present, Tylenol may be a better choice, although it is less effective.

5. Treatment of seizures is difficult in that most of the medicines used to treat seizures are porphyrinogenic. Benzodiazepines and intravenous $MgSO_4$ may be useful acutely. For chronic treatment, this scenario is one of the few in which bromides and paraldehyde are occasionally used. Gabapentin and vigabatrin may be safe, but clinical experience is limited because of the rarity of this disorder. Consultation with an epileptologist may be useful.

Key Treatment

- Patient education regarding the avoidance of precipitating factors (e.g., low-calorie diets, alcohol, and porphyrinogenics)

- Increased carbohydrate intake, orally or intravenously

- For acute exacerbations, intravenous hematin and pain relief

- Treatment of seizures remains difficult; therefore consultation with an epileptologist may be useful.

Follow-up

Prognosis is good if factors that may cause or exacerbate an attack are avoided. Recovery tends to occur over weeks; with severe attacks, however, recovery may be protracted or incomplete.

Bibliography

Elder GH, Hift RJ: Treatment of acute porphyria. Hosp Med 62:422–425, 2001.

Elder GH, Hift RJ, Meissner PN: The acute porphyrias. Lancet 349:1613–1617, 1997.

Gross U, Hoffmann GF, Doss MO: Erythropoietic and hepatic porphyrias. J Inherit Dis 23:641–661, 2000.

Nordmann Y, Puy H, Deybach JC: The porphyrias. J Hepatol 30(Suppl):12–16, 1999.

Tefferi A, Colgan JP, Solberg LA: Acute porphyrias: diagnosis and management. Mayo Clin Proc 69:991–995, 1994.

7 Genetically Determined Peripheral Neuropathies

Hazem Machkhas
Yadollah Harati

Peripheral neuropathies that have a hereditary basis range from conditions that selectively affect the peripheral nervous system (e.g., hereditary motor and sensory neuropathies) to conditions where peripheral nerve involvement is only one manifestation of a broader inherited syndrome (e.g., adrenomyeloneuropathy, Fabry disease, Friedreich's ataxia). Porphyrias are discussed in detail in another chapter and so are omitted here.

HEREDITARY MOTOR AND SENSORY NEUROPATHIES

The hereditary motor and sensory neuropathies (HMSNs) are also referred to by the original designation of hereditary neuropathies as Charcot-Marie-Tooth (CMT) neuropathies. The classification of these neuropathies is constantly being refined as new genes or loci are identified. This discussion is limited to the most common and well defined forms of each disorder.

1. Charcot-Marie-Tooth type 1 (HMSN I)—demyelinating
   a. Clinical features
      (1) Subdivided into CMT1A, CMT1B, CMT1C, and CMT1D, depending on genetic features, they all have essentially the same clinical characteristics.
      (2) Symptoms usually appear during the first or second decade of life. Electrophysiologic abnormalities may be detected as early as 2 years of age.
      (3) Characteristically, progressive weakness and atrophy in the distal lower limb muscle is the presenting symptom. Up to two-thirds of patients also have upper limb involvement.
      (4) Occasionally, foot deformities are the first clue to the diagnosis and consist of pes cavus or hammer toes.
      (5) Sensory symptoms are usually rare and typically minimal, although most patients have an abnormal sensory examination, with distal sensory loss.
      (6) Essential tremor is seen in one-third of patients.
      (7) Palpable enlarged nerves are seen in 50% of cases.
      (8) Deep tendon reflexes are typically absent at the ankles. As the disease progresses, 50% of patients have diffuse areflexia.

Key Signs: HMSN I—Demyelinating

- Onset before late teens
- Distal weakness and atrophy (lower then upper limbs)
- Neurogenic skeletal deformities
- Palpable nerves
- Depressed deep tendon reflexes

   b. Genetic features
      (1) Inheritance is autosomal dominant; 20% of cases are sporadic.
      (2) CMT1A is associated with mutations in the peripheral myelin protein-22 (*PMP-22*) gene on chromosome 17p11.2-12. Most cases have a duplication in that dosage-sensitive gene. In a small number of cases there is a point mutation in that gene. The normal function of *PMP-22* is not known nor is the mechanism by which duplication or point mutations in that gene lead to demyelination.
      (3) CMT1B is associated with mutations in the human myelin protein zero (*MPZ* or base pair) gene on chromosome 1q22-23. Mutations may be point mutations or small base pair deletions or duplications. Base pair, an integral myelin protein, is the major structural component of the peripheral nerve myelin. Mutations in base pair produce other phenotypes (including Dejerine-Sottas neuropathy—see below). A heterozygote state is typically associated with CMT1B.
      (4) CMT1C has not yet been linked to any locus.
      (5) CMT1D is associated with mutations in the early growth response 2 (*EGR2*) gene on chromosome 10q21.1-22.1. *EGR2* is presumed to play a role in regulating myelin genes in Schwann cells. CMT1D is a rare condition.

593

c. Laboratory features
  (1) Electrophysiologic testing reveals uniform slowing of nerve conduction velocities (NCVs), usually more prominent in the lower limbs. Typically, the slowing is more than 25% of normal in all nerves and does not correlate with the severity of the disease.
  (2) Nerve biopsy specimens reveal a significant reduction of myelinated nerve fibers. Semithin sections show many thinly myelinated fibers surrounded by so-called onion bulbs, which represent Schwann cell proliferation, induced by repeated demyelination and remyelination.
  (3) Genetic testing, if positive, confirms the diagnosis.

Key Tests: HMSN I—Demyelinating

• Electrophysiologic testing reveals significantly slowed nerve conduction velocity.

• Onion-bulb formations are seen in nerve biopsy specimens.

d. Treatment
  (1) Appropriate orthoses, as dictated by difficulties
  (2) Mechanized wheelchair or scooter, as needed

2. Charcot-Marie-Tooth type 2 (HMSN II)—axonal
  a. Clinical features
    (1) There are many subtypes of this axonal or neuronal form of HMSN, which are differentiated by genetic localization. This discussion is limited to the most common conditions: CMT2A, CMT2B, CMT2C.
    (2) Symptoms usually appear during the first or second decade of life, although some cases have been reported with onset during infancy for CMT2C and during the seventh decade for CMT2A and CMT2B.
    (3) Distal atrophy and weakness are prominent, mostly in the lower limbs. Upper limb involvement, if present, is much milder than with CMT1, except for CMT2C, where hand weakness and atrophy may be prominent.
    (4) CMT2C is characterized by vocal cord and laryngeal weakness or paralysis, heralded by such symptoms as hoarseness, stridor, and dyspnea.
    (5) Sensory symptoms are typically absent or minimal. Distal sensory loss may be present, more commonly in CMT2A and CMT2B.
    (6) Pes cavus and hammer toes may be present. Tremor is uncommon. Typically, there are no palpable nerves.

Key Signs: HMSN II—Axonal

• Onset before late teens

• Distal atrophy and weakness (lower limbs more than upper limbs)

• Neurogenic skeletal deformities

  b. Genetic features
    (1) Inheritance is autosomal dominant.
    (2) CMT2A has been mapped to chromosome 1p36. The gene is unknown.
    (3) CMT2B has been mapped to chromosome 3q13-22. The gene is unknown.
    (4) CMT2C has not been localized.
  c. Laboratory features
    (1) Electrophysiologic features reflect axonal degeneration and neuronal atrophy. Sensory nerve action potentials (SNAPs) are reduced or absent. Motor conduction velocities are normal or mildly slowed. Compound muscle action potentials (CMAPs) are absent or significantly reduced, more so in the lower limbs than the upper limbs.
    (2) Nerve biopsies reveal a significant reduction of myelinated nerve fibers. Teased nerve fibers demonstrate wallerian degeneration. Semithin sections demonstrate degenerated axons and small clusters of regenerating axons.

Key Tests: HSMN II—Axonal

• Electrophysiologic testing reveals reduced or absent SNAPs and CMAPs.

• Nerve biopsy reveals a significant reduction of myelinated nerve fibers.

  d. Treatment
    (1) Appropriate orthoses, as dictated by difficulties
    (2) Respiratory care and support as needed for CMT2C

Key Treatment: HSMN II—Axonal

• Respiratory care and support for CMT2C

3. Dejerine-Sottas disease (HMSN III)—demyelinating
   a. Clinical features
      (1) Dejerine-Sottas disease (DSD) is a rare disorder that is considered by some to be a severe phenotypic variant of CMT1, with which it shares considerable clinical, genetic, electrophysiologic, and pathologic features.
      (2) Onset is typically during infancy or early childhood. Severe cases manifest at birth with hypotonia, respiratory distress, and swallowing difficulties. Death usually ensues within a few weeks after birth.
      (3) In less severe cases, the first symptoms consist of delayed motor milestones. Ultimately, progressive weakness affects all limb muscles and even trunk muscles. Weakness may be so severe as to render patients wheelchair-dependent.
      (4) Sensory loss is prominent and may lead to ataxia.
      (5) Prominent sensorineural hearing loss may be present.
      (6) Deep tendon reflexes are usually absent.
      (7) Palpable enlarged nerves are common.
      (8) Skeletal deformities, including pes cavus, hammer toes, and scoliosis, may be prominent.

Key Signs: HSMN III—Demyelinating

- Onset during infancy or early childhood
- Neonatal onset: hypotonia, breathing and swallowing difficulties, early death
- Prominent weakness and sensory loss
- Absent deep tendon reflexes
- Prominent neurogenic skeletal deformities

   b. Genetic features
      (1) Inheritance is autosomal dominant.
      (2) DSD has been associated with mutations of *PMP-22* on chromosome 17p11.2-12 (duplication or point mutations), *P0* on chromosome 1q22-23 (point mutations or small base pair deletions/duplications), and *EGR2* on chromosome 10q21.1-22.1.
      (3) It is believed that the locations of the mutation in the various responsible genes determines the phenotypic expression of the disease (CMT1 compared with DSD).
   c. Laboratory features
      (1) Electrophysiologic testing reveals a uni-

form, severe slowing of nerve conduction velocities, typically less than 20 m/s in the arms and less than 10 m/s in the legs. Distal latencies may be greatly prolonged. CMAPs are usually reduced. SNAPs are typically absent.
      (2) Nerve biopsies reveal a marked reduction of myelinated nerve fibers. In the infantile form of the disease, semithin sections reveal axons with little, if any, myelin. Onion-bulb formation is not seen. The less severe forms of the disease demonstrate thinly myelinated fibers with classic onion-bulb formation. Teased nerves may demonstrate segmental demyelination.

Key Tests: HSMN III—Demyelinating

- Electrophysiologic testing reveals nerve conduction velocities (NCVs) less than 20 m/s in the arms and less than 10 m/s in the legs.
- Nerve biopsy reveals significant reduction of myelinated nerve fibers.

   d. Treatment
      (1) Appropriate orthoses, as dictated by difficulties
      (2) Mechanized wheelchair or scooter, as needed

4. Charcot-Marie-Tooth type 4—demyelinating
   a. Clinical features
      (1) CMT4 neuropathies are a genetically heterogeneous group of autosomal recessive, typically severe demyelinating neuropathies. Up to seven subtypes have been identified so far. This discussion is limited to the better-defined subtypes: CMT4A and CMT4B.
      (2) CMT4A has been described in Tunisia. Onset is before 2 years of age, with delayed motor milestones. Severe weakness and atrophy are noted distally in the limbs but ultimately progress to involve proximal muscles. Loss of ambulation is not uncommon during the late teens. Sensory loss is mild. Diffuse areflexia is seen. Skeletal deformities include pes cavus, hammer toes, and scoliosis.
      (3) Patients with CMT4B achieve their early milestones. Onset is at around 3 years of age and is heralded by a waddling gait or toe walking, reflecting various degrees of proximal and distal weakness; it is initially more prominent in the lower limbs but ultimately involves the upper limbs in

teenagers. Some patients require wheelchairs but most retain the ability to ambulate. Sensory loss is mild. There is diffuse areflexia. Skeletal deformities include pes cavus, hammer toes, and scoliosis. Death is typically before age 50 years.

b. Genetic features

  (1) Inheritance is autosomal recessive.

  (2) CMT4A has been mapped to chromosome 8q13-21.1. The gene is unknown.

  (3) MT4B has been mapped to chromosome 11q23 in some families. The gene product is myotubularin-related protein-2 (MTMR2). Other families have been mapped to chromosome 11p15. That gene is unknown.

c. Laboratory features

  (1) Electrophysiologic testing reveals uniformly slowed motor nerve conduction velocities, in the range of 20 to 30 m/s, occasionally slower. SNAPs are typically absent.

  (2) Nerve biopsies reveal a marked reduction of myelinated nerve fiber density. Semithin sections demonstrate many thinly myelinated axons with surrounding onion-bulb formation. A characteristic feature of CMT4B is the presence of fibers with excessively folded myelin loops.

d. Treatment

  (1) Appropriate orthoses, as indicated by difficulties

  (2) Mechanized wheelchair or scooter, as needed

5. X-linked Charcot-Marie-Tooth disease (CMTX)

a. Clinical features

  (1) Clinical features are similar to those of CMT1.

  (2) Symptoms appear in men during the first two decades of life and initially consist of weakness and atrophy in the distal muscles of the upper and lower limbs.

  (3) Sensory symptoms are minimal or absent, but significant distal sensory loss is seen on examination.

  (4) Deep tendon reflexes are diffusely diminished or absent.

  (5) Skeletal deformities, including pes cavus, hammer toes, and claw-hand, are common.

  (6) Typically, there are no palpable nerves.

b. Genetic features

  (1) Inheritance is X-linked dominant.

  (2) CMTX is associated with mutations in the connexin 32 gene on chromosome Xq13.

Connexin 32 localizes in peripheral nerves to the paranodal region and to the Schmidt-Lantermann incisures. It is believed to form gap junctions that connect the folds of Schwann cell cytoplasm, thus shortening the pathway for nutrients and ions to diffuse into the innermost layers of the myelin sheath and into the periaxonal cytoplasm.

c. Laboratory features

  (1) Electrophysiologic testing reveals findings suggestive of mixed demyelination and axonal degeneration. This includes uniform moderate slowing of motor nerve conduction velocities, with diminished amplitudes of CMAPs. SNAPs are reduced or absent.

  (2) Nerve biopsies reveal a significant reduction of myelinated nerve fibers. Semithin sections demonstrate axonal degeneration and regenerating clusters, as well as thinly myelinated fibers with onion-bulb formations.

d. Treatment

  (1) Appropriate orthoses, as indicated by weakness

  (2) Appliances for hand weakness

6. Hereditary neuropathy with liability to pressure palsies (HNPP)

a. Clinical features

  (1) Age at onset is variable, typically during the second or third decade, but it may be earlier or later.

  (2) Typical presentation is with painless numbness or weakness in the distribution of a single peripheral nerve or multiple nerves. The symptoms are often precipitated by minor trauma or compression (crossing the legs, leaning on elbows). Some patients present with painless brachial plexopathy. The focal symptoms usually resolve within weeks or months.

  (3) Occasionally, patients present with symptoms and signs of a progressive diffuse sensorimotor polyneuropathy.

  (4) Deep tendon reflexes may be normal or diffusely decreased.

 Key Sign: HNPP

• Intermittent painless mononeuropathy(ies)

b. Genetic features

  (1) Inheritance is autosomal dominant.

  (2) HNPP is associated with mutation in the

PMP-22 gene. Most cases (85%–90%) have a 1.5 Mb deletion at that locus. Approximately 5% to 10% of cases have point mutations.

c. Laboratory features

(1) Electrophysiologic testing may reveal focal slowing of conduction velocities in the affected nerves. Conduction block may be seen at sites of compression. The changes may also be diffuse and reflect a predominantly demyelinating sensorimotor neuropathy.

(2) Nerve biopsies reveal reduction of myelinated nerve fibers. Semithin sections demonstrate thinly myelinated fibers and sporadic axons with redundant myelination. The latter correspond to the sausage-like swellings, or tomacula, seen on teased nerve preparations, which gave the disease its original name, tomaculous neuropathy.

(3) Genetic testing may confirm the diagnosis. Screening for point mutations is now available in some specialized laboratories.

Key Tests: HNPP

- Focal slowing of NCV (with or without conduction block) in affected nerves

- Tomacula on nerve biopsy

d. Treatment

(1) Instruct patients to avoid pressure on elbows and knees.

(2) Apply appropriate orthoses, as indicated by difficulties.

HEREDITARY SENSORY AND AUTONOMIC NEUROPATHIES

The hereditary sensory and autonomic neuropathies (HSANs) comprise a group of rare disorders that have been divided into five subtypes. They are grouped according to their mode of inheritance and their clinical, electrophysiologic, and pathologic similarities. As causative genes continue to be identified, a more rational classification may emerge.

1. Hereditary sensory and autonomic neuropathy type I (HSAN I)

a. Clinical features

(1) It is the most common HSAN.

(2) Onset of symptoms is during the second to fourth decades, with burning and lancinating pain in the feet or painless foot ulcers.

(3) Sensory examination reveals loss of pain

and temperature predominantly (but not exclusively) initially in the feet and subsequently in the hands. Motor strength remains normal.

(4) Autonomic neuropathy is not present, although distally sweating is impaired.

(5) Deep tendon reflexes are absent at the ankles and depressed elsewhere.

(6) Skeletal deformities, including pes cavus and hammer toes, can be seen.

b. Genetic features

(1) Inheritance is autosomal dominant.

(2) HSAN I has been mapped to chromosome 9q22. The candidate gene is suspected to be the one encoding for serine palmitoyltransferase long chain base-1 (SPTLC-1), an enzyme that catalyzes the rate-limiting step in the biosynthesis of sphingolipids.

c. Laboratory features

(1) Electrophysiologic features have not been well defined. SNAPs are mildly reduced but may be absent. Motor conduction is usually normal, but mild slowing of conduction velocities may be seen. Distal muscles may show denervation potentials.

(2) Pathologically, a severe reduction in the number of myelinated and unmyelinated fibers is seen in peripheral nerve biopsies. Postmortem studies have shown that the degenerative changes extend proximally to the lumbar dorsal root ganglia and even the posterior columns.

d. Treatment

(1) Pain may be treated with appropriate medications for neuropathic pain.

(2) Foot ulcers must be treated aggressively to avoid osteomyelitis. Patients should be instructed to avoid situations that may increase the risk of foot ulcers (tight shoes, prolonged standing or walking).

Key Treatment: HSAN I

- Management of pain

- Aggressive treatment of foot ulcers to avoid osteomyelitis

2. Hereditary sensory and autonomic neuropathy type II (HSAN II)

a. Clinical features

(1) Typically presents at birth or during early childhood, at which point the child starts to display unusual insensitivity to pain.

(2) Painless foot ulcers and unrecognized fractures in the feet are common.

(3) Gross foot deformities become prominent, including Charcot arthropathy, clubbing, and loss of nails.

(4) Distal sensory loss may be so prominent as to interfere with fine motor activity despite typically preserved motor strength. All sensory modalities are affected, and sensory ataxia is common.

(5) Sweating is impaired distally in the limbs. Other autonomic manifestations include bladder dysfunction and impotence.

(6) Deep tendon reflexes are typically absent.

b. Genetic features

(1) Inheritance is autosomal recessive.

(2) Genetic linkage has not been established.

c. Laboratory features

(1) Electrophysiologic testing reveals a total absence of SNAPs. Motor nerve conductions are typically normal. Abnormalities, if present, are mild, and appear restricted to the peroneal nerve. Denervation potentials may be present distally in the lower limbs.

(2) Pathologically, peripheral nerve biopsies reveal a near-total absence of myelinated nerve fibers. Unmyelinated fibers are mildly reduced.

d. Treatment

(1) Foot ulcers must be treated promptly and aggressively.

(2) Appropriate foot care instructions (see above) must be provided.

(3) Distal lower limb orthopedic deformities may be surgically corrected.

Key Treatment: HSAN II

- Aggressive treatment of foot ulcers

- Surgical correction for lower limb orthopedic deformities

3. Hereditary sensory and autonomic neuropathy type III (HSAN III)

a. Clinical features

(1) This rare disorder, also known as Riley-Day syndrome or familial dysautonomia, is mostly seen in Ashkenazi Jews, where it has an incidence of 1 in 3700 live births.

(2) Typical onset is during infancy, with feeding difficulties leading to failure to thrive, episodic vomiting, unexplained bouts of fever, and the characteristic associated feature of alacrimia (tearless crying). Most children have a tendency to sweat excessively.

(3) Seizures and delayed developmental milestones may occur.

(4) On examination, muscle strength is usually normal, deep tendon reflexes are absent, and there is a diffuse reduction in painful sensation.

(5) Life span is shortened. One in four patients dies before the age of 10, usually from recurrent pneumonia.

Key Signs: HSAN III

- Failure to thrive

- Unexplained fevers

- Alacrimia

- Excessive sweating

- Recurrent pneumonia

b. Genetic features

(1) Inheritance is autosomal recessive.

(2) HSAN III had been mapped to chromosome 9q31, and the gene was recently discovered to be coding for IκB kinase complex-associated protein (IKAP), a protein suspected to have a role in the activation of genes crucial to the development of sensory and autonomic neurons.

c. Laboratory features

(1) Electrophysiologic testing reveals mild reductions of SNAPs. Motor conduction velocities are normal or slightly reduced.

(2) Pathologically, peripheral nerve biopsies reveal a marked reduction in the number of unmyelinated fibers and only a mild reduction in large myelinated fibers.

d. Treatment

(1) Provide adequate nutrient supplementation during early life (nasogastric or gastric tube feeding).

(2) Prevent and treat pneumonias.

(3) Provide ocular lubrication with artificial tears.

Key Treatment: HSAN III

- Nasogastric or gastric tube feeding

- Prevention and treatment of pneumonias

- Ocular lubrication with artificial tears

4. Hereditary sensory and autonomic neuropathy type IV (HSAN IV)

a. Clinical features

(1) This is a rare disorder, also known as congenital sensory neuropathy with anhydrosis or congenital insensitivity to pain with anhydrosis.

(2) It is typically heralded during infancy or early childhood by unexplained bouts of fever. It is related to an inability to sweat in the presence of elevated ambient temperatures, a feature that helps differentiate HSAN IV from HSAN III. The other main features are insensitivity to pain, which leads to oral and acral mutilation, developmental delay, and mental retardation.

(3) On examination, there is prominent diffuse loss of pain and temperature sensation. Muscle strength is normal, and deep tendon reflexes are preserved.

b. Genetic features

(1) Inheritance is autosomal recessive.

(2) HSAN IV is associated with mutations in the gene coding for the receptor tyrosine kinase of nerve growth factor (NTRK1) on chromosome 1q21-22. Defects in nerve growth factor signal transduction lead to failure of sympathetic ganglion neurons and nociceptive sensory neurons derived from the neural crest to survive.

c. Laboratory features

(1) Electrophysiologic findings may be unrevealing, with normal or mildly reduced SNAPs and normal motor conduction.

(2) Quantitative sensory testing reveals markedly abnormal heat and cold perception.

(3) Pathologically, peripheral nerve biopsies reveal near-total loss of unmyelinated and small myelinated fibers. Postmortem studies have shown the absence of small neurons in the dorsal root ganglia and severe reduction of small myelinated fibers in the dorsal roots.

d. Treatment

(1) Avoid exposure to elevated ambient temperatures.

(2) Oral and acral ulcers must be vigorously treated.

Key Treatment: HSAN IV

• Aggressive treatment of oral and acral ulcers

5. Hereditary sensory and autonomic neuropathy type V (HSAN V)

a. Clinical features

(1) This is the least common of the hereditary sensory and autonomic neuropathies. It is also known as congenital indifference to pain.

(2) Onset is during infancy or childhood. Patients fail to react appropriately to pain by withdrawal or crying. This failure to appreciate pain leads to the development of acral ulcers, painless fractures, and neurogenic arthropathy.

(3) On examination, there is absence of pain and temperature sensation in the limbs, with other sensory modalities being preserved. Motor strength and deep tendon reflexes are normal.

b. Genetic features

(1) Both autosomal dominant and recessive modes of inheritance have been described.

(2) Genetic linkage has not been established.

c. Laboratory features

(1) Electrophysiologic testing is unrevealing, with essentially normal sensory and motor conduction.

(2) Quantitative sensory testing is also normal.

(3) Pathologic features are not well established. Sural nerve biopsies have been reported to be normal or show a mild loss of small myelinated and unmyelinated fibers.

FAMILIAL AMYLOID POLYNEUROPATHIES

The classification of familial amyloid polyneuropathies (FAPs) has evolved. The original classification followed ethnically established clinical features, but biochemical and genetic advances have allowed a classification based on the mutated protein.

1. Transthyretin amyloidosis

a. Clinical features

(1) Age at onset is variable, ranging from the third to sixth decade of life.

(2) Although the clinical presentation varies, most patients classically have distal numbness in the lower limbs associated with stabbing, lancinating pain.

(3) Typically, significant autonomic dysfunction is present, manifesting as impotence, postural hypotension, constipation, or diarrhea.

(4) Amyloid deposits in other organs result in

vitreous opacities, nephropathy, and cardiomyopathy.

(5) Distal weakness and atrophy, mostly in the lower limbs, ultimately develops.

(6) Some patients have carpal tunnel syndrome as the only manifestation of peripheral nerve involvement.

Key Signs: Transthyretin Amyloidosis

- Distal painful numbness (feet more than hands)
- Autonomic dysfunction prominent
- Amyloid nephropathy and cardiomyopathy

b. Genetic features

(1) Inheritance is autosomal dominant.

(2) The gene is the one coding for transthyretin (*TTR*) on chromosome 18q11.2-12.1. The abnormal protein forms a β-pleated (amyloidogenic) sheet structure that deposits in affected tissues.

c. Laboratory features

(1) Electrophysiologic testing suggests axonal neuropathy, with reduced or absent SNAPs and reduced CMAPs. Median mononeuropathies at the wrists may be seen, even in asymptomatic individuals.

(2) Pathologically, the hallmark feature is the presence of amyloid deposits in nerve, skin, or rectal mucosa. The sural nerve demonstrates a decrease in myelinated nerve fibers.

(3) Routine blood studies may reflect other organ involvement, with elevated serum levels of urea nitrogen, creatinine, and liver enzymes.

d. Treatment

(1) Neuropathic pain may be treated with appropriate medications.

(2) Other organ involvement requires appropriate management.

(3) Liver transplantation halts the progression of the disease and improves the neuropathy clinically and electrophysiologically. Without treatment, transthyretin amyloidosis progresses to death within 10 to 15 years.

Key Treatment: Transthyretin Amyloidosis

- Pain management
- Appropriate management of other organ involvement
- Liver transplantation, which halts disease progression and alleviates the neuropathy

2. Apolipoprotein A-1 amyloidosis

a. Clinical features

(1) This is a rare disorder, described in two kindreds in Iowa and Italy.

(2) Onset of symptoms is usually during the thirties, with numbness and dysesthesias in the distal lower limbs that ultimately progress proximally.

(3) Muscle atrophy and weakness may be seen.

(4) Autonomic involvement is mild and mostly consists of gastroparesis. Impotence may be prominent and is due to direct deposition of amyloid in the testicles.

(5) Endocrine disturbances include hypothyroidism and adrenal insufficiency.

b. Genetic features

(1) Inheritance is autosomal dominant.

(2) It is caused by mutation in the apolipoprotein A1 gene on chromosome 11q23.

c. Laboratory features

(1) Electrophysiologic features are not well established.

(2) Pathologic features, in addition to the presence of amyloid, are not well defined.

d. Treatment

(1) Renal failure must be appropriately managed, ultimately with dialysis.

(2) Hormone replacement for endocrinopathies.

(3) Appropriate treatment of neuropathic pain.

3. Gelsolin amyloidosis

a. Clinical features

(1) Seen mostly in Finland, it occurs sporadically in the rest of the world.

(2) It is characterized by multiple cranial neuropathies, loss of skin turgor, and amyloid deposits in the corneal branches of the trigeminal nerve resulting in corneal lattice dystrophy.

(3) Peripheral neuropathy, when present, is mild.

b. Genetic features

   (1) Inheritance is autosomal dominant.

   (2) It is caused by mutations in the gelsolin gene on chromosome 9q32-34.

c. Laboratory features

   (1) Electrophysiologic testing reveals changes suggestive of an axonal neuropathy.

   (2) Pathologically, amyloid deposits are seen in skin and peripheral nerve biopsies.

OTHER INHERITED NEUROPATHIES

Many other inherited conditions have peripheral neuropathy as a dominant feature. They include several disorders of lipid metabolism, peroxisomal disorders, other inborn errors of metabolism, and hereditary ataxias. This discussion is limited to the most clinically relevant conditions.

1. Adrenomyeloneuropathy

   a. Clinical features

      (1) Adrenomyeloneuropathy (AMN) is an allelic disorder of the more commonly encountered adrenoleukodystrophy (ALD).

      (2) Age of onset is typically during the third decade. AMN is slowly progressive and normally does not affect life-span. It mostly affects men but may be seen in women.

      (3) It manifests as a slowly progressive spastic paraplegia, associated with a peripheral neuropathy.

      (4) Cerebral involvement may be seen and causes progressive cognitive decline. The presence of cerebral involvement is associated with rapid progression of weakness to disability.

      (5) Adrenal insufficiency is seen in 70% of men.

      (6) On examination, there is a combination of upper and lower motor neuron findings. Spasticity and weakness are confined to the lower extremities in most cases, with hyperactive deep tendon reflexes, extensor plantar responses, and distal sensory loss that may involve all modalities.

Key Signs: Adrenomyeloneuropathy

• Spastic paraplegia

• Peripheral neuropathy

• Adrenal insufficiency

b. Genetic features

   (1) Inheritance is X-linked recessive.

   (2) AMN is associated with mutations in the gene coding for a peroxisomal transmembrane adenosine triphosphate (ATP)-binding cassette (ABC) transporter, on chromosome Xq28.

c. Laboratory features

   (1) Electrophysiologic testing reveals nonspecific sensory and motor slowing of conduction velocities, with reduced amplitudes, suggesting an axonal neuropathy.

   (2) Imaging abnormalities are seen in most cases. Magnetic resonance imaging (MRI) of the brain reveals white matter demyelinating changes in up to 50% of cases. MRI of the thoracic spinal cord almost invariably reveals some degree of atrophy.

   (3) Cerebrospinal fluid (CSF) analysis is usually normal. The diagnostic value of this test is restricted to excluding other conditions, such as multiple sclerosis. Classic cases of adrenoleukodystrophy may have various CSF abnormalities, including increased immunoglobulin G synthesis.

   (4) Sural nerve biopsy is not routinely part of the diagnostic work-up. When done, it reveals a uniform reduction in myelinated fibers of all sizes. Other changes mostly indicate a process of axonal degeneration, with secondary demyelination and remyelination.

   (5) The most important diagnostic test is documentation of elevated serum levels of saturated unbranched very long chain fatty acids (VLCFAs). This finding does not differentiate ALD from AMN.

Key Test: Adrenomyeloneuropathy

• The most important diagnostic test is for elevated serum levels of very long chain fatty acids.

d. Treatment

   (1) Corticosteroid supplementation for adrenal insufficiency, if present.

   (2) Dietary restriction of VLCFAs.

   (3) Supplementation with "Lorenzo's oil" has been suggested but has never been proven to work.

   (4) Bone marrow transplantation may help in select cases.

2. Refsum's disease

a. Clinical features

(1) This is a rare peroxisomal disorder related to abnormal metabolism of phytanic acid.

(2) Characterized by a tetrad of features, including peripheral neuropathy, retinitis pigmentosa, ataxia, and elevated CSF protein.

(3) Onset is typically during the first two decades of life but may be later.

(4) Other features include sensorineural hearing loss, anosmia, and cardiac conduction abnormalities.

(5) The neuropathy may be relapsing-remitting or slowly progressive. Features include distal weakness and wasting in the lower limbs that later progresses to the upper limbs. There is distal sensory loss, and some patients have shooting pain in the feet. Deep tendon reflexes are reduced or absent.

Key Signs: Refsum's Disease

• Peripheral neuropathy

• Retinitis pigmentosa

• Ataxia

• Elevated CSF protein levels

b. Genetic features

(1) Inheritance is autosomal recessive.

(2) Associated with mutations in the phytanoyl-CoA α-hydroxylase gene on chromosome 10p13.

c. Laboratory features

(1) Electrophysiologic testing is invariably abnormal but with no consistent features. Changes of significant demyelination or predominant axonal degeneration may be seen.

(2) Sural nerve biopsy reveals a reduction in myelinated nerve fibers. Semithin sections reveal many thinly myelinated fibers with frequent onion-bulb formation.

(3) CSF analysis reveals markedly elevated protein levels, with a normal cell count.

(4) Phytanic acid levels are elevated, but that feature is not specific, as it may be seen with other peroxisomal disorders.

Key Tests: Refsum's Disease

• Electrophysiologic testing is abnormal.

• Sural nerve biopsy reveals a reduction in myelinated nerve fibers.

• CSF analysis reveals markedly elevated protein levels, with a normal cell count.

• Phytanic acid levels are elevated.

d. Treatment

(1) Early, accurate diagnosis is important, as this disorder is potentially treatable.

(2) Strict dietary restriction to exclude all precursors of phytanic acid, including dairy products and ruminant meat, usually results in lowering the phytanic acid levels and may result in arresting the progression of symptoms, including peripheral neuropathy.

Key Treatment: Refsum's Disease

• Early, accurate diagnosis is important because this disorder is potentially treatable.

3. Fabry's disease

a. Clinical features

(1) This is a slowly progressive, multiorgan disease with onset typically during the second decade.

(2) Neuropathy is often the presenting complaint, with episodic burning and stabbing pain in the hands and feet that over time may become constant. Despite the severity of symptoms, the examination is strikingly normal. Rare patients have minimal distal weakness and atrophy, as well as depressed ankle reflexes.

(3) Other organs involved include the brain (strokes, dementia, personality changes), skin (characteristic inguinal and genital angiokeratomas), kidneys (renal failure), eyes (cataracts), and heart (arrhythmias, myocardial infarction, heart failure).

(4) Female carriers may develop a mild painful sensory neuropathy.

b. Genetic features

(1) Inheritance is X-linked recessive.

(2) It is associated with mutations in the α-galactosidase gene on chromosome Xq21-22.

c. Laboratory features
 (1) Electrophysiologic testing is typically normal.
 (2) Sural nerve biopsy reveals a selective loss of small myelinated and unmyelinated nerve fibers.
 (3) Definitive diagnosis is made with the serum α-galactosidase assay.

d. Treatment
 (1) Painful neuropathy is treated with appropriate medications.
 (2) Cardiac and brain ischemic risks must be prophylactically treated with antiplatelet agents.
 (3) Renal failure may require hemodialysis. Successful renal transplantation corrects many of the abnormalities and increases survival.
 (4) Future direction of therapy is through enzyme replacement.

4. Tangier disease
 a. Clinical features
  (1) Rare disorder of lipoprotein metabolism, with variable age of onset and three distinct patterns of neurologic involvement.
  (2) First pattern (type I) is that of an asymmetrical peripheral neuropathy, often manifesting as multiple mononeuropathies.
  (3) Second pattern (type II) is that of a slowly progressive sensorimotor polyneuropathy, predominantly of the lower limbs.
  (4) Third pattern (type III) is that of a syringomyelia-like syndrome with dissociation between loss of pain/temperature and position/vibration in the upper limbs.
  (5) The dominant nonneurologic feature is the presence of enlarged, orange tonsils. Splenomegaly may be present.

b. Genetic features
 (1) Inheritance is autosomal recessive.
 (2) It is associated with mutations in the ATP-binding cassette transporter 1 (*ABC1*) gene on chromosome 9q22-31.

c. Laboratory features
 (1) Electrophysiologic testing varies depending on the clinical pattern. In types I and II, the changes are those of a predominantly axonal neuropathy. In type III, the changes are restricted to the upper limbs and include absent SNAPs.
 (2) Sural nerve biopsies reveal a reduction of myelinated and unmyelinated nerve fibers. Semithin sections show degenerated axons and small clusters of axonal regeneration.
 (3) Diagnosis is confirmed by demonstrating severely reduced or absent high-density lipoprotein (HDL) and decreased total cholesterol, with normal or elevated triglycerides, in plasma.

d. Treatment
 (1) No treatment alters the course of the illness.
 (2) Reduction of low-density lipoprotein (LDL) cholesterol may reduce the risk of heart disease.

Bibliography

Amato AA, Dumitru D: Hereditary neuropathies. In Dumitru D, Amato AA, Zwarts M (eds): Electrodiagnostic Medicine. Philadelphia, Hanley & Belfus, 2002, pp. 899–936.

Hund E, Linke RP, Willig F, Grau A: Transthyretin-associated neuropathic amyloidosis: pathogenesis and treatment. Neurology 56:431–435, 2001.

Watts GDJ, Chance PF: Molecular basis of hereditary neuropathies. Adv Neurol 88:133–146, 2002.

1 Brachial Plexopathies

Bashar Katirji

Anatomy

1. The brachial plexus is derived from the anterior rami of C5 through T1 spinal roots. Nerve fibers intertangle at multiple sites to form structures, which are usually divided into five components: roots, trunks, divisions, cords, peripheral (terminal) nerves (Fig. 1–1). Because the divisions are generally located underneath the clavicle, the brachial plexus may also be divided into two regions: *supraclavicular* (roots and trunks) and *infraclavicular* (cords and terminal peripheral nerves).

2. Nerve fibers from C5 and C6 roots combine to form the upper trunk, C8 and T1 roots combine to form the lower trunk, and the C7 root continues as the middle trunk. Behind the clavicle, each trunk divides into two divisions (anterior and posterior).

3. All three posterior divisions unite to form the posterior cord, the upper two anterior divisions merge to form the lateral cord, and the anterior division of the lower trunk run continues as the medial cord.

4. The terminal peripheral nerves are the main outflow of the brachial plexus to the upper limb. Two major nerves arise from each cord: The posterior cord gives rise to the radial and axillary nerves, the lateral cord gives rise to the musculocutaneous nerve and to the lateral head of the median nerve, and the medial cord divides into the ulnar nerve and the medial head of the median nerve. The lateral and medial heads combine to form the median nerve.

5. In addition to the terminal nerves, many nerves take off directly from the main component of the brachial plexus. Except for four supraclavicular nerves, all are infraclavicular (i.e., originate from the cords). Also, except for two pure sensory nerves, all others are pure motor nerves and innervate shoulder girdle muscles (Table 1–1).

Etiology and Clinical Features

Traumatic Brachial Plexopathies

1. Traumatic lesions are the most common brachial plexus lesions. They may be mild but often are devastating and result in significant disability.

2. Traumatic brachial plexopathies present acutely. They are due to vehicular accidents or sporting or occupational injuries; still others are iatrogenic. Based on their causation and mechanism, they are usually subdivided into the following groups.

   a. *Traction injuries* are the most common causes of supraclavicular plexopathies. Most are due to closed traction sustained during certain sporting activities or vehicular accidents. In these situations, the upper plexus is predominantly injured if the shoulder is forced downward while the upper limb is adducted or if the head and shoulder are forcefully distracted from one another. In contrast, the lower plexus is often affected with upward traction on a hyperabducted arm. Open injuries are much less common, such as those with gunshot or knife wounds.

   b. *Avulsion root injuries* are due to tearing of the anterior or posterior spinal roots from the spinal cord. They are the most severe types of traction injury, occurring mostly after high energy accidents such as motorcycle crashes. The C8 and T1 roots and, to a lesser extent, the C7 root, are most vulnerable. When T1 root is also injured, there is often an associated ipsilateral Horner's syndrome.

   c. *Obstetric paralysis* is a traction brachial plexus injury sustained by infants during the birthing process. Associated root avulsions are not uncommon. Predisposing factors include uncommon fetal presentations (e.g., breech), large fetus, difficult deliveries, the use of instrumentation, and maternal obesity and diabetes mellitus. Historically, these lesions are subdivided into *Erb's palsy* (when the predominant injury is to the upper plexus) and *Klumpke's paralysis* (when the predominant injury is to the lower plexus).

      (1) With an upper plexus injury, the child's arm hangs adducted and internally rotated at the shoulder and extended and pronated at the elbow. The biceps and brachioradialis reflexes are absent.

      (2) If the middle trunk is also involved with the upper plexus, the extensors of the elbow, wrist, and fingers are also weak, and the arm assumes a "waiter's tip" position.

      (3) With selective lower plexus injury, intrinsic

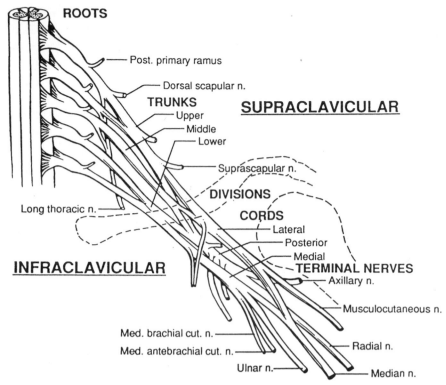

ROOTS

Post. primary ramus

Dorsal scapular n.

TRUNKS
Upper
Middle
Lower

SUPRACLAVICULAR

Suprascapular n.

DIVISIONS

CORDS
Lateral
Posterior
Medial

Long thoracic n.

INFRACLAVICULAR

TERMINAL NERVES
Axillary n.

Musculocutaneous n.

Med. brachial cut. n.
Med. antebrachial cut. n.
Ulnar n.

Radial n.

Median n.

Figure 1–1. Brachial plexus with its relation to the clavicle. (From Dyck PJ, Thomas PK: Peripheral Neuropathy, 3rd ed. Philadelphia, W.B. Saunders, 1993; with permission.)

hand muscles are weakened out of proportion to the long finger extensors, resulting in clawing of the hand (extension at the metacarpophalangeal joints and flexion at the proximal and distal interphalangeal joints).

d. *Postoperative brachial plexopathies* manifest after a surgical procedure, done under general anesthesia, on a portion of the body distant from the brachial plexus, such as abdominal surgery or craniotomy. It is caused by poor arm positioning on the operating table. The lesion has a predilection for the upper plexus, though pan-plexopathy may occur. Two special types of postoperative brachial plexopathies deserve special attention:

(1) *Post-median sternotomy plexopathies* occur after midline sternal splitting, usually for open-heart surgical procedures. The exact cause is still debated but is likely due to damage of the proximal lower trunk fibers (mostly extraspinal C8) by a fractured first thoracic rib as the anterior thorax is opened.

TABLE 1–1. MOTOR AND SENSORY NERVES ARISING DIRECTLY FROM THE BRACHIAL PLEXUS (EXCLUDING THE MAIN TERMINAL NERVES)

NERVE	ORIGIN	FUNCTION	DESTINATION
Dorsal scapular*	Anterior ramus of C5	Motor	Rhomboids (C5)
Long thoracic*	Anterior rami of C5–7	Motor	Serratus anterior (C5–7)
Suprascapular*	Upper trunk	Motor	Supraspinatus (C5–6) and infraspinatus (C5–6)
N. to subclavius*	Upper trunk	Motor	Subclavius (C5–6)
Lateral pectoral (lateral anterior thoracic)	Lateral cord	Motor	Pectoralis major and minor (C5–T1)
Subscapular (upper and lower)	Posterior cord	Motor	Teres major (C5–6) and subscapularis (C5–6)
Thoracodorsal	Posterior cord	Motor	Latissimus dorsi (C6–8)
Medial pectoral (medial anterior thoracic)	Medial cord	Motor	Pectoralis major and minor (C5–T1)
Medial cutaneous of arm (brachial cutaneous)	Medial cord	Sensory	Skin of medial arm (C8–T1)
Lateral cutaneous of forearm (antebrachial cutaneous)	Medial cord	Sensory	Skin of medial forearm (C8–T1)

*The only supraclavicular nerves.
From Katirji B: Electromyography in Clinical Practice: A Case Study Approach. St. Louis, Mosby, 1998; with permission.

(2) *Post-thoracic outlet surgery plexopathies* may occur during attempts to remove the first rib or perform a scalenectomy. The lower plexus most often is selectively involved.

e. *Pack palsy*, relatively rare, is due to brachial plexus compression by pack straps that traverse the shoulder. Although it most often involves the upper trunk, occasionally only the long thoracic or spinal accessory nerves are affected.

Neurogenic Thoracic Outlet Syndrome

The neurogenic thoracic outlet syndrome is discussed in Part XVI, Chapter 2, Neurogenic Thoracic Outlet Syndrome.

Neoplastic Brachial Plexopathies

1. Neoplastic brachial plexopathies are usually due to malignant tumors that reach the plexus via metastases or direct extension. Most are primary lung or breast cancer, but others are due to metastasis to the lung from other organs (e.g., colon, thyroid, testis). Because of anatomic proximity to the lung and breast, these lesions usually affect the lower plexus initially but may spread to involve the entire plexus.

2. The presentation is often subacute, with pain being the predominant feature. Pain usually involves the shoulder and radiates to the medial arm and forearm. Numbness is common and often correlates with the pain and extends into the medial hand. Weakness of hand and wrist muscles become apparent. Horner's syndrome may accompany this presentation.

3. *Pancoast syndrome* is a neoplastic plexopathy caused by an apical malignant lung neoplasm (called a superior sulcus tumor) that reaches the proximal lower plexus and adjacent vertebrae by direct extension. In sharp contrast to other neoplastic brachial plexopathies, the neurologic symptoms are usually the first manifestation of this malignancy.

Key Signs: Neoplastic Brachial Plexopathies

- Pain in the shoulder, medial arm, and forearm
- Numbness
- Weakness of hand and wrist muscles

Radiation Brachial Plexopathies

1. Radiation-induced brachial plexopathy may follow radiation therapy to the axilla, neck, or shoulder. The most common cause is radiation of the axillary lymph nodes in patients with breast carcinoma. Hence radiation-induced brachial plexopathy is most common in women and is usually unilateral.

2. Radiation damage to peripheral nerve elements is likely related to the dose of radiation, which may induce extensive loss of nerve fibers, myelin, obliteration of the vasculature, and fibrosis. Although all elements of the plexus may be affected, there is a predilection for the lateral cord and upper trunk.

3. Symptoms of brachial plexus injury usually appear after a latent period of 12 to 20 months, though occasionally longer symptom-free intervals occur. The onset is insidious, and the earliest manifestations are paresthesias in the index finger, middle finger, or thumb due to damage to the upper plexus. Pain is rare. Weakness of shoulder and elbow muscles appears later; and the paresthesias, sensory loss, and weakness progress slowly but relentlessly over several years.

Key Signs and Symptoms: Radiation Brachial Plexopathies

- Symptoms usually start after 12 to 20 months.
- Onset of the disease is insidious.
- Paresthesias in the index finger, middle finger, or thumb
- Weakness of shoulder and elbow muscles

Neuralgic Amyotrophy

1. Neuralgic amyotrophy is most likely an immune-mediated disorder that affects peripheral nerves of the upper limb and is not restricted to elements of the brachial plexus. This disorder has many synonyms, including idiopathic brachial plexitis, brachial neuritis, and Parsonage-Turner syndrome.

2. It is rare disorder with an estimated annual incidence of 1 to 2 cases per 100,000 population. It affects adults mainly, with a peak during the third decade of life. Men are affected twice as often as women.

3. Neuralgic amyotrophy is usually unilateral but sometimes bilateral and asymmetrical; rarely, it is recurrent. About half of the cases have a precipitating factor, such as upper respiratory infections, vaccinations, childbirth, or surgical procedures.

4. The illness often manifests with relatively abrupt shoulder and scapular pain, which reaches its maximum intensity quite rapidly and is usually

severe. Many patients visit emergency rooms for pain control. The pain is often worse at night and may extend into the arm and the antecubital fossa. The pain usually lasts for 1 to 2 weeks and is replaced by a mild, dull ache.

5. As the pain starts to subside during the first week, the patient notices upper limb weakness and wasting with minimal or no sensory symptoms. Upper plexus-innervated muscles are the most involved, resulting in weakness of shoulder muscles principally. The illness has also a tendency to affect motor nerves selectively, including the long thoracic nerve, axillary nerve, suprascapular nerve, musculocutaneous nerve, anterior interosseous nerve, and rarely the phrenic nerve.

6. In contrast to the sporadic form of neuralgic amyotrophy, a hereditary (usually autosomal dominant) form of neuralgic amyotrophy, linked to the distal long arm of chromosome 17q25, is characterized by recurrent bouts of neuralgic amyotrophy, which may start during childhood and is often associated with dysmorphic features (Table 1–2).

Key Signs: Neuralgic Amyotrophy

- Abrupt, intense shoulder and scapular pain, usually severe

- Pain usually lasts for 1 to 2 weeks.

- Following pain there is upper limb weakness and wasting with minimal or no sensory symptoms.

Diagnosis

1. The diagnosis of brachial plexus traumatic injuries depends on the history and neurologic examination, often supported by imaging and electrodiagnostic studies.

2. The clinical features of brachial plexopathies are similar to those of other focal peripheral nerve lesions, including pain, sensory loss, weakness,

TABLE 1–2. DISTINGUISHING FEATURES OF SPORADIC NEURALGIC AMYOTROPHY AND HEREDITARY NEURALGIC AMYOTROPHY

FEATURE	SPORADIC NEURALGIC AMYOTROPHY	HEREDITARY NEURALGIC AMYOTROPHY
Age	Adulthood	Onset is frequently during childhood
Sex	Males predominate	Males and females equally affected
Family history	Negative	Positive (dominant trait)
Pain	Prominent	Prominent
Recurrence	Rare (1–5%)	Common
Lower cranial nerve involvement	Exceedingly rare	Not uncommon
Associated findings	None	Dysmorphic features (e.g., cleft palate, canthal folds, syndactyly)

From Katirji B: Electromyography in Clinical Practice: A Case Study Approach, St. Louis, Mosby, 1998; with permission.

and reflex changes. The specific symptoms often depend on the etiology and severity of the brachial plexus lesion.

3. Localizing the element(s) injured in a brachial plexopathy is a major objective of the neurologic examination (Table 1–3), as the location of the lesion has diagnostic, therapeutic, and prognostic implications.

Electrodiagnosis

1. The most common pathophysiology encountered in brachial plexopathies is axonal loss. Typically, it is not accompanied by any focal conduction abnormalities caused by demyelination. In a small number of patients, however, demyelinating conduction block is prominent although usually accompanied by at least a minimal amount of axon loss.

2. The electrodiagnosis of brachial plexopathy requires a good grasp of the anatomy of the brachial plexus and its branches as well as the myotomal

TABLE 1–3. CLINICAL FINDINGS OF BRACHIAL PLEXOPATHIES

FINDING	UPPER PLEXUS*	MIDDLE PLEXUS	LOWER PLEXUS†
Weakness	Shoulder abduction Shoulder external rotation Elbow flexion Forearm supination Forearm pronation	Elbow extension Forearm pronation Wrist extension Wrist flexion	Finger abduction Finger adduction Finger extension Finger flexion
Sensory loss	Lateral shoulder, arm, forearm, thumb, index finger	Posterior arm and forearm, dorsum of hand, middle finger	Medial arm and forearm, medial hand
Hypoareflexia	Biceps and brachioradialis	Triceps	None

*Also with weakness of rhomboids and serratus anterior in avulsion root injuries.
†May be associated with Horner's syndrome in avulsion root injuries.

chart of all the muscles of the upper limb. Detailed motor and sensory nerve conduction studies (Table 1–4) and needle electromyography (EMG) provide valuable information. Because the lesions are often due to axonal loss, the amplitudes of the sensory and motor responses are informative, whereas the latencies and conduction velocities generally are not. To localize lesions accurately, each evoked sensory nerve action potential (SNAP), compound muscle action potential (CMAP), and sampled muscle is analyzed by checking them relative to their neural pathways through roots, trunks, cords, peripheral nerves, and branches.

3. Several important features of the electrodiagnostic

TABLE 1–4. UPPER EXTREMITY NERVE CONDUCTION STUDIES USEFUL FOR DETECTING AXON LOSS BRACHIAL PLEXOPATHIES (BASED ON AMPLITUDE CHANGES)

Upper Trunk
Median sensory (D1)
Lateral antebrachial cutaneous
Radial sensory (thumb base)
Musculocutaneous motor (biceps)
Axillary motor (deltoid)

Middle Trunk
Median sensory (D2)
Median sensory (D3)
Radial sensory (thumb base)*
Motor–none

Lower Trunk
Ulnar sensory (D5)
Medial antebrachial cutaneous
Ulnar motor (hypothenar)
Ulnar motor (FDI)
Median motor (thenar)
Radial motor (EIP)*

Lateral Cord
Median sensory (D1)
Median sensory (D2)
Median sensory (D3)
Lateral antebrachial cutaneous
Musculocutaneous motor (biceps)

Posterior Cord
Radial sensory (thumb base)
Posterior antebrachial cutaneous
Radial motor (EIP)
Radial motor (brachioradialis)
Axillary (deltoid)

Medial Cord
Ulnar sensory (D5)
Medial antebrachial cutaneous
Ulnar motor (hypothenar)
Ulnar motor (FDI)
Median motor (thenar)

Abbreviations: D, digit (D1, thumb; D2, index finger; D3, middle finger); FDI, first dorsal interosseous; EIP, extensor indices proprius. Recording points are bracketed with parentheses.
*Less reliable studies, mainly due to variations in root derivation.
From Katirji B, Kaminski HJ, Preston DC, et al (eds): Neuromuscular Disorders in Clinical Practice. Boston, Butterworth-Heinemann, 2002; with permission.

examination are extremely helpful for localization brachial plexopathies.

a. The SNAP amplitudes obtained with distal stimulation are the most sensitive nerve conduction study (NCS) indicator of lesions involving one or more elements of the brachial plexus. The SNAP amplitudes are normal in root lesions (i.e., lesions confined to the intraspinal canal). Hence they are not affected by preganglionic axonal loss lesions, including cervical radiculopathies and avulsion root injuries.

b. The median sensory fibers do not pass through the lower plexus. The thumb SNAP is innervated by C6 through the upper trunk, the index finger by C6 and C7 through the upper and middle trunks, and the middle finger by C7 through the middle trunk. All three SNAPs traverse the lateral cord to reach the median nerve.

c. The median motor fibers to the thenar muscles do not pass through the upper plexus. In contrast to the median fibers to the hand, the ulnar motor fibers and ulnar sensory fibers do not separate while traversing the plexus. They pass through the lower trunk and medial cord and continue through the ulnar nerve to their targets in the forearm and hand.

4. Myokymic discharges occur frequently on needle EMG of patients with *radiation plexopathies*. They are spontaneous, rhythmic, grouped repetitive discharges of the motor unit, with a firing frequency of less 2 Hz, producing a sound like marching soldiers on loudspeakers.

5. Certain electrodiagnostic (and neurologic) abnormalities are common in *neuralgic amyotrophy*. The following features are highly suggestive of this disorder and reinforce the patchy nature of the pathologic process:

a. Selective denervation of multiple motor peripheral nerves around the shoulder girdle (long thoracic, spinal accessory, suprascapular, axillary, and musculocutaneous nerves)

b. Partial proximal median mononeuropathy, affecting predominantly muscles innervated by the anterior interosseous nerve, without abnormalities in median SNAPs, CMAP, or thenar muscles

c. Denervation of specific muscles without affecting the main trunk of the supplying peripheral nerve. For example, the pronator muscle may be selectively denervated with sparing of other median innervated or other C6 or C7 innervated muscles. Similarly, the suprapinatus muscle may show prominent neurogenic changes, whereas the infraspinatus muscle and other C5 or C6 innervated muscles are normal.

Imaging Studies

1. Plain radiographs of the cervical spine, clavicle, shoulder, humerus, and chest are often required for traction injuries to exclude concomitant injuries.

2. The computed tomography (CT) scan is most useful for identifying hematomas in the brachial plexus with acute traumatic lesions. It has limited value for imaging the neural elements of the brachial plexus.

3. CT myelography of the cervical spine is valuable for assessing the cervical roots, including those involved in avulsion injuries. Traumatic meningoceles or obliteration of root sleeves are findings consistent with root avulsion.

4. Magnetic resonance imaging (MRI) of the brachial plexus is the imaging method of choice. It may delineate mass lesions in neoplastic cases but shows only diffuse thickening and enhancement without evidence of a mass in those with radiation plexopathy. Magnetic resonance neurography, including diffusion neurography and T2-based neurography, is a newly emerging technique that will possibly generate tissue specific images of nerves, analogous to angiograms.

Differential Diagnosis

1. The differential diagnosis of brachial plexopathies, in general, includes upper limb mononeuropathies, cervical radiculopathies, and orthopedic injuries (e.g., rotator cuff injuries).

2. In patients with postmedian sternotomies, the symptoms may be easily confused with ulnar neuropathies at the elbow, usually attributed to malpositioning the arm on the operating table.

3. In patients who received radiation to the axilla, neck, or shoulder area for treatment of a malignancy, a major part of the differential diagnosis is to distinguish radiation-induced plexopathy from a recurrent malignant neoplastic brachial plexopathy (Table 1–5). In general, chronic and painless upper brachial plexopathies are likely due to radiation injury, whereas subacute and painful lower brachial plexopathies are usually due to a malignant neoplasm. Moreover, the presence of myokymia on needle EMG strongly supports a diagnosis of radiation plexopathy rather than recurrent neoplastic invasion.

4. Neuralgic amyotrophy is often confused with acute cervical radiculopathy. In contrast to acute cervical radiculopathy, the pain of neuralgic amy-

TABLE 1–5. DIFFERENTIAL DIAGNOSIS BETWEEN RADIATION AND NEOPLASTIC BRACHIAL PLEXOPATHIES

Parameter	Radiation Plexopathy	Neoplastic Plexopathy
Onset	Insidious	Subacute
Pain	Absent	Common
Element involved	Upper plexus	Lower plexus
Myokymia on EMG	Present	Absent
MRI	Normal or thickening	Mass

otrophy is not exacerbated by the Valsalva maneuver, such as with coughing or sneezing, and is worse at night. The degree of atrophy and selective involvement of proximal peripheral nerve should raise the suspicion against cervical radiculopathy.

Treatment

1. Treatment of brachial plexopathies depends on an accurate diagnosis and identifying the etiology. In general, treatment may be conservative or surgical.

   a. Conservative treatment includes pain management, such as with tricyclic antidepressants and anticonvulsants. Neuralgic amyotrophy may require potent analgesics to control the pain during the acute phase. Physical and occupational therapy with a focus on active therapy and passive range of movement is necessary in all patients to improve muscle strength and prevent contractures.

   b. Surgical repair of the injured plexus elements in traumatic plexopathies may provide the only hope for recovery. Because the goal of surgical procedures is to restore motor function, intervention should not be delayed and should be done within 3 to 6 months after the injury. It should be done by surgeons with vast experience in nerve repair, particularly of the brachial plexus. Reconstructive orthopedic procedures may be useful palliative procedures.

2. There is no effective treatment for radiation-induced brachial plexopathies.

Key Treatment: Brachial Plexopathies

• Tricyclic antidepressants

• Anticonvulsants

• Physical and occupational therapy to improve muscle strength and prevent contractures

• Surgery

• No effective treatment for radiation-induced brachial plexopathies

Prognosis

1. The prognosis for the brachial plexopathies depends principally on the etiology, severity, and underlying pathophysiology (demyelinating conduction block or axonal loss). In general, recovery is more satisfactory with brachial plexus lesions that involve the upper plexus than the lower plexus and for those causing partial axonal loss compared to those causing total or near-total axonal loss.

2. Among all traumatic plexopathies, avulsion root injuries have the worse prognosis, as these patients have no hope for recovery, particularly when multiple roots are avulsed. The prognosis for children with obstetric paralysis is controversial but is always better with upper plexus lesions.

3. The prognosis for radiation-induced plexopathies is extremely poor, as the process usually is progressive, often leading to marked upper limb weakness and sensory ataxia.

4. The prognosis for neuralgic amyotrophy is generally good, although maximal motor recovery may require several years. Occasionally, there is residual weakness and atrophy.

Bibliography

Beghi E, Kurland LT, Mulder DW, Nicolosi A: Brachial plexus neuropathy in the population of Rochester, Minnesota, 1970–1981. Ann Neurol 18:320–323, 1985.

Ferrante M, Wilbourn AJ: Electrodiagnostic approach to the patient with suspected brachial plexopathy. Neurol Clin 20:423–450, 2002.

Filler A: Imaging of peripheral nerve. In Katirji B, Kaminski HJ, Preston DC, et al (eds): Neuromuscular Disorders in Clinical Practice. Boston, Butterworth-Heinemann, 2002, pp. 266–282.

Levin K, Wilbourn AJ, Maggiano HJ: Cervical rib and median sternotomy-related plexopathies: A reassessment. Neurology 50:1407–1413, 1998.

Tsairis P, Dyck PJ, Mulder DW: Natural history of brachial plexus neuropathy; Report of 99 cases. Arch Neurol 27:109–117, 1972.

Wilbourn AJ: Brachial plexopathies. In Katirji B, Kaminski HJ, Preston DC, et al (eds): Neuromuscular Disorders in Clinical Practice. Boston, Butterworth-Heinemann, 2002, pp. 884–906.

Wilbourn AJ: Thoracic outlet syndrome surgery causing severe brachial plexopathy. Muscle Nerve 11:66–74, 1988.

2 Neurogenic Thoracic Outlet Syndrome

Bashar Katirji

Definition

Neurogenic thoracic outlet syndrome (TOS) is a rare and chronic neurologic syndrome caused by compression of the lower brachial plexus by a congenital cervical rib or band.

Etiology

1. Neurogenic TOS (also named *true* or *classic neurogenic* TOS, or the *cervical rib and band syndrome*), is a nontraumatic supraclavicular plexopathy, described around the turn of the century by Thornburn and Howell, independently, but better defined more than 60 years later, by Gilliatt. Neurogenic TOS is usually caused by a congenital band originating from the tip of a rudimentary cervical rib or an elongated C7 transverse process and inserting into the first thoracic rib. This causes stretching and angulation of the T1 anterior primary ramus, or predominantly the T1 component of the lower trunk of the brachial plexus. Neurogenic TOS is associated with objective clinical and electrodiagnostic (EDX) evidence of peripheral nerve fiber injury, usually limited to the lower trunk of the plexus.

2. In contrast to the rare neurogenic TOS, a disputed TOS, also called *nonspecific* TOS, is much more frequently diagnosed and is surrounded by controversy. Here, pain or subjective sensory symptoms dominate the clinical picture but without objective neurologic or convincing EDX signs. In this situation, multiple compression sites have been advocated, resulting in many controversial "syndromes" and surgical procedures (Table 2–1). This form is beyond the scope of this chapter, but was recently debated (see Roos and Wilbourn).

Clinical Features

1. Neurogenic TOS is a unilateral disorder that affects almost solely women in their second to fourth decade.

2. Common complaints at presentation include intermittent, dull ache and sensory disturbance along the medial aspect of the forearm and hand. Atrophy of the thenar eminence, with or without hand weakness, may be also noted. Cramping of the hand that is exacerbated by upper limb activity is not uncommon. These symptoms may be traced back several years prior to presentation; some patients may have undergone carpal tunnel release, ulnar nerve transposition, or cervical laminectomy.

3. On clinical examination, atrophy is often restricted to the lateral thenar muscles or may involve the entire hand with a lateral thenar predominance. Similarly, the entire hand is weak, although the lateral thenar muscles may be noticeably the weakest. Sensory loss, often patchy, usually can be demonstrated along the medial forearm and arm (in the T1 distribution), as well as along the medial hand.

TABLE 2–1. THREE DISPUTED THORACIC OUTLET SYNDROMES

SYNDROME	SCALENUS ANTICUS SYNDROME	COSTOCLAVICULAR SYNDROME	HYPERABDUCTION SYNDROME
Proposed compression site	Interscalene triangle	Between first thoracic rib and clavicle	Between pectoralis minor tendon and/or between first rib and clavicle
Structures compressed	Subclavian artery or brachial plexus	Subclavian artery, subclavian vein, or brachial plexus	Subclavian/axillary artery, or brachial plexus
Suggested surgical procedure	Resection of scalenus anticus muscle	Resection of first thoracic rib	Resection of first thoracic rib and resection of pectoralis minor tendon

Adapted from Wilbourn AJ. Brachial plexus disorders. In Dyck PPJ, Thomas PK (eds), Peripheral Neuropathy, 3rd ed. Philadelphia, W.B. Saunders Company, 1993.

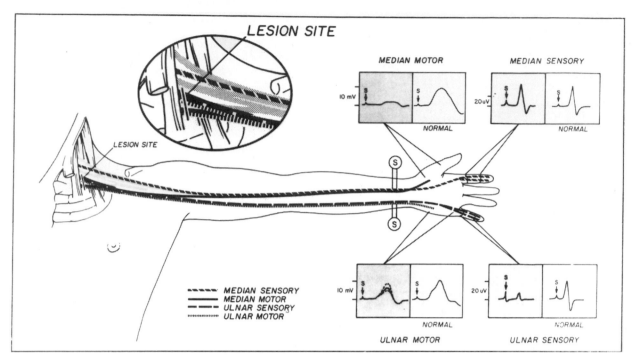

Figure 2–1. Neurogenic thoracic outlet syndrome showing the site of compression by the cervical rib or band and the abnormalities seen on routine nerve conduction studies. (From Wilbourn AJ, Controversies regarding thoracic outlet syndrome. Syllabus on controversies in entrapment neuropathies. American Association of Electrodiagnostic Medicine, Rochester, Minnesota, 1984, with permission).

Key Signs

- Intermittent, dull ache along the medial aspect of the forearm and hand

- Atrophy of the thenar eminence, with or without hand weakness

- Hand cramps

- Sensory loss of the medial arm, forearm and hand

Diagnosis

1. The diagnosis should be suspected in women who present with medial hand and forearm numbness and pain or thenar atrophy.

2. The EDX studies are often the mainstay in diagnosis, because neurogenic TOS is the result of a chronic axon-loss lower trunk brachial plexopathy.

   a. The findings on routine nerve conduction studies (NCS) in neurogenic TOS are pathognomonic (Fig. 2–1 and Key Findings). Because all ulnar sensory fibers, all ulnar motor fibers and the C8/T1 median fibers courses the lower

trunk and are subject to axonal loss, ulnar sensory nerve action potential (SNAP), ulnar compound muscle action potential (CMAP), and median CMAP are low in amplitude on routine NCS.

   b. Median CMAP is often the most severely affected routine NCS because the lesion commonly involves primarily the T1 anterior primary ramus, the major innervation of the lateral thenar muscles through the median nerve.

   c. An extremely sensitive finding in the diagnosis of neurogenic TOS is a low-amplitude or absent medial antebrachial cutaneous SNAP. The medial antebrachial cutaneous sensory fibers originate mainly from the T1 dorsal root ganglion and pass through the T1 anterior primary ramus and lower trunk and medial cord of the brachial plexus to innervate the skin of the medial forearm. This sensitive sensory NCS should be always part of the EDX evaluation of patients with possible neurogenic TOS.

   d. Needle electromyography examination often reveals motor unit action potentials with long duration and high amplitude with very limited amount of fibrillation potentials, consistent

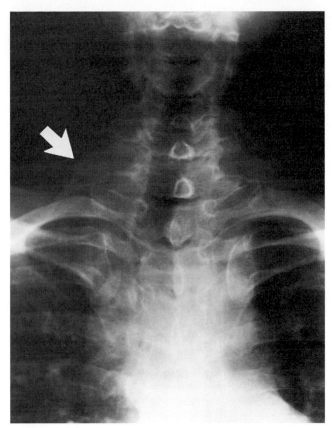

Figure 2–2. Cervical spine x-rays (anteroposterior view) revealing a rudimentary cervical rib on the right. (From Katirji B. Electromyography in Clinical Practice. St. Louis, Mosby, 1998, with permission).

with the chronic nature of compression in neurogenic TOS. This involves the T1 innervated muscles in general, most commonly the lateral thenar muscles (including abductor pollicis brevis), with lesser involvement of the interossei, abductor digiti minimi, adductor pollicis, flexor pollicis longus, and extensor indicis proprius.

Key Findings: Nerve Conduction Studies

I. Low-amplitude or absent medial antebrachial SNAP*

II. Low-amplitude ulnar SNAP

III. Low-amplitude median CMAP*

IV. Borderline/low-amplitude ulnar CMAP

V. Normal median SNAP

* The most consistent abnormalities.

SNAP: sensory nerve action potential; CMAP: compound muscle action potential.

Radiologic Features

1. Cervical spine x-rays typically show a cervical rib, a rudimentary cervical rib, or simply an elongated C7 transverse process (Fig. 2–2).

2. Other radiologic procedures are rarely indicated. Magnetic resonance imaging of the cervical spine is only useful when cervical radiculopathy is suspected.

Differential Diagnosis

1. The differential diagnosis of neurogenic TOS includes a severe carpal tunnel syndrome, ulnar neuropathy at the elbow, or low cervical radiculopathy (Table 2–2).

2. Other causes of lower trunk brachial plexopathies may also mimic neurogenic TOS. Brachial plexopathy after median sternotomy is acute and affects the C8 anterior ramus resulting in weakness of the hypothenar muscles and interossei. A lower trunk brachial plexopathy due to a Pancoast's tumor is often painful, and subacute with hand weakness but minimal atrophy.

Treatment and Prognosis

1. Once the diagnosis of neurogenic TOS is made, the brachial plexus should be explored surgically, preferably by a supraclavicular approach. The cervical band should be sectioned and, sometimes, the distal end of the cervical rib is removed.

2. Treatment of disputed TOS should be conservative, including physical therapy and pain management. Surgical intervention should only be considered in selected cases.

3. Surgical section of the cervical rib or band often relieves pain and sensory symptoms and halts the progression of weakness or atrophy. The prognosis for motor recovery is poor, however, and surgery does not reverse the hand atrophy once it has become advanced.

Key Treatment

• Surgical resection of cervical band and/or rib

• Conservative including physical therapy and pain management for disputed TOS.

• Surgical intervention in selected cases of disputed TOS.

TABLE 2–2. DIFFERENTIAL DIAGNOSIS OF NEUROGENIC THORACIC OUTLET SYNDROME

	CARPAL TUNNEL SYNDROME	CUBITAL TUNNEL SYNDROME	C8 RADICULOPATHY	T1 RADICULOPATHY	POST-MEDIAN STERNOTOMY BRACHIAL PLEXOPATHY	NEUROGENIC THORACIC OUTLET SYNDROME
Lesion site	Median nerve at the wrist	Ulnar nerve at the elbow	C8 intraspinal root	T1 intraspinal root	C8 anterior primary ramus component of lower trunk	T4 anterior primary ramus component of lower trunk
Mode of symptom onset	Subacute or chronic	Subacute or chronic	Acute, subacute, or chronic	Acute, subacute, or chronic	Acute (postoperative)	Chronic
Sensory loss distribution	Lateral three digits	Medial two digits	Medial two digits and medial forearm	Medial forearm and arm	Medial two digits and medial forearm	Medial two digits and medial forearm/arm
Muscle atrophy and/or weakness	Lateral thenars	Hypothenars, medial thenars, and interossei	Hypothenars, medial thenars, interossei, and long finger flexors	Lateral thenars	Hypothenars, medial thenars, interossei, and long finger flexors	Lateral thenars
Median SNAP	Abnormal	Normal	Normal	Normal	Normal	Normal
Ulnar SNAP	Normal	Abnormal	Normal	Normal	Abnormal	Usually abnormal
MAB SNAP	Normal	Normal	Normal	Normal	May be abnormal	Abnormal
Median CMAP	Abnormal	Normal	Normal	Normal or abnormal	Often normal	Abnormal
Ulnar CMAP	Normal	Abnormal	Normal or abnormal	Normal	Abnormal	Normal or abnormal

Abbreviations: SNAP: sensory nerve action potential; CMAP: compound muscle action potential; MAB: medial antebrachial.

Bibliography

Gilliatt RW, LeQuesne M, Logue V, Sumner AJ: Wasting of the hand associated with a cervical rib or band. J Neurol Neurosurg Psychiatry 33:615–624, 1970.

Nishida T, Price SJ, Minieka MM: Medial antebrachial cutaneous nerve conduction in true neurogenic thoracic outlet syndrome. Electromyogr Clin Neurophysiol 33: 285–288, 1993.

Roos DB, Wilbourn, AJ: Issues and opinions: Thoracic outlet syndrome. Muscle Nerve 22:126–138, 1999.

Wilbourn AJ: Brachial plexopathies, In Katirji B, Kaminski HJ, Preston DC, et al (eds). Neuromuscular Disorders in Clinical Practice. Boston, Butterworth-Heinemann, 2000. pp. 884–906.

Wilbourn AJ, Porter JM: Thoracic outlet syndromes. Spine: State of the Art Reviews 2:597–626, 1988.

3 Carpal Tunnel Syndrome and Other Median Neuropathies

Bashar Katirji
Ahmad Al-Khatib

ANATOMY

1. The median nerve is formed from fusion of its lateral and medial heads, which originate from the lateral and medial cords of the brachial plexus, respectively.

    a. The lateral head of the median nerve, composed of C6-7 fibers, innervates skin overlying the thenar eminence, thumb, index, and middle fingers and most of the motor fibers to the proximal median forearm muscles.

    b. The medial head of the median nerve, composed of C8–T1 fibers, supplies most of the motor fibers to the distal median muscles of the forearm and the hand as well as sensory fibers to the lateral half of the ring finger.

2. The median nerve descends in the upper arm without giving out any motor or sensory branches. In a small number of individuals a tendinous band stretches between a bony spur originating from the shaft of the medial humerus (ligament of Struthers) and the medial humeral epicondyle. In the antecubital fossa, the median nerve lies adjacent to the brachial artery. It then runs first underneath the lacertus fibrosus, a thick fibrous band that runs from the medial aspect of the biceps tendon to the proximal forearm flexor musculature.

3. In the forearm, the median runs between the two heads of the pronator teres before innervating the pronator teres, flexor carpi radialis, flexor digitorum sublimis, and in some individuals the palmaris longus muscles (Fig. 3–1).

4. In the proximal forearm, the anterior interosseous nerve is given off, innervating the flexor pollicis longus, flexor digitorum profundus to digits 2 and 3, and pronator quadratus muscles.

5. Proximal to the wrist the palmar cutaneous sensory branch originates and runs subcutaneously to supply sensation over the thenar eminence (Fig. 3–2).

6. At the wrist, the median nerve enters through the carpal tunnel, which is formed by carpal bones on the floor and sides, with the thick transverse carpal ligament forming the roof. In addition to the median nerve, nine flexor tendons to the digits and thumb enter the wrist through the carpal tunnel.

The median nerve divides in the palm into motor and sensory divisions.

    a. The motor division supplies the first and second lumbricals and then innervates the thenar muscles, including the opponens pollicis, abductor pollicis brevis, and superficial head of the flexor pollicis brevis.

    b. The sensory division supplies sensation to the index and middle fingers in addition to the medial thumb and lateral half of the ring finger. The index and middle fingers are both supplied by two digital branches each (one lateral and one medial), with the thumb and ring fingers receiving each one median digital branch only.

CARPAL TUNNEL SYNDROME (MEDIAN NEUROPATHY AT THE WRIST)

Definition

Carpal tunnel syndrome (CTS) is caused by compression of the median nerve in the carpal tunnel at the wrist.

Epidemiology

1. CTS is the most common entrapment neuropathy.

2. The prevalence of CTS in the United States is estimated at 125 cases per 100,000, and its incidence is estimated at 0.12 per 1000 person-years.

3. CTS symptoms peak at ages 55 to 64 years. The female/male ratio is about 2:1.

Etiology

1. Most cases of CTS are idiopathic or associated with chronic mechanical compression in an occupational or activity setting that involves repetitive hand use.

2. Other conditions associated with CTS include connective tissue disease (rheumatoid arthritis), endocrine disorders (diabetes, hypothyroidism, acromegaly), amyloidosis (familial and acquired), pregnancy, and any other conditions that cause edema.

3. Median neuropathy at the wrist may be a compli-

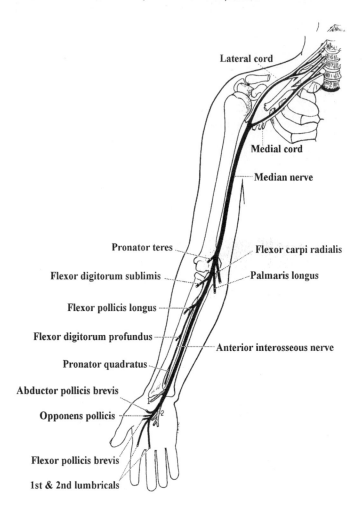

Figure 3–1. Anatomy of the median nerve. (From Haymaker W, Woodhall B: Peripheral nerve injuries. Philadelphia, W.B. Saunders, 1953, with permission.)

cation of wrist fracture (e.g., Colles fracture), anomalous muscle (e.g., palmaris longus), or a space-occupying lesion (e.g., ganglion, hemangioma, lipoma, neurofibroma, schwannoma).

4. Pathologic evaluation of the median nerve in CTS frequently shows edema, vascular sclerosis, fibrosis, and demyelination. In severe cases, there is wallerian degeneration with axonal loss probably due to nerve ischemia.

Symptoms

1. CTS is often bilateral, with the dominant hand usually more symptomatic.
2. Patients with CTS may present with a variety of sensory or motor symptoms.
   a. Pain and sensory disturbances
      (1) Sensory disturbances, which include paresthesia and diminished sensation, are usually localized to the hand and follow the median nerve distribution. However, some patients complain that the entire hand falls asleep.
      (2) The pain is usually in the wrist but may

radiate to the forearm, arm, or rarely the shoulder.
      (3) These symptoms are usually intermittent, often nocturnal, and provoked by either a flexed or an extended wrist posture such as when driving, typing, or holding a phone.
      (4) The symptoms are usually alleviated by shaking or wringing the hands.

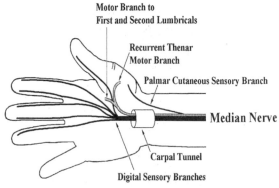

Figure 3–2. Anatomy of the carpal tunnel syndrome. (From Preston DC, Shapiro BE: Electromyography and Neuromuscular Disorders. Boston, Butterworth-Heinemann, 1998, with permission.)

(5) When sensory loss is severe, the patient may complain of decreased hand dexterity, such as difficulty buttoning a shirt.

b. Weakness and muscle wasting

(1) In advanced CTS, motor fibers may become involved resulting in hand weakness such as when opening jars or turning door-knobs.

(2) In such advanced cases, atrophy of the thenar eminence may become evident to the patient or may be brought to the patient's attention by family or friends.

Key Symptoms

- Often bilateral, with the dominant hand usually more symptomatic

- Paresthesia and diminished sensation

- Pain in the wrist that may radiate to forearm, arm, or rarely the shoulder

- Symptoms usually intermittent, often nocturnal, and provoked by either a flexed or an extended wrist posture (as when driving, typing, or holding a phone)

- Symptoms usually alleviated by shaking or wringing the hands

Physical Signs

1. Hypesthesia in the median nerve distribution in the hand involving the medial thumb, index, and middle or lateral ring finger (or any combination) is the most common finding. There is often sparing of sensation over the thenar area (innervated by the palmar cutaneous branch) and the medial aspect of the ring finger (innervated by the ulnar nerve).

2. Motor examination reveals weakness of thumb abduction and opposition and atrophy of the thenar eminence. These findings are present in more severe and advanced cases of CTS.

3. Two provocative maneuvers are extremely helpful for diagnosing CTS.

   a. Tinel's sign, where tapping over the median nerve at the wrist provokes paresthesia in the median nerve distribution

   b. Phalen's maneuver, where holding the wrist passively flexed for 30 seconds to 2 minutes provokes paresthesia in the median nerve distribution

Key Signs

- Hypesthesia involving medial thumb or the index, middle, or lateral ring finger

- Weakness of thumb abduction and opposition

- Atrophy of the thenar eminence

- Paresthesia (Tinel's sign, Phalen's maneuver)

Differential Diagnosis

CTS may mimic other disorders that can cause pain, numbness, tingling, and weakness in the hand.

1. C6-7 cervical radiculopathy. Clinically, neck pain radiating to the shoulder and arm and exacerbation of symptoms by neck movements are common symptoms of cervical radiculopathy and are not compatible with CTS. Proximal limb weakness and paresthesia are also common with cervical radiculopathy. On physical examination, the presence of abnormal biceps, brachioradialis or triceps reflexes, diminished power in proximal muscles, and sensory abnormalities in the palm or forearm are key differentiating features.

2. Median neuropathy at the elbow. Median neuropathy at the elbow is much less common than with CTS and is associated with sensory disturbance over the thenar eminence and weakness of median innervated muscles proximal to the carpal tunnel (e.g., flexor pollicis longus, pronator teres, pronator quadratus, flexor carpi radialis muscles).

3. Brachial plexopathy. Upper brachial plexopathy, involving the upper trunk or lateral cord causes numbness of the lateral fingers mimicking CTS. However, there is often associated reflex abnormalities (depressed or absent biceps or brachioradialis reflexes), sensory loss in the lateral forearm and arm, and weakness in proximal muscles (biceps, deltoid, spinati).

4. Central nervous system disorders. Transient ischemic attacks, seizures, and migraine may manifest with intermittent paresthesia in the hand but usually without hand or forearm pain.

5. Other conditions. CTS may be confused with other causes of wrist and hand pain including tenosynovitis, osteoarthritis, and Raynaud's disease.

Diagnosis

1. The clinical presentation and physical examination of CTS may be so classic that the diagnosis

can be made based on clinical grounds. Also, provocative tests, particularly Phalen's sign, are highly specific.

2. Electrodiagnostic testing is often useful for confirmation, particularly when the symptoms are atypical or mild, the findings are equivocal, or there is an overlapping disorder such as peripheral polyneuropathy or cervical radiculopathy.

3. Because the pathophysiology of CTS is typically demyelination, with evidence of secondary axonal loss in severe cases only, the hallmark of CTS is focal slowing of conduction at the wrist. Hence, median nerve conduction studies, and particularly distal latencies, are the most sensitive for confirming the diagnosis.

4. A common finding in CTS is prolongation of distal median motor and sensory latencies due to focal slowing of conduction across the carpal tunnel. In more severe cases and if the demyelination has resulted in conduction block or secondary axonal loss, the distal compound muscle action potential and sensory nerve action potential amplitudes are decreased as well. The median minimum F-wave latencies may also be prolonged, especially in comparison with the ulnar nerve.

5. Approximately 10% to 25% of patients have normal or borderline routine median sensory and motor nerve conduction studies. In these patients more sensitive tests are needed to confirm the diagnosis. Such tests are of two types: inching across the carpal tunnel, and internal comparison studies between the median nerve and an adjacent nerve of similar length and size in the same hand. The absence of a gold standard for the diagnosis of CTS precludes determining the exact sensitivity, specificity, or predictive value of any of these tests.

   a. Inching across the carpal tunnel. This study, described by Kimura, consists of serial stimulations of the median nerve from midpalm to distal forearm in 1 cm increments while recording antidromically from the index or middle finger. There is usually a latency change of 0.16 to 0.21 ms/cm. In patients with CTS, there is an abrupt latency increase across one or a few adjoining segments of more than 0.4 to 0.5 ms.

   b. The most common comparison studies (Fig. 3–3, Table 3–1) include

      (1) Median versus ulnar palm-to-wrist (palmar) mixed nerve latencies

      (2) Median versus ulnar wrist-to-digit 4 sensory latencies

      (3) Median (recording second lumbrical muscle) versus the ulnar (recording second palmar and dorsal interossei) distal motor latencies

      (4) Median versus radial wrist-to-thumb sensory latencies

6. Needle electromyography (EMG) is helpful for documenting any ongoing or past axonal loss and for excluding other conditions that may mimic CTS. In mild or early cases, needle examination of the thenar muscles is usually normal. The presence of active denervation or large reinnervated motor units in the abductor pollicis brevis and opponens pollicis indicates active or chronic denervation, respectively. These signs of axonal loss imply a more severe or advanced case.

7. Other tests maybe considered on an individual basis, depending on the suspicion of other conditions that may manifest as CTS.

   a. Laboratory screening tests (e.g., thyroid function test, rheumatoid factor, blood glucose)

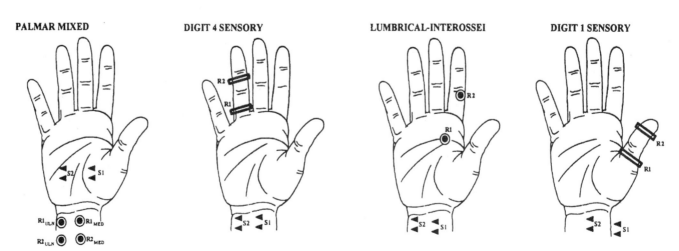

Figure 3–3. Internal comparison nerve conduction studies for diagnosing carpal tunnel syndrome. (Adapted from Preston DC, Shapiro BE: Electromyography and Neuromuscular Disorders. Boston, Butterworth-Heinemann, 1998.)

TABLE 3–1. COMMONLY USED INCHING AND INTERNAL COMPARISON NERVE CONDUCTION STUDIES FOR EVALUATION OF CARPAL TUNNEL SYNDROME

		STUDY			
PARAMETER	INCHING	MIXED NERVE PALMAR STUDIES	MEDIAN-ULNAR SENSORY LATENCY BETWEEN WRIST AND RING FINGER	MEDIAN-RADIAL SENSORY LATENCY BETWEEN WRIST AND THUMB	MEDIAN-ULNAR MOTOR LATENCY RECORDING 2ND LUMBRICAL-INTEROSSEI
Technique	Short segment (1 cm) incremental median sensory latency across the carpal tunnel	Palm stimulation of the median and ulnar nerves, recording at the wrist (8 cm distance)	Median and ulnar nerves stimulation at the wrist, recording the ring fingers (14 cm distance)	Median and radial nerves stimulation at the wrist, recording the thumb (10 cm distance)	Median nerve recording second lumbrical and ulnar nerve, recording the second palmar and dorsal interossei (9–10 cm distance)
Abnormal distal/ peak latency	Difference between consecutive segments > 0.4–0.5 ms	Median-ulnar latency difference > 0.4 ms	Median-ulnar latency difference > 0.4 ms	Median-radial latency difference > 0.4 ms	Median-ulnar latency difference > 0.4 ms

Adapted from Katirji B: Electromyography in Clinical Practice: A Case Study Approach. St. Louis, Mosby, 1998.

   b. Imaging studies with magnetic resonance imaging (MRI) to exclude a structural lesion (e.g., ganglion cyst, schwannoma, neurofibroma)

Treatment

1. Conservative management of CTS includes several axioms.
   a. Avoid or reduce all provoking factors, if possible.
   b. Correcting medical illness such as hypothyroidism or diabetes is often fruitful.
   c. Neutral wrist splint placement is the first course of treatment. Splint(s) should be worn on the symptomatic hand(s) during sleep. This is successful in about 50% of patients.
   d. Nonsteroidal antiinflammatory drugs (NSAIDs) are useful adjuncts, over a 2- to 3-week course, for temporary relief of CTS symptoms, especially pain, and to reduce swelling in the carpal tunnel.
   e. Oral corticosteroids, given for 1 to 2 weeks, effectively alleviate symptoms of CTS, but their benefits do not last more than several weeks.
   f. Local corticosteroid injection adjacent to the carpal tunnel [e.g., 40–80 mg of methylprednisolone (Depo-Medrol)] can provide immediate relief; it is more effective than oral corticosteroids, and its benefit is usually longer-lasting.
2. Surgical carpal tunnel release is recommended for patients who are symptomatic and have failed the above conservative measures and, among severe CTS cases, those associated with axonal loss or active denervation. This results in an improvement rate of 80% to 90%.

Key Treatment

- Avoiding or reducing all provoking factors
- Treating underlying illness (e.g., hypothyroidism or diabetes)
- Neutral wrist splint placement (first course of treatment)
- NSAIDs
- Oral corticosteroids
- Local corticosteroid injection adjacent to the carpal tunnel (e.g., 40–80 mg of Depo-Medrol)

Prognosis

1. The prognosis of CTS is usually good with either conservative or surgical treatment. Pain and paresthesia are usually the first symptoms that respond well to those measures.
2. The reversal of motor or sensory deficits depends on whether the underlying pathology is demyelination, axonal loss, or a combination of the two. Remyelination is usually complete within several weeks, but axonal loss recovers slowly over several months.
3. In severe cases, the recovery of motor and sensory function may be incomplete.

PROXIMAL MEDIAN NEUROPATHY AND ANTERIOR INTEROSSEOUS NEUROPATHY

1. Proximal median neuropathies are rare. They are usually caused by compression (e.g., from casting

or hematoma), trauma, or venipuncture. The proximal median nerve, especially the anterior interosseous nerve, may be involved in cases of neuralgic amyotrophy.

2. Proximal median nerve entrapment remains controversial. Potential sites of entrapment include the ligament of Struthers, a hypertrophied lacertus fibrosus, the pronator teres muscle, and the sublimis bridge.

3. The clinical features depend on the site of the lesion. Weakness may include some or all of the proximal median forearm muscles, resulting in weak pronation, wrist flexion, and long finger flexion particularly in digits 2 and 3, as well as the median innervated muscles in the hand.

4. Patients with selective anterior interosseous syndrome present with inability to flex the distal phalanx of the thumb and index finger, accompanied by weakness of pronation and no sensory loss. A characteristic compensatory posture occurs when the patient attempts to make the "OK" sign and is unable to flex the distal thumb and index fingers: hyperextension of the distal interphalangeal joint of the index finger and interphalangeal joint of the thumb.

Bibliography

Gerritsen AA, de Vet HC, Scholten RJ, et al.: Splinting vs surgery in the treatment of carpal tunnel syndrome: a randomized controlled trial. JAMA 288:1245–1251, 2002.

Gross PT, Tolomeo EA: Proximal median neuropathies. Neurol Clin 17:425–445, 1999.

Jablecki CK, Andary MT, So YT, et al.: Literature review of the usefulness of nerve conduction studies and electromyography for the evaluation of carpal tunnel syndrome. Muscle Nerve 16:1392–1414, 1993.

Preston DC: Distal median neuropathies. Neurol Clin 17:407–424, 1999.

Report of the Quality Standards Sub-Committee of the American Academy of Neurology: Practice parameter for carpal tunnel syndrome (summary statement) Neurology 43:2406–2409, 1993.

Rosenbaum RB, Ochoa JL: Carpal Tunnel Syndrome and Other Disorders of the Median Nerve. Boston, Butterworth-Heinemann, 1993.

ULNAR NEUROPATHY

Anatomy

1. The ulnar nerve derives its sensory and motor fibers from the C8 and T1 spinal nerves. These fibers pass first through the lower trunk and medial cord of the brachial plexus (Fig. 4–1). The ulnar nerve does not give off branches in the axilla or arm.

2. The ulnar nerve traverses the extensor surface of the elbow joint, in contrast to most major human peripheral nerves, which cross the flexor surfaces of large joints. This renders the nerve more vulnerable to trauma and compression at the elbow.

3. At the elbow level, the ulnar nerve crosses the ulnar (condylar or retroepicondylar) groove behind the medial epicondyle and then passes underneath the humeroulnar arcade (arcuate arcade, or Osborne's band) to enter the cubital tunnel. This aponeurosis is formed by the attachments of the flexor carpi ulnaris muscle to the olecranon and medial epicondyle. Its proximal edge is usually about 1.0 to 1.5 cm distal to the medial epicondyle. With elbow flexion, the distance between the olecranon and medial epicondyle increases by about 1 cm, and the medial elbow ligaments bulge. This results in tightening of the humeroulnar aponeurosis over the nerve and flattening of the concave surface of the ulnar groove.

4. In the forearm the ulnar nerve gives off several branches.
   a. Motor branches to the flexor carpi ulnaris and flexor digitorum profundus
   b. Two cutaneous sensory branches that reach the hand without passing through Guyon's canal at the wrist (see below)
      (1) Palmar cutaneous branch, which takes off at mid-forearm and innervates the proximal part of the ulnar border of the palm
      (2) Dorsal ulnar cutaneous branch, which arises 6 to 8 cm proximal to the ulnar styloid, winds around the ulna, and innervates the dorsal surfaces of the little and half of the ring fingers along with the ulnar side of the dorsum of the hand (Fig. 4–1)

5. At the wrist, the ulnar nerve enters the distal ulnar tunnel (Guyon's canal) where it divides into superficial (primarily sensory) and deep palmar (purely motor) branches (Fig. 4–1).
   a. The superficial branch innervates the palmaris brevis muscle and the palmar aspect of digit V and half of digit IV.
   b. The deep branch innervates the hypothenar muscles and enters the palm through the pisohamate hiatus, a musculotendinous attachment of the flexor brevis digiti minimi between the hook of hamate and the pisiform bone. In the hand, the ulnar nerve supplies all the dorsal and palmar interossei, third and fourth lumbricals, adductor pollicis, and a portion of the flexor pollicis brevis.

Epidemiology

1. Ulnar neuropathy is the second most common entrapment mononeuropathy (second to the carpal tunnel syndrome).

2. With improved orthopedic management of elbow injuries, there has been a decline in the frequency of ulnar neuropathies due to elbow deformity (tardy ulnar palsy).

3. Ulnar neuropathy around the elbow is the most common compressive neuropathy that occurs during anesthesia (followed by brachial plexopathy).

Etiology

1. Ulnar neuropathies may occur at the axilla, arm, elbow, wrist, or palm (Table 4–1).

2. Compression of the ulnar nerve in the elbow region occurs usually at one of the two following sites: the humeroulnar (arcuate) aponeurotic arcade or the ulnar (condylar) groove.
   a. *Ulnar neuropathy at the humeroulnar (arcuate) aponeurotic arcade (cubital tunnel syndrome)* is the most common cause of ulnar neuropathy. It should be suspected in patients with no history of trauma, elbow deformity, or arthritis. The ulnar nerve is compressed by the proximal edge of the humeroulnar (arcuate) aponeurosis. As outlined, during flexion, the distance between the olecranon and medial epicondyle increases by approximately 1 cm, which results in tightening of the ligament over the ulnar nerve. With flexion the medial collateral ligament also

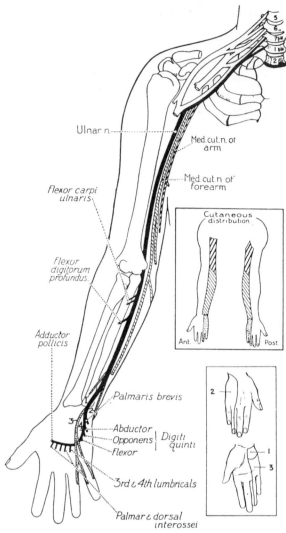

Figure 4–1. Anatomy of the ulnar nerve. *1*, palmar cutaneous branch; *2*, dorsal cutaneous branch; *3*, superficial cutaneous terminal branch; *4*, deep palmar motor terminal branch. (From Haymaker W, Woodhall B: Peripheral Nerve Injuries: Principles of Diagnosis. Philadelphia, W.B. Saunders, 1953, with permission.)

bulges out into the cubital tunnel, thus further compromising the ulnar nerve.

b. *Ulnar neuropathy at the ulnar (retroepicondylar) groove* is also common. It may be due to external pressure, trauma, elbow deformity, or a bony spur. Ulnar nerve subluxation and reduction during elbow flexion and extension, respectively, is a potential cause of repetitive ulnar nerve trauma.

3. *Tardy ulnar palsy* refers to a chronic ulnar neuropathy at the elbow that occurs years after elbow fracture or dislocation. This term is unfortunately misused, particularly by surgeons who often refer to any chronic ulnar neuropathy at the elbow as a tardy ulnar palsy.

4. Ulnar nerve compression at the elbow may occur during anesthesia, coma, intoxication, or pro-

longed bed rest. It often affects men and patients with thin habitus.

5. Ulnar neuropathy at the wrist is relatively rare, with compression by a ganglion accounting for one-half to one-third of cases. Other causes are listed in Table 4–1. Compression of the terminal motor branch at the pisohamate hiatus may occur spontaneously, or it may have an occupational or recreational origin (e.g., using hand tools or prolonged bicycling).

Clinical Features

1. Patients with ulnar neuropathy at the elbow usually presents with intermittent or persistent numbness and tingling of the little finger with variable degrees of hand weakness. Less commonly, patients present with hand weakness and wasting, particularly of the interossei, with no clear sensory symptoms. Pain is less common and, when present, is usually around the elbow.

2. The neurologic examination in patients with ulnar neuropathy at the elbow often reveals sensory impairment to light touch and to pinprick of the

TABLE 4–1. CAUSES OF ULNAR NERVE LESIONS

COMPRESSION SITE	ETIOLOGY
Axilla/upper arm	External pressure
	Crutch palsy
	Internal pressure
	Supracondylar fracture
	Supracondylar spur (Struthers' ligament)
Elbow—ulnar groove	External pressure
	Habitual elbow-leaning ("elbowing")
	Single event (anesthesia)
	Internal pressure
	Repetitive events (occupational repetitive flexion/extension)
	Chronic subluxation
	Elbow joint deformity
	Rheumatoid arthritis
	Valgus deformity
	Healed medial epicondyle fracture
	Mass (ganglion, bone spur, sesamoid bone)
	Fibrosis following trauma
	Idiopathic
Elbow—cubital tunnel syndrome	Internal pressure
	Entrapment by aponeurotic (arcuate) arcade*
Wrist palm—Guyon's canal/pisohamate	External pressure
	Occupational (e.g., hand tools)
	Recreational (e.g., bicycling)
	Internal pressure
	Mass (ganglion,† neuroma, lipoma, cyst, calcification, false aneurysm, giant cell tumor)
	Acute closed injury (fall on hand)
	Carpal bone fracture
	Entrapment

*Most common cause of ulnar neuropathy at the elbow.
†Most common cause of ulnar neuropathy at the wrist.

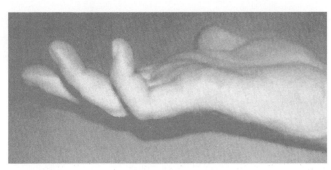

Figure 4–2. Ulnar clawing. (From Haymaker W, Woodhall B: Peripheral Nerve Injuries: Principles of Diagnosis. Philadelphia, W.B. Saunders, 1953, with permission.)

little finger and ulnar half of the ring finger. This impairment may be restricted to the palmar surface or the fingertips. Weakness of ulnar-innervated muscles in the hand (interossei and hypothenar muscles) predominates in ulnar nerve lesions across the elbow, whereas the forearm muscles are affected less often. The flexor digitorum longus to the fourth and fifth digits is assessed by flexing the distal interphalangeal joint of these digits.

3. Three signs are useful when assessing weakness of ulnar-innervated muscles in the hand.

   a. *Ulnar clawing* (*benediction posture*). Inspection of the hand at rest in patients with ulnar neuropathy may reveal hand clawing (Fig. 4–2), which manifests as

      (1) Hyperextension of the metacarpophalangeal joints of the little and ring fingers due to weakness of the third and fourth lumbricals, which allows the extensor digitorum communis to exert unopposed pull

      (2) Flexion of the interphalangeal joints of the same fingers due to the inherent flexion muscle tone of the flexor digitorum profundus and superficialis muscles, whose tendons are now stretched over the metacarpophalangeal joints owing to the above hyperextension

   b. *Wartenberg's sign.* With weakness of abduction of the little finger (due to weakness of the third palmar interosseous muscle), the finger has a tendency to get "hung up" when trying to place the hand in a pocket. On examination, the rested little finger also assumes an abducted posture.

   c. *Froment's sign.* The patient is asked to grasp a piece of paper between the thumb and second digit. Because of weakness of the adductor pollicis (ulnar nerve) and the normal flexor pollicis longus (median nerve), the patient flexes the thumb (i.e., uses the flexor pollicis

longus) as a substitute in an attempt to keep the paper from sliding (Fig. 4–3).

3. Examination of the elbow is often useful, particularly when it is compared to the asymptomatic limb. Elbow deformity or contracture may be useful clues. Palpation of the ulnar nerve at the ulnar groove may reveal nerve enlargement or tenderness. Tinel's sign, produced by percussing the nerve at the elbow, is often positive, but it may be also positive in healthy persons.

4. The manifestations of ulnar neuropathies at the wrist depend on the site of compression (Table 4–2).

   a. Sensation over the dorsum of the hand and the palmar portion of the hypothenar eminence is spared with all types of ulnar neuropathy at the wrist.

   b. One or both terminal ulnar branches (deep palmar motor and ulnar cutaneous) may be compressed at Guyon's canal, but only the deep palmar motor branch is compressed at the pisohamate hiatus.

Key Signs: Ulnar Neuropathies

- Intermittent or persistent numbness and tingling of the little finger, with a variable degree of hand weakness

- Neurologic examination often reveals sensory impairment to light touch and to pinprick of the little finger and ulnar half of the ring finger.

- Three signs are used to assess weakness of ulnar-innervated muscles in the hand.

  —Ulnar clawing (benediction posture)

  —Wartenberg's sign

  —Froment's sign

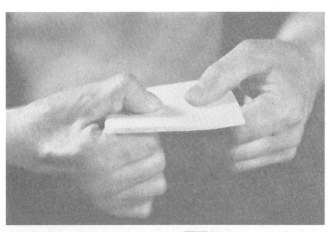

Figure 4–3. Froment's sign. (From Haymaker W, Woodhall B: Peripheral Nerve Injuries: Principles of Diagnosis. Philadelphia, W.B. Saunders, 1953, with permission.)

TABLE 4–2. ULNAR MONONEUROPATHIES AT THE WRIST

LESION SITE	NERVE AFFECTED	CLINICAL PRESENTATION
Proximal Guyon's canal	Main trunk of ulnar nerve *or*	Ulnar palmar sensory loss and weakness of all ulnar intrinsic hand muscles *or*
	Ulnar cutaneous branch	Ulnar palmar sensory loss only
Distal Guyon's canal	Deep palmar branch (proximal to branch to muscles the abductor digiti minimi)	Weakness of all ulnar intrinsic hand (interossei, ulnar lumbricals and hypothenars) without sensory loss
Pisohamate hiatus	Deep palmar branch (distal to branch to the abductor digiti minimi)	Weakness of ulnar intrinsic hand muscles with sparing of the hypothenar muscles and without sensory loss
Mid-palm (rare)	Deep palmar branch (distal to hypothenars)	Weakness of adductor pollicis; first, second and possibly third interossei only; sparing fourth interossei and without sensory loss

From Katirji B. Electromyography in Clinical Practice. St. Louis, Mosby, 1998, with permission.

• Examination of the elbow, comparing it with the asymptomatic limb. Deformity or contracture may be useful clues. Palpation of the ulnar nerve at the ulnar groove may show nerve enlargement or tenderness. Tinel's sign is often positive.

• Manifestations of ulnar neuropathies at the wrist depend on the site of compression.

Differential Diagnosis

1. Ulnar neuropathy at the elbow should be differentiated from ulnar neuropathy at the wrist, C8 radiculopathy, and lower brachial plexopathy (including neurogenic thoracic outlet syndrome).

2. The sensory findings are helpful for localization.

   a. Sensory loss of the dorsal surfaces of the little and ring fingers and the ulnar side of the hand (territory of the dorsal ulnar cutaneous nerve) or the palmar surface of the hypothenar eminence (territory of palmar cutaneous branch) excludes an ulnar lesion at the wrist.

   b. Sparing of sensation to the dorsal surfaces of the little and ring fingers and the ulnar side of the hand does not exclude an ulnar neuropathy at the elbow, as the fascicles of the dorsal ulnar cutaneous nerve may be spared at the elbow.

   c. Sensory loss that splits the ring finger (involves the medial half but not the lateral half) is pathognomonic of an ulnar nerve lesion and excludes a plexopathy or C8 radiculopathy.

   d. Sensory loss extending into the medial forearm (more than 5–6 cm above the wrist) is not compatible with an ulnar nerve lesion. The skin of the medial forearm is innervated by the medial antebrachial cutaneous nerve of the forearm, a branch of the medial cord of the brachial plexus. Abnormalities in this territory suggest a lesion of the lower plexus, the C8 or T1 roots, or the medial antebrachial nerve itself.

Laboratory Testing

1. Electrodiagnostic (EDX) studies are essential for accurate diagnosis, localization, and characterization of ulnar neuropathy at the elbow.

   a. Nerve conduction studies should include an ulnar sensory study, recording the little finger; a dorsal ulnar sensory study, recording the dorsum of the hand; an ulnar motor conduction study (including above- and below-elbow stimulation), recording the hypothenar muscles; and an ulnar motor conduction study (including above- and below-elbow stimulation), recording the first dorsal interosseus muscle. Median nerve sensory and motor conduction studies should also be done. Contralateral studies are often useful for comparison and for detecting bilateral lesions at the elbows.

   b. Needle electromyography (EMG) is useful for confirming an ulnar nerve lesion and assessing the extent of active (ongoing) denervation. In addition, in purely axonal ulnar nerve lesions (without focal or differential slowing, or conduction block), needle EMG is crucial for localizing the lesion to a particular segment of the nerve by establishing that muscles distal to the lesion are abnormal and muscles proximal to it are normal. The first dorsal interosseous, adductor digiti minimi, flexor carpi ulnaris, and ulnar part of the flexor digitorum profundus should be always sampled. Needle EMG is also important for excluding a C8 or T1 radiculopathy or a lower brachial plexopathy. Hence it is mandatory to sample other C8/T1/lower trunk muscles, such the abductor pollicis brevis or flexor pollicis longus (median nerve) and the extensor indicis proprius (radial nerve).

2. There are EDX limitations specific to the ulnar nerve that may render accurate localization of ulnar neuropathies to the elbow difficult.

   a. The ulnar nerve has a considerable degree of redundancy at the elbow, which influences surface measurements of nerve length and thus calculation of nerve conduction velocity. During extension the nerve is slack, resulting in falsely slowed conduction velocities because the impulses travel longer distances than estimated. Hence, it is recommended that ulnar nerve conduction and other measurements be made while the elbow is in the flexed position.

b. The ulnar motor fibers destined for the forearm muscles (flexor carpi ulnaris and flexor digitorum profundus) may be spared with ulnar neuropathy at the elbow (ulnar groove or cubital tunnel). This may be due, in part, to the location of the fascicles in the nerve trunk or to the exit site of the motor branch(es) in relation to the site of compression.

c. The dorsal ulnar sensory fibers may be spared in ulnar nerve lesions at the elbow owing to the fascicular nature of this lesion. Hence, an absent or low-amplitude dorsal ulnar sensory potential excludes a lesion at the wrist or hand, but a normal response does not exclude an ulnar lesion at the elbow.

d. Routine ulnar motor conduction studies recording hypothenar muscles may not reveal a localizing focal slowing, differential slowing, or conduction block. Thus, accurate localization of an ulnar nerve lesion to the elbow is not possible. Adding an ulnar motor conduction study recording of the first dorsal interosseous reveals such localizing features in about 10% to 20% of cases owing to the fascicular nature of the lesion at the elbow.

3. The EDX parameters required to diagnose an ulnar mononeuropathy at the elbow include one or more of the following abnormalities.

a. Decreased (>20%) motor amplitude from the below-elbow to the above-elbow stimulation site (in the absence of a Martin-Gruber anastomosis) when recording the hypothenar muscles, the first dorsal interosseous, or both

b. Conduction velocity slowing (>10 m/s) of the above-elbow to below-elbow segment compared with the below-elbow to wrist segment when recording the hypothenar muscles, the first dorsal interosseus, or both (using moderate elbow flexion of 70° to 90° and maintaining at least 10 cm distance across the elbow)

c. Significant change in the motor response configuration (dispersion) across the elbow

4. In ulnar neuropathy at the wrist, stimulating the ulnar nerve at the wrist and palm, and recording the first dorsal interosseous muscle improve EDX yield, by showing conduction block or focal slowing across the wrist.

5. X-ray films of the elbow and wrist are useful for patients with suspected fractures or dislocations, and they may reveal bony spurs in patients with chronic ulnar nerve lesions. Magnetic resonance imaging (MRI) of the wrist is extremely helpful for delineating compressive masses such as ganglia.

Key Tests: Ulnar Neuropathies

• Electrodiagnostic studies are essential for accurate diagnosis, localization, and characterization of ulnar neuropathy at the elbow.

• X-rays films of the elbow and wrist are useful for suspected fractures or dislocations and may also reveal bony spurs in chronic ulnar nerve lesions.

• MRI of the wrist is helpful for delineating compressive masses such as ganglia.

Treatment

1. Conservative management should be considered in patients with mild lesions, particularly those without axonal loss. Recommended measures include minimizing elbow flexion and avoiding external pressure.

a. Using elbow pads

b. Avoiding arm crossing while sitting

c. Using a book stand for prolonged reading

d. Holding the telephone in the asymptomatic hand only

e. Wrapping a towel loosely around the elbow during sleep or using elbow night splints

2. Surgical intervention may be necessary in patients with weakness due to ulnar nerve lesions at the elbow. It should be initiated before the occurrence of severe weakness or atrophy. Common surgical procedures include medial epicondylectomy, anterior transposition of the ulnar nerve, or simple decompression of the humeroulnar arcade.

3. Apart from eliminating occupational or recreational trauma (e.g., padding for bicycle palsy), surgical intervention is often necessary in patients with ulnar neuropathies at the wrists due to fractures, ganglia, or mass lesions. Similarly, patients who have progressive lesions with no apparent causes, surgical exploration of Guyon's canal extending into the pisohamate hiatus is often indicated.

Prognosis

1. Mild ulnar neuropathies at the elbow respond well to conservative treatment, and moderate and

severe lesions are often treated surgically. The surgical results from the various procedures are similar, with good outcomes in 70% of patients. Poor prognostic factors include diabetes, alcoholism, and end-stage ulnar nerve lesions.

2. The prognosis for ulnar neuropathy at the wrist with conservative treatment is generally good particularly when the EDX study reveals conduction block or slowing. Following surgical decompression, recovery is also relatively rapid because the lesion is distal and reinnervation to the target hand muscles is efficient.

Key Treatment: Ulnar Neuropathies

- Conservative management for mild lesions, particularly without axonal loss. Recommended measures include minimizing elbow flexion and avoiding external pressure.

- Surgery may be necessary for weakness due to ulnar nerve lesions at the elbow and should be initiated before severe weakness or atrophy occurs.

- Surgery is often necessary for ulnar neuropathies at the wrists due to fractures, ganglia, or mass lesions.

RADIAL NEUROPATHY

Anatomy

1. The radial nerve arises from the posterior cord of the brachial plexus after the takeoff of the axillary nerve. It contains fibers from all the contributing roots of the plexus (i.e., C5–T1).

2. In the upper arm, while lying medial to the humerus, the radial nerve supplies the triceps and anconeus muscles. The nerve passes obliquely behind the humerus, first between the lateral and medial heads of the triceps and then through the spiral groove, a shallow groove deep to the lateral head of the triceps muscle (Fig. 4–4). Before entering the spiral groove at mid-arm, it gives off three sensory branches.

   a. Posterior cutaneous nerve of the arm, which innervates the skin overlying the triceps muscle

   b. Lower lateral cutaneous nerve of the arm, which innervates the lateral half of arm

   c. Posterior cutaneous nerve of the forearm, which innervates the extensor surface of the forearm

3. The radial nerve pierces the lateral intermuscular septum below the deltoid insertion and enters the

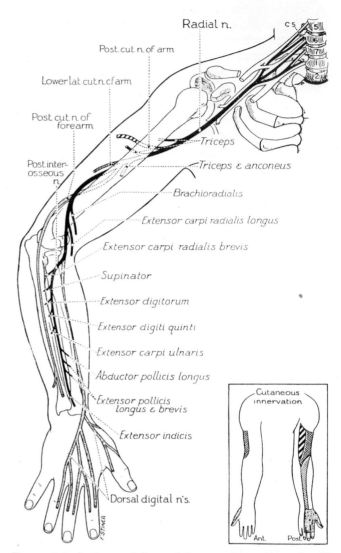

Figure 4–4. Anatomy of the radial nerve. (From Haymaker W, Woodhall B: Peripheral Nerve Injuries: Principles of Diagnosis. Philadelphia, W.B. Saunders, 1953, with permission.)

anterior compartment of the arm, where it innervates the brachioradialis, extensor carpi radialis longus, and extensor carpi radialis brevis.

4. Near the lateral epicondyle, the radial nerve enters the radial tunnel, which is bound by the capitulum of the humerus posteriorly, the brachialis muscle medially, and the brachioradialis and extensor carpi radialis anterolaterly. There, its divides into its terminal branches.

   a. The posterior interosseous nerve, a purely motor branch, innervates the supinator muscle and passes under a membranotendinous arch called the arcade of Frohse. It then travels in the forearm and innervates the rest of the wrist and finger extensors (extensor pollicis longus and brevis, abductor pollicis longus, extensor indicis, extensor carpi ulnaris, extensor digitorum communis, and extensor digiti minimi).

b. The superficial radial nerve, a purely sensory nerve that travels distally, becomes superficial at mid-forearm. It innervates the skin of the proximal two-thirds of the extensor surfaces of the thumb, index, middle finger, and half of the ring finger with the corresponding dorsum of the hand.

Etiology

1. Acute compression of the radial nerve at the spiral groove, where the nerve comes in close contact with the humerus, is the most common cause of radial neuropathy. Such compression often occurs during intoxication by alcohol or drugs (hence the terms Saturday night palsy and honeymoon palsy) or during anesthesia or coma. Other causes include humeral fracture, humeral callus, strenuous muscular effort, injection injury, and open trauma (gunshot or knife wound).

2. The radial nerve may be injured at the axilla in patients using crutches incorrectly or during shoulder surgery. Posterior interosseous neuropathy may be due to mass lesions (e.g., ganglion cysts, tumors) or rarely to nerve entrapment under the tendinous arcade of Frohse (radial tunnel syndrome).

3. Radial sensory neuropathy (cheiralgia paresthetica) is rare. It is often a complication of needle insertion but may be due to tight wristbands or wrist cuffing.

Clinical Features

1. Wrist drop is the most common presentation of proximal radial nerve palsy. With typical radial neuropathy at the spiral groove (Saturday night palsy), there is weakness of the wrist and finger extension and brachioradialis, with preservation of triceps and deltoid function. The brachioradialis, an elbow flexor, is best examined with the arm semipronated. Its weakness is often supported by the absence of the normal bulge with attempted flexion. The brachioradialis reflex is often absent, whereas the triceps jerk is normal. There is also often sensory loss in the dorsum of the hand in the radial territory.

2. Radial sensory neuropathy *(cheiralgia paresthetica)* manifests with sensory loss and variable pain in the radial distribution of the hand with no weakness.

Key Signs: Radial Neuropathies

• Wrist drop

• Sensory loss and variable pain in the radial distribution of the hand with no weakness, indicating radial sensory neuropathy (cheiralgia paresthetica)

Differential Diagnosis

1. Radial nerve lesions, causing wrist and finger drop, must be differentiated from lesions of the posterior interosseus nerve, lesions of the posterior cord of the brachial plexus, and severe C7 and C8 radiculopathies (Table 4–3).

2. The anatomy of the radial nerve renders diagnosing patients with wrist/finger drop relatively easy. Hence examining the following motor functions can help identify most patients with wrist drop: finger extension, wrist extension, elbow flexion with arm in semipronation (brachioradialis), elbow extension (triceps), and shoulder abduction (deltoid).

   a. A posterior interosseous nerve lesion causes weakened finger extension with no associated sensory loss. Characteristically, the lesion spares the brachioradialis (elbow flexion with forearm in semipronation), extensor carpi radialis longus (wrist extension), triceps (elbow extension), and deltoid (arm abduction). Because of sparing the strong extensor carpi radialis longus but weakness of the relatively weak extensor carpi ulnaris, there is often minimal wrist extensor weakness. Also, with attempted wrist extension, there is often radial deviation due to unopposed action of the extensor carpi radialis longus.

   b. A radial nerve lesion at the spiral groove spares the triceps and deltoid muscles. There is often associated radial sensory loss over the dorsum of the hand.

   c. A radial nerve lesion at the axilla spares the deltoid muscle. There is often associated radial sensory loss over the dorsum of the hand, frequently extending to the posterior forearm and arm (distribution of the posterior cutaneous nerves of the arm and forearm).

   d. A posterior cord brachial plexopathy causes weakened finger extension, wrist extension, elbow flexion with arm in semipronation (brachioradialis), elbow extension (triceps), and shoulder abduction (deltoid). The sensory loss

TABLE 4–3. DIFFERENTIAL DIAGNOSIS OF COMMON CAUSES OF WRIST/FINGER DROP

CRITERIA	RADIAL NEUROPATHY AT THE SPIRAL GROOVE	POSTERIOR INTEROSSEUS NEUROPATHY	SEVERE C7 AND C8 RADICULOPATHIES	POSTERIOR CORD BRACHIAL PLEXOPATHY
Clinical Diagnosis				
Common causes	Compression, humeral fracture, injection	Benign tumors, trauma, ? radial tunnel, arcade of Frohse	Disc herniation, spondylosis	Trauma, gunshot
Wrist extension	Weak	Normal	Weak	Weak
Finger extension	Weak	Weak	Weak	Weak
Radial deviation (during wrist extension)	Absent	Present	Absent	Absent
Brachioradialis	Weak	Normal	Normal	Weak
Triceps	Normal*	Normal	Weak	Weak
Wrist flexion, forearm pronation	Normal	Normal	Weak	Normal
Deltoid	Normal	Normal	Normal	Weak
Sensory loss distribution	Radial cutaneous with or without posterior cutaneous of forearm	None	Poorly demarcated to middle, ring, and little fingers	Radial cutaneous, posterior cutaneous of forearm and arm
Brachioradialis reflex	Absent or depressed	Normal	Normal	Absent or depressed
Triceps reflex	Normal*	Normal	Absent or depressed	Absent or depressed
Electrodiagnosis				
Radial motor study (recording EDC)	Low in amplitude or conduction block across the spiral groove	Low in amplitude	Normal or low in amplitude	Low in amplitude
Superficial radial sensory study	Low or absent*	Normal	Normal	Low or absent
Axillary motor study (recording deltoid)	Normal	Normal	Normal	Low in amplitude
Posterior interosseus muscles†	Abnormal	Abnormal	Abnormal	Abnormal
Brachioradialis	Abnormal	Normal	Normal	Abnormal
Other C7,8 muscles‡	Normal	Normal	Abnormal	Normal
Triceps	Normal*	Normal	Abnormal	Abnormal
Deltoid	Normal	Normal	Normal	Abnormal
Paraspinal muscles fibrillations	Absent	Absent	May be absent	Absent

*Extensor digitorum communis (EDC), triceps weakness, loss of triceps reflex, and triceps (and anconeus) denervation can occur when the radial lesion is more proximal (i.e., at the axilla); can be normal in purely demyelinating lesions or lesion of the posterior interosseous nerve.
†Lateral branch (extensor pollicis longus and brevis, abductor pollicis longus, extensor indicis) and medial branch (extensor carpi ulnaris, extensor digitorum communis, extensor digiti minimi).
‡Pronator teres, flexor pollicis longus, flexor carpi radialis in addition to the triceps, and anconeus.
From Katirji B: Electromyography in Clinical Practice. St. Louis, Mosby, 1998, with permission.

is similar to that seen with a high radial lesion but extends into the lateral arm (axillary nerve distribution).

Laboratory Investigations

1. EDX studies are essential for an accurate diagnosis and prognostication of patients with wrist drop and possible radial neuropathies.

2. EDX studies help differentiate radial nerve lesions from lesions of the posterior interosseus nerve, posterior cord of the brachial plexus, or the C7 and C8 roots (Table 4–3).

3. EDX studies are also useful for establishing the site of the radial lesion and excluding a distal lesion (e.g., posterior interosseus neuropathy) or a proximal lesion (e.g., posterior cord lesion).

4. There are two useful localizing findings for radial neuropathy at the spiral groove.

   a. Radial motor conduction block across the spiral groove

   b. Denervation (fibrillation potentials; decreased recruitment; long-duration, high-amplitude, polyphasic motor unit action potentials) of the brachioradialis or extensor carpi radialis longus (or both) with normal triceps, anconeus, and deltoid muscles

5. Another important role of the EDX examination is to determine the prognosis for radial nerve lesions based on the primary pathologic process. This can be achieved by studying the distal radial compound muscle action potential (CMAP) amplitude and area and the distal radial sensory nerve action potential (SNAP) amplitude. With axonal lesions,

the distal radial CMAP, stimulating at the elbow, is absent or low in amplitude/area, and the distal radial SNAP is often absent. However, in demyelinating lesions associated with conduction block, the distal radial CMAP and SNAP are normal on the symptomatic side. For a demyelinating lesion, comparing the CMAP amplitudes/areas and stimulating distal and proximal to the spiral groove is a good method for estimating the number of demyelinated fibers.

6. X-ray films of the humerus are useful in patients with fractures or callus formation. MRI may be useful in patients with slowly progressive radial nerve lesions.

Key Tests: Radial Neuropathies

- Electrodiagnostic studies
- X-ray films

Treatment

1. Acute compressive radial nerve lesions usually are treated conservatively. Active physical therapy, passive range of motion exercises, and wrist and finger splinting are essential for preventing flexion contractures of the wrist and fingers.

2. Surgical intervention is recommended for patients with severe axonal loss lesions, nerves in discontinuity, progressive radial palsies, or lesions showing no signs of reinnervation.

Key Treatment: Radial Neuropathies

- Acute compressive radial nerve lesions usually are treated conservatively with active physical therapy and passive range of motion exercises; splinting is essential for preventing flexion contractures of the wrist and fingers.

- Surgical intervention is undertaken for severe axonal loss lesions, nerves in discontinuity, progressive radial palsies, or lesions showing no signs of reinnervation.

Prognosis

1. Patients with a demyelinating radial nerve lesion recover rapidly within 6 to 8 weeks when further progression is prevented.

2. Patients with a partial axon loss lesion improve slowly over months. Those with severe or complete lesions often require surgical intervention and have a guarded prognosis.

 Bibliography

Brown WF, Watson BV: Quantitation of axon loss and conduction block in acute radial palsies. Muscle Nerve 15:768–773, 1992.

Cowdery SR, Preston DC, Herrmann DN, Logigian EL: Electrodiagnosis of ulnar neuropathy at the wrist: Conduction block versus traditional tests. Neurology 59:420–427, 2002.

Dellon AL, Hament W, Gittelshon A: Non-operative management of cubital tunnel syndrome: an 8-year prospective study. Neurology 43:1673–1677, 1993.

Ehrlich W, Dellon AL, Mackinnon SE: Cheiralgia paresthetica. J Hand Surg [Am] 11:196, 1986.

Jabley ME, Wallace WH, Heckler FR: Internal topography of the major nerves of the forearm and hand. J Hand Surg 5:1–21, 1980.

Katirji B, Dokko Y: Electrodiagnosis of deep palmar ulnar neuropathy at the pisohamate hiatus. Eur J Neurol 3:389–394, 1996.

Kincaid JC: The electrodiagnosis of ulnar neuropathy at the elbow. Muscle Nerve 11:1005–1015, 1988.

AXILLARY NEUROPATHY

Anatomy

1. The axillary nerve fibers originate from C5 and C6 spinal cord segments and pass through the upper trunk and the posterior cord of the brachial plexus.
2. Below the shoulder joint, the axillary nerve (also called the circumflex nerve) traverses the quadrilateral space, bounded superiorly by the teres minor muscle, inferiorly by the teres major muscle, medially by the long head of the triceps muscle, and laterally by the humeral neck.
3. The axillary nerve innervates motor fibers to teres minor and deltoid muscle. The posterior division ends in the upper lateral brachial cutaneous nerve, which innervates the skin overlying the deltoid (Fig. 5–1).

Etiology

1. Common causes of axillary neuropathy include shoulder trauma, anterior dislocation of the humeral head, hematoma associated with fracture, and surgery around the shoulder joint (Table 5–1). Other causes include nerve sheath tumor, neuralgic amyotrophy, and mal-positioning during anesthesia and sleep in prone position with arm raised above the head.
2. The pathology varies from mild neurapraxia (segmental demyelination) to severe axonal neuropathy.
3. Entrapment of the axillary nerve and the posterior humeral circumflex artery in the quadrilateral space by fibrous bands may occur, with trauma as a predisposing factor.

Clinical Findings

1. Axillary nerve lesion leads to weakness of shoulder abduction and extension and paresthesias over the lateral deltoid. In severe lesions, deltoid atrophy is common and can result in loss of muscle contour and flattening of the shoulder. Dysfunction of the nerve produces weakness of the teres minor muscle, which is seldom clinically significant be-

cause the supraspinatus muscle performs similar functions.

2. The quadrilateral space syndrome usually occurs in young athletes. The onset of symptoms is insidious and characterized by pain in the shoulder. The pain increases with shoulder abduction, external rotation, and flexion. External rotation and abduction for 1 minute may induce pain and alter the radial pulsation. In most patients, point tenderness and a trigger point identifies the quadrilateral syndrome. Weakness of the deltoid is uncommon but can be difficult to examine when pain in the shoulder is severe.

Key Clinical Findings: Axillary Neuropathy

- Weakness of shoulder abduction and extension
- Paresthesias over the lateral deltoid
- Deltoid atrophy in severe cases

Differential Diagnosis

1. Axillary neuropathy should be differentiated from C5 and C6 radiculopathies and from posterior cord lesion. Radial innervated muscles are weakened in posterior cord lesion. Weakness of biceps and brachioradialis and their depressed reflexes are common findings in C5 and C6 radiculopathies.
2. Musculoskeletal conditions such as rotator cuff tear, peri-arthropathies, and rupture of the deltoid muscle may present with shoulder pain and apparent weakness of the deltoid muscle, thus mimicking axillary nerve lesions.

Radiologic Findings

1. Plain x-ray and computed tomography (CT) scan are useful in traumatic axillary neuropathies. They are helpful in demonstrating fracture and dislocation of the humeral head and scapula, callus and osteophyte formation following trauma, and bone tumors. Magnetic resonance imaging (MRI) is useful in excluding rotator cuff tear and showing soft tissue masses.

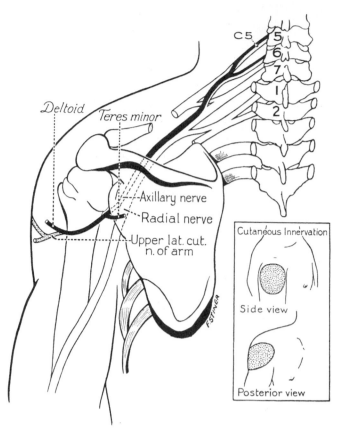

Figure 5–1. Anatomy of the axillary nerve. (From Haymaker W, Woodhall B: Peripheral Nerve Injuries. Principles of Diagnosis. Philadelphia, W.B. Saunders, 1953, with permission).

2. Axillary and posterior circumflex arteriograms are useful for detecting pseudoaneurysms. Posterior circumflex artery signal drop after arm abduction on the arteriogram is characteristic of quadrilateral space syndrome.

Laboratory Testing

1. Electrodiagnostic (EDX) evaluation in axillary mononeuropathy is restricted to needle electromyography (EMG) findings of the deltoid and teres minor muscles, which usually reveals fibrillation potentials and decreased recruitment of large motor unit action potentials (MUAPs).

2. Axillary motor conduction studies are important in prognosis. The axillary compound muscle action potential (CMAP), recording from the deltoid muscle, is usually normal in demyelinating lesions and low in axonal lesions.

3. Radial sensory nerve action potential (SNAP) and CMAP are reduced in amplitude in posterior cord lesions. Needle EMG shows fibrillation and large MUAPs in the radial nerve innervated muscles. In C5 or C6 radiculopathy, needle EMG reveals additional denervation in the biceps, brachioradi-

alis, supraspinatus, infraspinatus, or rhomboid muscles.

Treatment

1. The treatment of axillary neuropathies depends on the cause and severity, and on the duration of symptoms. The axillary nerve travels a short distance from its origin to the muscles, and recovery is usually expected within a few months.

2. Physical therapy to maintain shoulder range of motion and to strengthen shoulder muscles is the mainstay of conservative treatment.

3. Surgical treatment is reserved for mass lesions, severed nerve, delayed recovery, and, sometimes, decompression for quadrilateral space syndrome.

Key Treatment: Axillary Neuropathy

- Treatment depends on the cause and severity, and on the duration of symptoms

- Physical therapy

- Surgical treatment for mass lesions, severed nerve, delayed recovery, and, sometimes, decompression for quadrilateral space syndrome

Prognosis

1. Most blunt traumatic axillary neuropathies are due to neurapraxia; therefore, spontaneous recovery is expected. Neuralgic amyotrophy and quadrilateral space syndrome have good prognosis and rarely require surgical intervention.

2. In the absence of active physical therapy and good pain control, axillary neuropathy may result in frozen shoulder syndrome (adhesive capsulitis), a disabling complication in elderly patients.

TABLE 5–1. COMMON CAUSES OF AXILLARY MONONEUROPATHY

Trauma
  Shoulder dislocation
  Fracture of neck of humerus
  Blunt trauma
Iatrogenic
  During shoulder joint surgery
  Injection injury
Idiopathic
  Brachial plexitis (neuralgic amyotrophy)

Adapted from Katirji B. Electromyography in Clinical Practice. St. Louis, Mosby, 1988.

MUSCULOCUTANEOUS NERVE

Anatomy, Etiology, and Pathogenesis

1. The musculocutaneous nerve fibers originate from C5 and C6 spinal cord segments and pass through the upper trunk and lateral cord of the brachial plexus. The nerve pierces the coracobrachialis muscle and runs in the space between the brachialis and biceps muscles. The musculocutaneous nerve supplies motor fibers to coracobrachialis, brachialis, and biceps muscles. It ends as the lateral antebrachial cutaneous nerve, which innervates the skin of the lateral forearm to the thumb (Fig. 5–2).

2. The nerve is rarely injured in the arm but is commonly involved in a brachial plexus lesion, such as postoperative upper trunk brachial paralysis. Shoulder dislocation may rarely cause an isolated musculocutaneous injury. Strenuous exercise such as weight lifting may compress the nerve within the coracobrachialis muscle. Surgical operation around the shoulder or axilla may result in musculocutaneous neuropathy. Other traumatic causes include gunshot, stab wound, and blunt trauma. Nerve sheath tumors and lipomas are extremely rare causes of musculocutaneous neuropathy.

3. Isolated lesion of the lateral antebrachial nerve may occur with venipuncture, surgery, or blunt trauma to the antecubital fossa. The nerve may be entrapped by the lateral edge of the biceps tendon (Olson's point).

Clinical Findings

1. Musculocutaneous neuropathy presents with variable features depending on the location of the lesion.

   a. Proximal musculocutaneous neuropathy usually has predominant motor symptoms (weakness of elbow flexion) and variable sensory loss in the lateral forearm. Wasting is seen in chronic lesions. Pain may occur in the arm, elbow, or forearm.

   b. Distal musculocutaneous lesion (i.e., lateral antebrachial neuropathy) usually presents with radial forearm paresthesia. Tenderness to palpation or percussion, Tinel's sign at the elbow crease, and sensory loss in the lateral forearm may be present on examination. Relief of sensory symptoms after injecting local anesthetic at Olson's point may serve as a diagnostic test.

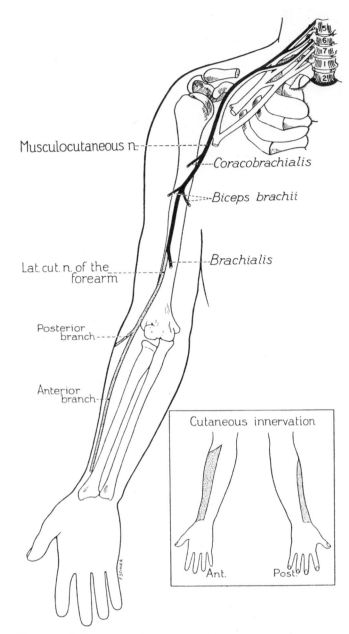

Figure 5–2. Anatomy of the musculocutaneous nerve. (From Haymaker W, Woodhall B: Peripheral Nerve Injuries. Principles of Diagnosis, Philadelphia. W.B. Saunders, 1953, with permission).

Key Clinical Findings: Musculocutaneous Neuropathies

- Features depend on the location of the lesion.

- Proximal musculocutaneous neuropathy: predominant motor symptoms (weakness of elbow flexion) and variable sensory loss in the lateral forearm

- Distal musculocutaneous neuropathy: radial forearm paresthesia, tenderness to palpation or percussion, Tinel's sign at the elbow crease, and sensory loss in the lateral forearm

Differential Diagnosis

1. Lateral cord and upper trunk brachial plexopathies and C5-C6 radiculopathies may mimic a musculocutaneous neuropathy. In addition to weakness of elbow flexion (biceps and brachialis), there is weakness of the deltoid, brachioradialis, and pronator teres in upper trunk lesions, and weakness of pronator teres and flexor carpi radialis in lateral cord lesions.

2. Rupture of biceps muscle tendon presents with pain, swelling, and weakness of elbow flexion. However, there is usually a mass in the arm consistent with contracted biceps muscle.

Laboratory Testing

1. EDX testing is the mainstay of diagnosing musculocutaneous neuropathy. Musculocutaneous CMAP, recording from the biceps muscle, is typically reduced in amplitude in the presence of clinical muscle weakness. Lateral antebrachial SNAP is reduced in amplitude or absent. Needle EMG usually show fibrillation potentials in the biceps and brachialis muscles.

2. Imaging has a limited use in musculocutaneous neuropathy. Plain x-ray and CT scan are useful in skeletal lesions, and MRI is better for soft tissue masses.

Treatment

1. Treatment is conservative with active physical therapy. Entrapment syndrome at the elbow requires modification of activity and/or posterior splint. Pain control with oral medication and injection with local anesthetics or steroids may be tried.

2. Gunshot wounds, stab wounds, fracture and dislocation, neoplasm, and, rarely, entrapment at the elbow may require surgical intervention. Tendon transplantation sometimes is useful for severe traumatic lesions.

Key Treatment: Musculocutaneous Neuropathies

- Conservative, with active physical therapy

- Oral medication, local injection with local anesthetics, or steroids for pain

- Surgical intervention for severe traumatic lesions and other serious conditions

Prognosis

1. The prognosis depends on the cause of the musculocutaneous nerve lesion. In general, a lesion responding to conservative therapy has a better prognosis. Postoperative neuropraxia has excellent prognosis.

SUPRASCAPULAR NEUROPATHY

Anatomy

1. The suprascapular nerve is pure motor nerve. Its fibers originate from C5 and C6 spinal cord segments and pass through the upper trunk.

2. The nerve emerges from the upper trunk, passes underneath the trapezius muscle and traverses the suprascapular notch beneath the superior transverse scapular ligament. The suprascapular nerve enters the supraspinous fossa, where it innervates the supraspinatus muscle. It continues through the spinoglenoid notch underneath the inferior transverse scapular ligament to enter the infraspinous fossa, where it innervates the infraspinatus muscle (Fig. 5–3).

3. Blunt trauma (from falls, motor vehicle accidents, and athletic injuries) is the most common cause of suprascapular neuropathy. Repetitive forceful shoulder movement, with scapular excursion articularly, in athletes such as baseball players, may cause entrapment at the suprascapular notch. Mass lesions at the suprascapular notch (such as ganglion), may compress the suprascapular nerve. Neuralgic amyotrophy may selectively affect the suprascapular nerve and the denervation may be restricted to one or both spinatus muscles.

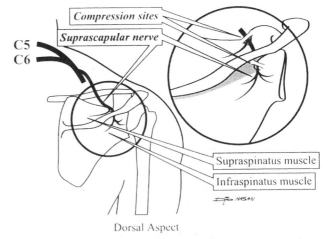

Figure 5–3. Anatomy of the suprascapular nerve. (From Staal A, van Gijn J, Spaans F: Mononeuropathies. Examination, Diagnsosis and Treatment. London, W.B. Saunders, 1999, with permission).

Clinical Findings

1. Suprascapular neuropathy usually affects men more than women. It is often unilateral and commonly affects the dominant limb.

2. Pain is the most common manifestation of suprascapular neuropathy; it is usually diffuse and poorly localizing to the shoulder. Pain may radiate to the neck and arm. The pain increases with traction on the nerve by active cross-body shoulder adduction of the extended arm.

3. Suprascapular neuropathy may also present with painless weakness or atrophy of the shoulder. Weakness usually involves both the supraspinatus and infraspinatus muscles if the lesion is high at the suprascapular notch. Weakness involves only the infraspinatus if the lesion is low, at the spinoglenoid notch. Examination may confirm weakness in shoulder abduction and/or external rotation.

Key Clinical Findings: Suprascapular Neuropathy

- Often, shoulder area pain that may radiate to neck and arm

- May present with painless shoulder weakness or atrophy

- Suprascapular notch lesion: usually supraspinatus and infraspinatus muscles are weak

- Spinoglenoid notch lesion: infraspinatus muscle only is weak

Differential Diagnosis

1. Many orthopedic conditions presenting with shoulder abduction impairment and pain simulate suprascapular neuropathy. These include rotator cuff syndrome, tendinitis of the supraspinatus muscle and frozen shoulder. MRI and needle EMG are useful to differentiate the lesion.

2. Clinical, EDX, and radiographic studies help to differentiate suprascapular neuropathy from C5-C6 radiculopathies and upper trunk brachial plexopathy, where there is also weakness of the deltoid, biceps, and brachioradialis, and a depressed or absent biceps reflex.

Laboratory Testing

1. MRI and ultrasound are useful in excluding structural lesions such as mass or ganglion, and ligament calcification. They are also helpful in assessing other causes of shoulder pain such as rotator cuff tear.

2. EDX testing should always include needle EMG because both the supraspinatus and infraspinatus muscles are easily accessible. Fibrillation and neurogenic MUAPs are the classical finding in axonal damage.

3. EDX testing helps to exclude C5-C6 radiculopathies by showing fibrillation potentials in deltoid, biceps, brachioradialis, and pronator teres, as well as the supraspinatus and infraspinatus. Cervical paraspinal muscles may also reveal fibrillation potentials. Upper trunk plexopathy characteristically shows also reduced or non-elicitable SNAP amplitudes in the lateral antebrachial or the median nerve. Neuralgic amyotrophy may be difficult to differentiate from entrapped suprascapular nerve. Neuralgic amyotrophy tends to be acute and associated with selective involvement of the infraspinatus or supraspinatus muscles.

Treatment

1. Treatment should be directed to the specific cause. Entrapment under the suprascapular or spinoglenoid notch can be treated conservatively with rest. If pain continues or muscle wasting is demonstrated, then surgical decompression is indicated. Cyst and ganglion can be treated with drainage under ultrasound or CT guidance.

2. With isolated infraspinatus weakness, the compression could be at the spinoglenoid notch, or more proximal at the suprascapular notch, affecting the suprascapular nerve fascicles to the infraspinatus muscle. Thus, surgical decompression at both levels is indicated.

Key Treatment: Suprascapular Neuropathy

- Treatment should be directed at the specific cause.

Prognosis

1. The prognosis depends in large part on the extent of axonal loss and the cause of the neuropathy.

2. Entrapment at the suprascapular or spinoglenoid notch treated successfully by surgical decompression has good prognosis with respect to pain control and recovery of muscle strength. Surgical treatment of ganglion cysts generally provides adequate pain relief but does not restore muscle strength.

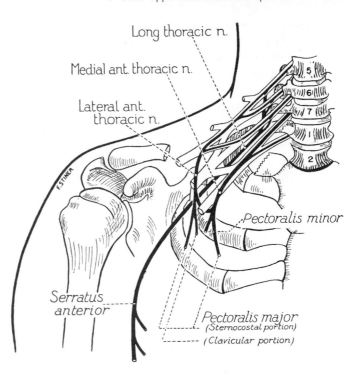

Figure 5–4. Anatomy of the long thoracic nerve. (From Haymaker W, Woodhall B: Peripheral Nerve Injuries. Principles of Diagnosis. Philadelphia, W.B. Saunders, 1953, with permission).

LONG THORACIC NERVE

Anatomy, Etiology and Pathogenesis

1. Fibers to the long thoracic nerve originate from the C5, C6, and C7 segments of the spinal cord. The nerve is a pure motor nerve to the serratus anterior muscle. The nerve courses down to, through, and anterior to the medial scalenus muscle and dorsal to the brachial plexus (Fig. 5–4).

2. Neuralgic amyotrophy often involves the long thoracic nerve. Varieties of athletic activities may damage the long thoracic nerve, including volleyball, tennis, professional ballet, and archery. Trauma from carrying heavy load on the back or pushing loads above the head or falling on outstretched hand can cause long thoracic neuropathy. Surgical operations such as first rib resection or scalenotomy may damage the long thoracic nerve.

Clinical Findings

1. Patients with long thoracic neuropathy usually present with difficulty with shoulder elevation such as combing their hair or shaving. Weakness may be associated with a dull ache in the shoulder.

2. Examination confirms winging of the medial border of the scapula, which limits shoulder abduction.

Key Clinical Findings: Long Thoracic Neuropathy

- Difficulty with shoulder elevation
- Dull ache in the shoulder
- Winging of the medial border of the scapula

Differential Diagnosis

1. Winging of the scapula as a result of serratus anterior muscle weakness may resemble trapezius muscle weakness.

   a. At rest, the scapular winging is striking in trapezius weakness, the shoulder sags significantly, and the scapula is displaced laterally from the midline. In contrast, with serratus anterior weakness, there is little change in the appearance of the shoulder girdle at rest, and the scapular translocation is medial.

   b. Shoulder abduction accentuates scapular winging with trapezius weakness, whereas with serratus anterior weakness, forward flexion of the shoulder (particularly to 45 degrees below horizontal) or protraction against resistance worsens the scapular winging.

2. C5-C6 radiculopathies, upper trunk brachial plexopathy, and myopathy (such as facioscapulohumeral muscular dystrophy) should be considered in the differential diagnosis of long thoracic neuropathy.

3. Scapular fracture and rheumatoid arthritis can cause rupture of the serratus anterior muscle at the level of insertion, which can present with similar winging of the scapula.

Laboratory Testing

1. Needle EMG is the mainstay of diagnosis of long thoracic neuropathy. Needle EMG of the serratus anterior muscle often shows fibrillation potentials and impaired recruitment of large MUAPs in long thoracic neuropathy.

2. EDX testing is also helpful to rule out C5 or C6 radiculopathies, upper trunk brachial plexopathy, and myopathy.

Treatment

1. Treatment should be directed to the underlying cause. Neuralgic amyotrophy is often self-limiting. Surgery should only be considered in cases of structural lesion or to stabilize the scapula after longstanding winging.

Key Treatment: Long Thoracic Nerve

- Treatment should be directed at the underlying cause.

Bibliography

Cahill BR, Palmer RE: Quadrilateral space syndrome. J Hand Surg 8:65, 1983.

Fritz RC, Helms CA, Steinbach LS, Genant HK: Suprascapular nerve entrapment: evaluation with MR imaging. Radiology 182:437, 1992.

Liveson JA, Bronson MJ, Pollack MA: Suprascapular nerve lesions at the spinoglenoid notch: report of three cases and review of the literature. J Neurol Neurosurg Psychiatry 54:241–243, 1991.

Mastaglia FL: Musculocutaneous neuropathy after strenuous physical activity. Med J Aust 145:153–154, 1986.

Wiater JM. Flatow EL: Long thoracic nerve injury. Clin Orthoped Rel Res 368:17–27, 1999.

6 Peroneal, Sciatic and Tibial Neuropathies

Bashar Katirji

ANATOMY

1. The sciatic nerve originates from the L4, L5, S1, and S2 spinal roots after the exits of the superior and inferior gluteal nerves. It is composed of a lateral division, named the *common peroneal nerve* or the *lateral popliteal nerve,* and a medial division named the *tibial nerve* or the *medial popliteal nerve.* Though enclosed in a common sheath, these two nerves are separate from the outset and do not exchange any fascicles.

2. The sciatic nerve leaves the pelvis via the sciatic notch, where the nerve lies in close relation with the piriformis muscle, a flat pyramidal muscle that originate at the front of the sacrum, the gluteal surface of the ilium, and the anterior capsule of the sacroiliac joint. The piriformis muscle, which externally rotates and abducts the hip while in the flexed position, leaves the pelvis via the greater sciatic foramen and inserts into the upper border of the greater trochanter. Usually, the sciatic nerve passes underneath the piriformis muscle; Sometimes, however, only the peroneal division passes through or above the piriformis muscle, and rarely the entire sciatic nerve pierces the piriformis muscle or passes above it.

3. In the thigh, the tibial component of the sciatic nerve innervates most hamstring muscles (semitendinosus, semimembranosus, and long head of biceps femoris), and supplies a branch to the adductor magnus, while the common peroneal component innervates the short head of biceps femoris only (Fig. 6–1A). Usually, the common peroneal and tibial nerves physically separate in the upper popliteal fossa. The common peroneal nerve travels laterally and sweeps around the fibular head to travel in the anterior leg, and the tibial nerve continues posteriorly in the midline to enter the calf (Fig. 6–1B).

4. The common peroneal nerve gives off the lateral cutaneous nerve of the calf, soon after its formation, which innervates the skin over the upper third of the lateral aspect of the leg (Fig. 6–2A). Then, the common peroneal nerve winds around the fibular neck and divides into its terminal branches, the deep and superficial peroneal nerves (Fig. 6–2B).

5. The deep peroneal nerve innervates the tibialis anterior, extensor hallucis, peroneus tertius, and extensor digitorum longus. Slightly proximal to the ankle joint, the deep peroneal nerve passes under the extensor retinaculum to innervate the extensor digitorum brevis and the skin of the web space between the first and second toes (Fig. 6–2A and B).

6. The superficial peroneal nerve gives motor branches to the peroneus longus and brevis. Then, it pierces the crural fascia approximately 10 cm proximal to the lateral malleolus, to become subcutaneous. It innervates the skin of the lower two thirds of the lateral aspect of the leg and the dorsum of the foot, except for the first web space (Fig. 6–2A and B).

7. Soon after it separates from the common peroneal nerve, the tibial nerve gives off its first branch, the sural nerve, a purely sensory nerve that innervates the skin over lateral aspect of the lower leg and foot including the little toe. In the upper calf, the tibial nerve dips underneath the tendinous arch of soleus muscle and innervates the gastrocnemius, soleus, tibialis posterior, flexor digitorum profundus, and flexor hallucis longus (Fig. 148–1B). At the ankle, the tibial nerve passes posterior to the medial malleolus and through the tarsal tunnel to enter the foot. There, the tibial nerve divides into its three terminal branches:

   a. the calcaneal branch, a purely sensory nerve, that innervates the skin of the sole of the heel

   b. the medial plantar nerve, which innervates the abductor hallucis, flexor digitorum brevis, and flexor hallucis brevis in addition to the skin of the medial sole and, at least, the medial three toes (Fig. 6–3)

   c. the lateral plantar nerve which innervates the abductor digiti quinti pedis, flexor digiti quinti pedis, adductor hallucis, and the interossei, in addition to the skin of the lateral sole and two lateral toes.

PERONEAL AND SCIATIC NEUROPATHIES

Epidemiology

1. Peroneal neuropathy is the most common compressive neuropathy in the lower limb. All age groups are equally affected, but the disorder is

more common in men. Most peroneal nerve lesions are unilateral, while bilateral lesions constitute about 10% of all the cases.

2. Among all peroneal neuropathies, lesions of the common peroneal nerve at the fibular neck are the most common. Selective deep peroneal neuropathies and proximal (high) common peroneal nerve lesions are much less common, each constituting about 5% of all peroneal nerve lesions. It is extremely rare for peroneal nerve lesions at the fibular neck to affect the superficial peroneal nerve only, without greater damage to the deep peroneal nerve.

3. Sciatic nerve lesions are rare. Sciatic nerve compression in the region of the piriformis muscle ("the piriformis syndrome") is a debated syndrome but it is an uncommon cause of buttock and leg pain ("sciatica")

Etiology and Pathophysiology

1. Peroneal mononeuropathies around the fibular neck are usually caused by nerve compression or by knee trauma (Table 6–1). In compressive

lesions, the common peroneal nerve is often trapped between an external object and the fibular neck.

2. Typically, the deep peroneal nerve is more severely affected than the superficial peroneal nerve, and, occasionally, only the deep peroneal nerve is compressed. This phenomenon is related to the topographical arrangement of the common peroneal nerve around the fibular neck. The exiting fascicles, forming the superficial branch, are placed laterally while the deep peroneal branch is located medially in direct contact with the fibula.

3. Partial lesions of the sciatic nerve in the upper thigh usually affect the lateral division (peroneal nerve) more than the adjacent medial division (tibial nerve). On rare occasions, the common peroneal nerve is the only nerve injured, leaving the tibial nerve completely intact. The greater vulnerability of the peroneal division of the sciatic nerve to physical injury has several causes:

a. The difference in the fascicular pattern of the perineurium between these two nerves in the upper thigh. The peroneal nerve has fewer and

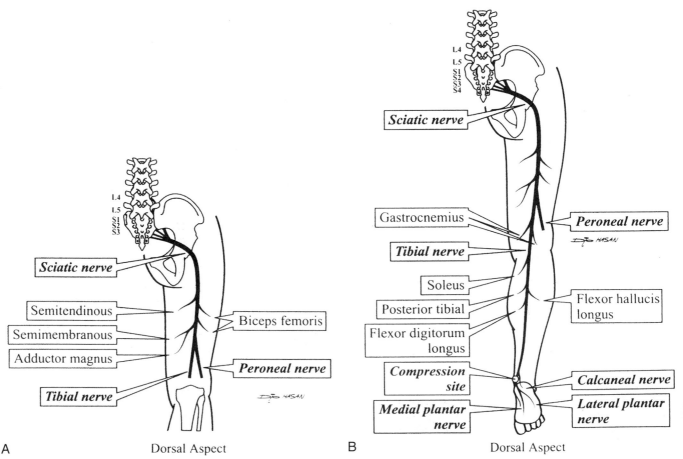

A Dorsal Aspect B Dorsal Aspect

Figure 6–1. *A.* The sciatic nerve in the thigh with its branches. *B.* The tibial nerve with its motor and terminal branches. (From Staal A, van Gijn J, Spaans F: Mononeuropathies. Examination, Diagnosis and Treatment. London, W.B. Saunders, 1999, with permission).

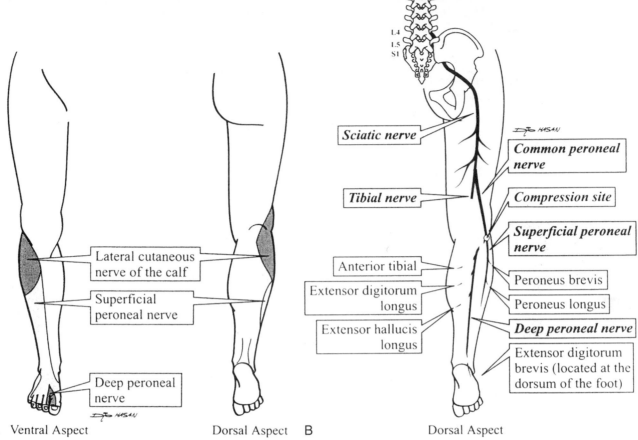

Figure 6–2. *A.* The common, deep, and superficial peroneal nerves with their motor branches. *B.* Cutaneous innervation of the branches of the common peroneal nerve. (From Staal A, van Gijn J, Spaans F: Mononeuropathies. Examination, Diagnosis and Treatment. London, W.B. Saunders, 1999, with permission).

larger fascicles with limited supportive tissue, while the tibial nerve is composed of many cushioning fascicles, well placed between the elastic epineurial tissue. This renders the peroneal division of the sciatic nerve more susceptible to external pressure.

b. The anatomical course of the common peroneal and tibial nerves; the peroneal nerve is taut and secured at the sciatic notch and fibular neck, whereas the tibial nerve is loosely fixed posteriorly. As a result, traction of the sciatic nerve in the upper thigh (such as during total hip replacement) will result in earlier and more extensive damage to the peroneal nerve than the tibial nerve.

4. Sciatic nerve lesions and high common peroneal nerve lesions are usually associated with total hip replacement, hip fracture/dislocation, femur fracture, gluteal injection, gluteal compartment syndrome, gunshot or knife wound, and acute compression during coma, drug overdose, intensive care unit, or prolonged sitting.

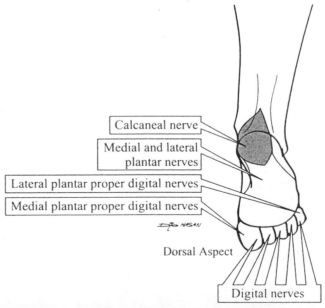

Figure 6–3. Cutaneous innervation of the sole and heel by the tibial nerve. (From Staal A, van Gijn J, Spaans F: Mononeuropathies. Examination, Diagnosis and Treatment. London, W.B. Saunders, 1999, with permission).

TABLE 6–1. CAUSES OF PERONEAL NERVE LESIONS AT THE FIBULAR NECK

Compression	Trauma	Mass Lesions
During anesthesia	Blunt	Extrinsic
Weight loss	Fibular fracture	Osteochondroma
Habitual leg crossing	Ligamental knee	Baker's cyst
Prolonged	joint rupture	Ganglion cyst
hospitalization	Knee dislocation	Hematoma
Prolonged bed rest	Tibio-fibular joint	Pseudoaneurysm
Anorexia nervosa	dislocation	Intrinsic
Coma	Ankle sprain	Schwannoma
Diabetes mellitus	Open laceration	Neurofibroma
Peripheral	Gunshot wound	Neurogenic
polyneuropathy	Animal bite	sarcoma
Prolonged squatting	Iatrogenic	
Yoga	Conventional knee	
Crop harvesting	surgery	
Childbirth	Knee joint	
Iatrogenic	replacement	
Knee cast	Arthroscopic knee	
Ankle-foot orthosis	surgery	
Pneumatic		
compression		
Anti-thrombotic		
stocking		
Bandage		
Strap		
Lithotomy position		
Intrauterine (with		
breech presentation)		

Clinical Features

1. Peroneal neuropathy at the fibular neck usually presents with an acute foot drop. Less often, the foot drop may be subacute, developing gradually over days or weeks. Subjective numbness, mostly on the dorsum of the foot, but occasionally extending into the lower lateral leg, is common. Pain, usually mild, is rare.

2. The neurologic examination of a patient with common peroneal neuropathy reveals weakness of ankle and toe dorsiflexion, and ankle eversion; ankle inversion, toe flexion, and plantar flexion are spared. A steppage gait may be evident in patients with significant foot drop. Deep tendon reflexes are normal. Hypesthesia or hyperesthesia to touch and pain is common and limited to the lower two thirds of the lateral leg and dorsum of foot. In some patients, Tinel's sign may be elicited by percussion of the peroneal nerve around the fibular neck. In selective deep peroneal nerve lesions, ankle eversion is normal and there is no sensory loss (except sometimes in the first web space).

Key Clinical Findings: Common Peroneal Neuropathy

• Weakness of ankle and toe dorsiflexion and ankle eversion

• Sensory change of lower two thirds of the lateral leg and dorsum of foot

• Tinel's sign

3. Common peroneal neuropathy in the upper thigh presents with foot drop with neurologic findings similar to lesions at the fibular neck. The only possible clinical sign is that the numbness in the lateral leg may extend into the knee, by following the distribution of the lateral cutaneous nerve of the calf (Fig. 6–2B). Although the short head of biceps femoris is weak with high common peroneal lesions, this muscle cannot be evaluated satisfactorily in isolation with manual muscle testing, because its function is often overshadowed by the more powerful hamstring muscles (semitendinosus, semimembranosus, and long head of biceps femoris), all innervated by the tibial nerve. Also, it cannot be palpated during such testing because of its location deep to the long head of the biceps femoris.

4. Sciatic mononeuropathy presents with weakness, pain, and sensory loss. Often foot drop dominates the picture, because the peroneal component is usually more affected than the tibial component. Careful examination often reveals weakness of knee flexion, plantar flexion, or ankle inversion. However, severe sciatic nerve lesions are associated with a flail foot (i.e., weak foot and ankle in all directions) and hamstring weakness. Foot pain and dysesthesia are common symptoms of sciatic nerve injuries and signs of reflex sympathetic dystrophy (allodynia with skin, nail and bone dystrophic changes) are not uncommon late manifestations of the nerve injury. The ankle jerk is usually depressed or absent and the sensory loss and dysesthesia involves the sole, the dorsum of the foot, and the lateral leg.

Key Clinical Findings: Sciatic Neuropathy

• Usually peroneal >tibial weakness (often foot drop)

• Foot pain and dysesthesias

• Sensory loss of the sole and dorsum of the foot and lateral leg

• Ankle jerk decreased or absent

Differential Diagnosis

1. The first step in the diagnosis of peroneal and sciatic neuropathy is to differentiate foot drop from a *flail foot*. Foot drop is defined as severe weakness of ankle dorsiflexion with intact plantar

flexion, while in a flail foot there is no or minimal ankle or foot movement in all directions, including severe weakness of ankle dorsiflexion, plantar flexion, and intrinsic foot muscles. In contrast to a flail foot, voluntary movement at or distal to the ankle occurs in foot drop because plantar flexion and the intrinsic foot muscles remain intact.

2. The clinical evaluation often leads to the correct diagnosis of peroneal neuropathy, particularly in the appropriate clinical setting. For example, a patient who awakens a prolonged surgical procedure such as craniotomy or coronary artery bypass surgery with a foot drop and normal plantar flexion most likely has a compressive peroneal nerve lesion at the fibular neck.

3. Unilateral peroneal neuropathy should be differentiated from L5 radiculopathy, sciatic nerve lesion or lumbosacral plexopathy (Table 6–2). In general, radicular pain and a positive straight leg test (Lasègue's sign) are common in L5 radiculopathy, may be present in sciatic nerve lesions, but are not seen in common peroneal mononeuropathy at the fibular neck. Weakness of ankle inversion, toe flexion or plantar flexion, or absent/depressed ankle jerk are inconsistent findings of peroneal nerve lesion.

4. Acute unilateral foot drop may be a manifestation of the *anterior compartmental syndrome of the leg,* in which increased pressure within a limited space (anterior leg compartment) compromises the perfusion, circulation, and function of the contents of that space. This may occur after limb trauma (crush, contusion, fractures), spontaneous bleeding into a compartment, or strenuous exercise such as running. A compartmental syndrome is a is a state of emergency and a tissue pressure above 60 mm Hg is usually diagnostic. Anterior compartmental syndrome of the leg often results in foot drop because the anterior compartment contains all muscles that functions as ankle and toe evertors (tibialis anterior, extensor hallucis, and extensor

digitorum longus). Characteristic findings of anterior compartmental syndrome not present in other causes of foot drop include:

a. Severe leg pain, out of proportion to what is anticipated from the clinical situation

b. Pain on flexion of toes and plantar flexion of ankle, which lead to passive stretch of the anterior compartmental muscles of the leg

c. A tenseness of the anterior compartmental fascia

5. Partial sciatic nerve lesions presenting with foot drop should be differentiated from peroneal mononeuropathy, lumbosacral radiculopathy, and lumbosacral plexopathy (Table 6–2). In contrast, severe sciatic nerve lesions pose little difficulty in diagnosis because the weakness involves all muscles along the knee and the hamstrings, and because the sensory loss below the knee spans both the peroneal and tibial distributions, sparing the medial leg (saphenous nerve distribution).

Laboratory Testing

1. Establishing the diagnosis of peroneal mononeuropathy may be based on clinical grounds, but often requires electrodiagnostic (EDX) confirmation. The EDX studies in patients with suspected peroneal neuropathy are extremely useful, with the following objectives:

a. Confirm that the foot drop is due to a lesion of the common or deep peroneal nerves, and exclude other causes of foot drop such as L5 radiculopathy and sciatic mononeuropathy.

b. Localize the site of the peroneal nerve lesion (common or deep peroneal nerve at fibular neck or common peroneal nerve in the upper thigh).

c. Define the lesion's primary pathophysiologic mechanism (demyelinating versus axonal versus mixed).

TABLE 6–2. DIFFERENTIAL DIAGNOSIS OF COMMON CAUSES OF FOOT DROP

	Common Peroneal Neuropathy at the Fibular Head	L5 Radiculopathy	Lumbar Plexopathy (Lumbosacral Trunk)	Sciatic Neuropathy (Mainly or Exclusively Peroneal)
Common causes	Compression (weight loss, perioperative, iatrogenic); blunt and open trauma	Disc herniation; lumbar spinal stenosis	Prolonged labor; pelvic fracture; hematoma	Hip surgery; injection injury; coma
Ankle inversion	Normal	Weak	Weak	Normal or mildly weak
Toe flexion	Normal	Weak	Weak	Normal or mildly weak
Plantar flexion	Normal	Normal	Normal	Normal or mildly weak
Ankle jerk	Normal	Normal (unless with S1)	Normal (unless with S1)	Normal or depressed
Sensory loss	Peroneal distribution only	Poorly demarcated, predominantly big toe	Well demarcated to L5 dermatome	Peroneal and lateral cutaneous of calf
Pain	Rare, deep	Common, radicular	Common, can be radicular	Can be severe

From Katirji B. Electromyography in Clinical Practice. St. Louis, Mosby, 1998, with permission.

d. Predict the prognosis and expected course of recovery.

e. Assess the presence and extent of reinnervation (in axonal loss lesions).

2. The EDX findings in peroneal neuropathies may reveal a demyelinative conduction block, axonal loss, or mixed patterns (Table 6–3). The axonal lesions may be further localized to the upper thigh or between the fibular and upper thigh, based on whether there is denervation of the short head of the biceps femoris or not. Selective deep peroneal neuropathies are much less common and often are axonal in type.

3. A proximal (high) common peroneal lesion often presents a diagnostic challenge because it imitates a lesion at the fibular neck. When the tibial component of the sciatic nerve is also involved, there is often sensory loss in the sole with weakness of plantar flexion, depressed/absent ankle jerk, asymmetrically low (or sometimes absent) sural sensory nerve action potential (SNAP) amplitude or abnormal H-reflex, borderline or low tibial compound muscle action potential (CMAP) amplitude, or neurogenic changes in tibial-innervated muscles (such as the gastrocnemius, tibialis posterior, or flexor digitorum longus). When the lesion affects the common peroneal nerve selectively, however, the clinical and EDX findings are identical to an axon loss distal common peroneal neuropathy. However, needle electromyogram (EMG) of the short head of biceps femoris, the only hamstring muscle innervated by the peroneal division of the sciatic nerve, reveals signs of denervation only in proximal (high) common peroneal mononeuropathies and is normal in distal lesions such as at the fibular neck. This muscle is difficult to examine in isolation on manual muscle testing, but is easily accessible to needle EMG examination.

Treatment

1. Ankle-foot orthosis, to improve gait and prevent ankle contractures and sprains, is indicated when the foot drop is profound, axonal, or expected to have a protracted course. Active foot exercises and passive range of movements are useful.

2. Patients with peroneal neuropathy associated with significant weight loss should be warned about leg crossing, and should wear protective knee pads, properly placed over the fibular head and neck, to prevent recurrent external compression.

3. Sciatic nerve lesions often require pain management with tricyclic antidepressants or anticonvulsants.

4. Patients with axon-loss peroneal nerve lesions

around the fibular neck should be observed for 4 to 6 months to allow for improvement by spontaneous reinnervation. Severe lesions often require sequential EDX examination to look for early evidence of reinnervation and follow its progression.

5. Surgical intervention for treatment of the peroneal nerve is indicated with nerve laceration or a mass lesion, and is often appropriate with progressive peroneal mononeuropathies and in severe axonal lesions with no clinical or EMG evidence of reinnervation 4 to 6 months from injury. Surgical interventions to treat the sciatic nerve are often indicated in patients with lacerations, trauma, or severe stretch injuries.

Key Treatment

Foot Drop
- Orthosis
- Active foot exercises

Sciatic Nerve Lesions
- Tricyclic or antidepressant anticonvulsants
- Surgery

Prognosis

1. Peroneal nerve injury may result in significant disability, mostly from foot drop, which may not recover completely or in a timely manner, particularly when axonal loss is severe.

2. Significant axonal loss, which carries a relatively poor prognosis, is present in about 80% of cases of nerve lesions (based on a low-amplitude distal peroneal motor response). This occurs independent of the mode of onset (i.e., in acute, subacute, or undetermined onset lesions) and applies equally to all compressive peroneal lesions, including perioperative cases. This finding is in contrast to the common belief that acute perioperative compressive peroneal lesions are due to neurapraxia (i.e., segmental demyelination) and should recover rapidly. Even patients with acute perioperative compressive nerve lesions at the fibular neck have a higher likelihood of harboring axon loss.

3. Compressive peroneal neuropathies at the fibular neck caused by demyelinative conduction block often have good prognosis with spontaneous recovery in 2 to 3 months as long as further compression is prevented.

4. The prognosis of sciatic nerve lesions is generally guarded and many patients are left with chronic

TABLE 6–3. ELECTROPHYSIOLOGIC PATTERNS OF PERONEAL MONONEUROPATHIES

Pattern	Site of Lesion	Frequency	Superficial Peroneal SNAP	Distal Peroneal CMAPs[a]	Conduction Block at Fibular Head	Focal Slowing Across the Fibular Head	Needle EMG of Peroneus Longus	Needle EMG of Biceps Femoris (Short Head)	Prognosis for Recovery
Conduction block	Fibular head	20%–30%	Normal	Normal	Present	Rare	Abnormal	Normal	Excellent
Axonal loss	Mid-thigh and fibular head[b]	45%–50%	Usually absent	Low amplitude or absent	Absent	Absent	Abnormal	Normal	Protracted
	Deep peroneal	5%	Normal	Low amplitude or absent	Absent	Absent	Normal	Normal	Fair
	Proximal[c]	<5%	Usually absent	Low amplitude or absent	Absent	Absent	Abnormal	Abnormal	Very poor
Mixed	Fibular head	25%–30%	Low amplitude or absent	Low amplitude	Present	Rare	Abnormal	Normal	Biphasic

Abbreviations: SNAP, sensory nerve action potential, CMAP, compound muscle action potential, EMG, electromyogram.
[a]Recording tibialis anterior and extensor digitorum brevis.
[b]Usually around the fibular head.
[c]High, proximal to the gluteal fold.
From Katirji B. Peroneal neuropathy. Neurol Clin 17:567-591, 1999, with permission.

foot pain. Patients with severe lesions have significant residual weakness while the weakness in partial lesions may improve significantly.

TIBIAL NEUROPATHIES (TARSAL TUNNEL SYNDROME)

Definition

Tarsal tunnel syndrome (TTS) is the most common tibial neuropathy. It is caused by compression of the tibial nerve or any of its three terminal branches under the flexor retinaculum.

Epidemiology

The incidence and prevalence of compression of the tibial nerve or one of its terminal branches at the ankle (TTS) in the general population is unknown. The disorder is clearly much less common than the carpal tunnel syndrome.

Etiology and Pathophysiology

Most cases are idiopathic, but ankle trauma, particularly sprains and fractures, arthritis and tenosynovitis of the ankle, ill-fitting footwear, or heel varus and valgus deformity may be associated with TTS.

Clinical Features

1. Tarsal tunnel syndrome usually presents with burning pain, which may worsen after prolonged standing or walking, and numbness in the sole of the foot and heel.

2. The neurologic examination reveals sensory impairment in the sole in the distribution of one or all of the terminal tibial branches (medial plantar, lateral plantar, or calcaneal). Tinel's sign, induced by percussion of the tibial nerve at the flexor retinaculum (behind the medial malleolus), is present in most patients.

Key Clinical Findings: Tarsal Tunnel Syndrome

- Burning pain worse after prolonged standing or walking
- Numbness in the sole of the foot and heel
- Tinel's sign

Differential Diagnosis

1. Tarsal tunnel syndrome may be difficult to distinguish from other common orthopedic and rheu- matologic conditions such as plantar fasciitis, stress fracture, arthritis, or bursitis. However, the pain in these conditions is usually worse in the morning, improves with walking, and is not associated with paresthesia or Tinel's phenomenon.

2. S1 or S2 radiculopathy may result in foot numbness or pain, which is often worse with walking or standing. However, there is usually low back and posterior thigh pain, depressed or absent ankle jerk, or weakness of gastrocnemius or glutei muscles.

3. Distinguishing patients with bilateral TTS from those with early sensory peripheral polyneuropathy may be difficult. A useful feature is that TTS is not commonly bilateral whereas peripheral polyneuropathy often affects both feet. Also, the sensory loss in polyneuropathy usually involves both the sole and the dorsum of foot and is rarely associated with Tinel's sign at the flexor retinaculum.

Laboratory Testing

1. Plain x-rays, tomogram, and bone scan are usually normal in TTS, but all are useful in revealing other causes of foot pain such as stress fracture or arthritis. Magnetic resonance imaging of the ankle may reveal a ganglion cyst, neuroma, or lipoma in the region of the flexor retinaculum.

2. Several EDX techniques are used to assess for TTS. Most of these involve assessing sensory or motor nerve fibers that traverse the medial or the lateral plantar nerves.

   a. Tibial motor nerve conduction studies, recording from the abductor hallucis (medial plantar nerve) and the abductor digiti quinti pedis (lateral plantar nerve) but are easy to perform, they are not sensitive. Prolonged medial and/or lateral plantar distal latencies are considered diagnostic.

   b. Mixed medial and lateral plantar nerve conduction studies are the counterparts of the median and ulnar palmar mixed studies performed for the evaluation of carpal tunnel syndrome. This test is more sensitive than the tibial motor distal latencies test. Asymmetric slowing of latency of the medial or lateral (or both) mixed nerve action potentials is considered abnormal. Unfortunately, it may be technically difficult to elicit these potentials in subjects with foot calluses, ankle edema, or foot deformities, or even in normal adults over 45 years of age.

   c. Sensory medial and lateral nerve conduction studies are extremely low in amplitude (and sometimes absent) in normal subjects and require signal averaging.

Treatment

1. Conservative treatment should be initiated and includes minimizing ankle edema by elevation and special stockings and control of heel valgus or varus with an orthotic insole or lateral foot wedge. Ill-fitting footwear should be eliminated. Nonsteroidal anti-inflammatory agents or local injection with long-acting corticosteroids may be also useful.

2. Surgical intervention is indicated in patients with identifiable mass lesions. Surgical release of the flexor retinaculum may be required in a small proportion of patients.

Key Treatment

- Minimizing ankle edema by elevation and special stockings, control of heel valgus or varus with an orthotic insole or lateral foot wedge

- Nonsteroidal anti-inflammatory agents or local injection with long-acting corticosteroids

- Surgery for identifiable mass lesions

Prognosis

1. Most patients improve without any sequela.
2. Some patients may not improve despite surgical

intervention or go on to develop chronic pain syndromes and features of reflex sympathetic dystrophy.

Bibliography

Galardi G, Amadio S, Maderna L, et al.: Electrophysiologic studies of tarsal tunnel syndrome. Diagnostic reliability of motor distal latency, mixed nerve and sensory nerve conduction studies. Am J Phys Med Rehab 73:193–198, 1994.

Katirji B: Peroneal neuropathy. Neurol Clin 17:567–591, 1999.

Katirji MB, Wilbourn AJ: High sciatic lesions mimicking peroneal neuropathy at the fibular head. J Neurol Sci 121:172–175, 1994.

Katirji MB, Wilbourn AJ: Common peroneal mononeuropathy: a clinical and electrophysiologic study of 116 lesions. Neurology 38:1723–1728, 1988.

Kim DH, Kline DG: Management and results of peroneal nerve lesions. Neurosurgery 39:312–319, 1996.

Oh SH, Meyer RD: Entrapment neuropathies of the tibial (posterior tibial) nerve. Neurol Clin 17:593–615, 1999.

Sourkes M, Stewart JD: Common peroneal neuropathy: a study of selective motor and sensory involvement. Neurology 41:1029–1033, 1991.

Yuen EC, Olney RK, So YT: Sciatic neuropathy: clinical and prognostic features in 73 patients. Neurology 44:1669–1674, 1994.

Yuen EC, So YT, Olney RK: The electrophysiologic features of sciatic neuropathy in 100 patients. Muscle Nerve 18:414–420, 1995.

FEMORAL NEUROPATHIES

Anatomy

1. The femoral nerve is formed by the combination of the posterior divisions of the ventral rami of L2, L3, and L4 spinal roots. Soon after its formation in the pelvis, it innervates the psoas muscle, which receives additional branches directly from the L3 and L4 roots. The femoral nerve passes between the psoas and iliacus muscles within the iliacus compartment which is covered by the tight iliacus fascia. Before crossing the inguinal ligament, the femoral nerve supplies the iliacus muscle.

2. The femoral nerve emerges from the pelvis after passing underneath the inguinal ligament in the groin and branches widely into

   a. terminal motor branches to the rectus femoris, quadriceps, and sartorius muscles

   b. three terminal sensory branches, the medial and intermediate cutaneous nerve of the thigh, which innervate the skin of the anterior thigh, and the saphenous sensory nerve, which innervates the skin of the medial surface of the knee and the medial leg (Fig. 7–1).

Epidemiology

1. The incidence and prevalence of femoral neuropathy is unknown.

2. Estimated frequencies of iatrogenic femoral nerve injury after certain procedures are as follows:

   a. 7% to 11% after abdominal hysterectomy

   b. 2% after total hip replacement

   c. 0.1% after femoral artery cannulation for cardiac catheterization resulting in retroperitoneal hemorrhage: The prevalence of retroperitoneal hemorrhage is about 0.5%, and about a third of such hemorrhages result in femoral nerve injury or a lumbar plexopathy.

   d. 2.8/100,000 deliveries during lithotomy positioning for vaginal delivery: This is likely underestimated and represents only patients with severe femoral nerve lesions necessitating neurologic consultations.

Etiology

1. Most femoral mononeuropathies are iatrogenic, and the femoral nerve is usually injured at one of two sites, the retroperitoneal pelvic space or the inguinal ligament.

2. Iatrogenic femoral neuropathy during pelvic surgical procedures is the most common cause of femoral nerve injury. This occurs most commonly during abdominal hysterectomy, but it may complicate radical prostatectomy, renal transplantation, colectomy, proctectomy, inguinal herniorrhaphy, lumbar sympathectomy, appendectomy, tubal sterilization, abdominal aortic repair, and a variety of other intraabdominal vascular, urologic or gynecologic operations. During these surgical procedures, the lateral blade of the retractor compresses the intrapelvic portion of the femoral nerve against the pelvic wall. Rarely, intrapelvic postoperative femoral lesions are caused by ischemia, retroperitoneal hematoma, or inadvertent laceration or suturing of the femoral nerve.

3. Femoral neuropathy associated with iliacus *or* retroperitoneal hematoma is not uncommon. Acute hemorrhage in the iliacus compartment may lead to a compartmental syndrome that results in iliopsoas muscle or femoral nerve ischemia or both. Occasionally, the hematoma is large and extends into the psoas muscle or retroperitoneal space, leading to more extensive injury of the lumbar plexus or the entire lumbosacral plexus. These hematomas are usually spontaneous as complications of anticoagulant therapy (heparin or warfarin), hemophilia, or other blood dyscrasias. They may also occur with ruptured abdominal aortic aneurysm, pelvic operations, or femoral artery (and less commonly femoral vein) catheterization for coronary, cerebral, and aortic angiography.

4. Femoral neuropathy due to lithotomy positioning used for vaginal delivery. The risk is higher with prolonged lithotomy positioning, particularly with extreme hip flexion and external rotation. These lesions are likely underestimated because most are mild and resolve rapidly. Similar femoral nerve lesions occur with other procedures in which the patient is placed in lithotomy position, such as vaginal hysterectomy, prostatectomy, and laparos-

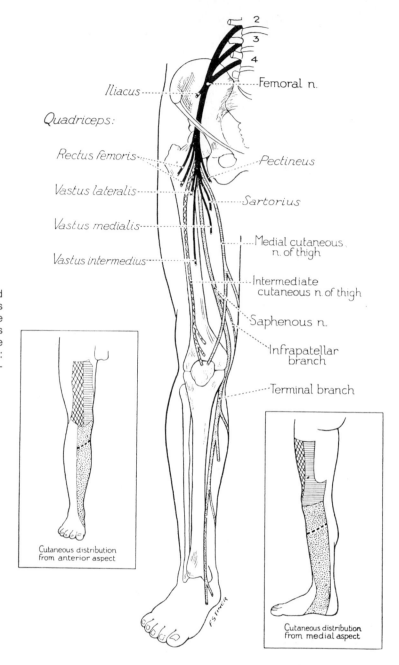

2
3
4

Iliacus
Quadriceps:
Rectus femoris
Vastus lateralis
Vastus medialis
Vastus intermedius

Femoral n.
Pectineus
Sartorius
Medial cutaneous n. of thigh
Intermediate cutaneous n. of thigh
Saphenous n.
Infrapatellar branch
Terminal branch

Cutaneous distribution from anterior aspect

Cutaneous distribution from medial aspect

Figure 7–1. The femoral nerve and its terminal motor and sensory branches and cutaneous distribution. The patterns of the cutaneous nerves are duplicated in the inserts. The broken line in the inserts represents the boundaries between the infrapatellar and terminal branches of the saphenous nerve. (From Haymaker W, Woodhall B: Peripheral Nerve Injuries. Principles of Diagnosis. Philadelphia, W.B. Saunders, 1953, with permission).

copy. During such positioning, the femoral nerve becomes compressed by the rigid inguinal ligament.

5. Other causes of femoral neuropathy include

   a. Surgical procedures of the hip joint, particularly revisions of total hip replacements and complicated reconstructions, where the femoral injury is due to misplacement of the anterior acetabular retractors during the procedure

   b. Pelvic masses (as in lymphadenopathy, abscess, cyst, enlarged iliac or aortic aneurysm, or tumor)

   c. Femoral nerve tumors such as neurofibromas,

schwannomas, and neurogenic sarcomas are relatively rare.

   d. Open nerve injuries such as penetrating gunshot and stab wounds, lacerations, and contusions associated with pelvic fractures

   e. Traumatic stretch may occur with hyperextension of the hip, such as in dancers, or with prolonged squatting such as during Yoga exercise.

6. The term *diabetic femoral neuropathy* is a misnomer and should be abandoned. Diabetic patients develop extensive peripheral nerve disease involving the lumbosacral plexus and spinal roots consistent with diabetic radiculoplexopathy, also

known as *diabetic amyotrophy* or *diabetic proximal neuropathy*. Although the brunt of weakness in these patients often falls on the quadriceps muscle, mimicking selective femoral nerve injuries, careful clinical and needle EMG examinations reveal more widespread involvement of thigh adductors, hip flexors, and, sometimes, foot dorsiflexors.

Clinical Features

1. Femoral nerve lesions usually present acutely with thigh weakness and anterior thigh and leg numbness. Patients frequently complain that their leg buckles underneath them; such buckling may lead to falls.

2. The neurologic examination reveals weakness of the quadriceps with absent or depressed knee jerk. Hip flexion weakness due to involvement of the iliopsoas muscle is important for localizing the site of the lesion. Usually, hip flexion is weak when the lesion is intrapelvic (such as during pelvic surgery) but normal when the lesion is at the inguinal region (such as during lithotomy positioning). However, evaluating hip flexion may be difficult in patients with pain such as following pelvic surgery or vaginal delivery, or with iliacus hematoma. Hypesthesia over the anterior thigh and medial calf is common.

3. Groin or thigh pain is usually mild in femoral nerve lesions. However, it may be severe when associated with iliacus or retroperitoneal hemorrhage. In such instances, the patient may keep the hip flexed and the reversed straight leg test will be positive.

Key Clinical Findings: Femoral Neuropathy

- Acute quadriceps and hip flexor weakness
- Numbness of the anterior thigh and medial calf
- Absent or decreased knee jerk

Differential Diagnosis

1. Femoral neuropathy should be differentiated from an upper lumbar (L2, L3, and L4) radiculopathy and lumbar plexopathy. The thigh adductors, innervated by the L2, L3, and L4 roots via the obturator nerve, are spared in femoral nerve lesion while they are often weak in upper lumbar radiculopathy or lumbar plexopathy. Also, weakness of the tibialis anterior, innervated by the L4 and L5 roots via the common peroneal nerve, may

occur with L4 radiculopathy or lumbar plexopathy, but not with femoral neuropathy.

2. The sensory manifestations in mild femoral nerve lesions may be confused with meralgia paresthetica. The latter causes sensory loss in the lateral thigh that does not extend beyond the knee.

Laboratory Evaluation

1. Imaging studies of the pelvis (computed tomography [CT] scan or magnetic resonance imaging [MRI]) should be obtained urgently in patients with acute femoral neuropathy and suspected iliacus or retroperitoneal hematoma, such as in the setting of anticoagulation, coagulopathy, or femoral vessel catheterization. CT or MRI of the pelvis will also be useful in patients with a suspected pelvic mass lesion or femoral nerve tumor.

2. The electrodiagnostic (EDX) testing in a patient with suspected femoral neuropathy is extremely useful for the following reasons:
   a. It confirms the presence of a selective femoral mononeuropathy.
   b. It excludes a lumbar plexopathy and radiculopathy.
   c. It localizes the site of femoral nerve injury.
   d. It predicts the prognosis by assessing the primarily pathophysiologic process (segmental demyelination or axonal loss).

3. On sensory nerve conduction studies, the saphenous sensory nerve action potential, which should be studied bilaterally for comparison, is often absent in femoral neuropathy and lumbar plexopathy but normal in L4 radiculopathy (intraspinal lesion proximal to the dorsal root ganglion; Table 7–1). This response may be normal in "purely" demyelinating femoral mononeuropathies and if the nerve conduction studies are done in the first 10 days from onset of an axon-loss femoral nerve lesion (prior to the completion of Wallerian degeneration).

4. On motor nerve conduction studies, femoral motor amplitude and/or area, obtained after 5 days from acute femoral nerve injury is the best estimate of the extent of axonal loss and prognosis.
   a. If the femoral motor amplitude and/or area are low or absent, the lesion is primarily axonal. Recovery is relatively protracted because it will depend on sprouting and reinnervation.
   b. If the femoral motor amplitude and/or area are normal (with significant reduction of motor unit action potential (MUAP) recruitment on needle electromyogram—EMG), the lesion is primarily demyelinating and the prognosis is

TABLE 7–1.   ELECTRODIAGNOSTIC DIFFERENTIAL DIAGNOSIS OF FEMORAL NEUROPATHY

	FEMORAL NEUROPATHY	LUMBAR PLEXOPATHY	LUMBAR RADICULOPATHY
Thigh adductors (hip adduction)	Normal	Denervation	Denervation
Tibialis anterior (ankle dorsiflexion)	Normal	Denervation[a]	Denervation[a]
Saphenous sensory nerve action potential[b]	Low or absent[c]	Low or absent[c]	Normal
Lumbar paraspinal fibrillation potentials	Absent	Absent	Usually present

[a] Abnormal in L4 radiculopathy/plexopathy only.
[b] May be technically difficult, particularly in elderly patients or if there is leg edema.
[c] Normal in purely demyelinating lesions and if tested <10 days after acute axon-loss lesions.
Adapted from Katirji B: Electromyography in Clinical Practice. St Louis, Mosby, 1998, with permission.

excellent because recovery is dependent on remyelination.

5. Needle EMG in femoral mononeuropathy reveals fibrillation potentials and decreased recruitment of MUAPs in the quadriceps muscle in all patients. In patients with intrapelvic lesions, similar changes are present in the iliacus muscle, which is normal in femoral lesions around the inguinal ligament. The thigh adductors (L2/L3/L4-obturator nerve) are normal in femoral neuropathy, whereas they often show neurogenic changes in patients with upper lumbar radiculopathy or plexopathy (Table 149–1). In L4 radiculopathy, neurogenic changes may be also be present in the tibialis anterior (L4/L5-common peroneal nerve).

Treatment

1. Patients with iliacus or retroperitoneal hematoma require emergent surgical drainage or aspiration. The evacuation should occur before signs of severe femoral nerve injury occur. There is ongoing controversy regarding the indication and timing of surgical evacuation of hematoma once a femoral nerve lesion has become severe. There is no evidence that surgical treatment improves the neurologic outcome in these patients.

2. A knee-ankle-foot orthosis is helpful for patients with severe weakness of the quadriceps to assist in walking and prevent falls.

3. Tricyclic antidepressants or anticonvulsants may be used for the delayed pain and hyperesthesia associated with femoral nerve lesions.

Prognosis

1. As outlined, the femoral motor amplitude is the best estimate of the extent of axonal loss and is the only independent factor influencing prognosis. In contrast, fibrillation potentials, which are highly sensitive (i.e., identified in patients with minimal axonal loss), are a poor quantitative measure of the extent of axonal loss.

   a. Patients with femoral motor amplitude on

motor nerve conduction studies more than 50% of the contralateral side improve within 1 year.

   b. Fewer than half the patients with an amplitude less than 50% of the contralateral side improve in the course of 1 year.

2. Despite the above, and compared to other axon-loss peripheral nerve lesions, axon-loss femoral nerve lesions carry a relatively good prognosis, because of the nerve's short length. The quadriceps, which is the most clinically relevant muscle, is proximal and relatively near the injury sites (the inguinal ligament or pelvis). These optimal conditions often lead to effective sprouting and reinnervation in axonal loss lesions.

3. Demyelinative femoral nerve lesions, as occur after childbirth or laparoscopy, often resolve in 2 to 3 months by remyelination.

4. Prevention of iatrogenic femoral nerve lesions is essential.

   a. Elimination of retractors, particularly self-retractors, during pelvic surgery decreases the incidence of postoperative femoral neuropathy.

   b. Avoidance of prolonged lithotomy positioning, particularly extreme hip flexion and external rotation, may prevent the occurrence of femoral neuropathies during childbirth and other gynecologic and urologic procedures.

OTHER LOWER LIMB NEUROPATHIES

Definition

1. The lower limb is innervated by two main large nerves, the sciatic nerve (with its common peroneal and tibial branches) and the femoral nerve.

2. There are several small nerves in the lower limbs, most of which are proximal sensory nerves. Exceptions are the obturator nerve, which is a motor nerve with a minor sensory contribution, and the saphenous nerve, which is distal.

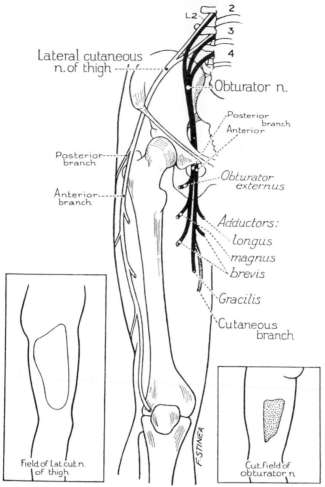

Figure 7–2. The lateral cutaneous nerve of the thigh and the obturator nerves. (From Haymaker W, Woodhall B: Peripheral Nerve Injuries. Principles of Diagnosis. Philadelphia, W.B. Saunders, 1953, with permission).

Anatomy

1. *The lateral cutaneous nerve of the thigh (lateral femoral cutaneous nerve)* is formed from sensory fibers originating from the ventral rami of L2, and L3 spinal roots. The nerve travels within the lower abdominal muscles, crosses the iliacus muscle, and passes underneath the inguinal ligament near its insertion at the anterior superior iliac spine. The lateral cutaneous nerve of the thigh pierces the fascia lata below the inguinal ligament and innervates the skin of the lateral thigh. The sensory territory of the lateral cutaneous nerve of the thigh does not extend beyond the knee, and seldom extends across the anterior or posterior midline of the thigh (Fig. 7–2).

2. *The ilioinguinal nerve* originates from L1 spinal root and follows the abdominal wall in much the same way as an intercostal nerve and innervates the lower abdominal muscles. Near the anterior superior iliac spine, the ilioinguinal nerve pierces the transverse and internal oblique muscles and

innervates a strip of skin along the inguinal ligament to the base of the penis and scrotum in men or the labia majora in women (Fig. 7–3).

3. *The genitofemoral nerve* is formed from the L1 and L2 spinal roots and divides near the inguinal ligament into femoral and genital branches. The femoral branch passes under the inguinal ligament and innervates a small area of skin on the anterior aspect of the thigh. The genital branch travels medially, with the ilioinguinal nerve, to supply the cremasteric muscle and the scrotum or labium majus (Fig. 7–3).

4. *The iliohypogastric nerve* originates from the L1 spinal root and crosses the lower border of the kidney. Near the iliac crest, it divides into two cutaneous terminal branches, a lateral branch that innervates a small strip of skin in the upper lateral buttock, and an anterior branch that innervates a small area of skin above the pubic symphysis.

5. *The saphenous nerve* is a terminal branch of the femoral nerve (see above). It travels in the thigh posteromedially from the femoral triangle through the subsartorial (Hunter's or adductor) canal. At the knee, it gives off the infrapatellar branch, which innervates the skin over the anterior surface of the patella. In the lower third of the leg, it divides into two terminal branches to innervate the skin of the medial surface of the knee, the medial leg, the medial malleolus, and a small area of the medial arch of the foot (Fig. 7–1).

6. *The obturator nerve* derives its fibers from the

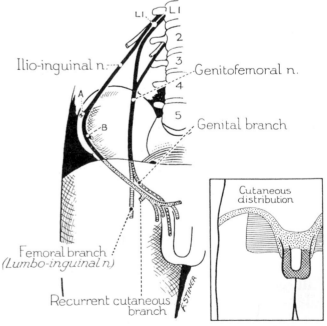

Figure 7–3. The ilioinguinal and genitofemoral nerves. A and B are motor branches to the abdominal muscles. (From Haymaker W, Woodhall B: Peripheral Nerve Injuries. Principles of Diagnosis. Philadelphia, W.B. Saunders, 1953, with permission).

TABLE 7–2. OTHER LOWER LIMB MONONEUROPATHIES

Nerve	Etiology	Clinical Features	Differential Diagnosis	Management
Lateral femoral cutaneous (meralgia paresthetica)	Entrapment at the inguinal ligament (idiopathic, pregnancy, obesity, diabetes, tight belt, large belt, beeper), pelvic mass, pelvic hematoma, or abdominal surgery	Paresthesia and pain (deep and superficial) in lateral thigh; exam: well-demarcated sensory impairment of the lateral thigh. Sensory conduction study is technically difficult	L3 or L2 radiculopathy; femoral neuropathy	Conservative, since most resolve in months; local steroids and anesthetic injections are sometimes helpful; decompression at the inguinal ligament is rarely required
Ilioinguinal (inguinal neuralgia)	Inguinal hernia repair, appendectomy, retroperitoneal mass or incision	Burning pain in the lower abdomen, groin radiating to the scrotum (in men) and upper thigh, worse with walking; exam: sensory disturbance along inguinal ligament	Genitofemoral neuropathy (diagnostic nerve block might be required), L1 or L2 radiculopathy, hip joint disease	Analgesia and nerve blocks in postoperative cases; rarely, surgical exploration
Genitofemoral	Appendectomy, inguinal hernia repair	Painful paresthesias in upper thigh, scrotum, and medial groin; exam: sensory disturbance in scrotum (in men) and upper thigh, absence of cremasteric reflex	Ilioinguinal neuropathy (diagnostic nerve block might be required), L1 or L2 radiculopathy, hip joint disease	Conservative
Iliohypogastric	Retroperitoneal mass or incision (nephrectomy)	Asymmetrical abdominal wall bulging and trivial sensory loss in suprapubic area	Ilioinguinal or genitofemoral neuropathy, L1 or L2 radiculopathy	Conservative
Saphenous	Surgery for varicose veins or removal of saphenous vein for coronary artery graft; knee surgery, entrapment at Hunter's canal	Numbness of medial thigh with variable pain; exam: sensory loss in medial thigh. Saphenous sensory conduction study is useful	L4 radiculopathy, mild femoral neuropathy	Conservative; exploration of Hunter's canal is rarely indicated
Obturator	Hip surgery, pelvic fracture, obturator hernia, malignant neoplasm	Leg weakness, pain, and paresthesias in thigh and inner leg; exam: weakness of thigh adductors	L2 and L3 radiculopathy, lumbar plexopathy, femoral neuropathy	Dependent on primary cause; surgical exploration is rarely required

Modified from Katirji B. Entrapments of the lower extremity. In Samuels MA, Feske S (eds), Office Practice of Neurology. Edinburgh, Churchill Livingstone, 1995, with permission.

ventral divisions of L2, L3, L4 spinal roots, in contrast to the femoral nerve, which originates from the dorsal divisions of the same roots. The obturator nerve passes along the medial edge of the psoas muscle and over the sacroiliac joint before it reaches the obturator canal. It is predominantly a motor nerve and innervates the obturator externus, gracilis, and thigh adductors, i.e., the adductor longus, adductor brevis, and adductor magnus (the latter receives additional innervation from the sciatic nerve). The obturator nerve sensory contribution is to a small area of skin on the inner thigh (Fig. 7–2).

Etiology, Clinical Features, Differential Diagnosis, and Treatment

1. The etiology, clinical features, differential diagnosis, and treatment of these uncommon nerves are listed in Table 7–2.

2. Disorders of the lateral femoral cutaneous nerve (meralgia paresthetica) are the most commonly encountered proximal leg sensory neuropathy in clinical practice.

3. Saphenous mononeuropathies are not uncommon, and occur mostly after venous stripping or saphenous vein harvesting for coronary artery bypass grafting.

Key Clinical Findings: Meralgia Paresthetica

- Variable pain, paresthesias, and numbness
- Involves the anterolateral thigh
- Often worse with standing or walking
- May be relieved by sitting down or flexing the hip

Laboratory Evaluation

1. Electrodiagnostic studies of these nerves, particularly sensory nerve conduction studies, are technically difficult or not feasible.

   a. There are no available nerve conduction studies for the evaluation of the ilioinguinal, iliohypogastric, genitofemoral, or obturator nerves.

   b. Sensory nerve conduction studies of the lateral femoral cutaneous nerve may be recorded antidromically or orthodromically, but potentials may be unevoked in a large proportion of healthy subjects. Hence, bilateral studies are essential for comparison purposes, and the most useful finding is an asymmetrically absent response on the symptomatic side. Somatosensory evoked potentials of the lateral femoral cutaneous nerve are also possible, but their sensitivity is low in meralgia paresthetica.

   c. Saphenous sensory nerve conduction studies are useful, but potentials may be unevoked in elderly or obese patients, or in edematous limbs. As with other technically difficult sensory nerve conduction studies, saphenous nerve conduction should be always studied bilaterally, and the most useful finding is an asymmetrically absent response on the symptomatic side. Saphenous sensory response is often absent or low in amplitude in patients with saphenous or femoral nerve lesions but normal in L4 radiculopathy.

   d. Needle EMG is most useful in excluding other causes of groin and proximal thigh pain and numbness such as lumbar radiculopathies or femoral neuropathies. Needle EMG of the upper lumbar paraspinal muscles is particularly useful in excluding a high lumbar radiculopathy.

      (1) In obturator neuropathy, needle EMG reveals fibrillation potentials and large MUAPs recruited rapidly in the thigh adductors. In contrast, needle EMG of the quadriceps, iliacus, and lumbar paraspinal muscles is normal.

      (2) Needle EMG of lower abdominal muscles in patients with ilioinguinal neuropathies may reveal denervation.

2. Patients with proximal lower limb sensory or obturator mononeuropathy with no clear cause should undergo a pelvic CT or MRI to exclude pelvic mass or malignancy.

Bibliography

Al Hakim M, Katirji MB: Femoral mononeuropathy induced by the lithotomy position: a report of 5 cases and a review of the literature. Muscle Nerve 16:891–895, 1993.

Goldman JA, Feldberg D, Dicker D, et al.: Femoral neuropathy subsequent to abdominal hysterectomy. A comparative study. Eur J Obstet Gynecol Reprod Biol 20:385–392, 1985.

Kopell HP, Thompson WAL, Postel AH: Entrapment of the inguinal nerve. N Engl J Med 266:16, 19, 1962.

Kuntzer T, van Melle G, Regli F: Clinical and prognostic features in unilateral femoral neuropathies. Muscle Nerve 20:205–211, 1997.

Kvist-Poulsen H, Borel J: Iatrogenic femoral neuropathy subsequent to abdominal hysterectomy: incidence and prevention. Obstet Gynecol 60:516–520, 1982.

Starling JR, Harms BA, Schroeder ME, Eichman PL: Diagnosis and treatment of genitofemoral and ilioinguinal entrapment neuralgia. Surgery 102:581–586, 1987.

8 Mononeuropathies During Pregnancy and Labor

Daniel W. Miller
Bashar Katirji

CARPAL TUNNEL SYNDROME

Definition

Entrapment of the median nerve at the wrist as it traverses the carpal tunnel, a bony canal roofed by the transverse carpal ligament, resulting in a clinical syndrome of painful upper limb paresthesias, sensory alterations, and variable weakness and atrophy of thenar muscles (see Part XVI, Chapter 3, Carpal Tunnel Syndrome and Other Median Neuropathies).

Epidemiology and Risk Factors

1. The incidence of pregnancy-related carpal tunnel syndrome (PRCTS) is about 1% to 10%. These figures compare to a reported prevalence of CTS in the general population of about 10%. Also, up to 50% of pregnant women will have nocturnal hand symptoms (though not necessarily a formal diagnosis of CTS).

2. PRCTS is diagnosed most frequently during the third trimester of pregnancy, but symptom onset occurs with equal frequency in each of the three trimesters.

3. The main posited risk factor for development of PRCTS is a prior history of PRCTS. Other factors include older age, excessive weight gain, generalized edema, and, possibly, pre-eclampsia.

Etiology and Pathophysiology

1. PRCTS presumably reflects the increase in body fluid that is commonly seen during pregnancy, resulting in median nerve compression in the carpal tunnel, demyelination, and ultimately (in severe cases) axonal loss. Hormonal factors may also play a causative role

2. Any of the numerous risk factors for CTS in general, such as repetitive stress, rheumatologic and endocrine conditions, local tumors, or a congenitally small carpal tunnel, must also be considered in the pregnant woman. Given the high frequency and female preponderance of CTS in the general population, some cases of PRCTS may be merely coincidental to pregnancy.

Clinical Findings

1. In general PRCTS resembles CTS of other etiologies. Paresthesias of hands, usually painful and worse at night, are the cardinal feature. Pain in hand, forearm, and even the upper arm may occur. Weakness of thenar eminence muscles (thumb opposition, abduction, and flexion) may be rarely reported.

2. In contrast to CTS of other etiologies, PRCTS may be associated with more severe pain, more hypesthesia, and diurnal persistence of symptoms.

3. Physical examination, as in CTS in general, may reveal sensory alterations in the median nerve territory. Tinel's sign and Phalen's sign are commonly noted. Weakness of thenar muscles and thenar atrophy may be noted in advanced cases. Wrist and hand swelling may be prominent.

Key Clinical Findings: Pregnancy-Related Carpal Tunnel Syndrome

- Paresthesias of hands, usually painful; condition usually worsens at night

- Pain in hand, forearm, and upper arm

- More severe pain, more hypesthesia, and diurnal persistence of symptoms than other CTS-related conditions

- Sensory alterations in the median nerve territory

- Tinel's sign and Phalen's sign

- Weakness of thenar muscles and thenar atrophy in advanced cases

- Wrist and hand swelling sometimes prominent

Differential Diagnosis

PRCTS should be differentiated from proximal median neuropathies, upper brachial plexopathies, or C6-C7 radiculopathies.

Laboratory Testing

1. Focal slowing of median nerve conduction across the wrist is the main abnormality on electrodiagnostic (EDX) testing.

2. As outlined in Part XVI, Chapter 3 (on Carpal Tunnel Syndrome), nerve conduction studies reveals prolonged median distal motor and sensory latencies, although more sensitive internal comparison studies (such as median-ulnar studies) help confirm the diagnosis. Needle electromyography (EMG) is done to look for evidence of denervation in thenar muscles, and exclude C6-C7 radiculopathy and proximal median neuropathy.

Treatment

1. PRCTS may be particularly painful necessitating symptomatic therapy. Treatment is usually conservative including wrist splinting (particularly overnight) and corticosteroid injections. Diuretics may also be useful, particularly when there is significant wrist edema.

2. Surgical decompression of the carpal tunnel by sectioning the transverse carpal ligament is indicated when severe pain is not responsive to conservative measures, when EDX studies indicate significant axonal loss and active denervation, or if the symptoms do not resolve within several months of delivery. Onset of symptoms before the third trimester or prior history of CTS symptoms is a good predictor for the ultimate need for surgical intervention.

3. Surgery generally yields good results where conservative measures fail.

Key Treatment: Pregnancy-Related Carpal Tunnel Syndrome

- Wrist splinting (particularly overnight)
- Corticosteroid injections
- Diuretics, particularly with significant edema
- Surgical decompression of the carpal tunnel by sectioning the transverse carpal ligament
- Surgery generally yields good results when conservative measures fail.

Prognosis and Complications

1. PRCTS usually, but not always, resolves after delivery within 4 to 6 weeks. This resolution typically takes somewhat longer in women who are breast-feeding (3 to 11 months) because of the prolonged use of the hand in a flexed position, which narrows the carpal tunnel diameter.

2. Untreated severe PRCTS may lead to residual neurologic disability. Axonal regeneration occurs at a slow pace relative to remyelination, and recovery may be incomplete.

3. PRCTS appears to predict an increased risk of CTS in future pregnancies.

Key Prognosis and Complications: Pregnancy-Related Carpal Tunnel Syndrome

- PRCTS usually resolves after delivery within 4 to 6 weeks.
- Condition may take longer to resolve in women who breast-feed.
- Untreated severe PRCTS may lead to residual neurologic disability.
- PRCTS appears to predict an increased risk of CTS in future pregnancies.

Prevention

1. It is unclear whether measures such as weight control and diuretic use during pregnancy would be effective in preventing PRCTS. Given the association of CTS in general with repetitive hand activities, pregnant women, particularly those with a prior history of PRCTS, should try to minimize such activities within reason.

2. Preventing pre-eclampsia might also reduce the risk of PRCTS.

MERALGIA PARESTHETICA

Definition

The clinical syndrome of paresthesias, numbness, or pain involving the anterolateral thigh, resulting from compression of the lateral femoral cutaneous nerve (see Part XVI, Chapter 7, Other Lower Limb Mononeuropathies).

Epidemiology and Risk Factors

1. Meralgia paresthetica is a relatively common mononeuropathy, and risk factors include prevalent conditions such as obesity and diabetes mellitus.

2. An increased incidence is noted in the third trimester of pregnancy, but symptoms may begin in the first trimester.

Etiology and Pathophysiology

1. The lateral femoral cutaneous nerve is a purely sensory nerve that arises from the second and third lumbar roots and courses either under or through the lateral aspect of the inguinal ligament just medial to the anterior superior iliac spine, to supply cutaneous sensation to a portion of the anterolateral thigh.

2. The nerve is vulnerable to compression as it passes near the anterior superior iliac spine.

3. Meralgia paresthetica is most commonly idiopathic, but a number of potential causes have been identified, including constrictive clothing or bandaging, surgeries (hernia repair, iliac bone harvesting), malignant nerve infiltration, and seat belt injury.

4. Pregnancy may predispose to the development of meralgia paresthetica by several mechanisms, including direct nerve compression by the gravid uterus, edema, and nerve stretch related to abdominal wall expansion and increasing lordosis.

5. Other contributing factors may also be present in the pregnant patient, such as tight waistbands or belts, preexisting obesity, or diabetes mellitus. Certain body positions (such as lying on the side of the entrapped nerve) may exacerbate symptoms in pregnant women.

Clinical Findings

1. Symptoms are localized to the anterolateral thigh and may include pain, paresthesias, and numbness. Often the initial painful dysesthesias are ultimately replaced by asymptomatic hypesthesia involving the same area.

2. Symptoms are often exacerbated by walking, standing, or thigh adduction, and may improve upon sitting. Touch may exacerbate dysesthesia, whereas rubbing the affected area frequently provides temporary relief.

Key Clinical Findings: Meralgia Paresthetica

- Pain, paresthesias, and numbness in the anterolateral thigh
- Painful dysesthesia often replaced by asymptomatic hypesthesia
- Symptoms often exacerbated by walking, standing, or thigh adduction; may improve when patient is sitting
- Touch may exacerbate dysesthesia; rubbing the affected area usually provides temporary relief.

Differential Diagnosis

Meralgia paresthetica should be differentiated from femoral neuropathy and L2-L4 radiculopathies (see Part XVI, Chapter 7, Other Lower Limb Mononeuropathies).

Laboratory Testing

1. Meralgia paresthetica is a clinical diagnosis, and ancillary studies are generally not necessary given a characteristic clinical picture.

2. The main indication for EDX studies in suspected meralgia paresthetica is to rule out L2-L4 radiculopathies and femoral neuropathies. The sensory potential of the lateral femoral cutaneous nerve is technically difficult; when done, it is usually absent on the symptomatic side.

Treatment

1. Pregnancy-associated meralgia paresthetica is only rarely severe enough to require pharmacologic or surgical intervention. Conservative measures such as wearing loose clothing may be of benefit in some patients. Attempting weight loss during pregnancy is impractical and may be detrimental to the fetus.

   a. Medical therapies include oral analgesics (such as acetaminophen), topical capsaicin or lidocaine, and local injection of hydrocortisone or anesthetic agents around the nerve.

   b. Surgical options include open decompression, nerve section, and medial transposition of the nerve. Potential risks to the fetus must be considered before advising surgery.

   c. Rarely, early induction of labor has been employed in refractory meralgia paresthetica.

Key Treatment: Meralgia Paresthetica

- Rarely requires pharmacologic or surgical intervention
- Conservative: Wearing loose clothing
- Pharmacologic: Oral analgesics (such as acetaminophen), topical capsaicin, and injection of hydrocortisone or anesthetic agents around the nerve
- Surgical: Open decompression, nerve section, and medial transposition of the nerve

Prognosis

1. In general, pregnancy-associated meralgia paresthetica gradually improves spontaneously after delivery. As with other compressive nerve processes, the rate and extent of recovery depend on whether the lesion is primarily demyelinating or instead involves axons to a significant degree.

2. Women with a history of the condition may be at increased risk of recurrence in subsequent pregnancies.

Key Prognosis: Meralgia Paresthetica

- Gradually resolves after delivery

- Increased risk of recurrence in subsequent pregnancies for women with a history of the condition

BELL'S PALSY

Definition

Bell's palsy is an acquired infranuclear facial palsy of sudden onset, occurring in isolation. It is the most common cause of isolated unilateral facial weakness.

Epidemiology and Risk Factors

1. Bell's palsy is two to four times more common among women of reproductive age than among men of the same age, and the recurrence rate (0.5% to 10% of patients) is twice as high among women. The incidence in women declines after age 50.

2. The incidence during pregnancy and the puerperium is 38 to 45 cases per 100,000 births per year. This is threefold higher than the incidence among non-pregnant, age-matched women.

3. Within pregnancy the risk of developing Bell's palsy is markedly greater in the third trimester and the first 2 weeks of the puerperium, with an incidence of 118 cases per 100,000 births per year.

Etiology and Pathophysiology

1. Many theories have been advanced to explain the increased incidence of Bell's palsy during pregnancy and the early puerperium.

   a. Extracellular fluid volume expands over the course of pregnancy and is maximal late, when Bell's palsy is most commonly seen. Consequent venous congestion within the bony facial canal may result in compression of the facial nerve, producing nerve dysfunction.

   b. Increased pressure within the facial canal may develop as a consequence of systemic hypertension. However, there is no demonstrated association between hypertension and Bell's palsy during pregnancy.

   c. Bell's palsy may represent an inflammatory demyelinating immune reaction to a viral infection (e.g., herpes simplex type 1). This reaction may occur in response to other viruses that are reactivated because of the immunosuppression of pregnancy, which is maximal near term.

   d. The hypercoagulable state of pregnancy may predispose to thrombosis of the vasa nervorum, resulting in an ischemic insult to the facial nerve.

Clinical Features

1. The clinical features of pregnancy-associated Bell's palsy do not differ significantly from those in nonpregnant individuals. The disorder is unilateral in 97% of cases, similar to the nonpregnant state.

2. There is acute onset of facial weakness, which may be preceded by pain in the ipsilateral cheek or ear, tinnitus, or fever.

3. The weakness involves the upper and lower facial muscles on the affected side. This result in flattening of the forehead and nasolabial fold, widening of the palpebral fissure, and asymmetry of smile and eye closure.

4. Associated features may include numbness of the ipsilateral face or tongue, drooling, dysgeusia, hyperacusis, and abnormalities of salivation and lacrimation.

Key Clinical Findings: Bell's Palsy

- Risk is three times higher during pregnancy.

- Risk is highest during the third trimester and the first 2 weeks postpartum.

- Unilateral in 97% of cases

- Acute lower motor neuron facial paresis

- Ipsilateral ear pain, altered taste, and hyperacusis

Differential Diagnosis

1. Central (supranuclear) lesions causing facial weakness usually spare the upper face, which distinguishes them from peripheral lesions such as Bell's palsy.

2. Other causes of isolated peripheral facial weakness should be excluded. These include diabetes melli-

tus, sarcoidosis, Herpes zoster (Ramsay Hunt syndrome), Lyme disease, and masses within the petrous bone, mastoid, middle ear, or cerebello-pontine angles.

Laboratory Testing

1. Bell's palsy is a clinical diagnosis with no specific or sensitive laboratory test. However, testing may be considered to rule out other causes of facial weakness.

2. EDX of the facial nerve provides prognostic information. Nerve conduction studies after 5 to 7 days are useful as follows:

   a. A low-amplitude facial motor response indicates an axon-loss lesion and poor prognosis.

   b. A normal facial motor response indicates a demyelinating lesion with excellent prognosis.

Radiologic Features

1. Magnetic resonance imaging may show gadolinium enhancement of the facial nerve or may be normal. Most imaging modalities are of uncertain safety in pregnancy and should probably not be employed in the routine evaluation of a typical Bell's palsy.

2. Imaging may be indicated when suspicion is strong for fracture, tumor, or other structural lesion as the cause of facial weakness, or when there is uncertainty as to whether the lesion is peripheral or central.

Treatment

1. As is the case in the nonpregnant patient, pregnancy-associated Bell's palsy usually improves to complete or near-complete recovery within weeks to a few months. Supportive care is always indicated, but the evidence for prednisone or acyclovir in pregnancy is not nearly so strong as it is in the nonpregnant population.

2. Supportive therapy includes patching of the involved eye (particularly overnight) and liberal use of lubricant eye drops, measures aimed at protecting the exposed cornea.

3. Uncontrolled clinical trials suggests that early use of prednisone in the non-pregnant patient with Bell's palsy may reduce pain. While prednisone is considered safe for both mother and fetus in late pregnancy, pregnant women receiving early treatment (60 to 80 mg/day for 5 to 10 days or 40 to 60 mg/day for 8 to 10 days) showed neither regimen to be superior to no treatment in duration of the deficit or degree of recovery.

4. Controlled data from nonpregnant patients suggests that the combination of acyclovir plus prednisone results in less denervation and a more complete recovery than prednisone alone. It has not otherwise been established as a standard treatment for pregnancy-associated Bell's palsy

5. Surgical decompression of the facial nerve is rarely indicated. Hypoglossal–facial nerve anastomosis has been performed to restore function in patients with persistent facial paralysis several months after onset.

Key Treatment: Bell's Palsy

- Complete or near-complete recovery usually within weeks to a few months after delivery

- Patching the involved eye (particularly overnight), and liberal use of lubricant eye drops for protecting exposed cornea

- Prednisone and acyclovir

Prognosis and Complications

1. Pregnancy-associated Bell's palsy generally has a favorable prognosis, with 90% of patients recovering completely. In one series, recurrent pregnancy-associated Bell's palsy and bilateral weakness were identified as predictors of incomplete recovery.

2. The time to complete recovery, averaging 7 weeks from onset, is somewhat less than in nonpregnant patients.

3. The extent of recovery depends on the extent of nerve injury. A normal facial motor response study performed after 5 to 7 days from onset of facial palsy indicates a 90% likelihood of complete recovery.

4. Aberrant regeneration of facial nerve fibers may result in synkinesis of voluntary facial movements, such as eyelid closure on smiling, or may lead to lacrimation occurring in conjunction with salivation (crocodile tears).

Key Prognosis: Bell's Palsy

- 90% of patients recover completely

- Time to complete recovery averages 7 weeks from onset

- Extent of recovery depends on the extent of nerve injury.

INTRAPARTUM MATERNAL LUMBOSACRAL PLEXOPATHY (LUMBOSACRAL TRUNK LESION)

Anatomy

1. The lumbosacral trunk (or cord) is formed primarily by the L5 root with a contributing branch from the L4 root (Fig. 8–1). It travels a relatively long distance in close contact with the ala of the sacrum adjacent to the sacroiliac joint.

2. The lumbosacral trunk is cushioned throughout its course by the psoas muscle, except at its terminal portion near the pelvic brim, where it lies in close contact with the bone. There, it is joined by the S1 root to form the sciatic nerve.

Etiology

1. Intrapartum maternal lumbosacral plexopathy is caused by lumbosacral trunk compression by the fetal head at the pelvic brim, where it is not protected by the psoas muscle.

2. Intrapartum maternal lumbosacral plexopathy is a manifestation of a cephalopelvic disproportion. It occurs mainly in short women but may be associated with delivering a large infant.

3. The progression of labor is often arrested because of the severe cephalopelvic disproportion, and in such cases almost all women ultimately deliver by cesarean section.

Clinical Findings

1. Intrapartum maternal lumbosacral plexopathy presents with foot drop, usually on the right. There is a variable buttock pain and numbness in the lateral leg and dorsum of the foot. Pain usually subsides within a few days.

2. The neurologic findings include weakness of ankle and toe dorsiflexion, ankle eversion, ankle inversion, and toe flexion. There is variable weakness of the glutei and hamstring muscles which resolves rapidly. Plantar flexion and ankle jerk are usually normal. Sensory loss is mainly in an L5 dermatomal distribution. Rarely, there are also sensory symptoms in an S1 distribution with a depressed or absent H-reflex.

Key Clinical Findings: Intrapartum Maternal Lumbosacral Plexopathy

- Foot drop, usually on the right
- Variable buttock pain and numbness in the lateral leg and dorsum of the foot
- Pain usually subsides within a few days.
- Weakness of ankle and toe dorsiflexion, ankle eversion, ankle inversion, and toe flexion

Differential Diagnosis

It is important to distinguish intrapartum maternal lumbosacral plexopathy from peroneal nerve compression or an L5 radiculopathy, because all may present with foot drop.

1. Intrapartum peroneal neuropathy at the fibular head is usually attributed to compression by leg holders, or to hand pressure or during squatting. Ankle inversion and toe flexion are preserved and the sensory loss is restricted to a common peroneal nerve distribution.

2. It is more difficult to separate a lumbosacral trunk lesion, such as seen in intrapartum maternal lumbosacral plexopathy, from L5 radiculopathy, because the weakness and sensory loss involves the L5 myotome and dermatome in both conditions. The appropriate clinical setting—i.e., intrapartum right foot drop in a short woman—and the lack of

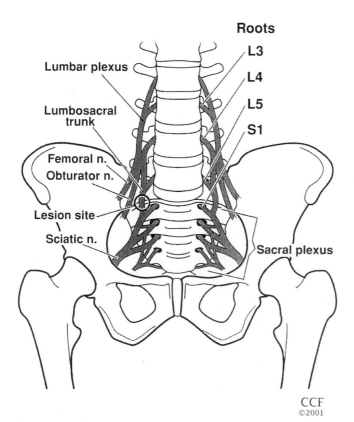

Figure 8–1. The lumbosacral plexus showing the lumbosacral trunk and the site of the compression by the fetal head causing intrapartum maternal lumbosacral plexopathy (Copyright © The Cleveland Clinic Foundation).

radicular pain are useful clinical findings. EDX studies are usually needed for final diagnosis.

Laboratory Testing

1. EDX studies are essential in the correct diagnosis of intrapartum maternal lumbosacral trunk lesions. Often the superficial peroneal sensory measurement is low in amplitude or absent, while the peroneal motor studies, recording tibialis anterior and extensor digitorum brevis, are normal. This is consistent with a proximal predominantly demyelinating lesion. The needle EMG reveals significant impairment of recruitment of motor units in an L5 distribution with normal lumbar paraspinal muscles.

2. Excluding a common peroneal lesion is an important task of the EDX studies. Those patients may have conduction block across the fibular head. Also, detecting weakness or denervation or both, in ankle inversion (tibialis posterior) or toe flexion (flexor digitorum longus), eliminates a peroneal neuropathy.

3. Excluding an L5 radiculopathy is a more difficult task because of the overlap between the innervation of the lumbosacral trunk and L5 root. A low-amplitude or absent superficial peroneal sensory response and normal lumbar paraspinal muscles are extremely useful clues in the diagnosis of an intrapartum maternal lumbosacral trunk lesion.

Treatment and Prognosis

1. Foot drop is treated by an ankle-foot orthosis and physical therapy.

2. The prognosis is very good in most patients, with recovery in about 2 to 5 months.

Key Treatment and Prognosis: Intrapartum Maternal Lumbosacral Plexopathy

- Treatment: Ankle-foot orthosis and physical therapy
- Prognosis: Very good with recovery in about 2 to 5 months

INTRAPARTUM FEMORAL NEUROPATHY

Etiology

1. Compression of the femoral nerve at the inguinal ligament may occur after prolonged lithotomy positioning, particularly with extreme hip flexion and external rotation. The nerve is often kinked under the inguinal ligament, but it may also be stretched by excessive hip abduction and external rotation.

2. These lesions are often associated with vaginal delivery, but they may occur with other procedures requiring lithotomy positioning such as vaginal hysterectomy, prostatectomy, and laparoscopy.

Epidemiology

1. Femoral neuropathy after vaginal delivery is likely underestimated since most are mild and resolve rapidly.

2. The reported incidence has declined, likely because of the increased use of cesarean section, from about 4.7% during the early 1900s to about 2.8/100,000 deliveries (0.0028%) currently.

Clinical Findings

1. The clinical presentation of femoral nerve lesions includes thigh weakness and anterior thigh and leg numbness.

2. Most cases are unilateral, but bilateral lesions may occur. Acutely, groin or thigh pain is usually mild, and a deep delayed pain and hyperesthesia are not uncommon. The neurologic examination reveals weakness of knee extension (quadriceps) with absent or depressed knee jerk. Thigh adduction and ankle dorsiflexion are, however, normal. Hip flexion is spared, but sometimes is difficult to examine accurately because of groin or abdominal pain related to the delivery or cesarean section. Hypesthesia over the anterior thigh and medial calf is common.

Key Clinical Findings: Intrapartum Femoral Neuropathy

- May occur after a prolonged lithotomy position
- Quadriceps weakness
- Numbness of the anterior thigh and medial leg
- Depressed or absent knee jerk
- Unilateral, although bilateral lesions may occur

Differential Diagnosis

1. Quadriceps weakness with absent/depressed knee jerk and sensory manifestations in the anterior thigh are manifestations shared not only by femoral neuropathy but also by an upper lumbar (L2, L3, and L4) radiculopathy (such as with disc herniation) and lumbar plexopathy (such as with

diabetic amyotrophy). Sparing thigh adduction and hip flexion are useful signs of a femoral nerve lesion at the inguinal ligament.

2. Sensory loss in the anterior thigh due to mild femoral neuropathy may occasionally be confused with meralgia paresthetica (lesion of the lateral femoral cutaneous nerve), which, as discussed earlier, is also common in pregnant women. The sensory loss in meralgia paresthetica is lateral, does not extend beyond the knee, and rarely crosses the anterior midline of the thigh. In contrast, the sensory loss in femoral nerve lesions is anterior and often extends beyond the knee to include the medial leg (saphenous distribution).

Treatment

The treatment of femoral mononeuropathies at the inguinal ligament following childbirth is conservative. Physical therapy and knee bracing are useful. There is no surgical indication for such lesions.

Key Treatment: Intrapartum Femoral Neuropathy

- Physical therapy and knee bracing

Prognosis

1. Compressive femoral mononeuropathies at the inguinal ligament after childbirth are usually

demyelinating and thus resolve within 3 to 4 months.

2. Iatrogenic femoral nerve lesions at the inguinal ligament may be prevented by avoiding prolonged lithotomy positioning and extreme hip flexion and external rotation.

Key Prognosis: Intrapartum Femoral Neuropathy

- Recovery within 3 to 4 months after childbirth

Bibliography

Al-Hakim M, Katirji MB: Femoral mononeuropathy induced by the lithotomy position. Muscle and Nerve 16:891–895, 1993.

Cohen Y, Lavie O, Granofsky-Grisaru S, et al.: Bell's palsy complicating pregnancy: a review. Obstet Gynecol Surv 55:184–188, 2000.

Katirji B, Wilbourn AJ, Scarberry SL, Preston DC: Intrapartum maternal lumbosacral plexopathy Muscle Nerve 26;340–347, 2002.

Rosenbaum RB, Donaldson JO: Peripheral nerve and neuromuscular disorders. Neurol Clin 12:465–466, 1994.

Seror P: Pregnancy-related carpal tunnel syndrome. J Hand Surg 23:98–101, 1998.

Stahl S, Blumenfeld Z, Yarnitsky D: Carpal tunnel syndrome in pregnancy: indications for early surgery. J Neurol Sci 136:182–184, 1996.

Stolp-Smith KA, Pascoe MK, Ogburn PL: Carpal tunnel syndrome in pregnancy: frequency, severity, and prognosis. Arch Phys Med Rehabil 79:1285–1287, 1998.-

1 **Manifestations of Myopathies**

Steven Lovitt
Yadollah Harati

Definition

A primary skeletal muscle disorder, independent of anterior horn cell, nerve, or myoneural junction function, and independent of etiology or inheritance

Symptoms

1. The cardinal symptom of myopathy is weakness. It is important to objectively confirm the presence of true muscle weakness because patients with other problems (e.g., depression, arthralgia, myalgia) also complain of weakness. A disorder of the neuromuscular junction (e.g., myasthenia gravis) may cause similar complaints. Of course, weakness due to a lesion at another point of the neuraxis, be it nerve, anterior horn cell, or upper motor neuron, should also be considered in the appropriate clinical setting. Most myopathies present with "limb-girdle" weakness consisting of proximal weakness of the arms and legs. Patients with proximal leg weakness commonly complain of difficulty ascending stairs; arising from a stool, chair, car, or toilet; or difficulty getting off the floor. If the arms are affected, patients may complain of difficulty combing hair, brushing teeth, applying makeup, or retrieving objects from a high shelf. It is important to remember that weakness in this distribution does not indicate a specific cause of the myopathy. However, when myopathy causes weakness in a non–limb-girdle distribution it is often a key diagnostic clue. For example, inclusion body myositis classically presents with weakness of the proximal legs and distal arms.

> ### Caveat
> - A key diagnostic clue is when myopathy causes weakness in a non–limb-girdle distribution (e.g., proximal leg and distal arm weakness in inclusion body myositis).

> ### Key Myopathies
> #### Presenting with Distal Weakness
> - Myotonic dystrophy
> - Nonaka myopathy
> - Miyoshi myopathy
> - Myofibrillar myopathy
> - Welander's myopathy
> - Markesbury-Udd myopathy
> - Liang myopathy
>
> #### Presenting with Scapuloperoneal Weakness
> - Facioscapulohumeral muscular dystrophy
> - Emery-Dreifuss muscular dystrophy
> - Acid maltase deficiency
>
> #### Presenting with Ptosis or Ophthalmoplegia
> - Ptosis, usually without ophthalmoplegia
>   —Myotonic dystrophy
>   —Congenital myopathies: nemaline, central core
>   —Desmin storage myopathy
> - Ptosis with ophthalmoplegia
>   —Oculopharyngeal muscular dystrophy
>   —Oculopharyngodistal myopathy
>   —Chronic progressive external ophthalmoplegia (mitochondrial myopathy)

2. Myalgias are a common reason for referral to a neuromuscular clinic. They are not usually due to myopathy, and myalgias without true muscle weakness are not expected with myopathy. However, myalgias can be seen as a feature of myopathy, especially sarcoidosis, hypothyroidism, inflammatory myopathy, toxic myopathy, and mitochondrial myopathy.

3. Cramps are another common reason for referral to a neuromuscular clinic. Cramps that occur during exercise may represent a metabolic myopathy, whereas cramps that occur at rest are unlikely to

be due to a myopathic disorder, although they may be due to denervation or a metabolic disorder such as hypoadrenalism, hypothyroidism, or renal insufficiency. Cramps may also be due to Isaac's syndrome or to stiff-person syndrome.

4. Masses are uncommon but when they occur may be due to inflammatory myopathy (especially trichinosis), granulomatous myopathy (due to sarcoidosis, thymoma, or inflammatory bowel disease), or neoplasia. More commonly, a muscle "mass" represents a ruptured tendon.

Clinical Findings

1. The most common objective finding is proximal weakness. The most commonly affected muscles are the neck flexor muscles, hip girdle and iliopsoas muscles, and shoulder girdle and biceps muscles. Mild degrees of weakness may be difficult to detect on examination. In such cases it is crucial to observe the patient arising from a low stool or the floor.

2. Facial weakness may be detected by having the patient whistle or forcefully close the lips or eyes against resistance. In patients with significant facial weakness ptosis, a tented lip, or a transverse smile may be present. Patients may be noted to "sleep with their eyes open." Distinctive facial features are present with some congenital myopathies and muscular dystrophies. Scapular winging should be excluded.

3. The presence of atrophy should be assessed, although it is not as common as in cases of denervation. Significant atrophy may be present in patients with chronic myopathy.

4. The muscle stretch reflexes tend to parallel the degree of muscle weakness, in contrast to that in patients with neuropathy, in whom they are generally decreased.

5. Grip and percussion myotonia should be sought if cramps or spasms are reported, as well as fasciculations and myokymia.

Key Signs

- Proximal weakness: watch the patient arise from a low stool or the floor.

- Facial weakness may be present.

- Exclude the presence of atrophy.

- Muscle stretch reflexes tend to parallel the degree of muscle weakness.

- With cramps and spasms, look for grip and percussion myotonia.

Clinical Investigations

1. Myopathy often causes an elevated creatine phosphokinase (CPK) level, although a normal CPK level does not exclude a myopathy. For example, a normal CPK level is commonly seen with inclusion body myopathy, corticosteroid-induced myopathy, alcoholic myopathy, and myopathy related to thyroid disease. Likewise, an elevated CPK level is not necessarily indicative of a myopathy. The CPK level may be elevated after trauma, whether from exercise, accidents, needle electromyography, or muscle biopsy. Moreover, it can be elevated in healthy African-American individuals. There is also a "familial hyper-CK-emia." The ALT AST levels are also abnormally high when the CPK level is significantly elevated. When this association is not recognized, the patient may be subjected to unnecessary evaluations including liver biopsy.

2. Electromyography is a complex study requiring skill on the part of the performing physician. Interpretation is often subjective and subject to technical error. A full explanation of the technique is beyond the scope of this chapter. Briefly, with myopathy the motor units are expected to be of small amplitude and short duration. Early recruitment may be present. Spontaneous activity, when present along with myopathic features, suggests an inflammatory process. Nerve conduction velocities are normal unless a neuropathy is superimposed.

3. Pathologic confirmation rests on the performance and interpretation of a muscle biopsy. Genetic testing, if available, may preclude the need for muscle biopsy. Interpretation should be performed by a neuromuscular specialist or a neuropathologist with adequate experience in neuromuscular pathology. Muscle biopsy is discussed in detail elsewhere in this text.

Key Tests

- CPK level

- ALT and AST levels

- Electromyography

- Muscle biopsy

2 Muscular Dystrophies

Hazem Machkhas

There has been an explosion in our knowledge about the molecular genetics of many muscular dystrophies. As genes and their products continue to be identified, the entire field of muscular dystrophies has been reclassified according to genotypes. This has given rise to the observation of marked genetic heterogeneity in many entities, where mutations in the same gene lead to a wide array of phenotypic expressions. It has also highlighted the depth of our ignorance regarding the complex interactions between the various molecules that regulate muscle function in health and in disease. A key component of the muscle membrane is the dystrophin–glycoprotein complex (DGC), which harbors many of the molecules that have revolutionized our understanding of muscular dystrophies (Fig. 2–1).

DYSTROPHINOPATHIES

Dystrophin is a 427-kDa protein expressed in skeletal, smooth, and cardiac muscles, as well as in the brain. It is bound to the cytoplasmic face of the muscle membrane, where it anchors the DGC. It probably plays a critical role in preserving plasma membrane stability during the process of contraction. It is the product of the largest gene yet identified (2.5 kb), located on chromosome Xp21.1. Dystrophin mutations result in two distinct phenotypes: Duchenne muscular dystrophy (DMD) is the more severe phenotype and results from an "out of frame" mutation that yields a nonfunctional protein, or one that is rapidly degraded. Becker muscular dystrophy (BMD) is less severe and results from an "in frame" mutation, yielding a truncated protein, with preserved C- and N- terminals, that is partially functional.

Duchenne Muscular Dystrophy

1. Genetics
   a. Mode of inheritance is X-linked recessive.
   b. It is characterized by a high mutation rate: Up to one third of isolated cases are due to new mutations.
   c. Incidence is 1 in 3500 live male newborns.
2. Clinical features
   a. Many children are normal at birth, although some display hypotonia.
   b. Most children manifest symptoms between 1 and 3 years, mostly as delayed milestones, abnormal gait, or inability to walk.
   c. Subsequent course is a relentless progression of weakness that culminates in death around the age of 20. Usually, ambulation becomes difficult at 8 to 10 years of age and is lost by 12 years, when wheelchair confinement begins.
   d. The features of the neurologic examination vary depending on the stage of the illness. At an early stage proximal weakness predominates, and muscles feel firm and rubbery. Pseudohypertrophy, especially of the calf muscles, is seen. As the disease advances, weakness and wasting become diffuse. Pseudohypertrophy usually disappears with loss of ambulation.
   e. Joint contractures typically appear at that time. Tightness of the heel cords may be seen when a child is still ambulatory and, unless corrected, seriously compromises independent walking.
   f. Scoliosis accelerates with the complete loss of ambulation. It results in a higher risk for developing respiratory infections, which may precipitate death.
   g. Mental retardation (IQ < 75) is seen in approximately 30% of children with DMD. Intellectual impairment is not progressive.
   h. Cardiac involvement is asymptomatic in most patients, although 90% have electrocardiographic changes, typically suggestive of right ventricular strain. Arrhythmias are rare. Congestive heart failure may be seen in end stages of the illness.

Key Signs: Duchenne Muscular Dystrophy

- Onset by 3 years of age
- Weakness initially proximal
- Pseudohypertrophy of calves
- Loss of ambulation by 12 years of age
- Scoliosis
- Mental retardation in 30%

3. Laboratory tests
   a. Several serum enzymes may be elevated, but the most sensitive is creatine kinase (CK), which in the early stages of the disease may be 50 to 100

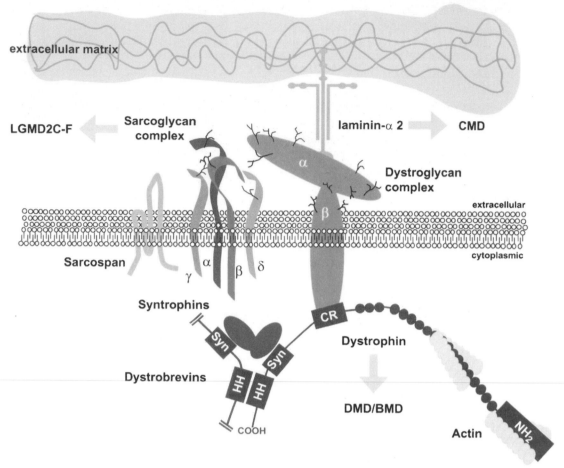

Figure 2–1. Dystrophin–glycoprotein complex. BMD, Becker muscular dystrophy; CMD, childhood muscular dystrophy; DMD, Duchenne muscular dystrophy. (From O'Brien KF, Kunkel LM: Dystrophin and muscular dystrophy: past, present, and future. Mol Genet Metab 74:75–88, 2001, with permission.)

times normal. Levels do not correlate with severity of disease.

b. Electrophysiology: Nerve conduction studies are typically normal. Electromyography (EMG) reveals characteristic but nonspecific "myopathic" units (i.e., low-amplitude short-duration polyphasic motor units).

c. Muscle biopsy reveals a chronic myopathy (changes commonly referred to as dystrophic). There is wide variation in fiber size and shape. Several fibers in various stages of necrosis are seen. There is extensive replacement of muscle fibers with connective and adipose tissues. Mild but definite inflammation is seen in a small number of biopsies. Immunostaining with dystrophin antibodies reveals total or near total absence of dystrophin.

d. Western blot analysis of muscle biopsy specimen reveals severely reduced or absent dystrophin.

e. DNA analysis may identify specific recognized

mutations (in up to 90% of cases), which allows unequivocal diagnosis.

Key Tests: Duchenne Muscular Dystrophy

• CK levels are 50 to 100 times normal

• Dystrophin is absent

4. Management
a. Prednisone, 0.75 mg/kg/day, has been shown to initially improve muscle strength, followed by slowing the progression of the illness, an effect that persisted after 3 years of follow-up.

b. Periodic stretching of the heel cords delays the onset of contractures and maintains independent ambulation.

c. Once contractures develop, surgical release of tendons (tenotomy) and fitting with the appropriate orthoses may prolong independent ambulation by up to 3 years.

d. Once the patient becomes wheelchair bound,

the risk of scoliosis can be reduced by the use of wheelchairs that allow optimal positioning of the back (vertical with a slight backward incline) and limbs.

e. Once progressive scoliosis develops, surgical correction can improve the respiratory status and restore comfort.

Key Treatment: Duchenne Muscular Dystrophy

• Prednisone slows progression.

Becker Muscular Dystrophy

1. Genetics
   a. Mode of inheritance is X-linked recessive.
   b. Incidence is much lower than that of DMD: approximately 3 per 100,000 live male newborns.
2. Clinical features
   a. BMD is a milder allelic disorder of DMD and thus shares with it a similar pattern of weakness, albeit milder, later in onset, and slower in its progression.
   b. Typically, the onset of symptoms is between 5 and 15 years of age, although some patients remain asymptomatic into their third or fourth decade.
   c. The earliest weakness is in the proximal lower extremity muscles. Calf hypertrophy is usually prominent.
   d. Most patients remain ambulatory into their late teens and some into the early twenties. This feature is crucial for distinguishing BMD from DMD on clinical grounds.
   e. With disease progression, weakness and wasting become generalized.
   f. Contractures and scoliosis appear with loss of ambulatory status.
   g. Intellectual impairment is infrequent. When present, it is mild.
   h. Cardiac involvement mostly consists of a dilated cardiomyopathy, which during the latter part of the illness produces congestive heart failure.

Key Signs: Becker Muscular Dystrophy

• Onset between 5 and 15 years of age

• Weakness is initially proximal

• Pseudohypertrophy of calves

• Ambulation retained into late teens, sometimes longer

• No mental retardation

3. Laboratory tests
   a. Serum CK levels, as in DMD, may be elevated 50 to 100 times normal, especially in the early stages.
   b. EMG reveals nonspecific myopathic changes.
   c. Muscle biopsy findings, on routine histochemistries, closely resemble those seen with DMD. However, dystrophin immunostaining and Western blot analysis reveal the presence of reduced amounts of dystrophin.
   d. DNA analysis allows detection of mutations in up to 65% of cases.

Key Tests: Becker Muscular Dystrophy

• CK levels are 50 to 100 times normal.

• Dystrophin is reduced.

4. Management
   a. There is no proof that prednisone works in BMD patients. Adequate studies have not been performed.
   b. Other palliative management measures are similar to those for DMD.

LIMB-GIRDLE MUSCULAR DYSTROPHIES

The syndrome of limb-girdle muscular dystrophy (LGMD) used to encompass a large number of patients with heterogeneous presentations who had the common feature of shoulder and pelvic girdle weakness distribution and whose disease did not fit any known muscular dystrophy syndrome. Identification of the components of the dystrophin–glycoprotein complex, as well as other genetic advances, have allowed better characterization of various disorders (Table 2–1). Most of these disorders, and the ones that have been well defined, are autosomal recessive (LGMD2). Autosomal dominant cases (LGMD1) represent only 10% of all cases. The autosomal recessive phenotype is uniformly more severe than the autosomal dominant phenotype.

1. Clinical features
   a. LGMD2D. Results from mutations in the α-sarcoglycan (also known as adhalin) gene (17q12-21.33). Clinical heterogeneity has been well documented, with some cases having a DMD-like severe course, and others having only mild weakness. Typically, the age of onset is 3 to 15 years, with the earliest symptoms being difficulty running and climbing stairs.

TABLE 2–1. LIMB-GIRDLE MUSCULAR DYSTROPHIES

Type of LGMD	Gene Locus	Protein
Autosomal Dominant		
LGMD (type 1)		
LGMD1A	5q22-24	Myotilin
LGMD1B	1q11-21	Lamin A/C
LGMD1C	3p25	Caveolin 3
Autosomal Recessive		
LGMD (type 2)		
LGMD2A	15q15-21	Calpain 3
LGMD2B	2p13	Dysferlin
LGMD2C	13q13	γ-Sarcoglycan
LGMD2D	17q12-21.33	α-Sarcoglycan
LGMD2E	4q12	β-Sarcoglycan
LGMD2F	5q33-34	δ-Sarcoglycan
LGMD2G	17q11-12	Telethonin
LGMD2H	9q31-33	?Ubiquitin ligase
LGMD2I	19q13	Unknown

Abbreviation: LGMD, limb-girdle muscular dystrophy.

Early onset is usually associated with rapid progression. Ultimately, all muscles become involved. Calf hypertrophy is common. Cardiac involvement is rare, and intelligence is usually normal. CK levels may be massively elevated, especially early in the disease. EMG shows nonspecific myopathic changes. Muscle biopsy shows a dystrophic pattern. Immunostaining for α-sarcoglycan reveals the deficiency. Note that dystrophin immunostaining may reveal a secondary absence. DNA analysis, if positive, unequivocally confirms the diagnosis.

b. LGMD2C. Results from mutations in the γ-sarcoglycan gene (13q13). Little is known about the full spectrum of this disorder, as only a few reports exist in the literature. These reports suggest a clinical picture similar to that of LGMD2D, with clinical heterogeneity, predominance of childhood onset, proximal lower limb weakness in the early stages, and lack of cardiac and intellectual involvement. Diagnostic testing follows the same guidelines as for LGMD2D.

c. LGMD2E. Results from mutations in the β-sarcoglycan gene (4q12). Typically, it has a milder phenotype than the previous two disorders, although some cases with a severe, rapidly progressive course have been reported. Age at loss of ambulation ranges from 12 to 38 years.

d. LGMD2F. Results from mutations in the δ-sarcoglycan gene (5q33-34). The few available case reports suggest a uniformly severe, DMD-like clinical picture. Ambulation is usually lost by 16 years, and death ensues at 19 to 20 years. There is a strong association with a dilated cardiomyopathy.

e. LGMD2B. Results from mutations in the dysferlin gene (2p13). Onset of weakness is usually during the late teens and starts in the pelvic girdle muscles. Progression is slow, with ultimate involvement of distal lower limbs muscles and the shoulder girdle. Transient calf hypertrophy may be seen. There is no associated cardiomyopathy. An intriguing observation is the association of dysferlin mutations with the completely distinct phenotype of Miyoshi myopathy (see later).

f. LGMD2A. Results from mutations in the calpain3 gene (15q15-21). The phenotype is quite distinct but of variable severity. Typical onset is during the mid to late teens, with symmetrical, selective weakness of the pelvic, scapular, and trunk muscles. Heel contractures appear early. There is no associated cardiomyopathy.

2. Approach to diagnosis

a. A rational approach to the diagnosis is one that employs historical, clinical, genetic, and histologic features.

b. The history and physical examination may be helpful in guiding the workup. For example, disorders with childhood onset are more suggestive of a sarcoglycanopathy, whereas those with onset during the late teens, especially when associated with some degree of distal muscle involvement, suggest a dysferlinopathy.

c. The family history is obviously important; a dominant pattern of inheritance suggests the rare type 1 LGMD.

d. Before further proceeding to pinpoint the diagnosis, a dystrophinopathy should be ruled out in all cases. This may be done by DNA analysis, and if negative, by performing Western blot or immunostaining on a muscle biopsy.

e. Once a dystrophinopathy has been excluded, immunostaining for other components is required. Some laboratories employ a shotgun approach, performing an entire screen for sarcoglycans, dysferlin, caveolin3, and calpain3. It is preferable to employ a more directed approach, guided by the clinical impression. Note that distinguishing among sarcoglycanopathies is difficult, as abnormalities in any of the components of the complex result in abnormal immunostaining for the other three.

DISTAL MYOPATHIES

Distal myopathies are also referred to as distal muscular dystrophies. They encompass a large number of well defined and less well defined entities that have in common a distal pattern of onset of weakness and the absence of a clear "dystrophic" pattern on muscle biopsies. This discussion is limited to the well defined conditions.

1. *Miyoshi myopathy.* The hallmark of Miyoshi myopathy (MM) is weakness and atrophy of the posterior compartment of the lower limbs. The age at onset is between 15 and 30 years, and the earliest complaint is an inability to get up on tiptoes. Typically, the condition slowly progresses to involve proximal muscles, and weakness ultimately becomes generalized. CK levels are massively elevated, especially early. Inheritance is autosomal recessive. The gene for MM has been mapped to the same dysferlin locus identified for LGMD2B. In some families the same mutation has been associated with both conditions, although siblings always express the same phenotype. This suggests that some modifying factors (probably genetic) play a role in determining the phenotype.

2. *Nonaka distal myopathy.* The onset of weakness and atrophy is in the anterior compartment of the lower limbs, and typically begins at 15 to 30 years of age. There is slow progression to severe diffuse weakness. CK levels are only moderately elevated. The gene has been mapped to 9p1-q1.

3. *Welander distal myopathy.* This condition presents late in life (over 40 years of age) with weakness in the extension of the index finger, followed by slow progression to the other hand extensor muscles and to muscle of the anterior and posterior compartments of the distal lower limbs. CK levels are mildly to moderately elevated.

4. *Late onset distal myopathy.* Also known as Markesbery distal myopathy, it presents late (over 40 years of age) with anterior distal weakness of the lower limbs. The illness slowly progresses to involve the upper limbs distally and the proximal lower limbs. CK levels are mildly elevated.

MYOTONIC DYSTROPHIES

Genetic advances have allowed identification, in addition to the classic myotonic dystrophy (DM) phenotype, of several related conditions that manifest as myotonia and weakness.

1. Myotonic dystrophy type 1 (DM1)

   a. With a prevalence of 2 to 14 per 100,000, this is one of the most common inherited neuromuscular disorders.

   b. It is inherited as an autosomal dominant disease, with a gene locus at 19q13.3. The mutation is a triplet (CTG) repeat expansion in the untranslated region of the gene coding for the myotonic dystrophy protein kinase (DMPK). The intergenerational expansion of the triplet repeat accounts for the phenomenon of *anticipation,* that is, earlier onset of symptoms, with increasing severity of the disease, in successive generations.

   c. The severe and rapidly fatal phenotype of congenital DM is transmitted maternally.

   d. Skeletal muscle manifestations usually start as grip and percussion myotonia followed by progressive weakness and wasting of the distal limb muscles and facial muscles. Dysphagia and dysarthria are prominent. Facial muscle weakness and temporal wasting give the face the classic "hatchet" appearance. Diaphragmatic and intercostal muscle weakness may result in respiratory insufficiency.

   e. DM1 is a multisystem disorder. Other organs that are involved include the heart (dilated cardiomyopathy, conduction defects, arrhythmias), gastrointestinal tract (constipation, diarrhea, megacolon), endocrine glands (hyperinsulinism, testicular atrophy), eyes (cataracts, retinal degeneration, extraocular weakness and myotonia), and central nervous system (intellectual impairment).

   f. Laboratory features include mildly to moderately elevated CK levels, myotonic discharges on electrophysiologic testing, and the occasional presence of myopathic motor units. Muscle biopsy reveals variation in fiber size and shape, type I fiber atrophy, excessive number of central nuclei, and abundant numbers of ring fibers and sarcoplasmic masses. DNA testing showing abnormal CTG expansion confirms the diagnosis.

   g. Treatment is symptomatic and mainly aims at reducing the severity of the myotonia. Phenytoin is the agent of choice. Other effective drugs (e.g., quinine or procainamide) may have undesirable cardiac side effects.

Caveat: DM1

- *Anticipation:* earlier onset of symptoms, with increasing severity of the disease, in successive generations

---

 Key Signs: DM1

- Diffuse weakness and wasting

- Myotonia

- Dysphagia and dysarthria

- Respiratory insufficiency

- Cataracts
- Cardiac conduction defects

Key Tests: DM1

- Increased CK levels
- Myotonic discharges on EMG

2. Proximal myotonic myopathy (PROMM)

   a. The concept of PROMM developed when it was noted that a small subgroup of patients with clinical features strongly suggestive of DM had a normal size CTG repeat at the DMPK locus.

   b. Weakness is typically proximal at onset, affecting neck flexors, arm abductors, and proximal lower limb muscles. Some patients have predominantly distal involvement, and some develop it later in the course of the illness. Facial muscles are typically not involved.

   c. Myotonia is seen in 50% of patients and is less pronounced than in DM1.

   d. Extramuscular involvement includes cataracts, cardiac arrhythmias, cognitive impairment, and gastrointestinal and endocrine abnormalities.

   e. Inheritance pattern is autosomal dominant. Neither the gene nor the gene locus has been identified.

3. Myotonic dystrophy type 2 (DM2)

   a. Refers to an entity closely resembling DM1. It has been observed in some families who did not have CTG expansion.

   b. Gene is mapped to a locus on 3q. "Anticipation" has been noted.

EMERY-DREIFUSS MUSCULAR DYSTROPHY

1. Genetics

   a. Two forms of inheritance have been described: X-linked recessive and autosomal dominant. The former is the more common. Both produce essentially identical phenotypes.

   b. The X-linked recessive form results from mutations in the STA gene on Xq28, which codes for a nuclear membrane protein called emerin.

   c. The autosomal dominant form results from mutations in the LMNA gene on 1q21, which codes for other nuclear membrane proteins: laminins A and C.

2. Clinical features

   a. First symptoms occur during the early teens and consist of contractures in the limbs and spine, where tightness in the spinal extensor muscles results in limited neck and trunk flexion.

   b. Weakness follows a humeroperoneal distribution, with striking wasting of biceps, triceps, and peroneal muscles and relative sparing of other muscles.

   c. Cardiac involvement is an important feature that is occasionally fatal. It may be seen in patients with minimal muscle weakness. Abnormalities include arrhythmias (including atrial paralysis), conduction defects, heart block, and dilated cardiomyopathy.

Key Signs: Emery-Dreifuss Muscular Dystrophy

- Contractures of limbs and spine
- Weakness and wasting
- Cardiomyopathy

3. Laboratory features

   a. CK levels are mildly to moderately elevated.

   b. EMG findings are nonspecific, mostly consisting of myopathic features.

   c. Muscle biopsy reveals chronic myopathic changes (variation in fiber size and shape, increased internal nuclei, fibrosis). Immunostaining for the appropriate nuclear membrane protein is typically abnormal.

   d. DNA analysis showing mutations in the emerin or laminin genes confirms the diagnosis.

FACIOSCAPULOHUMERAL MUSCULAR DYSTROPHY

1. Genetics

   a. Facioscapulotumeral muscular dystrophy (FSHD) is an autosomal dominant disorder. With an estimated prevalence of 1 in 20,000, it is one of the most common muscular dystrophies (third most common, after DMD and DM1).

   b. The gene for the disease maps to 4q35, where affected individuals were found to carry a small *Eco*RI fragment (<38 kb). The gene and its product have not been elucidated.

2. Clinical features

   a. Typical onset is during childhood to late teens, although some individuals are not affected until the fourth to fifth decades. Progression is invariably slow.

   b. In most cases, facial weakness is the initial

symptom. It results in an expressionless face, with inability to smile or close the eyes.

c. Concomitantly or soon after, patients develop shoulder girdle weakness, with marked inability to elevate the arms. Weakness of scapular muscles results in the characteristic winging of the scapula with attempts to elevate the arms.

d. With disease progression, wrist extensors and muscles of the anterior compartment of the legs become involved.

e. In 20% of cases, prominent pelvic girdle involvement is seen, leading ultimately to wheelchair confinement.

f. There are no associated cardiac or mental abnormalities. Some families display retinal telangiectasia or sensorineural hearing loss.

3. Laboratory features

a. CK levels are normal or mildly elevated.

b. EMG reveals nonspecific myopathic features.

c. Muscle biopsy shows "milder" myopathic features than most other muscular dystrophies. Endomysial inflammation is not uncommon.

OCULOPHARYNGEAL MUSCULAR DYSTROPHY

1. Genetics

a. Oculopharyngeal muscular dystrophy (OPMD) is typically inherited as an autosomal dominant trait with complete penetrance.

b. Initially mapped to 14q11, the gene for OPMD was recently identified as the gene that codes the poly(A) binding protein2 (PABP2). PABP2 is a nuclear protein with regulatory functions in polyadenylation of messenger RNA. The mutation is an extremely small GCG trinucleotide repeat expansion.

2. Clinical features

a. Typical onset is during late adulthood (fourth to sixth decades).

b. Earliest symptoms are ptosis and dysphagia. Ptosis may be asymmetrical early.

c. Restricted extraocular range of motion is seen in at least 50% of patients. It is typically moderate to severe but rarely reaches complete ophthalmoplegia.

d. Mild neck and limb weakness (predominantly proximal) may be seen later in the disease course, but it almost never leads to significant functional disability.

3. Laboratory features

a. CK is typically mildly elevated.

b. EMG reveals nonspecific myopathic changes.

c. Muscle biopsy reveals chronic myopathic changes and characteristic "rimmed vacuoles."

Bibliography

Bushby KMD: Making sense of the limb-girdle muscular dystrophies. Brain 122:1403–1420, 1999.

Dubowitz V: What is muscular dystrophy? Forty years of progressive ignorance. J R Coll Physicians Lond 34:464–468, 2000.

Dubowitz V, Kinali M, Main M, et al.: Remission of clinical signs in early duchenne muscular dystrophy on intermittent low-dosage prednisolone therapy. Eur J Paediatr Neurol 6:153–159, 2002.

Hartigan-O'Connor D, Chamberlain JS: Developments in gene therapy for muscular dystrophy. Microsc Res Tech 48:223–338, 2000.

Hoffman EP, Dressman D: Molecular pathophysiology and targeted therapeutics for muscular dystrophy. Trends Pharmacol Sci 22:465–470, 2001.

Mendell JR, Buzin CH, Feng J, et al.: Diagnosis of Duchenne dystrophy by enhanced detection of small mutations. Neurology 57:645–650, 2001.

3 Congenital Myopathies

Steven Lovitt
Yadollah Harati

Definition

Originally, the congenital myopathies referred to nonprogressive muscle diseases that were present at birth. As our understanding and recognition of muscle diseases has grown, this definition has fallen somewhat out of favor because some myopathies that fall under this classification are indeed progressive. An alternative inclusion criterion is the presence of a specific morphologic abnormality seen on muscle biopsy. Muscle biopsy is therefore required for establishing the diagnosis. Each condition has significant clinical heterogeneity; although they can present with neonatal hypotonia or delayed milestones, weakness may not be appreciated until later in life.

In contrast, the congenital muscular dystrophies were originally thought to represent a group of diseases that present with muscle weakness at birth or within a few months of life. Many of them are associated with joint contractures or central nervous system (CNS) abnormalities. This classification system is somewhat arbitrary, however, because other myopathies can present near or after birth (Duchenne muscular dystrophy) or can be associated with joint contractures (Emery-Dreifuss muscular dystrophy, Bethlem myopathy).

CONGENITAL MYOPATHIES

Central Core Disease

1. Symptoms

   a. Central core disease may present as neonatal hypotonia, and congenital hip dislocation may be present in such cases. Patients may also present with delayed motor development. In such cases the children may have difficulty walking, getting off the floor, or ascending stairs. A Gowers' sign is often present. Conversely, patients may be asymptomatic until later in life.

   b. Other skeletal abnormalities (e.g., pes cavus, scoliosis, clubfoot) are common.

   c. A significant number of patients have malignant hyperthermia, but it may not be recognized until surgery is performed, often for orthopedic reasons. Patients with central core disease should wear a medical alert bracelet to alert treating physicians to the potential for malignant hyperthermia.

   d. Weakness is usually not progressive.

2. Clinical findings

   a. Patients have proximal weakness of the legs and sometimes of the arms. The neck flexors and facial musculature may be mildly affected, but the remainder of the bulbar musculature is spared.

   b. Sensory examination is normal; muscle stretch reflexes may be normal or decreased.

Key Symptoms and Signs: Central Core Disease

- Neonatal hypotonia, congenital hip dislocation, delayed motor development, Gowers' sign

- Other skeletal abnormalities

- Malignant hyperthermia

- Proximal leg weakness and sometimes arm weakness; usually not progressive

3. Clinical investigations

   a. Creatine phosphokinase (CPK) level is normal or mildly increased.

   b. Nerve conduction velocity studies are normal. Electromyography (EMG) shows short-duration, small-amplitude polyphasic units without spontaneous activity.

   c. Muscle biopsy shows decreased central oxidative enzymatic activity, affecting type I fibers more than type II fibers. Because type I fiber predominance is often present, nearly all fibers may appear to be affected. The core occupies a significant portion of the muscle fiber on cross section and extends the entire length of the fiber on longitudinal section. Decreased staining can also be seen with the ATPase, myophosphorylase, and periodic acid-Schiff (PAS) stains.

Key Test: Central Core Disease

- Muscle biopsy shows decreased central oxidative enzymatic activity, affecting type I more than type II fibers. Because type I fibers often predominate, it may appear that almost all fibers are affected.

4. Genetics

   a. The causative gene has been mapped to chromosome 19q, but the underlying pathogenesis remains unknown.

   b. The ryanodine receptor gene localizes to the same region, which may explain the high rate of co-morbidity of these two conditions.

   c. Inheritance is autosomal dominant with variable expressivity.

NEMALINE MYOPATHY

1. Symptoms

   a. Patients usually present with neonatal hypotonia. Delayed motor development is common, especially walking. When respiratory distress is present, death can occur within days to months due to respiratory failure and pneumonia.

   b. During childhood, patients may be brought for evaluation owing to difficulty walking, arising form the floor, or ascending stairs.

   c. The childhood onset form is generally not progressive. Patients with the neonatal form acquire motor milestones if they do not have respiratory failure, although orthopedic complications may cause further delay.

   d. An adult form has been reported, which presents with a limb-girdle phenotype. These cases may be genetically distinct, because the weakness is progressive and not associated with the classic skeletal features of the pediatric form.

2. Clinical findings

   a. During infancy the only manifestation may be hypotonia.

   b. During childhood, adolescence, and adulthood patients have weakness most prominently in the proximal legs, neck flexors, distal legs. The muscle stretch reflexes are generally absent.

   c. Patients have significant facial weakness with a high-arched palate and micrognathia, often with "slack jaw." Although the pharyngeal and laryngeal muscles may be affected, ptosis and extraocular muscle involvement does not occur.

   d. Scoliosis, pectus excavatum, clubfoot, and pes cavus are common.

Key Symptoms and Signs: Nemoline Myopathy

- Hypotonia during infancy

- Weakness in the proximal arms and legs and the neck flexors

- Facial weakness with a high palate and micrognathia

- Scoliosis, pectus excavatum, clubfoot, pes cavus

3. Clinical investigations

   a. CPK level is usually normal.

   b. Nerve conduction velocity studies are normal. EMG shows short-duration, short-amplitude polyphasic units with early recruitment. Rare fibrillations may be present. Later in life a second population of high-amplitude, long-duration units may be present.

   c. Muscle biopsy shows typical "rods" manifesting as subsarcolemmal red clusters. Type I fibers are affected more commonly than type II fibers; because type I predominance is common, it may appear that nearly all fibers are affected. The increased variation in fiber size and shape that is characteristic of most myopathic processes is often absent, especially when the patient is young. Electron microscopy reveals that the rods arise from the Z disc.

Key Test: Nemoline Myopathy

- Muscle biopsy shows typical "rods" manifesting as subsarcolemmal red clusters, affecting type I more than type II fibers. Because type I fibers often predominate, it may appear that almost all fibers are affected.

4. Genetics

   a. In most families, transmission appears to be by way of autosomal dominant inheritance.

   b. In one family, a mutation in a gene encoding for α-tropomyosin was discovered. Further research may help explain if and how this mutation is causative. No other kinships have displayed this mutation, and the underlying pathogenesis remains unknown.

CENTRONUCLEAR MYOPATHY

1. Symptoms

   a. Patients present most commonly during infancy or early childhood. They frequently have delayed motor milestones, especially walking, but also have trouble ascending stairs and with other tasks that depend on the proximal musculature of the legs. Weakness of the neck flexor muscles, proximal arms, and facial muscles may be present as well. Ptosis and ophthalmoparesis are common and serve as key diagnostic clues for distinguishing this condition from other congenital myopathies.

b. The neonatal form of this disease presents with severe hypotonia, often necessitating respiratory support. Interestingly, facial and extraocular muscles are usually spared in this form of the disease. Most patients die within the first year of life from pneumonia or respiratory failure; those who do not die remain significantly weak. This particular subtype of centronuclear myopathy is sometimes called myotubular myopathy.

c. The least common form presents during the second or third decade of life. Patients present with limb-girdle weakness without ptosis or ophthalmoparesis.

2. Clinical findings

a. In the neonatal form, patients have severe hypotonia and occasionally ptosis with ophthalmoparesis.

b. Patients with the late infantile–early childhood form have predominantly proximal weakness with ptosis and ophthalmoparesis. Scoliosis, clubfoot, increased lumbar lordosis, and a marfanoid appearance may be present.

c. The late childhood–adult type presents with proximal weakness, with some patients displaying ptosis and ophthalmoparesis.

d. All patients have hyporeflexia or areflexia with a normal sensory examination.

Key Symptoms and Signs: Centronuclear Myopathy

- Ptosis and ophthalmoparesis are common and serve as key diagnostic clues for distinguishing this condition from other myopathies.

- Neonatal type: hypotonia

- Late infantile–early childhood type: predominantly proximal weakness with ptosis and ophthalmoparesis

- Late childhood–adult type: proximal weakness

- All patients have hyporeflexia or areflexia with a normal sensory examination.

3. Clinical investigations

a. Patients have a normal or mildly elevated CPK level.

b. Nerve conduction velocity studies are normal. EMG shows the typical myopathic features of short-duration, short-amplitude motor units. Positive sharp waves, fibrillation potentials, electrical myotonia, and complex repetitive discharges have all been reported and serve as important diagnostic clues for distinguishing

this myopathy from other congenital myopathies.

c. Muscle biopsy reveals that as many as 80% of muscle fibers contain internal nuclei. The nuclei are not necessarily in the exact center of the muscle fiber, particularly in those with the late childhood–adult subtype. Type I fibers are more affected than type II fibers; when type I fibers predominate, which is often the case, most fibers appear to have internal nuclei. Oxidative enzyme and PAS staining shows increased reactivity in the center of fibers, and the ATPase stain reveals corresponding absent staining. NADH staining may reveal a characteristic "spokes on a wheel" pattern.

Key Tests: Centronuclear Myopathy

- On EMG, positive sharp waves, fibrillation potentials, electrical myotonia, and complex repetitive discharges have all been reported and serve as important diagnostic clues for distinguishing this myopathy from other congenital myopathies.

- Muscle biopsy reveals that 80% of muscle fibers contain internal nuclei. Because type I fibers often predominate, it may appear that almost all fibers have internal nuclei.

4. Genetics

a. The neonatal subtype is transmitted by way of X-linked recessive inheritance.

b. The late infantile–early childhood form is most likely transmitted by way of autosomal recessive inheritance.

c. The late childhood–adult type is transmitted by way of autosomal dominant inheritance.

d. The underlying pathogenesis is unknown.

CONGENITAL FIBER TYPE DISPROPORTION

1. Symptoms

a. Patients present with infantile hypotonia and delayed motor milestones.

b. Patients usually improve as they grow older, although this is not necessarily so.

2. Clinical findings

a. Weakness and hypotonia may be significant.

b. Scoliosis, clubfoot, congenital hip dislocation, short stature, contractures, and high-arched palate are common.

Key Symptoms and Signs: Congenital Fiber Type Disproportion

- Weakness and hypotonia
- Scoliosis, clubfoot, congenital hip dislocation, short stature, high palate

3. Clinical investigations
   a. CPK level is usually normal
   b. EMG may be normal or may show myopathic changes of short-duration, short-amplitude motor units.
   c. Muscle biopsy shows a predominance of small type I fibers and may show type II fiber hypertrophy.

Key Test: Congenital Fiber Type Disproportion

- Muscle biopsy shows a predominance of small type I fibers and may show type II fiber hypertrophy

4. Genetics
   a. Mode of inheritance is unknown, although in some families autosomal dominant inheritance is suggested.
   b. Pathogenesis is unknown.

MULTICORE/MINICORE DISEASE

1. Symptoms and signs. Patients usually present with delayed motor milestones, although neonatal hypotonia has also been reported. The weakness tends to be mild and nonprogressive. Mild facial weakness may be present; ptosis and ophthalmoplegia rarely occur. Diaphragmatic weakness can lead to nocturnal hypoventilation. Scoliosis, clubfoot, high-arched palate, and a slender body habitus may be present.

Key Symptoms and Signs: Multicore/Minicore Disease

- Significant weakness and hypotonia
- Scoliosis, clubfoot, slender body, high palate

2. Clinical investigations. The CPK level is usually normal, and the EMG shows myopathic features. Muscle biopsy shows decreased central oxidative enzymatic activity. Importantly, the core does not extend the length of the fiber on longitudinal section, distinguishing this process from central core disease. Several cores may occur within the

same fiber, although this has been reported in central core disease as well. A type I fiber predominance is generally present, and the cores tend to occur in type I fibers, which may lead to the appearance that nearly all fibers are affected.

Key Test: Multicore/Minicore Disease

- Muscle biopsy shows decreased central oxidative enzymatic activity, affecting type I more than type II fibers. Because type I fibers often predominate, it may appear that almost all fibers are affected. The core does not extend the length of the fiber on longitudinal section.

3. Genetics. Both autosomal dominant inheritance and recessive inheritance have been reported, as have sporadic cases. The underlying pathogenesis is unknown.

CONGENITAL MUSCULAR DYSTROPHY

Merosin Deficiency (Merosin-Negative) Congenital Muscular Dystrophy

1. Symptoms and signs
   a. Patients with merosin deficiency congenital muscular dystrophy (CMD) commonly are hypotonic at birth and often have associated joint contractures.
   b. The arms and legs are both weak, proximally more than distally. Although the neck and facial muscles are often weak, extraocular muscles are spared, which helps distinguish this condition from centronuclear myopathy.
   c. Mental retardation does not occur, but about 20% develop seizures.

Key Symptoms and Signs: Merosin Deficiency CMD

- Hypotonia is present at birth, with associated joint contractures.
- Although neck and facial muscles are often weak, extraocular muscles are spared, which helps distinguish this condition from centronuclear myopathy.

2. Clinical investigations
   a. CPK level is usually elevated to three to four times normal, but even greater degrees of elevation can occur.
   b. EMG reveals myopathic changes of short-duration, low-amplitude motor units.
   c. Muscle biopsy shows dystrophic-appearing changes of increased variation in fiber size and

shape with replacement of portions of the muscle by adipose tissue and fibrous tissue. Areas of inflammation may be present.

d. Immunostaining for merosin reveals absence or reduction in reactivity, with complete absence correlating with a more severe phenotype.

e. Magnetic resonance imaging (MRI) scan of the brain often reveals abnormal T_2-weighted signals in the white matter, perhaps reflecting the absence of merosin in blood vessel walls.

Key Tests: Merosin Deficiency CMD

- CPK level is three to four times normal.

- Muscle biopsy shows dystrophic-appearing changes; immunostaining for merosin reveals absence or reduction in reactivity, with complete absence correlating with a more severe phenotype.

- MRI scan of brain reveals abnormal white matter.

3. Genetics

a. Both autosomal dominant and recessive inheritance have been reported.

MEROSIN-POSITIVE CONGENITAL MUSCULAR DYSTROPHY ("PURE CMD")

1. Symptoms and signs

a. Symptoms are similar to those of merosin deficiency CMD, although with a milder phenotype. Most patients can walk, and the symptoms are minimally progressive.

b. Joint contractures may occur, and patients may have a rigid spine.

c. Mental retardation and seizures do not occur.

Caveat: Pure CMD

- Symptoms are similar to those of merosin deficiency CMD but milder.

---

2. Clinical investigations

a. CPK level is elevated but less so than in merosin deficiency CMD.

b. MRI of the brain is normal.

c. EMG reveals myopathic changes of short-duration, low-amplitude motor units.

d. Muscle biopsy reveals dystrophic-appearing changes similar to that of merosin deficiency CMD, but immunostaining for merosin is normal. Some patients have been shown to have a deficiency in α-actinin-3.

Key Tests: Pure CMD

- CPK level is elevated.

- Muscle biopsy reveals dystrophic-appearing changes similar to those of merosin deficiency CMD, but immunostaining for merosin is normal.

- MRI of brain is normal.

3. Genetics

a. Inheritance appears to be autosomal recessive.

b. No genetic defect has been discovered.

Fukuyama-type CMD

1. Symptoms and signs

a. Mental retardation is present; seizures are common, either febrile or afebrile. Progressive hydrocephalus often occurs.

b. Patients have hypotonia and generalized weakness, including the facial musculature. Many patients are eventually able to sit unassisted, but only those with a mild phenotype can learn to walk.

c. Joint contractures are common.

d. Cachexia develops, and patients die near the end of the first decade of life.

Caveat: Fukuyama-type CMD

- The disease is rare outside Japan.

---

2. Clinical investigations

a. MRI reveals polymicrogyria with migrational deficits (type II lissencephaly).

b. CPK level is elevated; EMG shows myopathic changes.

c. Muscle biopsy shows variation in fiber size without hypertrophic fibers. A portion of the muscle is replaced by connective tissue. Endomysial necrosis and inflammation are common. Muscle fascicle involvement may be somewhat selective. Immunohistochemistry shows decreased activity for merosin- and dystrophin-associated proteins.

3. Genetics

a. Inheritance is autosomal recessive. The affected protein is futukin, with a chromosomal localization of 9q31-q33; its function is unknown.

b. The disease is rare outside Japan.

Muscle-Eye-Brain Disease (Santavuori CMD)

1. Symptoms and signs
   a. Patients are mentally retarded and have delayed motor milestones.
   b. Although patients have neonatal hypotonia and generalized weakness, survival into early adulthood is not unusual.
   c. Severe myopia and retinal dysplasia occur.

Key Symptoms and Signs: Santavuori CMD

- Mental retardation
- Delayed motor milestones
- Severe myopia and retinal dysplasia

2. Clinical investigations
   a. CPK level is mildly elevated.
   b. EMG shows myopathic changes.
   c. Visual evoked responses show giant potentials.
   d. MRI shows type II lissencephaly with a "cobblestone cortex."
   e. Muscle biopsy shows dystrophic changes. Immunohistochemistry shows decreased merosin activity.
3. Genetics
   a. Inheritance is autosomal recessive. The gene is located on chromosome 1p32-p34, but the exact gene has not yet been found.
   b. Pathogenesis is unknown.

Walker-Warburg Syndrome

1. Symptoms and signs
   a. Patients have seizures and severe mental retardation.
   b. Neonatal hypotonia is present.
   c. Retinal malformation occurs, and other ocular abnormalities (e.g., cataracts, microcornea, lens abnormalities, optic nerve hypoplasia or atrophy) are common.
   d. Type II lissencephaly is present; other cerebral malformations (e.g., vermal hypoplasia, hydrocephalus, occipital encephalocele, agenesis of the corpus callosum) are frequent.

Key Symptoms and Signs: Walker-Warburg Syndrome

- Mental retardation
- Seizures
- Neonatal hypotonia
- Ocular abnormalities
- Cerebral malformations

2. Clinical investigations
   a. MRI is grossly abnormal, with a "cobblestone cortex" appearance, along with the other abnormalities previously listed.
   b. CPK level is normal or mildly elevated.
   c. Muscle biopsy reveals mild dystrophic changes with normal immunohistochemical staining for merosin.
3. Genetics. The genetic locus is unknown. Linkage to the 1p32-p34 locus of muscle-eye-brain disease was recently excluded, confirming that these diseases are genetically distinct.

Bibliography

Carpenter S, Karpati G: Pathology of Skeletal Muscle, 2nd ed. Oxford, Oxford University Press, 2001.
Cormand B, Pinko H, Bayes M, et al.: Clinical and genetic distinction between Walker-Warburg syndrome and muscle-eye-brain disease. Neurology 56:1059–1074, 2001.
Dubowitz V: Congenital muscular dystrophy: an expanding clinical syndrome. Ann Neurol 47:143–144, 2000.
Flanigan KM, Kerr L, Bromberg MB, et al.: Congenital muscular dystrophy with rigid spine syndrome: a clinical, pathological, radiological, and genetic study. Ann Neurol 47:152–161, 2000.
Taratulo AL: Congenital myopathies and related disorders. Curr Opin Neurol 15:553–561, 2002.

4 Dermatomyositis and Polymyositis

Hazem Machkhas
Yadollah Harati

Dermatomyositis (DM) and polymyositis (PM) are acquired inflammatory myopathies that share many clinical features. Despite these similarities, the conditions have dissimilar pathogeneses, with the aberrant immune response in DM being mounted against intramuscular capillaries and small blood vessels and in PM against muscle fibers. The commonly held perception of DM as PM with a rash is inaccurate: In addition to having distinct immune pathogenic mechanisms, the conditions differ in some clinical aspects, their association with other diseases, and their response to treatment.

Differential Diagnosis

1. Overlap syndrome: systemic lupus erythematosus, rheumatoid arthritis, systemic sclerosis, Sjögren's syndrome, sarcoidosis, mixed connective tissue disease
2. Inclusion body myositis
3. Endocrine myopathies: steroids, hyperthyroidism, hypothyroidism, hyperparathyroidism
4. Toxic myopathies: alcohol, cholesterol-lowering agents, colchicine
5. Infectious myopathies: viral myositis, trichinosis, human immunodeficiency virus (HIV), human T-cell leukemia virus-1 (HTLV-1)
6. Limb-girdle muscular dystrophies
7. Metabolic myopathies: Glycogen storage disorders, lipid storage disorders

DERMATOMYOSITIS

1. Symptoms
   a. Most patients develop a characteristic rash, which accompanies but occasionally precedes the onset of muscle weakness.
   b. Subacute weakness appears in a pattern attributable to proximal muscle involvement, such as difficulty climbing up and down stairs, arising from a seated position, and raising arms above the head.
   c. Dysphagia is reported by 25% to 30% of patients. Facial muscles can be involved in extremely severe cases. Extraocular muscles are spared.
   d. The symptomatology for *juvenile dermatomyositis* differs slightly from that of the adult form. Onset may be insidious or fulminant. Peak incidence is between the ages of 5 and 10 years. In addition to the typical pattern of weakness, pain is a prominent complaint. Flexion contractures rapidly develop. Calcinosis of subcutaneous tissues occurs in up to 60% of cases.
   e. An unusual from of DM is *amyopathic dermatomyositis,* where patients have all the classic skin changes of DM but none of the overt muscle involvement. Some patients have subclinical evidence of the disease (on muscle biopsies), and most do not develop a myopathy until several years after appearance of the rash.

Key Symptoms: Dermatomyositis

- Limb weakness, proximal
- Rash

2. Clinical findings
   a. Classic heliotrope (violaceous) rash of the periorbital regions. In severe cases periorbital edema may be prominent.
   b. Erythematous rash of the face, neck, and upper trunk.
   c. Grotton's papules: erythematous changes of the knuckles with purplish or reddish, raised, scaly lesions. This finding is highly characteristic of DM.
   d. Dilated and deformed capillary loops at the base of the fingernails. Nailfold thrombi may be seen. These changes are best seen by nailfold capillary microscopy.
   e. Muscle weakness is predominantly in the proximal musculature, including the neck flexors. A lesser degree of distal weakness may be seen. Affected muscles are sometimes tender to palpation.
   f. Extramuscular manifestations may be seen.
   (1) Interstitial lung disease, which affects 5% to 10% of adult patients with DM. Typically insidious, but a rapidly progressive, occasionally fatal form can occur consisting of acute fever, dyspnea, and cough.

(2) Arthralgias, joint effusions, and contractures

(3) Necrotizing vasculitis, which may affect skin, muscles, gut (where it causes visceral ulcerations or perforation), kidneys, or lungs

(4) Cardiac involvement is rare. Conduction abnormalities, congestive heart failure, and myocarditis have been described.

g. Patients with DM have an increased risk of *cancer*. This is true only with the adult form of the disease. The risk has been estimated to be 5 to 10 times higher than that for the general population. Most common associated malignancies include non-Hodgkin's lymphoma and cancer of the ovary, lung, pancreas, stomach, colon, and rectum.

Key Signs: Dermatomyositis

- Proximal weakness
- Heliotrope rash
- Grotton's papules

3. Laboratory tests

a. Serum creatine kinase (CK) assay is the most sensitive blood test and is elevated in up to 90% of patients. CK levels do not correlate with disease activity or severity and should not be serially monitored to determine the response to therapy.

b. Other muscle enzymes levels are elevated: alanine aminotranferase (ALT), aspartate aminotransferase (AST), and lactate dehydrogenase (LDH).

c. Amylase levels may be elevated.

d. Several myositis-specific autoantibodies and myositis-associated autoantibodies have been identified in patients with DM. Their role in the routine diagnosis and management of patients remains limited, partly owing to their low incidence. The best described is the anti-Jo-1 antibody, which when present heralds coexisting interstitial lung disease and arthritis.

e. Other serologic abnormalities may be seen, including elevated antinuclear antibodies (ANA), rheumatoid factor (RF), and erythrocyte sedimentation rate (ESR); they typically indicate the presence of an associated connective tissue disorder.

f. Electrodiagnostic studies (electromyography/nerve conduction studies [EMG/NCS]) reveal normal nerve conduction and characteristic myopathic units on needle testing, including short-duration, low-amplitude, and polyphasic motor unit potentials. The extent of spontaneous activity (fibrillations and positive sharp waves) usually provides an indication of disease activity. Early recruitment is seen in weak muscles.

g. Muscle biopsy is paramount for confirming the diagnosis. In most patients with DM, muscle biopsy reveals the highly specific finding of perifascicular atrophy, resulting from microvascular ischemic injury. Inflammation is almost exclusively perivascular and reveals a predominance of B cells and CD4+ (T-helper) cells. Endothelial immunostaining for complement membrane attack complex (MAC) is another characteristic feature in DM muscle biopsies and may be the earliest pathologic abnormality.

Key Tests: Dermatomyositis

- Elevated serum CK
- EMG (myopathic units)
- Muscle biopsy (perifascicular atrophy, perivascular inflammation)

4. Treatment

a. Oral prednisone is the mainstay of therapy in juvenile and adult forms of DM. Nearly all patients in both subgroups respond. The initial dosage is 1.0 to 1.5 mg/kg/day (maximum 100 mg/day) taken as a single dose in the morning. After definite clinical improvement is documented and persists, the regimen is changed to alternate-day therapy. Subsequent tapering is slow and tailored to the patient's clinical course.

b. Pulse intravenous methylprednisolone has been shown to be effective, predominantly for juvenile DM. It has a more favorable side effect profile than does oral prednisone.

c. In both open-label and placebo-controlled trials, intravenous immunoglobulin (IVIG) has been shown to be effective in steroid-resistant DM. Most experts now use it as a second-choice drug after prednisone. An initial loading dose of 2 g/kg is given over 3 to 5 days followed by booster doses of 0.5 g/kg every 3 to 4 weeks. The duration of therapy is tailored to the individual's response.

d. Various cytotoxic agents, given individually or in combination, can be used in resistant cases. They include cyclophosphamide, azathioprine, methotrexate, and cyclosporin. Insufficient data exist to suggest that one drug is superior to another, although some reports suggest that cyclophosphamide, alone or in combination with cyclosporin, is the treatment of choice in patients with interstitial lung disease.

Key Treatment: Dermatomyositis

• Prednisone

• Intravenous immunoglobulin

POLYMYOSITIS

1. Symptoms
   a. As in DM, there is subacute symmetrical weakness attributable to proximal muscle involvement. Patients report difficulty climbing up or down the stairs, arising from a seated position, and raising arms above the head. Rarely, the disease presents in a fulminant fashion.
   b. Dysphagia is a common complaint.
   c. Respiratory failure is rare but may occur in the latter stages of undiagnosed or treatment-resistant cases.
   d. Up to 50% of patients have muscle pain or tenderness.

Key Symptoms: Polymyositis

• Limb weakness (weakness)

• Muscle pain and tenderness

2. Clinical findings
   a. Symmetrical, predominantly proximal muscle weakness, including neck flexors. Most patients have mild but definite distal muscle weakness.
   b. Extramuscular manifestations
      (1) Interstitial lung disease is seen at the same frequency as in DM.
      (2) Cardiac involvement is more common than in DM. Up to 25% of patients have myocarditis associated with conduction anomalies and congestive heart failure. Cardiac manifestations may precede the onset of weakness.
   c. The incidence of *cancer* in PM is much lower than in DM, but patients have an approximately twofold increased risk compared with the general population. Common associated malignancies include Hodgkin's lymphoma, non-Hodgkin's lymphoma, and lung and bladder cancer.

Key Sign: Polymyositis

• Proximal weakness

3. Laboratory tests
   a. As in DM, serum CK is the most sensitive test. Serum CK is elevated 5 to 10 times normal levels in 90% of patients and occasionally up to 50 times normal levels. CK levels do not correlate with disease activity and should not be serially monitored to guide therapy.
   b. ALT, AST, and LDH are also elevated.
   c. Amylase may be elevated.
   d. As in DM, myositis-specific and myositis-associated antibodies have been identified but are of limited diagnostic value.
   e. The ANA, RF, and ESR may be elevated and usually indicate the presence of coexisting connective tissue disease.
   f. Electrodiagnostic studies reveal the same abnormalities as those described for DM.
   g. Muscle biopsy is critical for adequate diagnosis. The pathologic hallmarks are scattered foci of endomysial inflammation and necrosis. The inflammatory reaction consists mostly of CD8+ T cells and macrophages. Myofibers in various stages of necrosis and some undergoing phagocytosis are scattered throughout the specimen. MAC deposits are not seen.

Key Tests: Polymyositis

• Elevated serum CK

• EMG (myopathic units)

• Muscle biopsy (endomysial inflammation, necrosis)

4. Treatment
   a. As in DM, prednisone is the first-line treatment. A high dosage of 1.0 to 1.5 mg/kg/day (maximum 100 mg/day) is maintained until adequate persistent clinical response is achieved, at which time conversion to every-other-day dosing is done, with subsequent slow tapering as guided by the patient's symptoms. Adequate patient education is paramount for minimizing the potentially hazardous side effects of prolonged prednisone therapy.
   b. IVIG has not been shown to be as effective as in DM.
   c. Azathioprine remains the second-line agent of choice in refractory cases and as a steroid-sparing agent. The typical dosage is 150 mg/

day. It is recommended that it be introduced gradually (50 mg/day for a week, then 100 mg/day for a week, then full dose) to avoid the typical hypersensitivity reaction (nausea, vomiting, flu-like symptoms). The therapeutic response is usually delayed 3 to 6 months.

d. Other cytotoxic agents can be used in refractory cases, including cyclophosphamide, cyclosporin, and methotrexate.

Key Treatments: Polymyositis

• Prednisone

• Azathioprine

Bibliography

Buchbinder R, Forbes A, Hall S, et al.: Incidence of malignant disease in biopsy-proven inflammatory myopathy. a population-based cohort study. Ann Intern Med 134: 1087–1095, 2001.

Dalakas MC: Inflammatory myopathies: recent advances in pathogenesis. Adv Neurol 88:253–271, 2002.

Hirakata M, Nagai S: Interstitial lung disease in polymyositis and dermatomyositis. Curr Opin Rheumatol 12:501–508, 2000.

Kissel JT: Misunderstandings, misperceptions, and mistakes in the management of the inflammatory myopathies. Semin Neurol 22:41–51, 2002.

Oddis CV: Current approach to the treatment of polymyositis and dermatomyositis. Curr Opin Rheumatol 12:492–497, 2000.

Inclusion body myositis (IBM) has become increasingly recognized since the 1980s and is currently the leading cause of acquired myopathy in patients over 50 years of age. Although most still classify it as an inflammatory myopathy, IBM distinguishes itself from the other inflammatory myopathies by several clinical and pathologic characteristics and by its resistance to therapy. It therefore deserves to be discussed separately, pending its possible reclassification as a leading cause of "degenerative myopathies." This discussion is limited to sporadic IBM. Hereditary inclusion body myopathy shares with sporadic IBM many clinical and pathologic features but is distinguished by being hereditary (autosomal dominant and recessive patterns of inheritance have been described) and by the lack of inflammation on muscle biopsy.

Epidemiology

1. Although accurate incidence and prevalence data are not available, there is a definite indication that the number of IBM cases has steadily increased in the recent past. This is likely due, however, to improved recognition and diagnosis of the condition.

2. Prevalence data are scarce and widely variable, ranging from 0.8 per 100,000 to 3.3 per 100,000 in two reports.

3. An incidence of 2.2 per million has been reported in Sweden.

4. The male/female ratio has also been reported to vary widely, from 1.3:1.0 to 6.5:1.0. A more likely figure is 2:1.

5. There is a delay of approximately 6 years between the onset of symptoms and an accurate diagnosis, mostly owing to patient delay in seeking medical attention.

6. In a recent large series from The Netherlands, the mean age at onset was 59 years for men (range 40–75 years) and 60 years for women (39–77 years), comparable to what has been previously reported. Mean age at death was 74 years for men and 77 years for women (comparable to that of the general population), suggesting that IBM has no negative effect on life expectancy.

Differential Diagnosis

1. Polymyositis (PM) and dermatomyositis (DM). In the past, most cases of IBM were misdiagnosed as

resistant PM. Although the clinical picture may overlap, IBM should be readily distinguishable from PM and DM based on muscle pathology.

2. Distal myopathies. These include especially the Welander and Nonaka variants, which display some of the pathologic features of IBM (rimmed vacuoles). However, the clinical syndromes are quite distinct.

3. Motor neuron disease (MND). In some series, IBM was misdiagnosed as MND in one of five cases. The syndromes may be distinguished clinically: IBM typically does not have muscle fasciculations and lacks the upper motor neuron findings (unless there is coexisting cervical spinal stenosis).

4. Oculopharyngeal muscular dystrophy (OPMD). It may have some of the pathologic findings of IBM (rimmed vacuoles). It can be distinguished clinically, with IBM lacking any ocular involvement.

5. Chronic inflammatory demyelinating polyradiculoneuropathy (CIDP). IBM may have some mild neuropathic changes on examination. Typically, CIDP progresses faster. Electrophysiologic testing should readily help differentiate the two conditions.

Clinical Features

1. The onset of weakness is insidious, and progression is extremely slow. This is probably the main reason for the delay in diagnosis: Patients assume that most of the early symptoms are due to old age or arthritis, so they seek medical attention only when independent ambulation becomes difficult or impossible.

2. At an early stage the weakness may be asymmetrical, in contrast to what is seen with most other myopathic processes. There are two main patterns of muscle involvement: one where weakness is mostly distal (finger flexors and foot extensors) and the other where there is selective weakness and atrophy of the quadriceps muscle (sparing the hamstrings) and the flexor compartment of the forearm (sparing the extensors). The latter pattern is almost pathognomonic of IBM. Quadriceps weakness causes the common complaint of sudden collapse of the knees, resulting in falls.

3. Dysphagia is a common complaint, seen in 30% to 60% of patients, especially during the latter stages of the illness.

4. Even though most patients do not have sensory complaints, up to 30% have some degree of distal sensory loss on examination and may also have electrophysiologic evidence of a polyneuropathy.

Key Symptoms

- Frequent unprovoked falls
- Difficulty rising from a chair
- Difficulty climbing up and down stairs
- Weakness of grip
- Dysphagia

Key Signs

- Distal weakness and atrophy
- Selective quadriceps and forearm flexor weakness

Laboratory Features

1. Serum creatine kinase (CK) levels may be normal (especially during the latter stages of the illness) or mildly elevated (less than 10-fold normal).
2. Electrophysiologic testing. Although rarely diagnostic, electrophysiologic testing may provide important clues to confirm the diagnosis.
   a. Nerve conduction studies. These are normal in most patients, although some display abnormalities of sensory conduction, mostly consisting of reduced amplitudes. Some patients also have abnormal motor nerve conduction, mostly in the lower limbs, consisting of mild slowing of conduction velocities and reduced amplitude.
   b. Needle electromyography (EMG). Even though IBM is a myopathy, needle testing reveals a mixture of "myopathic" and "neuropathic" EMG features. They consist of increased insertional activity and the presence of positive sharp waves and fibrillations (reflecting membrane irritability), short-duration small-amplitude motor unit action potentials (MUAPs) (so-called myopathic units), and long-duration large-amplitude MUAPs (so-called neurogenic units).
3. Pathology (muscle biopsy)
   a. Variation in fiber size and shape, a tendency for rounding of fibers, increased internal nuclei, and increased endomysial connective tissue are seen, all changes indicative of a chronic myopathy.

b. Varying degrees of endomysial inflammation may be seen, with inflammatory foci mostly occupied by CD8+ cells and macrophages.
c. Small clusters of dark small angular fibers (on NADH and nonspecific esterase), indicating neurogenic atrophy, are seen in almost all biopsy specimens.
d. Several fibers contain rimmed vacuoles lined with granular material. Rimmed vacuoles are not specific to IBM and may be seen in OPMD and some distal myopathies.
e. Some fibers have cytoplasmic eosinophilic inclusions, which give the disease its name.
f. Amyloid-positive deposits are seen in several muscle fibers. They appear as apple-green birefringent deposits seen with polarized light after staining with congo red.
g. On electron microscopy, nonbranching filaments (tubofilaments) measuring 15 to 18 nm in diameter are seen in areas adjacent to rimmed vacuoles.

Key Tests

- Normal or mildly elevated CK
- EMG: mixed myopathic and neuropathic findings
- Muscle biopsy: rimmed vacuoles, eosinophilic inclusions, mild endomysial inflammation, amyloid deposits

Pathophysiology

1. Immune mechanisms. Histologic and immunologic studies have shown that IBM shares many of the immunologic features of PM, suggesting that autoimmune mechanisms play an important role in its pathogenesis. However, IBM has remained strongly resistant to all immunomodulatory interventions. That, together with a host of nonimmune features that characterize IBM, has suggested that some of these immunologic features are secondary to other mechanisms.
   a. Role of cytotoxic T cells. The inflammatory cells that invade the endomysium in IBM consist of CD8+ cytotoxic T cells, which surround and attack nonnecrotic muscle fibers expressing major histocompatibility complex (MHC) class 1 antigens. T cells release cytokines and perforin granules, which, upon release, result in osmolysis and necrosis.
   b. Role of viruses. There is evidence that PM and IBM have an association with retroviruses. IBM has been described in the setting of

infections with human immunodeficiency virus (HIV) and human T-cell lymphotropic virus type I (HTLV-I). Viral antigens could not be detected within muscle fibers from these patients' muscle biopsies, although some of the endomysial macrophages harbored them.

2. Nonimmune mechanisms. There is increasing evidence that a degenerative process plays an important role in the pathogenesis of IBM. The strongest such evidence is the existence of Alzheimer-like proteins in the vacuolated muscle fibers, including accumulations of β-amyloid, β-amyloid precursor protein (β-APP), chymotrypsin, apolipoprotein E, ubiquitin, prion protein, and hyperphosphorylated tau protein. Along the same lines, it was observed that some IBM patients have an increased frequency of the apolipoprotein Eε4, similar to what is seen in Alzheimer disease. That latter feature has not been consistently documented. Finally, mitochondrial DNA deletions have been observed in up to 70% IBM muscle biopsies in one series.

Treatment

The perception of IBM as an untreatable disease remains despite the scarcity of controlled trials. One reason is that the risks of using an aggressive approach with chemotherapeutic agents in this elderly population have outweighed the benefits. Anecdotal reports of dramatic improvement with intravenous methylprednisolone and intravenous immunoglobulin (IVIG) continue to surface. IVIG was promising in at least one uncontrolled trial. However, when faced with the scrutiny of a double-blind, placebo-controlled design, IVIG alone or in combination with high dose oral prednisone failed to demonstrate any significant benefit. This grim picture should not discourage the treating physician, however, and a trial of steroids or IVIG is recommended in most patients, especially those with rapid progression, unless medically contraindicated.

Bibliography

Askanas V, Engel WK: Inclusion-body myositis and myopathies: different etiologies, possibly similar pathogenic mechanisms. Curr Opin Neurol 15:525–531, 2002.

Askanas V, Engel WK: Inclusion-body myositis: newest concepts of pathogenesis and relation to aging and Alzheimer disease. J Neuropathol Exp Neurol 60:1–14, 2001.

Badrising UA, Maat-Schieman M, van Duinen SG, et al.: Epidemiology of inclusion body myositis in The Netherlands: a nationwide study. Neurology 55:1385–1387, 2000.

Dalakas MC, Koffman B, Fujii M, et al.: A controlled study of intravenous immunoglobulin combined with prednisone in the treatment of IBM. Neurology 56:323–327, 2001.

Peng A, Koffman BM, Malley JD, Dalakas MC: Disease progression in sporadic inclusion body myositis: observations in 78 patients. Neurology 55:296–298, 2000.

6 Other Acquired Myopathies

Hazem Machkhas
Yadollah Harati

In addition to polymyositis (PM), dermatomyositis (DM), and inclusion body myositis (IBM), there are a host of other acquired myopathies, some inflammatory and others not, some amenable to therapy and others resistant. A detailed review of all these entities is beyond the scope of this chapter, and we limit this discussion to the ones that are most clinically relevant. The myositis associated with connective tissue disorders (overlap syndrome) is similar to PM and so is not discussed here.

OTHER IDIOPATHIC INFLAMMATORY MYOPATHIES

1. Focal myositis
   a. Clinical features
      (1) This is a rare disorder with variable age of onset.
      (2) Most common site of involvement is the leg, but any muscle can be involved.
      (3) It presents as an isolated, painful, and rapidly expanding muscle mass that mimics a tumor.
      (4) Rarely, it generalizes to become classic PM.

Key Sign: Focal Myositis

- Painful muscle mass

   b. Laboratory features
      (1) Serum creatine kinase (CK) is typically normal but may be mildly elevated.
      (2) Imaging of the area reveals edema within the muscle.
      (3) Biopsy of the involved area reveals an inflammatory myopathy with necrosis.

Key Test: Focal Myositis

- Normal CK

   c. Treatment
      (1) Occasionally, lesions resolve spontaneously.
      (2) Treatment with corticosteroids is invariably successful. Rarely, surgical excision is needed.

Key Treatment: Focal Myositis

- Treated with prednisone

2. Eosinophilic polymyositis
   a. Clinical features
      (1) Usually occurs in the setting of hypereosinophilic syndrome (HES).
      (2) Symptoms are insidious in onset and consist of myalgias and proximal weakness.
      (3) Other manifestations of HES can be seen in various combinations, including encephalopathy, peripheral neuropathy, myocarditis, pluritis, and pulmonary fibrosis.

Key Signs: Eosinophilic Polymyositis

- Insidious onset of painful proximal weakness

   b. Laboratory features
      (1) Persistent hypereosinophilia (1500 eosinophils/mm^3) is always present.
      (2) Serum CK is usually elevated, as are rheumatoid factor (RF) and the erythrocyte sedimentation rate (ESR).
      (3) Electrophysiologic testing reveals the myopathic features encountered with PM.
      (4) Muscle biopsy reveals a necrotic myopathy, with endomysial and perivascular foci of inflammation composed almost exclusively of eosinophils.

Key Test: Eosinophilic Polymyositis

- Elevated CK levels
- Persistent hypereosinophilia

   c. Treatment
      (1) Condition has a poor prognosis, with a 3-year survival of less than 20%.
      (2) Oral prednisone is used as a first-line drug, although studies have shown an inconsistent response to corticosteroids.
      (3) In cases of prednisone failure, aggressive

treatment with cytotoxic agents is advocated.

(4) Prompt identification and management of cardiac complications is required.

MYOPATHIES ASSOCIATED WITH INFECTIONS

1. Human immunodeficiency virus (HIV) infection

   a. Clinical features

      (1) An inflammatory myopathy has been described in the setting of acquired immunodeficiency syndrome (AIDS) but may also develop in the earlier stages of HIV infection.

      (2) Clinical features and presentations are identical to those of PM.

      (3) Differential diagnosis in this setting should include zidovudine (azidothymidine, or AZT) toxicity, HIV wasting syndrome, and other neuromuscular disorders that may occur in the setting of HIV infection, such as mononeuritis multiplex and chronic inflammatory demyelinating polyradiculoneuropathy.

   b. Laboratory features

      (1) Serum CK is invariably elevated.

      (2) Electrophysiologic testing reveals a nonspecific active myopathy, with features of membrane irritability, including fibrillations and positive sharp waves.

      (3) Muscle biopsy reveals a necrotic inflammatory myopathy. In approximately 50% of cases, nemaline rods are seen in some fibers.

   c. Treatment

      (1) Prednisone has been shown to be effective in reversing the myopathy but carries the risk of further immunosuppression in an already vulnerable population.

      (2) Intravenous immunoglobulin (IVIG) and plasma exchange are potentially safer but usually less effective alternatives.

      (3) If the patient is not already on antiretroviral medications, starting such therapy may prove effective in controlling the myopathy.

2. Trichinosis

   a. Clinical features

      (1) Trichinosis results from infection with the nematode *Trichinella spiralis* after eating infected, inadequately cooked meat, usually pork.

      (2) An inflammatory myopathy may ensue, usually preceded by diarrhea, which occurs within a week from ingesting the infected meat.

      (3) Myalgia and weakness appear a week after the infected meat has been consumed, usually accompanied by fever, maculopapular rash, and periorbital edema.

      (4) Some patients develop encephalopathy.

   b. Laboratory features

      (1) Serum CK levels are invariably elevated.

      (2) Eosinophilia is seen in most patients, and ranges from 5 to 90% of white blood cells.

      (3) Electrophysiologic testing reveals nonspecific myopathic changes.

      (4) Muscle biopsy reveals an inflammatory myopathy. A large sample enhances the possibility of identifying *Trichinella* larvae embedded in muscle fibers.

      (5) Serologic tests for the nematode are negative during the early stages of the infection but become positive later.

   c. Treatment

      (1) High-dose prednisone is recommended in all patients with weakness.

      (2) Concomitant anti-*Trichinella* therapy with albendazole is advised.

      (3) The illness may be fatal in patients who develop encephalopathy or severe cardiac myositis.

ENDOCRINE MYOPATHIES

1. Thyrotoxic myopathy

   a. Clinical features

      (1) Overt myopathy affects approximately 5% of patients with thyrotoxicosis.

      (2) Typically, there is insidious onset of painless proximal weakness and atrophy.

      (3) Some patients have selective severe involvement of the shoulder girdle, resulting in severe atrophy and scapular winging.

      (4) Occasionally bulbar, esophageal, and respiratory muscles are involved, resulting in dysphagia, dysphonia, and respiratory distress.

      (5) On examination, in addition to the weakness, one may see fasciculations and myokymia.

Key Signs: Thyrotoxic Myopathy

- Insidious painless proximal weakness
- Fasciculations and myokymia
- Bulbar and respiratory involvement common

b. Laboratory features

(1) Thyroid function studies are obviously abnormal, reflecting the hyperthyroid state.

(2) Serum CK levels are usually normal but may be slightly elevated.

(3) Electrophysiologic testing reveals nonspecific myopathic motor unit potentials. Some patients have fibrillations and fasciculations.

(4) Muscle biopsies are usually not part of the routine work-up of this condition. If obtained, they reveal nonspecific myopathy with scattered necrotic fibers.

c. Treatment

(1) The myopathy typically improves with restoration of the euthyroid state. Full recovery may take months. Reversal of weakness precedes the resolution of atrophy.

(2) Immunosuppression has been advocated for severe cases, but it is of dubious benefit and carries high risks.

Key Treatment: Thyrotoxic Myopathy

- Correcting the endocrinopathy resolves the myopathy.

2. Hypothyroid myopathy

a. Clinical features

(1) Whereas most hypothyroid patients develop muscle complaints, muscle weakness occurs in only one-third of cases.

(2) In addition to complaints related to proximal muscle weakness, patients complain of myalgias, cramps, and stiffness.

(3) Muscle atrophy is rare, and some patients actually develop muscle hypertrophy.

(4) Respiratory muscle involvement is rare.

(5) Rhabdomyolysis may develop.

Key Signs: Hypothyroid Myopathy

- Proximal muscle weakness
- Myalgias and cramps

b. Laboratory features

(1) Serum CK levels are markedly elevated (10 to 100 times normal).

(2) Thyroid function studies reveal low free thyroxine levels, with elevated thyroid-stimulating hormone (TSH) levels.

(3) Electrophysiologic testing is typically normal.

(4) Muscle biopsies are not routinely obtained. They are often normal. Abnormalities, when present, are nonspecific and include variation in fiber size and selective type II fiber atrophy.

Key Test: Hypothyroid Myopathy

- Elevated CK levels

c. Treatment

(1) The myopathy improves with restoration of the euthyroid state.

(2) Total resolution of symptoms may take up to 1 year.

Key Treatment: Hypothyroid Myopathy

- Correction of endocrinopathy resolves the myopathy

3. Hyperparathyroid myopathy

a. Clinical features

(1) A myopathy can develop in association with primary hyperparathyroidism and secondary hyperparathyroidism (osteomalacia).

(2) Typically, there is proximal muscle weakness and atrophy that is worse in the lower limbs.

(3) Some patients develop bulbar weakness resulting in dysphagia and hoarseness.

(4) Respiratory compromise is rare.

(5) The examination may reveal coexisting upper motor neuron signs, including hyperactive deep tendon reflexes and spasticity. Plantar response is typically flexor but may rarely be extensor.

b. Laboratory features

(1) Serum CK levels are usually normal.

(2) Serum calcium levels are elevated and serum phosphate levels low in patients with primary hyperparathyroidism. In those with secondary hyperparathyroidism, serum calcium levels may be low or normal.

(3) Electrophysiologic testing reveals myopathic motor units.

(4) Muscle biopsy, if done, may reveal nonspecific myopathic features. Occasionally, selective type II fiber atrophy is seen.

c. Treatment

(1) Symptomatic patients with primary hyperparathyroidism need to undergo surgical removal of the parathyroid gland, which results in near-total resolution of symptoms within a few months.

(2) Patients with secondary hyperparathyroidism usually respond to medical therapy with vitamin D and calcium supplementation. Similarly, symptoms resolve within a few months.

TOXIC MYOPATHIES

1. Myopathy associated with cholesterol-lowering agents

a. Clinical features

(1) Two major classes of drugs are involved: fibric acid derivatives (clofibrate, gemfibrozil) and 3-hydroxy-3-methyl-glutaryl–coenzyme A (HMG-CoA) reductase inhibitors (lovastatin, simvastatin, provastatin, atorvastatin, fluvastatin, cerivastatin).

(2) Myopathy is characterized by proximal muscle weakness, cramps, and prominent myalgias.

(3) Myoglobinuria is seen in some cases.

Key Signs: Myopathy Associated with Cholesterol-lowering Drugs

• Acute onset of painful proximal weakness

b. Laboratory features

(1) Serum CK levels are invariably elevated in patients with myopathy. Up to one-third of asymptomatic patients have transient increases in serum CK levels at some point during therapy.

(2) Electrophysiologic testing reveals nonspecific myopathic motor units.

(3) Muscle biopsy demonstrates necrotic myopathy of variable severity. Rarely, inflammatory myopathy with prominent necrosis pathologically similar to PM is seen.

c. Treatment

(1) Immediately discontinue the offending agent.

(2) Symptoms may take several months to resolve completely.

Key Tests: Myopathy Associated with Cholesterol-lowering Drugs

• Elevated serum CK level

• Significant necrosis on muscle biopsy

Key Treatment: Myopathy Associated with Cholesterol-lowering Drugs

• Immediate removal of the offending drug

2. Alcoholic myopathy

a. Clinical features. There are three distinct patterns of skeletal muscle involvement due to chronic alcohol abuse.

(1) Acute necrotizing myopathy. It results from sustained excessive alcohol use. Symptoms include acute muscle pain, tenderness, cramping, and weakness. Rhabdomyolysis with myoglobinuria and acute renal failure may be seen.

(2) Acute hypokalemic myopathy. It usually presents with acute generalized weakness in the absence of pain or cramps.

(3) Chronic alcoholic myopathy. This has an insidious onset and manifests as slow progression of proximal weakness, preferentially involving the lower limbs. The degree of weakness is variable. Often the weakness is incidentally found on examination.

b. Laboratory features

(1) Serum CK levels are markedly elevated in acute necrotizing myopathy and acute hypokalemic myopathy. They are typically normal in chronic alcoholic myopathy.

(2) Serum potassium level is extremely low in acute hypokalemic myopathy.

(3) There is no distinctive pattern on electrophysiologic testing for any of these conditions. Most patients with chronic alcohol use have coexisting axonal polyneuropathies, which produce findings of denervation and reinnervation on needle evaluation. There may be interspersed myopathic motor unit potentials.

(4) The muscle biopsy for acute necrotizing myopathy demonstrates significant necrosis throughout the sample. These changes are absent in acute hypokalemic myopathy, where the dominant picture is that of a vacuolar myopathy. Selective type II fiber atrophy is usually seen in patients with chronic alcoholic myopathy.

c. Treatment
(1) All patients require supportive medical care as needed, with nutritional supplementation.
(2) Correction of hypokalemia in acute hypokalemic myopathy results in resolution of symptoms.

Bibliography

Amato AA, Dumitru D: Acquired myopathies. In Dumitru D, Amato AA, Zwarts M (eds): Electrodiagnostic Medicine. Philadelphia, Hanley & Belfus, 2002, pp. 1371–1432.

Griggs RC, Mendell JR, Miller RG: Inflammatory myopathies. In Griggs RC, Mendell JR, Miller RG (eds): Evaluation and Treatment of Myopathies. Philadelphia, F.A. Davis, 1995, pp. 154–210.

Griggs RC, Mendell JR, Miller RG: Myopathies of systemic disease. In Griggs RC, Mendell JR, Miller RG (eds): Evaluation and Treatment of Myopathies. Philadelphia, F.A. Davis, 1995, pp. 355–385.

Horak HA, Pourmand R: Endocrine myopathies. Neurol Clin 18:203–213, 2000.

Pascuzzi RM: Drugs and toxins associated with myopathies. Curr Opin Rheumatol 10:511–520, 1998.

7 Glycogen and Lipid Storage Myopathies

Hazem Machkhas
Yadollah Harati

Glycogen and lipid storage myopathies fall under the larger heading of metabolic myopathies. Most neurologists shudder at the thought of having to meander in this vast wasteland of disorders with obscure and often difficult to pronounce names. This review seeks to dissipate this apprehension. Instead of exhausting the reader with a detailed listing of all glycogen and lipid storage disorders that result in myopathies, we discuss only the ones most likely to be encountered in clinical practice. Individuals interested in more details are referred to the Bibliography. Tables 7–1 and 7–2 provide a brief overview of the glycogen and lipid storage disorders that cause a myopathy.

GENERAL COMMENTS

1. Not all disorders of glycogen and lipid metabolism cause a myopathy.
2. In most of these disorders the symptoms are dynamic; that is, they appear or increase as the energy requirements of the muscles increase during exercise. Some disorders (e.g., acid maltase deficiency) present with static weakness.
3. Symptoms common to most entities include weakness, myalgias, cramps, and rhabdomyolysis.
4. The time of onset of symptoms is important. During the initial phase of muscle exercise, energy is produced predominantly through glycogen metabolism. As exercise is sustained, the energy source becomes the lipid stores. Accordingly, patients with glycogen storage disorders manifest symptoms within the first few minutes (no longer than 5 minutes) after exercise. Patients with lipid storage disorders become symptomatic approx-

TABLE 7–1. MYOPATHIC GLYCOGENOSES

DISORDER	MODE OF INHERITANCE	ENZYME DEFICIENCY
GSD II	Autosomal recessive	Acid maltase
GSD III	Autosomal recessive	Debrancher
GSD IV	Autosomal recessive	Brancher
GSD V	Autosomal recessive	Myophosphorylase
GSD VII	Autosomal recessive	Phosphofructokinase
GSD VIII	Autosomal recessive	Phosphorylase B kinase
GSD IX	X-linked	Phosphoglycerate kinase
GSD X	Autosomal recessive	Phosphoglycerate mutase
GSD XI	Autosomal recessive	Lactate dehydrogenase
GSD XII	Unknown	β-Enolase

Abbreviation: GSD, glycogen storage disease.

688

TABLE 7–2. LIPID STORAGE MYOPATHIES

Carnitine deficiency
Carnitine palmitoyl transferase deficiency
Carnitine-acylcarnitine translocase deficiency
Very-long-chain acyl-CoA dehydrogenase deficiency
Trifunctional protein deficiency
Short-chain acyl-CoA dehydrogenase deficiency
Short-chain hydroxy-acyl-CoA dehydrogenase deficiency

Abbreviation: CoA, coenzyme A.

imately 15 to 20 minutes after the onset of exercise.

5. Initial investigation in all patients with suspected myopathy of metabolic origin should include serum creatine kinase (CK), serum chemistries, thyroid function tests, forearm ischemic exercise test, electrophysiologic testing with electromyography and nerve conduction studies (EMG/NCS), and muscle biopsy.
6. The forearm ischemic exercise test is a useful (and painful) tool for confirming (but not fully excluding) glycogen storage disorders. The normal response is a concomitant increase in ammonia and lactate (three to four times normal). Glycogen storage disorders cause an uncoupling of this increase, with lactate levels remaining at baseline. Note that false-negative results may occur.

GLYCOGEN STORAGE MYOPATHIES (MYOPATHIC GLYCOGENOSES)

1. Acid maltase deficiency (type II glycogenosis, GSD II)
   a. Clinical features
      (1) GSD II is seen in three clinically distinct forms, depending on the age of onset.
      (2) The infantile form is characterized by progressive weakness and hypotonia during the first 3 months of life. Respiratory failure ensues. There is associated macroglossia, cardiomegaly, and hepatomegaly. It is invariably fatal, with death by 2 years of age.
      (3) The juvenile form presents during early childhood with delayed motor milestones, including walking. There is prominent proximal muscle weakness. Often the clinical picture is reminiscent of Duchenne

muscular dystrophy. It slowly progresses and ultimately involves the respiratory muscles. Organomegaly is rare. Death ensues between 20 and 30 years of age.

(4) The adult form manifests after 20 years of age, often as late as the mid-thirties. Slowly progressive, predominantly proximal weakness is the presenting symptom in most cases, although up to one-third present with respiratory insufficiency, occasionally acute. Organomegaly is uncommon.

Key Signs: Acid Maltase Deficiency (GSD II)

• Three distinct forms: infantile, juvenile, adult

• Respiratory failure sometimes the dominant feature of adult form

b. Laboratory features

(1) All three forms share similar features.

(2) Serum CK is elevated, most significantly in the infantile form. In some patients with the adult form, CK is normal.

(3) Electrophysiologic testing reveals normal nerve conduction studies, except in advanced cases where muscle atrophy results in low compound muscle action potentials (CMAPs). Needle examination reveals findings of membrane instability (fibrillation, positive sharp waves), including of the paraspinous muscles. Volitional contraction produces typical myopathic units (low amplitude, short duration).

(4) Muscle biopsy reveals prominent vacuoles throughout the cytoplasm that contain glycogen and lysosomes. In addition, nonspecific myopathic changes of variable severity are seen.

(5) Deficiency of α-glucosidase can be demonstrated in various tissues (including muscle) and urine.

(6) Forearm ischemic exercise test is normal.

Key Tests: Acid Maltase Deficiency (GSD II)

• Serum CK (elevated)

• EMG ("myopathic")

• Muscle biopsy (vacuolar myopathy)

• Ischemic exercise test (normal)

c. Genetic features

(1) All forms are inherited in an autosomal recessive fashion.

(2) It is associated with mutations in the acid maltase (α-glucosidase) gene on chromosome 17q23-25.

d. Treatment

(1) Supportive therapy is given for respiratory failure.

(2) In some patients (mostly those with the adult form), a high-protein diet has been associated with striking improvement in muscle strength and respiratory function.

Key Treatment: Acid Maltase Deficiency (GSD II)

• In some patients (mostly with the adult form), a high-protein diet has been associated with striking improvement in muscle strength and respiratory function

2. Debranching enzyme deficiency (type III glycogenosis, GSD III)

a. Clinical features

(1) Two forms of the disease are recognized: one that spares muscles (GSD IIIb) and the other (GSD IIIa) with muscle involvement.

(2) Muscle weakness in GSD IIIa may manifest during childhood (delayed milestones) or adult life (third to fourth decades).

(3) Weakness is predominantly proximal, but most patients ultimately have various degrees of distal weakness.

(4) A small number of patients have dynamic symptoms of exercise-induced fatigue and cramps.

(5) Notable hepatomegaly with abnormal liver enzymes is seen in all cases.

Key Signs: Debranching Enzyme Deficiency (GSD III)

• Weakness is predominantly proximal

• Hepatomegaly

b. Laboratory features

(1) Serum CK is elevated.

(2) Forearm ischemic exercise test is abnormal, with no increase in lactate levels.

(3) Electrophysiologic testing reveals normal nerve conduction studies in most patients,

although a superimposed peripheral neuropathy is seen in some. Needle testing reveals membrane instability (fibrillations, positive sharp waves) and myopathic motor units on volition.

(4) Muscle biopsy reveals vacuolar myopathy, with most vacuoles in a subsarcolemmal location, and intense staining with periodic acid-Schiff (PAS), indicating abundant glycogen.

Key Tests: Debranching Enzyme Deficiency (GSD III)

• Serum CK (elevated)

• EMG ("myopathic")

• Muscle biopsy (subsarcolemmal, PAS-positive vacuoles)

c. Genetic features

(1) Inheritance is autosomal recessive.

(2) It is associated with mutations in the debranching enzyme gene on chromosome 1p21.

d. Treatment

(1) Frequent small meals to avoid hypoglycemia

(2) High-protein diet

3. Myophosphorylase deficiency (type V glycogenosis, GSD V)

a. Clinical features

(1) It is also commonly known as McArdle's disease.

(2) Onset is typically during childhood; the cardinal feature is exercise intolerance associated with myalgias, easy fatigability, and later cramps.

(3) Most patients have the characteristic "second-wind" phenomenon, whereby a short period of rest at the onset of symptoms results in improved exercise tolerance.

(4) Myoglobinuria is a common complaint, and up to 25% of patients have at least one associated episode of renal failure.

(5) A fixed myopathy is seen at a later stage in as many as one-third of patients.

(6) A significant number of patients, although symptomatic during childhood with easy fatigability, do not seek medical attention until their late teens or early adult life,

when cramps or myoglobinuria become prominent.

Key Signs: Myophosphorylase Deficiency (GSD V)

• Exercise intolerance

• "Second-wind" phenomenon

• Myoglobinuria

b. Laboratory features

(1) Serum CK is elevated even between attacks.

(2) Forearm ischemic exercise test is abnormal, with no increase in lactate. If the clinical suspicion is high for GSD V, it is advisable not to perform this test or to perform it without inducing ischemia (exercise only), as some patients develop a compartment syndrome or myoglobinuria.

(3) Electrophysiologic testing reveals normal nerve conduction studies. Needle testing may be normal or reveal membrane instability (fibrillations and positive sharp waves) and myopathic motor units. There appears to be a correlation between the duration of the disease and the presence of abnormalities on needle evaluation.

(4) Muscle biopsy reveals PAS-positive subsarcolemmal vacuoles. Myophosphorylase reaction is absent. Myophosphorylase assay reveals absent or significantly reduced activity.

Key Tests: Myophosphorylase Deficiency (GSD V)

• Serum CK (elevated)

• Ischemic exercise test (abnormal)

• Muscle biopsy (subsarcolemmal, PAS-positive vacuoles)

c. Genetic features

(1) Inheritance is autosomal recessive.

(2) It is associated with mutations in the myophosphorylase gene on chromosome 11q13.

d. Treatment

(1) Avoid intense isometric exercises (weight lifting).

(2) Mild aerobic exercise may be helpful.

(3) High-protein diet may be helpful.

4. Phosphofructokinase deficiency (type VII glycogenosis, GSD VII)

a. Clinical features

   (1) Also known as Tarui's disease, this is a rare disorder.

   (2) Shares many of the clinical features of GSD V, including exercise-induced fatigue, myalgias, cramps, and weakness.

   (3) No "second-wind" phenomenon.

   (4) Myoglobinuria is uncommon but may occur.

   (5) Fixed myopathic weakness does not occur.

   (6) Most patients have episodic hemolysis and jaundice secondary to phosphofructokinase (PFK) deficiency in erythrocytes.

b. Laboratory features

   (1) Varying degrees of serum CK elevation are seen.

   (2) Mild anemia (hemolytic) is present with increased reticulocyte count.

   (3) Abnormal forearm ischemic exercise test.

   (4) Electrophysiologic features are not well defined owing to the small number of cases.

   (5) Muscle biopsy findings are identical to those of GSD V. The PFK reaction is absent, and the PFK assay reveals absent or severely reduced activity.

c. Genetic features

   (1) Inheritance is autosomal recessive.

   (2) It is associated with mutation in the gene coding for the muscle subunit of PFK, located on chromosome 12q13.3.

d. Treatment

   (1) Mild aerobic exercise may be helpful.

   (2) Correction of the anemia, unless severe, is neither helpful nor recommended.

LIPID STORAGE MYOPATHIES

1. Carnitine deficiency

a. Clinical features

   (1) Carnitine deficiency manifests in two major forms. Primary systemic carnitine deficiency is a Reye-like syndrome, where the systemic manifestations eclipse the muscle symptoms. We limit this discussion to primary muscle carnitine deficiency.

   (2) Onset is during childhood or teens, with progressive, predominantly proximal muscle weakness and atrophy.

   (3) Exercise intolerance and cramps may be seen.

   (4) Myoglobinuria is rare.

Key Signs: Carnitine Deficiency

• Progressive, predominant proximal muscle weakness

• Exercise intolerance

b. Laboratory features

   (1) Serum CK levels may be normal or significantly elevated.

   (2) Forearm ischemic exercise test is normal.

   (3) Serum carnitine levels are normal.

   (4) Electrophysiologic testing reveals normal nerve conduction studies. Needle testing reveals myopathic motor units. Rarely, evidence of membrane instability is noted.

   (5) Muscle biopsy reveals abnormal accumulation of lipid droplets throughout the muscle fibers, seen on staining with oil red O. Biochemical assay for carnitine reveals significantly reduced levels.

Key Tests: Carnitine Deficiency

• Oil red O stain (abnormal)

• Muscle biopsy (severely reduced muscle carnitine)

c. Genetic features

   (1) Inheritance is suspected to be autosomal recessive, although sporadic cases are numerous.

   (2) It is associated with mutations in the organic cation transporter (*OCTN2*) gene on chromosome 5q31-32.

d. Treatment

   (1) L-Carnitine supplementation may be helpful for restoring muscle strength.

   (2) Some reports have suggested a beneficial effect after treatment with prednisone, but this approach is not recommended.

2. Carnitine palmitoyl transferase (CPT) deficiency

a. Clinical features

   (1) CPT exists in two forms: CPT I and CPT II. CPT I deficiency is not associated with a myopathy. CPT II deficiency presents in three forms: infantile, late infantile, and adult. Only the latter, which is associated with a distinct myopathy, is discussed here.

   (2) Typical presentation is with exercise-induced cramps, myalgia, weakness, rhabdomyolysis, and myoglobinuria. Prolonged fasting may also induce attacks.

   (3) Fixed weakness is almost never seen. Pa-

tients are asymptomatic and have a normal examination between attacks.

Key Signs: CPT Deficiency

- Exercise-induced cramps and weakness
- Rhabdomyolysis

b. Laboratory features

(1) Serum CK is typically normal but may be elevated.

(2) Electrodiagnostic testing is normal.

(3) Muscle biopsy is normal, including oil red O stain.

(4) Biochemical analysis of muscle biopsy reveals CPT II deficiency.

Key Tests: CPT Deficiency

- Oil red O (normal)
- Muscle biopsy (*CPT2* deficiency)

c. Genetic features

(1) Inheritance is autosomal recessive, but for unknown reasons males are affected far more often than females.

(2) Associated with mutations in the *CPT2* gene on chromosome 1p32.

d. Treatment

(1) Avoidance of precipitating factors, such as prolonged fasting or sustained exercise of more than 30 minutes

(2) Frequent high-carbohydrate, low-fat, small meals

Bibliography

Cwik VA: Disorders of lipid metabolism in skeletal muscle. Neurol Clin 18:167–184, 2000.

Hirano M, DiMauro S: Metabolic myopathies. Adv Neurol 88:217–234, 2002.

Pourmand R: Metabolic myopathies: a diagnostic evaluation. Neurol Clin 18:1–13, 2000.

Tsujino S, Nonaka I, DiMauro S: Glycogen storage myopathies. Neurol Clin 18:125–150, 2000.

Vladutiu GD: The molecular diagnosis of metabolic myopathies. Neurol Clin 18:53–104, 2000.

8 Skeletal Muscle Channelopathies

Hazem Machkhas

Major strides have been achieved in microscopic electrophysiologic techniques that have allowed the identification of disorders involving voltage-gated skeletal muscle channels, the so-called channelopathies. This has allowed the grouping of various disorders previously classified as periodic paralyses or nondystrophic myotonias according to the respective ion channel disorder (Table 8–1). To date, the exact mechanisms that govern the phenotypic expression of various genotypes have not been elucidated. Inherited disorders related to defects in skeletal muscle voltage-gated sodium, calcium, and chloride channels have been identified.

SODIUM CHANNELOPATHIES

1. Hyperkalemic periodic paralysis (HyperKPP)
   a. Clinical features
      (1) Age of onset of symptoms is usually during the first decade of life, often infancy.
      (2) Earliest symptom in infants is the onset of weakness and hypotonia after crying.
      (3) As children get older, the full clinical picture develops, with episodic quadriparesis induced by cold, emotional stress, fasting, and rest after vigorous exercise. The weakness may last up to 3 hours. Some patients report an "aura" of heaviness in the legs preceding an attack.
      (4) Some patients are able to "walk off" an attack by maintaining a sustained level of mild exercise following strenuous activity.
      (5) Frequency of the attacks may diminish with age.

TABLE 8–1. SKELETAL MUSCLE CHANNELOPATHIES

Sodium Channelopathies *(SCN4A)*
Hyperkalemic periodic paralysis
Paramyotonia congenita (some families with periodic paralysis)
Potassium-aggravated myotonia
Hypokalemic periodic paralysis (uncommon)

Calcium Channelopathies *(CACNL1A3)*
Hypokalemic periodic paralysis

Chloride Channelopathies *(CLCN1)*
Autosomal dominant myotonia congenita (Thomsen's disease)
Autosomal recessive myotonia congenita (Becker's disease)

(6) Some patients, with age, develop a slowly progressive myopathy, with fixed proximal muscle weakness between attacks.
(7) Examination is typically normal between attacks, although a subgroup of patients has myotonia. The only finding other than weakness during an attack is a tendency for depression of deep tendon reflexes.

Key Signs: Hyperkalemic Periodic Paralysis

- Episodic quadriparesis
- "Walk-off" phenomenon
- Fixed myopathy possible
- Myotonia typically absent
- Potassium sensitivity

   b. Laboratory features
      (1) Serum potassium levels are normal between attacks. During an attack most patients initially have elevated serum potassium, which subsequently normalizes or falls into the hypokalemic range. Some patients remain normokalemic throughout the attack, but they are invariably potassium-sensitive and become weak if given potassium.
      (2) Serum creatine kinase (CK) may be normal or slightly elevated, even between attacks.
      (3) Electrophysiologic testing reveals normal nerve conduction studies. Needle electromyography (EMG) between attacks may be normal, although some patients display myotonic discharges. Cooling the limb may exacerbate the myotonic discharges. The "exercise test" consists of recording compound muscle action potentials (CMAPs) during and after a muscle is exercised. Typically, there is an initial increase in CMAP amplitudes followed by a decline to nearly half the baseline value. During an attack, muscles are electrically silent.
      (4) Muscle biopsies may be normal, or reveal nonspecific changes, including variation in fiber size, increased central nuclei, and cytoplasmic vacuoles.

c. Genetic features

(1) Inheritance is autosomal dominant with complete penetrance. Sporadic mutations have been described.

(2) HyperKPP is associated with mutations in the α subunit of the voltage-gated sodium channel (*SCN4A*) on chromosome 17q.

d. Treatment

(1) Most treatment issues revolve around preventing attacks. This can be achieved through a low-potassium high-carbohydrate diet and avoidance of fasting, strenuous activities, and exposure to cold.

(2) During severe attacks intravenous infusion of glucose, insulin, or calcium carbonate is indicated.

(3) Prophylactic treatment with acetazolamide, hydrochlorothiazide, or occasionally beta-blockers may reduce the frequency of attacks.

2. Paramyotonia congenita

a. Clinical features

(1) This disease is also known as Eulenberg disease. It is related to HyperKPP in that they are allelic disorders.

(2) Paramyotonia is defined as a paradoxical reaction to exercise. Whereby classic myotonia displays a warm-up phenomenon, sustained exercise in patients with paramyotonia worsens the muscle stiffness.

(3) Onset of symptoms may be during infancy, typically in the first decade.

(4) The main symptom is paramyotonia, which may be precipitated by rest after exercise, cold, and fasting. Certain muscle groups seem to have a predilection for this symptom, including facial, bulbar, and hand muscles.

(5) The disease is typically nonprogressive, and paramyotonia is the only symptom.

(6) Some families have, in addition to paramyotonia, a tendency to develop periodic attacks of paralysis, similar to what is seen in HyperKPP. In those patients, potassium challenge may precipitate an attack.

(7) Examination is typically normal between attacks. Some patients have subtle percussion myotonia.

Key Signs: Paramyotonia Congenita

• "Paradoxical" myotonia

• Weakness typically not present

b. Laboratory features

(1) Serum CK levels are normal or mildly elevated.

(2) Potassium levels are typically normal but may be elevated during an attack.

(3) Electrophysiologic testing reveals normal routine nerve conduction studies. Cooling the limb produces a drastic decrease in the CMAP amplitudes in most patients. Needle testing usually reveals myotonic discharges, which increase after cooling.

(4) Muscle biopsies are rarely indicated for the routine work-up of this condition. If done, they are typically normal. In the subgroup of patients who have coexisting periodic paralysis, intracytoplasmic vacuoles may be seen.

c. Genetic features

(1) Inheritance is autosomal dominant with high penetrance.

(2) This disorder is allelic to HyperKPP and maps to the same *SCN4A* gene, where multiple mutations have been identified.

d. Treatment

(1) Most patients do not require treatment because they have adapted their lifestyle to avoid situations that trigger the attacks of stiffness.

(2) Mexiletine and tocainide have been shown to prevent cold-induced stiffness and weakness. Mexiletine is usually better tolerated than tocainide.

(3) Hydrochlorothiazide is occasionally helpful for relieving myotonia.

3. Potassium-aggravated myotonia (PAM)

a. Clinical features

(1) It encompasses three disorders—myotonia fluctuans, myotonia permanens, acetazolamide-responsive myotonia—which are now recognized to represent a spectra of phenotypic expression of the same disorder.

(2) The main symptom is myotonia of variable severity, which may be induced by potassium ingestion, exercise, or fasting.

(3) There is no associated weakness.

(4) On examination, muscle strength is normal. There may be percussion myotonia.

Key Signs: Potassium-Aggravated Myotonia

- Myotonia
- No weakness

b. Laboratory features

(1) Serum CK levels are normal or mildly elevated.

(2) Electrophysiologic testing is significant only for the presence of myotonic discharges.

(3) Muscle biopsies are not required in this setting. There are few reports on the pathologic features of PAM. The available information suggests the absence of any distinct pathology.

c. Genetic features

(1) Inheritance is autosomal dominant.

(2) PAM is allelic to HyperKPP and paramyotonia congenita, and maps to the same *SCN4A* gene.

d. Treatment

(1) Low-potassium diet is recommended.

(2) Mexiletine is effective in most patients for reducing myotonia.

(3) In a subgroup of patients in whom mexiletine is ineffective, acetazolamide may reduce the myotonia.

4. Pathophysiology

a. The voltage-gated sodium channel is composed of α and β subunits. The β subunit is not associated with any known diseases in humans. The α subunit has four homologous domains (D1–D4), arranged around the ion pore of the membrane. Each domain contains six membrane-spanning hydrophobic segments (S1–S6). The S4 segment contains positively charged amino acids and acts as the voltage sensor. The cytoplasmic loop that connects D3 and D4 acts as the channel inactivation gate and works through a "ball-valve" mechanism to close the ion pore physically. As a wave of depolarization travels, it triggers a conformational change in the S4 segment, resulting in opening of the ion pore. After a set period of being open, the inactivation gate swings into place to block the ion pore physically. With repolarization, the channel returns to its resting (inactive) state, with repositioning of the inactivation gate to its original conformation.

b. The common abnormality in all *SCN4A* mutations has to do with alterations of normal channel inactivation.

c. *SCN4A* mutations that result in myotonia produce sodium channels that, after membrane depolarization, have a tendency to remain open later and more persistently. As sodium keeps leaking through these channels, repeated waves of depolarization are triggered, leading to an increase in membrane excitability and the clinical picture of myotonia.

d. *SCN4A* mutations that lead to paralysis produce sodium channels that have large, long-lasting currents. This results in a prolonged state of membrane depolarization, which causes sustained inactivation in all channels, including the wild-type channels, leading to membrane inexitability and thus the clinical feature of paralysis.

CALCIUM CHANNELOPATHIES: HYPOKALEMIC PERIODIC PARALYSIS

To date, hypokalemic periodic paralysis (HypoKPP) is the only muscle disorder definitely linked to primary disruption of the normal function of the voltage-gated skeletal calcium channel. Thyrotoxic periodic paralysis shares features with HypoKPP and is suspected to be due to a calcium channel mutation, although none has been documented so far.

1. Clinical features

a. HypoKPP is the most common form of periodic paralysis and has a prevalence of 1 in 100,000. There is a slight male preponderance.

b. Symptoms usually begin at puberty and rarely after age 20.

c. The main manifestation of the illness is recurrent attacks of painless paralysis. Triggers include strenuous exercise followed by rest or sleep, a carbohydrate-rich meal, alcohol, cold, and emotional stress. The attacks have a predilection to occur during the early morning hours.

d. Occasionally, patients are able to "walk off" an attack by engaging in mild exercise.

e. Respiratory muscles are usually, but not always, spared.

f. Attacks may last a few hours to more than a day.

g. On examination during the attack, there is flaccid weakness with absent deep tendon reflexes. The examination is normal between attacks. Some patients develop a fixed myopathy with permanent proximal muscle weakness later in life.

h. Diffuse myotonia is not part of this syndrome, although some patients have eyelid myotonia.

Key Signs: Hypokalemic Periodic Paralysis

- Episodic painless paralysis
- "Walk-off" phenomenon
- Attacks sometimes lasting more than 24 hours
- Myotonia typically absent

2. Laboratory features

a. Serum potassium levels are low during an attack and typically normalize with return of normal muscle strength.

b. Serum CK levels are elevated during an attack and normal or mildly increased between attacks.

c. There may be some electrocardiographic changes secondary to hypokalemia, including flattening of T waves and QT-wave prolongation.

d. Electrophysiologic testing reveals normal nerve conduction studies between attacks. During an attack, CMAPs are low or unobtainable. Needle evaluation is normal between attacks, except in patients who have developed a fixed myopathy, where myopathic motor units appear. During an attack there is evidence of membrane irritability, including fibrillations and positive sharp waves.

e. Muscle biopsy reveals striking but nonpathognomonic changes, including tubular aggregates and intracellular vacuoles, which have a predilection to occupy the center of the myofibril.

Key Tests: Hypokalemic Periodic Paralysis

- During an attack: low serum potassium and high serum CK levels
- Electrocardiographic changes secondary to hypokalemia
- Normal nerve conduction studies between attacks
- Muscle biopsy: tubular aggregates and intracellular vacuoles occupying the center of the myofibril

3. Genetic features

a. Inheritance is autosomal dominant, with reduced penetrance in women, which explains the slight male preponderance.

b. It is associated with mutations in the α-1 subunit of the dihydropyridine-sensitive voltage-gated muscle calcium channel (CACNL1A3) on chromosome 1q31-32.

c. A few families with HypoKPP have displayed mutations on SCN4A. The major clinical characteristic that differentiates those patients from those harboring CACNL1A3 mutations is their tendency to have increased frequency and severity of attacks in response to treatment with acetazolamide.

4. Pathophysiology

a. The voltage-gated calcium channel is homologous to the α subunit of the sodium channel. It consists of a complex of five polypeptide chains (α1, α2, β, δ, and γ). The central component of the complex is the α1 subunit, which acts as the ion-conducting pore. Similar to the sodium channel, the α1 subunit of the calcium channel consists of four homologous domains (D1–D4), each having six membrane-spanning segments (S1–S6). The S4 segment is highly charged and is presumed to act as the voltage sensor.

b. The voltage-gated calcium channel plays a central role in excitation-contraction coupling. It normally interacts with the ryanodine receptor on the sarcoplasmic reticulum membrane to initiate muscle contraction through a depolarization-triggered physical interaction that leads to the opening of the calcium slow-release channel in the sarcoplasmic reticulum.

c. The exact mechanism by which mutations in the voltage-gated calcium channel lead to periodic paralysis remains unknown.

5. Treatment

a. Therapeutic intervention during an attack depends on the severity of paralysis. Mild paralytic attacks need no treatment. Generalized paralysis should be treated with oral supplementation of potassium chloride. Intravenous potassium supplementation carries the risk of arrhythmogenic and potentially life-threatening hyperkalemia.

b. Prophylactic treatment initially focuses on avoiding precipitants of attacks, such as carbohydrate-rich meals and strenuous exercise.

c. First-line pharmacologic prophylaxis is acetazolamide, but it must be used with care in patients with hypoKPP secondary to SCNA4 mutations.

d. Other drugs with reported beneficial effects are dichlorphenamide, spironolactone, and triamterene.

CHLORIDE CHANNELOPATHIES

1. Autosomal dominant myotonia congenita (Thomsen's disease)
   a. Clinical features
      (1) Typically, symptoms start during infancy with painless myotonia, mostly of the facial muscle after crying.
      (2) With age, the dominant symptom is painless stiffness and myotonia of the limbs and face. In some patients the symptoms diminish with aging.
      (3) There is a striking "warm-up" phenomenon, with repeated contractions leading to reduced myotonia.
      (4) On examination, there is evidence of action and percussion myotonia. The rest of the examination is normal. Most patients appear extremely muscular, as if they regularly lift weights.

Key Signs: Thomsen's Disease

- Onset during infancy
- Painless myotonia

   b. Laboratory features
      (1) Serum CK is usually normal but may be slightly elevated.
      (2) Electrophysiologic testing reveals normal routine nerve conduction studies. Mild exercise may produce a transient increase in CMAP amplitude. Needle evaluation reveals myotonic discharges at rest and with volitional muscle contraction.
      (3) Muscle biopsy is not routinely indicated in this setting. If performed, it may show nonspecific variation in fiber size, increased internal nuclei, and some tubular aggregates.
   c. Genetic features
      (1) Inheritance is autosomal dominant.
      (2) It is associated with mutations in the muscle chloride channel gene (CLCN1) on chromosome 7q35.
2. Autosomal recessive myotonia congenita (Becker's disease)
   a. Clinical features
      (1) This is the more common form of myotonia congenita, with a prevalence of 1 in 20,000 to 1 in 50,000.
      (2) Age at onset of symptoms is later than with Thomsen's disease, usually 4 to 12 years.

However, the disease phenotype is much more severe.
      (3) Myotonia involves the lower limbs more than the upper limbs. More importantly, there is usually accompanying transient weakness, mostly in the lower limbs. With mild exercise, the stiffness and weakness may be improved.
      (4) Some patients develop a fixed weakness, more prominent in the distal muscles.
      (5) On examination, the same findings as in Thomsen's disease are documented. Some patients have distal weakness and atrophy.

Key Signs: Becker's Disease

- Onset during childhood
- Myotonia and transient weakness
- Fixed weakness may develop

   b. Laboratory features
      (1) Serum CK levels are typically elevated, more than in Thomsen's disease.
      (2) Electrophysiologic testing reveals normal routine nerve conduction studies. Mild exercise produces a mild transient increase in the CMAP amplitudes. Needle evaluation reveals profuse myotonic discharges in the proximal and distal limb muscles.
      (3) Muscle pathology is similar to that observed with the dominant form.
   c. Genetic features
      (1) Inheritance is autosomal recessive.
      (2) It is associated with mutations in the CLCN1 gene.
3. Pathophysiology
   a. Much less is known about the chloride channel than the sodium and calcium channels.
   b. The full structure of the chloride channel has not been elucidated. Although no definite voltage-sensing region has been identified, it is presumably a voltage-gated channel.
   c. Functionally, the chloride channel is responsible for the high resting membrane conductance of the skeletal muscle cells. Mutations result in

loss of function and reduced chloride conductance. How that leads to the phenotypic expression of the two forms of myotonia congenita is not known.

4. Treatment

    a. Most patients do not require treatment.

    b. In severe cases, a host of medications have been used with some success, including mexiletine, quinine, phenytoin, carbamazepine, verapamil, and diazepam. Mexiletine is usually the first-line treatment.

Bibliography

Davies NP, Hanna MG: The skeletal muscle channelopathies: basic science, clinical genetics and treatment. Curr Opin Neurol 14:539–551, 2001.

Meola G, Sansone V: Therapy in myotonic disorders and in muscle channelopathies. Neurol Sci 21(Suppl 5):S953–S961, 2000.

Renner DR, Ptacek LJ: Periodic paralyses and non-dystrophic myotonias. Adv Neurol 88:235–252, 2002.

1 Bacterial Meningitis

Karen L. Roos

Definition

Bacterial meningitis is an acute purulent infection in the subarachnoid space that is associated with an inflammatory reaction in the brain parenchyma and cerebral blood vessels that causes decreased consciousness, seizure activity, raised intracranial pressure, and stroke.

Epidemiology and Risk Factors

1. The most common causative organisms of community-acquired bacterial meningitis are *Streptococcus pneumoniae* and *Neisseria meningitidis*. Risk factors for pneumococcal meningitis include pneumonia, acute and chronic otitis media, alcoholism, diabetes, splenectomy, hypogammaglobulinemia, and head trauma with basilar skull fracture and cerebrospinal fluid (CSF) rhinorrhea.

2. In the past few years there has been an increase in the incidence of meningococcal infection on college campuses, and an increase in the incidence of meningococcal disease in North America and Europe caused by the emergence of a virulent strain of serogroup C, serotype 2a *N. meningitidis*. Individuals with deficiencies of any of the complement components are highly susceptible to invasive meningococcal infections.

3. There has been a major change in the epidemiology of pneumococcal disease, with the global emergence and increasing prevalence of penicillin- and cephalosporin-resistant strains of *S. pneumoniae*.

4. There has been a marked decline in the incidence of meningitis due to *Haemophilus influenzae* type b in children because of the success of the *Haemophilus influenzae* type b conjugate vaccine. *Haemophilus influenzae* remains a causative organism of bacterial meningitis in the older adult.

5. *Listeria monocytogenes* is a causative organism of meningitis in individuals with impaired cell-mediated immunity from acquired immunodeficiency syndrome, organ transplantation, pregnancy, malignancy, chronic illness, or immunosuppressive therapy.

6. *Staphylococcus aureus* and coagulase-negative staphylococci are predominant organisms causing meningitis as a complication of a neurosurgical procedure, and as a complication of lumbar puncture.

7. *Streptococcus agalactiae* or group B streptococcus is a leading cause of bacterial meningitis and sepsis in neonates, and is increasingly seen in older adults.

Etiology and Pathophysiology

1. The most common bacteria that cause meningitis, *S. pneumoniae* and *N. meningitidis*, initially colonize the nasopharynx by attaching to the nasopharyngeal epithelial cells.

2. The bacteria then either are carried across the cell in membrane-bound vacuoles to the intravascular space or they invade the intravascular space by creating separations in the apical tight junctions of columnar epithelial cells.

3. Once the bacteria gain access to the bloodstream, they are able to avoid phagocytosis by neutrophils and classical complement-mediated bactericidal activity because of the presence of a polysaccharide capsule.

4. Bacteria that are able to survive in the bloodstream then enter the CSF.

5. Bacteria can multiply rapidly within the CSF because of the absence of effective host immune defenses. Normal uninfected CSF contains few white blood cells and insufficient numbers of complement components and immunoglobulins for the opsonization of bacteria, an essential step for phagocytosis by neutrophils.

6. The critical event, however, in the pathogenesis of bacterial meningitis is the inflammatory reaction to the invading meningeal pathogen. It is not the pathogen itself that causes the neurologic complications.

7. The lysis of bacteria with the release of bacterial cell wall components in the subarachnoid space is the initial step in the induction of the inflammatory process and the formation of a purulent exudate in the subarachnoid space.

8. Components of bacterial cell walls, such as lipopolysaccharide molecules (endotoxin), a cell wall component of gram-negative bacteria, and teichoic acid and peptidoglycan, cell wall components of the pneumococcus, induce meningeal inflamma-

tion by stimulating the production of inflammatory cytokines and chemokines.

9. A number of pathophysiologic consequences result from the production of inflammatory cytokines, including:

a. Increased blood–brain barrier permeability resulting in

(1) Vasogenic cerebral edema

(2) Leakage of serum proteins and other molecules into the CSF, contributing to the formation of a purulent exudate

b. Recruitment of polymorphonuclear leukocytes from the bloodstream that contributes to the formation of a purulent exudate that

(1) Obstructs the flow of CSF through the ventricular system and diminishes the resorptive capacity of the arachnoid granulations in the dural sinuses, leading to obstructive hydrocephalus, communicating hydrocephalus, and interstitial edema.

(2) Surrounds and narrows the diameter of the lumen of the large arteries at the base of the brain, and inflammatory cells infiltrate the arterial walls, resulting in

(a) Vasculitis

(b) Cerebral ischemia

(c) Focal neurologic deficits

(d) Stroke

Clinical Features

1. The classic clinical presentation of bacterial meningitis is the triad of fever, headache, and stiff neck that is accompanied by lethargy, stupor or coma, and/or seizure activity.

2. Nuchal rigidity is present when the neck resists passive flexion and is the pathognomonic sign of meningeal irritation. Brudzinski's sign is positive when passive flexion of the neck results in spontaneous flexion of the hips and knees.

3. Seizure activity occurs in approximately 40% of patients.

4. Raised intracranial pressure is an expected complication of bacterial meningitis; it is the major cause of obtundation and coma in this disease.

5. The rash of meningococcemia begins as a diffuse erythematous maculopapular rash resembling a viral exanthum, but the skin lesions of meningococcemia rapidly become petechial. Petechiae are found on the trunk and lower limbs, in the mucous membranes and conjunctiva, and occasionally on the palms and soles.

Key Signs

Classic Clinical Presentation

- Fever, headache, and stiff neck accompanied by lethargy, stupor or coma, and/or seizure activity

Other Signs

- Nuchal rigidity

- Seizure (40% of those affected)

- Rash of meningococcemia: Rash resembling a viral exanthum that rapidly becomes petechial

Differential Diagnosis

1. The leading disease in the differential diagnosis of bacterial meningitis is viral encephalitis, including herpes simplex virus encephalitis and the arthropod-borne viral encephalitides.

2. Rocky Mountain spotted fever begins with high fever and headache, and a diffuse erythematous maculopapular rash that is similar in appearance to the early rash of meningococcemia. The rash of Rocky Mountain spotted fever typically begins on the wrists and ankles and then spreads. The petechiae of meningococcemia are most prominent on the trunk and lower limbs.

3. Tuberculous meningitis presents as either a subacute meningitis with fever, headache, night sweats, and malaise, or a fulminant meningoencephalitis with coma, raised intracranial pressure, seizure, and stroke.

4. Focal infectious intracranial mass lesions present with headache, fever (in only 50% of cases), a localizing neurologic deficit, and/or focal or generalized seizure activity.

5. Septic thrombosis of the superior sagittal sinus presents with fever, headache, lower limb weakness with bilateral Babinski's signs, and/or focal or generalized seizures.

6. The classical presentation of a subarachnoid hemorrhage is the explosive onset of a severe headache. Nuchal rigidity and vomiting are frequently present.

Key CSF Tests

- Gram's stain and bacterial culture

- Polymerase chain reaction (PCR) for herpes simplex virus DNA

- Herpes simplex virus immunoglobulin G

- Fungal smear and culture

- Cryptococcal antigen
- Acid-fast smear and tuberculosis culture
- TB molecular diagnostic test

Laboratory Testing

1. Blood cultures should be obtained.
2. The diagnosis of bacterial meningitis is made by examination of the cerebrospinal fluid. The classic CSF abnormalities in bacterial meningitis are as follows
   a. Increased opening pressure (>180 mm H_2O)
   b. A pleocytosis of polymorphonuclear leukocytes (10 to 10,000 cells/mm^3)
   c. Decreased glucose concentration (<45 mg/dL and/or CSF:serum glucose ratio <0.31)
   d. Increased protein concentration (>45 mg/dL)
   e. Gram's stain demonstrates organisms in >60% of untreated cases.
   f. Bacterial cultures are positive in >80% of cases.
   g. The latex particle agglutination test detects bacterial antigens of *Streptococcus pneumoniae*, *Neisseria meningitidis*, *Haemophilus influenzae* type b, *Streptococcus agalactiae* and *Escherichia coli* K1 strains.
   h. The limulus amebocyte lysate assay detects gram-negative endotoxin.
   i. PCR for bacterial DNA is available, but the sensitivity and specificity are unknown.

CSF Abnormalities in Bacterial Meningitis

- Opening pressure >180 mm H_2O
- White blood cells >10 to <10,000 cells/mm^3—neutrophils predominate
- Glucose <45mg/dL
- Protein >45 mg/dL
- Gram's stain positive in 70% to 90% of untreated cases
- Culture positive in 80% of cases

Radiographic Features

Cranial computed tomography (CT) and cranial magnetic resonance imaging (MRI) will demonstrate enhancement of the meninges post-contrast administration. In addition, there may be evidence of cerebral edema, ischemia, or infarction.

Treatment

1. Empiric antimicrobial therapy should be initiated immediately when the clinical presentation is suggestive of bacterial meningitis. Empiric therapy should include a combination of a third generation cephalosporin, either ceftriaxone or cefotaxime, or a fourth generation cephalosporin (cefepime) plus vancomycin plus acyclovir.
   a. Ampicillin and gentamicin should be added to the empiric regimen in patients in whom *Listeria monocytogenes* may be a causative organism.
   b. Doxycycline should be added to the empiric regimen when a rash is present to treat the causative agent of Rocky Mountain spotted fever, *Rickettsia rickettsii*.
   c. In hospital-acquired meningitis and particularly meningitis after neurosurgical procedures, empiric therapy should include a combination of vancomycin and ceftazidime.
2. Once the organism has been identified by Gram's stain or bacterial culture of CSF, and the results of antimicrobial susceptibility tests are known, antimicrobial therapy can be modified according to Table 1–1.
3. The American Academy of Pediatrics recommends the consideration of dexamethasone for bacterial meningitis in infants and children 2 months of age and older.
   a. The recommended dose is 0.6 mg/kg/day in 4 divided doses (0.15 mg/kg/dose) given intravenously for the first 4 days of antibiotic therapy.
   b. The first dose of dexamethasone should be administered before or at least with the first dose of antibiotic.

🔑 Key Treatment

- Empiric antimicrobial therapy should be initiated in any patient with a clinical presentation suggestive of bacterial meningitis.
- Antimicrobial therapy should not await CT or MRI or lumbar puncture.
- Blood cultures should be obtained.
- Empiric therapy should include a combination of a third- or fourth-generation cephalosporin plus vancomycin plus acyclovir.
- Ampicillin and gentamicin should be added to the empiric regimen in patients in whom *L. monocytogenes* may be the causative organism.

TABLE 1–1. ANTIMICROBIAL THERAPY OF BACTERIAL MENINGITIS

ORGANISM	ANTIBIOTIC TOTAL DAILY DOSE (DOSING INTERVAL)

Streptococcus pneumoniae	Ceftriaxone
	  Adult dose: 4 g/day (every 12 hours)
	  Child dose: 100 mg/kg/day (every 12 hours)
	
	or
	
	Cefotaxime
	  Adult dose: 12 g/day (every 4 hours)
	  Child dose: 200 mg/kg/day (every 4 hours)
	
	plus
	
	Vancomycin
	  Adult dose: 2 g/day (every 6 or every 12 hours)
	  Child dose: 40–60 mg/kg/day (every 6–12 hours)

Neisseria meningitidis	Penicillin G
	  Adult dose: 20–24 million U/day (every 4 hours)
	  Child dose: 0.2 million U/kg (q 4 hours)
	
	or
	
	Ampicillin
	  Adult dose: 12 g/day (every 4 hours)
	  Child dose: 200–300 mg/kg/day (every 4 hours)

Staphylococci
  Methicillin-sensitive
	Nafcillin
	  Adult dose: 12 g/day (every 4 hours)
	  Child dose: 150–200 mg/kg/day (every 4 hours)

Methicillin-resistant	Vancomycin
	  Adult dose: 2 g/day (every 6 or every 12 hours)
	  Child dose: 40–60 mg/kg/day (every 6 to 12 hours)
	± Intraventricular vancomycin
	  Adult dose: 20 mg/day
	  Child dose: 10 mg/day

Gram-negative bacilli (with the exception of Pseudomonas aeruginosa)	Cefotaxime or ceftriaxone

Pseudomonas aeruginosa	Ceftazidime
	  Adult dose: 8 g/day (every 8 hours)
	  Child dose: 150–200 mg/kg/day (every 8 hours)

Listeria monocytogenes	Ampicillin
	  Adult dose: 12 g/day (every 4 hours)
	  Child dose: 200–300 mg/kg/day (every 4 hours)
	+ Gentamicin
	  Adult dose: 6 mg/kg/day (every 8 hours)
	  Child dose: 6 mg/kg/day (every 8 hours)

Streptococcus agalactiae	Penicillin G
Haemophilus influenzae	Cefotaxime or ceftriaxone
Enterobacteriaceae	Cefotaxime or ceftriaxone

- Doxycycline should be added to the empiric regimen in patients with a rash.

- Ceftazidime is the third-generation cephalosporin of choice for neurosurgical patients and for patients with hospital-acquired meningitis.

Prognosis

The risk of death from bacterial meningitis is significantly associated with the following:

1. A decreased level of consciousness on admission
2. The onset of seizures within 24 hours of admission
3. Signs of increased intracranial pressure
4. Young age (infancy) and age over 50 years
5. The presence of a comorbid condition
6. The presence of shock and/or the need for mechanical ventilation
7. Delay in the initiation of treatment

Prevention

1. The Advisory Committee on Immunization Practices recommends that college freshmen be vaccinated against meningococcal meningitis with the tetravalent (MenA,C,W135,Y) meningococcal polysaccharide vaccine. MenC polysaccharide vaccine would also be effective.

2. During an outbreak of meningococcal disease, individuals who have not been previously vacci-

nated should be treated with chemoprophylaxis if they come into contact with the index case.

   a. Adults and adolescents are treated with rifampin 600 mg twice a day for 2 days.

   b. Children are treated with rifampin 10 mg/kg twice a day for 2 days.

3. Vaccination against the pneumococcus is recommended for four at-risk populations.

   a. Adults older than age 65 years

   b. Adults with chronic underlying diseases (cardiopulmonary diseases, renal diseases, diabetes mellitus, splenectomy, and CSF fistula)

   c. Immunocompromised patients older than 10 years

   d. Individuals with human immunodeficiency virus

Pregnancy

Rifampin should not be given to pregnant women.

 ## Bibliography

Durand ML, Calderwood SB, Weber DJ, et al.: Acute bacterial meningitis in adults: A review of 493 episodes. N Engl J Med 328:21–28, 1993.

Kornelisse RF, Westerbeek CML, Spoor AB, et al.: Pneumococcal meningitis in children: Prognostic indicators and outcome. Clin Infect Dis 21:1390–1397, 1995.

Roos KL: What I have learned about infectious diseases with my sleeves rolled up. Semin Neurol 22:9–15, 2002.

Roos KL: Acute bacterial meningitis. Semin Neurol 20:293–306, 2000.

Roos KL: Meningitis: 100 Maxims in Neurology. London, Arnold, 1996.

Simberkoff MS, Moldover NH, Rahal J Jr: Absence of detectable bactericidal and opsonic activities in normal and infected human cerebrospinal fluids: A regional host deficiency. J Lab Clin Med 95:362–367, 1980.

Tauber MG, Moser B: Cytokines and chemokines in meningeal inflammation: Biology and clinical implications. Clin Infect Dis 28:1–12, 1999.

2 Chronic Meningitis

Patricia K. Coyle

Definition

Chronic meningitis is a meningoencephalitis syndrome in which clinical and cerebrospinal fluid (CSF) abnormalities persist for 4 or more weeks.

1. Most patients with this diagnosis are worsening; they should not be recovering or steadily improving.

2. Although CSF pleocytosis is a hallmark of meningitis, in rare cases CSF is acellular and chronic meningeal inflammation is confirmed through neuroimaging or biopsy studies.

Epidemiology and Risk Factors

1. Chronic meningitis accounts for about 8% of meningitis cases.

2. Recognized risk factors are evaluated during the history and examination (Table 2–1).

3. Tuberculous (TB) meningitis occurs most often in adults in developed countries and in children in developing countries.

   a. Human immunodeficiency virus-1 (HIV-1) infection is a risk factor for TB meningitis.

   b. Contact risks for TB are members of minority groups, foreign born, the elderly, intravenous drug users, alcoholics, and chronic care facility residents.

4. Immunocompromise is a key risk factor for fungal meningitis. Major pathogens are *Cryptococcus neoformans*, *Coccidioides immitis*, *Candida albicans*, and *Histoplasma capsulatum*.

   a. Defective cellular immunity predisposes to cryptococcal meningitis, which occurs in 2% to 13% of patients infected with HIV-1.

   b. Risk factors for coccidioidal meningitis are extremes of age, male gender, non-Caucasian race, negative skin test, serum complement fixation antibody titer higher than 1:64, and pregnancy.

   c. Risk factors for candida meningitis (candida species are normal body flora) are prematurity, treatment with broad-spectrum antibiotics, hyperalimentation, indwelling catheter line, glucocorticoid therapy, underlying malignancy, neutropenia, abdominal surgery, diabetes mellitus, thermal injury, and parenteral drug use.

TABLE 2–1. RISK FACTORS FOR CHRONIC MENINGITIS

Prior or Concurrent Systemic Conditions/Infections
Tuberculosis
Mycotic infection
Malignancy
Sarcoidosis
Vasculitis
Collagen vascular disease
Diabetes mellitus (*Zygomycetes* infection)
Specific infection (*Brucella* sp., spirochetes, *Cysticercus*)

Exposures
Mycobacterium tuberculosis (contact)
Treponema pallidum (sexual contact)
Borrelia burgdorferi (*Ixodes ricinus* tick)
Leptospira (animals, urine-infected water)
Brucella (dairy products, farms, laboratory exposure)
Francisella tularensis (cats, rabbits, ticks)
Pseudoallescheria boydii (near-drowning)
Sporothrix (rose thorn prick)
Angiostrongylus cantonensis (raw fish, snails, vegetables)
Retroviruses (sexual contact, intravenous drug use, blood transfusions)

Geographic Residence/Travel
Borrelia burgdorferi (Northeast, Upper Midwest, Upper Pacific regions)
Mycotic infection
  Coccidioides immitis (Southwest)
  Histoplasma capsulatum (Ohio and Mississippi river valleys)
  Blastomyces dermatitidis (Mississippi river valley, Mid-Atlantic region)
  Paracoccidioides brasiliensis (Latin America)
Cysticercus
Angiostrongylus (Indo-Pacific)
Human T-cell lymphotrophic virus type-I (Caribbean, tropics, Japan)

Immunocompromised
Mycotic agent (*Aspergillus fumigatus*, *Candida*, *Coccidioides*, *Cryptococcus neoformans*, *Histoplasma*, *Zygomycetes*, *Pseudoallescheria boydii*)
Bacterial agent
  M. tuberculosis
  Listeria, *Nocardia* (cancer)
Parasitic agent (*Acanthamoeba*, *Toxoplasma*)
Viral agent
  Cytomegalovirus
  Echovirus, poliovirus (hypogammaglobulinemia)

Etiology and Pathophysiology

1. Causes of the chronic meningitis syndrome can be divided into infectious (Table 2–2) and noninfectious etiologies (Table 2–3). Despite extensive work-up, no cause is found in up to 33% of cases.

2. The major infectious causes are *Mycobacterium tuberculosis* (TB meningitis), followed by cryptococcal meningitis.

   a. There are approximately 4000 cases of TB meningitis annually in the United States.

b. TB meningitis should trigger assessment for HIV-1 infection.

c. Two *Cryptococcus neoformans* varieties cause cryptococcal meningitis. Variety *neoformans* (serotypes A and D) is found worldwide, and is responsible for meningitis in immunocompromised hosts. Variety *gattii* (serotypes B and C) is found in the tropics and subtropics in association with the eucalyptus tree, and is responsible for meningitis in immunocompetent hosts.

3. The major noninfectious causes are neoplastic meningitis, neurosarcoidosis, and vasculitis.

a. Neoplastic meningitis occurs in 10% to 15% of solid tumors (particularly adenocarcinomas of breast and lung, and malignant melanoma); 20% to 50% of hematologic (lymphoma, leukemia) malignancies, particularly high-grade non-Hodgkin's lymphoma; up to 33% of primary central nervous system (CNS) lymphomas; and 14% to 25% of malignant gliomas. Up to 30% of children with medulloblastoma, ependymoma, germ cell tumors, or neuroectodermal tumors will develop meningitis. There are rare cases of primary diffuse leptomeningeal gliomatosis.

b. There is a benign steroid-responsive meningitis for which no etiology has been established.

4. Overall, the most common causes of chronic

TABLE 2–2. CHRONIC MENINGITIS: INFECTIOUS CAUSES

Bacteria
Mycobacteria (*M. tuberculosis*; *M. avium*)
Spirochetes (*B. burgdorferi, Leptospira interrogans, Treponema pallidum*)
Agents causing sinus tracts (*Actinomycetes, Arachnia, Nocardia*)
Brucella
Tropheryma whippelii
Listeria monocytogenes
Neisseria meningitidis
Francisella tularensis

Mycoses
Common (*Cryptococcus, Coccidioides, Histoplasma, Candida*)
Uncommon (*Aspergillus, Blastomyces, Dematiaceous* sp., paracoccidioides, pseudoallescheria, *Sporothrix schenckii, Trichosporon beigelii, Zygomycetes*).

Parasites
Taenia solium (cysticercosis)
Acanthamoeba (granulomatous amebic meningoencephalitis)
Angiostrongylus (eosinophilic meningitis)
Toxoplasma gondii
Coenurus cerebralis
Schistosoma sp.

Viruses
Retroviruses (human immunodeficiency virus type 1 [HIV-1], human T-cell lymphotrophic virus type 1 [HTLV-1])
Enteroviruses (in the setting of hypogammaglobulinemia)
Herpes viruses

TABLE 2–3. CHRONIC MENINGITIS: NONINFECTIOUS CAUSES

Neoplasm
Neurosarcoidosis
Vasculitis
  Isolated CNS angiitis
  Systemic
Behçet's disease
Chemical meningitis
  Endogenous
  Exogenous
Chronic benign lymphocytic meningitis
Fabry's disease
Hypertrophic pachymeningitis
Systemic lupus erythematosus
Uveomeningoencephalitides
  Vogt-Koyanagi-Harada disease
  Sympathetic ophthalmia

meningitis are TB (up to 57%), followed by neoplastic meningitis (8%), and cryptococcal meningitis (7%).

5. Chronic meningitis in HIV-1-positive patients has a distinct set of causes (Table 2–4).

6. Chronic meningitis that causes a basilar exudate can lead to vasculitis of adjacent vessels, cranial nerve entrapment, and blockage of CSF pathways.

Clinical Features

1. There are variable combinations of fever, headache, meningismus, mental status changes, seizures, and focal neurologic deficits.

a. Immunocompromised hosts may have particularly subtle complaints.

b. *Listeria* meningitis often presents with change in mental status, fever, and headache. Up to 40% of patients lack meningismus, up to 27% have seizures, and up to 20% experience movement disorders (ataxia, myclonus, tremor).

2. The examination should focus on identifying extraneural involvement, the pattern of neurologic involvement, and potential biopsy sites.

3. Clinical features can suggest specific etiologies.

a. Prominent fever usually indicates infection.

b. Multilevel neuraxis involvement, with symptoms out of proportion to signs, suggests neoplastic meningitis.

c. Facial nerve involvement is seen with Lyme disease or sarcoidosis, while optic nerve involvement is seen with cryptococcal meningitis.

d. Prominent ocular involvement suggests Behçet disease, lymphoma, sarcoidosis, Vogt-Koyanagi-Harada disease, or *Angiostrongylus* infection.

e. Other suggestive clinical features are pulmonary disease (TB, sarcoidosis, histoplasma,

TABLE 2–4. ETIOLOGY OF CHRONIC MENINGITIS IN HIV-1 INFECTED INDIVIDUALS

HIV-1
Cryptococcus (in 2%–13%)
Other fungi
  Aspergillus (meningitis + abscess)
  Candida (< 1%)
  Coccidioides
  Histoplasma
  Sporothrix
  Zygomycetes (intravenous drug users)
Other pathogens
  Treponema pallidum
  Mycobacteria (Haitians, African Americans, intravenous drug
    users)
  Listeria
  Salmonella
  Streptococcus
  Prototheca wickerhamii (algae)
Neoplasm
  Metastatic systemic lymphoma
  Primary CNS lymphoma

blastomyces, or aspergillus infection), peripheral nerve involvement (Lyme disease, Fabry's disease, sarcoidosis), subcutaneous abscesses or draining sinus tracts (*Actinomyces, Nocardia, Blastomyces, Coccidioides* infection), joint involvement (Lyme disease), and sinus disease (zygomycetes).

4. The British Research Council divides TB meningitis into stages based on clinical features. Stage I indicates normal level of consciousness without focal deficits. Stage II indicates lethargy or altered behavior, meningismus, and minor deficits such as cranial nerve palsies. Stage III involves stupor or coma, seizures, abnormal movements, and severe deficits such as hemiparesis. TB meningitis tends to take a fairly rapid course over weeks.

5. Benign steroid-responsive meningitis manifests with depression, mild personality changes, headache, and malaise, without cranial nerve or focal deficits.

Differential Diagnosis

1. The major differential diagnostic considerations involve acute and subacute neurologic infectious syndromes that produce CSF pleocytosis: acute meningitis, encephalitis, and recurrent meningitis. Recurrent meningitis has distinct etiologies (Table 2–5). These syndromes are significantly different from chronic meningitis:
   a. More acute onset
   b. More fulminant course
   c. More prominent mental status changes, major parenchymal features, and minor meningeal features (encephalitis)

d. Distinct CSF profile: Very low glucose and high cell count with polymorphonuclear cells (septic meningitis); normal glucose and moderate mononuclear pleocytosis (aseptic meningitis); normal glucose with low-grade mixed pleocytosis (encephalitis).

e. Monophasic and self-limited course (acute meningitis and encephalitis); at least two discrete attacks, with normal clinical and CSF parameters in between (recurrent meningitis).

2. Other conditions can mimic chronic meningitis.
   a. Infections: Partially treated bacterial meningitis, parameningeal infection with an aseptic CSF reaction, subacute bacterial endocarditis
   b. Noninfectious etiologies: Brain tumor, giant cell arteritis, metabolic-toxic encephalopathy, paraneoplastic syndrome, postinfectious encephalitis/encephalomyelitis, systemic lupus erythematosus, subarachnoid hemorrhage, subdural hematoma.

Laboratory Testing

1. The goals of laboratory testing are twofold: Confirm the diagnosis (by CSF examination), and identify the etiology.
   a. Generally, multiple tests and repeat sampling are required.
   b. The work-up should be logical and extensive.
   c. Aggressive measures are justified in deteriorating patients.
   d. Laboratory tests are selected based on the

TABLE 2–5. CAUSES OF THE RECURRENT MENINGITIS SYNDROME

Anatomic defects
  Congenital
  Postoperative
  Trauma
Beçhet's disease
Chemical meningitis
  Endogeneous (cyst, tumor)
  Exogeneous (dye, drug)
Collagen vascular disease
Drug-induced hypersensitivity
Familial Mediterranean fever
Idiopathic (Mollaret's meningitis)
  Herpes simplex virus
  Other causes
Immune defects
  Antibody deficiency
  Complement deficiency
  Splenectomy
Migraine with pleocytosis
Parameningeal infection with seeding
Recurrent bacterial/viral infections
Sarcoidosis
Vogt-Koyanagi-Harada disease
Whipple's disease

history, examination, and suspected etiologies (Table 2–6).

2. Contrast brain magnetic resonance imaging (MRI) is usually done before lumbar puncture.

3. CSF is abnormal in virtually all patients. The characteristic picture is a mononuclear pleocytosis accompanied by low glucose (below 40 mg/dL, but not below 10 mg/dL), elevated protein, and normal or elevated opening pressure.

   a. Typically several lumbar punctures are done within the first few weeks to provide sufficient volumes.

   b. In addition to standard tests, useful selective tests include cultures, stains, and antibody; nucleic acid, antigen and metabolic product assays for infectious causes; cytology, autoantibodies, and angiotensin-converting enzyme (ACE) for noninfectious causes

   c. Yields from CSF culture, cytology, and stain studies are increased with large volumes and multiple samples. Pelleting of CSF can help to detect infectious causes

   d. CSF studies should be repeated if they are negative initially.

   e. CSF antibody levels should be measured as paired CSF and serum titers, to evaluate intrathecal organism-specific antibody production.

   f. Certain CSF cell patterns suggest specific etiologies. Less than 50 WBC/mm^3 suggest a noninfectious cause, or cryptococcal meninigitis in a HIV-1 infected individual. Oligoclonal bands and elevated IgG index suggest an infectious cause. A very high CSF protein level suggests TB or lymphomatous meningitis. In benign steroid-responsive meningitis, CSF abnormalities are mild (normal glucose, slight increase in cell count ranging from 7 to 380 WBCs, slight increase in protein), and CSF cultures are negative.

   g. Cisternal or even ventricular taps can be considered when lumbar CSF is consistently negative, particularly in the setting of a basilar meningitis.

   h. CSF cryptococcal antigen is positive in 83% to 93% of meningitis cases. In 14% to 59% of HIV-1-positive patients, CSF cell count and protein are normal.

   i. CSF cytology is positive in up to 80% to 90% of patients with neoplastic meningitis, but more than one lumbar puncture is required for this yield. Increasing CSF sample volume from 2.5 to 10.5 mL decreases the false-negative cytology rate from 32% to 3%. CSF tumor markers are being evaluated both for diagnosis and monitoring of disease activity. Recent studies

TABLE 2–6. KEY LABORATORY FINDINGS IN CHRONIC MENINGITIS

Cerebrospinal Fluid
- Major diagnostic test; abnormal in virtually 100%
- Many studies (both standard and selective) and multiple samples are required
- Suggestive pattern: mononuclear pleocytosis, low glucose, high protein
- Eosinophil predominance suggests parasitic infection (*Angiostrongylus, Cysticercus, Schistosoma*), *Coccidioides*, and noninfectious (chemical meningitis, lymphoma, polyarteritis nodosa) etiologies
- Neutrophil predominance suggests bacterial (*Actinomyces, Arachnia, Brucella, Listeria, Nocardia,* early *M. tuberculosis*), fungal (*Aspergillus, Blastomyces, Candida, Cladosporium, Coccidioides, Histoplasma, Pseudoallescheria, Zygomycetes*), parasites (*Acanthamoeba*), noninfectious (chemical meningitis, systemic lupus erythematosus, vasculitis) etiologies

General Blood Studies
- Complete blood count and differential, electrolytes (sodium), chemistries, vasculitis screen, angiotensin-converting enzyme (ACE), coagulation profile

Cultures
- Multiple sites (standard: blood, urine, sputum, CSF; selective: gastric washings, prostatic secretions, joint fluid, bone marrow, stool)
- Multiple (at least 3) times
- Check for variety of agents
- Samples optimized by first morning urine, deep sputum sample, large-volume CSF
- Require prolonged incubations, optimized techniques

Antibody Studies
- Paired CSF, serum (to assess intrathecal production)
- Most helpful for bacteria (*B. burgdorferi, Brucella, Leptospira, T. pallidum*), fungi (*Coccidioides, Histoplasma, Sporothrix*), parasites (*Cysticercus, Toxoplasma*), retroviruses
- Autoantibodies (collagen vascular disease)

Nucleic Acid Studies
- Most meaningful in CSF
- Useful for TB and certain other infections

Antigen Studies
- Most meaningful in CSF; occasionally done on blood or urine
- Useful for *Cryptococcus* (polysaccharide), *Aspergillus* (galactomannan), *Cysticercus*
- PPD + anergy panel (intermediate, then second strength)

Metabolic Products
- Most meaningful in CSF
- Useful for TB (tuberculostearic acid), *Candida* (arabinitol)

Imaging
- Neuroimaging abnormal in 60%
- May include contrast brain MRI or CT, occasionally spinal cord MRI (with very high CSF protein, clinical or radiologic evidence of involvement), MR spectroscopy, SPECT, PET
- Chest radiograph
- Angiography
- Gallium scan

Ancillary Tests
- Electrophysiologic
- Synovial fluid
- Pulmonary function tests

Biopsy
- Extraneural (skin, node, bone marrow)
- Leptomeningeal/brain (yield 20% to 39%)

report promising results for carcinoembryonic antigen, soluble CD27, cytokeratins, gastrin-releasing peptide, and lipid associated sialoprotein.

    j. For neurosarcoidosis, an elevated CSF ACE is most meaningful in the setting of normal serum ACE, relatively normal CSF cell count and protein parameters, or an elevated CSF to serum ACE index.

4. Cultures are sent from multiple sites (blood, CSF, urine, sputum), generally at at least three distinct time points. Cultures are tested for multiple agents.

5. Certain blood laboratory tests suggest specific etiologies.

    a. Hypernatremia due to diabetes insipidus suggests neurosarcoidosis.

    b. Hyponatremia with the syndrome of inappropriate antidiuretic hormone (SIADH), suggests TB meningitis.

6. Placement of skin tests should involve purified protein derivative (PPD) for TB, as well as an anergy panel. Nonreactive PPDs are repeated in 2 weeks.

7. The yield from extraneural biopsy is typically low (< 4%).

8. Leptomeningeal/brain biopsy is reserved for undiagnosed, especially deteriorating patients or those undergoing neurosurgical procedures. The overall yield is 20% to 39% (cortical biopsy has a low diagnostic yield [6%]). It is most helpful in noninfectious causes of chronic meningitis. For example, up to 70% of patients with primary CNS angitis will have an abnormal biopsy. Biopsy yield is enhanced by

    a. Use of contrast MRI guidance (47% vs 6%)

    b. Biopsy of an enhancing lesion (80% vs 9%)

    c. Suboccipital/pterional craniotomy

    d. Open biopsy to obtain >1 cm^2 tissue sample

    e. Full-thickness leptomeningeal biopsy

9. Diagnosis of TB meningitis depends on positive CSF culture or detection of specific CSF nucleic acid, antigen, or antibodies. Diagnosis of cryptococcal meningitis depends on positive CSF culture or antigen.

Radiographic Features

1. Suspected chronic meningitis patients should have neuroimaging prior to CSF analysis.

2. Neuroimaging is abnormal in almost 60% of patients (Table 2–7). Contrast MRI is the preferred neuroimaging test. It is particularly helpful to detect meningeal enhancement, basilar menin-

TABLE 2–7. KEY RADIOGRAPHIC FEATURES IN CHRONIC MENINGITIS

Hydrocephalus/Basilar Meningeal Exudate
Tuberculosis
Cysticercosis
Fungal meningitis
Neurosarcoidosis
Neurosyphilis

Focal Lesions
Abscess
Tumor
Infarction
Dural involvement (hypertrophic pachymeningitis)
Tuberculoma (more common in HIV-1-infected patients)

Chest Radiograph
Hilar adenopathy (sarcoidosis)
Lung lesion (tumor, granuloma, abscess)

gitis, associated vascular involvement, and associated structural lesions (tuberculoma, cryptococcoma, abscess, granuloma).

3. Chest radiograph is abnormal in 50% of TB meningitis cases.

Treatment

1. Empiric therapy is indicated in patients who are very ill, rapidly deteriorating, or in whom there is a reasonable presumptive etiology (Table 2–8).

    a. Empiric therapy generally involves anti-TB therapy, followed by broad-spectrum antibiotics (for unusual bacterium), antifungal agents, and finally a trial of glucocorticoids.

    b. Anti-TB therapy involves multiple drugs. Four drugs (isoniazid, rifampin, pyrazinamide, and ethambutol or streptomycin) are used during an induction phase of 8 weeks, followed by isoniazid and rifampin during the continuation phase. Treatment ranges from 6 to 24 months, depending on age, underlying conditions, clinical response, and drug resistance. Multi-drug-resistant strains (which have an extremely poor prognosis) require four to five anti-TB drugs.

TABLE 2–8. KEY TREATMENT FEATURES IN CHRONIC MENINGITIS

- Empiric therapy dictated by degree of illness, likely etiology
- Anti-TB therapy generally first approach
- Broad-spectrum antibiotics are generally the next approach
- Antifungal therapy reserved for immunocompromised hosts; worsening course without response to other agents; evidence for mycotic infection
- Glucocorticoids reserved for noninfectious etiologies, often as adjunctive therapy in serious meningitis cases or presumptive benign steroid-responsive meningitis
- Delay in therapy until initial studies return may be reasonable in patients with a mild course.

c. Broad-spectrum antibiotics involve penicillins or third-generation cephalosporins (such as ceftriaxone) for *Actinomyces* or spirochetal infections, doxycycline or rifampicin for *Brucella* infections, and streptomycin/gentamycin for *Francisella tularensis,* and ampicillin (with gentamycin added in very ill patients) for *Listeria.*

d. Toxicity of the proposed therapy is a factor. Antifungal empiric therapy is generally reserved for immunocompromised hosts, or deteriorating patients unresponsive to other treatment. Antifungal therapies include amphotericin B, fluorocytosine, flucytosine, fluconazole, and other agents (itraconazole, ketoconazole, voriconazole).

e. Cryptococcal meningitis is treated with amphotericin B plus flucytosine during the induction phase of 2 weeks, followed by fluconazole (400 to 800 mg a day) for an 8-week maintenance phase. Fluconazole can then be lowered to 200 mg a day for a year, depending on the underlying condition.

f. Lipid complex forms of amphotericin B are used in the setting of renal dysfunction.

g. Glucocorticoids and occasionally immunosuppressive agents may be used to treat chronic meningitis due to noninfectious etiologies.

2. Sometimes indefinite treatment is required.

a. HIV-1 patients with cryptococcal meningitis require lifelong maintenance therapy.

b. Coccidioidal meningitis is difficult to eradicate, and relapses are frequent. Treatment is often continued for years.

3. Because infection with *Coccidioides* or *Histoplasma* is so difficult to eradicate, amphotericin B can be used intrathecally (either by direct injection or via an Ommaya reservoir).

4. Supportive therapy (adequate oxygenation, fluid hydration, nutrition, control of fever, correction of electrolyte and other metabolic abnormalities) is important.

5. Recognition and optimal management of complications is important. Shunt placement may be necessary for symptomatic hydrocephalus or uncontrollable intracranial hypertension even without hydrocephalus.

6. Treatment of noninfectious chronic meningitis depends on the etiology.

a. Treatment of neoplastic meningitis involves intrathecal chemotherapy, high-dose systemic chemotherapy, radiation therapy, and optimal treatment of the underlying malignancy.

b. Treatment of neurosarcoidosis and vasculitis involves glucocorticoids and immunosuppressives.

c. Treatment of benign steroid-responsive meningitis involves glucocorticoids; patients improve within days of starting therapy.

PEARLS

- CSF mononuclear pleocytosis, low glucose, and increased protein

- Major infectious causes are *M. tuberculosis* and *Cryptococcus.* Major noninfectious cause are neoplasm, sarcoidosis, and vasculitis

- Prominent fever suggests an infectious cause

- Low-grade CSF pleocytosis (<50 WBC/mm^3) suggests a noninfectious cause: the major exception is the HIV-1 positive patient

Prognosis and Complications

1. The mortality rate of chronic meningitis generally ranges from 20% to 35%.

a. Mortality rate depends on the underlying etiology, and can be as high as 50%.

b. In patients in whom no etiology can be established, the mortality rate is only 5%. Duration of illness is reported up to 9 years, with little morbidity.

2. Appropriate antimicrobial therapy for infectious meningitis lowers the mortality and morbidity rates. Delay in diagnosis and delay in therapy contribute to morbidity and mortality.

3. General poor prognosis features include

a. Age extremes (the very young and very old)

b. Significant underlying disease process

c. Major complications

d. Poorly managed complications

4. Complications include SIADH/hyponatremia, increased intracranial pressure, hydrocephalus, seizure disorder, cerebrovascular events (arterial or venous thrombosis, vasculitis, vasospasm, aneurysm, subarachnoid hemorrhage) and rarely diabetes insipious. These complications are major morbidity determinants.

5. Untreated TB meningitis has a mortality rate of 100%; with appropriate treatment, it is decreased to 20% to 30%. Modern series may still average 50% mortality, however.

a. Stage I has a mortality rate of < 10%; stage II, 4% to 55%; and stage III, 37% to 87%.

b. A rare form of TB meningitis, seen in children with active pulmonary TB, spontaneously resolves within several weeks. It actually represents a self-limited serous or sterile meningitis.

c. Adjunctive glucocorticoid therapy may lower morbidity and mortality rates in more severe infection.

d. Prognostic factors in TB meningitis are illness severity at the time of diagnosis and start of treatment, under 5 years of age and over 50 years of age, coexistent miliary TB, chronic medical or alcohol problems, pregnancy, and complicating ischemic infarction.

e. Higher morbidity among children is associated with age under 20 months, ischemic infarction, and hydrocephalus. More than half of children with seizures develop a permanent seizure disorder. Neurologic sequelae are noted in 25% to over 50% of children, and in 0% to 50% of adults.

f. TB meningitis due to multi-drug-resistant strains is very rare; the outcome is unfortunately fatal.

g. In HIV-1 infected patients, mortality of TB meningitis increases with low CD4+ T cell count.

6. Features associated with poor prognosis in cryptococcal meningitis are infection with variety *gattii*; abnormal mental status on presentation; extremes of age; underlying malignancy, HIV-1 infection, or ongoing glucocorticoid therapy; positive extraneural cultures; high serum cryptococcal antigen titer; low sodium; no detectable serum antibody; and abnormal neuroimaging with mass lesions and ventricular enlargement.

a. CSF features associated with a less favorable prognosis: Positive India ink stain, elevated opening pressure, <20 WBC/mm^3, high cryptococcal antigen titer

b. Cryptococcal meningitis subset with severe disease: infection with variety *gattii*, subacute onset, multiple small ring-enhancing lesions, papilledema, high antigen titers in both serum and CSF. Prolonged antifungal therapy and surgical shunt placement are generally required.

c. Poor prognosis in HIV-1-infected patients: lethargy or obtundation at onset, high CSF antigen titer, low CSF WBC count; increased intracranial pressure associated with higher morbidity.

7. Poor prognosis in *Coccidioides* meningitis is associated with hydrocephalus, underlying disease, non-Caucasian race, and complications involving associated vasculitis or encephalitis.

8. Neoplastic meningitis has an especially poor prognosis, with average survival of 4 to 6 weeks. Optimal treatment increases survival to 3 to 5 months.

Prevention

1. In theory all infectious causes of chronic meningitis are preventable through immunprophylaxis (use of a safe and effective vaccine). The bacille Calmette-Guérin vaccine reduces risk for TB meningitis but is not used worldwide.

2. Prevention of immunocompromise (by minimizing transmission of HIV-1, use of immunosuppressive agents) can lower rates of TB and fungal meningitis.

Pregnancy

Pregnancy increases risk of infection with intracellular pathogens, influences selection of antimicrobials, and can affect morbidity and mortality.

1. *Listeria* infection is increased in pregnancy, particularly in the third trimester.

2. TB meningitis has a worse prognosis in pregnant women. Isoniazid is more likely to produce hepatitis, yet streptomycin is contraindicated by the risk of fetal vestibulocochlear nerve damage.

3. Pregnancy is a risk factor for *Coccidioides* infection.

Bibliography

Anderson NE, Willoughby EW, Synek BJL: Leptomeningeal and brain biopsy in chronic meningitis. Aust NZ J Med 25:703–706, 1995.

Charleston AJ, Anderson NE, Willoughby EW: Idiopathic steroid responsive chronic lymphocytic meningitis: Clinical features and long term outcome in 17 patients. Aust NZ J Med 28:784–789, 1998.

Cheng TM, O'Neill BP, Scheithauer BW, Piepgras DG: Chronic meningitis: The role of meningeal or cortical biopsy. Neurosurgery 34:590–595, 1994.

Gripshover BM, Ellner JJ: Chronic meningitis syndrome and meningitis of noninfective or uncertain etiology. In Scheld WM, Whitley RJ, Durack, DT (eds): Infections of the Central Nervous System, 2nd ed. Philadelphia, Lippincott-Raven Publishers, 1997, pp. 881–896.

Liliang P-C, Liang C-L, Chang W-N, et al.: Use of ventriculoperitoneal shunts to treat uncontrollable intracranial hypertension in patients who have cryptococcal meningitis without hydrocephalus. Clin Infect Dis 34:e64–e68, 2002.

Smith JE, Aksamit AJ: Outcome of chronic idiopathic meningitis. Mayo Clin Proc 69:548–556, 1994.

3 Encephalitis

Karen L. Roos

Definition

Encephalitis is an acute infection of brain parenchyma characterized by fever, headache, and an altered level of consciousness. This may be associated with focal or generalized seizure activity and focal or multifocal neurologic deficits.

Epidemiology and Risk Factors

1. Herpes simplex virus-1 (HSV-1) is the most common cause of acute sporadic encephalitis.

2. The arthropod-borne viruses, La Crosse virus, St. Louis encephalitis virus, Japanese encephalitis virus, eastern equine encephalomyelitis virus, western equine encephalomyelitis virus, Venezuelan equine encephalomyelitis virus, tick-borne encephalitis virus, West Nile encephalitis virus, Powassan virus, and Colorado tick fever virus all cause encephalitis during the time of the year when mosquitoes and ticks are biting.

3. Epstein-Barr virus (EBV) can cause encephalitis during the course of infectious mononucleosis, and it can establish latent infection in the central nervous system and then reactivate, causing encephalitis in the setting of immunosuppression.

4. Varicella-zoster virus may cause encephalitis during varicella or at the time of (or months after) an eruption of shingles.

5. Enteroviruses are the most common causative organisms of viral meningitis, but they may also cause a meningoencephalitis, particularly in individuals who have defective humoral immunity.

Etiology and Pathophysiology

1. Primary infection with HSV-1 usually occurs in the oropharyngeal mucosa and is either asymptomatic or associated with fever, pain on swallowing, and vesicular lesions on the buccal and gingival mucosa. After primary infection, HSV-1 is transported to the central nervous system by retrograde transneuronal spread of virus along a division of the trigeminal nerve. The virus establishes latent infection in the trigeminal ganglion. Reactivation of latent ganglionic infection with replication of virus leads to infection in the temporal cortex and limbic system structures.

2. The arthropod-borne viruses are inoculated into the host subcutaneously by a mosquito or tick bite, and then undergo local replication at the skin site and in adjacent muscle. A serum viremia disseminates virus to the central nervous system.

Clinical Features

1. The clinical picture of HSV-1 encephalitis is typically a subacute presentation of fever, hemicranial or generalized headache, behavioral abnormalities, focal seizure activity, and focal neurologic deficits, most often dysphasia or hemiparesis.

2. The clinical presentation of arboviral encephalitis depends, to some extent, on the specific virus. Symptoms usually begin with headache, fever, vomiting, and malaise, followed by confusion, increasing lethargy, and seizure activity.

   a. La Crosse virus is the most common cause of pediatric arboviral encephalitis in the United States. Focal neurologic deficits occur in 16% to 25% of children, and focal and generalized seizures occur in 42% to 62% of children.

   b. Most cases of encephalitis from St. Louis encephalitis virus occur in adults older than 50 years of age. The onset of encephalitis symptoms may be preceded by an influenza-like prodrome of malaise, myalgias, and fever. This is followed by symptoms of headache, nausea, vomiting, confusion, disorientation, stupor, tremor, and occasionally convulsions.

   c. West Nile virus encephalitis begins with a febrile, influenza-like illness with headache, sore throat, malaise, myalgias, fatigue, and conjunctivitis. There may be a maculopapular or roseolar rash. This is followed by symptoms of encephalitis. Some cases of encephalitis have been associated with an axonal neuropathy.

3. The encephalitis of chicken pox may occur prior to the onset of the rash of chicken pox but most often occurs approximately 7 to 10 days after the onset of the rash and is characterized by headache, fever, vomiting, seizures, and focal neurologic abnormalities.

4. Herpes-zoster-associated encephalitis typically presents with headache, malaise, and confusion days to weeks after the cutaneous eruption of zoster (shingles).

Key Signs

HSV-1 Encephalitis

- Subacute fever, hemicranial or generalized headache, behavioral abnormalities, focal seizure activity, and focal neurologic deficits, most often dysphasia or hemiparesis

Arboviral Encephalitis

- Headache, fever, vomiting, and malaise followed by confusion, increasing lethargy, and seizure activity

- Symptoms depend—to some extent—on the specific virus (e.g., La Crosse, St. Louis, West Nile).

Chicken Pox Encephalitis

- Headache, fever, vomiting, seizures, and focal neurologic abnormalities

- Signs most often occur 7 to 10 days after onset of the rash.

Herpes-Zoster-Associated Encephalitis

- Headache, malaise, and confusion days to weeks following the cutaneous eruption of shingles

Differential Diagnosis

The differential diagnosis of fever, headache and an altered level of consciousness (with or without seizure activity and/or focal neurologic deficits) is viral encephalitis, bacterial meningitis, rickettsial disease, fungal meningoencephalitis, tuberculous meningoencephalitis, septic dural sinus thrombosis, Rocky Mountain spotted fever, and ehrlichiosis.

Laboratory Testing

1. Herpes simplex virus: Examination of the cerebrospinal fluid in herpes simplex virus encephalitis reveals an increased opening pressure, a lymphocytic pleocytosis of 5 to 500 cells/mm^3, a mild to moderate elevation of the protein concentration, and a normal or mildly decreased glucose concentration.
   a. Cerebrospinal fluid (CSF) viral cultures for herpes simplex virus-1 are almost negative.
   b. The polymerase chain reaction (PCR) has become the "gold standard" for making a diagnosis of herpes simplex virus encephalitis.
   c. The cerebrospinal fluid should also be examined for antibodies against herpes simplex virus. These do not appear in the CSF until approximately 8 to 12 days after the onset of disease, and they increase significantly during the first 2 to 4 weeks of infection.

2. Arbovirus: The laboratory diagnosis of arboviral encephalitis is a serologic diagnosis and is based on demonstrating a fourfold or greater rise in viral antibody titer between acute and convalescent sera or by detecting virus-specific immunoglobulin M (IgM) antibody in serum.
   a. Examination of the cerebrospinal fluid in arboviral encephalitis demonstrates a lymphocytic pleocytosis, a normal glucose concentration, and a moderately elevated protein concentration. There may be a predominance of polymorphonuclear leukocytes early in infection, with a shift to a lymphocytic pleocytosis early in the disease course.
   b. Virus-specific IgM antibody can sometimes be demonstrated in cerebrospinal fluid.

3. Varicella-zoster: The diagnosis of varicella-zoster virus encephalitis is made by
   a. The detection of varicella-zoster virus DNA in CSF
   b. Varicella-zoster virus IgM antibodies in CSF
   c. A positive CSF viral culture.

4. Epstein-Barr virus: The diagnosis of encephalitis caused by Epstein-Barr virus is made by the detection of EBV DNA in CSF.

Key Tests: Cerebrospinal Fluid

- Cell count with differential diagnosis

- Chemistries

- PCR for HSV-1, HSV-2 DNA

- PCR for VZV DNA

- PCR for EBV DNA

- PCR for West Nile virus DNA

- Virus-specific IgM and IgG antibodies (HSV-1 and VZV)

Radiographic Features

1. The characteristic abnormality on magnetic resonance imaging scan (MRI) in herpes simplex virus-1 encephalitis is a high signal intensity lesion on T_2-weighted and fluid-attenuated inversion recovery (FLAIR) images in the medial and inferotemporal lobe extending up into the insula. A normal T_2-weighted and FLAIR MRI scan is evidence against the diagnosis of HSV-1 encephalitis.

2. The cranial MRI in arthropod-borne virus encephalitis is typically normal, with the exception of eastern and equine encephalomyelitis and Japa-

nese virus encephalitis, in which there are increased signal intensity lesions in the basal ganglia and thalami.

3. In varicella-zoster virus encephalitis, cranial MRI may reveal large and small ischemic and hemorrhagic infarctions of the cortical and subcortical gray and white matter, as well as spherical subcortical white matter lesions with the typical appearance of demyelination.

Treatment

1. Every patient with fever, headache, and an altered level of consciousness (with or without seizure activity and/or focal neurologic deficits) should be treated empirically with acyclovir, a third- or fourth-generation cephalosporin (ceftriaxone, cefotaxime, or cefepime) and vancomycin. Ampicillin and gentamicin are added to the empiric regimen when the patient has risk factors for *Listeria monocytogenes* meningitis. Doxycycline is added to the empiric regimen in the presence of an erythematous maculopapular rash that begins on the ankles and wrists (Rocky Mountain spotted fever), and in patients who are at risk for ehrlichiosis (history of a tick bite in an endemic area).

2. Herpes simplex virus encephalitis is treated with intravenous acyclovir in a dose of 10 mg/kg every 8 hours for 14 to 21 days.

3. The treatment of arboviral encephalitis is primarily supportive care with the management of seizures and increased intracranial pressure. Ribavirin has been used successfully in La Crosse virus encephalitis, and there are ongoing clinical trials.

4. Varicella-zoster virus encephalitis is treated with acyclovir 10 mg/kg every 8 hours for 21 days.

5. Epstein-Barr virus encephalitis is treated with acyclovir 10 mg/kg every 8 hours for 21 days.

Key Treatment

- Acyclovir
- Third- or fourth-generation cephalosporin (ceftriaxone, cefotaxime, or cefepime)
- Vancomycin
- Ampicillin and gentamicin
- Doxycycline

Prognosis and Complications

1. Herpes simplex virus encephalitis, if untreated, is fatal. Neurologic sequelae are related to the length of time between the onset of symptoms and the initiation of acyclovir. Patients who develop seizure activity will require long-term anticonvulsant therapy. The focal neurologic deficits tend to improve, but many patients are left with some degree of difficulty with language.

2. The prognosis of arboviral encephalitis depends on the specific arbovirus. Mortality from La Crosse virus encephalitis is low but a residual seizure disorder occurs in approximately 15% of patients. St. Louis virus encephalitis has a mortality of 10 to 20%, and approximately 10% of survivors experience sequelae of memory loss, chronic fatigue and headache. The mortality rate from Japanese encephalitis virus is in the range of 20 to 40%. The highest mortality rate in arboviral encephalitis is from eastern equine encephalomyelitis virus, and is 50 to 75% with survivors having a high incidence of neurological sequelae of seizures, spastic para- or quadraparesis, and cognitive and behavioral abnormalities.

Prevention

Japanese encephalitis virus is preventable by vaccination with three doses of the inactivated Japanese encephalitis virus vaccine. None of the other viral causes of encephalitis are preventable.

Pregnancy

Acyclovir is safe during pregnancy.

Bibliography

Campbell GL, Marfin AA, Lanciotti RS, Gubler DJ: West Nile virus. Lancet Infec Dis 2:519–529, 2002.

Johnson R: Arboviruses. In Johnson R (ed): Viral Infections of the Nervous System, 2nd ed. Philadelphia, Lippincott-Raven, 1998, pp. 109–124.

Redington JJ, Tyler KL: Viral infections of the nervous system, 2002: update on diagnosis and treatment. Arch Neurol 59:712–718, 2002.

Roos KL: Encephalitis. Neurol Clin 17:813–834, 1999.

Whitley RJ, Gnann JW: Viral encephalitis: familiar infections and emerging pathogens. Lancet 359:507–513.

4 Human Immunodeficiency Virus and Human T-lymphotropic Virus Type 1

Russell Bartt

HIV

Definition

Human immunodeficiency virus (HIV), a blood-borne pathogen, is an RNA virus that infects immune competent cells, predominantly CD4+ lymphocytes and macrophage/monocytes, replicates by reverse transcription, and results in profound immunodeficiency over time.

Overview

1. HIV infection is a dynamic process of viral replication, lymphocyte turnover, cytokines, chemokines, and other immune factors in continual flux.
2. Viral suppression with antiretroviral compounds used in combination can reduce viral replication, resulting in lower serum viral burden (viral load); stabilize or improve CD4+ lymphocyte levels; reduce the incidence of opportunistic infections; and improve survival.
3. HIV is prone to spontaneous errors in replication, or as a result of antiviral medication pressure, resulting in new strains. Recently, genomic testing of the HIV has become available allowing for, in part, selection of antiretroviral (ARV) medications based on strain of virus.
4. Acquired immunodeficiency syndrome (AIDS) is defined by a CD4+ lymphocyte count of 200 cells/ml or less, or by the presence of an opportunistic infection referred to as an AIDS-defining illness.

Epidemiology

1. HIV virus can be found in brain macrophages, monocytes, or microglia (the immune competent cells of the nervous system) in virtually all pathologic cases.
2. Clinically relevant neurologic disease occurs in a cross section of 20% to 55% of all HIV-infected persons and heralds the presence of HIV infection in 7% to 20% of those individuals.
3. The occurrence of neurologic complications is greater the longer one survives with HIV or with greater degrees of immunosuppression.

Neurologic Complications of Initial Infection

HIV enters the nervous system very shortly after initial infection. The initial infection may not be associated with a systemic illness or neurologic symptoms. However, some patients will have systemic symptoms or nervous system complications that can range from trivial to significant enough to seek medical attention. HIV antibodies may not be present at this time; therefore, serum HIV viral load by polymerase chain reaction (reverse transcriptase or rtPCR) in the serum can help in the diagnosis.

1. Aseptic meningitis: A lymphocytic pleocytosis occurs with mild or no hypoglycorrhachia. HIV-1 antibody testing by enzyme-linked immunosorbent assay (ELISA) or Western blot may be negative at this time. Treatment is supportive with analgesics and fluids. Occasionally, the meningitis is not self-limited, and initiation of anti-retroviral medications can help.
2. Acute inflammatory demyelinating polyneuropathy (AIDP): AIDP can be "triggered" by HIV seroconversion reaction, just as other infections can precede AIDP. In areas with high incidence of HIV, or in patients with risk factors, HIV needs to be considered in every AIDP patient. Treatment is the same as AIDP from any other cause.

HIV-ASSOCIATED DISEASE OF THE CENTRAL NERVOUS SYSTEM

HIV- Associated Dementia

Definition and Epidemiology

1. Dementia in HIV subjects has several names in the literature such as AIDS dementia, AIDS dementia complex, HIV encephalopathy. These terms denote the same condition now referred to as HIV-associated dementia (HIV-D). The term HIV-encephalitis is a term that should be limited to pathologic description of multinucleated giant cells in the brain with HIV.
2. HIV-D occurs in 15% of patients. The annual incidence is 5%, making HIV-D the fourth most common complication of HIV infection. The

incidence rate is dropping with better regimens; however, living longer with HIV may translate to a greater proportion of HIV patients with dementia. Some studies have reported an increasing prevalence of dementia.

3. Patients with longer duration of HIV infection, higher serum viral loads, and lower CD4 counts are at higher risk for the development of dementia.

Pathogenesis

The exact pathogenesis of HIV-D is not well defined. Neuronal infection by HIV does not play a role. Activated macrophages and soluble factors such as chemokines, cytokines, tumor necrosis factor α (TNF-α), metalloproteinases, and nitric oxide may induce neuronal dysfunction and, eventually, cell death.

Clinical Manifestations

Symptoms include apathy, poor concentration, social withdrawal, slowed thinking, poor memory, and decreased mental dexterity. Depression and anxiety may be co-morbid or may be misdiagnoses for HIV-D. Mania or bipolar disease may be presenting features of HIV-D in a minority of cases. Signs of mental slowing, decreased smooth pursuit, mild increase in tendon reflexes, and change in posture may be present and become more pronounced with progression of dementia. See HIV-Associated Dementia Staging.

HIV-Associated Dementia (AIDS Dementia Complex) Staging

- Stage 0: Normal

- Stage 0.5: Minimal or equivocal motor or cognitive dysfunction but without impairment of work or capacity to perform activities of daily living (ADLs)

- Stage 1 (mild): Unequivocal evidence or functional intellectual or motor impairment characteristic of ADC but with the ability to perform the more demanding aspects of work of ADLs. Can walk without assistance

- Stage 2 (moderate): Cannot work or maintain the more demanding aspects of work or ADLs. Can walk without assistance

- Stage 3 (severe): Major intellectual incapacity. Unable to carry on a complex conversation, with significant slowing or motor disablitiy requiring a person or a walker for assistance. Arm clumsiness as well

- Stage 4 (end stage): Nearly vegetative. Nearly or completely mute. Incontinence. Paraparetic or paraplegic

---

1. Confounding factors such as substance use, low educational level, and depression or mental illness make the certain diagnosis of HIV-D difficult. Neuropsychiatric testing is helpful in most cases and can be repeated at a later date to assess for interim change. Magnetic resonance imaging (MRI) demonstrates symmetric, increased intensity of the white matter on T_2-weighted sequences. These changes correlate with the severity of disease.

2. Cerebrospinal fluid HIV-viral load (CSF viral load), when elevated, increases the risk of HIV-D but does not predict the severity of disease. The presence of an elevated CSF viral load is not diagnostic. However, with ARV treatment there may be a drop in CSF viral load and associated with cognitive improvement.

Treatment and Prognosis

1. HIV-D is treatable. Mild to moderate dementia is, in part, reversible. Improvement of cognitive dysfunction, motor signs, and MRI imaging in response to ARV therapy can occur. A list of ARVs, emphasizing those that may have better CNS penetration, is given under Key Treatment.

 Key Treatment: HIV-D Antiretroviral Medications and Those with Presumed Better CSF Penetration (*)

Nucleoside Analogs

- Zidovudine/Retrovir (AZT, ZDV)*

- Didanosine/Videx (ddI)

- Zalcitabine/Hivid (ddC)

- Stavudine/Zerit (d4T)*

- Lamivudine/Epivir (3TC)*

- Abacavir/Ziagen (ABC)*

- Combivir (AZT/3TC)

- Trizivir (AZT/3TC/abacavir)*

Nucleotide Analog

- Adefovir dipivoxil/Preveon

Non-Nucleoside Reverse Transcriptive Inhibitors (RTIs)

- Nevirapine/Viramune*

- Delavirdine/Rescriptor*

- Efavirenz/Sustiva (DMP-266)

Protease Inhibitors

- Ritonavir/Norvir
- Saquinavir/Invirase, Fortovase
- Nelfinavir/Viracept
- Amprenavir/Agenerase
- Indinavir/Crixivan*
- Lopinavir, ritonavir/ Kaletra

2. Some patients who have undetectable viral loads in the serum may develop progressive cognitive changes. CSF viral loads in these patients can be elevated, indicating a lack of viral suppression in the intrathecal space. This "CNS escape" should prompt a change in antiretroviral therapy or intensification of the existing regimen.

HIV-Associated Myelopathy

Definition and Epidemiology

1. Spinal cord disease due to HIV is typically a subacute progressive condition with typical signs of myelopathy.

2. The true incidence of myelopathy is not known. A case-control study has shown no correlation with dementia, even though both are syndromes of the indirect effects of HIV infection of the central nervous system (CNS). On autopsy, 20% to 55% of AIDS cases have the pathologic changes of vacuolization and HIV-infected macrophages predominantly in the anterior horn and posterior columns.

Pathogenesis

Clinical and pathologic similarities with HIV-associated myelopathy and sub-acute combined degeneration (vitamin B_{12} deficiency) have been noted. Vitamin B_{12} is a cofactor for synthesis of methionine subsequent compounds. Chemokines and cytokines released by activated macrophages interfere with the donation of methyl groups from these compounds that are needed in myelin formation and repair. Viral loads in the CSF do not correlate clinically with HIV-associated myelopathy.

Clinical Features

Weakness and sphincter dysfunction predominate, with sensory symptoms or signs being less impressive. Rarely, a myelitis-like presentation can occur. A transverse myelopathy with a discrete sensory level is uncommon and should raise suspicion of an alternative diagnosis.

Key Signs: HIV-Associated Myelopathy

- Weakness and sphincter dysfunction

Treatment and Prognosis

Although vitamin B_{12} supplementation has not proved helpful, treatment with L-methionine is under evaluation. Anecdotes of clinical improvement in response to ARV therapy alone are reported, but infrequent.

Key Treatment: HIV-Associated Myelopathy

- L-methionine (under evaluation)

Common Opportunistic Diseases of the CNS

Although the incidence of opportunistic entities is decreasing in this era of better ARV therapy, these conditions continue occur. In general, the following disorders are more likely to occur with CD4 counts below 200 cells/ml. An algorithmic approach is provided in Figure 4–1.

1. *Toxoplasma gondii* encephalitis

   a. The most common cause of intracranial mass lesion(s) in patients with AIDS. Ingestion of *T. gondii* often results in latent infection. Immunosuppression then allows for activation from a latent (bradyzoite) state to active (tachyzoite) infection. Population seropositivity (positive immunoglobulin G—IgG—titer) in the United States is 10% to 40% with higher rates in Europe, Latin America, and Africa.

   b. The probability that brain lesion(s) are toxoplasmic encephalitis is increased in patients with lower CD4 counts, positive IgG titers, multiple lesions, and those not taking trimethoprim-sulfamethoxazole prophylaxis (typically taken to prevent *Pneumocystis carinii* pneumonia, but also prevents toxoplasmic encephalitis).

   c. Typically, multiple mass lesions are found predominantly at the gray–white matter junction and in the basal ganglia/thalamic region. Computed tomography (CT) scanning often reveals multiple ring-enhancing lesions, at times demonstrating a central enhancing nodule creating a "target" lesion. MRI may show additional lesions, especially in the posterior fossa. Severity depends on location and intensity of the immune response responsible for the

Figure 4–1. An algorithm for the evaluation and treatment of intracranial mass lesions in AIDS patients (Report of the Quality Standards Subcommittee of the American Academy of Neurology: Evaluation and management of intracranial mass lesions in AIDS Neurology 50:23, 1998, with permission).

vasogenic and cytotoxic edema. Rarely, a purely encephalitic form (without discrete lesions) can occur.

d. The subacute clinical presentations are variable, but commonly headache, confusion, fever are present. Seizures, and focal neurologic findings are seen in about one third to one half of all patients. Psychiatric presentations have also been described.

Key Signs: *Toxoplasma gondii* Encephalitis

- Headache
- Confusion
- Fever
- Seizures and focal neurologic findings occur in one third to one half of all patients

e. Diagnosis is typically made by response to therapy within 2 weeks by clinical and radiologic criteria. Indirect fluorescent antibodies (IFA), ELISA, and IgM titers may be used as well.

Key Tests: *Toxoplasma gondii* Encephalitis

- CT
- MRI
- IFA
- ELISA
- IgM titers

f. Therapy

(1) Sulfadiazine (4 to 6 mg daily) and pyrimethamine 200 mg times one dose, then 75–100 mg daily. Folinic acid (leucovorin) administration should be used to prevent pyrimethamine-induced myelosuppression, at 10–15 mg per day orally.

(2) Sulfa-sensitive patients can be treated with clindamycin (600 mg every 6 hours intravenously) in the place of sulfadiazine.

(3) Azithromycin and pyrimethamine or atovaquone have been used for patients intoler-

ant to the above regimens, although efficacy is less certain.

(4) Corticosteroids to treat cerebral edema are to be avoided if possible. Non-toxoplasmic lesions may respond, and therefore a clinical improvement does not differentiate between toxoplasmosis and other etiologies.

(5) Chronic suppressive therapy is necessary after acute treatment with daily maintenance sulfadiazine (or clindamycin) plus pyrimethamine. In patients with positive titers and CD4 counts < 100 cells/µl (but no history of toxoplasmosis) can use once daily trimethoprim-sulfamethoxazole or dapsone plus pyrimethamine.

Key Treatment: *Toxoplasma gondii* Encephalitis

- Sulfadiazine and pyrimethamine

- Clindamycin for sulfa-sensitive patients

2. Primary central nervous system lymphoma (PCNSL)

 a. The second most common focal brain lesion in AIDS, PCNSL is a consideration in all AIDS patients presenting with a focal brain lesion(s). As many as 20% of all HIV patients will eventually develop a lymphoma, most commonly PCNSL. A study of consecutive focal brain lesions in AIDS found over 25% to be PCNSL. Factors that can help distinguish *T. gondii* encephalitis from PCNSL are listed under Suspicious Factors for PCNSL.

Suspicious Factors for PCNSL

- Negative IgG titer for *Toxoplasma gondii*

- Patient taking oral prophylaxis for *Pneumocystis carinii* pneumonia

- Solitary lesion on CT scan or MRI

- Thallium 201 single-photon emission computed tomography (SPECT) scan showing persistent uptake on delayed images

- No response to anti-toxoplasma treatment after 10 days

---

 b. Lymphomas in HIV (and immunosuppression in general) are high-grade B-cell lymphomas. A combination of factors may contribute to the development of PCNSL such as decreased immune surveillance of cancerous cells, activation of oncogenes, and inhibition of tumor-suppressor genes. In particular, Epstein-Barr virus DNA is found in the PCNSL cells, in striking contrast to non-HIV associated lymphomas, and it is thought to play a role in oncogenesis.

 c. Clinical presentation with impairment of consciousness and focal neurologic findings. Seizures and cranial nerve findings occur in less than 25% of cases. Onset of symptoms is generally short, from days to a few weeks. Symptoms of fever, chills, night sweats, and weight loss are common.

Key Signs: PCNSL

- Fever, chills, night sweats, and weight loss

- Seizures and cranial nerve findings occur in less than 25% of cases.

 d. Often there are multiple lesions, although one third are solitary. A single lesion is four times more likely to be PCNSL than toxoplasmic encephalitis. Periventricular lesions or lesions at the gray–white matter junction are typical.

(1) A contrast-enhanced CT scan will often demonstrate a hypodense lesion with enhancement. However, isodense and hyperdense lesions can occur, and enhancement can be variable.

(2) MRI is preferred for better resolution.

 e. A patient with a focal brain lesion should receive therapy for toxoplasmic encephalitis. In patients with solitary lesions, those without titers to *Toxoplasma* and/or receiving prophylaxis with trimethoprim-sulfamethoxazole, PCNSL should be suspected. Evidence in favor of PCNSL includes:

(1) CSF (if safe to obtain) cytology showing neoplastic cells (only about 10% of cases)

(2) CSF polymerase chain reaction (PCR) positivity for EBV-DNA. (Sensitivity close to 90% and specificity over 95%.)

(3) Thallium 201 brain single photon emission computed tomography (SPECT) scanning demonstrating persistent uptake on delayed images. Toxoplasmic lesions do not. False negatives and false positives exist, but sensitivity and specificity are above 80%.

(4) Stereotactic or open biopsy of the mass proving PCNSL. Despite the methods listed

above, biopsy is necessary to provide treatment with diagnostic certainty.

Key Tests: PCNSL

- CT
- MRI
- Thallium 201 brain SPECT scanning
- Stereotactic or open biopsy of the mass

f. Treatment prolongs survival and lessen symptoms in patients with PCNSL. Therefore, as mentioned above, evaluation for PCNSL should be performed when there are factors that make toxoplasmic encephalitis less likely. Waiting 2 weeks to prove a non-response to *Toxoplasma* therapy obviously delays starting treatment for an aggressive brain neoplasm. Treatments include

(1) Whole brain irradiation: Usually lower doses are administered in AIDS patients (about 3,000 to 4,000 cGy). This may improve survival from 1–2 months (without radiation) to 3–4 months. Patients who do not receive radiation often die of progressive PCNSL, whereas irradiated patients often stabilize but die of infectious causes.

(2) Radiation and chemotherapy regimens including methotrexate alone or in combination with cyclophosphamide and procarbazine have shown mean survival of 2 years or more.

Key Treatment: PCNSL

- Same as toxoplasmic encephalitis for patients with focal brain lesions
- Whole brain irradiation (about 3,000 to 4,000 cGy)
- Radiation and chemotherapy regimens including methotrexate with or without cyclophosphamide and procarbazine

3. Progressive multifocal leukoencephalopathy (PML)

a. PML is caused by the JC virus (JCV), a virus that infects oligodendrocytes causing demyelinating lesions of the CNS. Before the HIV pandemic, PML was rare. Nearly all cases today are associated with AIDS. Infrequently, patients present with CD4 counts lower than 200 cells/μl and have a better prognosis.

b. Clinical features most often include weakness and possibly cognitive disturbance. Occasionally the disease focus will be in the brainstem with associated gaze disturbance and long tract signs. Headache or visual field abnormalities are sometimes seen. Spinal cord and optic nerve are not involved.

Key Signs: PML

- Weakness and possibly cognitive disturbance
- Headache or visual field abnormalities

c. On MRI, T_2-weighted hyperintensities are seen in the white matter and can involve basal ganglia or the thalamus as well. Solitary lesions may be seen. The absence of mass effect and enhancement is typical. Enhancement, present in a quarter of patients, is associated with a better prognosis.

d. JCV presence in spinal fluid by PCR of is sufficiently diagnostic (sensitivity about 80% and specificity >98%) and obviates the need for biopsy. All PCR results should be used in the appropriate clinical and radiologic context.

Key Tests: PML

- MRI
- PCR

e. Although many patients progress rapidly, about 1 in 10 patients may stabilize and have prolonged survival. Response to ARV medications has a beneficial effect on survival and anecdotes of apparent "resolution" are known. Trials with cytosine arabinoside and a pilot study with cidofovir have not clearly shown additional benefit.

Key Treatment: PML

- ARV medications

4. *Cryptococcus neoformans* (cryptococcal) meningitis

a. Although not exclusive to the immunocompromised patient, cryptococcal meningitis is a common fungal infection in HIV. Up to 10% of all AIDS patients may develop this complication.

b. Clinical onset is usually subacute, with progression of headache, fevers, nausea, vomiting, and even obtundation. Definite signs of meningismus may be lacking. Mass lesions (cryptococcomas) are infrequent but can appear as a mass lesion or a small enhancing nodule.

Key Signs: Cryptococcal Meningitis
- Headache
- Fever
- Nausea
- Vomiting
- Obtundation

c. Diagnosis can be made or highly suspected by a few means.
  (1) Cryptococcal antigen (CRAG) in the CSF has a sensitivity >91% and is therefore useful for prompt diagnosis. The use of this test in the serum can also be helpful in increasing suspicion in the appropriate syndrome.
  (2) India ink staining is quickly available and may be positive more often than culture.
  (3) Culture of *Cryptococcus* remains the "gold standard" in diagnosis.
  (4) Cell counts may be normal (especially in the very immunosuppressed). Opening pressures are frequently high and glucose low. Fortunately, completely normal lumbar puncture examinations are rare.
  (5) CT scanning is most often normal or shows only atrophy.
d. Treatment includes the use of amphotericin therapy, alone or in combination with flucytosine (5FC), followed by chronic suppressive therapy to prevent relapse.
  (1) Amphotericin 0.7mg/kg/day intravenously with or without 5FC at 100 mg/kg/day orally for the first 2 weeks has been shown to be effective. Lower doses of amphotericin have been used (0.4 mg/kg per day) with success, but most experts suggest the higher dose given the seriousness of the disease.
  (2) Fluconazole, 400 mg/day orally, alone can be effective but longer time to CSF sterilization is a concern. Generally used following initial amphotericin therapy for a total of 10 weeks of therapy.
  (3) Elevated intracranial pressure is an important factor in the acute mortality of cryptococcal meningitis and should be managed

aggressively with lumbar punctures. Intervals of 6 to 24 hours are recommended as long as pressures remain elevated, and each procedure should result in a normal closing pressure. Lumbar drains can be used.

Key Treatment: Cryptococcal Meningitis
- Amphotericin with or without flucytosine

  e. Mortality during the acute treatment of cryptococcal meningitis ranges from 10% to 25%, and the 12-month survival rate is 30% to 60%. Factors associated with a poor prognosis include:
    (1) Depressed level of consciousness upon presentation
    (2) CRAG >1:1024 dilutions in the CSF
    (3) Fewer than 20 cells/ml in the CSF
    (4) Elevated opening pressure

HIV-ASSOCIATED DISEASE OF THE PERPHERAL NERVOUS SYSTEM (PNS)

Distal Symmetric Polyneuropathy (DSP)

Definition and Epidemiology
1. DSP is the most common neurologic complication of HIV, affecting approximately one third of patients.
   a. There is an inverse relationship between the incidence of DSP and CD4 counts. In addition, certain medications can cause or contribute to DSP.
   b. With better antiretroviral therapy, patients are living longer with HIV infection and are exposed to more drug regimens. Therefore, the incidence of DSP may actually increase, unlike that of other HIV-induced complications.

Pathogenesis
No one mechanism of peripheral nerve injury has been defined.
1. HIV itself, gp120 protein, soluble inflammatory factors such as cytokines, chemokines, TNFα, and several interleukins have been proposed.
2. Neurotoxic ARVs (d4T, ddI, and ddC) or other neurotoxic medications such as dapsone, vincristine, and isoniazid can cause or contribute to neuropathy.
3. Nutritional factors, alcohol use, or other medical conditions such as diabetes mellitus or thyroid disease may also be responsible for neuropathy in these patients.

Clinical Features

Distal lower limb pain, paresthesias, burning, shooting or other neuropathic qualities may be present. Sensitivity and worsening of pain in the evening hours are often present.

1. Signs include distal impairment of sharp sensation and/or vibration and attenuation or absence of stretch reflexes at the ankle relative to the knee. However, these signs are not universal.

2. Overall, the symptoms and signs are consistent with a small-fiber neuropathy. The predominance of large-fiber symptoms (profound position and vibration loss) should raise suspicion of another etiology.

Key Signs: DSP

- Pain in the distal lower limbs

- Paresthesias, burning, shooting pain, or other neuropathic qualities

- Sensitivity and worsening of pain in the evening hours

Treatment and Prognosis

Treatment of DSP is largely symptomatic.

1. If neurotoxic drugs are present, dose reduction or discontinuation may result in improvement.

2. Early or intermittent symptoms can sometimes be controlled with anti-inflammatory medications or acetaminophen.

3. Consistent discomfort often requires the consistent use of adjunctive agents such as tricyclic antidepressants or anticonvulsants such as gabapentin or lamotrigine. Mexiletine (an antiarrhythmic) is sometimes of additional benefit. Opioids as needed or by consistent dosing (i.e., fentanyl patch) for more severe cases can prove helpful.

4. Often the objective signs and symptoms remain stable over years and infrequently progress to involve the upper limbs. Progression over weeks and to the upper limbs casts doubt on a sole diagnosis of HIV-associated DSP.

Key Treatment: DSP

- Anti-inflammatory medications or acetaminophen

- Tricyclic antidepressants or anticonvulsants such as gabapentin or lamotrigine

Chronic Inflammatory Demyelinating Polyneuropathy (CIDP)

1. Inflammatory demyelinating polyneuropathy, either acute (AIDP) or chronic (CIDP), can occur in HIV. AIDP, as mentioned above, can occur as a consequence of primary HIV infection.

2. CIDP typically occurs with existing HIV infection, with modest immune dysfunction but not the profound immunosuppression of AIDS. Often, CD4 cell counts are between 200 and 400 cells/ml.

3. Evaluations for monoclonal antibodies, B-cell dyscrasias, and autoimmune conditions are often unrevealing. Lumbar puncture should reveal a low pleocytosis if any, and an elevated CSF protein.

4. The diagnosis relies heavily on electrodiagnostic testing (nerve conduction studies and electromyography) revealing widespread, and at times multifocal, demyelinating features of CIDP.

Key Tests: CIDP

- Nerve conduction studies and electromyography

5. Unlike conventional therapy for CIDP, treatment with intravenous immunoglobulin or plasma exchange is recommended as solitary therapy, and immunosuppressive medications (corticosteroids or cytotoxic agents) should be avoided if possible.

Key Treatment: CIDP

- Intravenous immunoglobulin or plasma exchange

Opportunistic Infection of the PNS

1. Polyradiculitis
   a. Cytomegalovirus (CMV) is responsible for a rapid cauda equina syndrome in patients with profound immunosuppression. Pain and paresthesias in the lower legs with a progressive, flaccid paraparesis, areflexia, and sphincter dysfunction is the common presentation.

Key Signs: Polyradiculitis

- Pain and paresthesias in the lower extremities with progressive, flaccid paraparesis, areflexia, and sphincter dysfunction

   b. Typically, patients have CD4 counts lower than 50 cells/ml and are therefore susceptible to invasive CMV disease.

c. Lumbar puncture reveals a neutrophilic pleocytosis, and CMV culture and PCR should be performed.

Key Tests: Polyradiculitis

- Lumbar puncture
- CMV culture
- PCR

d. Intravenous anti-CMV medication should be instituted at recognition of this syndrome in a susceptible host to provide the best chance for recovery.

Key Treatment: Polyradiculitis

- Intravenous anti-CMV medication

2. Mononeuritis multiplex
   a. CMV may also result in a multifocal mononeuropathies in profoundly immunosuppressed patients as with polyradiculitis. Clinically, a classic subacute syndrome of successive mononeuropathies occurs with the associated deficit (motor and/or sensory for that territory).
   b. Electrodiagnostic testing is helpful in proving the multifocal nature of the condition. Axonal, demyelinating, or mixed features can be seen.

Key Test: Mononeuritis Multiplex

- Electrodiagnostic testing

c. A CD4 count lower than 50 cells/ml and this syndrome helps distinguish this from CIDP, as described above, and should prompt at least single-drug intravenous therapy with ganciclovir or foscarnet. Nerve biopsy may demonstrate CMV inclusions in the specimen. Long-term therapy is needed.

Key Treatment: Mononeuritis Multiplex

- Ganciclovir or foscarnet

HTLV-1

Definition and Epidemiology

1. Human T-lymphotropic virus type 1 (HTLV-1) is an RNA virus (retrovirus, like HIV) that is not as pathogenic. The Caribbean islands, Japan, equatorial Africa, and the southeastern United States are areas of higher seroprevalence. Clinical disease occurs in primarily two forms.
   a. Acute T-cell leukemia/lymphoma occurs in 2% to 4% of seropositive patients. This condition is aggressive, with a mean survival of less than a year.
   b. HTLV-1 associated myelopathy or tropical spastic paraparesis (HAM/TSP) occurs in 0.25% of seropositive individuals. Other factors such as environment and genetics may play a role in seropositive patients developing clinically relevant myelopathy.

Pathogenesis

Transmission of HTLV-1 is by blood and body fluid contact.

1. Sexual contact, intravenous drug use with sharing of needles, breast-feeding, and blood transfusions are common modes. Transmission is inefficient, and seroconversion may occur only after repeated exposures over time.
2. The mechanism of spinal cord dysfunction and vasculitis is mediated by cytotoxic CD8 lymphocytes and CD4 lymphocytes that express the pX protein (unique to HTLV).

Clinical Features

Systemic signs of infection are absent. Gradual onset of spasticity and progressive weakness with sphincter dysfunction and impotence are usually evident.

1. Backache, pain, and sensory symptoms in the lower limbs are often subjectively greater than objectively evident.
2. Like HIV-associated myelopathy, a discrete sensory level is unusual and should suggest a more focal disease process.
3. Co-infection with HIV and HTLV-1 is described, and both viruses should be sought in myelopathic patients because, as clinically, the two are difficult to separate.

Key Signs: HTLV-1

- Spasticity
- Progressive weakness with sphincter dysfunction and impotence
- Backache
- Sensory symptoms in the lower limbs

Treatment and Prognosis

Improvement of myelopathy with chronic corticosteroid treatment can demonstrate improvement, particularly in the early stages of disease. However, some patients will not respond or will worsen at a later time despite such treatment.

1. Interferon α, plasmapheresis, and intravenous immunoglobulin may also result in short-term improvement.

2. There is little clinical data using antiretrovirals. Zidovudine (AZT) has been shown to reduce serum HTLV-1 burden with high doses in the short term complicated by anemia in some patients. HIV protease inhibitors are not active against HTLV protease.

Key Treatment: HTLV-1

- Corticosteroids
- Interferon α
- Plasmapheresis
- Intravenous immunoglobulin

Bibliography

Antinori A, Ammassari A, De Luca A, et al.: Diagnosis of AIDS-related focal brain lesions. Neurology 48:687–694, 1997.

Berger JR, Levy RM (eds): AIDS and the Nervous System, 2nd ed. Philadelphia, Lippincott-Raven, 1997.

Berger JR (guest ed), Pascuzzi RM (ed): Neurologic complications of AIDS. Semin Neurol 19:105–233, 1999.

Clifford DB: AIDS dementia. Med Clin North Am 86:537–550, 2002.

Evaluation and management of intracranial mass lesions in AIDS. Report of the Quality Standards Subcommittee of the American Academy of Neurology. Neurology 50:21–26, 1998.

Mamidi A, DeSimone JA, Pomerantz RJ: Central nervous system infections in individuals with HIV-1 infection. J Neurovirol 8:158–167, 2002.

5 Brain and Spinal Abscess

John E. Greenlee

BRAIN ABSCESS

Definition

Brain abscesses are loculated infections within brain parenchyma. Brain abscess may occur as an isolated event or may be accompanied by other intracranial infections, including epidural abscess, subdural empyema, and meningitis. Abscesses may be single or multiple.

Epidemiology

Brain abscess is an uncommon condition, representing approximately 1 in 10,000 hospitalizations and 0.18% to 1.3% of autopsies. The incidence is higher under conditions of immunosuppression.

1. Peak age incidence is 30 to 45 years. Males predominate by a 2:1 ratio in most series.
2. Approximately 25% of brain abscesses occur in children, with the peak age being between 4 and 7 years. As in adult cases, there is a 2:1 male predominance.

Etiology, Pathophysiology, and Risk Factors

1. Brain abscesses most commonly arise by hematogenous spread of bacteria from an extracranial source of infection. Less frequently, brain abscess is caused by extension of infection from pericranial structures. Brain abscess may also result from penetrating head trauma or neurosurgical procedures.
2. Extracranial foci of infection associated with hematogenous brain abscess include lung abscess, bronchiectasis, or other chronic lung infections, and bacterial endocarditis. Brain abscess may also arise during bacteremia in diabetics, drug addicts, or patients with cyanotic congenital heart disease. Hematogenous abscesses are most common in the distribution of the middle cerebral artery followed by the anterior cerebral artery, and the posterior circulation. *Listeria* abscesses tend to involve brainstem.
3. The most common pericranial infection associated with brain abscess is sinusitis—in particular involving the frontal, ethmoidal, and sphenoidal sinuses. Chronic otitis media and mastoiditis,

although less common in the modern era, may also cause brain abscess. Occasionally, brain abscess may result from facial or dental infections.

   a. Abscesses arising from frontal or ethmoidal sinusitis tend to be located in the frontal lobes; those due to sphenoidal sinusitis may involve either frontal or temporal lobes.
   b. Abscesses arising from otitis or mastoiditis tend usually to involve the temporal lobes, the cerebellum, or, occasionally, the brainstem.
4. Brain abscesses usually form at the gray–white junction, where collateral blood supply is poorest and brain is most easily injured. The initial injury is an area of septic microvascular ischemia followed by focal encephalitis or "cerebritis" and development of an encapsulated abscess cavity. The capsule is usually thinnest on its medial aspect, and tends to enlarge inwardly, toward the ventricular system.
5. Death in brain abscess is almost always the result of brain herniation. This may be caused by the mass effect of the abscess and its surrounding cerebral edema; obstruction of ventricular outflow and hydrocephalus; or by ventricular rupture causing an abrupt rise in intraventricular pressure and meningitis.
6. Causative organisms
   a. Multiple organisms may be present simultaneously in brain abscess.
   b. Certain organisms are particularly common (see Key Causative Agents of Brain Abscess). These include aerobic, microaerophilic, and anaerobic streptococci, in particular members of the *Streptococcus milleri* group, (*Streptococcus intermedius* and *Streptococcus anginosus*). These may occur in any setting but are particularly common in abscesses arising from sinusitis or dental infections.
   c. *Staphylococcus aureus* is found in 10% to 15% of cases and is the most common organism associated with penetrating trauma or neurosurgical infections.
   d. *Bacteroides* species and enteric bacteria such as *Escherichia coli*, *Proteus* species, and *Pseudomonas* species are found in 20% to 40% of cases. Multiple organisms may be present, in particular in abscesses associated with sinusitis or otitis.
   e. Occasionally, brain abscesses in immunologi-

cally normal adults may be due to more unusual organisms such as *Listeria monocytogenes*, *Clostridium*, *Fusobacterium*, or *Actinomyces* species, or *Entamoeba histolytica*.

f. Brain abscesses in immunocompromised patients may be caused by *Enterobacteriaceae*, *Pseudomonas aeruginosa*, and *Nocardia asteroides*; fungi such as *Cryptococcus neoformans*, *Candida*, *Rhizopus* (*Mucor*), and *Aspergillus*. The most common cause of loculated intracranial infection in patients with AIDS is *Toxoplasma gondii*, followed by *Cryptococcus neoformans* and *Mycobacterium tuberculosis*.

g. Brain abscess in neonates is usually a complication of meningitis. The most common organisms in neonates are thus gram-negative organisms, such as *Escherichia coli* or *Proteus mirabilis*, or *Serratia marcescens*. *Citrobacter* species, in particular *Citrobacter diversus*, and *Salmonella* species, although unusual in adults, may be causes of brain abscesses in infants.

h. Isolates from brain abscess in older children most frequently include aerobic and anaerobic gram-positive organisms, *Bacteroides*, and less common anaerobic species such as *Fusobacterium*, and *Prevotella*.

Major Causative Agents of Brain Abscess

In Adults and Older Children

- Aerobic, anaerobic, and microaerophilic streptococci
- (*Streptococcus anginosus*, *Streptococcus intermedius*)
- Gram-negative aerobic bacteria
  - *Escherichia coli*, *Proteus* sp., *Pseudomonas* sp.
- *Staphylococcus aureus*
- *Bacteroides* species

In Immunosuppressed Adults

- *Nocardia asteroides*
- *Listeria monocytogenes*
- *Aspergillus* sp. and other fungi

In Acquired Immunodeficiency Syndrome

- *Toxoplasma gondii*
- *Cryptococcus neoformans* and other fungi
- *Mycobacterium tuberculosis*
- (Less common: *Nocardia asteroides*, *Listeria monocytogenes*)

In Infants

- Gram-negative enteric bacteria
  - *Citrobacter* sp.

Clinical Features

1. The classic triad of fever, headache or impairment of consciousness, and focal neurologic deficit is present in entirety in only a minority of patients. Patients with brain abscesses most often present with a history suggesting a rapidly or subacutely developing space-occupying lesion.

2. Headache is present in 75% of patients; nausea and vomiting, in about 50%. Fever is present in less than 50% of patients and may be mistakenly attributed to coexisting sinusitis or other infection.

3. Focal neurologic signs, although suggestive of abscess, are present in less than 50% of patients and may be subtle. Nuchal rigidity is present in 25% of cases. Papilledema is often absent.

4. Seizures occur in approximately one third of patients and are most frequently associated with frontal lobe abscesses.

5. In 75% of cases, symptoms will have been present for less than 2 weeks. However, the onset of symptoms may be so rapid as to suggest stroke or may develop over weeks to months in a manner more suggestive of brain tumor.

Key Symptoms and Signs

- Headache (75% of patients)
- Nausea and vomiting (50%)
- Fever (less than 50%)
- Focal neurologic signs of abscess (less than 50%)
- Nuchal rigidity (25%)
- Seizures—most frequently associated with frontal lobe abscesses (33%)
- Symptoms present for less than 2 weeks (75%)

Diagnosis

1. Brain abscess should be suspected in any patient presenting with history or findings suggesting an acutely or subacutely expanding intracranial mass lesion.

   a. Suspicion of brain abscess should be heightened if risk factors are present: these include sinusitis, otitis, cyanotic congenital heart disease, intravenous drug abuse, diabetes, or human immunodeficiency virus infection.

b. The diagnosis is supported by a history of rapidly progressing illness, focal neurologic signs, or fever, but these may be absent, and the patient's history may extend over weeks or months.

2. Laboratory findings

a. Only 10% of patients will have elevation of the white blood count to above 20,000 cells/mm^3. In 40% of cases the white blood count is normal.

b. The erythrocyte sedimentation rate (ESR) is usually either normal or elevated to less than 45–55 mm/hr.

c. C-reactive protein (CRP) may be elevated, including in cases where the ESR is normal; however, CRP may also occasionally be elevated in patients with brain neoplasms.

d. Blood cultures are positive in less than 10% of patients.

3. Radiologic studies

a. The diagnostic study of choice in suspected brain abscess is magnetic resonance imaging (MRI) with gadolinium enhancement. Diffusion-weighted MRI may be helpful in distinguishing between brain abscess, stroke, and intracranial tumor.

b. Contrast-enhanced computed tomographic (CT) scan may be used where MRI is not available. CT, however, may fail to detect small or posterior fossa abscesses. Sensitivity of CT can be enhanced by obtaining delayed films after contrast administration.

c. MRI and CT may remain abnormal for many weeks despite clinical recovery

4. Lumbar puncture is contraindicated where brain abscess is suspected.

a. Cerebrospinal fluid in brain abscess usually shows nonspecific changes and will not contain organisms unless the abscess has ruptured into the ventricles or subarachnoid space.

b. Loss of cerebrospinal fluid following the lumbar puncture may cause brain herniation within hours of the procedure; mortality following lumbar puncture in brain abscess may approach 20%.

c. Patients in whom there is question of meningitis versus brain abscess should be treated emergently with antibiotics (see Treatment, below), scanned, and then investigated with lumbar puncture only after abscess is ruled out.

Key Tests

- MRI with gadolinium enhancement
- Contrast-enhanced CT (if MRI is not available)*
- Blood cultures
- Cultures of sinuses or other pericranial foci of infection

*Sedation with close observation may be required in agitated patients.

Differential Diagnosis

Brain abscess with nuchal rigidity and without focal signs may resemble bacterial meningitis. Rapidly expanding brain abscesses may also be confused with stroke, intracranial hemorrhage, or, especially in a febrile patient, epidural abscess or subdural empyema. More slowly expanding abscesses may mimic brain tumors. Brain imaging is essential in establishing the diagnosis.

Treatment

1. Treatment of brain abscess involves surgery, antibiotic therapy, and treatment of complications

2. Surgical therapy

a. Brain abscess may be treated either by aspiration or by excision.

b. In recent years, stereotactic aspiration under CT or MRI guidance has been used more and more; it is less injurious to brain than excision or blind aspiration, and it effectively drains the purulent center of the abscess, allowing greater penetration of antibiotics into the abscess capsule. In some instances, stereotactic drainage may need to be repeated one or more times.

c. Excision should be considered if the abscess is large or resistant to repeated stereotactic drainage; it should be considered if ventricular rupture appears imminent.

2. Antibiotic therapy

a. Initial antibiotic therapy where there are no clues to the causative organism should be directed against *Staphylococcus aureus*, Gram-negative enteric bacteria, and *Bacteroides* species and should include nafcillin or oxacillin, ceftriaxone or cefotaxime, and metronidazole.

b. Vancomycin should be used in place of nafcillin or oxacillin if methicillin-resistant *Staphylococcus aureus* is suspected or if the patient is allergic to penicillin.

c. Penicillin or ampicillin should be added if *Listeria* is suspected and the patient is not receiving nafcillin or oxacillin.

d. Ceftazidime should be used in place of ceftriaxone or cefotaxime if *Pseudomonas aeruginosa* is suspected.

e. Treatment of brain abscess in patients with AIDS should include therapy for *Toxoplasma gondii*: pyrimethamine, sulfadiazene or clindamycin, and folinic acid. Concomitant antituberculous therapy may also warrant consideration. Brain biopsy should be considered if the abscess does not diminish in size during therapy for *Toxoplasma.*

f. Treatment of neonatal brain abscess should be directed against the organism isolated from an accompanying meningitis. In most cases, this will involve agents effective against gramnegative bacilli.

g. Duration of antibiotic therapy is determined by abscess behavior on MRI or CT but in general will be 8 weeks if antibiotic therapy is used alone and 4 weeks if antibiotic therapy is used in conjunction with surgical drainage. In selected, stable patients, antibiotic therapy may be completed on an outpatient basis, with careful MRI follow-up.

3. Treatment of brain abscess with antibiotic therapy only

a. Abscesses at the stage of cerebritis do not contain pus and are thus not amenable to drainage. Here, treatment is initiated with antibiotics alone.

b. Consideration may also be given to deferring surgery in favor or antibiotic therapy alone if the patient is neurologically stable and the abscess is less than 3 cm in diameter.

c. Abscesses may continue to enlarge despite antibiotic therapy. It is thus *imperative* to obtain a follow-up MRI or CT within 24 to 48 hours of initiation of therapy and at intervals of not more than 3 to 5 days during the first 2 weeks, moving ahead to surgery if the abscess enlarges.

4. Treatment of complications

a. Cerebral edema often accompanies brain abscess and may require hyperventilation, mannitol, or dexamethasone. Hyperventilation is carried out to a pco$_2$ of less than 28 Torr and is used only in the short term, because its efficacy rapidly wanes. Mannitol is given, following placement of a urinary catheter, as a 20% solution, initially as 0.5 to 1.0 g/kg body weight over 10 minutes, followed by 0.25 to 0.5 g/kg every 3 to 5 hours. Serum electrolytes and osmolality must be carefully followed during mannitol administration. Dexamethasone, given as an initial dose of 10 mg intravenously, followed by 4 mg every 4 to 6 hours, is effective in treating vasogenic edema and should be considered if there is need for control of intracranial pressure over time. Although there is theoretical concern that dexamethasone may reduce antibiotic penetration into the abscess, this does not appear to have been a problem in clinical practice.

b. Ventricular shunting may be required in hemispheric abscesses that occlude the foramen of Monro or in cerebellar abscesses that compress the fourth ventricle causing hydrocephalus.

c. Ventricular rupture remains one of the most feared complications of brain abscess, with a mortality rate approaching 80%. Survival has been reported, however, following aggressive surgical and antibiotic therapy.

d. Patients should be carefully followed for development of inappropriate secretion of antidiuretic hormone or diabetes insipidus: in such patients, administration of 5% dextrose without sodium may cause profound hyponatremia.

e. Subcutaneous heparin and/or pressure stockings should be considered to prevent deep venous thrombophlebitis and pulmonary embolism.

f. Seizure activity may require short-term treatment with lorazepam or diazepam, followed by intravenous fosphenytoin. Treatment with propofol or phenobarbital may be required if seizures are refractory to fosphenytoin.

Key Treatment

- Surgery
  - Stereotactic aspiration
  - Excision
- Antibiotics
  - Treatment depends on the organism (see text)
- Treatment of complications
  - Cerebral edema: Hyperventilation, mannitol, or dexamethasone
  - Hydrocephalus: Ventricular shunting
  - Deep venous thrombophlebitis and pulmonary embolism: Subcutaneous heparin and/or pressure stockings
  - Seizures: Lorazepam or diazepam, followed by intravenous fosphenytoin

Prognosis and Long-Term Complications

Patients who present fully alert almost invariably survive, and those who are stuporous but not comatose have a mortality of less than 10%. In contrast, mortality in patients who respond only to pain at presentation is 59%, and it is 82% in those without response to pain.

1. Mortality and morbidity are increased by delay in diagnosis, use of improper antibiotics, and inadequate surgical therapy.

2. Mortality is also higher in large, multiloculated or posterior fossa abscesses and is extremely high where there is intraventricular rupture.

3. Between 30% and 55% of patients with brain abscess suffer permanent deficits; these are incapacitating in 17% of patients. Morbidity is less in patients who are alert at presentation and tends to be less in patients successfully treated with antibiotics alone or with antibiotics plus aspiration.

4. Seizures occur in 35% of patients surviving brain abscess. These may begin as long as 12 months after treatment; early treatment with anticonvulsant medications may diminish the likelihood of subsequent seizures. Careful withdrawal of anticonvulsants may be considered after 2 years in patients who have seizures early in their course but remain seizure-free on anticonvulsant therapy and are without focal neurologic deficits or electroencephalographic abnormalities.

SPINAL ABSCESS

Etiology

1. Definition: Spinal abscesses (intraspinal abscess, intramedullary abscess) represents loculated infection within the parenchyma of the spinal cord. The condition must be differentiated from the more common condition of spinal epidural abscess and from spinal subdural empyema.

2. Epidemiology: Spinal abscess is rare, with fewer than 100 cases reported in the world literature.

3. Pathogenesis

   a. Approximately 50% of cases of spinal abscess develop as a consequence of bacteremia. Spinal abscess may be associated with identifiable systemic infections such as chronic lung infections or bacterial endocarditis. However, most cases of hematogenous spinal abscess arise following occult bacteremia without known focus.

   b. Nearly 50% of cases arise by extension of infection through anatomical abnormalities of the vertebral column and/or spinal cord. These include dermal sinuses, dorsal midline skin lesions, spinal bifida, and spinal dysraphism. Extension along a dermal sinus accounts for about 25% of cases.

   c. Patients developing spinal abscess in the setting of bacteremia tend to be over 40 years of age. Abscesses arising by direct extension usually occur in childhood.

   d. The sequence of events in development of spinal abscess—focal ischemic injury, localized infection, and liquefaction of the abscess cavity—is as described above for brain abscess.

4. Causative organisms

   a. Historically, spinal abscess has been associated with *Mycobacterium tuberculosis;* this remains a concern in immunosuppressed patients and in patients from developing countries.

   b. Nontuberculous bacteria causing spinal abscess include gram-negative organisms such as *Proteus* species or *Escherichia coli; Listeria monocytogenes; Staphylococcus epidermidis; Bacteroides* species; *Haemophilus* species; *Brucella* and *Pseudomonas. Staphylococcus epidermidis* is particularly common in cases arising from dermal sinuses or related spine defects. *Listeria* abscesses have involved the cervical spinal cord in 75% of cases.

Signs and Symptoms

1. Most patients with spinal abscess present with fever and neurologic symptoms. Approximately 60% will have back and/or radicular pain; 40% will have fever; 68% will have a combination of motor and sensory deficits; 24% will have motor deficits only; and 6% will have sensory rather than motor signs and symptoms.

2. Average time from onset of symptoms to presentation is 46 days. However, patients may present within 1 day of onset or may not present for over a year.

Key Signs and Symptoms

- Back and/or radicular pain (60% of patients)
- Fever (40%)
- Both motor and sensory deficits (68%)
- Motor deficits only (24%)
- Sensory rather than motor signs and symptoms (6%)
- Average time from onset of symptoms to presentation is 46 days

Diagnosis

1. As in brain abscess, MRI with gadolinium enhancement is the diagnostic procedure of choice.
2. CT or CT myelography may show widening of the cord or an intramedullary mass lesion. However, CT or CT myelography are much less sensitive than MRI and may appear falsely normal.
3. Blood cultures or cultures of suspected sinus tracts may prove useful in identifying the causative organism. White blood count and erythrocyte sedimentation rate may be essentially normal.

Key Tests

- MRI with gadolinium enhancement (procedure of choice)
- CT or CT myelography
- Blood cultures or cultures of suspected sinus tracts

Differential Diagnosis

Intramedullary spinal abscess must be differentiated from spinal epidural abscess or subdural empyema. Slowly developing cases may mimic intraspinal neoplasm or syrinx.

Treatment

1. Spinal abscess, like brain abscess, is treated with antibiotics and open surgery or aspiration.
2. No controlled trials exist of antibiotic therapy in spinal abscess. Initial treatment, based on reported cases would include vancomycin for *Staphylococcus epidermidis* plus ampicillin for *Listeria monocytogenes* plus cefotaxime or ceftriaxone for gram-negative coverage plus metronidazole for *Bacteroides*.
   a. Where *Staphylococcus epidermidis* is strongly suspected, consideration should be given to additional coverage with rifampin.
   b. Antituberculous therapy should be strongly considered in patients from developing countries or patients with AIDS.
   c. Antibiotic therapy may need to be modified based on results of abscess or other cultures.

Key Treatment

- Surgery or aspiration
- Antibiotics
  - Treatment depends on the organism (see text)

Prognosis

Over 90% of patients survive. However, 70% of patients suffer permanent neurologic deficits.

Bibliography

Barlas O, Sencer A, Erkan K, et al.: Stereotactic surgery in the management of brain abscess. Surg Neurol 52:404–410, 1999.

Calfee DP, Wispelwey B: Brain abscess. Semin Neurol 20:353–360, 2002.

Chan CT, Gold WL: Intramedullary abscesses of the spinal cord in the antibiotic era: Clinical features, microbial etiologies, trends in pathogenesis, and outcomes. Clin Infect Dis 27:619–626, 1998.

Murphy KJ, Brunberg JA, Quint DJ, et al.: Spinal cord infection: Myelitis and abscess formation. AJNR Am J Neuroradiol 19:341–348, 1998.

Saez-Llorens XJ, Uman MA, Odio CM, et al.: Brain abscess in infants and children. Pediatr Infect Dis J 8:449–458, 1989.

Wispelwey B, Dacey RG Jr, Scheld WM: Brain abscess. In Scheld WM, Whitley RJ, Durack D (eds): Infections of the Central Nervous System. New York, Raven, 1997, pp 463–493.

6 Spirochetal Infections (Neurosyphilis and Lyme Neuroborreliosis)

Harald Gelderblom
Andrew R. Pachner

NEUROSYPHILIS

Definition

1. Neurosyphilis (NS) is involvement of the central nervous system (CNS) during systemic infection with the causative agent of syphilis, the spirochete *Treponema pallidum* subspecies *pallidum*. Although NS was described extensively during the preantibiotic era, diagnostic criteria, optimal therapy, and response guidelines have not yet been satisfactorily established. Today, NS is most common during infection with the human immunodeficiency virus (HIV).

2. Its diversity, alteration of the disease spectrum due to widespread use of antibiotics, and possible concurrent neurologic manifestations of HIV infection frequently make NS more challenging now.

3. In most cases antibiotic treatment halts CNS tissue destruction. If the disease remains unrecognized, the consequences may be devastating.

Epidemiology and Risk Factors

1. Syphilis is predominantly a sexually transmitted disease, with an average incidence in the United States of 2.5 per 100,000 population (primary and secondary syphilis).

2. About 5% to 10% of patients with untreated primary infection develop clinically apparent CNS involvement. This percentage may be higher during infection with HIV.

3. Life expectancy in patients with untreated NS is reduced by approximately 20%.

4. The incidence of primary and secondary syphilis is influenced by sexual habits, drug consumption including alcohol abuse, social background, race, and ethnicity.

5. Syphilis is an independent risk factor for the acquisition and transmission of HIV. Patients with HIV are more likely to have a higher pathogen burden, have longer periods of infectivity during secondary syphilis, and to be at increased risk to develop clinically apparent NS.

Etiology

1. Spirochetes are of a higher phylogenic order than most bacteria. *T. pallidum* has a slow replication time, cannot be cultured ex vivo, and cannot be visualized by conventional microscopy.

2. Around 3 weeks after infection, a primary lesion develops (primary syphilis). A second bacteremic stage with generalized mucocutaneous lesions (secondary syphilis) is followed by a period of latent infection lasting up to decades (latent syphilis). About one-third of untreated patients develop reemerging clinical signs indicating active infection (tertiary syphilis), the most severe being symptomatic CNS disease or aortitis.

3. *T. pallidum* enters the CNS during the first stage and early second stage. In the CNS the spirochete induces direct meningeal inflammation, arteritis of small to medium-size vessels leading to fibrotic occlusion, and in late NS direct neuronal damage and loss.

Clinical Features

Neurosyphilis can be divided into several clinical syndromes that tend to cluster at different time points or stages in the natural history of untreated syphilis.

1. Early CNS involvement—limited to the meninges and vessels

   a. *Syphilitic meningitis* commonly presents 1 to 2 years after infection. Cranial neuropathies, which are common, and hydrocephalus, which is rare, are signs of basilar predominance. Hemispheric focal signs are possible. This stage resolves with effective therapy.

   b. *Meningovascular and cerebrovascular neurosyphilis* generally appears approximately 5 to 7 years after infection. Signs of supratentorial or infratentorial ischemia, predominantly in the middle cerebral artery (MCA) territory, and meningeal inflammation may be present. This form of NS may include episodic prodromal symptoms over weeks, stroke in evolution, and involvement of a variety of vascular territories, including those of the spine. Residual defects frequently remain after appropriate antibiotic treatment.

2. Late CNS involvement—parenchymatous NS

a. *General paresis* occurs at least 10 years after infection. A chronic, progressive, frontotemporal encephalitis, it starts with impairment of higher cortical functions, uniformly leading to dementia. During progression, symptoms mimicking any psychiatric disease, pupillary abnormalities, optic atrophy, and signs of cerebellar and pyramidal tract involvement may develop. Treatment halts progression in most cases but rarely leads to improvement. Although it used to be a common cause of admission to psychiatric facilities, it now is rare.

b. *Tabes dorsalis* usually becomes symptomatic 10 to 20 years after infection. Demyelination of dorsal columns, posterior nerve roots, and ganglia result in a characteristic lancinating pain, sensory ataxia, and bladder and bowel dysfunction. Pupillary abnormalities and optic atrophy are possible. Treatment halts progression in most cases but rarely leads to improvement.

3. *Gummatous neurosyphilis* can occur at any time during infection. Symptoms are due to compression by gummas arising from the pia mater. Gummas resolve after treatment.

4. *Asymptomatic neurosyphilis* is a relatively frequent form of NS. Despite no symptoms, cerebrospinal fluid (CSF) abnormalities typical for NS persist. There is a significant risk of developing symptomatic NS, especially during HIV infection and if the CSF cell count and total protein are high.

Key Signs: Neurosyphilis Syndromes

- Syphilitic meningitis
  - —Signs occurring 1 to 2 years after infection
  - —Cranial neuropathies
- Meningovascular and cerebrovascular neurosyphilis
  - —Signs occurring approximately 5 to 7 years after infection
  - —Signs of supratentorial or infratentorial ischemia (MCA territory) and meningeal inflammation

- General paresis
  - —Signs occurring 10 years after infection
  - —Chronic and progressive
  - —Impairment of higher cortical functions leading to dementia
  - —Symptoms mimicking any psychiatric disease
- Tabes dorsalis
  - —Signs occurring 10 to 20 years after infection
  - —Lancinating pain
  - —Sensory ataxia
  - —Bladder and bowel dysfunction
- Gummatous neurosyphilis
  - —Signs occurring any time after infection
- Asymptomatic neurosyphilis
  - —Asymptomatic, although CSF abnormalities for NS are typical

Differential Diagnosis and Laboratory Testing

1. The main guideline when diagnosing is to "remember syphilis." Questions to ask the patient concern a history of genital ulcerations, skin rashes compatible with secondary syphilis, treatment for syphilis in the past, psychiatric or neurologic disorders, and nonvenereal treponematoses.

2. If the patient's syndrome is compatible with NS, including ophthalmologic and otologic symptoms, if he or she belongs to a risk group for sexually transmitted disease (STD) or is HIV-infected, a search for *T. pallidum*-specific antibodies in the serum [hemagglutination tests such as the microhemagglutination-*T. pallidum* (MHA-TP), *T. pallidum* hemagglutination (TPHA), or fluorescent treponemal antibody-absorbed (FTA-ABS) test] should be performed. Nonreactivity excludes NS. Some laboratories or medical centers do not perform a treponemal assay unless there has been a positive reaginic assay such as a Venereal Disease Research Laboratory (VDRL) test or a rapid plasma reagin (RPR) assay. These assays are less expensive than treponemal assays and are helpful in patients with primary and secondary syphilis. They are less sensitive for NS, and a negative reaginic assay in the serum does not exclude NS. Moreover, reaginic assays have a relatively high rate of false-positive results, often called biologic false-positive (BFP) results.

3. If serologic testing is positive, CSF should be obtained. A characteristic CSF data pattern supports the diagnosis of NS (Table 6–1). Testing for *T. pallidum*-specific antibodies is the most specific and sensitive laboratory approach to the diagnosis of NS, but which test is the correct one to order is controversial. VRDL or RPR are usually used, but some believe they are not sensitive enough to exclude NS, especially late NS.

4. Sensitivity of polymerase chain reaction (PCR) protocols for detecting *T. pallidum* nucleic acid in the CSF is low. Prospective studies on the significance of a positive PCR for the diagnosis or for judging the treatment response are not available. Hence, to date, PCR is not a tool for NS diagnosis or for assessing therapeutic efficacy.

5. No serologic test can distinguish between syphilis and the nonvenereal treponematoses yaws, pinta, and endemic syphilis.

6. The clinical spectra of NS and symptomatic neurologic involvement during HIV infection overlap. Hence NS should be considered in any HIV-infected patient with neurologic symptoms. Studies indicate that patients with syphilis and HIV may be at an increased risk for treatment failure and for developing NS.

Treatment

1. Few controlled trials on the therapy of NS have been reported. Sound clinical data are lacking on the optimal dose, duration of treatment, and long-term efficacy of antimicrobials other than penicillin. Recommendations are still based partly on laboratory considerations, plausibility, expert opinion, case studies, and past clinical experience. The recommendations of long treatment courses take into consideration the slow replication time of *T. pallidum*.

2. The presently recommended treatment regimen for NS is high dose intravenous penicillin (see Key Treatment). Alternate regimens have not been proven to be as effective. Thus when penicillin allergy is suspected, skin testing and desensitization should be considered. Whether Jarisch-Herxheimer reactions occur in NS and, if so, how they should be treated are controversial issues. Certainly if such reactions occur, they must be rare.

Key Treatment: Neurosyphilis Syndromes

- Aqueous penicillin G (2 million to 4 million units IV q4h) for 10 to 14 days

- Outpatient treatment

  —Combination of intramuscular procaine penicillin (2.4 million units IM qd) plus oral probenecid (500 mg PO qid) for 10 to 14 days

  —Addition of intramuscular benzathine penicillin G (2.4 million units weekly for 3 weeks) has been recommended

- In case of penicillin allergy, confirmed by skin testing: desensitization

  —Doxycycline (200 mg PO bid) for 28 days and ceftriaxone (2 g IV qd) for 14 days are alternatives but have not been systematically studied.

TABLE 6–1.   CSF ANALYSIS OF PATIENTS WITH SYPHILIS

Indications for CSF Analysis*
When neurosyphilis is suspected
    Neurologic, ophthalmologic, otic, or psychiatric symptoms

To exclude asymptomatic neurosyphilis
    Tertiary-stage gummatous or cardiovascular disease
    Newly diagnosed *Treponema pallidum* infection with a duration
        > 1 year or unknown duration
    Active or latent syphilis in an HIV-infected patient
    Untreated or benzathine/penicillin-treated syphilis in the past

Treatment failure

CSF Pattern During Neurosyphilis
Total protein up to 200 mg/dL
Lymphocytic pleocytosis < 400/µl
Intrathecal IgG synthesis
Positive CSF VDRL in most patients

Abbreviations: CDC, Centers for Disease Control and Prevention; CSF, cerebrospinal fluid; HIV, human immunodeficiency virus; IgG, immunoglobulin G; VDRL, Venereal Disease Research Laboratory (test for syphilis).
*Based on CDC-recommended indications for CSF analysis; extended.

Prognosis

Treatment response can be defined as clinical improvement in early NS and lack of progression in late NS. Optimally, CSF is reexamined periodically. In most cases, after effective therapy an elevated cell count returns to normal in 3 to 12 months; protein, VDRL, intrathecal total immunoglobulins (Igs), and the *T. pallidum*-specific antibody index decline more slowly. Another helpful criterion is a decrease in the serum VDRL titer. Retreatment should be considered when clinical symptoms do not diminish or if there is no decrease in CSF parameters within the first 6 to 12 months. The threshold for retreatment may be lower in HIV-positive patients with NS.

LYME NEUROBORRELIOSIS

Definition

1. Lyme neuroborreliosis (LNB) is defined as the neurologic manifestations of Lyme borreliosis (LB), a multisystem disease involving joints, skin, and heart. LB is caused by the tick-transmitted spirochete *Borrelia burgdorferi sensu lato*.

2. The LNB syndromes are attributed to the early disseminated phase or the late phase of the disease, depending on the time elapsed since infection. The prevalence of syndromes differs for the United States, Europe, and Asia. The clinical spectrum of and the diagnostic criteria for late LNB are still a matter of debate.

Epidemiology and Risk Factors

1. LB is one of the most common vector-borne diseases in the United States, with currently about 15,000 cases being reported each year.

2. LB is endemic from Maryland to Maine and in Wisconsin/Minnesota, Northern California, and Oregon. Overseas, LB is endemic in central and eastern Europe, Sweden, China, and Japan.

3. The incidence of LB coincides with outdoor activity in woody, moist areas, mainly during late spring and summer. About 10% to 20% of individuals with LB develop LNB.

Etiology

1. LB is transmitted by ticks during their blood meal on the host.

2. Three species of *B. burgdorferi sensu lato* (*B. burgdorferi sensu stricto*, *B. garinii*, *B. afzelii*) have been characterized. Whereas *B. burgdorferi sensu stricto* is the only species found in the United States, *B. garinii* and *B. afzelii* cause most of the disease in Europe and are the only species found in Asia. Regional differences in clinical spectra of LB have been associated with the various species of *B. burgdorferi*.

3. *B. burgdorferi* persists in tissue and body fluids of the infected host in low numbers. Thus culturing *Borrelia* for diagnosis is not a sensitive test. The predominant mechanism of CNS pathogenesis in LNB is thought to be *B. burgdorferi*-mediated inflammation leading to altered function and tissue damage.

4. Many patients with LNB remember erythema migrans (EM), the hallmark of early infection. EM is a spreading circular red rash at the site of the tick bite and the most sensitive indicator of *B.*

burgdorferi infection. Starting weeks to months after infection, involvement of the CNS, joints (arthritis), muscles (myalgia), heart (atrioventricular block, carditis), and skin [acrodermatitis chronica atrophicans (ACA), disseminated EM], together with influenza-like symptoms (headache, fatigue, low-grade fever), indicate ongoing infection.

Clinical Features

1. Early LNB syndromes are subacute, occurring within days to several months after infection as either one or a combination of the following triad (a–c).

   a. Cranial neuropathy: predominantly facial nerve palsy. Along with Guillain-Barré syndrome, LNB is a frequent cause of bilateral facial nerve palsy.

   b. Meningitis (dominant in American LNB): clinical signs of chronic basilar meningitis. A dissociation between relatively mild complaints and significant CSF abnormalities is not uncommon.

   c. Radiculoneuropathy (dominant in European LNB): Leading symptom is severe radicular pain, refractory to analgesics and worsening at night, followed by sensory symptoms and paresis. Symptoms are asymmetrical and multifocal.

   d. Acute encephalomyelitis and Guillain-Barré syndrome are rare presentations of acute LNB.

2. Late LNB syndromes are rare and take a chronic, progressive course.

   a. Chronic progressive encephalomyelitis presents with spastic paraparesis or quadriparesis, occasionally with cerebellar involvement, cranial neuropathy, and cognitive impairment. It is rare, described only in Europe, and progresses over months to years.

   b. Lyme encephalopathy is usually mild, leading to cognitive disturbances, accompanied by symptoms such as malaise, fatigue, and occasionally arthralgias and sensory symptoms without objective clinical findings. It is mainly described in the United States and is the most vague of all LNB syndromes.

   c. Polyneuropathy and radiculopathy may be present in late LNB. Polyneuropathy is predominantly axonal. Symptoms are patchy, sensory, and usually without objective clinical findings. In Europe, an axonal polyneuropathy can be seen together with ACA.

Key Signs: Lyme Neuroborreliosis

Early LNB

- Cranial neuropathy

  —Facial nerve palsy

- Meningitis (American LNB)

  —Signs of chronic basilar meningitis

- Radiculoneuropathy (European LNB)

  —Severe radicular pain—refractory to analgesics and worsening at night—followed by sensory symptoms and paresis

  —Symptoms asymmetrical and multifocal

Late LNB

- Chronic progressive encephalomyelitis

  —Spastic paraparesis or quadriparesis, occasionally with cerebellar involvement

  —Cranial neuropathy

  —Cognitive impairment

- Lyme encephalopathy

  —Cognitive disturbances accompanied by malaise, fatigue, and occasionally arthralgias and by sensory symptoms without objective clinical findings

- Polyneuropathy and radiculopathy

  —Polyneuropathy, predominantly axonal

  —Symptoms patchy and sensory in nature, usually without objective clinical findings

---

Frequency of Lyme Neuroborreliosis Syndromes

- Meningitis: +++

- Cranial neuropathy–facial nerve palsy: +++

- Radiculoneuropathy: ++

- Polyneuropathy: +

- Chronic progressive encephalomyelitis: (+)

- Encephalopathy: (+)

Differential Diagnosis and Laboratory Testing

1. Evaluating CSF for inflammatory changes and *B. burgdorferi*-specific antibodies (Abs) is the major laboratory approach when LNB is suspected (Table 6–2).

   a. Searching for anti-*B. burgdorferi* Abs in the CSF is valuable for the differential diagnosis (Table 6–3). It is done by an enzyme-linked immunosorbent assay (ELISA), a sensitive test measuring Ab binding to *Borrelia*. The absence of anti-*B. burgdorferi* Abs in the CSF of patients with LNB is unusual. Europeans frequently search for intrathecal Ab production in the CSF, commonly seen with LNB. This requires measuring total serum and CSF IgG and IgM levels, measuring serum and CSF specific anti-*B. burgdorferi* Ab levels, and determining Ab indices based on relative percentages of specific Abs in CSF and serum.

   b. The PCR protocols for *B. burgdorferi* nucleic acids in the CSF have a sensitivity of 40% to 50% in patients with early Lyme meningitis but are much less sensitive in late LNB. In general, because of its cost, lack of standardization, and insensitivity, PCR is not clinically useful at this time.

2. Serum analysis shows that for LNB the Abs to *B. burgdorferi* are readily detectable in the serum. The most commonly used assay is the ELISA, although occasionally immunofluorescence assays (IFAs) are also used. The Centers for Disease Control and Prevention (CDC) has stated that because screening antibody assays in the serum are frequently false-positive an immunoblot must be used to confirm positivity of all ELISA-positive or IFA-positive specimens. In the United States evaluation by immunoblotting is based on criteria issued by the CDC in 1995. In Europe, criteria are usually evaluated for each kit, a difficult process because European strains are much more heterogeneous than American ones.

3. Diagnosis of *early LNB* is usually straightforward, with a characteristic clinical syndrome in an area

---

TABLE 6–2. CSF ANALYSIS FOR SUSPECTED LYME NEUROBORRELIOSIS

Indications for CSF Analysis
In every patient, where LNB is suspected
Reexamine only the patients with worsening of symptoms or without improvement 1 month after treatment in early LNB and 3–6 months after treatment of late LNB

Characteristic CSF Pattern in Lyme Neuroborreliosis
Total protein up to 100 mg/dL and higher; blood/CSF barrier dysfunction
Lymphomononuclear pleocytosis up to 1000/μL, usually 30 to 300/μL
Intrathecal IgM → IgA → IgG synthesis
Borrelia burgdorferi antibody: usually ↑↑ (exception: within the first weeks of infection)

Abbreviation: LNB, Lyme neuroborreliosis.

TABLE 6–3. DIFFERENTIAL DIAGNOSIS OF LYME NEUROBORRELIOSIS

Early Lyme Neuroborreliosis
Meningitis
   Viral meningitis
   Neurosyphilis
   Carcinomatous meningiosis
   Tuberculous meningitis
   Fungal meningitis
   Leptospirosis
   Relapsing fever
Facial nerve palsy
   Guillain-Barré syndrome
   Miller-Fisher syndrome
Radiculoneuropathy
   Disc compression
   Herpes zoster radiculitis

Late Lyme Neuroborreliosis
Encephalomyelitis
   Multiple sclerosis
   Neurosarcoidosis
Lyme encephalopathy
   Chronic fatigue syndrome
   Depression
   Polymyalgia rheumatica
   Conversion syndrome

endemic for LB during late spring to early fall, a history of EM, and systemic symptoms compatible with LB. The CSF is inflammatory with intrathecal synthesis of anti-*B. burgdorferi* Abs (Table 6–2). Bell's palsy may occur before seroconversion. Inflammatory CSF syndrome and influenza-like symptoms are helpful for differentiating LNB from idiopathic facial nerve palsy.

4. Diagnosis of *late LNB* is generally much more difficult. With the progressive encephalomyelitic syndrome of late LNB, the CSF cell count is lower than in early LNB. However, high concentrations of intrathecally synthesized *B. burgdorferi*-specific IgG are usually present.

Treatment

1. Antiinfective agents. Once the diagnosis of LNB has been established, the optimal antibiotic treatment is controversial, but a number of treatment regimens have been successful.

   a. For early facial nerve palsy without pleocytosis, doxycycline (200 mg PO bid) is given for 21 days.

   b. For all other LNB syndromes, ceftriaxone (2 g IV qd) for 14 to 28 days is the drug of choice. Penicillin G sodium (3.3 million units IV q4h) for 14 to 28 days and oral doxycycline (200 mg bid) for 21 days are alternatives.

2. Antiinflammatory agents. Within the first days of antibiotic therapy, nonsteroidal antiinflammatory drugs may help alleviate symptoms associated with inflammation, such as arthralgias, myalgias, and headache.

Key Treatment: Lyme Neuroborreliosis

Early Facial Nerve Palsy Without Pleocytosis

• Doxycycline (200 mg PO bid) for 21 days

Other LNB Syndromes

• Ceftriaxone (2 g IV qd) for 14 to 28 days (drug of choice)

• Penicillin G sodium (3.3 million units IV q4h) for 14 to 28 days

• Doxycycline (same as above)

• Nonsteroidal antiinflammatory drugs: administer early in antibiotic therapy for arthralgias, myalgias, and headache

Prognosis

1. For early LNB the response to antibiotic treatment is excellent.

2. For late LNB, clinical improvement frequently is slower and in some cases incomplete. However, many patients with "treatment-resistant late LNB" may not really have LB.

3. After appropriate treatment, some patients complain of persistent subjective symptoms, such as neurocognitive difficulties, musculoskeletal pain, and dysesthesias. In one large study, the frequency of these symptoms was similar in a group of age-matched subjects without LB. One well controlled study in these patients did not show any advantage of repeated antibiotic treatment compared to placebo, irrespective of persistent seroreactivity.

Bibliography

Coyle PK, Schutzer SE: Neurologic aspects of Lyme disease. Med Clin North Am 86:261–284, 2002.

Estanislao LB, Pachner AR: Spirochetal infections of the nervous system. Neurol Clin 17:783–800, 1999.

Klempner MS, Hu LT, Evans J, et al.: Two controlled trials of antibiotic treatment in patients with persistent symptoms and a history of Lyme disease. N Engl J Med 345:85–92, 2001.

Luger AF, Schmidt BL, Kaulich M: Significance of laboratory findings for the diagnosis of neurosyphilis. Int J STD AIDS 11:224–234, 2000.

Reiber H, Peter JB: Cerebrospinal fluid analysis: disease-related patterns and evaluation programs. J Neurol Sci 184:101–122, 2001.

Steere AC: Lyme disease. N Engl J Med 345:115–125, 2001.

MMWR Morb Mortal Wkly Rep 50:113–120, 2001.

7 Creutzfeldt-Jakob Disease

Joseph R. Zunt

Definition

Creutzfeldt-Jakob disease (CJD) is a transmissible spongiform encephalopathy (TSE) that can be sporadic, familial, or acquired through transplantation of infected materials or by eating food containing infected tissue (new variant CJD).

Epidemiology and Risk Factors

1. Sporadic CJD occurs in 0.5 to 1.0 per 1 million people.

   Accounts for 85% to 90% of cases of CJD

2. Familial CJD is transmitted in an autosomal dominant manner.

   a. Accounts for 5% to 15% of cases of CJD

   b. Occurs in Libyan Jews living in Israel, North African Jews living in France, as well as in people living in Chile or Slovakia

3. Acquired CJD is associated with introduction of infected materials into the host:

   a. CJD has been transmitted by infected dural grafts, corneal transplants, human pituitary extracts, and pericardial homografts.

   b. CJD has also been transmitted by neurosurgical procedures using instruments contaminated with CJD.

4. New variant CJD (nvCJD) is associated with the consumption of cattle that had consumed nervous tissue byproducts of cattle with bovine spongiform encephalopathy (BSE or "mad cow disease").

   a. Highest prevalence is in the United Kingdom, but cases have also been identified in Ireland and France.

   b. As of December, 2000, nearly 200,000 cases of BSE have been reported; the majority of cases occurring in the United Kingdom.

Etiology and Pathophysiology

1. All forms of CJD are caused by infectious proteins, called prions.

   a. Normal prions (PrP^C) are coded for by the *PRNP* gene located on chromosome 20, and can be degraded by proteinase.

   b. Prions associated with disease (PrP^{Sc}) are resistant to proteinase as well as treatments and procedures that inactivate other infectious agents, such as those using organic solvents, formaldehyde, ultraviolet light, gamma irradiation, and standard autoclaving.

   c. Exogenous PrP^{Sc} causes a conformational change in normal prion protein folding and induces spontaneous conversion of PrP^C to PrP^{Sc}.

2. Variations in *PRNP* are associated with increased risk of acquiring CJD.

   a. Familial CJD is associated with various mutations in the *PRNP* gene.

   b. All people who have developed nvCJD through consumption of infected cattle have been homozygous for methionine at codon 129 of the *PRNP* gene. The incubation period for nvCJD is unknown, but may be between 5 and 15 years.

3. Neuropathology of brains from patients with CJD reveals spongiform changes with neuronal loss and gliosis.

   a. Spongiform changes in patients with nvCJD are most common in the basal ganglia and thalamus.

   b. PrP^{Sc} aggregates into amyloid fibrils and causes neuronal dysfunction.

   c. Amyloid plaques are present in 10% of brains of patients with sporadic CJD, but are more common in patients with familial CJD and nvCJD.

Clinical Features

1. Mean age of onset of sporadic CJD is 60 years.

   a. 25% of patients will have a prodrome of anxiety, asthenia, insomnia, decreased appetite, and weight loss.

   b. 30% to 40% of patients will present with neurologic manifestations.

   (1) Early presentation may include a combination of confusion, cerebellar ataxia, and sensory dysfunction.

   (2) Late presentation may include a combination of behavioral abnormalities, dementia, stimulus-sensitive myoclonus, akinetic mutism, and visual dysfunction.

2. Mean age of onset of familial CJD is 48 years. The clinical presentation is similar to sporadic CJD.

3. The onset of iatrogenic CJD varies according to the mode of inoculation.

 a. Direct inoculation of CJD into the nervous system by an infected surgical instrument or implantation of infected tissue typically causes disease within 2 years. Dementia is common as the presenting symptom of iatrogenic CJD.

 b. Extracranial inoculation of CJD has an incubation period ranging from 2 to 40 years. Cerebellar dysfunction or personality change without dementia are common presenting symptoms of CJD in this group of patients.

4. Mean age of onset of nvCJD is 29 years.

 a. Sensory dysfunction and psychiatric symptoms are common at the time of presentation.

 b. Other neurologic signs, such as ataxia, cognitive impairment, involuntary movements, and incontinence, occur months after the initial presentation.

Key Signs

Sporadic and Familial CJD

- *Prodromal:* anxiety, asthenia, insomnia, decreased appetite, weight loss
- *Early:* confusion, cerebellar ataxia, sensory dysfunction
- *Late:* behavioral abnormalities, dementia, stimulus-sensitive myoclonus, dementia, akinetic mutism, visual dysfunction

Iatrogenic CJD

- Dementia with intracranial inoculation
- Cerebellar dysfunction and personality change without dementia with extracranial inoculation

New Variant CJD

- Sensory dysfunction and psychiatric symptoms common at presentation
- Ataxia, cognitive impairment, involuntary movements, and incontinence occur months after initial presentation

Differential Diagnosis

Differential diagnosis includes other infectious etiologies that can cause subacute cognitive impairment with neurologic dysfunction, such as subacute sclerosing panencephalitis, intoxication with bismuth, mercury, bromides or lithium, Whipple's disease, neurosyphilis, status epilepticus, HIV-associated dementia, and degenerative diseases such as Pick's disease.

Laboratory Diagnosis

1. Electroencephalography may be normal in early sporadic CJD. As the disease progresses, background activity slows, and 1 to 2 cycles/second triphasic waves appear.

2. Identification of the 14-3-3 protein in cerebrospinal fluid is sensitive (84% to 92%) and specific (92% to 99%) for sporadic CJD.

 a. False positive results are seen in patients with encephalitis and patients with stroke in the prior month.

 b. 14-3-3 protein is detected less often in patients with nvCJD.

3. Detection of PrP^{Sc} in tonsil tissue is sensitive and specific for nvCJD, but not for other forms of CJD.

Radiologic Features

In sporadic CJD, brain imaging may be normal or demonstrate atrophy.

Diffusion-weighted, proton-density weighted, or T_2-weighted magnetic resonance imaging may demonstrate increased signal in the basal ganglia and cortex.

Key Tests

- Electroencephalogram
- Magnetic resonance imaging with proton-density and diffusion-weighted imaging
- Cerebrospinal fluid testing for 14-3-3 protein
- Tonsil or brain biopsy for detection of PrP^{Sc}

Treatment

1. There is no known effective treatment for any form of CJD.

2. Branched chain polyamines can eliminate PrP^{Sc} from neuroblastoma cells.

Key Treatment

- None

Prognosis

All forms of TSE are uniformly fatal.

1. Median survival for patients with sporadic CJD is 4 months, and 90% of patients die within 1 year.

2. Median survival for patients with familial CJD approaches 2 years.

3. Median survival for patients with nvCJD is 16 months.

Prevention

1. There is no known prevention for sporadic or familial forms of CJD.

2. Adequate sterilization of surgical instruments can prevent iatrogenic CJD.

3. Human pituitary-derived growth hormone has been replaced by recombinant growth hormone.

 Bibliography

Alter M: How is Creutzfeldt-Jakob disease acquired? Neuroepidemiology 19:55–61, 2000.

Brown P: Drug therapy in human and experimental transmissible spongiform encephalopathy. Neurology 58:1720–1725, 2002.

Brown P, Will G, Bradley R, et al.: Bovine spongiform encephalopathy and variant Creutzfeldt-Jakob disease: Background, evolution, and current concerns. Emerg Infect Dis 7:6–16, 2001.

Prusiner SB: Shattuck Lecture–Neurodegenerative diseases and prions. N Engl J Med 344:1516–1526, 2001.

Weihl CC, et al.: Creutzfeldt-Jakob disease, new variant Creutzfeldt-Jakob disease, and bovine spongiform encephalopathy. Neurol Clin 17:835–859, 1999.

Zeidler M, Stewart GE, Barraclough CR, et al.: New variant Creutzfeldt-Jakob disease: Neurological features and diagnostic tests. Lancet 350:903–907, 1997.

8 Cerebral Malaria

Joseph R. Zunt

Definition

Cerebral malaria (CM) is an unarousable state of unconsciousness accompanied by the presence of asexual parasitemia (most often *Plasmodium falciparum*) with exclusion of other causes of an unconscious state, such as hypoglycemia, post-ictal sedation, or other central nervous system infection.

Epidemiology and Risk Factors

1. Malaria occurs in 300,000 to 500,000 people each year, and can be caused by *P. falciparum, P. vivax, P. ovale, or P. malariae. P. falciparum* is the most common cause of malaria and CM.

2. Malaria is endemic in Africa, Central and South America, and Southeast Asia. Each year, 25 to 30 million people from non-endemic countries travel through countries where malaria is endemic. Of these 25-30 million people, 10,000 to 30,000 will contract malaria.

Etiology and Pathophysiology

1. Cerebral malaria is likely due to the sequestration of red blood cells containing *Plasmodium* trophozoites and meronts within cerebral capillaries and venules. Sequestration provides an optimal environment for parasite growth and prevents destruction of infected cells by the spleen.

2. Petechial hemorrhages and endothelial activation are present in brains of persons who died with CM.

Clinical Features

1. Cerebral malaria is usually preceded by several days of nonspecific feverish symptoms, but it may occur within 24 hours of the first symptoms. Episodic fevers may be accompanied by diaphoresis, headache, malaise, arthralgias, myalgias, nausea, or dizziness.

2. Coma may develop subacutely or precipitously after a generalized seizure.

    a. Coma typically lasts 1 to 3 days.

    b. Signs of increased intracranial pressure, such as papilledema and meningismus, are uncommon.

3. Generalized seizures occur in 20% to 50% of patients.

    a. *P. falciparum* is most frequent species associated with seizures.

    b. In children, seizures are usually recurrent, and are often focal.

4. Cranial nerve dysfunction, such as horizontal or vertical nystagmus, ocular bobbing, or sixth nerve palsy is occasionally present.

5. Presence of retinal hemorrhages is associated with poor prognosis.

Key Signs

- Comatose state

- Seizures, often focal

- Episodic fevers accompanied by diaphoresis, headache, malaise, arthralgias, myalgias, nausea, or dizziness

- Cranial nerve dysfunction

Differential Diagnosis

1. Bacterial or tuberculous meningitis should be considered in the differential diagnosis of CM. Because many people with CM have elevated intracranial pressure, most experts recommend empiric treatment of suspected bacterial or tuberculous meningitis, unless neuroimaging demonstrates that a diagnostic lumbar puncture can be performed without risk of herniation.

2. Hypoglycemia and prolonged post-ictal unresponsiveness are common during malaria and should be excluded as causes of a comatose state.

Laboratory Diagnosis

1. Analysis of thick smears of blood with Giemsa staining is performed to detect parasitemia.

    a. If malaria due to *P. falciparum* is suspected, thick smears should be repeated every 6 to 8 hours for 3 days.

    b. If malaria due to other species of *Plasmodium* is suspected, thick smears should be obtained during febrile periods.

2. Analysis of thin smears of blood with Giemsa staining is performed to identify the species of *Plasmodium*.

3. Other serologic tests available outside the United States include the ParaSight-F and Immunochromotographic Malaria *P. falciparum* tests.

   a. Both tests are rapid, sensitive and specific, but expensive.

   b. False-positive ParaSight-F tests occur frequently in the presence of rheumatoid factor.

4. Lumbar puncture should be avoided during the comatose state of CM because increased pressure may result in herniation.

Radiologic Features

1. Computed tomography may demonstrate cerebral edema during the agonal stages of CM.

2. Magnetic resonance imaging (MRI) may reveal brain enlargement without edema. In fatal cases of CM, MRI often reveals transtentorial herniation.

Key Tests

• Thick and thin blood smears for parasitemia

• MRI or computed tomography of brain

Treatment

1. In areas where *P. falciparum* coexists with other species of *Plasmodium,* most experts suggest treating for *P. falciparum,* as this is the most harmful of the species.

2. Choice of treatment should be guided by the prevalence of chloroquine-resistant *P. falciparum* (CRPF) in the country where malaria was acquired.

   a. Most strains of *P. falciparum* in Southeast Asia and the Amazon region of South America are completely resistant to chloroquine.

   b. Sub-Saharan Africa has high rates of resistance in certain regions.

3. For non-CRPF, chloroquine can be used for treatment. For CRPF, quinine with doxycycline, mefloquine, or one of the newer antimalarials, such as halofantrine or one of the artemisinian derivatives, can be used.

4. For CM, treatment should include intravenous quinine.
   Quinine dosing: 7 mg salt/kg over 30 minutes, followed by 10 to 20 mg/kg over 4 hours, repeated every 8 to 12 hours

5. Concomitant treatment with steroids provides no

benefit, and may be associated with worse outcome.

6. Treatment of elevated intracranial pressure with mannitol has been associated with improved outcome.

Key Treatment

Non-CRPF

• Chloroquine

CRPF

• Quinine with doxycycline, mefloquine, or halofantrine or an artemisinian derivative

CM

• Intravenous quinine

Prognosis and Complications

1. Poor prognosis of CM is associated with longer duration of seizures, coma, hypoglycemia, or anemia.

2. Neurologic deficits after CM can resolve quickly, slowly, or not at all.

   a. Ataxia usually resolves rapidly.

   b. Hemiparesis or cortical blindness usually requires months to resolve.

   c. Children who have a spastic quadriparesis or are in a vegetative state usually die.

   d. Residual cognitive, behavioral, and language deficits occur, but the incidence is not known.

   e. The incidence of epilepsy after CM is not known.

Prevention

1. Prevention of CM requires prevention of malaria. Various forms of prevention are available, including insecticide-treated nets (ITN), topical insect repellents, protective clothing, and prophylactic medications.

   a. Permethrin is the active ingredient on ITN and must be reapplied every 4 months.

   b. The most frequently used prophylactic antimalarials are mefloquine, chloroquine, and doxycycline.

      (1) Mefloquine use is often associated with sleep disturbances, psychosis, and headache, but it is very effective in preventing malaria: 250 mg weekly, starting 1 week prior to departure and continued for 4 weeks after return.

(2) Chloroquine can cause neuropsychiatric side effects or rash, and should not be used for prophylaxis of CRPF: otherwise, 500 mg weekly starting 1 week prior to departure and continued for 4 weeks after return.

(3) Doxycycline is frequently associated with gastrointestinal and dermatologic side effects, and should not be taken by children or by women who are pregnant or breast-feeding: otherwise, 100 mg daily, starting 1 to 2 days prior to departure and continued for 4 weeks after return, with primaquine 26.3 mg/day given concomitantly during the final 2 weeks.

2. Antimalarial vaccines have unproven efficacy.

Preventive Measures

- Insecticide-treated nets

- Topical insect repellents: Permethrin

- Prophylactic antimalarial medications: mefloquine, chloroquine, and doxycycline

---

Pregnancy

1. Pregnant women are at greater risk of contracting malaria than are non-pregnant women.

   a. Malaria in pregnant women is associated with an increased risk of fetal death. Mefloquine and chloroquine are safe during preqnancy.

   b. Preventive treatment with topical insect repellents containing diethyltoluamide should be avoided because of the risk of teratogenicity.

   c. Doxycycline should be avoided during pregnancy or breast-feeding because it may cause damage to fetal or infant bones and teeth.

   d. Primaquine should be avoided because teratogenic effects have been demonstrated in rats.

2. Prophylactic measures, such as ITN and citronella-based topical repellents are safe during pregnancy and breast-feeding.

3. Treatment of malaria with chloroquine or mefloquine during pregnancy or breast-feeding has not been reported to cause adverse effects in fetuses or children.

Bibliography

Croft A: Malaria: Prevention in travelers. BMJ 321:154–160, 2000.

Malaguarnera L, Musumeci S: The immune response to plasmodium falciparum malaria. Lancet Infect Dis 2:472–478, 2002.

Newton CR, Warrell DA: Neurologic manifestations of Falciparum malaria. Ann Neurol 43:695–702, 1998.

Warrell DA, Molyneux ME, Beales PF: Severe and complicated malaria. Trans R Soc Trop Med Hyg 84(Suppl 2):1–65, 1990.

9 Neurocysticercosis

Joseph R. Zunt

Definition

1. Neurocysticercosis (NCC) is a parasitic infection caused by *Taenia solium* and is an important cause of epilepsy in developing countries.

2. Two types of infection with *T. solium* occur in humans: taeniasis, or tapeworm infection, which is caused by ingestion of cysts in undercooked pork; and cysticercosis, which is caused by the ingestion of *T. solium* eggs.

Epidemiology and Risk Factors

1. *T. solium* infection is endemic throughout South and Central America.

   a. In Brazil, the seroprevalence of antibodies to *T. solium* is 0.7% to 5.2%, with the highest rates in rural areas. In Mexico, Perú, and Ecuador, rates range between 5% and 11%.

   b. In other parts of the world, seroprevalence rates vary from 13% in Bali, to 2% to 4% in Korea, and 18% in Madagascar.

2. In the United States more than 80 million hogs are slaughtered under government inspection each year, in which fewer than 10 cases of cysticercosis are usually identified.

   a. Few states require health authorities to report cases of NCC.

   b. In California, NCC became a reportable disease in 1989. In the first year, 134 cases were reported, most of them in Hispanic immigrants. Three cases were identified in people who had never traveled outside the United States.

3. Travel to developing countries and household exposure to immigrants form endemic countries increase the risk of acquiring NCC.

   a. NCC has occurred in Orthodox Jews who had no exposure to pork products or travel outside the United States.

   b. Asymptomatic carriers of cysticercosis can transmit infection through contamination of food products.

Etiology and Pathophysiology

1. The life cycle of *T. solium* includes ova (eggs), oncospheres, and cysts (*Cysticercus cellulosae*).

   a. The definitive host is the human, who ingests *T. solium* larvae in undercooked pork, resulting in taeniasis.

   b. The larva requires a human intestinal tract to develop into a mature tapeworm and may reach 2 to 8 meters in length and live up to 20 years.

      (1) Each tapeworm elongates through the production of segments, proglottids, that mature as they develop distally and are metabolically independent of the worm.

      (2) The proglottids can break off singly or in chains to release eggs, which are passed into the environment with evacuation of feces.

      (3) The eggs are ingested by a pig, the intermediate host, where they hatch, become larvae, and migrate to brain, muscle, or eye tissue.

      (4) Humans may also become "accidental" intermediate hosts if eggs are ingested, either by auto-infection or through contact with an infected carrier, causing NCC. *T. solium* eggs have been found on the clothes, perianal skin and under the fingernails of infected carriers.

2. NCC typically begins as one or more areas of non-contrast-enhancing edema. These areas progress to become homogeneously contrast-enhancing lesions, then non-enhancing cystic lesions, then ring-enhancing cystic lesions with or without edema, and finally to complete resolution or calcification.

Clinical Features

1. Clinical symptoms of NCC typically begin years after the initial infection, when a host inflammatory response develops against *T. solium* antigens released during the death of the parasite.

2. Neurologic symptoms of cysticercosis may be acute, chronic, or relapsing and are determined by the location of the cysts within the neuraxis.

   a. Parenchymal cysts occur most frequently, and are typically associated with seizures or encephalitis.
   Dementia or behavioral abnormalities occur frequently.

b. Meningeal cysts are associated with arachnoiditis/meningitis.
   (1) May involve cranial nerves
   (2) If cysts proliferate at the base of the brain, basilar meningitis (racemose cysticercosis) occurs and is often associated with mental deterioration, coma, and death.
c. Ventricular cysts are most frequently found in the fourth ventricle.
   (1) If blockage of the sylvian aqueduct occurs, symptoms of intracranial hypertension (headache, vomiting) may develop.
   (2) Obstructive hydrocephalus is common.
d. Spinal cord cysts are uncommon.
   (1) May present as transverse myelitis, mass lesions, or nerve root irritation
   (2) Cysts are most frequently located in cervical cord.

3. Neurocysticercosis may mimic stroke, tumor, carotid artery occlusion, or intracerebral hemorrhage.
4. Extraneural cysticercosis may affect skeletal musculature, conjunctiva, or retina; it rarely occurs in persons with NCC.

Key Signs and Symptoms

- Seizure (60% of cases)
- Increased intracranial pressure (headaches, vomiting, papilledema) (25%)
- Meningitis (25%)
- Altered mental status (including dementia, stupor, or confusion) (15%)
- Focal neurologic deficit (hemiparesis or paraparesis, visual loss, or aphasia) (10%)
- Asymptomatic (10%)

Differential Diagnosis

Differential diagnosis of NCC includes other infections that can cause focal CNS lesions, such as miliary tuberculosis, and bacterial, fungal, or atypical organisms. In patients with AIDS, cryptococcoma, toxoplasmosis, and primary CNS lymphoma should be included in the differential diagnosis.

Laboratory Diagnosis

1. The diagnosis of NCC is usually obtained through a combination of neuroimaging and serology. Del Brutto and colleagues have proposed criteria for diagnosing NCC that combine histologic, radiographic, immunologic, and clinical evidence.
   a. Definitive diagnosis of NCC can be made if there is:
      (1) Histopathology diagnostic of NCC
      (2) Visualization of a scolex within a cystic lesion by computed tomography (CT) or magnetic resonance imaging (MRI)
      (3) Lesion(s) suggestive of NCC by neuroimaging
      (4) Clinical response to treatment of NCC, combined with serologic evidence of *T. solium* infection by serum immunoblot or cerebrospinal fluid enzyme-linked immunosorbent assay (ELISA)
   b. Other combinations of criteria can be used to diagnose NCC with lesser degrees of certainty.
2. Various tests can be used to diagnose NCC: immunoblot, ELISA, and immunoelectropheresis. The test of choice for diagnosis is the immunoblot on serum. Crossreactivity (false positives) may occur in persons infected with the intestinal tapeworm *Hymenolepis nana*.
3. Lumbar puncture: 50% of patients with NCC have a normal CSF formula; 40% have an elevated opening pressure, white blood cell count, or protein level.

Radiologic Features

1. CT imaging of people with NCC typically reveals single or multiple cysts with varying degrees of calcification, cyst wall enhancement, or surrounding edema.
2. Magnetic resonance imaging may identify cysts not visualized with CT, and is best for detecting the racemose form of NCC or the parasite's scolex.

Key Tests

- CT of brain
- MRI of brain
- Serologic testing with immunoblot or ELISA for *Taenia solium*
- Electroencephalogram

Treatment

1. Inactive infection is characterized by the presence of calcified lesions. Most experts agree that no anthelmintic treatment is necessary for asymptomatic persons with only calcified lesions. If seizures

are present, they should be treated with antiepileptic medications.

2. Transitional infection is characterized by ring-enhancing cysts with or without edema. The cyst is dying and treatment with anthelmintics is probably not necessary. Patients are often symptomatic but can be treated with antiepileptic medications.

3. Active infection should be treated with an anthelmintic, with or without concomitant steroids. Treatment of choice is praziquantel: 25 mg/kg every 2 hours for three doses, or albendazole: 15 mg/kg/day in two divided doses (max 800 mg/day) for 8 to 15 days.

   a. Non-contrast-enhancing edematous lesions

   b. Homogeneously contrast-enhancing lesions

   c. Cystic lesions without ring-enhancement or edema

4. Encephalitic NCC is characterized by numerous intraparenchymal cysts and diffuse cerebral edema.

   a. Most often seen in young girls

   b. Steroids and aggressive management of hydrocephalus are first-line therapies.

   c. Anthelmintics should not be given until after resolution of elevated intracranial pressure, because they may exacerbate inflammation.

5. Spinal cord lesions are uncommon and are often removed at the time of diagnostic surgery. Surgical extirpation is usually performed, but medical therapy alone may be sufficient.

6. Intraventricular lesions or racemose cysticercosis usually require surgical extirpation, but medical therapy can be effective. Ventricular shunting is indicated for cysts located in the fourth ventricle and is frequently necessary for cysts located in other parts of the ventricular system. Bacterial shunt infections occur more frequently in the setting of NCC.

7. Intraocular lesions usually require surgical extirpation, because inflammation occurring with medical treatment may result in loss of vision.

8. As cysticercosis is often spread to others by carriers of *T. solium*, close contacts of people with NCC should receive serologic testing for *T. solium*. Treatment of adult intestinal infection by *T. solium* is a single dose of niclosamide, an oral anthelmintic. Dosage is 1 g for children weighing 25 to 75 lb., 1.5 g for children over 75 lb., and 2 g for adults.

Key Treatment

- Anthelmintics

- No treatment necessary for asymptomatic patients with calcified lesions

- Antiepileptic medications for seizures

- Steroids and aggressive management for encephalitic NCC

- Extirpation for intraventricular lesions, racemose cysticercosis, and intraocular lesions

Prognosis and Complications

1. Prognosis of NCC varies with location of cysts. Intraventricular and encephalitic cysts are most commonly associated with poor outcome.

2. Seizures are the most common complication of NCC.

Prevention

Prevention of neurocysticercosis requires avoiding consumption of pork containing cysts that were not killed during the cooking process and food prepared by a food handler infected with *T. solium*.

Pregnancy

Praziquantel is safe during pregnancy and lactation; albendazole should not be used during pregnancy or lactation because it has teratogenic side effects.

Bibliography

Cuetter AC, Garcí-Bobadilla, Guerra LG, et al.: Neurocysticercosis: Focus on intraventricular disease. Clin Infect Dis 24:157–164, 1997.

Kelly R, Duong DH, Locke GE: Characteristics of ventricular shunt malfunctions among patients with neurocysticercosis. Neurosurgery 50:757–762, 2002.

Román G, Sotelo J, Del Brutto O, et al.: A proposal to declare neurocysticercosis an international reportable disease. Bull WHO 78:399–405, 2000.

White AC: Neurocysticercosis: A major cause of neurological disease worldwide. Clin Infect Dis 24:101–115, 1997.

1 Approach to Neck and Low Back Disorders

Michael W. Devereaux

Low back and neck pain disorders in combination are a pervasive problem in the industrialized word. Low back pain alone is the fifth most common reason for a physician office visit, with an estimated 15 million physician visits per year. There are wide variations in the care of neck and back problems, particularly for pain, which indicates physician uncertainty about the optimal approach. The purpose of this section is to help equip the busy clinician to diagnose and treat neck and low back problems effectively.

Epidemiology

1. Lifetime prevalence for a "significant" episode of low back pain is 60% to 90%. Lifetime prevalence for an episode of low back pain 2 weeks or more in duration is 13.8%.

2. Lifetime prevalence for an episode of sciatica lasting longer than 2 weeks is 1.6% (higher in some studies).

3. Lifetime prevalence of neck pain is less frequent than that of low back pain, probably 40% to 70% for "significant" pain.

4. Disability issues

   a. Low back pain is the most common cause for work-related disability in people less than 45 years of age.

   b. Low back pain is the most expensive cause of work-related disability in terms of workers' compensation and medical expenses, with estimates as high as $100 billion per year.

   c. Spinal pain is responsible for 25% of all lost work days.

   d. At any given time, 1% of the work force in the United States is temporarily disabled and 1% chronically disabled secondary to low back pain.

Epidemiology: Low Back Disorders

- Approximately 15 million physician visits per year (second leading symptom after upper respiratory infections)

- Leading cause for workers' compensation claims in the United States

---

- Total direct and indirect costs per year approximately $100 billion

---

Risk Factors

1. Risk factors are better established for low back pain than for neck pain, but certainly some risk factors are common to both.

Risk Factors: Low Back Pain

- Increasing age

- Heavy physical work, particularly long static work postures, heavy lifting, twisting, and vibration (e.g., from pneumatic drills)

- Psychosocial factors, including work dissatisfaction and monotonous work

- Depression

- Obesity

- Smoking

- Severe scoliosis (>80%)

- Drug abuse

- History of headache

---

2. A number of factors are commonly thought to increase risk but probably do not.

Low/Non Risk Factors: Low Back Pain

- Anthropometric status (height, body build)

- Posture including kyphosis, lordosis, and scoliosis less than 80%

- Minor leg length differences

- Gender

- State of physical fitness (although not a predictor of acute low back pain, fit individuals recover more quickly)

- Most radiographic structural lesions

Anatomic Considerations

1. Spinal column

   a. Composed of 7 cervical, 12 thoracic, 5 lumbar, and 5 fused sacral vertebrae along with 5 coccygeal bones

   b. Between each pair of vertebrae are two openings, the foramina, through each of which pass a spinal nerve, radicular blood vessels, and the sinuvertebral (recurrent meningeal) nerves (Fig. 1–1).

   c. The spinal canal is formed posterolaterally by the laminae and ligamentum flavum, anterolaterally by the pedicles, and anteriorly by the posterior surface of the vertebral bodies and intervertebral discs. The midsagittal diameter of the cervical cord is about 40% of the midsagittal diameter of the cervical canal. Cervical spondylosis with resultant narrowing of the canal coupled with hyperextension injury transiently narrowing the canal further can result in cervical cord ischemia and compression (myelopathy).

2. Facet joint

   a. True synovial joint

   b. Disorders of the facet joint may be a significant contributor to low back and neck pain.

3. Intervertebral disc

   a. It is comprised of a ring of elastic collagen, the annulus fibrosis, and surrounding gelatinous nucleus pulposus (Fig. 1–2).

   b. With aging, fibrous tissue replaces the highly elastic collagen fibers of the annulus fibrosis;

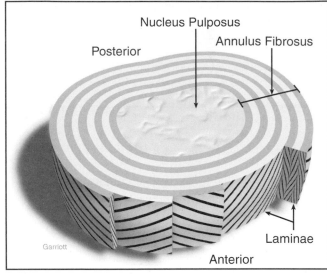

Figure 1–2. Anatomy of the intervertebral disc. (From Levin KH, Covington EC, Devereaux M, et al.: Neck and back pain. Continuum 7:1-208, 2001, with permission.)

and the nucleus pulposus becomes increasingly fibrotic, weakening the structure.

   c. There are no nociceptive nerve endings in the healthy disc. Herniation of the nucleus pulposus through the annulus fibrosis therefore does not in itself cause pain. Pain originates in structures in contact with the herniated disc as a result of direct compression and inflammation, secondary in part to the release of phospholipase A_2.

   d. Evidence suggests that there is ingrowth of nociceptive fibers into degenerated discs, which may be a source of chronic spinal pain. This point remains controversial.

4. Ligaments

   a. Posterior ligament: stretching from C1 to the distal sacrum along the posterior surface of the vertebrae and intervertebral discs. It progressively narrows as it descends in the lumbar spine, allowing lateral disc herniation to occur more readily in the lower lumbar spine.

   b. Ligamentum flavum: spans the space between the lamina. With aging, it can thicken and contribute to lumbar canal stenosis.

   c. A number of other less clinically significant ligaments contributes to the stability of the spinal column.

5. Muscles

   a. The extensor muscles are responsible for maintaining erect posture.

   b. Numerous individual muscles span the entire spine from occiput to sacrum and are known collectively as the erector spinae muscles. Deep

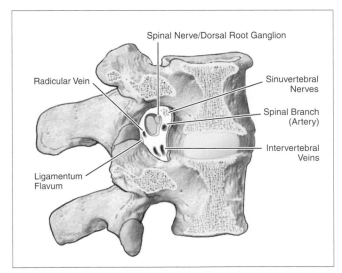

Figure 1–1. Anatomy of the spinal column. (From Levin KH, Covington EC, Devereaux M, et al.: Neck and back pain. Continuum 7:1-208, 2001, with permission.)

to the erector spinae is the transversospinalis muscle group.

c. The complicated extensor muscles function as a system of guy ropes that contribute to stability and motion. These muscles are most likely a principal source of acute back and neck pain. They are less often the cause of chronic localized lumbosacral spinal pain.

Pathophysiology of Neck and Back Pain

1. The precise etiology of neck and back pain in a given individual is usually elusive.

2. In the case of acute low back pain, a definitive diagnosis (source of pain) cannot be established in 85% of patients because of weak associations between symptoms, pathologic changes, and imaging results.

3. It is widely assumed that much nonradiating neck and low back pain is secondary to musculoligamentous injury, degenerative changes in the spine, or both.

4. Localized cervical and lumbosacral pain is mediated primarily through the posterior primary ramus and the sinuvertebral (recurrent meningeal) nerves.

   a. Sinuvertebral nerves supply structures within the spinal canal. They arise from the rami communicantes entering the spinal canal by way of the intervertebral foramina (Fig. 1–3).

   b. Branches of the posterior ramus provide sensory fibers to fascia, ligaments, periosteum, facet joints, and the paraspinous muscles.

5. Nonradiating neck and low back pain is probably most commonly caused by increased tension in the paraspinous muscles related to physical activity (e.g., lifting) or an injury (e.g., whiplash).

   a. Increased muscle tension can lead to avulsion of tendinous attachments of muscles to bony structures, rupture of muscle fibers, and tearing of muscle sheaths.

   b. Persistent use or overuse of a muscle group can result in pain and potentially tonic contraction (spasm).

   c. Although muscle spasm secondary to injury is generally thought to be a cause of pain, there is some controversy. There is a lack of electromyographic evidence of increased muscle activity in patients with pain allegedly secondary to spasm, raising the possibility that it is muscle edema secondary to injury rather than spasm that produces muscle "tightness" and fullness on examination.

6. Radicular pain is not mediated by the sinuvertebral nerves or the posterior rami but, rather, by the proximal spinal nerves.

   a. Two major factors are involved in the generation of radicular pain: compression and inflammation.

      (1) Compression of the nerve root produces local ischemia with possible alteration in axoplasmic transport and edema affecting the large mechanoreceptor fibers more, resulting in loss of inhibition of pain impulses carried by the unmyelinated fibers with resultant increased nociceptive input into the spinal cord (gate theory).

      (2) Inflammation, which may be neurogenic or immunologic at the site of compression, usually from herniated disc material, contributes to the generation of radicular pain.

7. In summary, low back and radiating radicular pain secondary to a herniated intervertebral disc are due to a combination of compression of the spinal nerve and inflammation (radiating pain) plus stimulation of nociceptive fibers of the sinuvertebral nerves in the lateral posterior ligament and in the dura of the nerve root sleeve, which produces localized neck and back pain.

History

1. Pain profile

   a. Onset. Patients presenting with a history of acute onset of neck and low back pain usually have a history of prior episodes of pain.

   b. Quality. Variable. Nonradiating back pain is often described as being deep and aching, whereas radicular pain is usually described as sharp, jabbing, or lancinating.

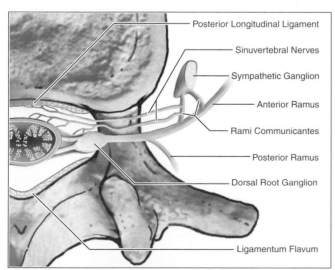

Figure 1–3. The sinu-vertebral nerves. (From Levin KH, Covington EC, Devereaux, M, et al.: Neck and back pain. Continuum 7:1-208, 2001, with permission.)

Posterior Longitudinal Ligament
Sinuvertebral Nerves
Sympathetic Ganglion
Anterior Ramus
Rami Communicantes
Posterior Ramus
Dorsal Root Ganglion
Ligamentum Flavum

c. Location. Musculoskeletal pain is usually localized to the paraspinous regions, sometimes spreading to the shoulders in the case of paracervical pain and sometimes to the flanks and buttocks in the case of lumbosacral pain. When cervical roots are involved, the pain radiates into the upper extremity. "High" lumbar (L2, L3) radiculopathic pain radiates into the anterior thigh. L4 radiculopathic pain radiates to the medial aspect of the leg distal to the knee. L5 and S1 radiculopathies (more than 90% of lumbosacral radiculopathies) produce pain radiating to the posterolateral thigh and posterolateral leg involving the foot (sciatica is defined as low back pain radiating distal to the knee).

d. Duration. Mechanical low back pain generally lasts days to several weeks. Radicular pain often resolves more gradually, over a period of 6 to 8 weeks.

e. Severity. Often difficult to assess. Radicular pain secondary to a herniated disc, although often severe, need not be.

f. Time of day. At onset, both cervical and lumbar radiculopathy are often present upon awakening in the morning. Nocturnal neck and back pain not relieved with recumbency raises the possibility of cervical or lumbar spine tumors and infection.

g. Associated symptoms. Cervical spine disorders causing localized and radiating pain into an upper extremity may also produce symptoms secondary to cervical myelopathy, including weakness and paresthesia in the lower extremities and bladder/bowel dysfunction. Back pain with abdominal/gastrointestinal (GI) symptoms raises the possibility of an intra-abdominal process producing back pain.

h. Aggravators of pain
(1) Valsalva maneuver (coughing, sneezing) can accentuate both cervical and lumbar pain.
(2) Lateral head movements most often to the side of pain can aggravate cervical radicular pain.
(3) Standing and sometimes sitting can aggravate lumbar radicular pain secondary to disc herniation.
(4) Continued or increased low back pain with recumbency raises the possibility of metastatic cancer to or infection of one or more vertebral bodies.

i. Factors that relieve pain. Supine position can relieve radiating pain secondary to cervical and lumbar disc herniation

j. Motor symptoms. If the patient complains of weakness, the history can help the clinician distinguish between weakness secondary to nerve root or spinal cord involvement and guarding secondary to pain. Specific complaints, such as foot drop, foot slapping, difficulty writing, difficulty lifting an arm, or a history of falls secondary to a lower extremity giving way, favor weakness rather than guarding.

k. Sensory disturbances. The presence and distribution of paresthesia by history may be even more useful than the sensory examination for determining the presence and site of radiculopathy.

2. Bladder and bowel disturbances. Cervical myelopathy and compression of the cauda equina can each produce symptoms suggestive of a neurogenic bladder.

3. Risk factors. Features that should lead to considering an immediate work-up include

a. Age over 50

b. Body temperature higher than 38°C

c. Neuromuscular weakness

d. Significant trauma prior to the onset of spine pain

e. Known malignancies

f. Pain with recumbency

g. Unexplained weight loss

h. Drug and alcohol abuse

Key Considerations for Pain Profile

• Onset

• Quality

• Location

• Duration

• Severity

• Time of day pain is experienced

• Associated symptoms

• Aggravators of pain (e.g., Valsalva maneuver, lateral head movements)

• Factors that relieve pain

• Motor symptoms

• Sensory disturbances

Physical Examination

1. General examination
   a. The presence of a low-grade fever in a patient with low back or neck pain may signal an infection involving the vertebral column, epidural space, or surrounding muscle.
   b. Inspection of the skin. Certain skin disorders, such as psoriasis, café-au-lait spots (neurofibromatosis), vesicles (herpes zoster), and needle marks (intravenous drug abuse), permit a specific diagnosis for nonspecific, nonradiating spinal pain or the symptoms/signs of radiculopathy.
   c. Rectal examination for sphincter tone is important.
   d. Abdominal examination looks for evidence of a disorder causing low back pain (e.g., presence of an abdominal bruit and pulsatile mass from an aortic aneurysm).
   e. Peripheral pulses help distinguish neurogenic from vascular claudication in the lower extremities.

Key Tests: General Examination

- Checking for low-grade fever
- Inspection of the skin
- Rectal examination for sphincter tone
- Abdominal examination
- Peripheral pulses

2. General neurologic examination for neck and low back
   a. Motor testing of each myotome, sensory testing of each dermatome, testing deep tendon reflexes, testing for pathologic reflexes (e.g., Babinski's sign, Hoffman sign)
   b. Coordination tests
   c. Both tests are essential when evaluating spinal problems.

Key Tests: General Neurologic Examination

- Motor testing of each myotome
- Sensory testing of each dermatome
- Deep tendon reflexes
- Testing for pathologic reflexes
- Coordination tests

3. Neurologic examination (low back pain)
   a. Inspect the low back for deformities, a pilonidal cyst, or a patch of hair suggesting spina bifida.
   b. Percussion over the spinous processes may aggravate pain secondary to malignancy or infection of the spinal column.
   c. Check the posture. Splinting with listing away from the painful lower extremity can signal lateral lumbar herniation. Listing toward the painful side can be due to medial disc herniation. In patients with neurogenic claudication, flexion of the trunk can relieve pain and paresthesia, whereas extension of the trunk can aggravate pain and paresthesia.
   d. Gait
      (1) Antalgic gait favoring one lower extremity can be due to lumbar radiculopathy.
      (2) Foot slap/drop secondary to weakness of dorsiflexors of the foot may be secondary to L5 radiculopathy.
      (3) Trendelenburg gait ("drop" of pelvis on the symptomatic side as foot is lifted) signals proximal muscle weakness.
   e. Neuromechanical tests are important adjuncts to the traditional neurologic examination in patients with low back pain and sciatica.
      (1) Straight leg raising test is sensitive for disc herniation causing lumbosacral radiculopathy. Pain is accentuated with elevation of 30° to 70°.
      (2) Bragard's test is done in conjunction with the straight leg raising test. If pain is generated with straight leg raising, the extremity is lowered slightly and then the foot is dorsiflexed. This recreates radicular pain in patients with lumbar disc herniation.
      (3) Prone straight leg raising test often reveals accentuation of pain in the anterior thigh as a result of "high" lumbar (L2, L3) radiculopathy.
      (4) Valsalva maneuver can accentuate lumbar radicular pain in the presence of spinal nerve compression and inflammation.
      (5) Patrick's (Faber) test is done by placing the lateral malleolus of the symptomatic lower extremity on the knee of the opposite extremity and then externally rotating the thigh. Pain is often aggravated with hip joint disease.
      (6) Waddell test reveals that if there is excessive discomfort to light pinching of the skin in the region of the low back pain a functional component may be involved.

Key Tests: Low Back Pain

- Inspection for deformities, pilonidal cyst, or patch of hair suggesting spina bifida

- Percussion over the spinous processes

- Posture tests (see text)

- Gait tests (see text)

- Neuromechanical tests

  —Straight leg raising test

  —Bragard's test in conjunction with straight leg raising test

  —Prone straight leg raising test

  —Valsalva maneuver

  —Patrick's (Faber) test

  —Waddell test

4. Neurologic examination (neck pain)

    a. Inspection of the head and neck looking for reduced spontaneous head movement, head tilt, neck deformity

    b. Gait assessment for spastic, ataxic gait, which signals possible cervical myelopathy

    c. Neuromechanical tests

       (1) Spurling test. The head is inclined toward the side of the painful upper extremity and then compressed downward. Pain and paresthesia radiating into the symptomatic extremity signals nerve root compression.

       (2) Traction test. Lifting the head may relieve cervical spinal nerve root compression, transiently reducing upper extremity pain and paresthesia.

       (3) Valsalva maneuver. It can accentuate the pain of cervical radiculopathy secondary to compression.

       (4) Lhermitte's test. Neck flexion can produce paresthesia, usually of the back in patients with myelitis.

       (5) Adson's and hyperabduction tests. Long used, they are unreliable for determining the presence of thoracic outlet compression. With the patient sitting erect and the upper extremities at the side (Adson test) or the symptomatic upper extremity abducted and extended (hyperabduction test), the radial pulse is palpated. The tests are positive if the pulse disappears and if paresthesia develops in the hand of the symptomatic extremity.

Key Tests: Neck Pain

- Inspection of head and neck

- Gait assessment

- Neuromechanical tests

  —Spurling test

  —Traction test

  —Valsalva maneuver

  —Lhermitte's test

  —Adson's and hyperabduction tests

Important Points in the Approach to Neck and Low Back Disorders

1. Approximately 85% of patients with acute, nonradiating low back pain and 60% with chronic low back pain cannot be given a precise pathoanatomic diagnosis. Although less well studied, the same is probably true for nonradiating neck pain. Thus diagnoses such as muscle strain or sprain and degenerative arthritis of the spine as a cause of pain are probably often incorrect.

2. Association between symptoms and spine imaging results is weak. Therefore, spine radiographs and other neuroimaging procedures are frequently not helpful for establishing an etiology in patients with nonradiating neck and low back pain.

3. Patients with low back and neck pain and a suspicion of underlying systemic illness are candidates for a more aggressive work-up early in the course of the pain. This includes patients older than 50 and those with a history of cancer, unexplained weight loss, injection drug use, chronic infection, or persistence of pain when recumbent.

4. Patients with neck and low back pain radiating into the extremities with associated paresthesia and weakness are candidates for an early diagnostic work-up.

5. Ninety percent of patients with nonspecific localized low back pain generally recover within several weeks. Although less well studied, this is probably also true for neck pain.

6. Natural history of disc herniation is also favorable, and improvement without surgery is the norm, usually within 6 weeks. The herniated portion of the disc tends to regress with time with partial or complete resolution of symptoms in

most patients within 6 months. Therefore even in patients with documented disc herniation, surgery should be delayed as long as the situation permits. An exception is the presence of significant weakness. Early surgery can be justified in this setting.

7. Most therapeutic modalities for acute, nonspecific, nonradiating neck and low back pain have not been proven to be particularly effective. This includes prolonged bed rest, physical therapy, cervical collars and back braces, the application of heat and cold, "blocks" (e.g., epidural), acupuncture, traction, spinal manipulation, and transcutaneous electrical nerve stimulation (TENS).

8. Medications. The judicious short-term use of analgesic medications for severe pain can be helpful. NSAIDs are effective for symptom relief, but their benefit must be weighed against potential side effects. Muscle relaxants are of marginal value.

9. Physical therapy (exercise) is not helpful during the acute phase of back and neck pain, although it can be useful after recovery for preventing recurrences of acute pain and for treating chronic low back pain (neck and back schools).

10. Chronic low back pain is best treated with a regular exercise program; medications such as the tricyclic antidepressants can prove beneficial. Repeated spinal blocks of one type or another should be avoided. Chronic pain programs can be useful for treatments aimed at physical and psychological rehabilitation, with an emphasis on return to activities of daily living.

11. There is conflicting evidence from clinical trials regarding the effectiveness of spinal surgery for patients who have chronic low back pain or neck pain in the absence of evidence of cervical myelopathy, radiculopathy, neurogenic claudication, or spondylolisthesis. Surgery for this population of patients should be recommended with great trepidation.

Origin and Treatment of Low Back Pain

• About 85% of patients with acute, non-radiating low back pain cannot be given a precise pathoanatomic diagnosis.

• Association between symptoms and imaging results is weak.

• Few treatments have been scientifically validated.

Bibliography

Cherkin D, Deyo R, Battie M, et al.: A comparison of physical therapy, chiropractic manipulation, and provision of an educational booklet for the treatment of patients with low back pain. N Engl J Med 339:1021–1029, 1998.

Deyo RA, Weinstein JA: Low back pain. N Engl J Med 344:363–370, 2001.

Groen G, Balget B, Drukker J: Nerves and nerve plexuses of the human vertebral column. Am J Anat 188:282–296, 1997.

Hart L, Deyo R, Cherkin D: Physician office visits for low back pain. Spine 20:11–19, 1995.

Levin KH, Covington EC, Devereaux M, et al.: Neck and back pain. Continuum 7:1–208, 2001.

Malmivarra A, Hakkinen U, Aro T, et al.: The treatment of acute low back pain—bed rest, exercise or ordinary activity? N Engl J Med 332:331–335, 1995.

Techniques and Principles

1. Radiography
   a. Plain radiographs define the bony anatomy but do not visualize neural structures such as nerve roots and spinal cord.
   b. Plain radiographs are usually immediately available in emergency departments, and can quickly exclude trauma or serious bony disease.

2. Computed tomography (CT)
   a. This technique visualizes bony structures and neural structures such as spinal nerve roots and spinal cord.
   b. Images of the neural structures are easily degraded by movement, obesity, and contiguous bony structures.

3. Magnetic resonance imaging (MRI)
   a. This technique is the single best imaging procedure for the identification of structural defects causing damage to neural structures arising within the spinal canal.
   b. The resolution is several millimeters, and it is more precise than other procedures, although bony structures are less well visualized than with the previously mentioned techniques.

4. Myelography
   a. This technique employs plain radiography after instillation of a radiopaque contrast medium within the spinal canal, by way of lumbar or high cervical puncture.
   b. The technique is invasive, but does permit visualization of the spinal cord, spinal nerve roots, and their relationship with contiguous bony structures such as facet joints, uncovertebral joints, and neural foramina.
   c. Myelography is not a first choice for diagnostic testing because of its invasiveness and the technical difficulty of the procedure.

5. CT-myelography
   a. When conventional myelography is followed by CT scanning, the combined technique provides a level of diagnostic resolution that may surpass MRI.
   b. Because of the invasive nature of myelography it is not a first choice test, but may be used when MRI is contraindicated or when MRI results are inconclusive.

6. Electrodiagnosis
   a. Nerve conduction studies are performed by delivering electrical stimuli percutaneously over major nerve trunks and recording the subsequent sensory nerve responses and the muscle responses.
      (1) When spinal nerve root fibers are transected or severely damaged, motor nerve fibers degenerate. As a result, the muscle responses recorded during motor nerve stimulation are reduced in amplitude.
      (2) When sensory nerve fibers are damaged in the spinal canal (as with radiculopathy), degeneration of the nerve fibers does not occur, because the sensory nerve cell bodies reside distal to the point of spinal nerve root damage in the spinal canal. Because these sensory ganglia remain connected to their distal nerve fibers, degeneration of the sensory axons does not occur, and the measured response from sensory nerve stimulation remains normal.
   b. The needle electrode examination involves the insertion of a recording needle electrode into one or more muscles of the symptomatic extremity. This is the most sensitive part of the EMG study for the diagnosis of radiculopathy.
      (1) Acute changes consistent with radiculopathy are unlikely to appear during the needle electrode examination until at least 3 weeks after the onset of weakness.
      (2) Fibrillation potentials require 3 or more weeks to develop after transection of a nerve trunk innervating the recorded muscle.
   c. EMG studies can be useful to establish that weakness is due to nerve damage, as opposed to weakness resulting from reduced effort or pain.
   d. The needle electrode examination can distinguish between recent and chronic axon loss, as well as between axon loss and conduction block along spinal nerve root fibers.

7. Discography
   a. This procedure is a controversial diagnostic test

during which fluid with or without a contrast medium is injected into a vertebral disc presumed to be causing pain. The development of pain reproducing the patient's symptoms is used by some physicians to identify the diseased disc and the level at which to perform spinal fusion.

   b. An antibiotic is often instilled at the time of fluid injection to minimize the risk of postprocedure discitis.

8. Selective nerve root localization

   a. This procedure is a controversial diagnostic technique that has been recommended when there is lack of agreement between clinical and neuroimaging findings in regard to symptoms of radiculopathy, when there is atypical limb pain, and when there is a history of failed surgery at the spinal level where symptoms persist.

   b. The localization procedure is performed under fluoroscopic guidance, using a spinal needle through which a nonionic contrast medium is instilled in the extraspinal neural foramen to outline the selected nerve root.

   c. This may be followed by instillation of a combination of anesthetic and long-acting corticosteroid to further assess the relationship between the patient's pain and the identified nerve root pathology.

Key Tests: Diagnostic Tests for Neck and Back Pain

Imaging Techniques

• Plain radiographs of the spine

• CT of the spine

• MRI of the spine

• CT-myelography

• Discography

• Selective nerve root localization

Electrophysiologic Techniques

• Nerve conduction studies

• Needle electrode examination

Indications

1. Diagnostic testing should be considered in the setting of neck and back pain when there are symptoms or signs of neurologic dysfunction for which a structural cause of nerve root or spinal cord damage is sought.

2. Less commonly, diagnostic testing may be indicated in the setting of chronic or progressive spine pain in the absence of neurologic symptoms or signs.

3. In general, when the symptoms or disability are such that surgical intervention is warranted based on the clinical picture, or when other treatable conditions need to be ruled in or out, then diagnostic testing is valuable.

4. The presence of unexplained neurologic symptoms or signs suggesting cervical or thoracic myelopathy is a strong indication for imaging techniques such MRI or CT-myelography.

5. Plain radiography

   a. Spine radiographs are performed most often in the setting of acute trauma. A recent study showed that the likelihood of a positive finding in this setting is extremely low in the absence of neurologic symptoms or signs.

   b. Spine radiographs are useful as part of a general radiographic bone survey to identify osteosclerotic or lytic bone lesions that could indicate plasmacytoma, multiple myeloma, or metastatic disease.

   c. Spine radiographs are useful in the identification of certain rheumatologic causes of spine pain, such as ankylosing spondylitis, Paget's disease, and diffuse idiopathic skeletal hyperostosis.

6. Computerized tomography

   a. CT imaging is indicated for the diagnosis of structural lesions causing neurologic symptoms and signs of radiculopathy or myelopathy.

   b. For uncomplicated spine pain, CT imaging is not recommended for symptoms of less than 7 weeks duration, according to a practice guideline published by the American Academy of Neurology.

   c. CT imaging may be the study of choice for patients in whom MRI studies are contraindicated.

7. Magnetic resonance imaging

   a. MRI studies have the same indications as CT studies, and are performed because of their superior ability to resolve soft tissue and neural structures.

   b. Furthermore, MRI studies are indicated for the evaluation of osteomyelitis, disc space infections, and intraspinal soft tissue collections due to infection, hemorrhage, or malignancy.

8. CT myelography

 a. This procedure is valuable in patients for whom MRI studies are inconclusive, or in situations where a CT study is inconclusive and MRI studies are contraindicated.

 b. It is especially useful in the assessment of the relationship between spinal nerve roots and the bony neural foramina.

9. Electromyography

 a. Electrodiagnostic studies are useful to support the presence or absence of peripheral nerve damage as the result of spinal nerve root disease.

 b. EMG studies are most useful in the presence of a motor deficit on neurologic examination.

 c. Nerve conduction studies are indicated primarily to exclude other neuromuscular disorders that may mimic radiculopathy. The H-reflex can be a useful nerve conduction study when assessing the patient for the presence of an S1 radiculopathy.

 d. The needle electrode examination is most likely to be useful in the presence of clinical weakness. This procedure will help distinguish weakness due to spinal nerve root damage from other causes of weakness, such as other neuromuscular disorders, central nervous system disorders, and non-neurologic causes of weakness.

 e. The needle electrode examination should be performed after at least 3 weeks have passed since the onset of weakness, as fibrillation potentials (the major manifestation of acute denervation) do not reliably develop before that time.

10. Discography

 a. There is disagreement regarding the value of and indications for this procedure.

 b. The North American Spine Society has produced a position statement regarding indications for lumbar discography:

 (1) For further evaluation of demonstrably abnormal discs to help assess the extent of abnormality or correlate the abnormality with clinical symptoms

 (2) For persistent severe symptoms when other diagnostic tests have failed to reveal a clear localization and source of pain

 (3) For assessment of failed surgery patients to determine if there is a painful pseudarthrosis of a symptomatic disc in a posteriorly fused segment

 (4) For assessment of disc for fusion to

determine if the discs within the proposed fusion segment are symptomatic

 (5) For assessment of minimally invasive surgery candidates to confirm the appropriate anatomic architecture for the proposed technique.

11. Selective nerve root localization

 a. There is disagreement regarding the value of and indications for this procedure.

 b. Proponents of this technique recommend it when there is lack of agreement between clinical and neural imaging findings in regard to symptoms of radiculopathy, when there is atypical limb pain, and when there is a history of failed surgery at the spinal level where symptoms persist.

Key Signs: Indications for Diagnostic Testing

- Spinal trauma
- Neurologic symptoms or signs of radiculopathy
- Neurologic symptoms or signs of myelopathy
- Chronic spine pain

Contraindications

1. Radiography: Contraindicated in pregnant women and in others who are at risk from exposure to radiation.

2. Computed tomography: Like radiography, this technique is relatively contraindicated in pregnant women.

3. MRI

 a. This technique does not expose patients to radiation, but because the effects of high magnetic fields on the fetus have not been defined, there is a relative contraindication to its use in pregnant women.

 b. MRI studies are contraindicated in patients with cardiac pacemakers, implanted defibrillators, cochlear implants, and other indwelling devices whose mechanism can be altered by applying a magnetic field.

 c. Patients who have metal debris in the eye should not be subjected to MRI studies.

 d. MRI studies are also contraindicated in patients who have undergone placement of clips for treatment of cerebral aneurysms. Caution is also recommended in the presence of intracranial clips made of metals said to be made of MR-compatible materials, such as titanium.

e. The contrast medium gadolinium is generally well tolerated; hypersensitivity reactions are rare.

4. CT-myelography
   a. Noniodinated and nonionic contrast media now eliminate most contraindications to this procedure.
   b. Lumbar and cisternal puncture is contraindicated in patients with a bleeding diathesis, such as thrombocytopenia (platelet count less than 50,000), and hereditary and acquired coagulopathy.

5. EMG
   a. As already noted, the needle electrode examination is contraindicated in patients with a bleeding diathesis.
   b. Nerve conduction studies are contraindicated in patients with indwelling defibrillators unless such devices can be turned off during the procedure.

6. Discography: This procedure is contraindicated in the presence of systemic or local infection, and in patients with a bleeding diathesis.

7. Selective nerve root localization: This procedure is contraindicated in the presence of systemic or local infection, and in patients with a bleeding diathesis.

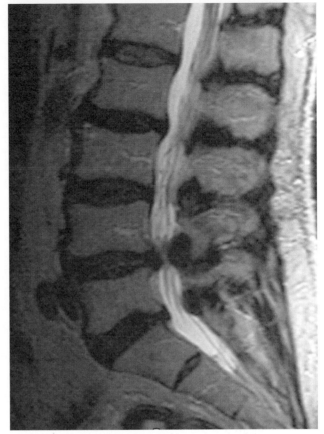

Figure 2–1. T_2-weighted sagittal MRI scan of the lumbar spine demonstrating severe canal stenosis at the L4–5 level.

Key Indications: Contraindications for Diagnostic Testing

- Pregnancy for radiographic procedures
- Coagulopathy/thrombocytopenia for invasive studies
- Indwelling electrical devices, such as cardiac or other pacemakers, defibrillators, for MRI studies
- Indwelling cardiac defibrillator for nerve conduction studies

---

Abnormal Findings

1. Imaging studies
   a. Bone and disc changes
      (1) Canal stenosis may occur at the cervical, thoracic or lumbar levels (Fig. 2–1). This may occur on the basis of disc protrusion, thickening of the posterior longitudinal ligament or ligamentum flavum, congenital shortening of the pedicles, or degenerative facet joint hypertrophy. Canal stenosis may result in spinal cord compression at the cervical and thoracic levels, or cauda equina compression at the lumbar levels.

      (2) Neural forminal stenosis may occur as the result of several pathological processes:
         (a) Far lateral disc protrusion
         (b) Degenerative arthritic change causing osteophyte formation at the facet joints or uncovertebral joints.
   b. Disease directly affecting neural structures
      (1) Spinal cord
          Findings may include demyelination, malignancy, hemorrhage, and infection.
      (2) Spinal nerve roots
          Findings may include schwannoma, neurofibroma, infection, and hemorrhage.

2. EMG
   a. Nerve conduction studies
      (1) Loss or asymmetry of the tibial H-reflex suggests S1 root disease, but may also occur in tibial or sciatic neuropathy.
      (2) With severe T1, C8, or C5–6 radiculopathy, one may see reduction of the compound muscle action potential (CMAP) amplitude when recording over the abductor pollicis brevis, abductor digiti minimi/first dorsal interosseus, or deltoid/biceps muscles, respectively.

(3) With severe S1, L5, or L3–4 radiculopathy, one may see reduction of the CMAP amplitude when recording over the abductor hallucis, extensor digitorum brevis/tibialis anterior, or rectus femoris muscles, respectively.

b. Needle electrode examination

(1) The presence of fibrillation potentials in muscles sharing a single nerve root innervation supports recent or ongoing motor nerve fiber axon loss (denervation) in a root distribution.

(2) The presence of enlarged motor unit action potentials (MUAPs) in muscles sharing a single nerve root innervation suggests chronic reinnervation in a root distribution that has previously undergone denervation.

(3) The presence of reduced numbers of rapidly firing MUAPs with maximal voluntary muscle contraction in the absence of fibrillation potentials and enlarged MUAPs suggests the presence of conduction block along nerve fibers in a single nerve root, without chronic or active motor axon loss.

3. Discography

a. The main abnormality diagnosed with discography is internal disc disruption, which is associated with little or no alteration of the external contour of the disc. There is disagreement whether internal disc disruption represents a pathological entity that produces pain or other symptoms.

b. Discography may also identify the presence of a pseudarthrosis or a painful transition disc.

4. Selective nerve root localization: May identify a compressed nerve root within the neural foramen and may show the degree to which a facet or uncovertebral joint osteophyte is compressing a nerve root sleeve.

Complications

1. CT myelography, EMG, discography, and selective nerve root localization are invasive techniques. Intra-thecal hemorrhage may occur with those techniques entering the spinal canal, and EMG needles can produce intramuscular hemorrhage and, rarely, compartment syndromes. These complications are extremely unlikely in the patient who has no bleeding diathesis.

2. Infections such as meningitis and discitis are rare with discography.

3. Spinal headaches may occur after CT myelography.

Key Complications: CT Myelography, EMG, Discography, Nerve Root Localization

- Intrathecal hemorrhage with CT myelography, discography, nerve root localization

- Intramuscular hemorrhage (EMG needles)

- Spinal headaches (CT myelography)

Bibliography

American Academy of Neurology: Practice parameters: Magnetic resonance imaging in the evaluation of low back syndrome (summary statement). Report of the quality standards subcommittee of the American Academy of Neurology. Neurology 44:767–770, 1994.

Guyer R, Ohnmeiss D: Contemporary Concepts in Spine Care—Lumbar Discography: Physician's statement from the North American Spine Society Diagnostic and Therapeutic Committee. Spine 20:2048–2059, 1995.

Hoffman JR, Mower WR, Wolfson AB, et al.: Validity of a set of criteria to rule out injury to the cervical spine in patients with blunt trauma. National Emergency X-Radiography Utilization Study Group. N Engl J Med 343:94–99, 2000.

Levin KH: Electrodiagnostic approach to the patient with suspected radiculopathy. Neurol Clin 20:397–421, 2002.

Nachemson AL Johnsson E (eds): Neck and Back Pain. The Scientific Evidence of Causes, Diagnosis, and Treatment. Philadelphia, Lippincott Williams & Wilkins, 2000.

3 Radiculopathy and Cauda Equina Syndrome

Eugene Dulaney

Definitions

1. Radiculopathy: Any disease process affecting the spinal nerve roots. Nerve roots contain either motor (ventral root) or sensory (dorsal root) axons, which pass through the subarachnoid space between the spinal cord and the neural foramina. The dorsal and ventral roots enter the neural foramina, where they merge to form the spinal nerves. Therefore, disease processes injuring spinal roots must be localized within either the spinal canal or the neural foramina. Note that dorsal and ventral roots may be affected simultaneously or individually. Injury to multiple roots is termed *polyradiculopathy.*

2. Cauda equina syndrome: The cauda equina comprises the lumbar and sacral nerve roots extending below the termination of the spinal cord at the L1–L2 level. The term *cauda equina syndrome* is applied to polyradiculopathy affecting these roots.

3. Spondylosis: A degenerative disorder of the spine characterized by intervertebral disc degeneration, overgrowth of vertebral end plates, hypertrophy of the facet joints, and hypertrophy and calcification of the spinal ligaments. Spondylotic changes are ubiquitous in the adult population, and are an expected part of the aging process. These changes can produce nerve root compression, as described below.

Etiology and Pathophysiology

1. The etiology of radiculopathies can be either spondylotic or nonspondylotic. Radiculopathies due to spondylosis are most common.

2. Spondylotic radiculopathies

   a. Impingement by disc material

   (1) Herniation of the nucleus pulposis of an intervertebral disc into the spinal canal can produce signs and symptoms of radiculopathy. The anatomic relationship of discs and nerve roots usually leads to injury of the root exiting at the level of a cervical disc herniation and the root exiting at the level below a lumbar disc herniation. Note, however, that large lumbar disc herniations can compress several nerve roots within the cauda equina simultaneously.

   (2) Compression is believed to injure nerve roots either directly or by producing local ischemia. In addition, the nucleus pulposus is rich in prostaglandins, which incite an inflammatory response in adjacent roots, contributing to radicular pain.

   b. Nerve roots can also be affected by osteoarthritis of the spinal facet joints, which can project into the foramina and the lateral spinal canal. Facet joint disease is often present at multiple levels and may produce signs and symptoms referable to several nerve roots.

   c. Abnormal anteroposterior narrowing of the spinal canal is referred to as *spinal stenosis.* This narrowing may be produced acutely by large central disc herniations. More commonly, a combination of congenital shortness of the spinal pedicles, hypertrophy of the ligamentum flavum, and osteophytes from the facet joints result in chronic, progressive stenosis. In the cervical region, spinal stenosis usually produces myelopathy as well as radiculopathy. In the lumbar region, spinal stenosis is the most common cause of cauda equina syndrome.

3. Nonspondylotic radiculopathies

   a. This heterogeneous group of diseases, the most common of which are listed in Table 3–1, are beyond the scope of this chapter. Only spondylolisthesis will be discussed here.

   b. Spondylolisthesis is the anterior displacement of a vertebra over the one beneath it. It may be secondary to spondylolysis (a congenital or acquired defect in the pars interarticularis of the vertebral body), and in these cases is termed *isthmic spondylolisthesis.* Isthmic spondylolisthesis is most common at L5–S1, and less so at L4–L5. Spondylolisthesis can also occur as a result of facet joint remodeling in an elderly patient in whom there is an intact pars interarticularis. This is most common at the L4–L5 level. Spondylolisthesis may result in L5 and S1 radiculopathy and cauda equina syndrome.

4. Demyelination vs. axonal loss

   a. Another way of categorizing radiculopathies is to distinguish the mechanism of injury at the

TABLE 3–1. CAUSES OF NONSPONDYLOTIC RADICULOPATHY

Structural Lesions
Spondylolisthesis
Epidural hematoma
Epidural endometriosis
Arachnoid and synovial cysts

Infection
Epidural abscess
Osteomyelitis
Herpes zoster
Herpes simplex
Syphilis
Lyme disease
Cytomegalovirus (in patients with immunosuppression)

Neoplastic Lesions
Metastatic tumors
Meningiomas
Schwannomas and neurofibromas of nerve roots
Neoplastic meningitis

Arteriovenous Malformation (Dural and Intradural)
Inflammatory Disorders
Sarcoidosis
Vasculitis

Endocrine/Metabolic Disorders
Diabetic radiculopathy
Osteoporosis with vertebral fracture
Epidural lipomatosis
Acromegaly
Paget's disease

Traumatic/Toxic
Vertebral fracture
Nerve root avulsion
Nerve root toxicity from spinal anesthesia

cellular level. Nerve roots may be compromised by injury to the nerve cell axons themselves or to the myelin sheath surrounding them. Distinguishing between axonal loss and demyelination is of practical importance for judging the severity or radiculopathies and their prognosis for recovery.

b. Demyelination: Because myelin is more susceptible to injury than are the axons themselves, many compressive radiculopathies begin as demyelinating lesions. Loss of myelin may block axonal transmission of action potentials. Nevertheless, Schwann cells are able to regenerate myelin quickly, and demyelinating radiculopathies have the potential to resolve fully within days or a few weeks. The chance of long-term neurologic deficits is negligible.

c. Axonal loss: Lesions that compromise axons carry a poorer prognosis. Axonal regeneration is slow (approximately 1 mm per day, or 1 inch per month), and is often incomplete. Axonal loss can be prominent in severe compressive lesions, as well as in vasculitis, some infections, and malignant meningitis. If there is complete compromise of both axons and myelin, as in nerve root avulsions, recovery is not possible.

d. The most practical way to determine the degree of axonal loss in radiculopathies is by electromyography.

Epidemiology and Risk Factors

1. Cervical spondylotic radiculopathy

   a. The annual incidence in one large Mayo Clinic study was 83/100,000 (male to female ratio of 1.7).

   b. Frequency of cervical disc herniations with radiculopathy is as follows:

      (1) C6–C7 (compressing C7 root) 45% to 60%

      (2) C5–C6 (C6 root) 20% to 25%

      (3) C8–T1 (C8 root) and C4–C5 (C5 root) <10% each

2. Lumbar spondylotic radiculopathy

   a. In the U.S. population, the cumulative lifetime incidence of an episode of sciatica is 1.6%.

   b. Symptomatic disc herniations are most common at L4–L5 and L5–S1. These account for approximately 95% of lumbar herniations.

3. Risk factors for spondylotic radiculopathy

   a. The major risk factor is aging. Other reported risk factors include smoking, chronic cough, heavy lifting, and heavy physical labor, including twisting and exposure to vibration.

   b. Recent genetic studies have shown that certain variations in the collagen IX gene sequence are a risk factor for lumbar disk disease. Collagen IX is present in the annulus fibrosus and nucleus pulposus of intervertebral discs.

Clinical Features

1. Sensory symptoms

   a. Classically, "radicular" pain is sharp and lancinating, and radiates from the spine into the dermatomal distribution of the affected root. It may be triggered or aggravated by maneuvers that place traction on the roots, such as lateral movement of the neck, bending at the waist, or a Valsalva maneuver. Table 3–2 lists typical patterns of pain radiation in radiculopathy. Unfortunately, nerve root pain does not always follow these rules. It may be constant, aching, and present more diffusely throughout a limb. Whatever the specifics, pain is usually the most prominent symptom of radiculopathy.

   b. *Sciatica* is a term frequently misused both by

clinicians and patients. It refers to pain radiating from the low back into one or both legs, *below the knee*. Sciatica is relatively specific for L4, L5, and S1 radiculopathies. Pain radiating into the lower limb above the knee is frequently musculoskeletal in origin, although high lumbar radiculopathies (L2, L3) can cause pain radiating into the anterior thigh.

c. Spinal (or "neurogenic") claudication is usually a symptom of lumbar spinal stenosis. Patients with this condition report aching pain in the lower limbs precipitated by walking or standing. There is usually associated numbness and paresthesia. Symptoms are often reliably encountered after a specific duration of activity, similar to vascular claudication (see below). The pathophysiology is believed to be compression of the cauda equina and consequent nerve root ischemia in the area of stenosis, which is increased by spinal extension in the standing position, and reduced by spinal flexion.

d. Sensory loss and paresthesia are frequently reported in the dermatome of the affected nerve root. The distribution of the paresthesia is often more useful in identifying which nerve root is compromised than is the sensory examination itself.

2. Motor symptoms

a. Weakness is usually a less prominent complaint than pain and sensory symptoms, and when present reflects more severe nerve root injury. It is more frequent for clinicians to detect mild weakness of which the patient is not aware than for patients to present weakness as a complaint.

b. Patients with severe and longstanding radiculopathy may become aware of atrophy of affected muscles. Uncommonly, they may experience fasciculations in affected muscles, al-though these are more typical for motor neuron disease (see below).

3. Signs

a. Typical patterns of sensory, motor, and reflex abnormalities for the most common radiculopathies are noted in Table 3–2.

b. Loss or suppression of reflexes is a highly sensitive diagnostic sign in radiculopathy, and it is often the only objective abnormality found on the neurologic exam.

c. Muscle atrophy may be seen in chronic radiculopathy, but it is usually not prominent because most muscles are inervated by several nerve roots.

d. Certain provocative maneuvers (e.g., the Spurling test and straight leg raise test) are of benefit in the diagnosis of radiculopathy. These are reviewed in detail in Part XIX, Chapter 2, Diagnostic Testing for Neck and Back Disorders.

Differential Diagnosis

1. Musculoskeletal conditions

a. The vast majority of patients with spine pain do not have radiculopathy. However, pain from spinal structures, such as facet joints and vertebral bodies may be referred to the proximal limbs. Absence of neurologic deficits and lack of a dermatomal distribution of pain suggests a musculoskeletal cause.

b. Myofascial pain syndrome and occasionally fibromyalgia may present with pain that mimics radiculopathy. Myofascial pain syndrome produces localized pain, most often around the shoulder and hip. It is characterized by trigger points in muscle, which cause radiation of pain when pressure is applied. Patients with fibromyalgia complain of widespread muscle pain

TABLE 3–2. KEY SYMPTOMS AND SIGNS ASSOCIATED WITH COMMON RADICULOPATHIES

Root	Pain Distribution	Dermatomal Sensory Loss	Prominent Affected Muscles	Affected Reflex
C5	Shoulder, anterior arm	Lateral arm	Deltoid, biceps	Biceps, brachioradialis
C6	Lateral arm and forearm, into first and second fingers	Lateral forearm and hand, 1st and 2nd fingers	Deltoid, biceps	Biceps, brachioradialis
C7	Lateral arm and extensor surface of forearm	3rd finger	Triceps, finger extensors	Triceps
C8	Medial arm and forearm, into fourth and fifth fingers	Medial forearm and hand, 4th and 5th fingers	Intrinsic hand muscles	Finger flexors
Thoracic	Band-like, extending from spine to midline	Band-like, extending from spine to midline	Abdominal muscles	Superficial abdominal
L3	Anterior thigh and patella	Distal anterior thigh and knee	Quadriceps, adductors	Patellar
L4	Anterior thigh and medial calf	Medial calf	Quadriceps, adductors	Patellar
L5	Lateral thigh and calf, dorsal foot	Lateral calf, dorsal foot	Tibialis anterior, extensor hallucis	None
S1	Posterior thigh and calf, plantar surface of foot	Posterior calf, plantar surface of foot	Gastrocnemius, toe flexors	Achilles

and exhibit multiple tender points distributed over the body. Neurologic deficits are not present in either condition.

2. Nerve and plexus lesions can cause pain and sensory-motor deficits similar to those produced by nerve root lesions. Certain problems in the differential diagnosis of peripheral nervous system lesions are common, such as L5 radiculopathy vs. peroneal neuropathy, or C8 radiculopathy vs. ulnar neuropathy vs. lower trunk brachial plexopathy. In general, accurate anatomical localization depends on neurologic examination, as the patterns of neurologic deficits seen in radiculopathies, plexopathies, and mononeuropathies are distinctly different. In difficult cases, electromyography can be very helpful in anatomic localization.

3. Spinal cord lesions

   a. Lesions affecting the lower tip of the spinal cord (the conus medullaris) can mimic cauda equina lesions. The conus medullaris syndrome typically presents with sphincter disturbances, impotence, and symmetric sensory loss in S3–S5 dermatomes (saddle anesthesia). Cauda equina lesions are less often symmetric and more often painful. Mass lesions, however, often impinge on both conus and cauda. Neuroimaging can define the site of pathology.

   b. Syringomyelia is a cystic degenerative process affecting the central spinal cord, most commonly in the cervical region. Involvement of lower motor neurons leads to muscle weakness and atrophy. Damage to sensory pathways within the spinal cord typically produces both neuropathic pain and loss of pain and temperature sensitivity, with preservation of touch and position. Both sensory and motor findings are localized to the affected spinal segment. This pattern is not consistent with radiculopathy, and should prompt imaging of the spinal cord.

4. Motor neuron disease

   a. Painless weakness and muscle wasting are the typical features of diseases affecting lower motor neurons, such as amyotrophic lateral sclerosis (ALS). These are usually generalized conditions affecting all spinal segments, but they can present in a single limb.

   b. Helpful diagnostic features in motor neuron disease include lack of radicular pain and sensory loss, the presence of findings in the distribution of several roots, and prominent fasciculations. Upper motor neuron findings such as hyperreflexia are typically found in the weak and wasted limbs of patients with ALS. Magnetic resonance imaging (MRI) of the affected spine segment is normal in motor neuron disease.

5. Visceral pathology

   a. Pain from the viscera is carried to the spinal cord by autonomic afferent fibers that course through the dorsal roots. Thus, visceral pain may be referred in a segmental (not strictly dermatomal) pattern. The skin in areas of referred pain may be hypersensitive, but sensory loss does not occur.

   b. Examples of referred pain include cardiac pain referred to the left chest and arm, renal pain referred to the costovertebral angle, and pain from an abdominal aortic aneurysm referred to the low back.

   c. The absence of typical features of nerve root pathology such as weakness, reflex loss, sensory loss, and a dermatomal distribution of pain aids in making the correct diagnosis.

6. Vascular claudication may be confused with spinal (neurogenic) claudication.

   a. Pedal pulses should be absent in patients with vascular claudication.

   b. Leg pain in vascular claudication is due to muscle ischemia, and is typically produced by walking or other exertion. In contrast, the leg pain of spinal claudication is due to nerve root compression, and may occur with simply maintaining a standing position. Symptoms of spinal claudication are usually improved by flexion at the waist.

   c. Paresthesia is typical for spinal claudication, but not vascular claudication.

   d. Both spinal claudication and vascular claudication are diseases of late life and may occur together in the same patient. Laboratory testing can help determine the relative contributions of each disease process. Arterial Doppler ultrasound studies can confirm the presence of peripheral vascular disease. Neuroimaging and electromyography can confirm the presence of polyradiculopathy.

Diagnostic Testing

1. Neuroimaging plays a very important role in the diagnosis and management of radiculopathy. This subject is covered in more depth in Chapter 2 in this section, but certain points must be emphasized:

   a. MRI is usually the imaging procedure of choice. It can visualize all elements of the spine, including the nerve roots themselves.

   b. Computed tomography (CT) of the spine has accuracy similar to MRI in detecting disk herniation and spinal stenosis. It is less satisfactory in detecting abnormalities of soft tissues, such as infection and neoplasia. This is a useful technique for patients with implanted medical devices, who are not candidates for MRI, or for those who cannot tolerate MRI.

c. CT coupled with myelography may detect pathology missed by MRI or CT alone. It is an invasive test, and for this reason is reserved only for difficult diagnostic situations.

d. Plain radiographs are almost valueless in the diagnosis of radiculopathy, and their routine use is discouraged.

e. Imaging studies frequently uncover spondylotic changes unrelated to patients' symptoms and signs. It is important to interpret imaging findings conservatively, and to correlate them with clinical and electromyographic data.

2. Electromyography and nerve conduction studies (collectively referred to as EMG) are highly useful in the diagnosis of radiculopathy. They serve the purpose of localizing lesions within the peripheral nervous system (e.g., to root, plexus, or nerve), as well as determining lesion severity and chronicity. The nuances of performing and interpreting EMG studies are discussed in Part II, Chapter 2. It is generally accepted that EMG should be performed on any patient in whom history, examination, and imaging fail to provide a clear anatomic localization, as well as on most patients being considered for surgery.

3. Somatosensory evoked potentials have been the subject of considerable interest in years past. They have been replaced in the diagnosis of radiculopathy by modern imaging and EMG techniques.

4. Cerebrospinal fluid (CSF) analysis is helpful in diagnosing certain causes of radiculopathy, including infectious and inflammatory disorders and neoplastic meningitis. CSF findings in these conditions are discussed in Part II, Chapter 1.

5. Genetic testing is presently a subject for research, but has the potential to become a clinical tool. Certain variations in the collagen IX gene have been shown to be risk factors for lumbar disc disease, as discussed above under Etiology and Risk Factors. Further understanding of the genetic influence on spondylosis may lead to more effective therapy and prevention.

Key Tests

- MRI or CT of the spine

- EMG of affected limbs

- CT-myelography in selected cases

Treatment

1. Overall approach

   a. The goals in treating radiculopathy are to relieve suffering, prevent disability, and avoid exposing the patient to useless or even harmful interventions. An approach to treatment of spondylotic radiculopathy is outlined in this section. Treatment of nonspondylotic radiculopathy is dependent on the underlying disease, and is outside the scope of this chapter.

   b. Is treatment emergent? Some nerve root lesions may require inpatient admission, neuroimaging, and prompt consultation with a surgeon. Emergent treatment is often required in the following settings:

      (1) Radiculopathies producing disabling or progressive weakness. For reasons discussed above, prognosis for recovery declines once axonal loss has occurred. Prompt surgical decompression may prevent or minimize axonal loss.

      (2) Bowel or bladder dysfunction: These symptoms are typically encountered in the setting of cauda equina syndrome. Prompt decompression may allow return of function.

      (3) Intractable pain: Radicular pain may be severe enough to require bedrest and parenteral opiates. The severity of radicular pain correlates poorly with other clinical features such as weakness and sensory loss, and pain may be the major complaint.

2. Nonoperative management

   a. Suspected disc herniation

      (1) In patients with pain alone or mild neurologic deficits, the prognosis is favorable, and conservative treatment may suffice. For example, only 10% of patients with sciatica have severe enough pain at 6 weeks for surgery to be considered. MRI studies have shown that disc herniation can partially or completely regress with time.

      (2) Nonsteroidal antiinflamatory drugs (NSAIDs) are useful for pain management, but their benefit must be weighed against their risks. Muscle relaxants may be helpful for some patients, but selection criteria are unclear. Severe pain may require a limited course of opiates.

      (3) Epidural corticosteroids have been shown to yield short-term improvements in pain and sensory loss in patients with sciatica, but they do not improve level of function or reduce the need for surgery. Trials of

systemic corticosteroids are inconclusive, although short courses of oral steroids are frequently prescribed.

(4) In patients with sciatica, a randomized trial comparing bedrest for two weeks vs. activity ad lib showed no benefit from bedrest. Patients with radiculopathy should be advised to remain as active as possible, although heavy lifting, twisting, and bodily vibration should be avoided.

(5) Use of a soft cervical collar for patients with cervical radiculopathy is of uncertain benefit. If used, it should be limited to a 2- to 3-week period.

(6) Cervical traction is also of uncertain benefit for cervical radiculopathy. Lumbar traction is probably useless.

b. Spinal stenosis
 (1) In contrast to disk herniation, spinal stenosis is usually a slowly progressive condition.
 (2) Use of NSAIDs and other analgesics is appropriate. Patients should be encouraged to remain physically fit. Water aerobics and the use of a stationary bicycle are often tolerated well by individuals with spinal claudication.

3. Alternative therapies
 a. Acupuncture and massage may provide symptomatic benefit for patients with radiculopathy, although this is uncertain.
 b. Spinal manipulation is not recommended. There is no evidence to support its benefit in patients with radiculopathy or spinal stenosis. In contrast, acute worsening of radiculopathy and development of cauda equina syndrome have been reported as complications.

Key Treatment: Nonoperative Therapy

- Nonsteroidal anti-inflammatory drugs
- Muscle relaxants
- Opiates
- Epidural corticosteroids

4. Surgery
 a. Accepted indications for surgery on spondylotic radiculopathy include
  (1) Progressive or severe weakness, or bowel/bladder dysfunction
  (2) Persistent sensory or motor deficit after 4 to 6 weeks of conservative therapy
  (3) Persistent radicular pain (not neck or back pain alone) after 4 to 6 weeks of conservative therapy
  (4) Spinal claudication that is persistent and disabling
 b. The purpose of surgery is to relieve pressure on the roots, within either the spinal canal or the neural foramina. Several procedures are available.
  (1) Standard surgery for disc herniation involves creation of a hole in the lamina (partial laminectomy) and removal of the extruded portion of a disc (discectomy). Frequently, discectomy is performed under an operating microscope, a procedure termed microdiscectomy. Results of discectomy and microdiscectomy are comparable.
  (2) Disc material may also be approached percutaneously, either through a trochar (percutaneous automated discectomy) or by vaporization with a laser (laser discectomy). These procedures have the advantage of reduced soft tissue injury and allow for more rapid rehabilitation, but they have not proved as effective as standard discectomy.
  (3) Percutaneous arthroscopic discectomy permits a percutaneous approach but also allows local pathology to be visualized. It is a promising procedure that may someday prove as effective as standard discectomy.
  (4) Surgical treatment of spinal stenosis requires decompressive laminectomy. If the stenosis is due to spondylolisthesis, spinal fusion may be added.

Indications for Surgical Referral

A structural lesion causing

- Disabling or progressive weakness
- Bowel or bladder dysfunction
- Persistent sensory or motor deficit despite conservative therapy
- Persistent radicular pain despite conservative therapy
- Spinal claudication

 Bibliography

Carette S, Leclaire R, Marcoux S, et al.: Epidural corticosteroid injections for sciatica due to herniated nucleus pulposis. N Engl J Med 336:1634–1640, 1997.

Hall, H: Surgery: Indications and options. Neurol Clin North Am 17:113–129, 1999.

Jensen MC, Brant-Zawadzki MN, Obuchowski N, et al.: Magnetic resonance imaging of the lumbar spine in people without back pain. N Engl J Med 331:69–73, 1994.

Paassilta P, Lohiniva J, Goring HHH, et al.: Identification of a novel common genetic risk factor for lumbar disk disease. JAMA 285:1843–1849, 2001.

Porter RW: Spinal stenosis and neurogenic claudication. Spine 21:2046–2052, 1996.

Radhakrishnan K, Litchy WJ, O'Fallon WM, Kurland LT: Epidemiology of cervical radiculopathy: A population-based study from Rochester, Minnesota, 1976 through 1990. Brain 117:325–335, 1994.

Storm PB, Chou D, Tamargo RJ: Lumbar spinal stenosis, cauda equina syndrome, and multiple lumbosacral radiculopathies. Phys Med Rehabil Clin N Am 13:713–733, 2002.

Vroomen PCAJ, deKrom MCTFM, Wilmink JT, et al.: Lack of effectiveness of bed rest for sciatica. N Engl J Med 340:418–423, 1999.

SPONDYLOSIS

Definition

Spondylosis refers to the degenerative changes that occur in the spine, including degeneration of joints, intervertebral discs, and their associated ligaments.

Epidemiology

1. Altogether, 60% of women and 80% of men have osteophytes in vertebral bodies by age 49.
2. By 79 years of age, approximately 95% of both genders have spondylosis.
3. In the cervical region, osteophytes may compress the spinal cord and cause cervical spondylotic myelopathy (CSM). This is the most common cause of spinal cord dysfunction in persons older than age 55 in North America.
4. In a prospective study in the United Kingdom, 23.6% of 585 patients with tetraparesis or quadriparesis had CSM.

Anatomy

Also see Part XIX, Chapter 1.

1. Vertebrae are adjoined anteriorly by the intervertebral disc and posteriorly by apophyseal joints, which are synovial in type.
2. During childhood the superior and inferior surfaces of the vertebral bodies are covered with a layer of hyaline cartilage, the center of which persists in adult life. The periphery ossifies to form a ring that fuses to the body of the vertebra by the third decade.
3. During childhood the disc consists of a firm peripheral annulus fibrosus surrounding a gelatinous nucleus pulposus. The annulus is made up of collagenous fibers, and the nucleus has a mucoid stroma of a gel containing water held in polysaccharide complexes.
4. Although the intervertebral disc is primarily responsible for the support and strength of the vertebral joints, it is supplemented by the anterior longitudinal ligament, facet joints and capsules, ligamentum flavum, and interspinous and supraspinous ligaments and in the lumbar region by the

lumbodorsal fascia. Muscles of the trunk, primarily the paraspinal muscles, contribute to the support of the spine.

5. The periphery of the disc contains blood vessels that disappear between 5 and 10 years of age. Healthy discs contain no nociceptive nerve endings; but portions of the vertebral bodies, anterior surface of the spinal dura, and the posterior and anterior longitudinal ligaments receive sensory nerve fibers. The annulus fibrosus (outer one-third) contains nerve fibers from the sinuvertebral system, but there is no proof that they are nociceptive.

Pathophysiology

1. Static mechanical factors result in a reduction of the spinal canal diameter and spinal cord compression.

   a. Intervertebral discs dry out with age, resulting in loss of disc height and bulging of the annulus. These changes predispose to increased movement of the vertebral bodies. The resulting stress on the apophyseal joints leads to typical osteoarthritic changes, with thinning of articular cartilage and osteophyte formation. Osteophytes develop on the edges of the vertebral body secondary to traction of the annulus on the periosteum, resulting in sclerosis.

      (1) Osteophytes form mostly in the anterior direction of vertebral bodies because the anterior longitudinal ligament is weak.

      (2) Osteophytes growing in the dorsolateral direction cause narrowing of the intervertebral foramen and, if severe enough, can compress the exiting spinal nerve root.

      (3) If cervical vertebral osteophytes develop in the anterior section of the facet joints, they may compress the vertebral artery from the medial direction. This is important with regard to chiropractic manipulation, where osteophytes in the facet joints may result in dissection of the vertebral artery.

      (4) In the lumbar spine, osteophytic enlargement of the superior articular process of the facet joint causes narrowing of the lateral recess and compression of the nerve root.

Osteophyte enlargement of the inferior articular process of the facet joint causes narrowing of the central spinal canal and may result in central spinal stenosis.

b. The ligamentum flavum may stiffen and buckle into the spinal cord dorsally.

2. A dynamic mechanical factor (i.e., normal motion of the cervical spine) superimposed on static mechanical factors may aggravate spinal cord compression.

a. During flexion the spinal cord lengthens, resulting in stretching over ventral osteophytic ridges.

b. During extension the ligamentum flavum may buckle into the spinal cord, causing a reduction of the space available for the spinal cord.

3. Spinal cord ischemia plays a role in the development of myelopathy in the later stages.

Symptoms

1. Cervical spondylosis

a. Patients commonly complain of neck stiffness and unilateral or bilateral deep, aching neck, arm, and shoulder pain. Some experience crepitus in the neck with movement; brachialgia (dull achy feeling in the upper limbs); and numbness or tingling in the hands if the exiting cervical nerve roots are compromised by foraminal narrowing.

b. CSM occurs when osteophytes protrude into the spinal canal.

(1) The most characteristic symptom is weakness or stiffness in the lower extremities. Weakness or clumsiness of the hands in conjunction with the lower extremities is typical.

(2) Involvement of the posterior tracts results in an ataxic broad-based gait.

(3) Loss of sphincter control is rare and occurs in the late stages of spondylotic myelopathy, although patients may complain of slight urinary hesitancy earlier.

c. With a hyperextension injury, such as with whiplash, there is further reduction in the diameter of the already stenotic cervical spinal canal.

d. Sudden death from respiratory failure may occur if the C3-4 spinal cord level is compressed, as these nerve roots innervate the diaphragm.

e. Dysphagia may result from compression of the esophageal lumen by large anterior osteophytes.

2. Osteophytes in the lumbar region without compromise of neural elements can produce

a. Dull aching localized back pain and stiffness

b. Symptoms exacerbated by general activity, bending, standing, twisting, or lifting

c. Back pain relieved by decreased activity and rest

Key Symptoms: Spondylosis

- Neck stiffness and unilateral or bilateral deep, aching neck, arm, and shoulder pain

- Symptoms exacerbated by general activity, bending, standing, twisting, or lifting

- Cervical spondylotic myelopathy

—Weakness or stiffness in the lower extremities

—Weakness or clumsiness of the hands in conjunction with the lower extremities

Clinical Findings

1. Usually the neurologic examination is normal.

2. If nerve root(s) or the spinal cord (or both) are compressed, neurologic signs and symptoms occur.

a. Cervical spondylotic myelopathy

(1) Flexion of the neck may cause a generalized "electric shock-like" sensation down the center of the back referred to as Lhermitte's sign.

(2) Valsalva maneuver (e.g., coughing, sneezing, straining) may provoke or aggravate radicular pains. Rotation and lateral bending of the head toward the affected side (Spurling's test) increase symptoms, as this motion further decreases the foraminal area.

(3) Motor weakness, often with fasciculations, is seen in 61% to 68% of symptomatic patients, particularly in those with chronic radicular complaints.

(4) When the upper extremity is involved, a "myelopathy hand" may occur. The fourth and fifth fingers gradually abduct and flex when the patient is asked to maintain finger extension and adduction (finger escape sign) owing to weakness of intrinsic hand muscles. There may be accompanying atrophy. In this setting the patient cannot open and close the hand rapidly. The normal rate is 20 hand closures or more in 10 seconds.

(5) Hyperreflexia with ankle clonus and upgoing toes is characteristic of CSM. The

biceps and brachioradialis reflexes (C5-6) may be depressed or absent, whereas the triceps reflex (C7) is brisk. This pattern is pathognomonic of cord compression due to cervical spondylosis at the C5-6 interspace. A stiff or spastic gait is also characteristic but occurs in the later stages.

(6) Loss of vibratory and position senses may occur, particularly in the feet.

Key Signs: Spondylosis

- Neurologic examination is frequently normal.

- Cervical spondylotic myelopathy

  —Flexion of the neck may cause a generalized "electric shock-like" sensation down the center of the back (Lhermitte's sign).

  —Valsalva maneuver may provoke or aggravate radicular pains.

  —Motor weakness—often with fasciculations—is seen in 61% to 68% of symptomatic patients.

  —"Myelopathy hand"

  —Hyperreflexia with ankle clonus and upgoing toes

  —Loss of vibratory and position senses, particularly in the feet

- Clinical symptoms do not correlate well with radiographic findings.

Differential Diagnosis

1. Symptomatic cervical and lumbar spondylosis must be differentiated from other causes of localized and referred radicular pain (see Part XIX, Chapter 3).
2. A number of conditions present with a myelopathic picture mimicking CSM, including amyotrophic lateral sclerosis (ALS), multiple sclerosis, hereditary spastic paraplegia, intrinsic or extrinsic tumors of the spinal cord, spinal cord infarction, and syringomyelia. Intracranial pathology, such as tumors, arteriovenous malformation, or hydrocephalus, should be ruled out.

Diagnostic Studies

1. Plain radiography of the spine is of little value as an initial diagnostic procedure except in patients with a history of trauma, malignancy, fever or recent infection, intravenous drug use, a compromised immune system (e.g., prolonged steroid

use), low back pain not improved with recumbency, or unexplained weight loss.

a. The normal adult cervical canal is more than 17 mm in anteroposterior (AP) diameter in the midsagittal plane.

b. Cord impingement begins when the spinal canal is 10 to 13 mm.

c. A canal with an AP diameter of less than 10 mm represents absolute stenosis and is strongly correlated with spinal cord compression.

2. Magnetic resonance imaging (MRI) is the standard test for imaging the spine. Aside from being noninvasive, it provides excellent resolution of disk and neural elements, assesses the degree of spinal canal stenosis, and can identify intrinsic spinal cord lesions that also present with myelopathy (e.g., tumors, demyelination).

3. The combination of computed tomography (CT) with myelography yields more information than either alone. CT more accurately assesses the amount of canal compromise because it is superior to MRI for evaluating new bone formation (osteophytes).

4. Electromyography (EMG) is helpful for assessing denervation, confirming neurologic findings, localizing the site of the lesion, and differentiating peripheral versus central compression, plexopathy, ALS, or other overlapping conditions that may mimic CSM.

Key Tests: Spondylosis

- Plain radiographs are of little use as an initial diagnostic procedure.

- MRI is the standard technique for imaging the spine.

- CT

  —Accurately assesses the amount of canal compromise

  —Evaluates new bone formation better than MRI

- Electromyography

  —Helpful for determining the presence and extent of radiculopathy

  —Helpful for excluding disorders that may mimic root disease

Treatment

1. Because of the often benign course of cervical and lumbar spondylosis, nonsurgical management is recommended initially for patients with radicu-

lopathy and mild myelopathy (i.e., with upper or lower extremity symptoms but still able to perform everyday tasks).

2. Optimal pain management is desirable.

a. Nonsteroidal antiinflammatory drugs (NSAIDs) are the safest, most effective medication when used situationally for neck and low back problems of mechanical origin. Chronic usage should be discouraged given the modest benefits and significant side effects.

b. Acute flare-ups may respond to a short course of oral steroids in patients who do not have any medical contraindications (e.g., diabetes, peptic ulcer disease).

c. Muscle relaxants are less useful and often produce sedation.

d. Opioids may be used for short periods of time in severe cases but may result in misuse and dependence.

e. Tricyclic antidepressants are useful for chronic pain.

3. Directed rehabilitation including exercises (i.e., flexibility, strengthening, aerobic training), even in patients with radicular symptoms, can be beneficial and cost-effective. Physical therapy is a key component of any multimodality pain clinic program. Referral to a pain management program may be best, as studies have shown that pain clinics produce demonstrable, long-lasting changes in pain intensity and emotional outlook and restore functional capacity.

a. With acute flare-ups, physical therapy is initiated with passive modalities. Treadmill walking, cycling, and aquatic exercises are also tolerated during this phase.

b. After the acute symptoms have subsided, active modalities, including stretching, dynamic, and strengthening exercises, are recommended.

c. Aerobic training is useful or should be encouraged.

4. Surgical decompression is necessary when there is evidence to suggest moderate to severe myelopathy. With moderate myelopathy secondary to CSM, there is involvement of both arms and legs and both lower limbs in lumbar spondylosis with a resultant effect on the performance of daily activities. Patients with severe myelopathy require aids for ambulation and are often confined to chair, bed, or home.

a. Anterior surgical approaches are increasingly used for moderate to severe CSM, as they permit direct visualization when removing osteophytes and disc material for decompression of the cervical spinal cord. If fusion is done, it

predisposes to degeneration of adjacent segments, most often below the fusion site. The failure rate increases with the number of levels attempted.

b. Laminectomy, from a posterior approach, may be necessary for multiple level decompression for cervical or lumbar spinal pathology. Neurologic deterioration after laminectomy is attributed to development of latent instability of the spine with resultant kyphotic spinal deformities.

Key Treatment: Spondylosis

- Conservative management with pain control and physical therapy is the first line of treatment.

- Drugs for pain management

  —NSAIDs

  —Oral steroids

  —Muscle relaxants

  —Opioids

  —Tricyclic antidepressants

- Surgical intervention may be necessary for cases of intractable pain, poor quality of life, neurologic deficits, and corresponding pathology on imaging studies.

Prognosis

1. Favorable outcome from surgery is no better than 50%.

2. Predictors of less favorable surgical outcomes include severe preoperative neurologic deficits and abnormal signal changes in the spinal cord, spinal cord atrophy seen on MRI, or both.

3. Favorable prognostic indicators include less than 1 year duration of neurologic symptoms and young age at presentation.

LUMBAR FACET PAIN

Definition

The facet syndrome is purported to be the result of degenerative change of the facet (zygapophyseal) joints with narrowing of the adjacent vertebral foramina in the superior and inferior dimensions.

768 • XIX Neck, Back, and Spinal Cord Disorders

Epidemiology

The incidence of facet syndrome is uncertain, as the clinical manifestations are nonspecific. Some even debate its existence.

Anatomy

1. Facet joints are paired synovial joints that join the vertebral arch of one vertebra to the arch of the next vertebra.

2. The medial branches of the posterior rami of the spinal nerve innervate the facet joint just after exiting the intervertebral foramen. Typically, the joint is innervated from a branch at the same level and a branch originating from the foramen above.

3. An extensive distribution of small nerve fibers and free and encapsulated nerve endings exist in the lumbar facet joint capsule, including nerves containing substance P, a putative neuromodulator of pain.

Etiology

1. Traumatic: accompanied by inflammation of the capsule, producing interfacet pressure and subsequent pain. This may exist without any corresponding radiologic abnormality.

2. Pathologic: due to degeneration and thinning of the intervertebral discs. This permits an approximation of the articular facet surfaces with reduction of the intrafacet joint space, which becomes roughened and sclerosed.

3. Postural: During extreme ranges of flexion and unguarded movements, posterior spinal muscles are overextended resulting in damage to spinal structures such as the facet joints of the low back.

Pathophysiology

1. Facet joints are highly innervated structures that are subject to high stress and strain.

2. Acute traumatic strain on the facet joint capsule could lead to acute or subacute low back pain.

3. The resulting tissue damage or inflammation can cause prolonged nociceptor excitation. This peripheral sensitization can lead to sensitization of neurons in the spinal cord (central sensitization), contributing to persistent pain. Additionally, release of substance P from nerve terminals contributes to the cycle of chronic pain.

Key Etiology and Pathophysiology: Lumbar Facet Pain

- Facet syndrome is the result of degenerative changes in the facet (zygapophyseal) joints with subsequent narrowing of the adjacent vertebral foramina.

- Trauma, degenerative changes, and poor posture are the main causes of this syndrome.

- The resulting tissue damage, inflammation, or both can cause prolonged nociceptor excitation that leads to sensitization of the spinal cord, contributing to persistent pain.

Clinical Features

1. Most common symptoms are
   a. Hip and buttock pain
   b. Cramping lower extremity pain confined to the thigh
   c. Low back stiffness, especially in the morning or with inactivity
   d. Absence of paresthesia or motor weakness
2. Signs include
   a. Local paralumbar tenderness
   b. Pain on spine hyperextension
   c. Hip, buttock, or back pain on straight leg raising
   d. Absence of neurologic signs
   e. Absence of root tension signs

 Key Symptoms and Signs: Lumbar Facet Pain

- Hip and buttock pain
- Cramping lower extremity pain confined to thigh
- Low back stiffness, especially in the morning or with inactivity
- Local paralumbar tenderness
- Pain with spinal extension

Diagnostic Studies

1. CT scans provide the radiographic detail necessary for accurate delineation and diagnosis of facet joint abnormalities that may or may not correlate with the presence of clinical symptoms.

2. Diagnosis of facet syndrome is confirmed by provocation and relief of pain with facet joint/

medial branch posterior ramus injection. Therapeutic blocks are of unproven value.

Key Tests: Lumbar Facet Pain

- CT scans

- Diagnosis confirmed by provocation and relief of pain following injection in the facet joint/medial branch posterior ramus

Treatment

1. Conservative management is the first line of treatment. Optimal pain management is the goal. Exercises for strengthening the abdominal and gluteal muscles, stretching the hamstrings, and postural correction are helpful.

2. Percutaneous radiofrequency neurotomy provides lasting pain relief, which offers support for the existence of the facet joint syndrome.

Key Treatment: Lumbar Facet Pain

- Conservative management with pain control and physical therapy is the first line of treatment.

- Percutaneous radiofrequency neurotomy is done when conservative therapy fails.

Bibliography

Barnsley L, Lord SM, Wallis BJ, Bogduk M: Lack of effect of intraarticular corticosteroids for chronic pain in the cervical zygapophyseal joints. N Engl J Med 330:1047–1050, 1994.

Cavanaugh JM, Ozatkay AC, Yamashita HT, King AI: Lumbar facet pain: biomechanics, neuroanatomy and neurophysiology. J Biomech 29:1117–1129, 1996.

Fouyas IP, Statham PF, Sandercock PA: Cochrane review on the role of surgery in cervical spondylotic radiculomyelopathy. Spine 27:736–747, 2002.

Levin KH, Covington EC, Devereaux M, et al.: Neck and back pain. Continuum 7:1–208, 2001.

Lord S, Barnsley L, Wallis BJ, et al.: Percutaneous radiofrequency neurotomy for chronic zygapophyseal-joint pain. N Engl J Med 335:1721–1726, 1996.

Moran R, O'Connell D, Walsh MG: The diagnostic value of facet joint injections. Spine 13:1407–1410, 1988.

Wahlig JB, McLaughlin MR, Subach BR, et al.: Management of low back pain. Neurologist 6:326–337, 2000.

Young WF: Cervical spondylotic myelopathy: a common cause of spinal cord dysfunction in older persons. Am Fam Physician 62:1064–1070, 2000.

Myofascial Pain Syndrome and Sacroiliac Joint Dysfunction

Jennifer S. Kriegler

MYOFASCIAL PAIN SYNDROME

Definition

1. Myofascial pain syndrome (MPS) is defined as a pain disorder involving pain referred from trigger points within myofascial structures, either locally or distant from the pain. The trigger point may be localized to a single muscle group or occur in multiple muscles.
2. A trigger point (TrP) is defined as a localized tender area within a taut band of skeletal muscle or its associated fascia.

Epidemiology

1. TrPs are extremely common.
2. They may be the most common cause of neck and low back pain.

Etiology

1. May occur without apparent trauma
2. Can also follow trauma (e.g., whiplash injury or lumbar spine surgery) or occupational overuse

Clinical Features

1. Tenderness in a taut muscle band containing the trigger point
   a. A taut band is a palpable rope-like hardening of a muscle due to a group of tense muscle fibers.
   b. TrPs can be active (a hyperirritable focus within a taut band that is tender on palpation and refers pain in a characteristic pattern unique to the muscle) or latent (a subclinical TrP that does not spontaneously cause pain but elicits a zone of muscle-specific referred pain on palpation).
2. Pain may be local or referred.
   a. Local pain is usually an aching sensation.
   b. Myofascial pain is often referred to a site some distance from the TrP in a pattern characteristic for each muscle. The patient may report numbness or paresthesias rather than pain.

3. Local twitch or contraction of a taut band may be elicited by snapping, palpation, or penetration with a needle.
4. Patient's pain may be reproduced with digital stimulation.
5. There may be weakness without atrophy.
6. Range of motion may be restricted.
7. Injection of local anesthetic abolishes pain.

Key Symptoms: Myofascial Pain Syndrome

- Local or regional pain
- Trigger points
  —Tenderness in a taut muscle band
  —Referred pain due to stimulation
  —Reproduction of patients' pain by digital stimulation
  —Weakness without atrophy
  —Possibly restricted range of motion
  —Injection of local anesthesia abolishes pain

Differential Diagnosis

Includes radiculopathy, entrapment neuropathy, and joint pathology

Treatment

1. Medications may be of benefit, such as nonsteroidal antiinflammatory drugs (NSAIDs), analgesics (avoiding long-term use of habituating opiate agonists), antidepressants, and muscle relaxants.
2. TrP injections may be useful using a combination of local anesthetic and a steroid preparation, local anesthetic alone, or steroid alone. They may be done in conjunction with physical therapy and deep pressure massage.
3. Physical and occupational therapy: stretching, strengthening exercises, deep pressure massage, soft tissue mobilization, passive measures such as heat, cold, and ultrasound
4. Medical acupuncture

Key Treatment: Myofascial Pain Syndrome

- NSAIDs
- Analgesics
- Antidepressants
- Muscle relaxants
- TrP injections
- Stretching
- Strengthening exercises
- Deep pressure massage
- Soft tissue mobilization
- Passive measures such as heat, cold, and ultrasound
- Acupuncture

Prognosis

Most patients respond within 2 months after appropriate treatment, but a small number have chronic pain refractory to treatment.

SACROILIAC JOINT DYSFUNCTION

Anatomy

1. Iliolumbar ligament stabilizes L5.
2. Upper and lower sacroiliac (SI) ligaments hold the two SI joints in proper alignment, acting as anchors.
3. Superficial lumbodorsal facia transfers the forces of walking across the pelvis and back.
4. Ligaments crisscross.
5. Paraspinous muscles, gluteus maximus, and hamstrings attach to the SI ligaments.

Physiology

1. SI ligaments support the mechanics of walking.
2. They also support upright posture.
3. If SI ligaments become lax, the bony structures are not held in alignment. Muscles then contract to compensate, leading to poor posture and pain.
4. There is little movement in ligaments.
5. Minor trauma (e.g., lifting injury, motor vehicle accident) can rupture ligaments, causing a popping sensation and local pain, with or without radiating pain.

Basic Neurologic Examination

1. Standing forward bending: abnormal if one posterosuperior iliac spine (PSIS) is higher than the other. Supine, the patient has a leg length discrepancy, representing an iliac shift.
2. Ligamentous stress tests: performed with the patient supine
   a. Straight leg raising: evaluates nerves, ligaments, and muscles
   b. Forced hip flexion: stresses the iliolumbar ligament. Posterior stress with hip in 90° of flexion stresses the lower SI ligaments, reproducing pain.
   c. Palpation: Ligaments are superficial. Palpation is painful if ligaments are injured and mildly uncomfortable if the ligaments are normal. The iliolumbar ligament is palpated along the iliac crest lateral to the L5 spinous process. Upper SI ligaments are below the PSIS.

Clinical Features

1. Pain is present that increases with walking, sitting, or standing and improves with position change.
2. Iliolumbar ligament refers pain to the groin and hip.
3. SI ligaments refer pain down the back and lateral aspects of the leg.

Treatment

1. Physical therapy to stabilize SI joint
2. Stretching and strengthening exercise
3. NSAIDs
4. SI joint injection
5. Surgical stabilization

 Bibliography

Kriegler JS: Fibromyalgia. In Katirji B, Kaminski H, Preston D, et al (eds), Neuromuscular Disorders in Clinical Practice. Boston, Butterworth Heinemann, 2002.

Moldofsky H, Wong MTH, Lue FA: Litigation, sleep. symptoms and disabilities in post-accident pain (fibromyalgia). J Rheumatol 20:1935–1940, 1993.

Ravin TH: An in-depth look at the sacroiliac joint. Part I, pp. 1–3 and Part II, pp. 4–6. Neuropractice, 1996.

Simons DG, Travel JG, Simons LS: Myofascial Pain and Dysfunction: The Trigger Point Manual, 2nd ed. Baltimore, Williams & Wilkins, 1999.

Wolfe F, Anderson J, Harkness D, et al.: Health status and disease severity in fibromyalgia: results of a six-center longitudinal study. Arthritis Rheum 40:1571, 1997.

Wolfe F, Smythe HA, Yunus MB, et al.: The American College of Rheumatology 1990 criteria for the classification of fibromyalgia: report of the multicenter criteria committee. Arthritis Rheum 33:160, 1990.

6 Treatment of Chronic Neck and Back Pain

Edward C. Covington

Definition

1. Back pain is the second most common reason for medical office visits and the most common reason for workers' compensation.

2. It is essentially universal, but back-related disability is epidemic. In the United States, 2% of the work force has compensable back pain at any given time.

3. The lifetime prevalence of significant neck pain is probably 40% to 70% at a given time; approximately 9% of men and 12% of women have neck complaints.

4. Most spine pain results from degenerative and traumatic factors. Other causes, including neoplastic, infectious, and systemic inflammatory conditions, will not be addressed here.

5. Much treatment is ineffective, and it is regionally idiosyncratic. For example, in the United States, which has 4.6 times the population of the United Kingdom, the medical costs for lower back pain (LBP) are 11 times greater, there are 18 times more MRIs (magnetic resonance imaging scans), 11 times more spine operations, and 23 times more fusions. Patients tend to be dissatisfied in both systems.

6. The pathophysiology of spine pain is unexplained in most cases. Most people with symptoms have few findings, and most of those with findings have no symptoms. Over half of asymptomatic people have disc bulges on MRI; 2% have disc protrusions, and 1% have disc extrusions. In people under the age of 60 years who have never had back pain, 20% may have herniated discs.

Identification of Risk for Adverse Outcome

Because chronicity is determined by orthopedic, psychological, and social factors, management of spine disability must consider more than spine pathology. Although 90% of acute LBP patients return to work within 3 months, continuous or recurrent pain affects 30% to 40%, and neck pain after vehicle accidents persists in 24%. In acute radicular pain with disc prolapse/protrusion, application for retirement was best predicted by depression and work hassles. The only somatic predictor was degree of disc displacement—the less the displacement, the worse the outcome. The best predictors of back-related absenteeism are prior back problems, job dissatisfaction, poor performance appraisals, feeling underpaid, and lower socioeconomic status. Chronicity is also associated with nonorganic findings, leg pain, self-rated disability, multiple recurrences, current and prior compensation and litigation, and workers' compensation involvement.

1. Chronic pain syndrome
   It is important to distinguish chronic pain from chronic pain *syndrome* (CPS), defined by the Social Security Administration as intractable pain of ≥ 6 months duration, with
   a. Marked alteration of behavior with depression or anxiety
   b. Marked restriction in daily activities
   c. Excessive use of medication and frequent use of medical services
   d. No clear relationship to organic disorder
   e. History of multiple, non-productive tests, treatment, and surgeries

2. Most CPS patients have preexisting psychopathology and disability that is disproportionate to objective illness. By contrast, spine patients with little psychopathology had more findings, but much less impairment.

3. Psychological factors in chronic pain
   a. Cognitions: Pain is increased and causes more dysfunction when it is mysterious or is thought to presage disaster. "Catastrophic" interpretations of pain and self-perceptions of helplessness increase disability.
   b. Incentives: Illness behaviors may increase without a direct relation to nociception in response to positive reinforcers (caretaking, drugs, money) and avoidance of noxious situations. Disability can be a form of pain behavior because it is strongly influenced by incentives and disincentives for vocational recovery.
   c. Fear of injury engenders inactivity, deconditioning, and susceptibility to strains/sprains. This cycle is a prominent and easily treatable cause of regression and dysfunction.
   d. Psychiatric illness in chronic pain
      (1) The prevalence of depression varies from 10% to 83%. Because the depression usu-

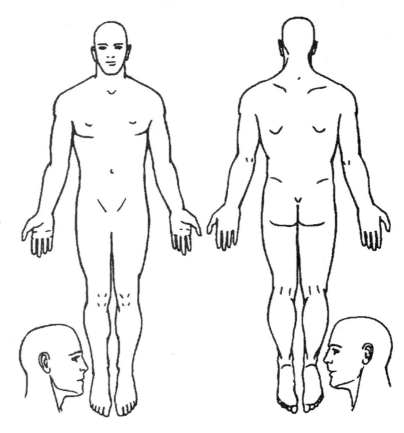

Figure 6–1. Sample illustration used for pain drawings.

ally results not only from pain but also from loss of activities and perceived helplessness, it responds to rehabilitation.

(2) Anxiety amplifies pain and provides disincentives for recovery. Tension promotes muscle contractions and other physiological responses that worsen pain. Anger may play a critical role in chronic pain, and those preoccupied with external blame have reduced treatment response.

(3) Addictive disorders promote pain behavior, hyperalgesia, and regression. Probably 23% of chronic pain patients have active medication misuse or dependency, with 9% in remission.

(4) *Psychogenic pain* is a controversial concept that is supported by the presence of multiple pains in somatization disorder. Hypochondriasis, dementia, psychosis, and factitious disorder may also present with pain. New onset of conversion/somatization in the elderly is rare, and often heralds dementia.

(5) Malingering is not a psychiatric illness. It is thought to be uncommon, based on little data.

(6) Personality disorders predispose to CPS. Parents of CPS patients often have chronic

pain, depression, or alcoholism, and developmental histories often include neglect, loss, abuse, molestation, and excessive early responsibility.

Diagnosis

1. History

   a. Pain description includes severity, quality, and exacerbating and relieving factors.

   b. Pain drawings help identify such patterns as radiculopathy, Herpes zoster, peripheral neuropathy, or post-stroke pain (Fig. 6–1). They usually highlight anatomically understandable locations or more diffuse areas in fibromyalgia, connective tissue disease, and endocrinopathies. Bizarre, multiple locations, and pain outside the body suggest functional components.

   c. Impairments in work, recreation, chores, socialization, self-care, and sexuality should be noted. Down time (hours spent reclining), shut-in status, living in night clothes are significant. The concordance between dysfunction and identified pathology is of major diagnostic importance.

   d. Emotional symptoms—e.g., depression, anxiety, and irritability—should be elicited. Posttraumatic stress disorder is suggested by "re-experiencing" (flashbacks, nightmares), anxiety with startle response, and avoidance of situations reminiscent of the original trauma.

e. Addiction is suggested by moodiness, forgetfulness, irritability, incoordination, multisourcing, rapid dose escalation, and reports of lost or stolen medicines. Tolerance and withdrawal are expected with chronic opioids and do not indicate addiction, the essence of which is captured by the "3 C's":

(1) Craving/compulsive use

(2) Loss of control (inability to regulate the amount consumed)

(3) Continued use despite adverse consequences

f. It is important to distinguish pseudoaddiction, in which drug-seeking behaviors result from inadequate treatment.

g. Psychogenic symptoms are suggested by nonphysiologic signs and behavioral inconsistencies. Patients may be dramatic, may deny nonmedical problems, and may be cheerful despite severe disability, or they may be depressed. An inability to discuss nonsomatic issues suggests a component of psychogenic pain.

h. Response of family and friends should ideally consist of appropriate support with neither rejection nor excessive caretaking.

i. Stresses, most commonly work, family, and entitlement agencies, should be noted. An absence of nonmedical stresses suggests the presence of denial.

j. Litigation/disability income: Disability income may be less relevant than being in the process of obtaining it, which requires demonstration of dysfunction and pain. It is hard to get well while trying to prove how sick one is.

k. Collateral information helps confirm histories that are weakened by poor recollection, drug-impaired understanding, and the need to portray oneself favorably. Other people close to the patient may disclose substance abuse, functional impairment, depression, or suicide threats.

Items for History

- Pain: severity, modifiers, quality
- Impairment
- Emotional response
- Gains/losses
- Stress

---

1. Examination

a. Physical

(1) It is important to note whether findings are consistent among themselves, with known pathology, from time to time, and from observer to observer.

(2) Waddell's nonphysiologic signs in LBP patients correlate with psychopathology, excessive health care utilization, and poor treatment response.

b. Mental status examination should note apparent distress and autonomic arousal (moist palms, tight facial muscles, rapid pulse). Pain behaviors and their appropriateness should be recorded, along with somatic preoccupation and affect, including its appropriateness to the level of pain and disability. Medication intoxication is important to note, as is inordinate dependence on companions, often shown by looking to them for answers or presenting questionnaires in another person's handwriting. Brief assessment of cognitive function and general knowledge may clarify disincentives for employment. Inordinate blame, anger, and external locus of control are notable.

c. Testing with self-assessment instruments for pain severity (0–10 scale), mood (e.g., Beck Depression Inventory), and functional impairment (Pain Disability Index, Roland-Morris, Oswestry Questionnaire) can expedite evaluation and provide documentation of treatment response.

Key Indications: Mental Status Concerns with Spine Pain

- Distress
- Pain behaviors
- Somatic preoccupation
- Locus of responsibility
- Medication effects
- Affect, appropriateness to pain, disability
- Dependence on companions
- Cognition
- Blame/anger

---

2. Regional anesthesia: Diagnostic nerve blocks may identify nociceptive pathways, pain mechanisms (e.g., sympathetic), and anatomic sources of pain (e.g., facet joints, brain).

3. Discography: Reproduction of typical pain by contrast injection into a degenerated disc, when

such injection into adjacent discs does not reproduce pain, may identify "discogenic pain" and suggest possible benefit from fusion or intradiscal thermocoagulation.

Treatment

The plethora of treatments for chronic spine pain is testimony to the frequent failure of all treatments to provide relief. Given the multifactorial nature of such pain, combined parallel treatments may be required. Pain perception may require medications, nerve blocks, or transcutaneous electrical nerve stimulation (TENS); depression may respond to psychotherapy and education; and deconditioning to behavior modification, and work hardening.

1. Prevention of chronicity: Early aggressive intervention reduces disability, as does rapid resumption of normal activities. A program of exercises, ergonomic education, relaxation and coping skills training reduces absenteeism, pain, anxiety, fatigue, and insomnia. Impeding access to specialists and diagnostic studies, so that patients must spend months demonstrating illness, is counterproductive.

2. Education: The fact that uncertainty worsens pain and disability poses a special challenge in spine pain, given its ambiguous pathophysiology, the disparate terminology of various disciplines, and the attribution of symptoms to imaging findings that are common in asymptomatic patients. It is essential to educate patients about their pathology, if known, the current inability of medicine to explain most spine pain, its typically benign nature, and the difference between hurt and harm—so that they are not inappropriately deterred from reconditioning programs that may at first increase pain. Education must include family members lest they inadvertently promote regression.

3. Exercise and physical reconditioning: The clinical picture of chronic LBP is largely attributable to deactivation with attendant impairments in flexibility, strength, and endurance. Similar, though usually less marked, changes occur with neck pain. Deactivation increases pain and precludes healthy distractions. It seems obvious that pain treatment must include rehabilitation, yet this aspect of care is often neglected.

4. Massage: Although the mechanism is unclear, there is evidence that massage is beneficial. It was equal to acupuncture acutely and was superior at 1 year. It was initially superior to a self-care educational program.

5. Transcutaneous electrical neurostimulation: Early efficacy of TENS is well supported, but most studies show reduced benefit over time.

Because most studies are poor and not all studies have shown benefit, there is a lack of convincing evidence in chronic pain. Purchasers of TENS units perceive improvement in pain, work, home, and social activities, and decreased use of physical therapy, occupational therapy, chiropractic, and medications.

6. Manipulation: Studies in back patients, often not of good quality, generally demonstrate some benefit from osteopathic and chiropractic manipulation, with reduced need for analgesics and other therapies. Patient satisfaction is high, perhaps in part because of unambiguous explanations, time, and 'touch.' Manipulation is less demonstrably beneficial for neck pain.

7. Acupuncture: Demonstrated to be analgesic in humans and animals, lasting benefit of acupuncture for chronic pain remains to be proved.

8. Epidural steroid injections are superior to placebo in the short term, but study outcomes differ as to whether steroids are superior to local anesthetics or muscle relaxants. Reviews are inconclusive as to long-term benefit. Number-needed-to-treat calculations suggest that for 1 person with LBP/sciatica to obtain 75% relief for 1 to 60 days, 6 need to be treated. For 1 to obtain 3 to 12 months of 50% relief, 11 would have to be treated.

9. Intradiscal electrothermal annuloplasty (IDET): The belief that discogenic pain results from annular tears or internal disc disruption led to treatment with percutaneous thermal coagulation of the disc (as selected by provocative discography). Preliminary studies report benefit at 1 year with few complications. The rationale for IDET is challenged by findings that the site of annular tears on discography does not correlate with the site of the patient's pain.

10. Facet denervation via radiofrequency medial branch neurotomy is useful for whiplash-induced pain that originates in the facet joint, some cervicogenic headaches, and pain of lumbar facet origin. Complications are few.

11. Spinal cord stimulation: Most studies of back pain (usually with radicular component) report ≥ 50% relief in > 50% of patients; however, study quality is marginal. Response as measured by patient satisfaction and pain relief is considerably better than that reflected in return to work.

12. Back "schools" provide exercises and education concerning spine health. They are effective for chronic LBP patients and reduce functional impairment.

13. Pharmacotherapy: Traditional pharmacotherapy relies on central analgesics (opioids) and peripheral analgesics (nonsteroidal anti-inflammatory

drugs—NSAIDs) and is most effective in nociceptive pain. Neuropathic pains, which result from injury to neural tissue, perineural inflammation, or other causes of neural sensitization, may respond better to antidepressants, anticonvulsants, or other agents.

a. Nonsteroidal anti-inflammatory drugs

 (1) Especially useful for inflammatory and bone pain. Discs may leak substances that produce perineural inflammation, perhaps explaining benefit in some neuropathic pains.

 (2) Evidence of efficacy in acute spine pain is better than for chronic pain.

 (3) Various NSAIDs appear equally effective.

 (4) Gastrointestinal complications of NSAIDs are the most prevalent category of adverse drug reactions in the United States and cause 16,500 deaths annually. NSAIDs that selectively inhibit cyclooxygenase-2 are less likely to produce these effects, due to sparing inhibition of cytoprotective mucosal prostaglandins.

b. Chronic opioid therapy (COT)

 (1) Opioids are most helpful in dull, aching, visceral pain, and less so for quick, sharp pains and skin pains. Sedating doses are often required to relieve deafferentation pain and some types of allodynia.

 (2) While efficacy for *acute* spine pain is unquestioned, usefulness in *chronic* pain is less clear. Fears that tolerance would eliminate analgesic efficacy proved to be overly pessimistic, and COT has recently become widely supported. The literature in spine pain consists mostly of case series, which are generally positive.

 (3) Naturally long-acting (methadone) or sustained-release preparations are less addicting and probably more efficacious.

 (4) COT has been successful even in people with addictive disorders. Patients who abuse the treatment tend to do so early. Those who are active in AA, have stable support systems, and who lack a history of polysubstance abuse tend to fare better.

 (5) Enthusiasm for COT is tempered by (a) reports of pain reduction following opioid *elimination,* (b) studies showing only transient benefit in myofascial and rheumatic pain, and (c) evidence of opioid-induced hyperalgesia after chronic use. There may be a dissociation between efficacy and satisfaction. Patient and family satisfaction with intrathecal opioids was excellent despite a six-fold increase in opioid requirement after 4 years, little pain reduction, persistent marked functional impairment, and numerous side effects.

 (6) Risks

  (a) Iatrogenic addiction from opioid use for *acute* pain is rare, although relapse of a prior addictive disorder may not be. *Pseudoaddiction* is easily confused with true addiction. Iatrogenic addiction in *chronic* use also seems rare, but the incidence is unknown because most studies are short term.

  (b) Functional impairment is not found after decades of methadone use by heroin addicts. They are safe to drive and work. Opioid-induced functional impairment should be weighed against the potential impairment from anticonvulsants, antidepressants, and unrelieved pain.

 (7) Conclusions: Some people are harmed by chronic opioids; others are helped. We lack good predictors, beyond the idea that CPS, being due in large part to nonnociceptive factors, will respond poorly. A 6-month trial of COT is low risk, with the caveat that treatment should be terminated unless clear improvements in pain and quality of life are demonstrated.

Key Treatment: Chronic Opioid Therapy

Monitor the 5 "A's":

• Analgesia

• Affect

• Activity level

• Adverse effects

• Aberrant behaviors

c. Atypical analgesics

 (1) Antidepressants are analgesic in neuropathic pain, fibromyalgia, migraine prophylaxis, and perhaps visceral hyperalgesia. Studies reporting the best efficacy used full therapeutic doses. Tricyclic antidepressants are greatly superior to selective serotonin reuptake inhibitors (SSRIs) for pain, and venlafaxine may have tricyclic benefits with SSRI-like side effects. Early studies suggested that antidepressants are *not* effective for spine pain;

however, a more recent study found benefit in LBP from maprotiline (≤150 mg/day). Thus the role of antidepressants in spine pain is unclear. Analgesia has not been shown with trazodone, bupropion, and several SSRIs.

(2) Antiepileptic drugs have demonstrated efficacy for neuropathic pain—e.g., radiculitis, arachnoiditis, and post-laminectomy syndrome—but not for nociceptive axial pain. Useful agents include those that (a) block fast-acting Na⁺ channels (carbamazepine), (b) increase GABA effects (valproate, tiagabine), (c) interfere with excitatory amino acids (topiramate), and (d) attenuate transport through calcium channels on second-order neurons (gabapentin). Relative efficacy of various anticonvulsants and antidepressants is largely unknown.

(3) Antiarrhythmics may inhibit discharge in animal neuromas and relieve allodynia from cord injuries. Mexiletine, a lidocaine analogue, has been used for various neuropathic pains. Experimental support is equivocal but is strongest in studies using high doses. A trial of IV lidocaine probably predicts response. Other antiarrhythmics are rarely used because of proarrhythmic effects. These agents have diminished in popularity as anti-epileptic drugs have shown improved efficacy.

(4) Neuroleptic agents were reported to reduce neuropathic pain in old uncontrolled studies, usually in combination with tricyclic antidepressants. The lack of good data coupled with the risk of tardive dyskinesia has relegated them to last-resort status for most pains. There are no studies of use in axial pain.

d. Muscle relaxants, by and large, do not affect muscles, but are sedatives or central analgesics. They appear equally effective for acute spine pain but not for chronic spine pain. Most are benign, except that carisoprodol is addictive. Baclofen reduces spasticity, especially when given intrathecally. Tizanidine relieves pain due to spasticity, and may also have nonspecific analgesic activity. In *acute* LBP it relieved spasm better than diazepam, but there are no studies in chronic LBP. Cyclobenzaprine, a tricyclic, reduces pain in fibromyalgia.

14. Biofeedback training/relaxation therapies: With the aid of visual or audio feedback, patients can learn to regulate such functions as digital temperature, surface electromyogram (EMG), and palmar sweating. This provides generalized relaxation and pain reduction. Paraspinal EMG feedback is commonly used with chronic LBP patients. Effects are similar to those of relaxation training, self-hypnosis, and meditation, with which it is often combined. Such techniques may improve pain, function, mood, health care utilization, and catastrophic thinking. In a multidisciplinary pain rehabilitation program, chronic pain patients generally rate biofeedback and exercises as the most helpful program components. Most studies of such relaxation treatments as Progressive Muscular Relaxation find pain reduction but do not demonstrate superiority to other treatments.

15. Behavior modification: Withdrawal of social reinforcers of "pain behavior," and consistently rewarding such "wellness behaviors" as exercising and conversing about nonmedical issues demonstrably lead to improvements in pain and in psychological and physical function. Compared with cognitive therapy, operant treatment produced greater immediate effects on medication intake and functional impairment. Although this is not easily provided in an office practice, family members can be educated about the advantages of attending more to the person and less to the symptoms. At the same time, the person's life situation can be reviewed to determine whether disincentives to recovery can be replaced with rewards.

16. Cognitive–behavioral therapies, which trains spine patients to identify, challenge, and alter automatic maladaptive thinking patterns, is consistently shown to improve activity and psychological function. Studies find reductions in pain and medication use and improvements in mood, pain behavior, and function.

17. Multidisciplinary pain programs (MDP): Typically range from a few hours a week to inpatient in intensity. They typically attempt to replace "sick role" behaviors with normal activities. Such programs are indicated when appropriate treatments in less intensive settings fail to produce functional restoration or when there is an inability to cope with residual pain. Typically the clientele of such programs is more than two thirds spine pain patients (Table 6–1). Extensive studies confirm improved pain, function, affect, drug use, and health care utilization. Vocational recovery is often achieved, but less reliably than other treatment goals. Effects are stable over time and typically include 14% to 60% pain reduction; up to 73% decrease in opioid use; and dramatic increases in activity levels, with 43%

TABLE 6–1. COMMON MULTIDISCIPLINARY PAIN PROGRAM COMPONENTS

Reconditioning physical therapy	Nerve blocks	Treatment of psychiatric comorbidity
Operant conditioning	Biofeedback/ relaxation training	Detoxification/ weaning
Medications	TENS	Chemical dependence treatment
Education	Psychotherapies	Coping skills training

more participants working after treatment than before; a 90% reduction in physician visits, fewer surgeries; 65% fewer hospitalizations; and 35% fewer disability applications. MDPs return 50% to 150% more people to work than surgery, and 2.6 times more than spinal cord stimulation. Cost–benefit analysis suggested that MDP treatment results in a savings of over $10,500 the first year, with greater savings in subsequent years, based on 1995 dollars. Each person saved from total permanent disability results in a savings of $350,000 in disability benefits over that person's earning lifetime. The necessary and sufficient components and duration of MDPs are unclear. They are less useful in people with "needs" to remain disabled, e.g., those who see their jobs as dangerous or intolerable, who lack skills, and who are in the process of applying for disability income.

18. Self-help groups: Spine patients benefit from mutual support, the understanding of those who have "been there," and encouragement to optimize quality of life despite pain, rather than deferring life while seeking a cure. The American Chronic Pain Association supports such groups, provides information on existing chapters, and helps to set up new chapters.

Treatment Failures

There is a residual group of chronic spine pain patients for whom all rational treatments have failed. Some have severe spinal pathology, while others are unable to rehabilitate for psychiatric reasons. Heroic efforts to correct pathology of questionable relevance to their pain typically make them worse. Some respond, at least for a time, to intrathecal analgesics, and spinal cord stimulation helps some, but for many we have no acceptable answer. Chronic opioids (long half-life) may provide comfort and should be used, where possible, as an incentive to promote life activities. Beyond this, support may be all that can be provided.

Conclusions

Early identification of patients at risk for chronicity is critical, as this group accounts for most of the human and economic costs as well as the best opportunities for preventive intervention. Pain and disability in chronic spine pain are multifactorial, reflecting organic, psychological, and socioeconomic issues; therefore treatment must address all of these domains. The overall chronic pain experience typically involves pain, affective suffering, loss of function, and behavioral abnormalities. Each of these elements may require specific interventions. The evidence is compelling that even patients who have failed all reasonable and surgical treatments can have excellent outcomes, in terms of function and quality of life, after intensive multidisciplinary treatment.

B Bibliography

Covington EC: A pain medicine approach to chronic low back pain. Continuum. 7:112–140, 2001.

Hasenbring M, Marienfeld G, Kuhlendahl D, Soyka D: Risk factors of chronicity in lumbar disc patients. A prospective investigation of biologic, psychologic, and social predictors of therapy outcome. Spine 19:2759–2765, 1994.

McQuay HJ, Moore RA, Eccleston C, et al.: Systematic review of outpatient services for chronic pain control. Health Technol Assess 1:1–135, 1997.

Van Tulder MW, Koes BW, Bouter LM: Conservative treatment of acute and chronic nonspecific low back pain. A systematic review of randomized controlled trials of the most common interventions. Spine 22:2128–2156, 1997.

Vingard E, Mortimer M, Wiktorin C, et al.: Seeking Care for Low Back Pain in the General Population: A Two-Year Follow-up Study: Results From the MUSIC-Norrtalje Study. Spine 27:2159–2165, 2002.

1 Inflammatory Spondyloarthropathies

Richard B. Rosenbaum
Kimberly L. Goslin

Definition

1. Ankylosing spondylitis (AS) is the prototypic inflammatory spondyloarthropathy, characterized clinically by the inflammatory type of low back pain and radiographically by evidence of sacroiliitis.

2. Reactive arthritis (formerly known at Reiter's syndrome), psoriatic arthritis, and arthritis associated with inflammatory bowel disease are additional examples of spondyloarthropathies.

3. Extraspinal features of spondyloarthropathies can include peripheral inflammatory arthritis of a few large joints or of multiple symmetrical joints, particularly distal interphalangeal joints; enthesopathies (inflammation of tendon insertions, such as Achilles' tendinitis or sausage digits); mucocutaneous lesions, such as oral ulcers, psoriasis, keratoderma blenorrhagica, or urethritis; inflammatory eye disease, particularly iritis; and cardiac disease, classically aortitis leading to aortic insufficiency.

Epidemiology

1. Ankylosing spondylitis has a prevalence in the United States of about 1:500. Psoriatic arthritis is common, affecting about one-tenth of patients with psoriasis. Reactive arthritis and spondyloarthropathy with inflammatory bowel disease are less common.

2. For AS, the ratio of clinically affected men to women is 3:1, and men tend to have more severe spinal disease. When women are affected, they often have peripheral manifestations such as acral arthritis or uveitis.

3. Symptoms usually begin before age 40 years.

Etiology and Pathophysiology

1. A genetic predisposition is important, usually associated in AS with the presence of HLA-B27.

2. A preceding antigenic challenge, such as an infection with Shigella, Salmonella, Yersinia, Campylobacter, or Chlamydia in reactive arthritis, may begin a process of molecular mimicry leading to autoimmune disease.

Clinical Neurologic Findings

1. Inflammatory low back pain is a diagnosis based on history. No specific physical findings reliably diagnose sacroiliitis. Limitation of lumber flexion (Schober's test) does not distinguish spondyloarthropathy from other forms of low back pain. Advanced spondyloarthropathy results in limited chest expansion or increased kyphosis.

2. Spinal cord compression is the most devastating neurologic complication of inflammatory spondyloarthropathies. Patients with chronic spinal ankylosis are at risk for spinal fractures, particularly in the cervical spine after relatively mild trauma. Less common causes of spinal cord compression disk and vertebral body destruction, usually in the low thoracic or high lumbar spine, spinal canal stenosis, or atlantoaxial joint dislocation (discussed in more detail in Part XX, Chapter 4, Rheumatoid Arthritis).

3. Posterior diverticuli of the lumbar arachnoid are an unusual but distinctive later complication of inflammatory spondyloarthropathies. The neurologic presentation is insidious evolution of cauda equina dysfunction.

4. A mild symmetric proximal myopathy, characterized by normal or mild elevation of creatine kinase, normal or minimally abnormal electromyogram, and nonspecific noninflammatory changes on muscle biopsy, sometimes occurs in patients with psoriatic arthritis or advanced spondyloarthropathy.

Key Clinical Findings

- Inflammatory low back pain
- Spinal cord compression
- Lumbar radiculopathy due to arachnoid diverticuli
- Mild myopathy

779

Key Signs of Inflammatory Low Back Pain

- Insidious onset of low back and buttock pain
- Duration greater than 3 months
- Prominent night pain and morning stiffness
- Limitation of spinal motion

Differential Diagnosis

1. Mechanical and nonspecific causes of back pain are much more common than spondyloarthropathies.

2. Most patients with clinical characteristics of inflammatory low back pain do not have demonstrable spondyloarthropathies.

Laboratory Findings

1. The histocompatibility antigen, HLA B-27 is present in about 90% of patients with AS, and to a lesser extent in patients with reactive arthritis, psoriatic arthritis, and arthritis with inflammatory bowel disease. It is present in about 9% of white Americans, of whom only about 5% eventually develop spondyloarthropathy.

2. When eye symptoms are present, slit-lamp examination may confirm a diagnosis of iritis.

Imaging Findings

1. Pelvic anteroposterior radiographs are the usual method of demonstrating sacroiliitis but may be negative in mild cases. Pelvic computed tomography (CT) scanning may increase sensitivity but decrease specificity.

2. Spinal radiographs in advanced spondyloarthropathy can show characteristic changes of squaring of vertebral bodies, calcified syndesmophytes bridging disc spaces, and calcification of spinal ligaments.

3. Lumbar spine magnetic resonance imaging or CT scanning are important in the evaluation of patients with cauda equina dysfunction and are sensitive for arachnoid diverticuli.

Treatment

1. Inflammatory low back pain often responds symptomatically to treatment with nonsteroidal anti-inflammatory drugs.

2. Sulfasalazine for peripheral arthritis and tumor necrosis factor inhibitors are treatment options for more severe disease.

3. No treatment has been shown to prevent progression of the spondyloarthropathy

4. Management of spinal fractures or spinal cord compression requires neurosurgical consultation

5. Treatment of cauda equina syndrome in patients with lumbar diverticuli is challenging. Surgical resection of the diverticuli usually does not improve cauda equina dysfunction. Lumbar-peritoneal shunting has been tried with possible success.

Prevention

No preventive measures are known. Patients with advanced spondyloarthropathy should be educated to avoid spinal trauma and to consult their physicians after spinal trauma, even if apparently mild.

Key Treatment and Prevention

- Nonsteroidal anti-inflammatory drugs
- Sulfasalazine and tumor necrosis factor inhibitors
- Neurosurgical consultation
- Treatment cannot prevent progression of the disease
- No preventive measures are known

Bibliography

Ginsburg WW, Cohen MD, Miller GM, Bartleson JD: Posterior vertebral body erosion by arachnoid diverticula in cauda equina syndrome: an unusual manifestation of ankylosing spondylitis. J Rheumatol 24:1417–1420, 1997.

Sieper J, Braun J, Rudwaleit M, et al.: Ankylosing spondylitis: an overview. Ann Rheum Dis 61 (Suppl 3):III8–III18, 2002.

Weinstein P, Karpman RR, Gall EP, et al.: Spinal injury, spinal fracture, and spinal stenosis in ankylosing spondylitis. J Neurosurg 37:609–616, 1982.

2 Systemic Lupus Erythematosus

Richard B. Rosenbaum
Kimberly L. Goslin

Definition

1. Systemic lupus erythematosus (SLE) is a multi-system, inflammatory autoimmune disease. The American College of Rheumatology classification criteria require that a patient have at least four of the factors shown in the box from Table 2–1 below.
2. The disease may have varied permutations of the classification criteria, has a wide range of severity, and often has a relapsing-remitting course spanning months or years.

Epidemiology

1. Prevalence in the United States is perhaps 1:2500.
2. Female:male ratio is between 7 and 9 to 1.
3. Onset is usually before age 50; patients with a later onset may have a different course.
4. SLE is more common, and perhaps more severe, in some groups, among them, black women.
5. A positive family history is obtained in 10% to 20% of patients with SLE; the concordance in monozygotic twins is 20% to 30%.

Etiology and Pathophysiology

1. The basic immunologic abnormality is production of autoantibodies by B cells and T cell–mediated autoimmunity.
2. Varied mechanisms contribute to varied neurologic manifestations:
   a. Noninflammatory central nervous system (CNS) microangiopathy associated with microinfarcts
   b. Immune complex deposition
   c. Correlation of specific autoantibodies with specific neurologic syndromes

TABLE 2–1. AMERICAN COLLEGE OF RHEUMATOLOGY CLASSIFICATION CRITERIA FOR SYSTEMIC LUPUS ERYTHEMATOSUS

Malar rash	Oral ulcers	Hematologic disorder
Discoid rash	Serositis	Immunologic disorder
Photosensitivity	Renal disorder	Antinuclear antibodies
Arthritis	Neurologic disorder*	

*The criteria for neurologic disorder officially include only seizures and psychosis, but SLE can cause numerous other neurologic syndromes.

d. Coagulation abnormalities with antiphospholipid antibodies causing stroke
   e. Vasculitis, rarely affecting the CNS but often affecting peripheral nerves, causing distal symmetric axonal neuropathy or mononeuritis multiplex

Clinical Neurologic Findings

If carefully studied, most patients with SLE will develop some form of neurologic dysfunction during the course of their illness. The neurologic manifestations of SLE are extremely varied.

1. Seizures, either generalized or partial, occur in over one-tenth of patients with SLE. Seizures can be treated with standard anticonvulsants, including those reported to cause drug-induced SLE syndromes. Seizures by themselves are not an indication for aggressive immunosuppression; the need for anti-inflammatory therapy is assessed based on findings of systemic or CNS inflammation including results of neurologic examination and of neuroimaging.
2. Psychosis or delirium can develop acutely in patients with SLE. These patients must be carefully assessed for alternative causes of encephalopathy, such as opportunistic infections, metabolic disturbances, drug toxicity, or focal brain lesions. Magnetic resonance imaging (MRI), single photon emission computed tomography (SPECT), or antibody studies such as antiribosomal P antibodies are often abnormal in these patients but lack sensitivity and specificity. Once an alternative cause has been excluded, the psychosis or delirium of SLE is usually treated with steroids and sometimes other forms of immunosuppression.
3. Cognitive changes in areas such as attention, memory, and visuospatial function are detectable by psychometric testing in a significant minority of patients with SLE, even if they have never had clinical evidence of other forms of CNS dysfunction. Patients with SLE also have an increased incidence of affective disorders.
4. Headache, either migraine or tension type, is common in patients with SLE. Rarer causes of headache in patients with SLE include specific CNS syndromes such as stroke, meningitis, or pseudotumor cerebri.

5. Stroke or transient ischemic attacks (TIA) can occur in patients with SLE via numerous mechanisms including small-vessel ischemic infarcts, hypercoaguability associated with antiphospholipid antibodies, and cardiogenic emboli. Rare mechanisms of stroke include thromboses in larger intracranial or extracranial arteries, thrombotic thrombocytopenic purpura, intracranial hemorrhages, or cerebral venous thrombosis. Patients with SLE who develop a stroke or TIA need a careful investigation of the stroke mechanism as the basis for therapeutic decisions, such as the need for anticoagulation or immunosuppression.

6. Varied movement disorders have been described in patients with SLE. Chorea, the most common of these, occurs in less than 1% of patients with SLE and is often associated with the presence of antiphospholipid antibodies.

7. Meningitis can be caused by SLE and follow a chronic or recurrent course. The cerebrospinal fluid (CSF) in these cases shows mild leukocytic pleocytosis. CSF glucose is usually normal; CSF protein may be increased. Infectious and drug-induced meningitis are important in the differential diagnosis. Pseudotumor cerebri and hydrocephalus are rare complications of SLE.

8. Cranial neuropathies and brainstem syndromes occur uncommonly in patients with SLE. For example, less than 1% of patients with SLE develop optic neuropathy. Trigeminal neuropathy is discussed in more detail in Part XX, Chapter 5, Progressive Systemic Sclerosis. Peripheral facial palsy may occur. Internuclear ophthalmoplegia can be caused by brainstem stroke or inflammation. Other cranial neuropathies are even rarer in patients with SLE.

9. Acute or subacute transverse myelitis occurs in less than 1% of patients with SLE.

10. Peripheral neuropathy is clinically important in a small minority of patients with SLE, even though the incidence of abnormal nerve conduction studies is much higher. Patients may develop a mild distal symmetric axonal vasculitic neuropathy, usually late in the illness. Patients with SLE may also develop carpal tunnel syndrome. Acute or chronic demyelinating neuropathies, Miller Fisher syndrome, mononeuritis multiplex, or autonomic neuropathies have all been observed in patients with SLE.

11. Inflammatory myopathy develops in some patients with SLE, and SLE should be investigated as a possible cause whenever a patient presents with polymyositis or dermatomyositis.

12. Myasthenia gravis or Eaton-Lambert myasthenic syndrome can occur in patients with SLE.

Key Clinical Findings

- Seizures, generalized or partial
- Psychosis or delirium
- Cognitive changes
- Headache, either migraine or tension type
- Stroke or transient ischemic attack
- Movement disorders (e.g., chorea)
- Meningitis
- Cranial neuropathies and brainstem syndromes (e.g., optic neuropathy, facial palsy, internuclear ophthalmoplegia)
- Transverse myelitis
- Peripheral neuropathy
- Inflammatory neuropathy
- Myasthenia gravis or Eaton-Lambert myasthenic syndrome

Differential Diagnosis

1. Neurologic disease secondary to other systemic factors, including opportunistic CNS infections, drug toxicities, stroke due to hypertension or bleeding diathesis, complications of uremia or pulmonary failure, should always be considered in the differential diagnosis of patients with SLE and neurologic findings.

2. Clinical relatives of SLE

   a. Mixed connective tissue disease may have features of SLE, inflammatory myopathy, and progressive systemic sclerosis. Neurologic complications are similar to those of classic SLE except for a higher incidence of inflammatory myopathy and, probably, of trigeminal sensory neuropathy (see Part XX, Chapter 5).

   b. Primary anti-phospholipid antibody syndrome is associated with venous and arterial thromboses, spontaneous abortions, and thrombocytopenia. Whether associated with an autoimmune disease such as SLE or in the primary syndrome, patients with antiphospholipid antibodies have increased risk of stroke and may present with chorea or myelopathy.

   c. Drug-induced SLE: A number of drugs, including many of the anticonvulsants can cause a syndrome of antinuclear antibodies with joint manifestations or serosis. Neurologic manifestations are unusual in drug-induced lupus.

PEARL

LE is a multisystem, autoimmune inflammatory disease. The diagnosis rests on establishing:

- the involvement of multiple organ systems

- detecting autoantibodies

- excluding other diagnoses

The presence of antinuclear antibodies is not by itself sufficient to establish the diagnosis.

Laboratory Findings

1. Antinuclear antibodies (ANA) are present in almost all patients with SLE but have low specificity because they are also present in patients with many other inflammatory diseases and in 2% to 30% of the normal population. If a patient has a positive test for antinuclear antibodies, serum should be tested for specific subsets of ANA. Anti-double-stranded DNA antibodies are highly specific for SLE and are present in 30% to 80% of patients with SLE. Anti-Smith antibodies are also specific for SLE and are present in 15% to 40% of patients with SLE. Anti-RNP (ribonucleoprotein) antibodies are sensitive for mixed connective tissue disease.

2. CSF findings: A significant minority of patients with SLE and neurologic syndromes have abnormal spinal fluid, most commonly showing only mild leukocytosis or protein elevation. CSF examination can not confirm or refute the diagnosis of CNS SLE, but it is particularly important to exclude alternative diagnoses such as opportunistic CNS infections.

3. Specific autoantibodies

   a. Antiphospholipid antibodies are more common in SLE patients who have neurologic findings than in those who have no evident neurologic disease. Clues to the presence of antiphospholipid antibodies include elevated partial thromboplastin time (PTT), prolongation in more sensitive coagulation tests such as the kaolin clot time or Russell viper venom test, or biologically false-positive serology for syphilis.

   b. Antiribosomal P protein antibodies are present in the serum of perhaps 5/6 of patients with psychosis or depression due to SLE but have low specificity.

   c. Antineuronal antibodies in serum or spinal fluid have been associated in research studies with manifestations such as psychosis but are currently not a clinically useful test.

PEARL

Treatment of neurologic findings in a patient who has SLE is dependent on diagnosis and delineation of the nature and pathophysiology of the patient's neurologic dysfunction.

Imaging Findings

1. In patients with SLE who experience specific stroke or infectious syndromes, MRI or CT brain scanning can be helpful in delineating focal brain lesions. In addition, MRI brain scans of patients with SLE often show abnormalities, including multifocal white matter lesions and brain atrophy. These abnormalities are most common in patients with neurologic manifestations of SLE but can also be found in many patients with SLE who have no clinical or psychometric evidence of CNS disease.

2. SPECT brain scanning can demonstrate multifocal abnormalities of cerebral blood flow in most patients who have CNS manifestations of SLE and in a significant minority of patients with lupus who do not have evidence of CNS dysfunction.

3. Positron emission tomography (PET) brain scanning and MR techniques such as spectroscopy and magnetic transfer imaging have shown abnormalities in SLE patients in research studies but are currently not clinically useful.

Treatment

1. Acute syndromes such as psychosis, transverse myelitis, or focal cerebritis are usually treated with steroids. In patients with more severe neurologic deficits steroids may be used in higher doses or supplemented with other immunosuppressants such as cyclophosphamide.

2. Patients who have had an ischemic stroke or TIA are often given antiplatelet or anticoagulant medication as prophylaxis against additional strokes. Anticoagulation with warfarin is often chosen in these patients if they have antiphospholipid antibodies.

3. Symptomatic treatment is needed for individual syndromes such as seizures, migraine, or movement disorders.

Key Treatment

- Steroids for psychosis, transverse myelitis, and focal cerebritis

- Antiplatelet or anticoagulant medication for ischemic stroke or TIA

- Symptomatic treatment for seizures, migraine, or movement disorders

Prevention

No preventive measures are known.

Pregnancy

1. Women with antiphospholipid antibodies are at risk for miscarriage; aspirin or low-dose heparin treatment decreases the risk.

2. Women with SLE or primary antiphospholipid antibody syndrome who develop chorea may experience worsening of the chorea during pregnancy or while taking oral contraceptives.

Bibliography

Feinglass EJ, Arnett FC, Dorsch CA, et al.: Neuropsychiatric manifestations of systemic lupus erythematosus: diagnosis, clinical spectrum, and relationship to other features of the disease. Medicine 55:323–339, 1976.

Hanly JG: Evaluation of patients with CNS involvement in SLE. Balliere's Clin Rheumatol 12:415–431, 1998.

Johnson RT, Richardson EP: The neurological manifestations of systemic lupus erythematosus. Medicine 47:337–369, 1968.

Nadeau SE: Neurologic manifestations of connective tissue disease. Neurol Clin 20:151–178, 2002.

Omdal R, Mellgren SI, Goransson L, et al.: Small nerve fiber involvement in systemic lupus erythematosus: a controlled study. Arthritis Rheum 46:1228–1232, 2002.

Toubi E, Khamashta MA, Panarra A, et al.: Association of antiphospholipid antibodies with central nervous system disease in systemic lupus erythematosus. Am J Med 99:397–401, 1995.

3 Sjögren's Syndrome

Richard B. Rosenbaum
Kimberly L. Goslin

Definition

1. Sjögren's syndrome is an autoimmune disease manifest primarily by inflammation of exocrine glands, such as the lacrimal and salivary glands.

2. Lacrimal gland disease can cause dry eyes (xerophthalmia). Salivary gland disease can cause dry mouth (xerostomia). Sicca syndrome is the combination of xerophthalmia and xerostomia

3. Diagnostic criteria vary. Stricter criteria require objective evidence of sicca and either a positive minor salivary gland biopsy or a positive anti-SSA or anti-SSB antibody.

4. Sjögren's syndrome can have varied systemic manifestations including arthralgias, generalized symptoms such as fever and weight loss, dry skin or mucous membranes, thyroiditis or hypothyroidism, interstitial nephritis, vasculitis, anemia, lymphoma or pseudolymphoma, hypergammaglobulinemia or monoclonal gammopathy, and pulmonary or gastrointestinal dysfunction.

Epidemiology

1. The perceived prevalence of Sjögren's syndrome is heavily dependent on the diagnostic criteria used. Prevalence has been placed as high as 3% but is much lower if strict criteria for inflammation and autoimmunity are used.

2. Women are more frequently affected than men, and prevalence increases with increasing age.

3. Most patients with Sjögren's syndrome have an associated rheumatic disease such as rheumatoid arthritis (RA); these patients are classified as having secondary Sjögren's syndrome.

4. Primary Sjögren's syndrome is less common than secondary Sjögren's syndrome, but most instances of neurologic complications occur in patients with secondary Sjögren's syndrome.

Etiology and Pathophysiology

1. The autoimmune inflammatory response in Sjögren's syndrome includes infiltration of affected exocrine glands by B and T lymphocytes. T lymphocyte infiltration of dorsal root ganglia has been observed in patients with Sjögren's syndrome and sensory neuronopathy.

2. The pathogenic role of autoantibodies in Sjögren's syndrome is poorly understood. Anti-SSA or anti-SSB antibody levels correlate poorly with neurologic manifestations. Anti-neuronal antibodies have been identified in brain tissue of some patients who have Sjögren's syndrome and neurologic illness.

Clinical Neurologic Findings

1. The incidence of central nervous system (CNS) dysfunction due to Sjögren's syndrome is low. Alexander and colleagues described a wide variety of neurologic syndromes in patients with Sjögren's syndrome, including cognitive and affective illnesses; focal or multifocal recurrent neurologic illnesses mimicking relapsing-remitting multiple sclerosis; and myelopathies. However, these associations are unusual.

2. Patients with Sjögren's syndrome may be at increased risk for recurrent headaches, usually unassociated with specific neuropathology. However, recurrent aseptic meningitis is a rare manifestation of primary Sjögren's syndrome. In other patients with Sjögren's syndrome, asymptomatic meningeal inflammation can occur.

3. Trigeminal sensory neuropathy can occur in association with Sjögren's syndrome, as it does with progressive systemic sclerosis (see Part XX, Chapter 5, Progressive Systemic Sclerosis). Optic neuritis is rarely associated with Sjögren's syndrome.

4. Familiar peripheral nerve manifestations of Sjögren's syndrome include symmetric distal sensory or sensorimotor neuropathy, autonomic neuropathy, and carpal tunnel syndrome.

5. Sensory neuronopathy is a distinctive syndrome characterized by large fiber sensory dysfunction, causing asymmetric sensory loss on trunk or limbs. Patients can have tendon areflexia, sensory ataxia, and autonomic dysfunction. In this rare syndrome patients may meet diagnostic criteria for Sjögren's syndrome but do not manifest other systemic evidence of primary Sjögren's syndrome.

6. Polymyositis or dermatomyositis can occur in patients with Sjögren's syndrome. An unusual cause of muscle weakness associated with Sjögren's syndrome is hypokalemic paralysis due to renal tubular acidosis.

PEARL

Patients with Sjögren's syndrome may display a wide variety of central nervous system manifestations; however, only a small minority of these patients are clinically affected.

Differential Diagnosis

1. The sicca syndrome can be attributed to Sjögren's syndrome only if the patient has evidence of inflammation and autoimmunity.

2. Sicca and signs of autoimmunity can occur in some patients with infections such as hepatitis C or human immunodeficiency virus.

3. Patients with a clinical diagnosis of multiple sclerosis may have symptoms of sicca but rarely have Sjögren's syndrome.

Key Diagnostic Criterion

- The diagnosis of Sjögren's syndrome requires not only the presence of sicca syndrome but also demonstration of an inflammatory autoimmune illness, often with varied systemic manifestations.

Laboratory Findings

1. Many patients with Sjögren's syndrome have serologic evidence of autoantibodies; rheumatoid factor, anti-SSA (Ro), and anti-SSB (La) antibodies are each present in up to 70% of patients with Sjögren's syndrome; positive antinuclear antibodies (ANA) are even more common. None of these autoantibodies are specific for Sjögren's syndrome.

2. Eye dryness can be quantified by Schirmer's test. Keratitis due to dry eyes can be evaluated by slit-lamp examination using rose Bengal or fluorescein dyes.

3. Minor salivary gland biopsies, if interpreted with strict criteria, can have a specificity over 90% and sensitivity over 60% for diagnosis of Sjögren's syndrome.

4. Some patients with Sjögren's syndrome and neurologic symptoms have nonspecific abnormalities of the cerebrospinal fluid (CSF) such as mononuclear pleocytosis, increased protein, increased intrathecal production of immunoglobulin (IgG), or oligoclonal bands.

Key Laboratory Findings

- Serologic evidence of autoanitbodies

- Specificity over 90% and sensitivity over 60% with minor salivary gland biopsies

- Nonspecific CSF abnormalities such as mononuclear pleocytosis, increased protein, increased intrathecal production of IgG, or oligoclonal bands.

Imaging Findings

1. Magnetic resonance brain scans can show multifocal deep and subcortical cerebral white matter lesions in patients with Sjögren's syndrome, even if they have no clinical manifestations of CNS disease

2. Technetium-99–hexamethyl propylene-amine-oxime (HMPAO)-single photon emission computed tomography abnormalities have been described in some patients with Sjögren's syndrome.

Treatment

When patients with Sjögren's syndrome develop neurologic syndromes, various steroid and immunosuppressive regimens are often tried, with more aggressive drugs and higher doses reserved for patients with greater neurologic impairment; however, data permitting assessment of these therapies are scant.

Key Treatment

- Various steroid and immunosuppressive regimens

- Aggressive regimens and higher doses for patients with greater neurologic impairment

- Data assessing these therapies are scant.

Prevention

No preventive measures are known.

Bibliography

Alexander E: Central nervous system disease in Sjögren's syndrome. Rheum Dis Clin North Am 18:637–672, 1992.
Coates T, Slavotinek JP, Rischmueller M, et al.: Cerebral white matter lesions in primary Sjögren's syndrome: a controlled study. J Rheumatol 26:1301–1305, 1999.

Fox RI, Tornwall J, Maruyama T, et al.: Evolving concepts of diagnosis, pathogenesis, and therapy of Sjogren's syndrome. Curr Opin Rheumatol 10:446–456, 1998.

Govoni M, Bajocchi G, Rizzo N, et al.: Neurological involvement in primary Sjögren's syndrome: clinical and instrumental evaluation in a cohort of Italian patients. Clin Rheumatol 18:299–303, 1999.

Griffin JW, Cornblath DR, Alexander E, et al.: Ataxic sensory neuropathy and dorsal root ganglionitis associated with Sjögren's syndrome. Ann Neurol 27:304–315, 1990.

Lindvall B, Bengtsson A, Emerudh J, Eriksson P: Subclinical myositis is common in primary Sjögren's syndrome and is not related to muscle pain. J Rheumatol 29:717–725, 2002.

Definition

1. Rheumatoid arthritis (RA) is a chronic symmetric inflammatory polyarthritis.

2. Classification criteria for RA (American College of Rheumatology) require presence of at least four of the following (The first four criteria must be present for at least 6 weeks):

   a. Morning stiffness

   b. Objective arthritis of three or more joints

   c. Objective arthritis of at least one hand joint

   d. Symmetrical arthritis

   e. Subcutaneous rheumatoid nodules

   f. Serum rheumatoid factor (RF)

   g. Radiographic evidence of erosions or juxta-articular demineralization on hand films.

Epidemiology

1. Approximately 1% of the population has RA, with an annual incidence of new cases of approximately 300 cases per million population.

2. Woman are affected twice as often as men.

3. The peak age of onset is between 40 and 60 years old.

Etiology and Pathophysiology

1. RA is an autoimmune disease characterized by soft tissue inflammation leading to destruction of bone and cartilage.

2. Neurologic complications of RA can be caused by nerve, spinal cord, or brainstem compression directly by inflamed, proliferative synovium called *pannus* or by joint instability resulting from the inflammatory process.

3. Less common mechanisms of neurologic injury are compression of nervous system tissue by rheumatoid nodules or development of immune complex–mediated vasculitis.

Clinical Neurologic Findings

1. Carpal tunnel syndrome occurs with increased incidence in patients with RA, particularly if they have inflammation of the digital flexor tendons in the wrist. Other focal nerve compressions due to local synovial inflammation can also occur in patients with RA.

2. Mild sensory distal symmetrical axonal neuropathy occurs in some patients with chronic RA.

3. Spinal cord, brainstem, or vertebrobasilar artery compression due to atlantoaxial joint dislocation is a feared, late complication of RA.

4. Head and neck pain are common in patients with chronic RA, especially in those with disease of the atlantoaxial joint.

5. Mononeuritis multiplex can occur when RA progresses to rheumatoid vasculitis. This is discussed further in Part XX, Chapter 10, Neurologic Manifestations of the Vasculitides.

6. Rheumatoid pachymeningitis is a very rare syndrome of focal meningeal inflammatory thickening, sometimes with evidence of granulomas or rheumatoid nodules. Neurologic manifestations vary, depending on which portions of the neuraxis are compressed or irritated by the inflammatory tissue.

Key Clinical Findings

- Carpal tunnel syndrome

- Peripheral neuropathy

- Spinal cord or brainstem compression due to atlanto-axial dislocation

- Head and neck pain

- Mononeuritis multiplex due to rheumatoid vasculitis

Laboratory Findings

1. RF is present in the serum of between 70% and 90% of patients with RA, in many patients with other inflammatory diseases, and in at least 2% of the general population.

2. Antinuclear antibodies (ANA) are present in between 25% and 75% of patients with RA.

Imaging Findings

Cervical spine lateral radiographs, including flexion and extension views, are useful for detecting atlantoaxial joint dislocation. A gap of greater than 3 mm between the anterior atlas and the dens is abnormal; a gap of less than 14 mm between the posterior atlas and the dens places the patient at high risk for spinal cord compression. Vertical position of the dens in relation to the skull must also be evaluated. Magnetic resonance imaging of the cervical spine is the preferred method to further characterize abnormalities in patients with abnormal cervical spine radiographs or clinical neurologic deficits.

Treatment

1. Anti-inflammatory and immunosuppressive treatment of RA can prevent progression of the disease and is likely to reduce the incidence of neurologic complications in the future.
2. Carpal tunnel syndrome in patients with RA can improve after successful anti-inflammatory treatment of flexor tenosynovitis. If the carpal tunnel syndrome is severe enough to require surgical therapy, some patients will need flexor tenosynovectomy at the time of carpal tunnel surgery.
3. Surgical treatment of atlantoaxial dislocation is indicated when it causes spinal cord or brainstem compression and probably in certain patients at high risk for compression, such as those with a dens-posterior atlas gap less than 14 mm.

Key Treatment

• Anti-inflammatory and immunosuppressive drugs

Prevention

No preventive measures for RA are known. In patients with advanced RA who undergo surgery, cervical spine radiographs including flexion and extension views should be obtained prior to anesthesia induction to plan protection of the spine during intubation and surgery.

Bibliography

Dreyer SJ, Boden SD: Natural history of rheumatoid arthritis of the cervical spine. Clin Orthop 366:98–106, 1999.

Nakano KK: The entrapment neuropathies of rheumatoid arthritis. Orthop Clin North Am 6:837–860, 1975.

Rosenbaum R: Neuromuscular complications of connective tissue diseases. Muscle Nerve 24:154–169, 2001.

Sivri A, Guler-Uysal F: The electroneurophysiological evaluation of rheumatoid arthritis patients. Clin Rheumatol 17:416–418, 1998.

5 Progressive Systemic Sclerosis

Richard B. Rosenbaum
Kimberly L. Goslin

Definition

1. Progressive systemic sclerosis (PSS) is characterized by excessive fibrosis, microvascular disease, and autoimmunity.

2. Systemic manifestations include subcutaneous calcinosis, Raynaud's phenomenon (present in 90% of patients), gastrointestinal disturbances, especially disordered esophageal motility, sclerodermatous skin, and telangectasias–the *CREST syndrome,* occurrence of these five elements without other systemic manifestation of PSS.

3. Other systemic manifestations include pulmonary fibrosis or pulmonary hypertension, electrocardiographic abnormalities, arthralgias and tenosynovitis, and scleroderma renal crisis. There is an association between CREST and primary biliary cirrhosis.

Epidemiology

1. Prevalence in the United States is about 70 per 1 million, with an incidence between 5 and 15 per million person-years.

2. The ratio of affected woman to men is between 3 and 5 to 1.

3. The peak age of onset is 50 to 60 years old.

Etiology and Pathophysiology

The pathophysiology of neurologic complications of PSS is poorly understood.

Clinical Neurologic Findings

1. Trigeminal sensory neuropathy occurs in about 4% of patients with PSS. The evolution of facial sensory symptoms is usually insidious and favors the second and third divisions of the trigeminal nerve but may spread to the first division. The neuropathy is more often bilateral than unilateral. Trigeminal motor function is spared.

2. Myopathy, characterized by mild symmetric proximal weakness, is present in most patients with PSS. This is termed *simple* myopathy when accompanied by normal findings or mild abnormalities

of creatine kinase, electromyogram, and muscle biopsy. Perhaps one-eighth of patients with PSS develop full manifestations of inflammatory myopathy.

3. Migraine may be more common in patients with PSS than in the general population.

4. Clinical peripheral nervous system disease is uncommon in patients with PSS. Reported associations include carpal tunnel syndrome, distal symmetric axonal neuropathy, mononeuritis multiplex, plexopathies, and asymptomatic nerve conduction abnormalities

5. Cerebral vasculopathy may be a very rare manifestation of PSS.

Key Clinical Findings

- Trigeminal sensory neuropathy
- Myopathy
- Headache
- Autonomic neuropathy (usually subclinical)
- Cutaneous sensory loss (usually subclinical)

Differential Diagnosis

1. Trigeminal sensory neuropathy can also occur in patients with systemic lupus erythematosus, particularly in the mixed connective tissue disease variant, or with Sjögren's syndrome.

2. When patients with PSS develop renal crisis, they often have malignant hypertension, with resulting central nervous system (CNS) manifestations.

3. For most patients with PSS who develop CNS illnesses, such as seizures, strokes, multiple sclerosis, or encephalopathy, the CNS illness is not pathogenically linked to the PSS

Laboratory Findings

1. ANAs are present in 40% to 90% of patients with PSS. The anticentromere pattern of ANA is present in perhaps one quarter of patients with PSS, particularly those with milder disease; they

are occasionally seen in patients with isolated Raynaud's syndrome but are otherwise relatively specific for PSS or CREST.

2. Patients with PSS may have subclinical abnormalities of cutaneous sensation detectable by von Frey hair testing or by examining terminal cutaneous axons in skin biopsies.

3. Autonomic laboratory testing in patients with PSS may demonstrate subclinical deficiencies of autonomic function.

Imaging Findings

There are no specific neuroimaging abnormalities in patients with PSS.

Treatment

1. There is no specific therapy for the neurologic complications of PSS.

2. Cases reports suggest that steroid therapy of PSS may increase the risk that the patient will develop scleroderma renal crisis.

Prevention

No preventive measures are known.

Key Treatment and Prevention

• There are no specific therapies or preventive measures for neurologic complications of PSS.

Bibliography

Farrell DA, Medsger TA Jr.: Trigeminal neuropathy in progressive systemic sclerosis. Am J Med 73:57–62, 1982.

Hietaharju A, Jääskeläinen S, Hietarinta M, et al.: Central nervous system involvement and psychiatric manifestations in systemic sclerosis (scleroderma): clinical and neurophysiological evaluation. Acta Neurol Scand 87: 382–387, 1993.

Hietaharju A, Jääskeläinen S, Kalimo H, et al.: Peripheral neuromuscular manifestations of systemic sclerosis (scleroderma). Muscle Nerve 16:1204–1212, 1993.

Lee P, Bruni J, Sukenik S: Neurological manifestations in systemic sclerosis (scleroderma). J Rheumatol 11:480–483, 1984.

Straub RH, Zeuner M, Lock G: Autonomic and sensory neuropathy in patients with systemic lupus erythematosus and systemic sclerosis. J Rheumatol 23:87–92, 1996.

Stummvol GH. Current treatment options in systemic sclerosis (scleroderma). Acta Med Austriaca 29:14–19, 2002.

6 Fibromyalgia

Richard B. Rosenbaum
Kimberly L. Goslin

Definition

1. Fibromyalgia is a syndrome of chronic, widespread musculoskeletal or soft tissue pain. To meet the American College of Rheumatology classification criteria for the diagnosis, a patient must have tenderness to palpation at 11 or more of 18 specific points: bilaterally at the occiput, low neck, trapezius, supraspinati, second costochondral junctions, lateral forearms distal to the lateral epicondyles, upper outer glutei maximi, greater trochanters, and medial knees.

2. The validity of tender points as diagnostic criteria is debated, but the existence of many patients with the clinical syndrome of fibromyalgia is well-known.

Epidemiology

1. Fibromyalgia reportedly occurs in 1% to 5% of the adult population, but prevalence rates just over 10% have been found in some selected populations.

2. Prevalence is 5 to 8 times higher in women than in men.

3. Whites may be more affected than non-whites.

Etiology and Pathophysiology

1. The cause of fibromyalgia is unknown.

2. Patients with fibromyalgia have been investigated for abnormal metabolism of neurotransmitters such as substance P or serotonin; neuroendocrine changes; sleep disturbances; and numerous other mechanisms, but no consistent pathophysiologic model is established.

3. The role of trauma as a cause of fibromyalgia is debated.

Clinical Findings

1. The pain and tenderness of fibromyalgia are chronic, lasting over 3 months, and widespread, occurring bilaterally, above and below the waist, and axially.

2. Patients with fibromyalgia have multiple symptoms: a partial list may include fatigue, stiffness, non-restorative sleep, headaches, autonomic disturbances, paresthesias, cognitive complaints, and mood disorders.

3. Fibromyalgia does not cause objective abnormalities detectable by neurologic examination.

Key Clinical Findings

- Chronic musculoskeletal or soft tissue pain
- Widespread tender points at specific locations
- Varied somatic symptoms

> **NOTE**
> Fibromyalgia does not cause abnormalities that are detectable by neurologic examination.

Differential Diagnosis

1. Myofascial pain syndromes are characterized by more localized musculoskeletal pain, often associated with focal trigger points.

2. Depending on the clinical presentation, patients with prominent myalgias may merit evaluation for polymyalgia rheumatica, inflammatory myopathy, or metabolic myopathies.

3. Fibromyalgia can occur secondary to other well-defined pathologies such as autoimmune and inflammatory diseases, infections, malignancies, thyroid disease, or drug reactions.

4. Depression or somatoform pain disorders are included in the differential diagnosis of many patients with fibromyalgia.

Laboratory Findings

1. Fibromyalgia by itself is not associated with abnormalities on standard blood tests, such as CBC, sedimentation rate, C-reactive protein, creatine kinase, and autoantibody tests.

2. Fibromyalgia is not associated with abnormalities on routine electrodiagnostic tests.

3. Muscle biopsy of patients with fibromyalgia shows no specific abnormalities but may show nonspecific changes such as atrophy of type II muscle fibers.

Key Laboratory Findings

- Abnormalities on routine clinical laboratory or neuroimaging studies
- Muscle biopsy may show nonspecific changes such as atrophy of type II fibers

Imaging Findings

Fibromyalgia is not associated with abnormalities on neuroimaging studies.

Treatment

1. Tricyclic antidepressants may improve sleep or decrease pain for some patients. Selective serotonin release inhibitors (SSRIs) antidepressants are tried for some patients. Neither tricyclic nor SSRI antidepressants relieve tender points.

2. Nonsteroidal anti-inflammatory drugs or cyclobenzaprine may deserve therapeutic trials in individual patients.

3. Some patients with fibromyalgia seem to benefit from cognitive behavior therapy aimed at improving coping skills or improving physical fitness.

Key Treatment

- Tricyclic or SSRI antidepressants
- Nonsteroidal anti-inflammatory or cyclobenzaprine for certain patients
- Cognitive behavior therapy

Prognosis and Complications

1. Fibromyalgia is not a progressive disease, and symptoms regress spontaneously in some patients, but complete recovery is not common.
2. Fibromyalgia is a significant cause of disability claims.

Prevention

No preventive measures are known.

Bibliography

Bohr T: Problems with myofascial pain syndrome and fibromyalgia syndrome. Neurology 46:593–597, 1996.
Goldenberg DL: Controversies in fibromyalgia and related conditions. Rheum Dis Clin North Am 22:219–410, 1996.
Littlejohn GO, Walker J: A realistic approach to managing patients with fibromyalgia. Curr Rheumatol Rep 4:286–292, 2002.
Russell IJ: Fibromyalgia syndrome. In Mense S, Simons, DG, Russell IJ (eds): Muscle Pain. Understanding its nature, diagnosis, and treatment. Philadelphia, Lippincott Williams & Wilkins, 2001, pp. 289–337.
White KP, Carette S, Harth M, Teasell RW: Trauma and fibromyalgia: is there an association and what does it mean? Semin Arthritis Rheum 29:200–216, 2000.

7 Behçet's Disease

Richard B. Rosenbaum
Kimberly L. Goslin

Definition

1. Behçet's disease (BD) is a systemic inflammatory disorder, classically described as a triad of uveitis and oral and genital ulceration.

2. The International Study Group for Behçet's Disease diagnostic criteria require oral ulceration as well as at least two of the following: recurrent genital ulceration, eye lesions, skin lesions, and a positive pathergy test (see later, under Laboratory Tests).

3. Neuro-Behçet's is the term used when neurologic involvement occurs.

Epidemiology and Risk Factors

1. BD is a rare condition in general, but it is most common in the Mediterranean countries and Asia. The highest prevalence is in Turkey (80–370/100,000) and the lowest prevalence is in Western countries such as the United States (0.12/100,000).

2. Onset is typically in the third and fourth decades of life.

3. In countries where the disease is prevalent, it is associated with HLA-B51. In these regions, the incidence of HLA-B51 is significantly higher among patients with BD than in those without the disease (55% versus 10%)

Etiology and Pathophysiology

1. The cause of BD is not known. Epidemiologic findings suggest that genetic and environmental factors contribute to the development of the disease.

2. Pathophysiologic mechanisms leading to clinical manifestations include:

   a. Small vessel vasculitis, which is the primary lesion in BD, though vessels of all sizes, both arteries and veins, may be affected

   b. Hyperfunction of neutrophils, leading to tissue injury

   c. Autoimmune mechanisms as a primary or secondary event

   d. Hypercoagulability with thrombotic complications

Clinical Findings

1. Oral ulceration is required for the diagnosis and is frequently the initial manifestation. Other mucocutaneous lesions include erythema nodosum, genital ulcers, and mucosal ulceration of the gastrointestinal tract mainly in the terminal ileum and cecum.

2. Ocular symptoms occur in 60% to 80% of patients with BD, and are the presenting feature in 20% of patients. In one series, two thirds of the patients had uveitis, which is often recurrent, bilateral but asymmetric. The hallmark of Behçet's associated uveitis is hypopyon, or pus in the anterior ocular chamber. Retinal vasculitis is especially characteristic of Behçet's disease.

Key Clinical Findings

- Oral ulcers
- Genital ulcers
- Skin lesions
- Eye involvement
- Joint involvement
- Thrombophlebitis
- Central nervous system involvement
- Gastrointestinal involvement
- Constitutional disturbances such as malaise, fatigue, weight loss

3. Neurologic manifestations

   a. 10% to 40% of patients with BD have neurologic disease (Neuro-Behçet's). Neurologic symptoms generally occur 4 to 6 years after onset of BD, but they can be the initial clinical manifestations. Neurologic involvement is relapsing-remitting, primary progressive, or secondary progressive.

   b. Headache is common in BD; it can occur secondary to intracranial disease or can be a nonspecific systemic symptom.

   c. There are three distinctive neurologic syndromes.

      (1) Cerebral venous thrombosis, often with increased intracranial pressure. This is seen

in up to 25% of patients with neuro-Behçet's. It can present with headache, visual changes, altered mental status, seizures, or rarely stroke. Papilledema is often present on examination.

(2) Chronic meningitis or meningoencephalitis. This may present with headache, fever, meningeal signs, altered mental status, cranial neuropathies, or seizures.

(3) Relapsing-remitting multifocal encephalitis. Focal inflammatory lesions occur, with a predilection for the brainstem. The cerebellum and cortex are relatively spared. Symptoms and findings are related to the site of involvement; pyramidal tract abnormalities are common.

Key Neurologic Findings

- Pyramidal signs
- Papilledema
- Cerebellar signs
- Cranial nerve palsies
- Optic atrophy
- Dysarthria
- Pseudobulbar signs
- Optic neuropathy
- Sensory findings
- Seizures

Differential Diagnosis

1. When neurologic manifestations predominate, multiple sclerosis must be considered in the differential diagnosis, though the pattern of brain lesions usually differs for the two diseases. Other causes of meningitis and encephalitis should be ruled out.

2. When ocular and mucocutaneous lesions are present, inflammatory bowel disease, other HLA-B27 related syndromes, and sarcoidosis should be considered.

Laboratory Tests

1. There are no specific tests for BD. Nonspecific acute phase reactants such as erythrocyte sedimentation rate and C-reactive protein are usually elevated.

2. Cerebrospinal fluid (CSF) findings are variable.

CSF pressure is often elevated when venous sinus thrombosis occurs. If a patient has meningitis or encephalitis, CSF pleocytosis with mixed neutrophils and lymphocytes can be present. The CSF protein can also be elevated. Increased immunoglobulin indices have been reported, and oligoclonal bands rarely occur.

3. The pathergy test is one of the diagnostic criteria for Behçet's disease. A sterile needle is used to prick the patient's forearm. The results are judged as positive when the puncture causes an aseptic erythematous nodule or pustule that is more than 2 mm in diameter, within 24 to 48 hours.

Radiologic Features

1. Magnetic resonance imaging (MRI) is more sensitive than computed tomography for revealing central nervous system (CNS) involvement. With focal encephalitis, high-intensity focal lesions can be seen on T_2-weighted images, often with abnormal enhancement. The most prevalent lesion involves the midbrain, extending into the basal ganglia. When meningitis occurs, MRI can show enhancement and thickening of the meninges.

2. MR-venography is a useful, noninvasive test for detecting venous sinus thrombosis.

Treatment

1. Inflammatory eye disease: Steroids are often effective orally or by periocular injection. For severe refractory eye disease, many cytotoxic agents such as azathioprine, chlorambucil, and cyclophosphamide have been used to help prevent recurrent ocular attacks. Cyclosporine may be particularly beneficial, but it also has increased neurologic toxicity in patients with BD. Colchicine has some efficacy in preventing uveitis.

2. Mucocutaneous lesions: Dapsone and thalidomide (doses 100 to 300 mg/day) are beneficial for some mucocutaneous lesions. Colchicine has been used but is rarely helpful. Steroids may be necessary for refractory mucocutaneous lesions.

3. Treatment of the neurologic complications of BD.

   a. Aseptic meningitis with encephalitis can be self-limited and not require specific therapy. However, there is usually a good response to steroids.

   b. Venous sinus thrombosis is usually treated with chronic anticoagulation with heparin and then coumadin.

   c. Relapsing-remitting multifocal encephalitis requires more aggressive treatment. Steroids at doses up to 100 mg/day are used. Other cytotoxic agents have been tried with varying success. Chronic progressive CNS disease is relatively resistant to current therapies.

Key Treatment

Eye Disease

• Steroids

• Cytotoxic agents

• Cyclosporine

Mucocutaneous Lesions

• Dapsone and thalidomide

• Steroids

Neurologic Complications

Aseptic Menigitis with Encephalitis

• Steroids, but condition can be self-limiting

Venous Sinus Thrombosis

• Long-term use of heparin and then coumadin

Multifocal Encephalitis:

• Steroids at doses up to 100 mg/day

Prognosis and Complications

1. Despite treatment, about 25% of patients with ocular lesions eventually become blind.
2. Early age of onset and male sex are risk factors for serious ocular and neurologic symptoms.
3. The prognosis for dural sinus thrombosis is good.
4. In one large series following patients for 3 years after acute focal encephalitis, most patients became symptom-free, 28% experienced further attacks, and 14% were disabled as a consequence of the absence of recovery or the development of progressive disease.

Bibliography

International Study Group for Behçet's Disease: Criteria for diagnosis of Behçet's disease. Lancet 335:1078–1080, 1995.

Kidd D, Steuer A, Denman A.M, and Rudge P: Neurologic complications in Behçet's syndrome. Brain 122:2183–2194, 1999.

Rosenbaum RB, Campbell SM, Rosenbaum JT: Clinical Neurology of Rheumatic Diseases. Boston, Butterworth-Heinemann 1996, pp. 292–298.

Serdaroglu P: Behçet's disease and the nervous system. J Neurol 245:197–205, 1998.

St n C: A famous Turkish dermatologist, Dr. Hulusi Behcet. Eur J Dermatol 12:469–470, 2002.

Yazici H, Yurdakul S, Hamuryudan V: Behçet's syndrome. Curr Opin Rheumatol 11:53–57, 1999.

Richard B. Rosenbaum
Kimberly L. Goslin

8 Sarcoidosis

Definition

1. Sarcoidosis is a multisystem granulomatous disease of unknown etiology. Pulmonary features typically dominate, but virtually any organ can be affected. The diagnosis rests on identifying the characteristic pattern of organ involvement, demonstrating noncaseating granulomas by biopsy, and ruling out other causes of granulomatous disease.

2. *Neurosarcoidosis* is the term used when there is neurologic involvement.

Epidemiology and Risk Factors

1. There is a worldwide distribution, but certain ethnic groups, among them African Americans and northern Europeans have a higher incidence. The incidence for African Americans is 81.8/100,000 as opposed to 7.6/100,000 for white Americans.

2. The highest incidence is in the 20- to 40-year age group.

3. There is a slight female predominance.

Etiology and Pathophysiology

1. The cause of sarcoidosis is not known

2. The pathologic hallmark of sarcoidosis is noncaseating granulomas that are composed of multinucleated giant cells and epithelioid cells.

3. Multiple mechanisms contribute to the clinical manifestations, including

    a. Mass effect of the granulomas

    b. Immune complex vasculitis

    c. Metabolically active granulomas

Clinical Features

1. Systemic manifestations

    a. Virtually any organ can be affected, but the lungs are the most common site of involvement. The chest x-ray is abnormal in more than 90% of individuals with sarcoidosis. Involvement may be asymptomatic or present with dyspnea, cough, pneumothorax, or hemoptysis.

    b. Approximately 35% of patients with sarcoidosis have skin involvement. Erythema nodosum is the most common manifestation.

    c. Ocular disturbances occur in 25% to 40% of patients with sarcoidosis, but may be relatively asymptomatic. Dry eyes are a frequent complaint. Uveitis is the most common disturbance, occurring in 25% of patients. A formal eye examination is recommended for all patients at the time of diagnosis.

    d. Cardiac and renal involvement are infrequent. Arthritis occurs in 20% of patients. Constitutional symptoms are common.

2. Neurologic manifestations

    a. 5% to 16% of patients with sarcoidosis have clinical evidence of neurologic involvement, and in 50% this occurs before there is evidence of systemic disease. Sarcoidosis can affect any part of the nervous system, but it has a predilection for the base of the brain.

    b. One or more cranial neuropathies occur in about one half of cases of neurosarcoidosis. Facial neuropathy is the most common neurologic manifestation of sarcoidosis and the most common cranial neuropathy, occurring in 25% to 50% of patients with neurosarcoidosis. One third of cases are bilateral. The optic nerve is the second most commonly involved cranial nerve.

    c. Aseptic meningitis occurs in up to 25% of patients with neurosarcoidosis. It may present with headache and stiff neck. It is often associated with cranial neuropathies or other focal neurologic dysfunction. Granulomata involving meninges are most common at the base of the brain.

    d. Seizures occur in 5% to 22% of patients with neurosarcoidosis. They can be focal or generalized.

    e. Hydrocephalus can be secondary to obstruction of cerebrospinal fluid (CSF) flow due to granulomatous disease within the ventricles or the cerebral aqueduct.

    f. Localized granulomatous masses have been found in every part of the central nervous system (CNS) and can be indistinguishable from other space-occupying masses.

    g. Patients with extensive CNS sarcoidosis can develop cognitive impairment with a wide variety of neuropsychiatric symptoms: im-

797

paired memory, poor concentration, hallucinations, and disturbances of mood or affect.

h. Hypothalamic-pituitary dysfunction is a characteristic feature of neurosarcoidosis. The hypothalamus rather than the pituitary is the most common pathologic site of involvement.

i. Any region of the spinal cord may rarely be involved in sarcoidosis

j. Peripheral neuropathy occurs in 9% to 20% of patients with neurosarcoidosis, particularly later in the disease course. A slowly progressive, distal, symmetrical axonal pattern is most common. Polyradiculitis, mononeuritis multiplex, and a clinical picture identical to Guillain-Barré syndrome also occur.

k. Clinical myopathy is rare, occurring in 1% of patients with neurosarcoidosis, but granulomata can be found on muscle biopsy in over 50% of patients with sarcoidosis.

l. Headache is common in sarcoidosis. It can occur secondary to intracranial disease or can be a nonspecific systemic symptom.

Key Neurologic Signs

- Cranial neuropathies
- Peripheral neuropathies
- Meningitis
- Hypothalamic dysfunction

Differential Diagnosis

1. Infectious diseases caused by fungi and mycobacteria, and processes such as Crohn's disease can also cause a granulomatous response.

2. When neurosarcoidosis occurs without systemic manifestations of the disease, the differential diagnosis is much broader and depends on the site of neurologic involvement.

Laboratory Tests

1. Angiotensin converting enzyme (ACE) is elevated in 70% of patients with sarcoidosis, but it can be elevated in a number of other conditions as well. Serum ACE levels may be normal in neurosarcoidosis.

2. Hypercalciuria and, less commonly, hypercalcemia occur as a result of granulomas that produce calcitriol, the active form of vitamin D.

3. In neurosarcoidosis CSF analysis generally reveals elevated protein level and mild lymphocytosis. The

CSF glucose is occasionally reduced. Intrathecal immunoglobulin G synthesis may be increased, but oligoclonal bands are rare. ACE levels in the CSF may be elevated. The sensitivity of CSF ACE levels for detecting neurosarcoidosis has not been firmly established.

4. Anergy skin testing demonstrates cutaneous hyporeactivity to common antigens in up to 50% of patients with sarcoidosis.

5. Biopsy of involved tissue such as lymph nodes, lung, conjunctiva, skin, and meninges reveals the characteristic noncaseating granulomas.

Key Laboratory Findings

- Increase in serum ACE
- Increase in serum lysozyme
- Increase in β_2 microglobulin
- Hypercalciuria
- Hypercalcemia (rarely)
- CSF abnormalities in neurosarcoidosis
  - Pleocytosis, predominantly lymphocytes
  - Increase protein
  - Increase ACE level
  - Increase in immunoglobulin G synthesis
  - Oligoclonal banding (rarely)

Radiologic Features

1. Chest x-ray is abnormal in more than 90% of patients with sarcoidosis. There may be bilateral hilar adenopathy, pulmonary infiltrates, or pulmonary fibrosis.

2. Magnetic resonance imaging (MRI) with gadolinium is the modality of choice for imaging CNS disease. Possible MRI findings include periventricular white matter abnormalities, meningeal enhancement with meningitis, space-occupying lesions, or hydrocephalus.

3. Radionuclide scans with gallium 67 have been used to measure disease activity, although the test is nonspecific.

Treatment

1. Not all sarcoidosis requires treatment, as the disease sometimes remits spontaneously. Most authorities agree that the following are indications for systemic treatment: nervous system involvement, hypercalcemia, rapidly progressive pulmo-

nary sarcoidosis, myocardial involvement, and uveitis (when topical treatment fails).

2. Prednisone is the mainstay of treatment. Different dosing regimens have been used. A dose of 0.5 to 1.5 mg/kg is usual. Duration of therapy depends on response; a slow taper is recommended to reduce relapses.

3. Because the disease is often chronic, corticosteroid sparing agents have been tried with success, including cyclosporine, azathioprine, methotrexate, cyclophosphamide, and chlorambucil. Whole-brain irradiation therapy has also been used for treatment-resistant CNS disease.

 Key Treatment

- Prednisone
- Corticosteroid-sparing agents such as cyclosporine, azathioprine, methotrexate, cyclophosphamide, and chlorambucil

Prognosis and Complications

1. Remissions occur in nearly two thirds of patients, although relapses are common.

2. Prognosis in neurosarcoidosis depends on the nature of neurologic involvement. Cranial neuropathies and acute meningitis have a better prognosis than encephalopathy or cerebral mass lesions and seizures.

3. Mortality rates vary from 5% to 8%. The main cause of death is pulmonary complications. Sudden death from cardiac involvement also occurs.

 Bibliography

Belfer MH, Stevens RW: Sarcoidosis: a primary care review. Am Fam Physician 58:2041–2050, 1998.

Gullapalli D, Phillips LH: Neurologic manifestations of sarcoidosis. Neurol Clin 20:59–83, 2002.

Puryear DW, Fowler AA: Sacoidosis: a clinical overview. Compr Ther 22:649–653, 1996.

Rosenbaum R, Campbell S, Rosenbaum J: Clinical Neurology of Rheumatic Diseases. Boston, Butterworth-Heinemann, 1996, pp. 385–397.

Sharma OP, Sharma AM: Sarcoidosis of the nervous system. Arch Intern Med 151:1317–1321, 1991.

Zjicek JP, Scolding NJ, Foster O: Central nervous system sarcoidosis—diagnosis and management. Q J Med 92:103–117, 1999.

Temporal Arteritis and Polymyalgia Rheumatica

Richard B. Rosenbaum
Kimberly L. Goslin

Definitions

1. Temporal arteritis (TA) and polymyalgia rheumatica (PMR) are inflammatory conditions that frequently occur in the same patient.

2. TA is a systemic vasculitis affecting large and medium-sized elastic arteries. The American College of Rheumatology classification criteria for TA require that a patient have at least three of the following:

    a. Age at disease onset greater than 50 years

    b. New headache

    c. Temporal artery abnormality on examination

    d. Erythrocyte sedimentation rate (ESR) higher than 50 mm/hour

    e. Temporal artery biopsy showing mononuclear infiltrate or granulomatous inflammation
    These criteria result in a diagnosis with a sensitivity of 93.5% and specificity of 91.2%.

3. PMR is a syndrome of polyarticular low-grade synovitis. Diagnostic criteria are less defined than for TA and include

    a. Patient older than 50 years of age

    b. Aching and morning stiffness for at least 1 month affecting at least two of the following areas: shoulders and upper arms, hips and thighs, neck, and torso.

    c. Findings of a systemic reaction such as elevated ESR higher than 40 mm/hour

    d. Exclusion of other disease processes such as rheumatoid arthritis

    e. No objective muscle disease

    f. Some definitions have included a rapid response to small doses of corticosteriods, such as 10 to 15 mg of prednisone daily.

Epidemiology and Risk Factors

1. TA and PMR occur in similar patient populations. Mean age of onset for both is age 70; rarely before age 50. Incidence increases with age. For TA, 2.1/100,000 for ages 50 to 59 years; 49/100,000 for ages above 80 years. PMR has an incidence of 52.5/100,000 in persons aged 50 years or older.

2. Female:male ratio is 2:1.

3. There is an association with HLA-DR4 with both conditions.

4. There is overlap between the two conditions: 50% to 60% of patients with TA have signs of PMR, and 15% to 25% of people with PMR have concurrent TA (15% to 33% of people with PMR have evidence of TA on temporal artery biopsy).

Etiology and Pathophysiology

1. The causes of TA and PMR are not known; both genetic and environmental factors may be involved.

2. Humoral and cellular immune systems have been implicated in the pathogenesis of TA and PMR.

3. The main pathologic mechanism underlying the clinical manifestations of TA is a vasculitis affecting medium-sized and large elastic arteries. Thrombosis may develop at the sites of active inflammation, resulting in ischemic complications. Arteries originating from the arch of the aorta are affected to the greatest degree, but almost any artery of the body may be affected. The highest incidence of severe involvement has been noted in the superficial temporal arteries, vertebral arteries, ophthalmic and posterior ciliary arteries. Intracranial arteries are infrequently involved.

4. The main pathologic mechanism thought to underlie the clinical manifestations of PMR is synovitis.

TEMPORAL ARTERITIS

Clinical Findings

1. Constitutional symptoms of fever, malaise, fatigue, and weight loss are frequent early manifestations of TA. PMR may also occur early in the disease course. Jaw claudication is particularly specific for TA and occurs in 15% to 30% of patients with this disorder. Thoracic aneurysms and dissection of the aorta occur as a late complication.

2. Neurologic involvement is diverse and common.

    a. Headache is the most frequent initial symptom and occurs in 90% of patients at some time during the illness. The headache type varies, but is often marked, boring, lancinating, and localized to the temporal or occipital regions of the scalp. Temporal artery tenderness and scalp swelling may occur. Any patient over 50 years of age with a new headache pattern should be evaluated for TA (also see Part IX, Chapter 8, Facial Numbness).

b. Visual symptoms may include diplopia, ptosis, and visual loss. Visual loss is caused by ischemia of the optic nerve or tracts secondary to arteritis of the branches of the ophthalmic or posterior ciliary arteries. If initially present unilaterally, involvement of the contralateral eye may occur within 1 to 2 weeks if treatment is not started.

c. Stroke is a well described but uncommon complication; average incidence is less than 5%. Arteritis has a predilection for the vertebral artery and rarely involves intracranial portions of arteries.

d. Peripheral neuropathy occurs in 14% of patients with biopsy-proven TA. All patterns of peripheral nerve involvement have been observed, including generalized polyneuropathy, mononeuropathy, and mononeuritis multiplex. Carpal tunnel syndrome is the most common mononeuropathy in TA.

e. TA can cause any cranial neuropathy. Optic neuropathy (described under visual symptoms, 2b, above) is the most common cranial neuropathy. Objective abnormalities of eye movement occur in up to 6% of patients with TA. Trigeminal involvement, with numbness of one side of the tongue occurs secondary to lingual artery ischemia. Facial neuropathy has been reported in isolated cases. Up to one third of patients with TA complain of dizziness. Rarely, auditory nerve ischemia results in acute onset of vertigo and hearing loss.

Key Clinical Features: Temporal Arteritis

- New or different headache

- Jaw claudication, facial pain, trismus

- Constitutional symptoms: anorexia, malaise, weight loss, fever

- Limb claudication, aortic arch syndrome

- Visual symptoms: amaurosis fugax, diplopia

- Polymyalgia rheumatica

- Temporal artery tenderness, scalp swelling

POLYMYALGIA RHEUMATICA

Clinical Findings

1. Constitutional symptoms are present in more than 50% of patients.

2. Arthralgias and myalgias can develop abruptly or evolve over weeks to months. Profound axial stiffness, pain, and aching that affects neck, back, shoulder girdle, and hips occur. Symptoms often begin asymmetrically, but usually become bilateral. Morning stiffness is prominent.

3. 15% to 25% of patients with PMR develop clinical TA.

4. In the absence of TA, neurologic complications are rare. There is no true muscle involvement, though atrophy occurs in later stages secondary to disuse. Carpal tunnel syndrome can occur secondary to synovitis.

Key Clinical Findings: Polymyalgia Rheumatica

- Arthralgia and myalgia

- Profound axial stiffness, pain, and aching that affects neck, back, shoulder girdle, and hips

- Symptoms often asymmetric but become bilateral

- Morning stiffness prominent

- 15% to 25% of patients with PMR develop clinical TA.

Differential Diagnosis

1. The differential diagnosis for TA includes other vasculitic processes such as Takayasu arteritis, polyarteritis nodosum, and Wegener's granulomatosis.

2. Anterior ischemic optic neuropathy has several nonarteritic causes such as diabetes and hypertension.

3. The differential diagnosis for PMR includes malignancy, acute and chronic infections, thyroid disorders, osteoarthritis, rheumatoid arthritis, and myositis of varied causes. Endocarditis may present with prominent musculoskeletal symptoms and elevated ESR early in the course of the disease.

Laboratory Tests

1. Hematologic tests in TA and PMR are similar. A markedly elevated ESR is characteristic of both, with levels usually greater than 100 mm/hour.

2. CSF is normal in most patients with TA and PMR.

CSF pleocytosis can occur in the unusual cases of TA involving intracranial arteries.

3. Synovial fluid analysis in PMR can show mild inflammation.

4. Because of the patchy nature of the vasculitis in which there may only be "skip lesions," at least 4 cm of the temporal artery should be obtained during biopsy. Biopsy before or soon after starting steroid therapy is important, but arteritis can be present even after 2 weeks of therapy. Sensitivity of the biopsy is 60% to 80%. A patient with PMR who does not have any other signs or symptoms of TA does not require a biopsy.

Key Laboratory Findings: TA and PMR

- Elevated ESR, usually >100 mm/hr

- Mild normochromic normocytic anemia

- Mild thrombocytosis

- Increase in acute phase reactants

- Mild liver function test abnormality, particularly alkaline phosphatase.

- CSF is usually normal; mild pleocytosis can occur with intracranial arteritis.

Radiologic Features

1. In cases of TA complicated by stroke, focal abnormalities will be present on brain magnetic resonance imaging or computed tomography scans.

2. Angiography is nonspecific for TA and can show focal narrowing in the temporal arteries.

3. Color duplex ultrasonography is a modality that is being used more and more to identify focal areas of arterial stenosis or occlusion.

Treatment

1. TA responds promptly to steroids. Patients suspected of having TA should begin therapy immediately. A variety of treatment protocols have been used. Generally an initial dose of 40 to 60 mg/day of prednisone is adequate. If there are visual symptoms, some advocate parenteral pulse methylprednisolone, 1000 mg/daily for 3 to 5 days, and then oral steroids. The effective starting dose should be continued until all reversible symptoms and findings have gone, and laboratory tests have reverted to normal or near normal. The steroid taper should be slow to allow for monitoring symptoms and ESR. If TA is unresponsive to steroids, the diagnosis should be questioned. A

variety of steroid sparing agents including methotrexate have been used with variable results.

2. PMR also responds promptly to steroids. Generally lower doses are required than for TA. An initial dose of 15 to 20 mg of prednisone per day is recommended. Dramatic improvement can be expected within a week. After symptoms subside, a slow taper is suggested to allow close monitoring of symptoms and ESR. Some advocate use of nonsteroidal anti-inflammatory agents rather than steroids for mild PMR symptoms.

Key Treatment: TA and PMR

Temporal Arteritis

- Steroids

- Methylprednisolone and oral steroids for visual symptoms

Polymyalgia Rheumatica

- Steroids

- Nonsteroidal anti-inflammatory agents for mild PMR

Prognosis and Complications

1. TA is generally self-limited over several months to several years. Visual loss is the most feared complication. Prognosis depends on prompt treatment.

2. Even without treatment, PMR generally resolves within 2 to 4 years. PMR, in the absence of TA, is not generally associated with serious complications.

3. Relapse after discontinuation of steroids can occur for both TA and PMR.

Bibliography

Hunder GG: Giant cell arteritis and polymyalgia rheumatica. Med Clin North Am 81:195–216, 1997.

Hunder GG, Bloch DA, Michel BA, et al.: The American College of Rheumatology 1990 Criteria for the Classification of Giant Cell Arteritis. Arthritis Rheum 33:1122, 1990.

Meskimen S, Cook TD, Blake RL: Management of giant cell arteritis and polymyalgia rheumatic. Am Fam Physician 61:2061–2067, 2000.

Nordborg E, Nordborg C, Malmvall B, et al.: Giant cell arteritis. Rheum Dis Clin North Am 21:1013–1024, 1995.

Rosenbaum RB, Campbell SM, Rosenbaum JT: Clinical Neurology of Rheumatic Diseases. Boston, Butterworth-Heinemann, 1996, pp. 273–287.

Salvarani C, Cantini F, Boiardi L, Hunder GG: Polymyalgia rheumatica and giant-cell arteritis. N Engl J Med 347:261–271, 2002.

10 Neurologic Manifestations of the Vasculitides

Richard B. Rosenbaum
Kimberly L. Goslin

Definition

1. Vasculitis is a disease process that results from inflammation directed against the walls of blood vessels or against an agent embedded within the wall of a blood vessel.

2. Neurologic manifestations may occur secondary to systemic vasculitis or as a result of an organ-specific vasculitis affecting the nervous system.

3. The systemic vasculitides can be classified based on size of the blood vessels affected: small, small-medium overlap, medium, large (see "Classification" box below).

   a. Small-vessel vasculitis is a relatively homogeneous syndrome with multiple causes. Nearly every case of small-vessel vasculitis is an immune complex–mediated hypersensitivity vasculitis. Henoch-Schönlein purpura, cryoglobulinemia, and serum sickness are characteristic examples. Skin involvement such as palpable purpura is the most common manifestation.

   b. Examples of vasculitis involving the small to medium-sized vessels include Wegener's granulomatosis and Churg-Strauss vasculitis. Wegener's granulomatosis presents as a triad of upper and lower respiratory tract involvement, focal segmental glomerulonephritis, and disseminated necrotizing vasculitis. Churg-Strauss syndrome is also a necrotizing vasculitis and is characterized by asthma, allergic rhinitis, and eosinophilia.

   c. Polyarteritis nodosa (PAN) is the prototypical medium-vessel vasculitis. It is a necrotizing vasculitis with systemic illness and multiorgan involvement such a glomerulonephritis and mononeuritis multiplex.

   d. The large-vessel vasculitides include temporal arteritis (discussed in detail in Part XX, Chapter 9, Temporal Arteritis and Polymyalgia Rheumatica) and Takayasu's arteritis, a granulomatous giant cell panarteritis predominantly affecting the aorta and its main branches.

4. The organ-specific vasculitides affecting the nervous system include primary central nervous system angiitis and nonsystemic vasculitic neuropathy. By definition, patients with these disorders do not have evidence of vasculitis outside of the nervous system and often present a diagnostic dilemma. Diagnosis usually requires biopsy.

Classification of Systemic Vasculitis Based on the Size of Blood Vessels Principally Involved

Small

Hypersensitivity Vasculitis

- Serum sickness
- Drugs/chemicals
- Infections
- Henoch-Schönlein purpura
- Cryoglobulinemia
- Rheumatic diseases
- Malignancy

Medium-Small Overlap

- Wegener's granulomatosis
- "Microscopic" polyarteritis nodosa
- Churg-Strauss vasculitis

Medium

- Polyarteritis nodosa
- Kawasaki disease

Large

- Temporal arteritis
- Takayasu's arteritis
- Buerger's disease

Epidemiology and Risk Factors

1. Vasculitis is an infrequent disorder.

2. The overall annual incidence of vasculitis (excluding temporal arteritis) is estimated to be 31 to 47 cases/million.

Etiology and Pathophysiology

1. The primary immunopathogenic events that initiate vascular inflammation are poorly understood.

2. Blood vessels respond to inflammation in a limited number of ways, and the clinical manifestations are the result of these specific responses.

   a. Vascular inflammation leads to swelling, fibrosis, and occlusion of the vessel lumen, resulting in ischemia.

   b. When the wall of the vessel becomes sufficiently inflamed, it may weaken, resulting in aneurysm formation or hemorrhage.

   c. Local and systemic inflammation with release of cytokines and other inflammatory mediators can produce secondary effects such as fever, weight loss, anemia, or elevation of acute phase reactants.

Clinical Findings

1. Systemic vasculitis presents clinically with several syndromes

   a. Multiorgan disease

   b. Systemic illness/fever of unknown origin

   c. Multiple or unusual ischemic events

   d. Organ-specific syndromes such as palpable purpura and mononeuritis multiplex.

2. Neurologic manifestations of systemic vasculitis

   a. Neurologic involvement is often prominent with the small/medium-vessel overlap syndromes and the medium-vessel syndromes. For example, at initial clinical presentation 10% of patients with PAN have signs or symptoms referable to the central nervous system, and 5% have peripheral neuropathy. Neurologic complications occur in 22% to 54% of patients with Wegener's granulomatosis and in 62% of patients with Churg-Strauss vasculitis. Neurologic involvement is uncommon with the pure small-vessel vasculitides.

   b. Mononeuritis multiplex is a syndrome that is strongly suggestive of vasculitis. In this type of vasculitic neuropathy multiple nerves are affected in a stepwise progression. Dysfunction of an individual nerve begins suddenly and reaches maximum severity within days. The neuropathy is frequently painful. Nerves are often affected in the proximal limbs rather than at typical sites of compression neuropathy. Legs are more frequently affected than arms. Mononeuritis multiplex occurs commonly in PAN, particularly early in the illness. It is also common in Wegener's granulomatosis.

   c. In patients with vasculitis a distal symmetrical sensorimotor polyneuropathy is more common than mononeuritis multiplex. It is found in up to 57% of patient with cryoglobulinemia and

50% of patients with PAN. Of course, vasculitis accounts for only a small fraction of cases of distal symmetric polyneuropathy.

   d. Many patients with vasculitis complain of myalgias and have vasculitis evident on the muscle biopsy, but few have clinical myopathy.

   e. Cranial neuropathies occur with many types of vasculitis. They are among the most common neurologic complications of Wegener's granulomatosis. In this disorder cranial nerves may be injured by granulomata in the respiratory tract or the orbit. Cranial nerve involvement is also well-described in patients with PAN, either in isolation or as part of mononeuritis multiplex.

   f. Stroke can occur as a complication of vasculitis. 10% of patients with PAN experience stroke sometime during their illness, although it is rarely an initial symptom of the disease. Stroke is a well-described, but uncommon complication of the large-vessel vasculitides. Small-vessel vasculitis is rarely associated with stroke. Of the causes of small-vessel vasculitis, Henoch-Schönlein purpura is the most likely to be associated with stroke.

   g. Cognitive dysfunction occurs with the medium- and large-vessel vasculiditis, but is rarely associated with small-vessel vasculitis. Nearly 25% of patients with PAN have mental status changes including confusion, disorientation, delirium, and disturbances of consciousness.

   h. Focal or generalized seizures can occur secondary to vasculitis involving the central nervous system (CNS). In one series, up to 11% of patients with PAN had seizures.

   i. Headache is a frequent symptom accompanying vasculitis of all types. Headache is not necessarily evidence of intracranial disease but instead may be a nonspecific systemic symptom.

3. Primary CNS angiitis

   a. Headache and mental status abnormalities are the most common early manifestations of this disease. The headache may be severe but has no pathognomonic features. Abnormal mental status is present in nearly three fourths of patients at initial evaluation. Seizures occur in up to one fourth of patients. Coma and focal findings such as weakness occur later in the illness.

   b. Systemic symptoms are usually absent, but a minority of patients have constitutional complaints.

   c. The mechanisms underlying these presentations can include multiple cerebral infarcts, meningitis with leptomeningeal vasculitis, increased intracranial pressure, and hydrocephalus.

4. Nonsystemic vasculitic neuropathy
   a. May present as mononeuritis multiplex, mononeuropathy, or distal peripheral neuropathy
   b. Systemic symptoms are usually absent, but a minority of patients have constitutional complaints.
   c. Vasculitic changes may also be present on muscle biopsy specimens and is not evidence of systemic vasculitis.
   d. Vasculitic neuropathy may rarely be an initial manifestation of systemic vasculitis. When this occurs, other manifestations are usually evident within 1 year.

Key Clinical Findings

Systemic Vasculitis

- Multiorgan disease
- Systemic illness/fever of unknown origin
- Multiple or unusual ischemic events
- Organ-specific syndromes such as palpable purpura and mononeuritis multiplex

Neurologic Manifestations

- Mononeuritis multiplex
- Polyneuropathy
- Cranial neuropathies
- Stroke
- Cognitive dysfunction
- Seizures
- Headache

Primary CNS Angiitis

- Headache and mental status abnormalities
- Constitutional complaints in a minority of patients

Laboratory Testing

1. Systemic vasculitis
   a. There are no specific laboratory tests, though acute-phase reactants are frequently elevated. An exception is the antineutrophil cytoplasmic antibody (ANCA), which is fairly specific for Wegener's granulomatosis.
   b. The diagnosis of vasculitis often requires a tissue biopsy to document inflammation of blood vessel walls. Small-vessel vasculitis virtually always presents with skin lesions, and skin biopsy will be diagnostic. Medium-vessel vas-culitis is usually best diagnosed by biopsy of a clinically involved organ (muscle, nerve, skin, or other tissue).
   c. Angiography is particularly important for confirmation of large-vessel vasculitis where the arteries are often too large for biopsy to be done routinely. The abnormalities observed are nonspecific.
   d. Magnetic resonance imaging (MRI) and computed tomography (CT) studies sometimes show nonspecific focal abnormalities, particularly when stroke is associated with the vasculitis.

2. Primary CNS angiitis
   a. Patients generally have normal findings or mild nonspecific abnormalities on systemic blood studies.
   b. About four fifths of patients have abnormal CSF with elevated protein levels or mildly elevated cell counts.
   c. Angiographic findings are nonspecific and may be normal in over one third of patients. This disorder typically affects small arteries and veins but may also involve larger intracerebral arteries.
   d. MRI or CT can show focal abnormalities that sometimes enhance with gadolinium. These are seen most frequently in the cortex or deep white matter, but also may occur in subcortical white matter.
   e. A CNS biopsy including leptomeninges and brain parenchyma is frequently necessary for the diagnosis but may be negative in up to 30% of cases of primary CNS angiitis.

3. Nonsystemic vasculitic neuropathy
   a. Serologic studies show normal findings or a mild elevation of the erythrocyte sedimentation rate (ESR).
   b. Spinal fluid analysis shows normal cell counts; protein levels may be elevated.
   c. Sural nerve biopsy is usually necessary for the diagnosis and confirms vasculitic involvement.

Treatment

1. Treatment of systemic vasculitis has several components.
   a. Identification of the vasculitic syndrome and avoidance of the specific antigen when possible
   b. Treatment of the underlying condition
   c. Assessment of multiorgan damage and treatment of secondary complications such as renal failure and hypertension

d. Corticosteroids often in combination with cytotoxic agents such as cyclophasphamide

2. There are no controlled trials regarding treatment of primary CNS angiitis and nonsystemic vasculitic neuropathy. In case reports, however, a good response to steroids or to cytotoxic agents has been reported.

Key Treatment

Systemic Vasculitis

• Identify the vasculitic syndrome.

• Treat the underlying condition.

• Assess multiorgan damage and treat secondary complications.

• Administer agents such as corticosteroids, often with cytotoxic agents.

CNS Angiitis and Nonsystemic Vasculitic Neuropathy

• Steroids or cytotoxic agents

Bibliography

Calabreses LH: Therapy of systemic vasculitis. Neurol Clin 15:973, 1997.

Ferro JM: Vasculitis of the central nervous system. J Neurol 245:766–776, 1998.

Nadeau SE: Neurologic manifestations of systemic vasculitis. Neurol Clin 20:123–150, 2002.

Nadeau SE: Diagnositc approach to central and peripheral nervous system vasculitis. Neurol Clin 15:759–777, 1997.

Rosenbaum RB, Campbell SM, Rosenbaum JT: Clinical Neurology of Rheumatic Diseases. Boston, Butterworth-Heinemann, 1996, pp. 237–318.

1   Hypoventilation, Hypoxia, and Carbon Monoxide Poisoning

G. Bryan Young

HYPOXIA-ISCHEMIA

Definition and Classification

Hypoxia is a decrease in oxygen delivery to tissues, whatever the cause. *Ischemia* is a decrease in the blood flow to an organ. *Hypoxemia* is a decrease in the oxygen-carrying capacity of the blood. Hypoxia is often accompanied by ischemia or decreased tissue perfusion. With respect to brain function, ischemia is more important pathophysiologically, in that it is much more commonly responsible for neuronal death. The following classification system gives the principal types of these disorders:

1. Focal ischemia (ischemic stroke)
2. Generalized ischemia or hypoxia

    a. Ischemic hypoxia: Complete disruption of blood flow, usually from cardiac arrest

    b. Oligemic hypoxia (partial ischemia): Incomplete reduction of blood flow that may generalized or focal

    c. Anoxic hypoxia: Arterial oxygen concentration is zero

    d. Hypoxic hypoxia: Arterial oxygen tension is reduced below the threshold level of 40 mm Hg

    e. Anemic hypoxia: Oxygen delivery to tissue is reduced because of reduced ability of the blood to carry oxygen. The example discussed is carbon monoxide poisoning.

    f. Histiotoxic hypoxia: Poisoning of the mitochondrial system involved in oxidative metabolism. The main example is cyanide poisoning. Inherited mitochondrial encephalopathies (e.g., MELAS: mitochondrial encephalopathy with lactic acidosis and stroke) can also produce this type of energy failure.

ETIOLOGY

Epidemiology

1. Cardiac arrest: The overall 1-year survival rate for initially unconscious survivors resuscitated from cardiac arrest has been variably quoted to be between 10% and 25%. Anoxic-ischemic enceph-

alopathy is the principal cause of mortality in 30% to 40% of those who die; only 3% to 10% return to their previous lifestyles, including employment. Well under 1% survive in a persistent vegetative state.

2. In the United States, 550,000 strokes occur annually.

    NOTE: To avoid overlap with other material in the following sections, generalized ischemic encephalopathy after cardiac arrest will be emphasized.

Pathophysiology

1. Certain neurons show a "selective vulnerability" to anoxic-ischemic insults.

    a. The large cell layers (3, 5, and 6) of the neocortex

    b. CA1 and end folium (CA4-6) of the hippocampus are especially vulnerable.

    c. Purkinje cells of the cerebellum, putamen, caudate, and thalamus

2. Trans-synaptic degeneration may affect thalamic nuclei and brainstem nuclei such as the inferior olivary complex

3. The pathogenesis of anoxic-ischemic encephalopathy is incompletely understood. Several hypotheses have been proposed.

    a. Excitotoxic damage from excitatory amino acids (notably glutamate and aspartate)

    b. Disturbance in neuronal calcium homeostasis (possibly related to excitotoxic amino acids)

    c. Damage from oxygen-derived free radicals

    d. The no-reflow phenomenon: Lack of capillary perfusion after restoration of cerebral blood flow

    e. Neuronal sodium–potassium pump and energy failure

4. Many of these insults relate to damage after reperfusion. There are some problems with each of these in serving as a complete explanation for neuronal death; it is likely that a number of mechanisms operate together. Delayed neuronal death may result from an influx of calcium ions

807

into the neuronal cytoplasm. This results in activation of

a. Various enzymes that cause proteolysis of the cytoskeleton

b. Protein kinase C, leading to further calcium entry into the cell

c. Phospholipase C, responsible for the generation of inositol triphosphate, which in turn causes release of ionized calcium from internal stores

d. Diacylglycerol, which activates protein kinase C

e. Phospholipase A_2, which contributes to free radical production

f. Calcium/calmodulin–dependent protein kinase II causing more glutamate release

g. The inducible form of nitric acid synthetase that leads to the formation of nitric oxide, which interacts with superoxide, producing a highly toxic free-radical species

Clinical Features

After resuscitation from cardiac arrest, certain factors are prognostically helpful.

1. Recovery of purposeful movements within the first 24 hours is favorable.

2. Coma lasting more than 3 days carries a greater than 90% risk of poor outcome.

3. Levy et al. (1985) found that independent existence did not occur with absence of pupillary light reflexes at the time of initial evaluation. Only one of the 93 patients studied who had no response or decorticate or decerebrate posturing to stimulation at 24 hours recovered.

4. Longstreth's group (1983) found that the following four variables on admission gave a positive predictive value for awakening of 0.84: motor response, pupillary light response, spontaneous eye movements, and/or elevated serum glucose

5. Edgren and colleagues (1994) found that predictive accuracy at resuscitation for poor outcome ranged from 52% to 84%. At 3 days clinical predictors for poor outcome using the Glasgow Coma Scale and Glasgow-Pittsburgh Coma Scale were reliable for poor outcome (severe cerebral disability, persistent vegetative state [PVS], or death), with absence of motor response being the best predictor. Unless there is considerable compromise of brainstem function, one cannot make a certain early prediction of an outcome of PVS or death in coma using clinical predictors alone.

Key Signs

- Examine responsiveness and cranial nerve function; document especially pupillary reaction and motor response within and after 24 hours of resuscitation

- Myoclonic seizures: Note distribution, axial structures, associated eye opening

Laboratory Testing

1. Somatosensory evoked potentials (SSEPs): The cortical N20 response to median nerve stimulation approaches the ideal prognostic test. The absence of the N20 response from median nerve stimulation is specific but is not especially sensitive for a hopeless prognosis. The lack of this response shows nearly 100% specificity for an outcome no better than PVS, but many patients with a preserved N20 response die without recovery of consciousness. The electroencephalogram (EEG) must be compared to this as a prognostic test.

2. EEG

a. The neurons that are the most sensitive to generalized ischemic damage are those of the cerebral cortex generating postsynaptic potentials that are recorded from scalp EEG. The EEG is flat during resuscitation; this may persist for several hours after circulation is restored. EEG rhythms in the very young, e.g., neonates and premature infants, may take longer to recover than in older patients. Thus, as a general rule, it is better to wait 24 hours or more from the event until the first EEG, unless seizures are suspected.

b. EEGs performed after the first day of arrest may show deteriorating patterns associated with a fatal outcome. This is supported by experimental models in which it has been shown that the phenomenon of "delayed neuronal death" may take more than 24 hours to develop. However, one must be wary that such later suppression is not related to drugs, shock, or sepsis.

c. There is general agreement that certain EEG patterns found after cardiac arrest are strongly associated with an poor neurologic outcome: generalized suppression; generalized burst-suppression; generalized periodic patterns, especially with epileptiform activity; and alpha or alpha-theta pattern coma. With the exception of complete generalized suppression, however, there have been isolated reports of rare patients who have recovered conscious awareness with these EEG patterns.

3. Other potential tests. Various tests are either less available or have not been evaluated sufficiently: biochemical tests (e.g., lactate or creatine kinase concentrations in the cerebrospinal fluid [CSF]), nuclear magnetic resonance (NMR) spectroscopy with quantitative measures of "neuronal metabolites" (e.g., N-acetyl aspartate), and cerebral blood flow and metabolic positron emission tomographic (PET) studies (e.g., measuring glucose metabolism). None has proved superior to the SSEPs mentioned above.

Prognostic Points: Coma after Resuscitation from Cardiac Arrest

- The two main clinical predictors of poor outcome are absence of pupillary light reflex and motor response (absent/decorticate or decerebrate posturing) at 24 hours.

- With intact brainstem reflexes, the absence of N20 potential with SSEPs or a flat (isolelectric) EEG after 24 hours indicates a poor prognosis.

Management

Along with optimal general care, it is important to minimize ongoing or subsequent brain damage.

1. Prevent hyperglycemia and hyperthermia.

2. Maintain adequate blood pressure: Because of loss of autoregulation, adequate systemic blood pressure is essential; hypertension, however, may lead to cerebral edema.

3. Achieve normal arterial concentrations of oxygen and carbon dioxide: Excessive oxygen may contribute to increased free radical damage; hypocapnia decreases cerebral perfusion and hypercapnia increases intracranial pressure.

4. Myoclonic status epilepticus after resuscitation from cardiac arrest is usually but not always associated with failure to recover awareness. It should be treated. Valproic acid and clobazam are often effective in stopping the seizures, allowing for a more definitive prognostic assessment.

Bibliography

Binnie CD, Prior PF: Electroencephalography. J Neurol Neurosurg Psychiatry 57:1308, 1994.
Edgren E, Hedstand U, Kelsey S, et al.: Assessment of neurological prognosis in comatose survivors of cardiac arrest. Lancet 343:1055, 1994.
Kuriowa T, Bonnekoh P, Hossmann K-A: Prevention of postischemic hyperthermia prevents ischemic injury of CA_1 neurons in gerbils. J Cereb Blood Flow Metab 10:550, 1990.
Levy DE, Caronna JJ, Singer BH, et al.: Predicting outcome from hypoxic-ischemic coma. JAMA 253:1420, 1985.
Longstreth W, Diehr P, Inui TS: Prediction of awakening after out-of-hospital cardiac arrest. N Engl J Med 308:1378, 1983.
Safar P, Behringer W, Bottiger BW, Sterz F: Cerebral resuscitation potentials for cardiac arrest. Crit Care Med 30:S140, 2002.
Thomassen A, Wernberg M: Prevalence and prognostic significance of coma after cardiac arrest outside intensive care and coronary care units. Acta Anesth Scand 23:143, 1979.
White BC, Grossman LI, Krause GS: Brain injury by global ischemia and reperfusion. Neurology 43:1656, 1993.
Zandbergen ED, de Haan RJ, Stoutenbeek CP, et al.: Systematic review of early prediction of poor outcome in anoxic-ischaemic coma. Lancet 352:1808, 1998.

HYPERCARBIA

Definition

Hypercarbia is defined as a carbon dioxide (CO_2) concentration in the arterial blood (Pa_{CO_2}) more than 60 mm Hg. Only marked elevations of Pa_{CO_2} affect brain metabolism and function.

Etiology

There is usually a background of chronic pulmonary problems with acute decompensation. This often relates to neuromuscular disorders (diminished ventilatory movements) or to diminished central ventilatory drive from an intercurrent illness, a sedative or narcotic drug. These allow for an increase in Pa_{CO_2}.

Pathophysiology

1. Brain cells are freely permeable to carbon dioxide (CO_2), but not to ions, including hydrogen (H^+) and bicarbonate (HCO^-_3). Thus, abrupt increases in arterial or capillary CO_2, associated with decreased pulmonary ventilation produce an intracellular acidosis. CO_3 and intracellular water form carbonic acid (H_3CO_3). The acidosis is understood by referring to the Henderson-Hasselbalch equation.

$$pH = pKa + \log[HCO^-_3] / \log [H_2CO_3].$$

2. Hypoventilation is usually associated with hypoxemia, but if oxygen is supplemented in a patient with an insensitive respiratory center, the Pa_{CO_2} can increase to high concentrations without hypoxemia. This can produce an encephalopathy.

3. Carbon dioxide narcosis is associated with an increase in cerebral blood flow; however, there is

no change in the cerebral metabolic consumption of oxygen or energy metabolism, except for a reduction of phosphocreatine (PCr) in the brain. This decrease in PCr is associated with an increase in the lactate/pyruvate ratio. Both the PCr decrease and the lactate/pyruvate increase are likely due to intracellular acidosis from the effect of increased carbonic acid on enzyme systems

4. Additional metabolic changes include increased glucose-6-phosphate and fructose-6-phosphate and decreases in tricarboxylic acid (TCA) cycle and amino acid pools. There is a state of substrate depletion for the TCA cycle with carbohydrate metabolism that is compensated for by increased amino acid oxidation. This leads to increased intracellular ammonia and hence glutamine concentration (Siesjö et al., 1976). **It is speculated these biochemical changes may alter normal neuronal function.**

5. These changes occur acutely; there is likely greater intracellular buffering of the effects of chronic respiratory acidosis. Intracranial hypertension can result from the increased cerebral blood flow, however.

Clinical Features

1. Early symptoms of CO_2 toxicity include diffuse headache, followed by impairment of conscious level through impaired attention to coma. There may be considerable fluctuations in the degree of obtundation.

2. Brainstem reflexes are spared, but pupils may be miotic. Exceptionally, with the combination of hypoxemia and hypercarbia, an early herniation syndrome may produce pupillary nonreactivity, sometimes unilaterally.

3. Coarse tremor, asterixis, and multifocal myoclonus are very common. Paratonic rigidity and extensor plantar responses are also frequently observed.

4. Chronic hypercarbia may be associated with papilledema from the increase in intracranial blood volume because of arterial dilatation and increased brain blood flow.

Key Signs

- Headache, impairment of consciousness (initially attention)

- Evidence of chronic lung disease/hypoventilation

- Papilledema in extreme cases

Laboratory Testing

1. Arterial or capillary blood gas determination usually reveal a $Paco_2$ level higher than 70 mm Hg and often higher than 90 mm Hg. Oxygenation of the arterial blood is usually reduced because of the hypoventilation.

2. Cerebrospinal fluid is under increased pressure.

3. The electroencephalogram shows diffuse slowing.

Treatment

1. Forced ventilation
2. Correction of the underlying precipitant or cause

Prevention

1. Patients with chronic lung disease or neuromuscular disorders are at risk. Caution should be used in prescribing medications that may reduce ventilatory effort in these patients.

2. Prompt therapy of systemic disorders such as hypokalemia, infections, and other metabolic or toxic disorders.

Key Tests and Treatment

- $Paco_2$ >70 mm Hg can be associated with impaired consciousness and raised intracranial pressure.

- Clinical features are of a metabolic encephalopathy.

- Treatment is forced ventilation.

- Prevent by avoiding administering excessive O_2 or sedative drugs to those at risk for hypoventilation.

 Bibliography

Austen FK, Carmichael MW, Adams RD: Neurologic manifestations of chronic pulmonary insufficiency. N Engl J Med 257:579, 1957.

Borgrström L, Norberg K, Siesjö BK. Glucose consumption in rat cerebral cortex in normoxemia, hypoxia and hypercapnia. Acta Physiol Scand 96:569, 1976.

Siesjö BK, Folbergrova J, MacMillan V: The effect of hypercapnia upon intracellular pH in the brain, evaluated by the bicarbonate-carbonic acid method and from the creatine phosphokinase equilibrium. J Neurochem 19:2483, 1972.

HYPOCARBIA

Definition

Hypocarbia is the lowering of the arterial carbon dioxide concentration to less than 35 mm Hg. This almost always relates to increased ventilation.

Pathophysiology

1. Arterial carbon dioxide concentration ($Paco_2$) is closely linked to cerebral blood flow (CBF). As the carbon dioxide concentration decreases, so does CBF.

2. Hyperventilation to a $Paco_2$ of 22 mm Hg will reduce CBF by 40%. This may mildly compromise cerebral function and causes diffuse slowing of the electroencephalogram (EEG).

Clinical Features

1. Hyperventilation alone is never sufficient to cause coma, but a mild encephalopathy may occur.

2. Hyperventilation may be associated with either a metabolic acidosis or a respiratory alkalosis. However, coma may be related to other disease processes (Table 1–1).

Laboratory Testing

1. Blood gas determination: Hypoapnea and respiratory alkalosis or metabolic acidosis

2. Tests for underlying conditions (Table 1–1).

Treatment

1. Hypocarbia itself usually does not require treatment.

2. Treatment of the underlying condition (Table 1–1).

Clinical Point

• Hypoventilation ($Paco_2$ < 40 mm Hg) alone never causes coma; look for an associated condition

---

TABLE 1–1. CONDITIONS ASSOCIATED WITH HYPERVENTILATION

Metabolic Acidosis	Respiratory Alkalosis
Uremia	Cardiopulmonary problems
Diabetic ketoacidosis	Psychogenic, e.g., panic attacks
Lactic acidosis, including sepsis	Hepatic failure
Salicylate poisoning	Sepsis (early)
Other poisons: Ammonium chloride, paraldehyde, ethylene glycol, methanol	Salicylates (early), dinitrophenol, theophylline, stimulants

Bibliography

Gerace RV: Poisoning. In Young GB, Ropper AH, Bolton CF (eds): Coma and Impaired Consciousness: A Clinical Perspective. New York, McGraw-Hill, 1998, pp. 457–467.
Kety SS, Schmidt CF: The effect of active and passive hyperventilation on the cerebral blood flow, cerebral oxygen concentration, cardiac output and blood pressure in normal young men. J Clin Invest 25:107, 1946.

CARBON MONOXIDE POISONING

Definition

Carbon monoxide (CO) is an odorless, colorless, poisonous gas that is formed by the incomplete combustion of carbon compounds.

Etiology and Epidemiology

1. CO intoxication is the most common form of serious anemic hypoxia, causing death in at least 3500 Americans yearly.

2. Most CO exposure occurs in accidental poisoning at home, either from building fires or from incomplete combustion by furnaces or gas leaks.

3. Other cases include attempted suicide by exposure to automobile exhaust or domestic cooking fumes.

4. Approximately 35% of fire victims have concomitant exposure to CO and cyanide (CN) gas.

Pathophysiology

The toxic effects of CO are due to tissue hypoxia from inactivation of the oxygen-carrying capacity of hemoglobin.

1. Carbon monoxide combines, with an affinity 200 times greater than oxygen, with hemoglobin to form carboxyhemoglobin.

2. Carboxyhemoglobin also prevents the release of oxygen from oxyhemoglobin.

3. The concentration of carboxyhemoglobin in the blood is a function of CO in the inhaled gas and the duration of exposure.

4. Hypoxia from CO usually is accompanied by cerebral ischemia and lactic acidosis.

5. Free radical production and lipid peroxidation have been demonstrated experimentally in rats.

6. CO may also be a mitochondrial poison, especially when there is co-exposure to cyanide (e.g., with wood fires).

7. Patients with delayed deterioration usually have symmetrical damage to deep cerebral white matter, with or without necrosis of the globus pallidus.

Clinical Features

1. The acuity depends on the concentration of CO in the inspired air: 0.05% CO in the inspired air for longer than 1 hour produces a concentration of carboxyhemoglobin of 30% to 50%

    a. High concentrations of CO may produce abrupt coma without warning.

    b. Lower concentrations cause a more protracted prodrome to coma.

2. Mild chronic exposure may result in headache; shortness of breath on exertion or at rest, or vague flulike symptoms; and sometimes bleeding diatheses, fever, and hepatomegaly.

3. Early acute symptoms: Generalized, throbbing headaches; confusion; irritability; dizziness; visual disturbances; nausea; and vomiting. Exertion may produce loss of consciousness.

4. An exposure for 1 hour at concentrations of = 0.1% of CO in inspired air will result in serum carboxyhemoglobin concentrations of 50% to 80% and coma, brainstem compromise with ventilatory failure, convulsions and, usually, death.

5. Physical examination: The most characteristic sign is a cherry-red discoloration of the lips and mucous membranes (not always present).

6. Neurologic examination: Comatose patients may show focal neurologic signs; some may progress to impairment of brainstem function and cranial nerve, including pupillary reflexes.

7. Delayed neurologic deterioration, following improvement, occurs in about 12% of patients who present in coma.

    a. This deterioration begins 2 days to 3 weeks after initial resuscitation.

    b. Acute confusional state accompanied by behavioral change or apathy; cognitive changes including agnosia and apraxia.

    c. This may be followed by severe deterioration in responsiveness with extrapyramidal features or a state resembling akinetic mutism.

    d. Coma may develop and can be followed by a persistent vegetative state.

Key Signs

- Headache, lethargy, vomiting, confusion progressing to stupor then coma
- Cherry-red color of lips and mucous membranes.

Prognosis

1. The prognosis is worse for patients who present in coma: At least 50% are left with severe motor and cognitive deficits.

2. Motor disability involves akinetic mutism, extrapyramidal complications with parkinsonian rigidity, akinesia, spasticity, and lateralized weakness.

3. Cognitive problems include apathy, defective memory, apraxia, visual agnosia, executive frontal lobe dysfunction, and impairments in concentration, attention, perception, and calculation.

Laboratory Testing

1. A blood carboxyhemoglobin concentration test should be done; a level higher than 20% is significant.

2. Arterial or capillary blood gases can help in the assessment of the severity of the hypoxemia insult and resultant metabolic acidosis.

3. Computed tomographic (CT) and magnetic resonance imaging (MRI), especially with the fluid attenuated inversion recovery (FLAIR) pulse imaging, have a role in determining prognosis. Early changes in the basal ganglia and white matter may be found.

Key Tests

- Carboxyhemoglobin: >20% is significant
- Arterial or capillary blood gases
- Baseline CT or MRI of brain

Management

1. Because the half-life of carboxyhemoglobin is inversely proportional to the pressure of oxygen in the inspired air, it follows that 100% oxygen should be promptly delivered. The airway should be secured; endotracheal intubation should be performed if the patient is unconscious. Assisted ventilation may also be necessary.

2. Hyperbaric oxygen is not necessary for patients without impaired consciousness.

3. The use of hyperbaric oxygen seems advisable for comatose CO-poisoned patients. In the face of CO-intoxication, its use seems safe even in infants and in pregnancy.

4. Patients should be monitored carefully in an ICU.

Cerebral edema is a risk and any deterioration should prompt a CT scan. Baseline CT scanning is probably worthwhile in comatose patients, once stabilized.

Prevention

The main prevention of CO intoxication involves fire prevention and the use of smoke detectors and carbon monoxide detectors in homes and buildings.

Key Treatment

- Give 100% oxygen to noncomatose victims of CO poisoning.

- Use hyperbaric oxygen with comatose patients with CO poisoning.

- Monitor patients for cerebral edema, delayed deterioration.

Bibliography

Gajdos PH, Korach JM, Conso F, et al.: Epidemiological investigation of acute carbon monoxide poisoning (A-CMP) in the Hauts-De-Seine department. Results of a 3 year survey. Intensive Care Med 14:324, 1988.

Ginsberg MD: Carbon monoxide intoxication: Clinical features, neuropathology and mechanisms of injury. Clin Toxicol 23:281, 1985.

Moore SJ, Norris JC, Walsh DA, Hume AS: Antidotal use of methylhemoglobin forming cyanide antagonists in concurrent carbon monoxide/cyanide intoxication. J Pharmacol Exp Ther 242:70, 1987.

Murata T, Itoh S, Loshino Y, et al.: Serial cerebral MRI with FLAIR sequences in acute carbon monoxide poisoning. J Comput Assist Tomogr 19:631, 1995.

Parkinson RB, Hopkins RO, Cleavinger HB, et al.: White matter hyperintensities and neuropsychological outcome following carbon monoxide poisoning. Neurology 58:1525, 2002.

Raphael J-C, Elkharrat D, Jars-Guinestre M-C, et al.: Trial of normobaric and hyperbaric oxygen for acute carbon monoxide intoxication. Lancet 2:414, 1989.

Vieregge P, Klostermann W, Blümm RG, Borgis KJ: Carbon monoxide poisoning: Clinical, neurophysiological, and brain imaging observations in acute disease and follow-up. J Neurol 236:478, 1988.

HEPATIC FAILURE

Definition and Classification

Hepatic failure and its associated encephalopathy can be classified into two distinct clinical entities, acute hepatic failure and chronic liver disease.

1. Acute hepatic failure
   a. Encephalopathy and coagulopathy within 6 months of the onset of acute liver disease. A subcategory, fulminant hepatic failure, usually refers to the development of cerebral dysfunction within 8 weeks of the initial development of the liver disorder.
   b. Evolutionary time course of onset is dependent on etiology.
      (1) Acute hepatic failure over a period of 1 week or less suggests a toxic cause.
      (2) Acute hepatic failure of more than 4 weeks is characteristic of viral hepatitis.
2. Chronic liver disease: Evolves over a longer time, with a fluctuating course or relapses. It is related to a combination of hepatocellular failure and portal-systemic shunting in which blood is diverted from the hepatic portal to the systemic circulation.

Etiology

1. See Table 2-1.
2. Chronic hepatic encephalopathy in North America is most commonly related to chronic alcoholism, but it may follow any condition that acutely damages the liver and disturbs its architecture to allow portal-systemic shunting of blood.

Epidemiology and Significance

Acute liver failure affects over 2000 persons per year in the United States. All are encephalopathic. The mortality is nearly 80%. Chronic hepatic encephalopathy occurs, conservatively, in about 1/3000 persons.

Pathophysiology

The detailed biochemical mechanisms have not been firmly established or entirely explained. Several hypothetical mechanisms and toxic chemicals have been proposed.

1. Increased benzodiazepine receptor activity. Increased endogenous benzodiazepine-like substances (endozepines) described in hepatic coma. Flumazenil, an antagonist of the γ-aminobutyric acid (GABA) A receptor may produce a transient improvement in the encephalopathy.
2. Ammonia: There is a rough correlation of the encephalopathy with serum and brain ammonia concentration.
3. Abnormalities of neurotransmission: The increased ratio of aromatic to branched amino acids may alter the balance of neurotransmitters derived from these; also, increased levels of octopamine, a putative false neurotransmitter
4. Mercaptans: These organic thio-alcohols inhibit urea cycle enzymes and contribute to hyperammonemia. They also depress mitochondrial respiration in liver and brain; some have direct membrane effects.
5. Short-chain fatty acids: Free fatty acids are increased in the plasma of patients with hepatic coma. This may lead to reduced cellular redox potentials in mitochondria. The enzymes involved in urea and glutamate synthesis are inhibited, and sodium–potassium ATPase activity is reduced. A

TABLE 2-1.   PRINCIPAL CAUSES OF ACUTE LIVER FAILURE

CAUSE	AGENT RESPONSIBLE
Viral hepatitis*	Hepatitis A, B, C, D, and E
	Herpes simplex virus
Drug-induced liver injury	Acetaminophen
	Idiosyncratic reactions
Toxins	Carbon tetrachloride
	Amanita phalloides
	Phosphorus
Vascular events	Ischemia
	Veno-occlusive disease
	Heatstroke
	Malignant hyperthermia
Miscellaneous	Wilson's disease
	Acute fatty liver of pregnancy
	Reye's syndrome
	Lymphoma
	Status epilepticus in children (rare) (Decell et al., 1994)†

*Accounts for more than 80% of cases in North America.
†Decell MK, Gordon JB, Silver K, Meagher-Villemure K: Fulminant hepatic failure associated with status epilepticus: Three cases and a review of potential mechanisms. Intensive Care Med 20:375–378, 1994.
From Lee WM: Acute liver failure. N Engl J Med 329:1862, 1993, with permission.

synergistic role with ammonia in producing impairment of brain function is possible.

6. Manganese intoxication. Mn is increased in the corpus striatum in hepatic encephalopathy. The mechanism for Mn neurotoxicity is not known, but in excess amounts it is a known cellular toxicant that can impair transport systems, mitochondrial and other enzyme activities, and membrane receptor function.

7. Phenols, free radicals, and copper have also been proposed to affect the brain in hepatic encephalopathy.

Clinical Features

1. Fulminant hepatic failure
   a. Delirium with delusions and hyperkinesis occurs commonly in fulminant hepatic failure and may precede icterus.
   b. Typically, the agitated confusional state (stages I and II) within hours is followed by stupor with preserved arousal (stage III) and then coma (stage IV). Mania has been described in children with the acute phase. Mortality is directly related to the encephalopathic grade.
   c. Patients with cerebral edema (about 80% of those with stage IV coma) frequently show a widened pulse pressure and bradycardia (Cushing's response), decortication, decerebration, and herniation.

2. Portal-systemic (chronic) hepatic encephalopathy
   a. Abnormalities on neuropsychological tests precede the clinical syndrome. Visuospatial and perceptuo-motor tasks are impaired and are followed by deficits in concentration and attention.
   b. With portal-systemic encephalopathy, the progression from stage I to stage IV (see above) is more gradual, variable, and potentially reversible than with acute hepatic failure.
   c. Hyperventilation and respiratory alkalosis, probably due to stimulation of the respiratory center by peptides from the gut, are almost universal. Hyperthermia is a near-terminal event, unless it is due to a complication such as infection.
   d. Asterixis is common; an intention or postural-action tremor occasionally appears. Frontal lobe signs (e.g., sucking, grasp, and palmomental reflexes) are common. Extrapyramidal features, including parkinsonian rigidity, sometimes occur. *Gegenhalten,* or paratonic rigidity, is almost universal. Dysarthria occurs in stage II; this can deteriorate into unintelligible speech. Some patients have an ataxic gait. With

deep coma, "false localizing signs" may appear. These include hemiparesis, ocular bobbing, skew deviation, dysconjugate eye movements, or tonic downward deviation of the eyes. Multifocal myoclonus occurs late and is not as common in hepatic failure as in renal failure. Convulsive seizures are found only in advanced encephalopathy or in complications such as hypoglycemia.
   e. The diagnosis of hepatic encephalopathy is helped by the almost universally present jaundice and stigmata of liver disease, including spider nevi, fetor hepaticus, enlarged or shrunken liver, signs of portal hypertension, parotid enlargement, clubbing and palmar erythema.

Key Signs

- Signs of chronic liver failure: Spider nevi, portal hypertension

- Acute liver failure: Usually jaundiced

- In both acute and chronic: Respiratory alkalosis, impaired attention and alertness (from delirium to coma), asterixis, tremor, multifocal myoclonus

Laboratory Testing

1. Biochemistry: The most sensitive and specific confirmatory test of hepatic encephalopathy is elevated CSF glutamine concentration. However, this is not commonly available and lumbar puncture is hazardous if there is an associated coagulopathy. The diagnosis of hepatic encephalopathy is strengthened by the demonstration of abnormal liver function tests. These reflect the acuity and severity of the problem, as well as provide information that is helpful in management. With acute hepatocellular damage, there is marked elevation of serum transaminase values. Serum bilirubin and alkaline phosphatase concentrations are increased. As mentioned above, a respiratory alkalosis accompanies hepatic encephalopathy. Serum glucose should be monitored; hypoglycemia relates to defective gluconeogenesis as well as to elevated serum insulin levels from inadequate uptake of insulin by the failing liver. Serum glucose is often depressed in acute liver failure and in Reye's syndrome, but seldom in chronic hepatic encephalopathy. Hypokalemia and hyponatremia are common.

2. Hematology: Severe coagulopathy is common. This relates in part to the defective synthesis of coagulation factors II, V, VII, IX, and X, causing

elevation of the prothrombin time (or INR) and partial thromboplastin time. Antithrombin III is decreased, platelet counts are usually less than 100,000/mm³, and platelet function is altered.

3. Electroencephalogram (EEG): Shows the progression of abnormalities often seen in other metabolic encephalopathies. Mild cases are associated with intermittent or persistent diffuse theta waves (>4 and <8 Hz frequencies). With further progression, triphasic waves or frontally predominant intermittent, high-amplitude, rhythmic delta waves (<4 Hz frequencies) are seen. These subside and are followed by diffuse, persistent arrhythmic delta waves and then by suppression with progressive deepening of coma. Epileptiform discharges, spikes or seizures, either multifocal or diffuse, occur in acute, rapidly progressive or very advanced (usually), ultimately fatal chronic hepatic encephalopathy.

Radiographic Features

1. Neuro-imaging: In chronic hepatic encephalopathy, computed tomographic (CT) scans show widened sulci over the frontal lobes, a narrowed third ventricle, even in patients without any history of alcoholism. Neuroimaging tests, CT or magnetic resonance imaging (MRI), may also demonstrate cerebral edema, especially in patients with stages III and IV fulminant hepatic encephalopathy, and will exclude other structural lesions, such as subdural hematomas.

   The globus pallidus shows an increase in signal on the T_1-weighted MRI in most patients with cirrhosis, but the intensity of the globus pallidus does not correlate with the severity of the hepatic encephalopathy. This increase is reversible following normalization of the biochemical derangements or following successful hepatic transplantation.

Key Tests

- Abnormal liver function tests
- Respiratory alkalosis on blood gas testing
- EEG: Triphasic waves
- Increased T_1 signal in globus pallidus on MRI (with portal-caval encephalopathy)

Management

1. Acute and chronic hepatic failure with encephalopathy
   Manage in ICU and monitor level of consciousness, watching for systemic conditions including systemic inflammation, infection, hypoglycemia, coagulopathies, pulmonary shunting. Chart temperature, pulse, intake and output, daily weights, and chest examination. Serum urea, glucose, bilirubin, electrolytes, hemoglobin, white cell and platelet count should be checked daily. 10% glucose should be administered as necessary for hypoglycemia. Serum electrolytes must be appropriately monitored and managed. If platelets drop below 50,000/mm³, platelet transfusion may be necessary. Fresh-frozen plasma is warranted only for active bleeding problems. Because infection is a common life-threatening complication, surveillance and prompt therapy are essential.

2. For patients with chronic liver disease, it is essential to aggressively determine and treat/eliminate the precipitant. Sepsis and gastrointestinal bleeding may not be obvious and require careful investigation and treatment.

3. The patient should be monitored for cerebral edema and any increase in intracranial pressure (ICP). Coagulopathy often makes most invasive methods of continuously monitoring intracranial pressure hazardous, but the epidural monitor may be an effective compromise. ICP monitoring should be considered for patients with grade 3/4 hepatic encephalopathy who are at high risk for cerebral edema. Monitoring is especially useful in the preoperative and postoperative period in patients with acute liver failure undergoing liver transplantation. If invasive monitoring is not feasible, transcranial Doppler monitoring of cerebral blood flow may be useful. Increased velocity is an indication of advanced edema and raised ICP, however. A CT scan of the head is recommended to exclude intracranial hemorrhages and to provide a rough evaluation of brain edema.

   a. Elevation of the head of the bed by 45 degrees has been recommended in the management of raised ICP. However, this is hazardous, as elevations of greater than 20 degrees reduce cerebral perfusion pressure.

   b. Medical management of elevated ICP: Mannitol administration is useful for cerebral edema and increased ICP, at least for patients with stage III encephalopathy. A rapid infusion of 100 to 200 mL of 20% mannitol is administered; this can be repeated. Tachyphylaxis, or rapidly developing tolerance, occurs with mannitol; therefore, it is a temporary measure. Dexamethazone is not effective in hepatic encephalopathy. Although hyperventilation may reduce ICP, it further reduces brain perfusion. It was not helpful in a trial for ICP management in acute liver failure. Pentobarbital coma or thiopental may help control ICP in desperate situations when mannitol is no longer effective or not possible because of renal impairment, e.g., to buy time before liver transplantation. Anesthetic barbiturates often eliminate the clinical evaluation of coma, but such patients are in deep coma in any case. Hypotension must be prevented. The prevention/treatment of massively raised ICP should take precedence over concerns about drug clearance in this situation.

4. General management for both acute and chronic hepatic failure

   a. Reduce ammonia production from the gastrointestinal tract by bowel clearance with enemas, lactulose or lactilol, and antimicrobials (e.g., neomycin, tetracycline, vancomycin, or metronidazole)

   b. Maintain caloric intake with carbohydrate to prevent protein catabolism and ammonia production; dietary protein should be stopped initially and glucose given (drinks, gastric or intravenous infusions) at 1600 calories per day.

   c. Prothrombin times should be checked and additional vitamin K administered if necessary. Fresh frozen plasma may be necessary in the face of active bleeding and a hepatic-related coagulopathy unresponsive to vitamin K. B-complex vitamins and potassium supplements for hypokalemia should be provided.

5. The use of infusions of branched-chain amino acids, levodopa or bromocriptine or flumazenil may benefit some patients in the short term.

6. Flumazenil was found to have an inconsistent effect in a series of seven children with encephalopathy secondary to fulminant hepatic failure: only one transiently improved in level of consciousness. A definitive randomized controlled study is needed to evaluate the role of flumazenil.

7. Occasionally the occlusion of portacaval anastomoses or esophageal varices is beneficial, the latter to stop gastrointestinal bleeding as well as to reduce shunting of blood past the liver.

8. Liver transplantation is appropriate for selected patients with acute hepatic failure. The survival rates are now over 70%. Keays and colleagues (1991) at King's College in London recently prepared guidelines for liver transplantation in acute hepatic failure (Table 2–2).

9. Charcoal hemoperfusion and prostaglandin E_1 have not improved outcomes over standard care in controlled trials. Despite some experimental

TABLE 2–2. CRITERIA FOR CONSIDERATION OF LIVER TRANSPLANTATION IN ACUTE LIVER FAILURE

Acetaminophen Toxicity
pH< 7.3 (regardless of coma grade)
or
Prothrombin time >100 seconds and serum creatinine >3.4 mg/dL (300 µmol/L) in patients with grade III or IV encephalopathy

All Other Causes
Prothrombin time >100 sec (regardless of coma grade), or any three of the following (regardless of coma grade):
Age <10 years but >40 years
Liver failure caused by non-A, non-B hepatitis, halothane-induced hepatitis, or idiosyncratic drug reactions
Duration of jaundice before the onset of encephalopathy >7 days
Prothrombin time >50 seconds
Serum bilirubin > 300 µmol/L (17.5 mg/dL)

support for improvement in hepatocellular regeneration, a controlled trial of insulin and glucagon proved unsuccessful in the treatment of fulminant hepatic failure.

10. Other procedures such as hepatocyte transplantation and bioartifical liver devices are promising. Intrasplenic hepatocellular transplantation in portacaval shunted rats improves locomotor activity. Extracorporeal hybrid bioartificial livers with porcine hepatocytes and charcoal filters can carry or "bridge" patients until a transplant is possible. According to a preliminary report, patients tolerate the procedure well and show an improvement in level of consciousness, intracranial pressure, cerebral perfusion pressure, and plasma biochemistry.

 Key Treatment

• Decrease ammonia production: low protein, high calorie diet; purge the bowel with lactulose

• Search for and treat underlying conditions/accompaniments: sepsis, gastrointestinal bleeding, coagulopathies, electrolyte disturbances

• Watch for and treat cerebral edema (especially with acute liver failure)

• Liver transplant: see Table 2–2: Criteria for Consideration of Liver Transplantation in Acute Liver Failure

 ## Bibliography

Blei AT: Cerebral edema and intracranial hypertension in acute liver failure: Distinct aspects of the same problem. Hepatology 13:376, 1991.
Brock J, Buckley N, Gluud C: Interventions for paracetamol (acetaminophen) overdose (Cochrane Review). Cochrane Review). Cochrane Database Syst Rev 3:CD003328, 2002.

Chapman RW, Forman D, Peto R, et al.: Liver transplantation for acute hepatic failure. Lancet 335:32, 1990.

Keays R, Potter D, O'Grady J, et al.: Intracranial and cerebral perfusion pressures before, during and immediately after orthotopic liver transplantation for fulminant hepatic failure. Q J Med 79:425, 1991.

Lee WM: Acute liver failure. N Engl J Med 329:1862, 1993.

Lockwood AH: Hepatic encephalopathy. Neurol Clin 20: 241–246, 2002.

Naylor CD, O'Rourke K, Detsky AS, et al.: Parenteral nutrition with branched-chain amino acids in hepatic encephalopathy: A meta-analysis. Gastroenterology 97: 1033, 1989.

Ribeiro J, Noprdlinger B, Ballet F, et al.: Intrasplenic hepatocellular transplantation corrects hepatic encephalopathy in portacaval-shunted rats. Hepatology 15:12, 1992.

RENAL FAILURE

Definition

Renal failure can be defined as a deterioration in kidney function that allows a build-up of nitrogenous wastes in the body. Neurologic disorders in patients with renal failure include uremic encephalopathy (acute and chronic), uremic neuropathies and myopathy, complications of therapy for uremia, and systemic disorders.

Etiology

Renal failure can be divided into pre-renal (diminished perfusion), intrinsic kidney disease and postrenal (outlet obstruction). At least half the cases of acute renal failure relate to surgery or trauma, others are due to medical conditions or complications of pregnancy. Ischemia, nephrotoxins, or, less commonly, rhabdomyolysis or hemolysis (with release of nephrotoxic myoglobin or hemoglobin into the plasma) are common underlying mechanisms for these etiologies to produce kidney failure.

Chronic renal failure is most commonly the result of glomerulonephritis. Other causes include renal damage from hypertension or diabetes, chronic infections, interstitial nephritis and hereditary causes, especially polycystic kidney disease.

Epidemiology

1. About 5% of hospitalized patients develop acute renal failure. This is often reversible.

2. End-stage chronic renal failure: 133 per million population require regular dialysis therapy or renal transplantation.

Pathophysiology

1. Renal disease can affect neurologic function either directly, through the effects of retained uremic toxins, or indirectly through complications of renal failure or its treatment.

2. Some systemic disorders may affect both the kidneys and the brain.

3. The specific uremic neurotoxin has not been identified, but it is unlikely that a single retained chemical species will account for uremic encephalopathy for all patients. Uremic neurotoxins could alter

   a. Neurotransmitter and synaptic function

   b. Enzymes

   c. The sodium–potassium pump mechanism

   d. Transcription from DNA to messenger RNA

   e. Phosphodiesterase and phosphoinositide functions

   f. Phosphate transfer in various enzymes and microtubular function.

Clinical Features

1. Acute renal failure (ARF): There are few specific features that differentiate uremic encephalopathy from other metabolic encephalopathies. However, the following combination suggests uremia, after the exclusion of exogenous agents:

   a. An encephalopathy with hyperventilation from a metabolic acidosis

   b. Excitability, including prominent myoclonus (usually multifocal but occasionally with action) or seizures (usually generalized). Tetany may also be found.

2. Chronic renal failure (CRF)

   a. Encephalopathy: In CRF signs and symptoms are less florid or fulminant than in ARF.

      (1) Lethargy and fatigability, problems concentrating, slowness in thinking and impaired memory function. More detailed neuropsychological studies have shown impairment in complex cognitive functions, including spatial synthesis and other visuoperceptual tasks, logical-grammatical and mathematical operations.

      (2) Headaches, sleep disturbances, dysarthric speech, and abnormal hormonal (including sexual) functions

      (3) Motor phenomena (common)

         (a) Tremor

         (b) Myoclonus: multifocal or synchronous

         (c) Asterixis

         (d) Paratonic rigidity

         (e) Primitive reflexes (rooting, grasp and snout)

(f) A coarse, irregular postural-action tremor: Best seen on supporting the limbs against gravity or on reaching for something

(g) Seizures: Usually generalized convulsions will occur as a near-terminal event, preceded by coma, in very advanced, untreated uremia or if a complication arises, e.g., stroke or metabolic upset, leading to a sudden change in acid-base or electrolyte composition, or to hypocalcemia

(4) Uremic meningitis

(a) May complicate chronic uremic encephalopathy

(b) Consciousness is not seriously compromised, but patients exhibit nuchal rigidity and positive Kernig's sign.

b. Uremic polyneuropathy: By the time end-stage renal disease is reached, 50% of patients have polyneuropathy. It tends to stabilize during treatment by chronic hemodialysis or peritoneal hemodialysis and then regularly improves with successful renal transplantation.

(1) The earliest and most prevalent symptoms are restless legs syndrome, muscle cramping, and distal paresthesias. (The burning foot syndrome, caused by a deficiency of the water-soluble B vitamins that are washed out during the hemodialysis procedure, is now rarely seen because of proper vitamin supplementation.)

(2) In more severe neuropathies, distal weakness (most marked in the legs), a stocking-glove loss of sensation to all modalities (pain, temperature, touch, vibration, position and fine discriminative sensory function), and an unsteady gait occur.

(3) The earliest signs of uremic polyneuropathy are loss of vibration sense in toes and reduction of deep tendon reflexes, beginning with ankle jerks.

c. Myopathy in uremia

(1) Relatively acute forms of myopathy associated with renal failure are those caused by water and electrolyte disturbances. If muscle weakness occurs in acute attacks, periodic paralysis associated with potassium disturbance should be considered. Hypocalcemia may occur and become manifest as tetany, but this is rare because of the often associated acidosis in renal failure.

(2) A more chronic myopathy may be induced as a complication of steroid therapy.

Key Signs

- Encephalopathy: fluctuating confusion, apathy; spontaneous and stimulus-sensitive myoclonus, asterixis, hyperventilation (metabolic acidosis), seizures

- Polyneuropathy: restless legs, burning feet, distal sensory impairment, distal wasting, loss of ankle jerks

Differential Diagnosis

The chief conditions to be considered in uremic myopathies are

1. The nonspecific cachexia associated with chronic renal failure

2. Wasting of proximal limb muscle associated with underlying bone disease that is due to either secondary hyperparathyroidism or aluminum accumulation. Needle electromyography reveals no clear-cut abnormalities, the creatine kinase levels are usually normal, and biopsy reveals some atrophy of type 2 muscle fibers.

Laboratory Testing

1. Biochemistry: In chronic renal failure the serum creatinine is 2.2 mg/dL (195 μmol/L) or higher. This represents a greater than 80% reduction of kidney function or a glomerular filtration rate below 20 mL/minute

2. EEG

a. Routine EEG may be normal with mild encephalopathy

b. Then intermittent bursts of low-voltage theta waves (>4 and <8 Hz rhythmic waves)

c. With more severe encephalopathy the EEG shows slowing of frequencies and an increase in amplitude. Bursts of rhythmic delta waves (<4 Hz waves) are common, especially on arousal from sleep; triphasic waves may be superimposed on background slowing.

d. Increased excitability: A photomyogenic response (muscle twitches of the face coincident with light flashes) or photoparoxysmal (generalized epileptiform discharges in response to photic stimulation). Bursts of irregular generalized spike and wave activity may also occur spontaneously during the recording.

3. Electromyography (EMG)

a. Nerve conduction velocity decreases in parallel with renal function, as measured by the creatinine clearance test. Compound muscle and sensory nerve action potential amplitudes decrease because of dispersion from secondary demyelination or fallout of larger myelinated axons from a primary axonal degeneration

b. Needle electromyography: Even with axonal neuropathy, fibrillation potentials and positive sharp waves may be relatively absent in human uremic muscle, possibly because of the inhibition of extrajunctional acetylcholine receptors. This may also explain failure of collateral reinnervation of muscle, which is dependent on the presence of these receptors. Thus, there may be little spontaneous activity, and motor unit potentials may be decreased in number, small in size, but polyphasic, suggesting a myopathy (as noted below).

c. Computer analysis: Reduced number of motor unit potentials

d. H-reflex and F-wave studies, which measure conduction on motor fibers both proximally and distally, have shown some prolongation of latencies in up to 85% of patients in end-stage renal failure, particularly those undergoing chronic hemodialysis.

4. Cerebrospinal fluid: May show up to 250 lymphocytes/mm^3 and up to 1.0 g/L (100 mg/dL) protein concentration

Radiologic Features

1. Neuroimaging is usually unhelpful. Cerebral atrophy may accompany dehydration

2. MRI may show reversible changes (low signal intensity T_1-weighted and high signal on T_2-weighted scans) in the periventricular white matter, basal ganglia, and internal capsule. These disappear or vary with dialysis.

Treatment

1. Conservative treatment involves preserving and facilitating remaining renal function, controlling uremic toxins with diet, treating the symptoms of seizures with anti-epileptic medications, and so on.

2. When end-stage renal disease has been reached, the patient is placed on either chronic hemodialysis or peritoneal dialysis.

3. Kidney transplantation has been shown to produce a much better quality of life than dialysis, and is much more cost-effective.

Key Tests

- Glomerular filtration rate usually <20mL/minute

- Blood urea nitrogen usually > 80 mg% (>30 mmol/L); serum creatinine

- Usually >6.0 mg% or >530 mmol/L

- Tests to establish pre-renal (volume depletion) and post-renal (obstructive) from renal disease

- Check serum electrolytes, calcium, phosphate, acid-base balance

- EEG: Intermittent rhythmic delta; triphasic waves

- EMG: Nerve conduction velocity, compound muscle and sensory nerve action potential amplitudes decrease. Needle electrode studies may show decreased motor unit potentials and mild, if any, denervation. Findings are due to an axonal polyneuropathy.

RELATED CONDITIONS

Dialysis Dementia

1. Occurrence: This clinical syndrome was initially described in clusters of patients on chronic hemodialysis, although a similar syndrome may occur in patients on peritoneal dialysis or those receiving orally ingested aluminum-containing phosphate binders.

2. Etiology and pathogenesis: The condition is related to an accumulation of aluminum in the brain. This interferes with a number of neuronal processes and may even cause neurofibrillary degeneration. The condition is progressive and fatal unless treated vigorously.

3. Clinical features

a. An initial nonfluent speech disturbance (aphasia plus dysarthria)

b. Involuntary motor phenomena (especially myoclonus and seizures)

c. Gait disturbance (apraxia or ataxia)

d. Mental changes: Initially apathy and behavioral changes, combined with speech and writing errors; confusional states appear transiently shortly after dialysis; memory failure, poor attention, disorientation; psychotic behavior, apraxia, and dyscalculia have been noted. Eventually the patient becomes bedridden, incontinent, and stuporous.

e. Associated features: Fracturing osteodystrophy and a severe, refractory microcytic anemia

Key Signs: Dialysis Dementia or Aluminum Intoxication

- Hesitant speech with aphasic errors

- Gait ataxia, apraxia, or both

- Myoclonus

4. Laboratory testing

a. EEG: Frequent "projected" bursts of rhythmic delta activity, triphasic waves, or irregular generalized epileptiform discharges

b. Serum aluminum levels are helpful but often not definitive. Although serum aluminum levels of <50 µg/L are unlikely to be associated with dialysis dementia, occasional cases have may have low levels. Bone aluminum measurements and the desferoxamine infusion test are further refinements.

Key Tests: Dialysis Dementia or Aluminum Intoxication

- EEG: Shows abortive generalized spike wave, projected activity, or triphasic waves despite adequate dialysis

- Plasma aluminum: Markedly elevated

- Urinary aluminum: Increased with desferoxamine infusion test

5. Management

a. With first symptoms of the condition, the patient should be withdrawn from all sources of aluminum (especially in dialysate, aluminum-containing antacids).

b. Desferoxamine, a chelating agent for aluminum, can be given safely on an intermittent or long-term basis. This can help arrest progression of the disorder and may reverse many of the features.

c. Symptomatic therapy with anti-epileptic drugs such as phenytoin or valproate may be necessary. Although benzodiazepines may have a transiently beneficial effect on the clinical features, their long-term usefulness has not been demonstrated.

Key Management: Dialysis Dementia

- Remove aluminum exposure if diagnosis suspected

- Desferoxamine treatment if diagnosis confirmed

- Symptomatic anti-epileptic drug therapy: Valproate or phenytoin

Dialysis Dysequilibrium

1. Definition: Dialysis dysequilibrium, a syndrome with a close temporal relationship to hemodialysis treatment, occurs mainly during or after the initial dialysis treatment in patients with chronic renal failure.

2. Etiology

a. Osmotic mismatch between the plasma and brain, with relatively lower osmolality in the blood than in the brain during dialysis

b. Intracellular acidosis in the brain

3. Clinical features: Begin either during or immediately after the dialysis treatment

a. Mild: Headache, nausea, vomiting, restlessness or drowsiness and muscle cramps, variably accompanied by disorientation and tremors

b. Moderate: Disorientation, somnolence, asterixis, and myoclonus

c. Severely affected patients develop an acute organic psychosis, coma, or generalized convulsions.

Key Signs

- Encephalopathic features during or just after dialysis therapy

- Syndrome is most common in uremic patients who are just starting hemodialysis therapy after having been managed conservatively

4. Laboratory testing

a. EEG: bursts of slow-frequency waves, higher voltage and slower with increasing severity of the encephalopathy, against an abnormal, mildly slowed or markedly dysrhythmic background. Generalized epileptiform activity may be found in patients with seizures. The EEG returns to normal with resolution of the encephalopathy.

b. The cerebrospinal fluid becomes acidotic during attacks.

5. Prevention

a. Use slower blood flow rates in dialysis by increasing the osmolality of the dialysate with the addition of urea, sodium, mannitol, or glycerol, or with the use of hemofiltration followed by dialysis or peritoneal dialysis.

b. Glycerol prevents the intracellular acidosis. Substituting bicarbonate for acetate in the dialysate has also been recommended.

Key Management

- Suspect dialysis dysequilibrium if central nervous system symptoms arise during or just after dialysis

- CSF acidosis during attack

- Prevent by using slower flow rates and increasing osmolality of dialysate

Subdural Hematoma in Hemodyalized Patients with Uremia

1. Incidence: Subdural hematomas, found in 1% to 3.3% of patients on hemodialysis, sometimes associated with anticoagulant therapy, can occur at any age in uremia. The hematomas are large in about 10% of cases; most show fresh bleeding with evidence of older hemorrhage. Iatrogenic and intrinsic uremic coagulopathies likely both contribute.

2. Clinical features
   a. Usually present with headache and tenderness of the head to percussion.
   b. Often decreased alertness and cognition or (apparent) emotional depression. (These are common features in uremia, so subdural hematomas can easily be overlooked.)
   c. Focal signs predominate in some patients; hemiparesis or a language disturbance may occur.
   d. Gait apraxia in older patients with subdural hematoma is common.

3. Radiologic testing
   Diagnosis is easily made with CT (beware of the isodense subdural hematoma, however) or MRI scans.

4. Management
   Treatment is usually surgical drainage. Occasional patients can be managed conservatively, but they require close follow-up.

Key Tests: Subdural Hematoma

- Suspect in any patient on hemodialysis who develops headaches, focal signs, gait problems, or cognitive decline
- CT or MRI of the head

Wernicke's Encephalopathy

1. Epidemiology: Wernicke's encephalopathy occurs in those dialyzed patients who are too ill to eat or who repeatedly vomit and are placed on intravenous solutions that do not contain thiamine. Uremic patients with hyperkalemia may be most at risk, as glucose boluses are often given to reduce the serum potassium concentration.

2. Clinical features: In some patients the classical features of ophthalmoplegia, nystagmus, encephalopathy, and ataxia may not all be present. Without the ocular findings there is great difficulty in differential diagnosis unless Wernicke's enceph-

alopathy is considered. Some patients may present with an encephalopathy and hypothermia (presumably from hypothalamic involvement).

Key Signs: Wernicke's Encephalopathy

- Ophthalmoplegia (gaze or single nerve), nystagmus, ataxia, encephalopathy
- All cardinal features may not be present.
- Consider the diagnosis in the hypothermic patient with impaired consciousness.

3. Prevention: Ensure vitamin supplementation in patients on dialysis therapy or those who are eating poorly.

4. Treatment: Prompt therapy with thiamine, 50 mg parenterally, followed by daily doses for several days, should be given as soon as the diagnosis of Wernicke's encephalopathy is even considered.

Key Treatment

- Supplement all patients on dialysis with thiamine.
- Give extra thiamine if encephalopathy, hypothermia, ataxia, or ocular movement abnormalities occur.

Rejection Encephalopathy

1. Incidence: Rejection encephalopathy affects mainly patients between 10 and 38 years of age, usually within the first few months after renal transplantation.

2. Etiology and pathogenesis: The release of cytokines may be of pathogenetic importance.

3. Clinical features: Symptoms include headache, confusion, or convulsions along with systemic features of graft rejection.

4. Management: The condition is treated symptomatically, mainly with anti-epileptic drugs and increased immunosuppression to combat the graft rejection response. The prognosis is usually favorable.

Key Treatment: Rejection Encephalopathy

- Enhanced immunosuppressive therapy if diagnosis is likely and other causes excluded

Infections

1. Classification: Infections of the central nervous system (CNS) can be divided into viral, fungal,

and bacterial. Predisposing factors, besides the immunosuppression, include diabetes, intravascular lines, uremia, and urinary catheters.

   a. Viral infections peak between 1 and 6 months after transplantation and include cytomegalovirus (can cause retinitis, blindness, and an encephalitis) and Epstein-Barr virus. Progressive multifocal leukoencephalopathy, caused by the JC picornavirus, may occur after many months or years of immunosuppression. Hepatitis C virus infection may cause an encephalopathy indirectly if hepatic failure occurs.

   b. Opportunistic fungi are mainly *Aspergillus fumigatus* and *Nocardia asteroides*. *Cryptococcus neoformans* may cause infection later in the course.

   c. The main bacterial infection is *Listeria monocytogenes*. *Mycobacterium tuberculosis* may cause infections late in the course.

2. Clinical features: Initial symptoms and signs of CNS infection may be dampened by the anti-inflammatory effects of the immunosuppressive therapy, so a high index of suspicion needs to be maintained.

3. Laboratory testing: CSF analysis, including polymerase chain reaction testing on the CSF (e.g., for the JC virus and *M. tuberculosis*); special stains and cultures are sometimes helpful.

4. Radiologic features: CT or MRI with contrast

Key Tests: Opportunistic Infections

- Neuroimaging (CT, MRI)
- CSF analysis

5. Management
   Recruitment of expert microbiological expertise is recommended. Treatment is targeted to the specific underlying infection.

Post-Transplant Lymphoproliferative Disorder

1. Definition and classification: Proliferation of B lymphocytes with disorders ranging from monoclonal gammopathy to B cell lymphomas of the CNS

2. Laboratory testing: Brain biopsy (stereotaxic) is usually necessary (see Radiologic Testing).

3. Radiologic testing: Lymphomas tend to be periventricular and multiple, with uniform contrast enhancement on CT and indistinct or fuzzy margins.

Key Tests: Suspect Central Nervous System Lymphoma

- MRI or CT of head
- Stereotaxic brain biopsy

4. Management: The condition may respond initially to radiation and chemotherapy, but the overall prognosis is usually poor.

Bibliography

Bolton CF, Young GB: Neurological Complications of Renal Disease. Boston, Butterworths, 1990.

Fraser CL: Neurologic manifestations of the uremic state. In Arieff AI, Griggs RC (eds): Metabolic Brain Dysfunction in Systemic Disorders. Boston, Little, Brown, 1992, pp. 139–166.

Jagadha V, Deck JHN, Halliday WC, et al.: Wernicke's encephalopathy in patients on chronic peritoneal dialysis or hemodialysis. Ann Neurol 21:78, 1987.

Ok E, Ünsal A, Çelik A, et al.: Clinicopathological features of rapidly progressive hepatitis C virus infection in HCV antibody negative renal transplant recipients. Nephrol Dial Transplant 13:3103, 1998.

Okada J, Yoshikawa K, Matsuo H, et al.: Reversible MRI and CT findings in uremic encephalopathy. Neuroradiology 33:524, 1991.

Raskin NH: Neurological complications of renal failure. In Aminoff MJ (ed): Neurology and General Medicine, 3rd ed. New York, Churchill Livingstone, 2001, pp. 293–306.

3 Vitamin Deficiency and Toxicity

Russell C. Packard

Definition

1. Vitamin deficiency in modern society results mainly from poverty, food faddism, drug misuse, chronic alcoholism, or prolonged parenteral feeding.

2. Although lack of these trace substances are generally associated with megavitamin deficiency syndrome, health enthusiasm has reached such a passionate pitch that some neurotoxic syndromes result from megavitamin therapy.

Vitamin Deficiency Etiology

- Poverty

- Food faddism

- Drug misuse

- Chronic alcoholism

- Prolonged parenteral feeding

Vitamin A Deficiency/Toxicity

1. Normal function: Vitamin A is a fat-soluble vitamin derived from β-carotene. It has a hormone-like feature that is necessary for normal vision, reproduction, and resistance to infection.

2. Etiology

   a. Primary vitamin A deficiency is usually caused by prolonged dietary deprivation. It is endemic in areas such as southern and eastern Asia, where rice, a food devoid of carotene, is the staple.

   b. Secondary vitamin A deficiency may occur when there is inadequate conversion of carotene to vitamin A, or when there is interference with absorption, storage, or transport of vitamin A.

   c. Toxicity may occur as an acute or chronic problem from excessive intake of vitamin A.

3. Clinical features: Deficiency

   a. The severity of the effects of vitamin A deficiency is inversely related to age. Growth retardation may occur in children.

   b. Inadequate intake or utilization of vitamin A can cause impaired dark adaptation and night blindness.

   c. Pathognomonic changes of deficiency are confined to the eye. The earliest change is rod dysfunction. With progression, blindness can occur.

4. Clinical features: Toxicity

   a. Early signs of toxicity of vitamin A may include sparse coarse hair, dry rough skin, and cracked lips.

   b. Vitamin A toxicity eventually results in a syndrome of increased intracranial pressure, severe headaches, blurred vision, and sixth nerve palsy. Gradual papilledema develops. The mechanism for the development of increased intracranial pressure is unknown.

   c. A rash may develop.

   d. Birth defects have been reported in the children of pregnant women taking large doses of vitamin A (usually for the treatment of acne).

 Key Clinical Findings: Vitamin A Deficiency and Toxicity

Deficiency

- Severity of effects inversely related to age

- Growth retardation may occur in children

- Impaired dark adaptation and night blindness

- Pathognomonic changes affecting the eye; blindness can occur.

Toxicity

- Early signs include sparse coarse hair, dry rough skin, and cracked lips

- Syndrome of increased intracranial pressure, severe headaches, blurred vision, and sixth nerve palsy; papilledema can develop

- Rash

- Birth defects

---

5. Prognosis and treatment: Prognosis is excellent for adults and children. Symptoms and signs of deficiency or toxicity will often improve within weeks of vitamin A supplementation or discontinuation.

Key Treatment: Vitamin A Deficiency and Toxicity

- Symptoms and signs of deficiency or toxicity often improve within weeks of supplementation or discontinuation.

Vitamin D Deficiency/Toxicity

1. Normal function: Facilitates intestinal absorption of calcium and phosphorus and mineralization of bone.

2. Etiology

   a. Inadequate exposure to sunlight and/or low dietary intake are usually the cause of deficiency. Nutritional rickets is rare in the United States.

   b. A malabsorption syndrome may cause deficiency in some cases.

3. Clinical features: Deficiency

   a. In children there is a defective calcification of growing bone (rickets).

   b. In adults, the changes are similar but are not confined to the ends of the long bones. This demineralization leads to osteomalacia.

   c. Hypocalcemia may occur and lead to tetany.

4. Clinical features: Toxicity

   a. Toxic effects have occurred in adults receiving 2500 μg/day for several months. This causes mobilization of bone calcium and phosphorus, leading to an elevation in serum calcium.

   b. Early symptoms are anorexia, nausea, and vomiting, followed by polyuria, polydipsia, weakness, and anxiety. Generalized weakness can occur.

   c. Where there is bone demineralization and degeneration, nerve root and spinal cord compression can occur.

   d. Meningeal symptoms and trigeminal neuralgia are two additional symptoms.

   e. If renal impairment occurs, a secondary encephalopathy may result.

Key Clinical Findings: Vitamin D Deficiency and Toxicity

Deficiency

- Children: Defective calcification of growing bone (Rickets)

- Adults: Same as children but the effects—not confined to ends of the long bones—lead to osteomalacia

- Possible hypocalcemia, leading to tetany

Toxicity

- Mobilization of bone calcium and phosphorus

- Anorexia, nausea, and vomiting, followed by polyuria, polydipsia, weakness, and anxiety

- Possible nerve root and spinal cord compression

- Meningeal symptoms and trigeminal neuralgia

- Encephalopathy possible if renal impairment occurs

Prognosis and Treatment

1. With adequate calcium and phosphorus intake, osteomalacia and uncomplicated rickets can be cured. Rickets and osteomalacia occurring from defective vitamin D production do not respond to nutritional supplementation.

2. Treatment of toxicity consists of discontinuing vitamin D, providing a low calcium diet, and giving corticosteroids. Kidney damage or metastatic calcium deposits may be irreversible.

Key Treatment: Vitamin D Deficiency and Toxicity

- Osteomalacia and uncomplicated rickets can be cured with adequate calcium and phosphorus intake.

- Toxicity: discontinue vitamin D; provide a low-calcium diet and corticosteroids

Vitamin E Deficiency/Toxicity

1. Normal function: A fat-soluble vitamin that acts as an antioxidant and as a scavenger for free radicals.

2. Etiology

   a. In children and adults malabsorption generally underlies vitamin E deficiency. Some cases may be genetic.

   b. Relatively large doses of vitamin E have been taken by some people for extended periods without apparent harm. In large amounts, vitamin E can antagonize vitamin K and prolong the prothrombin time.

3. Clinical features: Deficiency

   a. Dietary deficiency of vitamin E is rare in the

Western world. Malabsorption or a genetic metabolic defect may produce deficiency.

   b. Neurologic manifestations include

     (1) Absent or depressed tendon reflexes

     (2) Ataxia

     (3) Dysarthria and disorders of eye movements

     (4) Loss of position sense and vibratory sense

     (5) Loss of pain sensation

     (6) Muscle weakness

4. Clinical features: Toxicity

   a. Adults have taken relatively large doses without harm.

   b. Occasionally muscle weakness, fatigue, nausea, and diarrhea may develop.

   c. The most significant effect is antagonism to vitamin K action and prolong the prothrombin time, which results in a potentiation of oral anticoagulants.

Key Clinical Findings: Vitamin D Deficiency and Toxicity

Deficiency

• Absent or depressed tendon reflexes

• Ataxia

• Dysarthria and disorders of eye movements

• Loss of position sense and vibratory sense

• Loss of pain sensation

• Muscle weakness

Toxicity

• Occasional muscle weakness, fatigue, nausea, and diarrhea

• Antagonism to vitamin K action and potentiation of oral anticoagulants.

5. Treatment of vitamin E deficiency

   a. For malabsorption causing overt deficiency, 50 to 100 IU orally should be given daily.

   b. Much larger doses of vitamin E (up to 1000 IU per day in divided doses) are required to treat early neuropathy or to overcome defects of absorption or transportation. This dose in older patients can ameliorate the deficiency and arrest the neuropathy.

Thiamine Deficiency

1. Normal function: Works as a coenzyme and participates in carbohydrate metabolism. May have a specific role in neurons independent of its function in general metabolism. It is present in axonal membranes.

2. Etiology

   a. Primary thiamine deficiency is caused by inadequate dietary intake, particularly in people subsisting on rice.

   b. Secondary thiamine deficiency may occur in pregnancy, impaired absorption, or prolonged diarrhea.

   c. Alcoholism is associated with a combination of decreased intake, increased requirements, and impaired absorption.

3. Clinical features

   a. Early deficiency produces fatigue, irritation, poor memory, sleep disturbance, precordial pain, anorexia, and constipation.

   b. Peripheral neuropathy changes are bilateral and symmetric, involving predominantly the lower limbs. Paresthesias occur in the toes and burning sensations in the feet. There may be leg pain.

   c. Loss of reflexes, beginning at the ankles

   d. Loss of vibratory sense and position sense may occur.

   e. Continued deficiency results in atrophy of the calf and thigh muscles.

   f. Wernicke's encephalopathy is an acute syndrome characterized by inattentiveness, lethargy, ataxia, and abnormal eye movements. Alcoholism is the most common cause. If left untreated, the condition is fatal in 10% of cases. Wernicke's encephalopathy often merges into a mixed Wernicke-Korsakoff syndrome.

Key Clinical Findings: Wernicke's Encephalopathy

• Acute syndrome

• Global confusion

• Inattentiveness

• Disorientation

• Truncal ataxia

• Abnormal eye movements

   g. Korsakoff's syndrome also results from thiamine deficiency and is primarily an amnestic syndrome. Memory is usually impaired for anterograde (recent) events and retrograde (months to years ago) events. The patient may be alert and attentive but may confabulate. Insight is impaired. Even with treatment, only 25% of Korsakoff amnesia cases improve.

Key Clinical Findings: Korsakoff's Syndrome

- Primarily amnestic syndrome
- Both anterograde and retrograde symptoms
- Patient is relatively alert and attentive
- Confabulation may or may not occur
- Poor insight
- Less than 25% improve with treatment

Key Clinical Findings: Thiamine Deficiency

- Peripheral neuropathy
- Wernicke's encephalopathy
- Korsakoff's syndrome

4. Laboratory findings
   a. A low red blood cell transketolase is a sensitive indicator of tissue stores of thiamine.
   b. There may be elevated blood pyruvate and lactate.
   c. Diminished urinary thiamine excretion (less then 50 μg per day) is also consistent with thiamine deficiency.
   d. Serum thiamine levels lack sensitivity and are usually not helpful.

5. Treatment
   a. Oral thiamine can be given for mild polyneuropathy.
   b. Wernicke-Korsakoff syndrome is treated with thiamine 50 to 100 mg intramuscularly or intravenously for 3 days, followed by 50 mg of oral thiamine daily. If the patient requires glucose, thiamine should also be given to avoid worsening of the condition.
   c. Other B-complex vitamins will often be low and require supplementation. Daily multivitamin therapy should also be given.
   d. Magnesium should be given for the usual concomitant hypomagnesium state.

Niacin (Nicotinic Acid) Deficiency

1. Normal function: *Niacin* is the generic term for nicotinic acid. It is an essential coenzyme in cellular intermediary metabolism of fat, carbohydrate, and amino acids.

2. Etiology
   a. Primary deficiency of niacin in the diet occurs when maize (Indian corn) forms a major part of the diet.
   b. Secondary deficiency occurs in diarrhea, cirrhosis, and alcoholism.
   c. Prolonged isoniazid (INH) therapy and carcinoid tumors can also deplete niacin.

3. Clinical features: Deficiency
   a. Pellagra is characterized by cutaneous rashes, mucous membrane inflammation, central nervous system (CNS) and nonspecific gastrointestinal symptoms. Symptoms may appear alone or in combination.
   b. CNS symptoms
      1. Organic psychosis: Characterized by memory impairment, disorientation, confusion, and delirium. Sometimes paranoia occurs.
      2. Encephalopathy: Characterized by clouding of consciousness, cogwheel rigidity, uncontrollable sucking and grasping reflexes
   c. Niacin deficiency must be distinguished from other causes of stomatitis, glossitis, diarrhea, and dementia. If these features are all present together, the diagnosis is straightforward.

Key Clinical Findings: Niacin Deficiency

- Pellagra
- Organic psychosis (characterized by memory impairment, disorientation, confusion, and delirium)
- Encephalopathy (characterized by clouding of consciousness, cogwheel rigidity, uncontrollable sucking and grasping reflexes)

4. Treatment
   a. A balanced diet is needed because other B-vitamins are usually also deficient.
   b. Supplemental niacinamide 300–500 mg/day can be given only in divided doses.
   c. Niacinamide is preferred because niacin can cause flushing, itching, and burning side effects.
   d. If oral therapy is precluded, niacin may be given by injection.

Vitamin B₆ (Pyridoxine)

1. Pyridoxine is a water-soluble vitamin that is converted by pyridoxal kinase and pyridoxine phosphate oxidase to the active form, pyridoxal phosphate, which is a coenzyme involved in decarboxylation and transamination reactions.

2. Toxicity
   a. May occur with megadoses (2–6 g/day for

several months). Often abused by women using pyridoxine for premenstrual symptoms.

   b. Clinical features are progressive sensory ataxia and profound impairment of lower limb position sense and vibratory sense. Ankle jerks are absent. Rare muscle weakness.

3. Deficiency

   a. Causes a mixed distal symmetric polyneuropathy

   b. Patients treated for tuberculosis with INH may develop a deficiency because INH inhibits pyridoxine phosphorylation. The neuropathy can be treated by administration of 50 mg or more of pyridoxine daily. The neuropathy can be prevented by daily doses of 6 to 50 mg of pyridoxine.

Vitamin B$_{12}$ Deficiency

1. Normal function

   a. Vitamin B$_{12}$ (cobalamin) functions in nucleic acid metabolism and is the cofactor involved in defective DNA synthesis. It may also be a cofactor involved in altered myelin synthesis and repair.

   b. Vitamin B$_{12}$ is available in meat and animal protein foods. Its absorption is complex, requiring intrinsic factor from the gastric mucosa.

   c. Liver vitamin B$_{12}$ stores are normally sufficient to sustain physiologic needs for 3 to 5 years.

2. Etiology

   a. Inadequate absorption from lack of intrinsic factor is the major cause. This may have an autoimmune basis because antibodies to gastric parietal cells are found in 90% of cases.

   b. Inadequate diet is rare but can occur in breast-feeding mothers and with severe malnutrition.

   c. Inadequate utilization can occur in liver disease or malignancy. Malabsorption states may also be a cause.

3. Clinical features

   a. About 80% of adult-onset pernicious anemia is attributed to lack of gastric intrinsic factor from atrophic gastritis. This is a megaloblastic anemia that develops from impaired DNA synthesis, which causes red blood cell enlargement because of defective cell maturation.

   b. About 40% of all patients with pernicious anemia will have some neurologic symptom or signs. Neurologic involvement may be present even in the absence of anemia, especially in the elderly.

   c. Peripheral nerves are primarily involved, followed by spinal cord changes in the posterior and lateral columns.

     (1) This has been known as "combined degeneration of the spinal cord" or "combined system disease."

       (a) Pathology involving the spinal cord and peripheral nerves will show features of both myelopathy and peripheral neuropathy.

       (b) Upper motor neuron symptoms include hyperreflexia and Babinski's sign.

       (c) Magnetic resonance imaging (MRI) may show T$_2$-signal change in the posterior columns of the spinal cord.

   d. The most common neurologic symptom is burning and/or painful sensations in the feet and, sometimes, the hands.

   e. There may be sensory ataxia. Almost all patients show loss of vibratory sense and position sense in the lower limbs. A positive Romberg sign is noted.

   f. Lhermitte's phenomenon (flexion of the neck, producing paresthesias down the spine or across the shoulders) may be present.

   g. Mental signs

     (1) May range from change in personality to dementia

     (2) May present without other neurologic involvement

   h. Other symptoms include visual loss from optic neuropathy; orthostatic hypotension; anosmia; and impaired taste.

Key Clinical Findings: Vitamin B$_{12}$ Deficiency

- Peripheral neuropathy (acroparesthesias)
- Subacute combined degeneration of the spinal cord
- Dementia
- Rarely, optic neuropathy

4. Evaluation

   a. In a patient with signs and symptoms of cobalamin deficiency, a cobalamin assay should be ordered. A normal cobalamin level does not fully exclude vitamin B$_{12}$ deficiency, however, and the range of normal can vary depending on assay type.

   b. If the vitamin B$_{12}$ assay is less than the lower limit of normal, intrinsic factor antibodies should be measured. In pernicious anemia, evidence of an autoimmune process is often found.

c. The Schilling test measures absorption of radio-active vitamin B_{12} with and without intrinsic factor, but it is technically difficult and not always reliable. It probably is not necessary if antibodies to intrinsic factor are found, although it does help with determination of malabsorption states.

d. In patients with low-normal vitamin B_{12} levels, methylmalonic acid (MMA) and homocysteine levels should be tested.

Treatment

a. Vitamin B_{12} is administered by intramuscular injection, 1000 μg daily for a week, followed by weekly doses for a month. Patients then generally have one injection per month for life.

b. Oral replacement is an alternative for patients who cannot tolerate IM injections or if they are not practical. The recommended dose is 1000 μg daily (i.e., 1 mg).

c. Paresthesias are often the first symptoms to improve. Corticospinal abnormalities are slower to respond. About half of the patients will continue to have some abnormality on neurologic exam.

d. Sometimes a therapeutic trial of vitamin B_{12} is the only way to show neurologic symptoms to be actually related to deficiency.

Key Treatment: Vitamin B_{12} Deficiency

- 1000 μg/day for a week, intramuscularly; weekly doses for one month; one injection/month for life

- 1000 μg/day (1 mg), orally, if injections are impractical or cannot be tolerated

Bibliography

Beers MH, Berkow R (eds): Vitamin deficiency, dependency, and toxicity. In the Merck Manual of Diagnosis and Therapy, 17th ed. Nutley, New Jersey, Merck & Co, 1999, pp. 35–51.

Kinsella LJ, Riley DE: Nutritional deficiencies and syndromes associated with alcoholism. In Goetz CG, Pappert EJ (eds): Textbook of Clinical Neurology. Philadelphia, W.B. Saunders, 1999, pp. 798–818.

Kane AB, Kumar V: Environmental and nutritional pathology. In Cotran RX, Kumar V, Collins T (eds): Robbins Pathologic Basis of Disease, 6th ed. Philadelphia, W.B. Saunders, 1999, pp. 436–450.

Rowland LP, Worrell BP: Nutritional disorders: Vitamin B_{12} deficiency, malabsorption and malnutrition. In Rowland LP (ed): Merritt's Neurology, 10th ed. Philadelphia, Lippincott Williams & Wilkins, 2000, pp. 896–901.

Ward PC: Modern approaches to the investigation of vitamin B12 deficiency. Clin Lab Med 22:435–445, 2002.

Wilson DJ: Vitamin deficiency and excess. In Fauci AS, Braunwalk E, et al (ed): Harrison's Principles of Internal Medicine, 14th ed. New York, McGraw-Hill, 1998, pp. 480–489.

Stuart R. Chipkin
Erik A. Cohen
Brian W. Smith

4 Endocrine Disorders

HYPOTHYROIDISM

Definition

1. A clinical state characterized by reduced/impaired thyroid hormone action usually due to decreased thyroid gland production of thyroxine (T_4). Subclinical hypothyroidism is an asymptomatic state in which free T_4 levels are normal and thyroid stimulating hormone (TSH) is only mildly elevated.

Epidemiology and Risk Factors

1. Primary hypothyroidism is a common condition. Overall frequency is approximately 0.5% to 1.0%.
2. Over age 65 years, frequency increases to 6% to 10% of women and 2% to 3% of men.

Risk Factors

1. Age
2. Female gender
3. Other autoimmune diseases (including myasthenia gravis) or polyglandular failure
4. Positive family history

Etiology and Pathophysiology

1. The most common cause of primary hypothyroidism is autoimmune thyroid disease (Hashimoto's thyroiditis or chronic lymphocytic thyroiditis). It may also occur after transient hyperthyroidism, postablative hypothyroidism, or after thyroidectomy that is drug induced (propylthiouracil or methimazole, lithium, iodine, inorganic, or organic amiodarone).
2. Secondary (lack of TSH) or tertiary (lack of hypothalamic thyrotropin releasing hormone [TRH]) hypothyroidism: thyrotropin (TSH) deficiency rarely occurs as an isolated finding. May be due to pituitary tumors (see Part XXIII, Chapter 5), Sheehan's syndrome, infiltrative disorders of the pituitary, hypophysitis, or after severe head trauma with basal skull fracture or cavernous sinus thrombosis. Tertiary hypothyroidism is very rare.

Clinical Findings

1. Cognitive and behavioral changes: fatigue, apathy, inattention and slowness that may suggest depression. Myxedematous patients present with florid psychosis or "myxedema madness." Coma develops in up to 1% of patients with myxedema, usually in association with a superimposed infection, surgery, or trauma.
2. Myopathy: muscle weakness, cramps, pain, and stiffness. Muscle weakness is usually not severe and tends to affect proximal muscles of the shoulder and pelvic girdles. Symptoms are often worse at night, and muscle fatigue is more likely to be associated with prolonged, repetitive movements.
3. Reflex changes: in up to 77% of hypothyroid patients, the relaxation phase of deep tendon reflexes may be prolonged. Once thought to be pathognomonic of hypothyroidism, this finding is also caused by hypothermia, diabetes, parkinsonism, pernicious anemia, and several drugs.
4. Seizures: occur with a higher than expected frequency. The electroencephalogram shows slowing of the dominant rhythm and decreased amplitude.
5. Cranial nerve dysfunction: sensorineural hearing loss occurs in 50% to 85% of hypothyroid patients. The mechanism may be cranial nerve VIII compression due to temporal bone hypertrophy by glycosaminoglycan deposition. Ptosis occurs in 50% to 75% and appears to be secondary to diminished sympathetic tone of Mueller's muscle. This can be reversed by local administration of phenylephrine. Visual field defects may occur from secondary pituitary enlargement with resultant chiasmal compression. Pseudotumor cerebri has been seen in hypothyroidism and at initiation of replacement therapy.
6. Muscle hypertrophy: unusual finding in hypothyroid myopathy. Hoffman's syndrome is defined as

the combination of hypothroidism with muscle stiffness, cramps, and muscular enlargement in adults. The pattern of weakness and muscular enlargement in children with hypothyroidism is known as Kocher-Debré-Sémélaigne syndrome.

7. Ataxia: can be the presenting sign of myxedema and is similar to that found in alcoholic cerebellar degeneration

8. Peripheral neuropathy: the most common mononeuropathy is median nerve dysfunction or carpal tunnel syndrome that develops secondary to accumulation of glycosaminoglycans in the extracellular connective tissue, perineurium, and endoneurium. Sensory polyneuropathy (usually painful paresthesias) and cramping of the hands and feet are common complaints in hypothyroidism. Recurrent laryngeal nerve paralysis from thyroid enlargement may occur from compression of the nerve between the cervical spine and the trachea. Extraglandular thyroid cysts can cause a similar picture. The sympathetic chain traverses the neck within the common carotid sheath and may be compressed or invaded by thyroid masses. Reports describe Horner's syndrome caused by extension of the thyroid to involve the eighth thoracic vertebral body and compression of the sympathetic chain.

9. Myxedema coma: a rare manifestation of myxedema occurring in fewer than 1% of cases. The classic presentation includes hypothermia (80%), areflexia, slow shallow respirations, bradycardia, and hypotension. The entire constellation of symptoms takes months to develop but an acute stressor, i.e., myocardial infarction or infection may precipitate rapid deterioration.

10. Systemic features: may include constipation, hypothermia, hyperlipidemia, pernicious anemia, hyponatremia, dry cool skin, menorrhagia, and hyperprolactinemia

Key Clinical Findings

- Dry, coarse skin
- Periorbital puffiness
- Swelling of hands and feet
- Weakness, fatigue, lethargy
- Cold intolerance
- Constipation
- Menstrual irregularities
- Bradycardia
- Goiter

Differential Diagnosis

Nephrotic syndrome, chronic nephritis, neurasthenia, depression, euthyroid sick syndrome; congestive heart failure, dementia from other causes

Laboratory Testing

Total or free serum thyroxine (T_4) decreased; TSH elevated in primary disease. In severe hypothyroidism, anemia, elevated cholesterol, creatinine phosphokinase, lactate dehydrogenase, aspartate aminotransferase, hyponatremia.

Key Laboratory Findings

- Decreased total and free T_4
- Elevated TS (primary)

Radiographic Features

1. Enlarged heart on chest x-ray (often due to pericardial effusion)

2. Occasional evidence of large goiter (tracheal deviation, substernal mass)

3. Decreased radioactive iodine uptake

Treatment

Dose: 1.6 to 1.8 mcg/kg of ideal body weight. Patients who are elderly or have coronary artery disease should be started on 25 mcg by mouth daily.

Key Treatment

- Levothyroxine

Prognosis and Complications

With early treatment, striking improvement in appearance and mental function.

Possible Complications

Myxedema coma—(life-threatening complication of hypothyroidism); increased susceptibility to infection; megacolon; organic psychosis with paranoia; adrenal crisis with treatment of hypothyroidism in patients with concomitant Addison's disease; infertility; hypersensitivity to opiates. Pregnancy and postpartum replacement therapy may need adjustment.

Bibliography

Tonner DR, Schlechte JA: Neurologic complications of thyroid and parathyroid disease. Med Clin 77:251–263, 1993.

Horak HA, Pourmand R: Endocrine myopathies. Neurol Clin 18:203–213, 2000.

HYPERTHYROIDSIM

Definition

Excessive amounts of thyroid hormones. Subclinical hyperthyroidism is an asymptomatic state in which thyroid hormones remain within normal ranges but TSH levels are decreased.

Epidemiology

1. Hyperthyroidism is present in 1:1000 women and 1:3000 men in the United States.
2. May present at any age but incidence peaks in the third and forth decades.

Risk Factors

1. Positive family history
2. Female gender
3. Other autoimmune disorders
4. Iodide repletion after iodide deprivation

Clinical Findings

1. Behavioral: an excess of thyroid hormone causes irritability, emotional lability, hyperalertness, exhilaration, and euphoria. The hyperthyroid patient may overreact to trivial disruptions, leading to prolonged bouts of crying or insomnia. In the elderly, apathy and fatigue are often the only symptoms ("apathetic hyperthyroidism"). Psychotic behavior may be unmasked in susceptible individuals. There is no characteristic feature that distinguishes the psychiatric changes of hyperthyroidism from other psychotic conditions.
2. Corticospinal tract disease: presents with progressive weakness and urinary or fecal incontinence. The physical examination may reveal spasticity weakness, muscle atrophy, hyperreflexia, clonus, and Babinski and frontal release signs. As is true for myopathy, the degree of thyroid hormone elevation does not correlate with corticospinal tract signs, and these resolve with treatment of the hyperthyroidism.
3. Seizure: incidence in thyrotoxic patients range from 1% to 9%. Seizures usually occur in patients with an underlying seizure disorder.
4. Involuntary movements–tremor: as many as 97% of patients with hyperthyroidism have accompanying tremor, most commonly in the hands and fingers. The frequency of the movements is the same as that in physiologic tremor; however, the amplitude of the tremor is increased. The pattern of the tremor is the same as that seen with anxiety or pheochromocytoma (due to increased sympathetic tone). It is increased by emotional strain and can be effectively treated with propranolol.
5. Hyperthyroid chorea: rare. Dopamine agonists have been shown to exacerbate (and antagonists to ameliorate) choreiform movements. Dopamine receptor sites may be hypersensitive. Beta blockade is an effective treatment, which suggests beta-adrenergic mediation of the movement disorder. Increased sympathetic activity may be due to catecholamine receptor augmentation by thyroxine or by increased sensitivity. The chorea associated with hyperthyroidism can also be abolished with haloperidol. Chorea ceases once the euthyroid state is achieved.
6. Ophthalmic findings: the ocular findings associated with hyperthyroidism fall into two groups. Lid lag and retraction, widened palpebral fissures, and decreased frequency of blinking are mediated by adrenergic mechanisms and usually respond to beta blockade. The second group is caused by pathologic changes in the orbit and its contents. These are seen specifically with Graves' disease and include exophthalmos, ophthalmoplegia, swelling of the orbital contents and lids, corneal ulceration, and visual impairment caused by optic neuropathy. These signs do not disappear with the administration of adrenergic blocking agents or with achievement of the euthyroid state. Although usually bilateral, Graves' disease is the most common cause of unilateral exophthalmos. Exophthalmos can precede clinical thyroid disease. The ocular abnormalities are mediated by increases in mucopolysaccharides, water, connective tissue, and chronic inflammatory cells representing an autoimmune attack directed against orbital antigens. Changes in orbital fat and degenerative changes of intraocular muscles also occur. Indications for orbital decompression are compressive optic neuropathy unresponsive to steroids, exposure keratopathy, and cosmesis. Computerized tomography (CT) is useful in distinguishing thyroid ophthalmopathy from other orbital conditions. The most difficult condition to distinguish is orbital myositis, in which there is tendon enlargement, proptosis, and less prominent muscle enlargement.

7. Thyrotoxic periodic paralysis (TPP): thyrotoxic patients may suffer recurrent attacks of weakness primarily affecting proximal musculature and sparing bulbar and respiratory muscles and sphincters. Attacks may last minutes to days and are precipitated by carbohydrate loads, muscle cooling, or rest after exercise. Serum potassium is usually decreased during the attacks but may be normal. There are a number of differences between TPP and familial hypokalemic periodic paralysis (FHPP). TPP occurs after age 20, (FHPP <16), mostly in males (6 to 1 in TPP versus 3 to 1 in FHPP), more often in Asians. Normalization of thyroid function cures TPP, whereas thyroid status has no effect on the familial form.

8. Myasthenia gravis: approximately 5% of patients with myasthenia gravis will have hyperthyroidism, and in about 75% of those, thyroid symptoms appear before or with the onset of myasthenia. Less than 1% of patients with Graves' disease will develop myasthenia. However, the prevalence rate is 30 times greater than the prevalence of myasthenia gravis in the general population. Coexistence of the two disorders may lead to a more severe expression of the myasthenia, and correction of the hyperthyroidism is not always accompanied by improvement in the myasthenia. In some cases, myasthenia worsens after the subject becomes euthyroid. Diagnosing myasthenia may be complicated in the hyperthyroid patient because both conditions cause muscle weakness. Only an electromyogram done at maximal effort will differentiate normal and thyrotoxic patients.

9. Systemic: signs and symptoms of hyperthyroidism include tachycardia, cardiomegaly, heart failure, atrial fibrillation (resulting in embolic strokes), weight loss, abnormal liver function tests, skin changes (classically warm, moist, and velvety) impaired fertility in women, impotence and gynecomastia in men, weight loss, and aversion to heat.

Key Clinical Findings

- Nervousness (85%)
- Increased sweating (70%)
- Heat intolerance (70%)
- Palpitations and tachycardia (75%)
- Dyspnea (75%)
- Warm and moist skin (72%)
- Goiter (less common in elderly)
- Lid lag

Differential Diagnosis

1. Anxiety, malignancy, diabetes, pregnancy, menopause, and pheochromocytoma
2. Muscle spasticity, hyperreflexia and weakness includes spinal cord tumors, craniocervical junction abnormalities, motor neuron disease, spinocerebellar degeneration, and hyperthyroidism.

Laboratory Testing

1. T_4 above normal limits, TSH below normal limits, triiodothyronine (T_3) above normal limits. Increased thyroid RAIU in hyperthyroidism, Graves' disease, toxic multinodular goiter, and toxic adenoma. Decreased thyroid radioactive iodine uptake (RAIU) in thyroiditis, subacute, silent, and postpartum, exogenous thyroid hormone use, and exogenous iodine excess.
2. Approximately two thirds of hyperthyroid patients (most commonly young women) exhibit abnormalities on electroencephalography (EEG). Typical findings include generalized slow wave activity, increased alpha frequency, and, rarely, focal spike or slow waves.

Key Laboratory Findings

- Elevated free T_4
- Elevated free T_3
- Decreased TSH
- Increased RAIU (Graves' disease)
- Decreased RAIU (thyroiditis)

Radiologic Features

Thyroid radioiodine scan; diffuse homogeneous uptake confirms Graves' disease; may reveal heterogeneous uptake in toxic multinodular goiter, a single hot nodule (toxic adenoma), or a cold nodule (coexistent possible neoplasm).

Treatment

Antithyroid drugs (thionamides); propylthiouracil (PTU) and methimazole. Radioactive iodine (RAI ^{131}I): can be first-line therapy or for patients who have not achieved remission after 18 months of antithyroid drug therapy. Total or subtotal thyroidectomy is rarely performed. Propranolol alleviates the beta-adrenergic symptoms of hyperthyroidism. Initial dose is 20 to 40 mg orally every 6 hours; dosage is gradually increased until symptoms are controlled.

Prognosis and Complications

With proper diagnosis and treatment, prognosis is good. Hypothyroidism usually occurs after radioiodine treatment. Severe ophthalmopathy can cause visual loss or diplopia.

Bibliography

Bulens C: Neurologic complications of hyperthyroidism. Arch Neurol 38:669–670, 1981.

ADRENAL INSUFFICIENCY–HYPOADRENALISM

Definition

Adrenal hypofunction from primary, secondary, or tertiary causes resulting in inadequate secretion of glucocorticoids and (if primary) mineralocorticoids.

Epidemiology and Risk Factors

1. Incidence/prevalence of approximately 4:100,000. All age groups are affected, most commonly in the third to fifth decade. There is a slightly greater female to male predominance.
2. Risk factors: family history of autoimmune disease. (About 40% of patients have a relative with an associated disorder.) Other risk factors include history of taking steroids for prolonged periods (up to 1 year in the past), with either sudden cessation or precipitous stress, including severe infection, trauma, or surgical procedures.

Etiology and Pathophysiology

1. Addison's disease (primary adrenocortical insufficiency) is differentiated from secondary (pituitary failure) and tertiary (hypothalamic failure) causes. Two most common causes of primary adrenal insufficiency are autoimmune (often as part of a polyglandular autoimmune syndrome) and tuberculous.
2. Infections: tuberculosis, fungal, AIDS associated.
3. Adrenoleukodystrophy: an X-linked peroxisomal disorder causing accumulation of very long chain fatty acids in the adrenal cortex, testes, brain, and spinal cord.
4. Medications: steroidogenesis inhibitors (ketoconazole). Inducers of cortisol metabolism (rifampin, phenytoin, phenobarbital).
5. Secondary and tertiary adrenal insufficiency. Suppression of the hypothalamic pituitary adrenal (HPA) axis from exogenous glucocorticoids. Tumors or infarction of the pituitary or hypothalamus resulting in ACTH deficiency.
6. Other causes may include sarcoidosis, amyloidosis, and hemochromatosis.

Clinical Findings

1. Cognitive and behavioral: estimates of psychiatric symptoms in Addisonian patients range from 35% to 70%. Patients are irritable and depressed and may be psychotic or suffer acute confusional states that may progress to coma.
2. Neuromuscular: withdrawal from chronic steroid therapy can result in benign intracranial hypertension, but whether Addison's disease produces pseudotumor has not been established. Cases of papilledema and encephalopathy have been seen in combination with adrenal insufficiency.
3. Myopathy: between 25% and 50% of patients with adrenal insufficiency have generalized weakness, muscle cramping, and fatigue, all of which usually resolve with glucocorticoid replacement. The electromyogram (EMG), muscle enzyme tests, and the muscle biopsy are usually unremarkable. Hyperkalemic periodic paralysis may develop in patients with adrenal insufficiency. Adrenal insufficiency may cause electrolyte disturbances that may lead to intractable seizures.
4. Adrenoleukodystrophy: may present with psychiatric symptoms, often including mania, psychosis, or cognitive impairment. Neurologic deterioration including gait disorders and white matter changes on magnetic resonance imaging (MRI) may be severe or mild (particularly in heterozygote women). Symptoms mimic multiple sclerosis and can occur years after the onset of adrenal insufficiency.
5. Systemic: clinical features may include orthostatic hypotension, dizziness, weight loss, abdominal pain, anorexia, chronic diarrhea, nausea, vomiting, hyponatremia, hyperkalemia, azotemia, decreased cold tolerance, hyperpigmentation (primary adrenal insufficiency only), and loss of body hair in women.

Key Clinical Findings

- Weakness, fatigue
- Weight loss
- Dizziness: low blood pressure, orthostatic hypotension

- Anorexia, nausea, vomiting
- Abdominal pain
- Chronic diarrhea
- Hyperpigmentation (primary only)

Differential Diagnosis

Other forms of shock (e.g., septic, hemorrhagic, cardiogenic). Hyperkalemia seen with gastrointestinal bleeding, rhabdomyolysis, hyperkalemic paralysis, acetylcholinesterase (ACE) inhibitors, or spironolactone. Hyponatremia seen in hypothyroidism, diuretic use, heart failure, cirrhosis, vomiting, and diarrhea. Unexplained weight loss, weakness, and anorexia may be mistaken for occult cancer. Nausea, vomiting, diarrhea, and abdominal pain may be misdiagnosed as intrinsic gastrointestinal disease.

Laboratory Testing

Hyponatremia, hyperkalemia, azotemia, elevated serum calcium, metabolic acidosis, low cortisol level, elevated ACTH level, moderate neutropenia, eosinophilia, relative lymphocytosis, anemia. Diagnostic testing: low-dose rapid ACTH stimulation test: cosyntropin 1 mcg intravenously is administered with cortisol levels measured preinjection and 30 minutes postinjection. Patients with Addison's disease have low to normal values that do not rise.

Key Laboratory Findings

- Hyponatremia
- Hyperkalemia
- Failure to respond to cosyntropin on ACTH stimulation test

Treatment

Medications: for chronic adrenal insufficiency: hydrocortisone 15 to 20 mg orally each morning upon rising and 10 mg at 4 or 5 o'clock each afternoon is the usual dosage. Fludrocortisone 0.05 to 0.2 mg orally once/day (primary disease only). Acute adrenal insufficiency: hydrocortisone 100 mg intravenously followed by 10 mg/hour infusion. Intravenous glucose, saline, plasma expanders. For acute illnesses (fever, stress, minor trauma), double the patient's usual steroid dose.

Key Treatment

- Hydrocortisone or equipotent glucocorticoid
- Fludrocortisone

Prognosis and Complications

With adequate replacement therapy, life expectancy approximates normal. Active tuberculosis or fungal disease responds to specific chemotherapy. Possible complications: hyperpyrexia, psychotic reactions, complications from underlying disease, over or under steroid treatment, hyperkalemic paralysis (rare), Addisonian crisis.

Bibliography

Grinspoon SK, Biller BMK: Laboratory assessment of adrenal insufficiency. J Clin Endocrinol 79:923–931, 1994.

CUSHING'S DISEASE AND SYNDROME

Definition

Clinical abnormalities associated with chronic exposure to excessive amounts of cortisol.

Etiology and Pathophysiology

1. The most frequent cause is prolonged use of exogenous glucocorticoids.
2. Seen in all age groups.
3. Afflicts females more often than males.

Risk Factors

1. Any medical problem requiring prolonged use of corticosteroids
2. Pituitary tumor–Cushing's disease–overproduction of ACTH
3. Adrenal mass–Cushing's syndrome–autonomous overproduction of cortisol
4. Neuroendocrine tumor (e.g., bronchial carcinoid). (Rare—overproduction of either ACTH or corticotropin)

Clinical Findings

1. Behavioral: nearly 70% of individuals with Cushing's syndrome demonstrate some psychiatric changes. Depression is the most common distur-

bance and frank psychotic behavior may occur in up to 15% of patients. A schizophreniform disorder has been described in Cushing's syndrome but is more common in the later stages of the disease. Formal neuropsychological testing reveals diffuse cognitive impairment in two thirds of patients. Paradoxically, excessive exogenous steroid intake usually produces mania, although depression may also occur. Psychiatric symptoms usually resolve with lowering of corticosteroid level.

2. Spinal cord: rare reports of spinal cord compression after prolonged steroid therapy secondary to the accumulation of epidural fat. Tapering of the steroids resulted in disappearance of the fat without improvement of the myelopathy.

3. Cranial nerves: impaired visual acuity is the most common ophthalmologic complaint in patients with pituitary adenomas extending beyond the sella turcica. In Cushing's disease, up to 70% show some degree of optic atrophy and up to 90% show visual field defects usually bitemporal hemianopsia. MRI appears to be the procedure of choice in identifying adenoma.

4. Myopathy: between 2% and 80% of patients with Cushing's disease develop significant muscle weakness, whereas 2% to 21% of patients receiving chronic steroid therapy develop weakness severe enough to limit ambulation. The onset is usually insidious, occurring most frequently after 4 weeks of glucocorticoid use, with greater involvement of legs than arms and sparing of cranial nerve innervated muscles. Myalgias may accompany the weakness. Creatine kinase and aldolase are usually normal. Women are twice as likely to develop steroid myopathy as men.

Although any of the commonly used glucocorticoid preparations can cause steroid myopathy, fluorinated steroids, triamcinolone, betamethasone, and dexamethasone appear more likely to produce weakness.

The findings of EMG are variable. Usually a myopathic pattern with normal insertional activity and motor units of low amplitude and short duration are found. Occasionally, fibrillation potentials are noted. Muscle biopsy typically shows selective atrophy of type II (fast-twitch) muscle fibers. Type IIb fibers appear to be more susceptible to steroid-induced atrophy than type IIa fibers. Motor nerve axons and nerve terminals appear normal. Muscle spindles are atrophied only in fast-twitch muscles.

5. Systemic: general features include central obesity, facial rounding (moon facies), supraclavicular fullness, dorsocervical fullness (buffalo hump), hirsutism, purple striae on the abdomen, superfi-

cial fungal infections, impaired glucose tolerance or diabetes mellitus, and kidney stone formation.

Key Clinical Findings

- General: central obesity, facial rounding (moon facies), supraclavicular fullness, dorsocervical fullness–buffalo hump.
- Facial adiposity and plethora
- Emotional lability
- Wide purple striae on abdomen
- Proximal muscle weakness
- Glucose intolerance
- Hypertension
- Easy bruising with subcutaneous thinning
- Hirsutism and acne
- Supraclavicular fullness

Differential Diagnosis

Obesity, diabetes mellitus, hypertension; adrenogenital syndrome; hypercortisolism secondary to alcoholism (pseudo-Cushing's).

Laboratory Testing

Twenty-four-hour urinary cortisol; dexamethasone suppression test; inferior petrosal sinus sampling (± CRH) for ACTH.

Key Laboratory Findings

- Non-suppressed cortisol after overnight dexamethasone suppression test
- Increased 24-hour urinary free cortisol

Radiologic Features

If pituitary tumor suspected, pituitary MRI scan; if adrenal disease suspected, adrenal computed tomography (CT) scan; if ectopic ACTH secretion suspected, chest CT scan.

Treatment

1. Depends on etiology. Surgery is the treatment of choice, persistent disease may require radiation, drug therapy, or repeat surgery. Surgical measures: primary hypersecretion of ACTH: transsphenoidal

microsurgery. Radiation therapy as an adjunct for patients not cured. Adrenocortical tumors: surgical removal when possible; if adrenocortical carcinoma, prognosis is poor. Ectopic ACTH production: removal of the neoplastic tissue; metastatic spread makes surgical cure unlikely/impossible; bilateral adrenalectomy.

2. Treatment of steroid myopathy: consists primarily of reducing the steroid dose to the lowest possible level. Converting to a nonfluorinated steroid and to an alternate-day regimen may also help. Phenytoin may reduce steroid induced weakness, possibly by accelerating glucocorticoid degradation. Severe dietary restriction may accelerate the muscle wasting associated with glucocorticoid treatment. However, protein supplementation of a normal diet does not appear to reverse steroid myopathy or protect against its development. Steroid myopathy is accelerated in association with muscle disuse and may be partially prevented by exercise (even passive range of motion). Androgens can partially antagonize the catabolic actions of glucocorticoids, but as yet, anabolic steroids have not been very successful in treating steroid myopathy.

Prognosis and Complications

Usual course: chronic with cyclic exacerbations and rare remissions. Guardedly favorable prognosis with surgery but depends on source. Possible complications. Osteoporosis. Increased susceptibility to infections. Hirsutism. Pregnancy: can cause exacerbation of Cushing's Disease.

Bibliography

Anagnos A, Ruff RL, Kaminski HJ: Endocrine neuromyopathies. Neurol Clin 15:673–696, 1997.
Miller JW, Crapo L: The medical treatment of Cushing's syndrome. Endocr Rev 14:443, 1993.

PHEOCHROMOCYTOMA

Definition

Pheochromocytomas are rare tumors of chromaffin cells in the adrenal medulla or in extra-adrenal sympathetic ganglia that secrete catecholamines causing hypertension and other symptoms.

Epidemiology and Risk Factors

Pheochromocytomas are found in 0.01% to 0.1% of the hypertensive population. They may occur at any age and have a peak incidence in the third and fourth decades. The tumor occurs with equal frequency in both sexes in the adult, whereas 60% of children affected are male. Multiple tumors (adrenal and extra-adrenal) are more common in children (35% of cases) than in adults (8%). Approximately 10% of pheochromocytomas are familial and greater than 70% of these are bilateral.

Risk Factors

1. Familial pheochromocytoma
2. Multiple endocrine neoplasia types IIA and B
3. Neurofibromatosis: a neurocutaneous disease with two distinct forms. Type 1 (von Recklinghausen's disease) is characterized by multiple hyperpigmented macules and neurofibromas. Type 2 is marked by eighth nerve tumors, often accompanied by other intracranial or intraspinal tumors.
4. Von-Hippel-Lindau syndrome: one of the neurocutaneous syndromes. Characterized by headache, loss of vision, unilateral ataxia, dizziness, retinal detachment, and papilledema.

Etiology and Pathophysiology

The majority of pheochromocytomas arise from the adrenal medulla (90%) and the organ of Zuckerhandl (8%). Norepinephrine is the predominant catecholamine produced. Less than 10% of pheochromocytomas are malignant. These are more often extra-adrenal and dopamine secreting.

Clinical Findings

1. The clinical manifestations of pheochromocytoma are presented in the accompanying list of Key Clinical Findings. Common symptoms include: headache (72% to 92%), sweating (60% to 70%), palpitations with or without tachycardia (51% to 73%), nervousness (35% to 40%), weight loss (40% to 70%), chest or abdominal pain (22% to 48%), nausea with or without vomiting (26% to 43%), weakness or fatigue (15% to 38%).
2. Neurologic symptoms: the outstanding symptom is headache, which is almost always paroxysmal in nature and peaks within minutes. It is of severe intensity and throbbing in quality, often associated with nausea and vomiting. It frequently awakens patients in the early morning and prompts them to rise because the upright position is typically more comfortable. Coughing, sneezing, bending, and straining commonly aggravate the pain. The headache is bilateral, affecting the occipital, nuchal-occipital, and frontal-occipital regions. An important feature is the short duration of these headaches. In 50% of patients the pain lasted less

than 15 minutes, and in 70% its duration was less than 1 hour.

3. Visual abnormalities occur in 11% of patients and may include visual loss during attacks, scintillating scotomata synchronous with every heartbeat, or "snowy vision" (wavy lines or black spots) before the eyes.

4. Numbness and paresethesias may affect the hands, arms, face, perioral region, and scalp, and are almost always bilateral. Occasionally a secondary hyperventilation state accounts for this phenomenon.

5. A feeling of weakness or exhaustion can be present toward the end of an attack, and it lingers.

6. Generalized convulsions have been reported, occasionally occurring repeatedly in temporal relationship with other paroxysmal symptoms. In case reports of patients with seizures the blood pressure was persistently and markedly increased. In no case were the convulsions attributable to intracranial metastases.

7. Case reports of cerebral infarction and intracerebral hemorrhage have been described. Most of these patients have severe persistent hypertension when their stroke occurred.

 Key Clinical Findings

- Paroxysmal spells
- Pressure, sudden increase in blood pressure
- Pain, headache, chest and abdominal pain
- Perspiration
- Palpitation
- Pallor

Differential Diagnosis

1. Vasodilating headache, intracranial tumor, diencephalic-autonomia epilepsy, hypertensive encephalopathy, focal arterial brain disease, and anxiety state

2. Vasodilating headache (cluster headache). Cluster headaches tend to focus about or behind one eye, whereas pheochromocytoma headache is usually bilateral or occipital. Vegetative changes from cluster headache (tearing of the eye, watering of the nose, or facial sweating and flushing) tend to be unilateral. With pheochromocytoma, pallor is more common than flushing and sweating; it tends to occur diffusely about the waist. Nausea is uncommon with cluster headache and common with pheochromocytoma.

3. Intracranial tumor: periodic ventricular obstruction can be seen with pheochromocytoma. Both pheochromocytoma and intracranial tumor can reveal choked optic discs with hemorrhages on funduscopic examination. However, the hypertensive features seen in the fundi of patients with pheochromocytoma are not seen with increased intracranial pressure. An abnormally slow pulse rate in the presence of hypertension suggests increased intracranial pressure; however the distinction is not entirely reliable. Sudden "drop attacks" with momentary weakness in the legs or brief episodes of unconsciousness would be more suggestive of ventricular obstruction.

4. Diencephalic-autonomic epilepsy with exclusively autonomic manifestations is rare but can be deceptively similar in content to the episodic symptoms of pheochromocytoma. The common symptoms of pheochromocytoma are rarely seen in epilepsy. Quick onset and cessation, along with short duration of attacks are seen in both conditions. Marked variation in the duration of episodes is a distinctive feature of pheochromocytoma. Loss of consciousness suggests an epileptic cause, but occasionally a patient with pheochromocytoma will faint or even have a grand mal convulsion at the height of an attack. The electroencephalogram has only limited usefulness in the differential diagnosis.

5. Hypertensive encephalopathy: Pheochromocytoma is capable of causing malignant hypertension and inducing hypertensive encephalopathy. However, the distinct periodicity of symptoms caused by pheochromocytoma, severe and transient, is not typical of hypertensive encephalopathy. Transient amaurosis and confusion, common in encephalopathy, are extremely rare with pheochromocytoma.

6. Focal arterial brain disease: The general features of intermittent cerebral ischemia resemble the episodic dysfunction caused by pheochromocytoma, but the symptoms themselves differ. Symptoms of pheochromocytoma represent an exaggeration rather than an absence of function. In contrast, focal cerebral ischemia is marked by a decrease or absence of function, such as weakness, numbness, aphasia, diploplia, ataxia, and visual field defects. Many of these symptoms are unilateral and primarily somatic, unlike the systemic autonomic nervous system excess that is typical of pheochromocytoma.

Laboratory Testing

Elevated 24-hour urine catecholamines including metanephrine/normetanephrine. Elevated plasma catecholamines especially normetanephrine. The 24-hour urine vanillylmandelic acid (VMA) test is insensitive and is no longer recommended for diagnosis of pheochromocytoma.

Key Laboratory Tests

- Elevated 24-hour urine or plasma catecholamines

Radiologic Features

1. More than 95% of pheochromocytomas are intra-abdominal. MRI is the preferred imaging modality over CT. Iodine 123: M-iodobenzylguanidine (MIBG) scintigraphy can detect tumors that are widespread, functional, and small. Indium 111: octreotide scan is also useful.

Key Radiologic Tests

- Abdominal MRI
- Iodine 123: metaiodobenzylguanidine scan
- In-111: pentetreotide scan

Treatment

Surgical resection is definitive therapy. Combined alpha- and beta-adrenergic blockade is required preoperatively. Initiate alpha-blockade first: Phenoxybenzamine 10 mg daily and increase by 10 to 20 mg every 2 days as needed to control blood pressure and paroxysmal spells (.5 to 1.0 mg/kg daily). Beta-blockade after alpha-blockade is established. Propranolol 10 mg every 6 hours initially; increase as necessary to control tachycardia. Acute hypertensive crises should be treated with phentolamine or nitroprusside intravenously. Metyrosine (Demser), an inhibitor of norepinephrine synthesis, provides symptomatic relief; however, severe CNS side effects limit its use in patients who fail standard therapy. Radiation and combination chemotherapy yield only transient success in treating malignant pheochromocytoma.

Key Treatment

- Alpha blockade before beta blockade
- For hypertensive crisis: nitroprusside, phentolamine. Intraoperatively: intravenous fluids.

Prognosis and Complications

1. For benign disease, cure rates approach 85% and 5-year survival rates average 95%. For malignant pheochromocytoma, the 5-year survival rate is below 50%. Hypertensive crisis may also occur intraoperatively if adequate adrenergic blockade is not achieved.

2. Preoperative complications: preoperatively, beta-adrenergic blockade alone may result in more severe hypertension due to the unopposed alpha-adrenergic stimulation; beta-adrenergic blockade is initiated at low doses to avoid the possible side effect of pulmonary edema in the patient with catecholamine myocardiopathy.

3. Intraoperative complications: intraoperatively, very careful attention must be paid to anesthesia and fluid management. Patients are typically volume contracted and may experience hypotensive crisis when pheochromocytoma is removed. Because 5% to 10% of pheochromocytomas recur, urine or plasma catecholamines should be obtained 2 to 3 months after surgery and thereafter once a year for 2 to 5 years.

Bibliography

Bravo EL, Gifford RW: Pheochromocytoma: diagnosis, localization, and management. N Engl J Med 311:1298, 1984.
Young WF Jr: Pheochromocytoma 1926–1993. Trends Endocrinol Metab 4:122, 1993.

CARCINOID SYNDROME

Definition

Carcinoid syndrome is a symptom complex characterized by paroxysmal vasomotor disturbances, diarrhea, and bronchospasm. It is caused by the action of amines and peptides (serotonin, bradykinin, histamine) produced by tumors arising from neuroendocrine cells.

Epidemiology

Carcinoid tumors are found incidentally in 0.5% to 0.75% of autopsies.

Etiology and Pathophysiology

Carcinoid tumors are principally found in the following organs: appendix 40%, small bowel 20% (15% in the ileum), rectum 15%, bronchi 12%, esophagus, stomach, colon 10%, ovary, biliary tract, pancreas 3%. Although uncommon, carcinoid tumors are important because they can secrete a variety of vasoactive materials. These tumors metastasize with a frequency of 15% to 40% but have a relatively indolent course, making control of the syndrome important. Carcinoid tumors do not usually produce the syndrome unless liver metastases are present. All neurologic complications occur in patients with metastatic tumors.

Neurologic Complications

1. Approximately 40% of patients with metastatic tumors have neurologic complications.

2. Metastatic disease with epidural spinal cord compression is the most frequent neurologic complication. It is usually associated with vertebral bone lesions and may be the first manifestation of the tumor.

3. Intracranial, leptomeningeal, and brachial plexus metastases also occur, usually secondary to primary tumors of the lung.

4. Sagittal sinus thrombosis, carcinoid myopathy, and seizures have also been reported.

Systemic Features

1. Cutaneous flushing (75% to 90%): usually starting in the face, then spreading to the neck and upper trunk. These red-purple flushing episodes last from a few minutes to hours (longer-lasting flushes may be associated with bronchial carcinoids). Flushing may be triggered by emotion, alcohol, or foods, or it may occur spontaneously. Dizziness, tachycardia, and hypotension may be associated with the cutaneous flushing.

2. Diarrhea (>70%) often associated with abdominal bloating and audible peristaltic rushes

3. Intermittent bronchospasm (25%), characterized by severe dyspnea and wheezing

4. Facial telangiectasia

5. Tricuspid regurgitation from carcinoid heart lesions

Key Clinical Findings

- Cutaneous flushing

- Dizziness, tachycardia, hypotension

- Diarrhea

- Intermittent bronchospasm

- Facial telangiectasia

Differential Diagnosis

The carcinoid syndrome must be distinguished from idiopathic flushing; patients with idiopathic flushing are more often younger females with a long duration of symptoms including palpitations, syncope, and hypertension.

Laboratory Testing

The biochemical marker for carcinoid syndrome is increased 24-hour urinary 5-hydroxyindoleacetic acid (5-HIAA), a metabolite of serotonin (5-hydroxytryptamine). False elevations can be seen with ingestion of certain foods (banana, pineapple, eggplant, avocado, walnuts) and certain medications (acetaminophen, caffeine, guaifenesin, reserpine); therefore patients should be on a restricted diet and should avoid these medications when the test is ordered.

Key Laboratory Findings

- Increased 24-hour urinary 5-HIAA

Radiographic Features

Chest x-ray examination is useful to detect bronchial carcinoids. CT scans of abdomen or a liver and spleen radionuclide scan is useful to detect liver metastases (palpable in >50% of cases). Iodine 123–labeled somatostatin can detect carcinoid endocrine tumors with somatostatin receptors. Scanning with radiolabeled octreotide can visualize previously undetected or metastatic lesions.

Treatment

Surgical resection of the tumor can be curative if the tumor is localized or palliative and results in prolonged asymptomatic periods if metastases are present. Surgical manipulation of the tumor can, however, cause severe vasomotor abnormalities and bronchospasm (carcinoid crisis). Percutaneous embolization and ligation of the hepatic artery can decrease the bulk of the tumor in the liver and provide palliative treatment of tumors with hepatic metastases.

Control of Clinical Manifestations

Diarrhea usually responds to diphenoxylate with atropine (Lomotil). Flushing can be controlled by the combination of H1 and H2 receptor antagonist (diphenhydramine 25 to 50 mg orally every 6 hours and ranitidine 150 mg twice daily). Somatostatin analogs are effective for both flushing and diarrhea in most patients. Bronchospasm can be treated with aminophylline and/or albuterol. Subcutaneous somatostatin analogues (octreotide 150 μg subcutaneously three times daily) have been used successfully for long-term control of symptoms in patients with unresectable neoplasms.

Prognosis and Complication

Prognosis varies with the stage and location of the tumor. Carcinoids of the appendix and rectum have a low malignancy potential and rarely produce the clinical syndrome; metastases are also uncommon if the primary lesion is smaller than 2 cm in diameter.

Complications

1. Right-sided congestive heart failure; monitor with echocardiography.

2. Pellagra: supplemental niacin therapy may be useful because the tumor uses dietary tryptophan for serotonin synthesis.

Bibliography

Caplin ME, Buscombe JR, Hilson AJ, et al.: Carcinoid tumour. Lancet 352:799, 1998.

Kulke MH, Mayer RJ: Carcinoid tumors. N Engl J Med 340:898, 1999.

Lederman RJ, Bukowski RM, Nickerson P: Carcinoid myopathy (abstr). Neurology 35 (Suppl 1):165, 1985.

Patchell RA, Posner JB: Neurological complications of systemic cancer. Neurol Clin 3:729–750, 1985.

Patchell RA, Posner JB: Neurologic complications of carcinoid. Neurology 36:745–749, 1986.

HYPONATREMIA

Definition

Serum sodium of less than 135 mmol/L (mEq/L)

Etiology

There are certain risk factors for development of symptomatic hyponatremia.

1. Age over 75 years
2. Use of certain drugs (e.g., thiazide diuretics)
3. Female sex
4. Below-average body weight
5. Rate and extent of the decrease in serum sodium concentration (e.g., with loss of sodium in perspiration and rapid replacement with water in marathon runners)
6. Serious underlying illness

Epidemiology

Hyponatremia has an incidence of about 1% and a prevalence of about 3% among inpatients in general hospitals. Hyponatremia constitutes the most common electrolyte disturbance and is associated with a number of diseases (mentioned in Pathophysiology, below).

Pathophysiology

1. Hyponatremia may be hypo-osmolar or not. When it is not, the cause may be
   a. Osmotic: hyperglycemia, mannitol
   b. Artifactual: hyperlipidemia, hyperproteinemia
2. Hypo-osmolar hyponatremia can be divided according to volume status. Hypovolemic hyponatremia may be caused by loss of fluid or blood through the gastrointestinal tract, urinary tract (often with secretion of atrial natriuretic factor or loss of aldosterone effect), skin, blood loss from various sites or from third space sequestration (e.g., ascites with hypoproteinemia may be associated with contraction of the vascular volume). This stimulates secretion of antidiuretic hormone (ADH) as volume replacement has precedence over osmolality. Normovolemic or hypervolemic hyponatremia is usually related to inappropriate secretion of ADH or drugs that cause this effect.

   Most cases of hyponatremia arise from an excess of solvent relative to solute. This occurs when the kidney does not excrete dilute urine, which may be related to
   a. Inappropriate secretion of ADH, which is seen with a number of disorders
   b. Insufficient glomerular filtrate reaching distal parts of the nephron, which is related either to decreased glomerular filtration rate or to increased proximal tubular reabsorption of fluid and sodium
   c. Defective sodium transport in the diluting parts of the nephron or excessive water reabsorption
3. Neurologic complications
   a. The main neurologic effects relate to cellular swelling. If hypo-osmolar hyponatremia develops quickly, the brain does not have time to adjust (by diminishing its solute concentration), and cellular swelling occurs.
      (1) Volume or stretch sensors may involve the cytoskeleton, which has connections with the cell membrane and membrane channels. Thus specific stretch-sensitive ion channels can open fairly quickly.
      (2) If severe, cellular swelling can increase intracranial pressure and produce tissue ischemia.
   b. The ionic composition of the brain is altered, and changes in neurotransmitter function follow.
   c. Partial depolarization of nerve cells, related to the extrusion of potassium, occurs, which makes them hyperirritable. There is thus a reduced threshold for firing action potentials and an increased tendency for seizures.

Clinical Features

1. The patient is much more likely to be symptomatic if the hyponatremia develops acutely or subacutely and if the serum sodium is less than 125 mmol/L. In some chronic cases, the mental changes are due to the underlying condition (e.g., hypothyroidism)

rather than the hyponatremia. If symptomatic, it causes a metabolic encephalopathy consisting of

    a. Inappropriate behavior

    b. Confusion

    c. Headache

    d. Speech problems

    e. Vomiting

    f. Tremor

    g. Lethargy, weakness, malaise

    h. Muscle twitches and cramps

    i. Seizures

2. With overly rapid correction of hyponatremia or an abrupt rise in serum osmolarity, there is a risk of central pontine or extrapontine myelinolysis (CPM).

    a. Most cases of CPM occur after fairly prompt correction of hyponatremia at rates higher than 20 to 30 mmol/L over 3 days or more than 12 mmol/L/day.

    b. The condition occurs mainly in ill, hospitalized patients. Patients may develop confusion, coma, and then, in full-blown cases, pseudobulbar palsy and quadriparesis (locked-in syndrome).

    c. The actual mechanism of the demyelination is uncertain, but several hypotheses have been advanced.

        (1) There is osmotic damage to the capillary endothelium, exposing the brain to myelinotoxic factors in the plasma or vasogenic edema (or both). Plasminogen in the plasma could become activated, forming plasmin, which in turn hydrolyzes the myelin.

        (2) The edema itself may cause demyelination. This possibility has led to further speculation that the white matter of the pons becomes "choked" by the grid-like arrangement of fibers.

        (3) Patients with systemic illness may not be able to increase the cellular idiogenic concentration to match the changing osmolality of the plasma during the treatment of hyponatremia.

Key Signs: Hyponatremia

- Hyponatremia: lethargy, impaired cognition, impaired alertness, tremor, seizures

- Central pontine myelinolysis: quadriparesis with pseudobulbar palsy or locked-in syndrome

Laboratory Testing

The main laboratory tests are for serum electrolytes. In selected cases it wise to determine the serum or plasma osmolality (to exclude artifactual hyponatremia). This, combined with clinical assessment, is usually sufficient to classify the hyponatremia as hypovolemic, normovolemic, or hypervolemic. For hypovolemic conditions, ancillary tests include serum urea, creatinine, and hemoglobin determinations.

Radiologic Features

There are no specific radiographic findings except for cerebral edema in extreme cases and CPM in patients with this complication. The white matter change is best visualized with T_2-weighted magnetic resonance imaging (MRI).

Key Tests: Hyponatremia

- Assay the serum electrolytes and determine serum osmolality.

- Assess volume status clinically

- Syndrome of inappropriate secretion of ADH (SIADH)? Check urinary sodium concentration and urinary osmolality.

- Tests for underlying cause: Include thyroid and porphyrin screening tests.

Management

1. Management of hyponatremia depends on the underlying cause and the neurologic complications exhibited by the patient. The patient's hyponatremia should be categorized as hypovolemic, normovolemic, hypervolemic, or normo-osmolar. The specific underlying disorder should then be determined using clinical and laboratory means described in standard medical texts. Correcting the underlying disorder usually corrects the hyponatremia.

2. Asymptomatic patients with hypotonic hyponatremia who are hypervolemic or normovolemic are treated with volume restriction to 1.0 L/day and can be corrected at a maximum rate of 1.5 mmol/L/day (Ayus and Arieff, 1993). It can be supplemented with normal saline in amounts that create an increase in serum sodium of less than 12 mmol/day.

3. Management of acutely symptomatic patients is controversial. However, those with seizures and cerebral edema require more active treatment than water restriction alone. In these extreme and rare

circumstances, prompt therapy with mannitol or hypertonic saline with a loop diuretic should be administered such that the correction is no faster than 0.5 to 1.0 mmol/L/h or 20 mmol/L during the first day. Electrolytes must to be checked hourly with prompt reporting facilities.

4. If possible, it is best not to correct the serum sodium too quickly or to bring it to normal values. It is important to give just enough to get the serum sodium concentration in the range of 130 mmol/L and not to strive for prompt normalization of serum electrolytes, which could put the patient at greater risk for central nervous system (CNS) demyelination than the rapid sodium elevation. Karp and Laureno (1993) suggested striving for a level of less than 10 mEq/L for the first 24 hours and less than 21 mEq/L over the first 48 hours. Studies on acutely hyponatremic animals showed that an increase of more than 12 mmol/L/day may produce CPM if this rate of increase continues for 2 to 3 days.

5. Water restriction, if too vigorous, may be associated with complications. Treatment of hypovolemic shock may become necessary and may force a more rapid rise in osmolality than planned. The use of half-normal saline might be considered in this circumstance.

Prevention

It is better to avoid excessive water administration (but avoid volume depletion), thiazide diuretics, or drugs that may produce a syndrome of inappropriate ADH administration for those at risk (see Etiology).

Key Treatment: Hyponatremia

- Determine the classification and underlying cause of hyponatremia.

- Avoid overly rapid correction of hyponatremia (<10 mEq/L/24 h), except in an emergency, to prevent CPM.

Bibliography

Al-Salman J, Kemp D, Randall D: Hyponatremia. West J Med 176:173, 2002.
Ayus JC, Arieff AI: Pathogenesis and prevention of hyponatremic encephalopathy. Endocr Clin North Am 22:425, 1993.
Fraser CL, Arieff AI: Fatal central diabetes mellitus and insipidus resulting from untreated hyponatremia: a new syndrome. Ann Intern Med 112:113, 1990.
Karp BI, Laureno R: Pontine and extrapontine myelinolysis: A neurologic disorder following rapid correction of hyponatremia. Medicine (Baltimore) 72:359, 1993.
McKee AC, Winkelman M, Banjer B: CPM in severely burned patients: relationship to serum hyperosmolality. Neurology 38:1211, 1988.
Millious HJ, Liamis GL, Elisaf MS: The hyponatremic patient: A systemic approach to laboratory diagnosis. CMAJ 166:1056, 2002.
Mulloy AI, Caruana RJ: Hyponatremic emergencies. Med Clin North Am 79:155, 1995.
Pesantes-Morales H: Volume regulation in brain cells: cellular and molecular mechanisms. Metab Brain Dis 11:187, 1996.
Tien R, Arieff A, Kucharczyk RK, et al.: Hyponatremic brain damage: is central pontine myelinolysis common? Am J Med 92:513, 1992.
Wijdicks EFM, Larson TS: Absence of postoperative hyponatremia syndrome in young, healthy females. Ann Neurol 35:626, 1994.

HYPERNATREMIA

Definition

Hypernatremia, an increase in serum sodium concentration above 145 mmol/L, relates to a deficit of water relative to sodium and indicates general hypertonicity of body fluids.

Epidemiology

Acute/subacute hypernatremia with neurologic manifestations occurs predominantly in extremely young infants and the elderly. It may occur in patients of intermediate ages, especially in the presence of a net loss of water, iatrogenic or self-induced salt loading, and obtundation or inability to express needs or to satisfy thirst.

Pathophysiology

Table 5–1 lists the main mechanisms for hypernatremia.

TABLE 5–1.   MECHANISMS FOR HYPERNATREMIA

Water Loss
Extrarenal
  Skin: insensible perspiration
  Lungs
Renal
  Nephrogenic diabetes insipidus
Hypothalamic dysfunction including pituitary apoplexy

Water Loss with Sodium Loss
Extrarenal
  Skin: sweat
Renal
  Osmotic diuresis
Sodium gain
  Excessive sodium administration
  Adrenal hyperfunction (hyperaldosteronism, Cushing syndrome)

Clinical Features

1. Neurologic signs and symptoms relate to loss of the volume of cells in the CNS.

2. With hypernatremia, potent homeostatic mechanisms in the brain prevent neuronal and glial shrinkage by increasing the intracellular concentrations initially of sodium, potassium, and chloride followed in about 10 hours by an increase in organic substances, especially *myo*-inositol, glutamate, glutamine, and taurine. Thus only acute hypernatremia, with insufficient time for this adjustment, causes neurologic problems.

3. Neurologic complications

   a. Increased muscular tone: paratonic rigidity

   b. Subdural hematomas: due to brain shrinkage and tearing of bridging veins

   c. Capillary and venous congestion: bleeding with multiple microscopic hemorrhages; macroscopic subcortical, intracerebral, and subarachnoid hemorrhages; venous sinus or cortical vein thromboses

   d. Seizures sometimes result from the vascular complications, but they mainly occur during the rehydration phase of patients with chronic hyponatremia, in response to acute osmotic swelling of cells after administration of fluids of lower osmolality than that of the patient's serum and brain.

   e. Acute hypernatremia, seen especially in children, is associated with seizures and variably impaired consciousness.

Key Signs: Hypernatremia

- Encephalopathy with acute hypernatremia, especially in children

- Seizures, mainly with vascular complications or during rehydration with fluid shifts

- Dehydration with decreased skin turgor

- Chronic hypernatremia: often not associated with encephalopathy

Laboratory Testing

1. Serum electrolyte determination establishes the presence of hypernatremia. The cause should be apparent from the clinical setting.

2. Electroencephalographic (EEG) changes are nonspecific, consisting of diffuse slowing that reverses after uncomplicated correction. Epileptiform discharges are not seen with acute or chronic hyponatremia in the absence of vascular complications.

Radiologic Features

Intracranial hemorrhagic complications (see above) can be visualized with computed tomography (CT) or MRI scanning.

Management

1. Water deficit is calculated based on total body water (60% of body weight in nonobese patients).

2. If there is an associated volume deficit (i.e., combined water and sodium loss), replacement should begin with normal (0.9%) saline solution. Volume deficits must be replaced first.

3. Only profound acidosis, with pH less than 7.15, should be treated with sodium bicarbonate.

4. If the neurologic syndrome of acute hypertonicity predominates, replacement should start with half-normal (0.45%) saline. It is best to avoid reductions of plasma osmolality of more than 2 mOsm/L/h. Pure glucose solutions should be avoided, as the brain does not have time to adjust to the resultant shift of water into the intracellular compartment.

5. Serum electrolytes should be monitored every 2 to 4 hours during acute therapy.

6. Underlying disease process should be sought and treated. It is vital to give corticosteroids promptly to patients with pituitary apoplexy.

Key Treatment: Hypernatremia

- Calculate fluid loss and replace volume with 0.9% (normal) saline.

- If neurologic syndrome predominates, use 0.45% saline, reducing it at ≤ 2 mOsm/h.

- Identify and treat underlying disease.

Bibliography

Kahn A, Brachet E, Blum D: Controlled fall in natremia and risk of seizures in hypertonic dehydration. Intensive Care Med 5:27, 1979.

Pesantes-Morales H: Volume regulation in brain cells: cellular and molecular mechanisms. Metab Brain Dis 11:187, 1996.

Riggs JE: Neurologic manifestations of electrolyte disorders. Neurol Clin 20:227, 2002.

Snyder NA, Arieff AI: Neurologic manifestations of hypernatremia. In Arieff AI, Griggs RG (eds): Metabolic Brain Dysfunction in Systemic Disorders. Boston, Little, Brown, 1992, pp. 87–106.

Swanson PD: Neurological manifestations of hypernatremia. In Vinken PJ, Bruyn GW (eds): Handbook of Clinical Neurology, vol. 28. Amsterdam, North-Holland, 1976, pp. 443.

HYPERKALEMIA

Definition

Serum potassium concentration of more than 5.5 mEq/L (5.5 mmol/L)

Etiology

1. Renal failure: Potassium homeostasis is largely dependent on renal function; hence, clinically significant hyperkalemia is usually seen with renal failure.
2. Adrenal insufficiency occurs, especially with lack of the mineralocorticoid hormone aldosterone.
3. Acidosis with or without insulin deficiency may also be associated with hyperkalemia.

Epidemiology

Hyperkalemia is a common complication of renal failure. Other causes are relatively rare.

Pathophysiology

1. Potassium homeostasis is largely dependent on renal function. With renal failure, hyperkalemia results from failure of the kidney to excrete potassium. The situation can be exacerbated when renal blood flow is compromised, as in hypovolemia with hypotension.
2. Aldosterone fosters potassium excretion by the kidney, in exchange for sodium; hence aldosterone deficiency may lead to hyperkalemia.
3. Because potassium accompanies insulin-mediated glucose entry into cells and acidosis drives potassium out of cells, hyperkalemia is common in diabetic ketoacidosis.
4. Because potassium is concentrated in cells, cell lysis (e.g., hemolysis, rhabdomyolysis), especially combined with renal impairment, can produce acute hyperkalemia.
5. Other causes of or contributors to hyperkalemia are arginine infusion (potassium driven out of cells), beta-blockers (catecholamines foster movement of potassium into cells), hyperosmolality, hypovolemia, and hyperkalemic periodic paralysis.

Clinical Features

1. Cardiac complications of hyperkalemia eclipse any neurologic complications: cardiac arrhythmias, heart block, and atrial asystole; then ventricular complexes deteriorate followed by ventricular fibrillation or asystole.
2. Hyperkalemia is sometimes associated with diffuse muscle weakness and fatigability, most strikingly associated with adrenal insufficiency. Rarely, hyperkalemia can produce a flaccid quadriparesis that mimics an acute motor polyneuropathy.
3. Hyperkalemia does not appear to have significant CNS complications. Patients commonly are lethargic or nervous, but these symptoms may relate to the associated underlying diseases rather than to the potassium concentration.

Key Signs: Hyperkalemia

- Cardiac conduction problems or arrhythmias
- Diffuse muscle weakness, especially with associated adrenal insufficiency
- Lethargy

Laboratory Tests

1. Serum potassium determination should be accompanied by other tests to determine the underlying cause [e.g., renal failure, adrenal insufficiency, serum glucose, and blood gas (acid-base) determination].
2. Electrocardiographic monitoring to detect atrial or ventricular arrhythmias or heart block is wise.

Treatment

1. Mild hyperkalemia (serum potassium < 6.5 mEq/L) often resolves with treatment of the underlying cause.
2. Moderate or severe hyperkalemia requires more vigorous therapy. Calcium infusion counteracts the effects of hyperkalemia on cardiac and muscle membranes. Serum potassium can be reduced by infusion of glucose and insulin. Sodium bicarbonate may also help.
3. Cation exchange with sodium polystyrene sulfonate enemas can be undertaken.
4. For renal failure, hemodialysis or peritoneal dialysis can be used to lower the serum potassium level.

Prevention

1. In patients with renal failure, it is important to avoid dehydration and potassium administration.

2. In patients with adrenal failure, provide adequate mineralocorticoid and glucocorticoid replacement (e.g., at times of stress).

3. In other patients prevent dehydration, ensure good renal output, prevent diabetic ketoacidosis, and avoid drugs (see above) that may precipitate hyperkalemia.

4. Avoid conditions that precipitate hyperkalemic periodic paralysis. Have the patient eat frequent small meals rich in carbohydrates, use a low-potassium diet, and avoid strenuous exercise and exposure to cold.

Key Treatment: Hyperkalemia

- Emergency treatment of severe hyperkalemia (>7.0 mEq/L) includes infusions of calcium, glucose, and insulin; ion exchange resin enemas; and dialysis

Bibliography

Bia MJ, DeFronzo RA: Extrarenal potassium homeostasis. Am J Physiol 240:F257, 1981.

Knochel JP: Neuromuscular manifestations of electrolyte disorders. Am J Med 72:521, 1982.

Knoll GA, Sahgal A, Nair RC, et al.: Renin-angiotensin system blockade and the risk of hyperkalemia in chronic hemodialysis patients. Am J Med 112:110, 2002.

HYPOKALEMIA

Definition

Serum potassium concentration less than 3.5 mEq/L (mmol/L)

Etiology and Pathophysiology

1. Excessive losses through the gut or kidney (due to various disorders, some iatrogenic)

2. Diminished dietary intake

3. Shift of potassium into cells (as with hypokalemic periodic paralysis, insulin effect, or systemic alkalosis)

Epidemiology

Hypokalemia is the most common electrolyte disturbance.

Clinical Features

1. The main neurologic complication is muscular weakness. It begins at a potassium level of about 3.0 mEq/L (mmol/L), but concentrations of 2.5 mEq (mmol/L) or less are associated with significant proximal weakness. Typically, cranial nerve innervated muscles are spared. Rhabdomyolysis may develop with concentrations below 2.0 mEq/L (mmol/L).

2. Exceptionally, an encephalopathy develops, but it rarely progresses to coma.

Key Signs: Hypokalemia

- Muscular weakness

- Encephalopathy (rarely)

Differential Diagnosis

1. Myopathy: polymyositis, endocrine myopathy (especially Cushing's disease), acute necrotizing alcoholic myopathy

2. Hypokalemic periodic paralysis

3. Myasthenia gravis

4. Guillain-Barré syndrome with acute paralysis

Laboratory Testing

It is axiomatic that serum potassium be assayed. Other tests may reveal the underlying cause, although clinical features offer the main clues to etiology and guide investigative tests.

Management

1. The underlying cause should be determined and addressed.

2. When mild, oral supplementation is usually sufficient; but with ongoing losses (e.g., diarrhea) or when hypokalemia is profound, parenteral administration is necessary.

Key Treatment: Hypokalemia

- Identify the underlying cause and correct it.

- Replace potassium orally or parenterally.

Bibliography

Raymond KH, Kunau RT: Hypokalemic states. In Maxwell MH, Kleeman CR, Narins RG (eds): Clinical Disorders of Fluid and Electrolyte Metabolism, 4th ed. New York, McGraw-Hill, 1987, pp. 519–529.

Riggs JE: Nerologic manifestations of electrolyte disturbances. Neurol Clinics 20:227, 2002.

Welfare W, Sasi P, English M: Challenges in managing profound hypokalemia. BMJ 324:269, 2002.

HYPERMAGNESEMIA

Definition

Normal serum magnesium level ranges from 1.3 to 2.1 mEq/L (0.8–1.3 mmol/L; 2–3 mg/dL). Values over 2.1 mEq/L therefore constitute hypermagnesemia, although clinical symptoms begin at 4 mEq/L.

Epidemiology

Hypermagnesemia is almost certainly underrecognized. A survey in an Oklahoma VA hospital revealed elevated serum magnesium levels in 59 of 1033 samples (5.7%). Of these, physicians had requested serum magnesium determinations in only 7 (12%).

Pathophysiology of Clinically Significant Hypermagnesemia

1. Significant hypermagnesemia mainly occurs in the context of renal failure and magnesium administration. Magnesium may be administered as a cathartic or as an antihypertensive (e.g., as treatment for pre-eclampsia or eclampsia).
2. Hypermagnesemia has been reported in cases of laxative or antacid abuse (or both).
3. Magnesium excess reduces the metabolic rate of glucose utilization in both the gray and white matter of the rat spinal cord.

Clinical Features

1. Oral ingestion of excessive magnesium may cause gastrointestinal irritation and diarrhea. Hypotension may occur that is usually mild, although it can be marked if hypovolemia is also present.
2. Loss of deep tendon reflexes usually precedes the mental status changes and occurs at 5 to 6 mEq/L.
3. CNS depression develops at 8 to 10 mEq/L. Indeed, neuromuscular paralysis may precede clinical recognition of encephalopathy. Lethargy and confusion, however, are common early manifestations. High serum levels (e.g., >9 mEq/L) may also

cause parasympathetic paralysis in addition to coma, neuromuscular paralysis (including cranial nerve innervated and respiratory muscles), and areflexia. At times it mimics a brainstem stroke.
4. Context: renal failure and encephalopathy with weakness and areflexia, with or without palsy of cranial nerve innervated muscles.

Key Signs: Hypermagnesemia

- Suspect hypermagnesemia in a patient with impaired renal function who has diarrhea and depressed deep tendon reflexes with or without encephalopathy.

Laboratory Testing

1. Serum magnesium determination is essential. However, because magnesium is mainly intracellular, the serum level gives only a rough estimate of the total body burden of magnesium.
2. EEG slowing is found with serum magnesium concentrations above 15 mEq/L.
3. Electromyography (EMG) may reveal a presynaptic defect in neuromuscular transmission. Compound muscle action potential amplitudes are reduced; and there is a decremental amplitude of response to muscle nerve stimulation at low rates and a marked amplitude increase following brief exercise or high stimulation rates.

Key Tests: Hypermagnesemia

- Serum magnesium is higher than 5 mEq/L.
- EMG may show presynaptic defect in neuromuscular transmission.
- EEG slowing is seen with serum magnesium levels higher than 15 mEq/L.

Treatment

1. Because the effects of magnesium on the neuromuscular junction are the most life-threatening, and because these actions are antagonized by calcium, treatment of magnesium intoxication includes calcium gluconate administration. The usual dose is 10 mL of a 10% solution, which can be repeated as necessary to overcome neuromuscular blockade. Hemodialysis may be necessary to lower the serum magnesium concentration in extremely symptomatic patients, especially in the presence of renal failure.

2. Supportive care, particularly concerning ventilatory function in the intensive care unit (ICU), may be necessary. Blood pressure support, especially optimizing the blood volume, may be necessary if the patient is hypotensive.

Key Treatment: Hypermagnesemia

- Calcium infusion, hemodialysis (if serum magnesium is extremely high and encephalopathy or paralysis develops)

- Supportive care in ICU: especially for ventilatory support, airway protection, and treatment of arterial hypotension

Bibliography

Castelbaum AR, Donofrio PD, Walker FO, et al.: Laxative abuse causing hypermagnesemia, quadriparesis and neuromuscular conduction defect. Neurology 39:746, 1989.

Riggs JE: Neurologic manifestations of electrolyte disturbances. Neurol Clinics 20:227, 2002.

Rizzo MA, Fisher M, Lock JP: Hypermagnesemic pseudocoma. Arch Intern Med 153:1130, 1993.

Whang R, Ryder KW: Frequency of hypomagnesemia and hypermagnesemia: Requested vs. routine. JAMA 263:3063, 1990.

Zwerling H: Hypermagnesemia-induced hypotension and hyperventilation. JAMA 266:2374, 1991.

HYPOMAGNESEMIA

Definition

Serum magnesium level of less than 1.7 mg/dL

Epidemiology

Because magnesium is abundant in most foods, its deficiency in normal persons is rare. In hospitals, however, the estimated percentage of patients with low amounts of body magnesium ranges from 4% to 47%. The prevalence is highest in acute care settings, especially the ICU.

Pathophysiology

1. Neurologic features are usually present only with a serum concentration of less than 0.8 mEq/L.

2. Because only 10% of the body's magnesium is extracellular, the estimate of total body magnesium deficiency may be grossly inaccurate. A low serum concentration usually reflects a severe body deficit in magnesium, although the serum magnesium level may be normal despite a general body deficiency.

Clinical Features

1. Neurologic manifestations are similar to those of hypocalcemia and include hyperexcitability, muscle cramps, tetany (with positive Chvostek and Trousseau signs), hyperreflexia, and seizures.

2. Other clinical features that have been described include vertigo, nystagmus, dysphagia, athetoid movements, and focal signs such as hemiparesis and aphasia. An acute organic brain syndrome with psychiatric manifestations may develop.

3. In children, problems occur mainly during the neonatal period and early infancy. Deficiency may be caused by decreased intestinal absorption and impaired renal reabsorption, neonatal hepatitis, and maternal conditions (vomiting, diabetes mellitus, use of diuretics, excessive lactation). Seizures, tetany, hyperirritability, and impaired consciousness are the main features.

4. There may be serious cardiac complications, including arrhythmias and congestive heart failure refractory to standard therapy.

Key Signs: Hypomagnesemia

- Hyperexcitability: muscle cramps, tetany, hyperreflexia, seizures

- Less commonly: encephalopathy, movement disorder, dysphagia, vertigo, paresis

Laboratory Testing

1. In addition to the serum magnesium concentration, there are other methods of estimating magnesium deficiency. A simple physiologic test is the measurement of magnesium excretion in a 24-hour urine collection. If the value exceeds 24 mg in 24 hours, there is evidence of renal magnesium wasting. If 12 mg or less is excreted, magnesium deficiency is highly likely.

2. Measuring magnesium in erythrocytes or leukocytes offers a more accurate assessment of the total body deficit. This assay is not commonly available, however.

Key Tests: Hypomagnesemia

- Serum magnesium
- 24-hour urine collection
- Cerebrospinal fluid (CSF) magnesium in selected cases

Treatment

1. Parenteral magnesium is needed when convulsions occur. With such symptomatic magnesium deficiency, the average body deficit is 12 to 24 mg/kg body weight. This should be replaced by magnesium sulfate as a 50% solution, given in divided doses intravenously or intramuscularly for a total dose of 8 to 12 g of magnesium sulfate or 0.8 to 1.2 g of elemental magnesium. About 50% is lost in the urine.

2. When giving magnesium supplements, one should be aware of possible problems.

   a. Caution should be used in the presence of renal failure because magnesium toxicity may quickly develop.

   b. Serum magnesium and deep tendon reflexes should be closely monitored.

   c. Calcium should be available as a treatment in the event of hypermagnesemia. Hypocalcemia often accompanies hypomagnesemia, so calcium supplementation is usually needed. Potassium supplements are also often needed in the presence of magnesium deficiency.

Prevention

Prophylaxis by adding magnesium at 100 to 200 mg/day to parenteral nutrition helps prevent hypomagnesemia in the ICU. A diet rich in magnesium allows more gradual replacement of magnesium stores. Correction of risk factors (alcoholism, hypophosphatemia, diabetes) may prevent excessive urinary losses.

Key Treatment: Hypomagnesemia

- For convulsions due to hypomagnesemia, give MgSO₄ IV or IM as a 50% solution in divided doses for a total of 8 to 12 g in the average adult.
- Monitor the blood pressure.
- Give calcium and potassium supplements.

Bibliography

Al-Ghamdi SMG, Cameron EC, Sutton RAL: Magnesium deficiency: pathophysiologic and clinical overview. Am J Kidney Dis 24:737, 1994.
Geven WB, Monnens LAH, Willems JL: Magnesium metabolism in childhood. Miner Electrolyte Metab 19:308, 1993.
Leicher CR, Mezoff AG, Hyams JS: Focal cerebral deficits in severe hypomagnesemia. Pediatr Neurol 7:380, 1991.
Sutton R, Dirks JH: Disturbances of calcium and magnesium metabolism. In Brenner BM, Rector FR (eds): The Kidney, 4th ed., vol. 1. Philadelphia, WB Saunders, 1991, pp. 841–887.
Whang R, Hampton EM, Whang DD: Magnesium homeostasis and clinical disorders of magnesium deficiency. Ann Pharmacother 28:220, 1994.

HYPERCALCEMIA

Definition

Serum calcium concentration above the normal range of 8.5 to 10.5 mg/dL (2.12–2.62 mmol/L)

Epidemiology

An increase in serum calcium concentration sufficient to cause alteration of CNS function is not uncommon in certain populations (e.g., 5% of patients with cancer). Hypercalcemia has a prevalence of 0.5% among hospitalized patients.

Etiology and Pathophysiology

1. See Table 5–2.
2. Calcium plays a vital role in neurotransmitter release, in the activation of intracellular processes that result from neuronal excitation, and in electrical stabilization of neuronal membranes. A high extracellular concentration of calcium decreases membrane permeability and reduces its excitability.
3. Early generalized weakness and fatigability are related to reduced neuromuscular excitability.

Clinical Features

1. The severity of neurologic features depends on the serum concentration, the acutness of the hypercalcemia, and the associated medical conditions.
2. Mental status abnormalities commonly occur with serum calcium concentrations above 14 mg/dL (3.2 mmol/L). They consist of behavioral changes (ranging from personality changes to severe organic psychosis) and confusion progressing to lethargy, stupor, and coma. The clinical features

TABLE 5–2. CAUSES OF HYPERCALCEMIA

Disruption of Normal Bone–Extracellular Fluid Equilibrium
Metastatic tumor*
Multiple myeloma*
Lymphoma
Hyperthyroidism
Immobilization in a young individual or those with underlying
    disease, (e.g., Paget's disease)

Excessive Parathyroid Hormone*
Primary hyperparathyroidism
Nonparathyroid tumor producing parathormone-like substance,
    (e.g., lung, breast, kidney)
Lithium therapy
Familial hypocalciuric hypercalcemia

Excess Vitamin D
Hypervitaminosis D
Sarcoidosis (increased formation of 1,25-dihydrocholecalciferol)
Idiopathic hypercalcemia of childhood

Other
Adrenal insufficiency
Thiazide administration
Milk-alkali syndrome
Hypervitaminosis A

*Most common causes.

are those of diffuse or bihemispheric encephalopathy.

3. Convulsions occur occasionally.

4. Ocular palsies (including internuclear ophthalmoplegia), muscular wasting, weakness, and areflexia are seen occasionally.

5. Commonly associated problems include marked dehydration, abdominal pains, renal calculi, and metabolic bone disease. Renal insufficiency (prerenal, renal, or obstructive uropathy) may contribute to the acute picture.

Key Signs: Hypercalcemia

- Encephalopathy: psychosis, behavioral changes, confusion, impaired alertness to coma (worsening with increasing serum calcium concentration)

- Severe cases: seizures, areflexia, and ocular movement problems

Laboratory Testing

1. Ionized calcium is the physiologically active component of extravascular calcium. Calcium is largely protein-bound; the concentration of the ionized unbound portion is 1.16 to 1.32 mmol/L.

2. With hypoproteinemia, it is important to correct the serum albumin concentration or to determine the ionized calcium concentration.

Treatment

1. It is important to identify the underlying cause and treat it, if possible. The decision to treat should be based on the patient's anticipated quality of life and personal preferences, the diagnosis, and the prognosis of the underlying cause (often cancer). Hypercalcemia secondary to parathyroid adenoma, however, is cured with surgery.

2. Once a decision is made to treat, it is usually best not to correct the hypercalcemia rapidly. The first step is to correct dehydration or perform volume replacement with intravenous saline. Potassium supplements are also usually needed.

3. Subsequent specific treatment involves the correction of hypercalcemia over the next 24 to 48 hours.

    a. A loop diuretic and further infusion of saline, after the intravascular volume is adequate, enhance renal clearance of calcium.

    b. An intravenous biphosphonate drug (e.g., pamidronate or clodronate) is considered the drug of choice.

    c. Plicamycin (mithramycin), which inhibits bone resorption, is often effective but has significant dose and dose duration toxic effects on the liver, bone marrow, coagulation system, and kidneys. Gallium nitrate can be used as an alternative to plicamycin.

    d. Corticosteroids and calcitonin usually have a modest, or transient, effect at best on controlling the hypercalcemia of malignancy.

    e. Calcitonin can help acutely while waiting for the effects of the biphosphonate.

    f. Peritoneal dialysis or hemodialysis has been used to treat hypercalcemia due to secondary hyperparathyroidism in patients with chronic renal failure.

Prevention

To prevent recurrence of the hypercalcemia, the malignant process must be controlled. Acute primary hyperparathyroidism requires surgical removal of the offending gland. Oral phosphate is effective in many patients but is tolerated by few.

Key Treatment: Hypercalcemia

- Severe acute hypercalcemia [serum calcium > 14 mg/dL (3.2 mmol/L)] may require corticosteroids, calcitonin, biphosphonate, hemodialysis or peritoneal dialysis, and loop diuretics when the blood volume is adequate.

- Treat the underlying cause, if possible.

Bibliography

Fisken RA, Heath A, Bold AM: Hypercalcemia: a hospital survey. Q J Med 196:405, 1984.
Heath DA: Hypercalcaemia in malignancy. BMJ 298:1468, 1989.
Nussbaum SR: Pathophysiology and management of hypercalcemia. Endocrinol Metab Clin North Am 22:343, 1993.
Patten BM, Pages M: Severe neurologic disease associated with hyperparathyroidism. Ann Neurol 15:453, 1984.
Riggs JE: Neurologic manifestations of electrolyte disturbances. Neurol Clinics 20:227, 2002.
Wang CA, Guyton SW: Hyperparathyroid crisis: clinical and pathological studies of 14 patients. Ann Surg 190:782, 1979.
Waxman J: Hypercalcemia: a new mechanism for old observations. Br J Cancer 61:647, 1990.

HYPOCALCEMIA

Definition

Serum calcium less than 8.15 mg/dL (2.12 mmol/L)

Etiology

See Table 5–3.

Epidemiology

About 10% of patients in ICUs have hypocalcemia after correcting for the serum albumin levels and ionized calcium concentrations. A considerably smaller number are symptomatic.

Pathophysiology

1. The ionized portion can be altered by a change in pH; for example, with acidosis, protein binding is lessened and the percentage of the free fraction is increased. Conversely, with respiratory alkalosis, the protein binding is increased and the free fraction is less, sometimes producing tetany.
2. Calcium homeostasis is regulated by secretion of parathyroid hormone (PTH). The parathyroid glands are sensitive to the plasma concentration of ionized calcium; and secretion is prompt if the calcium concentration falls. PTH causes increased resorption of calcium from the kidney and gastrointestinal tract as well as increased mobilization of calcium from bone. A component of this situation is PTH-mediated renal conversion of 25-hydroxyvitamin D to 1,25-hydroxyvitamin D. A deficiency of either PTH or vitamin D can produce hypocalcemia. PTH secretion is inhibited by severe hypomagnesemia or hypermagnesemia.
3. Extracellular calcium ions have a stabilizing effect

TABLE 5–3. CAUSES OF HYPOCALCEMIA

Specific Cause	Mechanism
Hypoparathyroidism	
Postsurgical	Reduced PTH secretion
Autoimmune disease	Reduced PTH secretion
Infiltrative (e.g., cancer, hemochromatosis, sarcoid	Reduced PTH secretion
Irradiation	Reduced PTH secretion
Severe hypomagnesemia	Inhibits PTH secretion
Vitamin D deficiency	
Inadequate intake; severe liver or kidney disease	Decreased formation of 25 or 1,25-hydroxyvitamin D
Acute complexing or sequestration of calcium	
Acute pancreatitis	Sequestration of ionized calcium in an acute situation (PTH secretion cannot compensate)
Rhabdomyolysis	
Massive tumor lysis	
Phosphate infusion	
Toxic shock syndrome	
Acute severe illness	
Alkalosis	
Increased osteoblastic activity	
Hungry bone disease	Postparathyoidectomy
Osteoblastic metastases	Prostate or breast cancer
Anticalcemic agents	
Biphosphonates	
Plicamycin	
Calcitonin	
Gallium nitrate	
Phosphate	
Antineoplastic agents	
Asparaginase	
Doxorubicin	
Cytosine arabinoside	
WR2721	
Cisplatin	
Other drugs	
Ketoconazole	
Pentamidine	
Foscarnet	

Abbreviation: PTH, parathyroid hormone.

on the neuronal membrane. When reduced in concentration, the membrane is hyperexcitable because of this membrane effect and the decrease in calcium-mediated potassium conductance.
4. Intracellularly, calcium is required for the activity of many enzymes and for maintaining the integrity of cells. With hypoparathyroidism the concentration of intracellular calcium is reduced by 10% in the cerebral cortex but by about 35% in the white matter.

Clinical Features

1. Although the threshold for neurologic symptoms is not well defined, life-threatening complications frequently develop when the ionized portion falls to less than 2 mg/dL (0.5 mmol/L).
2. Seizures, usually of the generalized convulsive type, are the main complications of acute, severe hypocalcemia. They are more likely to occur in patients with preexisting seizure disorders. Mental

changes include depression, agitation, hallucinations, and psychosis; but these changes are nonspecific. Tetany with carpopedal spasm may occur, along with muscle spasms and cramps, paresthesias, and weakness.

3. The most important clinical signs are those of neuromuscular irritability: increased deep tendon reflexes and positive Chvostek and Trousseau signs.

4. Pseudotumor cerebri (benign intracranial hypertension) with papilledema may complicate hypoparathyroidism.

5. Many of the classic clinical signs and symptoms of hypocalcemia are absent or blunted in the ICU because of the use of drugs with paralyzing, sedating, and antiepileptic properties.

Key Signs: Hypocalcemia

- Seizures: usually generalized convulsions
- Hyperexcitability: brisk deep tendon reflexes and positive Chvostek and Trousseau signs

Laboratory Testing

The calcium concentration varies with the serum albumin; generally, for each 1.0 g/L decrease in albumin, the serum calcium decreases by 0.8 mg/dL (0.02 mmol/L). Normal ionized serum calcium is 4.1 to 5.1 mg/dL (1.02–1.27 mmol/L). When there is rapid chelation by blood transfusions and rhabdomyolysis or pancreatitis, the extent of protein binding varies unpredictably; it is important to measure the ionized serum calcium.

Management

1. All patients with signs or symptoms of hypocalcemia should be treated. Patients with seizures and impaired consciousness require emergency treatment. Etiology-specific therapy is ideal.

2. Emergency management of hypocalcemia involves prompt administration of calcium gluconate: 10 to 20 ml of 10% calcium gluconate, containing 93 mg of elemental calcium, administered intravenously over 10 minutes. A more rapid infusion may cause cardiac irregularity. A continuous infusion can follow. An infusion of 15 mg/kg increases the serum calcium level by 2 to 3 mg/dL; 11 ampoules are required for a 70 kg man to achieve this increase.

3. Chronic management requires correction of the underlying cause. In the case of hypoparathyroidism, lifetime supplementation is necessary. The mainstay of treatment is vitamin D. Orally administered, elemental calcium supplements (e.g., 1.0–1.5 g of elemental calcium per day in the form of calcium carbonate, citrate, lactate, gluconate, or glubionate is usually required as well. With malabsorption syndromes there may be malabsorption and deficiency of vitamin D itself. Large doses of vitamin D may be required, leading to the risk of vitamin D intoxication.

4. Hypocalcemia due to magnesium deficiency does not respond to calcium supplementation alone but does recover following magnesium replacement. As a corollary, it is generally wise to measure the serum magnesium whenever hypocalcemia is found and to correct any deficiency.

Key Treatment: Hypocalcemia

- Emergency treatment (e.g., for convulsions or tetany) requires calcium infusion.
- Always investigate and treat the underlying cause.

Bibliography

Carlstedt F, Lind L: Hypocalcemic syndromes. Crit Care Clin 17:503, 2001.

Eastell R, Heath H III: The hypocalcemic states: their differential diagnosis and management. In Coe FL, Favus MJ (eds): Disorders of Bone and Mineral Metabolism. New York, Raven Press, 1992, pp. 571–585.

Kapoor M, Chan GZ: Fluid and electrolyte disturbances. Crit Care Med 17:503, 2001.

Tohme JF, Bilezikian JP: Hypocalcemic emergencies. Endocrinol Metab Clin North Am 22:363, 1993.

Zaloga GP, Chernow B, Cook D, et al.: Assessment of calcium homeostasis in the critically ill patient: the diagnostic pitfalls of the Mclean Hastings nomogram. Ann Surg 202:587, 1985.

HYPOPHOSPHATEMIA

Definition

Serum phosphate of less than 2.5 mg/dL (< 0.83 mmol/L). Severe hypophosphatemia, during which symptoms relevant to the serum phosphate concentration appear, is reserved for a serum phosphate level of less than 1.5 mg/dL (0.5 mmol/L).

Etiology

See Table 5–4.

Epidemiology

1. Mild hypophosphatemia is common, but symptomatic hypophosphatemia is uncommon. It is

TABLE 5–4. CAUSES OF SEVERE HYPOPHOSPHATEMIA

Chronic alcoholism and alcoholic withdrawal
Dietary deficiency and phosphate binding antacids
Severe thermal burns
Recovery from diabetic ketoacidosis
Hyperalimentation
Nutritional recovery syndrome
Marked respiratory alkalosis
Therapeutic hyperthermia
Neuroleptic malignant syndrome
Recovery from exhaustive exercise
Renal transplantation
Acute renal failure
Shock with replacement with high volumes of glucose solutions

probably encountered less than five times per year in most ICUs in tertiary care hospitals.

2. Hypophosphatemia can be easily overlooked or not considered because its symptoms are mimicked by other, more common disorders (see below).

Pathophysiology

All levels of the nervous system can be clinically affected in hypophosphatemia. The cause of CNS dysfunction in hypophosphatemia is uncertain. Possibilities include

1. Inadequate oxygenation of tissues due to red blood cell 2,3-diphosphoglycerate (2,3-DPG) dysfunction.

2. Associated hyperventilation (e.g., with hyperammonemia, hypoxemia, or decreased 2,3-DPG) may cause reduced cerebral blood flow and further compromise of cerebral energy metabolism.

3. Altered neurotransmitter function has been found in an animal model, but uncertainty exists because the animal may have been hypotensive.

4. In clinical practice, there are often coexisting disorders that may also cause an encephalopathy (e.g., alcoholism with infections, pancreatitis, hypomagnesemia, hepatic failure). It may be difficult to recognize the main factors causing the impaired consciousness. There is a synergistic effect in some cases, although each may produce encephalopathy individually.

Clinical Features

1. An acute confusional state with irritability and apprehension may be present. Lethargy, distal paresthesias, dysarthria, and abnormal respiratory patterns are sometimes early features.

2. Reversible coma can occur, with or without seizures. We have also seen hypophosphatemia mimic brain death in a trauma patient who received large amounts of a glucose solution. The

cranial nerve areflexia and paralysis of movements were reversed by phosphate administration.

3. Variable motor abnormalities include athetosis, ballismus, myoclonus, ataxia, asterixis, weakness, paralysis with areflexia (peripheral), and a Guillain-Barré-like syndrome.

4. A syndrome of impaired eye movements, confusion, and ataxia, closely resembling Wernicke's encephalopathy, has been noted. This can be a diagnostic problem when treating alcoholics or the nutritionally deprived. Hypophosphatemia should be considered in patients with the clinical picture of Wernicke's encephalopathy who fail to respond to thiamine.

Key Signs: Hypophosphatemia

- Encephalopathy: impaired consciousness, seizures
- Movement disorders
- Impaired ocular movements

Differential Diagnosis

1. Encephalitis
2. Wernicke's encephalopathy
3. Acute hypercalcemia
4. Nonketotic hyperglycemia
5. Drug intoxication (e.g., phencyclidine)

Laboratory Testing

Serum phosphate should be monitored every day to once weekly during hyperalimentation in ICUs.

Management

1. When replacing phosphate, it is best to stop the hyperalimentation program temporarily or reduce calorie supplementation until the neurologic symptoms clear. This is often essential for prompt recovery; phosphate supplementation alone may not affect the clinical condition for some time.

2. In most cases it is unclear whether hypophosphatemia reflects a total body deficiency of phosphorus. In previously healthy patients who have become acutely ill, it is unlikely that there is phosphate deficiency. In the nutritionally deprived, however, such a deficit is likely. In milder cases the need for phosphate supplementation can be determined by the history; a review of medications, nutrition, and therapy; blood gas determinations; and urinary phosphorus and creatinine levels

(calculation of the fractional excretion of phosphate).

3. If supplements are needed and the patient is able to take fluids orally, it is safest to give milk, which contains 0.9 mg of phosphorus per milliliter. Other oral phosphate solutions are available. Parenteral administration of 9 mmol of phosphorus in 77 mM NaCl solution over 12 hours to provide 4 mg/kg body weight over this time has been implemented.

Prevention

1. Hyperalimentation fluids should be checked for phosphate content and phosphate added to meet the daily requirements. Magnesium supplementation should also be considered, as magnesium deficiency contributes to further excessive loss of phosphate in the urine.

2. Complications of phosphate administration include hyperphosphatemia, hypomagnesemia, hypocalcemia, hyperkalemia (if potassium salts of phosphate are used), metabolic acidosis, and volume excess with intravenous solutions. Oral treatment may cause diarrhea. It is thus important to monitor the serum phosphate and other electrolytes and calcium during therapy.

Key Treatment: Hypophosphatemia

• Suspect hypophosphatemia in patients with encephalopathy, abnormal movements, or paralysis who are on parenteral nutrition and in those who are nutritionally deprived.

• Replace phosphate in the form of milk or oral or parenteral phosphate compounds.

Bibliography

Bhaskaran D, Massry SG, Campese VM: Effect of hypophosphatemia on brain catecholamine content in the rat. Miner Electrolyte Metab 13:469, 1987.

Hicks W, Hardy G: Phosphate supplementation for hypophosphatemia and parenteral nutrition. Curr Opin Clin Nutr Metab Care 43:227, 2001.

Knochel JP: The pathophysiology and clinical characteristics of severe hypophosphatemia. Arch Intern Med 137:203, 1977.

Knochel JP, Montanari A: Central nervous system manifestations of hypophosphatemia and phosphorous depletion. In Arieff AI, Griggs RC (eds): Metabolic Brain Dysfunction in Systemic Disorders. Boston, Little, Brown, 1992, pp. 183–204.

Prins JG, Schrijver H, Staghouwer JH: Hyperalimentation, hypophosphatemia and coma. Lancet 1:1253, 1973.

Vannatta JB, Whang R, Papper S: Efficacy of intravenous phosphate therapy in the severely hypophosphatemic patient. Arch Intern Med 141:885, 1981.

Young GB, Amacher AL, Paulseth JE, et al.: Hypophosphatemia vs. brain death. Lancet 1:617, 1982.

TABLE 5–5. CAUSES OF HYPOGLYCEMIA

Postprandial Hypoglycemia
Glucose-induced
Fructose, galactose, leucine-induced (pediatric patients)

Fasting Hypoglycemia
Hepatic disease
Excess insulin from tumor (insulinoma)
Deficiency of growth hormone, cortisol
Renal failure
Sepsis
Alcoholism
Drugs (see Table 5-6)
Exogenous insulin
Malnutrition
Heart failure
Tumors that secrete insulin-like growth factor-1 (IGF$_1$)
  Sarcomas
  Mesotheliomas
  Hepatomas

HYPOGLYCEMIA

Definition

Serum glucose less than 2.5 mmol/L (40 mg/dL)

Etiology

See Tables 5–5 and 5–6.

Epidemiology

1. The etiologies vary from center to center; but the largest group, comprising 37% to 88% in various series, consists of diabetics on insulin.

TABLE 5–6. DRUGS (OTHER THAN INSULIN) REPORTED TO CAUSE HYPOGLYCEMIA

Acetaminophen
Acetylsalicylic acid
Amphetamine
Chloramphenicol
Dextropropoxyphene
Dicumarol
Dispyramide
Ethylenediaminetetraacetate
Halofenate
Haloperidol
Hypoglycine
Kerola (herb)
Manganese
Monoamine oxidase inhibitors
Onion extract
Orphenadrine
Oxytetracycline
Pentamidine
Phenothiazines
Phenylbutazone
Quinine
Sulfa drugs

2. About one fifth of insulin-dependent diabetics suffer significant hypoglycemic attacks. The prevalence of diabetes in the population is probably 0.2% to 1.0%, so it is a common problem.

Pathophysiology

1. Mild hypoglycemia may produce alterations in neural function without altering the functions of receptors and lower-order processing. Similarly, energy failure is usually late and incomplete; and cerebral blood flow and the oxygen supply are maintained. Because of the shortage of glucose, lactic acidosis does not occur unless glucose is replaced.

2. Hypoglycemia itself can cause neuronal death (e.g., diffusely in the neocortex, hippocampus, caudate, and putamen).

3. Extracellular calcium concentration decreases profoundly, and intracellular calcium increases before energy stores are depleted; this suggests that neuronal death is calcium-mediated, with activation of free radicals and various autodestructive enzymes. This may be due to release of aspartate and quinolinic acid. Seizures may contribute to brain damage.

Clinical Features

1. Principal clinical effects of hypoglycemia relate to CNS dysfunction. However, sympathetic autonomic responses to hypoglycemia related to epinephrine release are often prominent and constitute important clues to the diagnosis of early hypoglycemia. They include cold perspiration, tachycardia, palpitations, and associated anxiety. These signs can be prevented by beta-adrenergic blocking agents such as propranolol.

2. The CNS manifestations of hypoglycemia can be divided into confusion or delirium, seizures, focal defects, motor manifestations, and stupor or coma.

   a. Confusion and altered behavior represent the mildest form of acute hypoglycemic encephalopathy. Decreased attention and concentration and impaired orientation and memory are typical. Behavior can be bizarre, suggesting an acute psychiatric illness or drunkenness.

   b. Seizures are usually of the generalized convulsive type, commonly manifesting as status epilepticus, with EEG spikes indicating a corti-

cal origin. Multifocal seizures evolving to generalized convulsions occur occasionally.

   c. Focal neurologic signs, especially hemiplegia and aphasia (mimicking stroke) are occasionally encountered. The lateralized signs may occur without reduced consciousness and resolve promptly with glucose administration. Choreiform or athetoid movements may also accompany hypoglycemia and resolve promptly with intravenous glucose.

   d. Severely damaged individuals may remain in a persistent vegetative state or permanent coma, or they may die of complications.

Key Signs: Hypoglycemia

- Acute encephalopathy with confusion, seizures
- Focal signs occasionally
- Associated signs of sympathetic overactivity: perspiration, tachycardia

Treatment

1. Acute, severe hypoglycemia requires vigorous, sustained treatment, especially with insulin or oral hypoglycemic drug overdose. Give a bolus of 25 to 50 g of a 50% glucose solution followed by a steady intravenous infusion. Monitor the serum glucose at least hourly. In cases of insulin overdose, a considerable glucose infusion may be needed (e.g., 30% concentration).

2. Determine the cause of the hypoglycemia (see Tables 5–5 and 5–6).

3. Insulinoma is best treated surgically. Medical treatment with diazoxide can help prevent further hypoglycemic attacks until surgery is performed.

4. Idiopathic postprandial hypoglycemia and alimentary hypoglycemia are best treated by dietary management (e.g., small, frequent meals).

Prevention

1. In diabetics, prevention of severe hypoglycemic reactions consists of educating the patients and relatives, selecting specific therapy for specific patients, and estimating the degree of metabolic control necessary.

2. Instruct the family about first aid for hypoglycemia and the advisability of a Medic-Alert bracelet.

Key Treatment: Hypoglycemia

- Treat vigorously with glucose supplementation and monitor frequently for at least a day.

- Further prevention requires control of the cause or use of frequent, small meals.

Bibliography

Auer RN, Siesjö BK: Biological differences between ischemia, hypoglycemia and epilepsy. Ann Neurol 24:699, 1988.

Basdevant A, Costagliola D, Lanöe JL, et al: The risk of diabetic control: a comparison of hospital versus general practice supervision. Diabetiologia 22:309, 1982.

Dazzi D, Taddei F, Gavarini A, et al.: The control of blood glucose in the critical diabetic patient: a neuro-fuzzy method. J Diabetes Complications 15:80, 2001.

Fujioka M, Okuchi K, Hiramatsu K-I, et al.: Specific changes in human brain after hypoglycemic injury. Stroke 28:584, 1997.

Malouf R, Brust JCM: Hypoglycemia: causes, neurological manifestations and outcome. Ann Neurol 17:421, 1985.

Wallis WE, Donaldson I, Scott RS, et al.: Hypoglycemia masquerading as cerebrovascular disease (hypoglycemic hemiplegia). Ann Neurol 18:510, 1985.

HYPERGLYCEMIA

Definition and Classification

Hyperglycemia [serum glucose level higher than 140 mg/L (7.8 mmol/L)] can occur in two main contexts.

1. Diabetic ketoacidosis (DKA)
2. Nonketotic hyperglycemia (NKH)

Pathophysiology

1. Hyperglycemia is rarely associated with impaired consciousness if the serum glucose values are less than 300 mg/dL (16.7 mmol/L) in DKA or 600 mg/dL (33 mmol/L) plus hyperosmolality.
2. Hyperglycemia can arise from an increase in exogenous glucose, gluconeogenesis, or glycolysis. The lack of insulin or insulin effect fosters hyperglycemia by preventing glucose entry into cells, which in turn leads to alteration of the hormone balance that worsens regulation of carbohydrate metabolism.

Etiology

Hyperglycemia can arise from increased intake of exogenous glucose or from gluconeogenesis or glycolysis. Lack of insulin or insulin resistance fosters hyper-glycemia by preventing glucose entry into cells. This in turn leads to an alteration in hormone balance that worsens regulation of carbohydrate metabolism.

Epidemiology

Hyperglycemia is common, forming the principal definition of diabetes. It has a prevalence of 0.2% to 1.0% in the United States population.

Pathophysiology

1. Impaired consciousness correlates with the degree and rapidity of the hyperosmolality in patients and animals.
   a. Cellular dehydration or volume loss has been proposed as the main mechanism.
   b. An electrophysiologic study in animals showed that electrical activity of the reticular formation was affected by the osmolality.
   c. Acetoacetate, but not β-hydroxybutyric acid, in high concentrations in DKA may produce impaired consciousness and decreased cerebral oxygen utilization.
   d. Seizures may relate to a decrease in brain concentration of γ-aminobutyric acid (GABA), an inhibitory neurotransmitter. Such a decrease is due to defective production of GABA by mitochondria. This situation occurs in NKH but not DKA.
   e. There is preliminary evidence of altered mono-amine activity in the CNS in the presence of hyperglycemia: Serotonin turnover is increased in DKA; and there is reduced metabolism of norepinephrine, dopamine, and serotonin.
2. Cerebral edema during treatment of hyperglycemia probably results from a shift of water from plasma into brain cells when the serum osmolarity is suddenly reduced while treating a hyperosmolar, hyperglycemic state. The brain osmolarity, which had been upwardly adjusted during the hyperglycemic state, cannot adjust to match such a sudden change–hence the importance of gradual correction of hyperosmolar states.

Clinical Features

1. Premonitory symptoms include polyuria, polydipsia, increased thirst, malaise, lethargy, and weakness. Abdominal pain is frequent, but its pathogenesis is obscure.
2. Physical examination includes a search for the following.
   a. Dehydration and blood volume contraction
   b. Dry mucous membranes; decreased tissue turgor

c. Orthostatic hypotension with flat jugular veins; possibly tachycardia

d. DKA is usually associated with tachypnea and hyperventilation (Kussmaul's respiration) related to the metabolic acidosis. Acetone may give the breath a fruity odor. With NKH the hyperventilation and acetone breath are absent.

3. Hyperglycemia with impaired consciousness may occur apparently spontaneously or in the context of serious systemic metabolic stress (e.g., burns, infections, pancreatitis, corticosteroid or other drug therapy, dialysis). In some of the latter cases, the systemic stressor may contribute to the encephalopathy.

4. Focal signs of CNS dysfunction occur commonly with NKH, including hemiplegia, aphasia, and even brainstem signs. Movement disorders, including dystonic posturing, can occur. Seizures, usually focal but not invariably associated with a clear sensorium, are common. Focal tonic seizures, movement-induced or kinesigenic seizures, and epilepsia partialis continua have been reported. Features are often prolonged, recurrent, and variable, appearing in several discrete episodes during an episode of NKH.

Key Signs: Hyperglycemia

- Unexplained acute, variable focal seizures or dystonia

- Variably impaired consciousness (related to osmolality)

- History of diabetes mellitus

- Dehydration without ketosis

Laboratory Testing

1. Serum glucose is elevated, usually to more than 350 mg/dL (19 mmol/L) in patients with impaired consciousness. Glucosuria is generally present.

2. Patients with DKA show an increase in acetone and ketone bodies (acetoacetic acid and β-hydroxybutyric acid), increased anion gap (serum bicarbonate ≤ 10 mmol/L). Blood gas assays show metabolic acidosis with ventilatory compensation.

3. Patients with NKH are a heterogeneous group with severe hyperglycemia, hyperosmolality, and little ketone production. With time, there is a spontaneous decrease in serum glucose, with the glucose loss due to glucosuria, glucose metabolism, and fluid shifts from the intracellular compartment.

4. Hemoglobin, hematocrit, serum urea, and plasma proteins are commonly elevated, reflecting blood volume contraction. Serum sodium is usually decreased. Serum potassium concentration may be normal, increased, or decreased.

Key Tests: Hyperglycemia

- Suspect nonketotic hyperglycemia in patients with unexplained impaired consciousness, new focal or generalized seizures, or movement disorders.

- Serum glucose, serum osmolality, capillary blood gases (including pH), and urinary ketones may be helpful.

- Check for dehydration: elevated hemoglobin and serum urea.

Treatment

1. Restoration of blood volume with normal saline should take priority, especially if the patient is severely dehydrated. Glucose administration should be avoided.

2. Insulin administration is necessary to stop the gluconeogenesis and glycolysis that have been contributing to the vicious cycle of hyperglycemia and, in the case of DKA, ketone body production. To prevent cerebral edema and elevated intracranial pressure, it is usually sufficient to stop giving insulin in the acute situation before the serum glucose is lowered to 250 mg/dL (14 mmol/L).

3. For potassium deficiency, replacement with KCl can be started at about 10 mmol/h and then adjusted according to the urine output and the need.

Prevention

Cerebral edema should be sought during correction of hyperglycemic states. If the patient's level of consciousness or pupillary reactivity deteriorates, a CT scan may confirm this possibility. Judicious use of mannitol is sometimes (but rarely) necessary.

Key Treatment: Hyperglycemia

- Correct the dehydration.

- Gradually reduce the serum glucose with repeated doses of regular insulin.

- Replace potassium during treatment.

Bibliography

Hennis A, Corbin D, Fraser H: Focal seizures and non-ketotic hyperglycemia. J Neurol Neurosurg Psychiatry 55:195, 1992.

Lebovitz HE: Diabetic ketoacidosis. Lancet 345: 767, 1995.

Rowland NE, Bellush LL: Diabetes mellitus: stress, neuro-chemistry and behavior. Neurosci Biobehav Rev 13:199, 1989.

Schurr A: Bench-to-bedside review: A possible resolution of the glucose paradox of cerebral ischemia. Crit Care 6:330, 2002.

Tachibana Y, Yasuhara A: Hyperosmolar syndrome and diffuse CNS dysfunction with clinical implications. Funct Neurol 1:140, 1986.

Uribarri J, Carrol HJ: Neurologic manifestations of diabetic coma. In Arieff AI, Griggs RC (eds): Metabolic Brain Dysfunction in Systemic Disorders. Boston, Little, Brown, 1992, pp. 107–127.

HYPOTHERMIA

Definition and Classification

1. Overall definition: a body temperature less than 35°C

2. Hypothermia is also classified by severity: mild (32°–35°C), moderate (28°–32°C), severe (< 28°C).

3. Hypothermia may also be acute (minutes), subacute (hours), or chronic (days) depending on the time of development.

Etiology and Epidemiology

1. In hospitals in inner cities, patients who collapse indoors are usually elderly, are living alone, have an underlying systemic illness, and fall to the floor in poorly heated residences.

2. Patients admitted from outside their place of residence are younger.

3. Those from cities are often acutely intoxicated alcoholics.

4. Those exposed during recreational activities (e.g., skiing, hiking) are usually young and in otherwise good health. Profound hypothermia resulting from prolonged exposure to extremely cold temperatures is more likely in this group.

Pathophysiology

Hypothermia may also have other causes.
1. Excessive heat loss: cold weather or immersion in cold water

2. Abnormal heat conservation and reduced heat production: hypothyroidism, hypoglycemia (substrate depletion), hypopituitarism, hypoadrenalism, uremia, spinal cord transection above T1, peripheral neuropathy, autonomic neuropathy, certain drugs (alcohol, barbiturates, neuroleptics)

3. Defective heat regulation: hypothalamic lesions, including Wernicke's encephalopathy; strokes; tumors; head trauma; congenital abnormalities (e.g., Shapiro syndrome)

Pathophysiology

1. Hypothermia is a disturbance in the net regulation of heat production and heat loss, weighted toward the latter. It can result from defective homeostatic regulation, reduced metabolism (including diminished cellular metabolism and shivering), or increased heat loss due to exposure to extreme cold or impaired cardiovascular response, especially loss of vasomotor tone.

2. Acute hypothermia is usually the result of submersion in cold water, subacute hypothermia often results from cold air; and chronic hypothermia relates to underlying disease with disordered or insufficient autoregulation.

3. For each 1°C decrease in body temperature, metabolic processes slow and cerebral blood flow diminishes about 6%. At 28°C the metabolic rate falls to half normal. At less than 25°C the patient appears dead and has asystole. Perfusion falls in a pressure passive manner along with systemic blood pressure. Electroencephalographic (EEG) synaptic activity fails.

4. Both intrinsic and extrinsic coagulation systems are affected by hypothermia. Platelet function becomes ineffective because thromboxane B_2 is inhibited. Fibrinolytic activity is increased. A heparin-like substance is released. Enzyme activities necessary to initiate and maintain platelet-fibrin clots are reduced, resulting in an increased bleeding tendency. These features produce a disseminated intravascular coagulation-like syndrome but with a marked hemorrhagic tendency. It can be aggravated in the hypothermic trauma patient, who may require massive transfusions for blood loss.

Clinical Features

1. General features of mild hypothermia include shivering, tachycardia, tachypnea, diuresis, and peripheral cyanosis. With hypothermia the trunk and normally warm regions (e.g., axillae and groins) are cold. A low-reading thermometer should be used to measure the rectal temperature. The patient with chronic hypothermia may resemble one with hypothyroidism, with a puffy face, slow hoarse speech, and mental changes. The skin has a doughy consistency.

2. Neurologic features with mild hypothermia are dysarthria, ataxia, and amnesia.

3. With worsening, the pulse gets weaker and slower, shivering ceases, respirations are slow and shal-

low, and the patient becomes extremely pale. Deep tendon reflexes are increased above 32°C; hyporeflexia occurs between 26°C and 32°C, and areflexia is present below 26°C. Confusion worsens sometimes to delirium, and muscular rigidity develops.

4. Further deterioration leads to stupor or coma. Coma does not usually occur above 28°C. (Other causes for coma should be sought if the patient is comatose with a core temperature higher than 28°C.)

5. The pupils may become fixed to light; the heart may develop ventricular fibrillation without palpable pulse or audible heartbeat.

Key Signs: Hypothermia

- Hypothermia and pallor
- Dysarthria, ataxia, amnesia, confusion, coma
- Slow, weak pulse
- Shallow, slow respirations

Differential Diagnosis

1. Hypothyroidism (myxedema coma)

2. Wernicke's encephalopathy

3. Drug intoxication

4. Ventilatory failure with hypercarbia (CO_2 narcosis)

Laboratory Testing

1. The EEG develops evolutionary changes, with generalized slowing beginning at 30°C; it then changes to a burst-suppression pattern by 20° to 22°C and becomes flat at 18°C.

2. Evoked responses are less affected. At 29°C, waveforms are delayed by 33% but are still identifiable. Latencies lengthen progressively to unrecordable levels as 19°C is approached, and waveforms may disappear altogether.

3. Cardiac abnormalities occur with progressive hypothermia: obscured P waves; prolonged PR, QRS, and QT intervals; atrial fibrillation; ventricular dysrhythmias. Ventricular fibrillation may develop at 28°C.

4. Serum potassium should be checked, as hyperkalemia is a common accompaniment. A coagulation screen should probably be performed.

Key Tests: Hypothermia

- Core body temperature determination
- Thyroid function tests: rule out hypothyroidism
- Serum potassium
- Coagulation status

Prevention

Prevention of hypothermia involves dressing warmly in cold weather, avoiding adverse weather, maintaining adequate nutrition, maintaining adequate indoor temperatures, and arranging for regular checks on elderly patients in cold weather. Patients with quadriplegia, who cannot conserve heat by vasoconstriction or increase heat production by shivering, are especially at risk of hypothermia if exposed to cold environmental temperatures.

Management

1. As a general policy, patients found in an acute hypothermic situation should not be pronounced dead until they are assessed after rewarming to at least 33°C core temperature. It is important not to give up prematurely during resuscitative efforts.

2. Rewarming should be done expectantly, watching for serious cardiac arrhythmias, an afterdrop (a drop in core body temperature associated with conduction of heat away from the core while rewarming surrounding cold tissues and vasodilatation), and hypotension.

3. Simple rewarming techniques should begin in the field: removing wet, cold clothing; covering with warm, dry blankets; administering warmed intravenous (IV) fluids.

4. Active internal rewarming using IV fluids and warmed medical air (core rewarming) should be used only when the temperature is less than 32°C. The latter should be increased to 40° to 42°C to prevent afterdrop. It is safest to perform vigorous rewarming in an intensive care unit (ICU) setting because of cardiovascular instability or complications. Other methods to increase the core temperature more rapidly include use of cardiopulmonary bypass, continuous arteriovenous rewarming, and irrigation of the gastrointestinal tract or body cavities.

5. Monitoring the core temperature with an esophageal temperature probe or pulmonary artery catheter should be considered for more accurate measurements.

6. Cardiovascular support in the ICU is required.

7. In frail, elderly individuals the rewarming should be done gradually to avoid cardiovascular collapse: a rewarming rate of no more than 0.5°C per hour has been recommended.

8. Treating the underlying cause should be done in concert with rewarming. The administration of thiamine, antibiotics, or drug antagonists need not wait for temperature correction.

Key Treatment: Hypothermia

• (Gradual) internal and external rewarming when the temperature is less than 32°C

• Monitor blood pressure, electrocardiogram, and serum potassium in ICU

• Treat arrhythmias, hyperkalemia, hypotension

Bibliography

Altus P, Hickman JW, Nord HJ: Accidental hypothermia in a healthy quadriplegic patient. Neurology 35:427, 1985.

Bracker MD: Environmental and thermal injury. Clin Sports Med 11:419, 1992.

Fritsch DE: Hypothermia in the trauma patient. AACN Clin Issues 6:196, 1995.

Keim SM, Guisto JA, Sullivan JB Jr: Environmental thermal stress. Ann Agric Environ Med 9:1, 2002.

MacDonnell JE, Wrenn K: Hypothermia in the summer. South Med J 84:804, 1991.

Oung CM, Ebglish M, Chiu RC, et al: Effect of hypothermia on hemodynamic responses to dopamine and dobutamine. J Trauma 33:671, 1992.

Schaller MD, Fischer AP, Perret CH. Hyperkalemia. a prognostic factor during severe hypothermia. JAMA 264: 1842, 1990.

Woodhouse P, Keatinge WR, Coleshaw SR: Factors associated with hypothermia in patients admitted to inner city hospitals. Lancet 2:1201, 1989.

HYPERTHERMIA

Definition

With hyperthermia that causes neurologic impairment, the rectal temperature is usually higher than 41.1°C, although fever can be considered any body temperature higher than 37°C.

Etiology

Table 6–1 provides an effective approach to determining causation.

TABLE 6–1. DISORDERS OF HEAT PRODUCTION

Disorders of Heat Production
Exertional hyperthermia
Heat stroke (exceptional)
Malignant hyperthermia of anesthesia
Neuroleptic malignant syndrome
Lethal catatonia
Thyrotoxicosis
Pheochromocytoma
Salicylate intoxication
Drug abuse (especially cocaine and amphetamines)
Delirium tremens
Status epilepticus (especially convulsive type, occasionally with complex partial seizures)
Generalized tetanus

Disorders of Diminished Heat Dissipation
Heat stroke (classic)
Extensive use of occlusive dressings
Dehydration
Autonomic dysfunction
Use of anticholinergic medications
Neuroleptic malignant syndrome*
Cervical spinal cord lesions (plus hot environment)

Disorders of Hypothalamic Function
Neuroleptic malignant syndrome*
Cerebrovascular accidents
Encephalitis
Sarcoidosis and granulomatous infections
Trauma

*Mixed mechanisms.

Epidemiology

1. The incidence of severe hyperthermia is highest during hot summer months. During a summer heat wave in the United States, the death count may exceed 1200 persons.

2. The elderly poor are the most vulnerable.

3. Clusters of cases of hyperthermia may occur during military exercises, fun runs, and other activities in hot weather.

Pathophysiology and Pathology

1. Temperatures higher than 42°C cause decreased cerebral metabolism and EEG slowing.

2. Hyperpyrexia may impair neurologic function by a number of mechanisms.

   a. Interleukin-1 and other cytokines may have a direct effect on the central nervous system (CNS) in patients who have conditions in which cytokines are generated.

   b. The brain concentration of extracellular glutamate, an excitotoxic neurotransmitter, is directly related to temperature. Excessive amounts may cause an encephalopathy, including seizures.

   c. Systemic abnormalities are hypoglycemia, hypophosphatemia, extreme electrolyte disturbances, uremia and other end-organ damage.

d. Hemorrhages may occur in various organs, including the brain. These and microscopic infarctions relate to endothelial damage and disseminated intravascular coagulation (DIC). Areas showing maximal damage include the cerebellar cortex, cerebral cortex, thalamus, and striatum.

Clinical Features

See Table 6–2.

Laboratory Testing

1. Hematologic abnormalities: hemoconcentration, thrombocytopenia, leukocytosis, DIC
2. Electrolyte abnormalities: potassium initially decreased and then increased during late stages, hypocalcemia, hypophosphatemia, hypomagnesemia
3. Acid-base disturbances: respiratory alkalosis early, metabolic acidosis late
4. Hypoglycemia

TABLE 6–2.   MANIFESTATIONS OF HEATSTROKE

System	Manifestation
Central nervous	Confusional state (delirium)
	Seizures (status epilepticus)
	Oculogyric crisis
	Stupor
	Coma
	Cerebellar damage
	Hemiplegic episodes
Cardiovascular	Tachycardia
	Hypertension
	Hypotension (shock)
	Acute left heart failure
Pulmonary	Hyperventilation
	Pulmonary edema
	Pulmonary infarction
Renal	Acute nephropathy
	Chronic interstitial nephritis
Hematologic	Pupura; bleeding into various organs, including CNS
Gastroenterologic	Diarrhea and vomiting
	Hematemesis and melena
Endocrine	Hypoglycemia
Musculoskeletal	Muscles contracted and rigid; myoglobinuria

From Hart LE, Sutton JR: Environmental considerations for exercise. Clin Cardiol 5:246, 1987, with permission.

5. Myoglobinuria, elevated muscle enzymes, proteinuria, and microscopic hematuria are common complications. Hepatic dysfunction and renal failure are the first evidence of multiorgan failure and may contribute to the encephalopathy.

Key Tests: Hyperthermia

- Core body temperature determination
- Complete blood count and DIC screen
- Serum electrolytes, calcium, magnesium, phosphate, glucose, blood urea nitrogen, liver function tests
- Urine screen for blood/hemoglobin/myoglobin

Treatment

1. Treatment should begin on site using cooling therapy and hydration with intravenous fluids. Removing clothing and cooling with a fan and a fine, warm spray are simple, effective methods for instituting prompt therapy. They can prove lifesaving.
2. Meticulous electrolyte, cardiovascular, and neurologic monitoring is necessary as soon as the patient reaches medical care.
3. Further cooling with ice-water baths may be necessary in severe cases. Phenothiazines help reduce shivering. Antipyretics may assist in resetting the hypothalamus if the problem relates to fever, as described above.
4. Parkinsonian crisis related to abrupt withdrawal of dopaminergic agents may be treated by reinstituting antiparkinsonian treatment with dopaminergic agonists.
5. Antiepileptic drug therapy involves standard therapy for status epilepticus.

Prevention

1. Exercise caution with heat exposure, especially in the very young, the very old, the obese, and those lacking acclimatization.
2. Predisposing conditions include autonomic neuropathy (especially with diabetes mellitus), the use of anticholinergic drugs, skin diseases associated with impaired sweating, and the use of diuretics. Such individuals should exercise caution: Avoid running in hot, humid weather, and seek shade, adequate hydration, and air-conditioning.

Key Treatment: Hyperthermia

- Cooling: external and internal
- Investigation and treatment of underlying cause
- Symptomatic correction of abnormal biochemistry, hydration

Bibliography

Hart LE, Sutton JR: Environmental considerations for exercise. Clin Cardiol 5:246, 1987.

Heatstroke: United States, 1980. MMWR Morb Mortal Wkly Rep 30:277, 1981.

Kielblock AJ: Strategies for the prevention of heat disorders with particular reference to the efficacy of body cooling procedures. In Hales JRS, Richards D (eds): Heat Stress, Amsterdam, Excerpta Medica, 1987, pp. 489.

Kornhuber J, Weller M, Riederer P: Glutamate receptor antagonists for neuroleptic malignant syndrome and akinetic parkinsonian crisis. J Neural Transm 6:63, 1993.

Martinez M, Devenport L, Saussy J, Martinez J. Drug-associated heat stroke. South Med J 95:799, 2002.

Simon JF: Hyperthermia. N Engl J Med 328:483, 1993.

Sutton JR, Bar-Or O: Thermal illness in fun running. Am Heart J 100:778, 1980.

7 Alcoholism

Yuen T. So

Epidemiology and Risk Factors

1. The lifetime prevalence of alcoholism in the U.S. adult population is about 14%. It ranks after smoking and obesity as the third leading preventable cause of death.

2. A genetic predisposition has been demonstrated by studies of identical twins, adoption studies, and families of individuals with early-onset alcoholism. First-degree relatives of alcoholics, for example, are seven times more likely to be affected than the general population.

3. Neurologic complications are among the most serious adverse effects of alcoholism.

Etiology and Pathophysiology

1. Malnutrition is prevalent in people with alcoholism. One reason is the frequent occurrence of malabsorption in chronic alcoholics. Another is the so-called empty calories provided by alcohol. Thirty ounces of an 86-proof alcoholic beverage contain 2250 calories or nearly 100% of the adult daily requirement but provide only negligible amount of protein, vitamins, and other nutrients.

2. Excessive alcohol is directly toxic to the nervous system, as adequate diet or even nutritional supplements do not prevent many neurologic complications of alcoholism.

3. The diverse neurologic manifestations may be subdivided into three categories.

   a. Acute intoxication due to the pharmacologic effects of ethanol

   b. Withdrawal syndrome from sudden abstinence in individuals who have developed physical dependence on alcohol

   c. A varied group of potentially irreversible neurologic disorders secondary to prolonged alcohol abuse

4. Alcoholism has associated protean neurologic manifestations. Both the central and peripheral nervous systems are vulnerable.

5. The clinical presentations are probably governed by genetic, nutritional, and other environmental factors. Multiple neurologic abnormalities commonly occur in a single patient [e.g., alcoholic neuropathy in conjunction with some type of central nervous system (CNS) involvement].

Clinical Features

1. Acute intoxication

   a. Acute effects may include euphoria, dysphoria, disinhibition, drowsiness, belligerence, or aggression.

   b. In nonalcoholic individuals acute intoxication may occur at serum concentrations as low as 50 to 150 mg/dL.

   c. At higher serum concentrations, lethargy, stupor, coma, or even death from respiratory depression and hypotension occur.

   d. The lethal serum level varies, as tolerance develops with chronic use. Many alcoholics appear sober at a serum level of 500 mg/dL, whereas the same level is often fatal in nonalcoholic individuals.

Key Signs and Symptoms

- Euphoria, dysphoria, disinhibition, drowsiness, belligerence, or aggression

- Acute intoxication occurs at variable serum concentrations as tolerance develops with chronic use

- At high serum concentrations, lethargy, stupor, coma, or death from respiratory depression and hypotension

2. Alcohol withdrawal

   a. A withdrawal syndrome of CNS hyperexcitability or delirium tremens may result from sudden cessation or reduction of drinking in individuals with established alcohol dependence.

   b. Withdrawal symptoms commonly begin 6 to 8 hours after abstinence and are most pronounced at 24 to 72 hours.

   c. Generalized tremulousness appears first, followed by insomnia, agitation, delirium, auditory or visual hallucinations, or other perceptual disturbances.

   d. These symptoms are often accompanied by autonomic hyperactivity, such as tachycardia, profuse sweating, hypertension, and hyperthermia.

   e. Generalized tonic-clonic seizures, or withdrawal seizures, occur in some individuals,

865

typically 6 to 48 hours after the last drink. Seizures may occur singly or in a brief cluster.

f. Status epilepticus, though rare, is an important and potentially life-threatening complication.

g. Seizures sometimes occur in the midst of active drinking or more than a week after alcohol ingestion, suggesting pathogenic mechanisms other than withdrawal per se.

Key Signs and Symptoms

- CNS hyperexcitability or delirium tremens resulting from sudden cessation or reduction of drinking

- Generalized tremulousness, insomnia, agitation, delirium, auditory or visual hallucinations, or other perceptual disturbances

- Above symptoms often accompanied by autonomic hyperactivity, such as tachycardia, profuse sweating, hypertension, and hyperthermia

3. Wernicke-Korsakoff syndrome

a. Of the neurologic disorders due to chronic alcohol abuse, Wernicke-Korsakoff syndrome is probably the most important because of its serious consequences and the need for prompt recognition and treatment.

b. Wernicke-Korsakoff syndrome refers to two separately recognized disorders that often occur together. Wernicke encephalopathy and Korsakoff psychosis are successive stages of thiamine deficiency caused by alcohol abuse.

c. Both Wernicke encephalopathy and Korsakoff psychosis are caused by thiamine deficiency commonly encountered in alcoholics. The disorders, however, are not limited to alcoholism. All malnourished individuals with increased metabolic demand are at risk.

d. Wernicke encephalopathy is an acute or subacute encephalopathy characterized by apathy, disorientation, lethargy, and drowsiness. On examination, patients may have nystagmus, abducens or conjugate gaze palsies, and gait ataxia. The initial clinical picture may be masked by signs of alcohol withdrawal or overt delirium tremens. If the underlying thiamine deficiency is untreated, the encephalopathy may progress to stupor, coma, and death.

e. Korsakoff syndrome typically emerges as the acute symptoms and signs of Wernicke encephalopathy subside. It is a disorder of memory, characterized by an inability to recall the events of a period a few years before the onset of illness (retrograde amnesia) and an inability to learn new information (anterograde amnesia).

Confabulation is often present; and most, though not all, patients have limited insight into their memory dysfunction.

Key Signs

Wernicke Encephalopathy

- Disorientation, lethargy, drowsiness

- Nystagmus, abducens or conjugate gaze palsies

- Gait ataxia

Korsakoff Syndrome

- Retrograde amnesia

- Anterograde amnesia

- Confabulation

4. Alcoholic dementia

a. Apart from Wernicke-Korsakoff syndrome, mild cognitive impairment is frequently encountered in detoxified alcoholics.

b. Partly reversible brain shrinkage occurs with alcoholism. Brain atrophy, especially from loss of subcortical white matter, is seen. Computed tomography (CT) and magnetic resonance imaging (MRI) also may show enlargement of the cerebral ventricles and sulci.

c. Radiologic changes are also seen in nondemented alcoholic subjects and therefore are not specific enough for clinical diagnosis.

d. Although a direct neurotoxic effect of alcohol is suspected, there is a possibility that coexisting nutritional deficiency, head trauma, and liver disease may play a significant role.

5. Alcoholic neuropathy

a. This is likely to be the most prevalent neurologic syndrome of alcoholism. The most common neuropathic syndrome is a distal predominantly sensory or sensorimotor polyneuropathy.

b. Tingling or burning pain over the soles and toes is often the presenting symptom. If severe, the paresthesia interferes with sleep, wearing shoes, and ordinary walking. As the disease progresses, loss of sensation becomes more pronounced; and neuropathic pain may paradoxically diminish in severity.

c. Examination reveals abnormally elevated sensory thresholds to vibration, temperature, and pinprick. Atrophy of the intrinsic foot muscles and mild weakness are sometimes seen. Ankle tendon reflexes are diminished or absent.

d. Neuropathy varies widely in severity. Advanced

cases are seen rarely. In these patients, examination may demonstrate gait disturbances, widespread areflexia, weakness, Romberg sign, and severe sensory loss.

e. Neuropathy may also lead to autonomic insufficiency, as impotence, sweating abnormalities, and orthostatic hypotension are sometimes recognized.

f. Rare variants include a neuropathic joint due to deafferentation ("Charcot" joint) and hoarseness due to recurrent laryngeal neuropathy.

g. The cause of this neuropathy is not clear, though nutritional deficiency and direct alcohol neurotoxicity may play some role.

Key Signs and Symptoms

- Tingling or burning pain over the soles and toes
- Abnormally elevated sensory thresholds to vibration, temperature, and pinprick
- Diminished or absent ankle reflex

6. Subacute cerebellar degeneration

a. This is a slowly progressive cerebellar degeneration, preferentially affecting the anterior and superior vermis.

b. The resulting syndrome is a wide-based gait and an inability to tandem walk.

c. Limb ataxia is uncommon. If present, it is seen primarily in the legs, with the arms involved minimally if at all.

d. Some patients present more acutely. Mild gait instability may be present for some time only to deteriorate suddenly after binge drinking or an intercurrent illness.

e. Like alcoholic neuropathy, the cause of cerebellar degeneration is unknown.

Key Signs

- Truncal/gait ataxia with minimal or no limb ataxia

7. Acute or chronic myopathy

a. This most commonly manifests as a chronic, painless syndrome of proximal muscle wasting and weakness. As many as half of alcoholic patients have histologic evidence of myopathy on muscle biopsy, although overt weakness and elevation of serum creatine kinase (CK) are less common.

b. There is a wide range of severity of chronic myopathy. Mild cases of chronic myopathy are not surprisingly often unrecognized.

c. The skeletal myopathy may coexist with alcoholic cardiomyopathy.

d. A less common manifestation is an acute syndrome of severe muscle pain and tenderness, proximal weakness, and markedly elevated serum CK. If severe, rhabdomyolysis and myoglobinuria may lead to hyperkalemia and secondary renal failure.

Key Signs

- Proximal muscle wasting and weakness

8. Less common manifestations

a. A disorder of cerebral function, alcoholic pellagra, has been attributed to a deficiency of nicotinic acid or tryptophan. The disease has become rare since the widespread practice of supplementing cereals and bread with niacin. Initial symptoms are mood changes and neurasthenia that may progress to lethargy and confusion. Examination may show spastic paresis, paratonia, or myoclonus.

b. Marchiafava-Bignami syndrome is a rare but well documented disorder. It is a distinct syndrome of corpus callosum degeneration. The clinical presentation is varied. Some patients present with psychomotor slowing, incontinence, frontal release signs, and wide-based gait. Dysarthria, hemiparesis, apraxia, or aphasia may also be present. Occasional patients present in stupor or coma. MRI or CT may reveal lesions in the corpus callosum and anterior commissure, and less commonly the centrum semiovale.

9. Disorders not directly related to nutritional deficiency or neurotoxicity of alcohol

a. Alcoholic patients are prone to traumatic injuries of the brain and the peripheral nerves.

b. CNS complications include subdural and epidural hematoma, cerebral contusion, and post-traumatic epilepsy.

c. Compressive neuropathies may appear after prolonged unconsciousness, such as radial neuropathy at the spiral groove leading to wrist drop (Saturday night palsy), and peroneal nerve neuropathy at the fibular head or sciatic neuropathy in the gluteal region. Each leads to foot drop.

d. Rapid changes in serum electrolyte concentration, especially rapid correction of severe hyponatremia, are associated with central pontine myelinolysis. This is a disease of pontine white matter that causes dysarthria, paraparesis, or quadriparesis. Some patients also have symmetrical extrapontine lesions in the cerebral white matter, striatum, thalamus, and cerebellum.

e. End-stage liver disease due to alcoholic cirrhosis can present with encephalopathy, tremors, myoclonus, and asterixis.

f. Other causes of dementia associated with alcoholism include recurrent head trauma and hepatocerebral degeneration.

Differential Diagnosis

1. Acute encephalopathy

   a. The differential diagnosis of unexplained encephalopathy in an alcoholic subject should include Wernicke-Korsakoff syndrome, postictal confusion, electrolyte disturbances, and decompensated alcoholic liver disease, all of which are commonly encountered in this patient population.

   b. These patients are also at increased risk of head trauma and infection. Therefore other causes of structural, metabolic, infectious, or toxic encephalopathy should be considered.

   c. Prompt diagnosis of Wernicke-Korsakoff syndrome is critical, as delayed replacement of thiamine may lead to irreversible deficits or even death.

   d. Classic triad of encephalopathy, oculomotor palsy, and gait ataxia in Wernicke's encephalopathy may not be present to a full degree.

   e. In at-risk subjects, thiamine replacement should precede glucose infusion. Increased metabolic demands, glucose infusion, and sudden resumption of dietary intake after a period of malnourishment are risk factors for precipitating acute symptoms of Wernicke's encephalopathy.

   f. Alcoholism may coexist with other substance abuse.

2. Gait ataxia

   a. The gait ataxia of Wernicke's encephalopathy presents acutely.

   b. The more common alcoholic cerebellar degeneration is recognized by its subacute course. It is a predominantly truncal ataxia, with little or no limb involvement.

   c. Other causes (e.g., drug intoxication, cerebellar ischemia or hemorrhage, posterior fossa neoplasms or abscesses, infectious cerebellitis, hypothyroidism, paraneoplastic cerebellar de-

generation) should be considered through appropriate history, radiologic, and laboratory studies.

3. Peripheral neuropathy

   a. The clinical syndrome of alcoholic polyneuropathy is indistinguishable from the neuropathies associated with a wide range of common systemic disorders.

   b. Differential diagnosis includes diabetes mellitus, uremia, drugs, hypothyroidism, acquired immunodeficiency syndrome (AIDS), and many others.

   c. Diagnosis of alcoholic polyneuropathy depends on

      (1) Presence of an appropriate syndrome (i.e., a distal, symmetrical, predominantly sensory neuropathy)

      (2) Exclusion of other causes

      (3) Documentation of improvement with abstinence

   d. Disulfiram, a drug used for alcoholism rehabilitation, sometimes causes a neuropathy at doses higher than 125 mg/day.

Laboratory Testing

1. Blood alcohol at a level of 100 mg/dL raises serum osmolality by 22 mOsm/L. Serum osmolality thus provides a convenient measure of acute intoxication.

2. Initial evaluation of patients with acute neurologic symptoms should also include complete blood count, blood coagulation parameters, serum electrolytes, liver function tests, blood urea nitrogen (BUN), creatinine, bilirubin, toxicology screen, and arterial blood gases.

3. Prompt imaging of the brain is indicated when focal neurologic findings or unexplained encephalopathy is present.

4. After imaging studies, evaluation of unexplained encephalopathy may also include cerebrospinal fluid (CSF) examination for evidence of infection or subarachnoid blood.

5. Electromyography and nerve conduction studies are useful for characterizing neuropathy or myopathy.

6. Serum vitamin B_{12} and thyroid function tests are useful for evaluating neuropathy, serum CK for assessing acute or chronic myopathy, and thyroid function tests in individuals with chronic myopathy or cerebellar ataxia.

Radiologic Features

1. Mild, diffuse atrophy of the cerebral and cerebellar hemispheres is common, but this finding is too nonspecific for diagnosis.
2. MRI signal abnormalities of the corpus callosum and anterior commissure suggest Marchiafava-Bignami syndrome.
3. An important role of radiologic studies is to exclude other disorders that may mimic the neurologic syndromes associated with alcoholism.

Key Tests

- Serum osmolality
- Patients with acute neurologic symptoms: blood count, blood coagulation parameters, serum electrolytes, liver function tests, BUN, creatinine, bilirubin, toxicology screen, arterial blood gases
- MRI for focal neurologic findings or unexplained encephalopathy
- Electromyography and nerve conduction studies
- Serum vitamin B_{12} and thyroid function tests

Treatment

1. Management of alcohol intoxication and delirium tremens is primarily supportive.
2. All patients should be given supplements of parenteral thiamine and other vitamins.

PEARL

- Administer thiamine before glucose to avoid precipitating Wernicke's encephalopathy.

---

3. Delirium tremens may be treated with benzodiazepines (chlordiazepoxide 25–100 mg PO or IV, with a maximum of 300 mg over the first 24 hours), β-adrenergic antagonists (oral atenolol 50–100 mg/day) or α_2-adrenergic agonists (oral clonidine 0.1–0.4 mg four times per day). Cardiopulmonary parameters should be closely monitored.
4. Withdrawal seizures that are self-limited do not require specific anticonvulsant treatment.
5. Status epilepticus requires aggressive treatment with benzodiazepines and anticonvulsants as well as treatment of systemic complications.
6. The dysesthesia of peripheral neuropathy responds partially to tricyclic antidepressants and anticonvulsants (e.g., desipramine or amitriptyline 50–150 mg at bedtime; carbamazepine 400–1200 mg/day; or gabapentin 900–1800 mg/day).
7. Social support is needed for patients with significant cognitive deficits due to Korsakoff's syndrome or other causes.

Key Treatment

- Primarily supportive
- Parenteral thiamine and other vitamins
- Delirium tremens
  —Chlordiazepoxide
  —Oral atenolol
  —Oral clonidine
- Status epilepticus
  —Benzodiazepines, anticonvulsants, and treatment of systemic complications
- Dysesthesia (caused by peripheral neuropathy)
  —Desipramine or amitriptyline
  —Carbamazepine or gabapentin
- Social support for those with significant cognitive deficits from Korsakoff's syndrome or other causes

Prognosis and Complications

1. Neurologic dysfunction can be expected to improve partially with abstinence from alcohol and correction of malnutrition. The degree of recovery depends on the severity and chronicity of the disorder.
2. In patients with painful neuropathy, dysesthesias sometimes persist years after the initial manifestation.

Pregnancy

1. Prenatal exposure to excessive alcohol impairs fetal growth and leads to the fetal alcohol syndrome. Affected infants have short stature, microcephaly, and dysmorphic facies characterized by short palpebral fissures, thin upper lip, long flat philtrum, and flat midface.
2. Speech delay, learning disabilities, hyperactivity, and mental retardation are common in older children.

Bibliography

B

Caine D, Halliday GM, Kril JJ, Harper CG: Operational criteria for the classification of chronic alcoholics: identification of Wernicke's encephalopathy. J Neurol Neurosurg Psychiatry 62:51–60, 1997.

Chang PH, Steinberg MB: Alcohol withdrawal. Med Clin North Am 85:1191–1212, 2001.

Charness ME, Simon RP, Greenberg DA: Ethanol and the nervous system. N Engl J Med 321:442–454, 1989.

Diamond I, Messing RO: Neurologic effects of alcoholism. West J Med 161:279–287, 1994.

Monforte R, Estruch R, Valls-Sole J, et al.: Autonomic and peripheral neuropathies in patients with chronic alcoholism: a dose-related toxic effect of alcohol. Arch Neurol 52:45–51, 1995.

Victor M: Alcoholic dementia. Can J Neurol Sci 21:88–99, 1994.

Metals, Organic Solvent, and Pesticide Intoxication

Karen I. Bolla

LEAD (INORGANIC)

Epidemiology and Risk Factors

1. Occupational and environmental sources: automobile manufacturing and repair, bookbinding, cement-plastic mixing, dentistry, dyes, enamels, etching, stained glass making, paints, paper milling, pharmaceuticals, firing range instruction, printing, welding, pipe fitting, lithography, plastics, plumbing, pottery/ceramics, refineries, automobile emissions, (petroleum), rubber, shoe manufacturing and repair, and storage batteries.

2. More than 1 million workers have been exposed to lead.

Etiology and Pathophysiology

1. The most common routes of absorption of lead are by inhalation and ingestion.

2. Lead exposure is associated with changes in neurotransmitters (dopamine), inhibition of the *N*-methyl-D-aspartate (NMDA) receptor complex, punctate brain hemorrhages, dilation of vessels and ventricles, histologic changes in hippocampus and cerebellum, and demyelinization of peripheral nerves.

Clinical Features

A variety of symptoms are associated with lead exposure and differ depending on the length and intensity of exposure. Change in mental status, delirium, seizures, and unconsciousness are sequelae of acute high-level exposure.

Key Clinical Findings: Chronic Mild-to-Moderate Lead Toxicity

Physical Complaints

- Headaches
- Weakness
- Fatigue
- Vomiting
- Tremor
- Abdominal pain
- Constipation
- Sensorimotor polyneuropathy
- Scotopic visual effects
- Changes in auditory threshold
- Hypertension
- Anemia
- Reduced sperm counts and motility

Cognitive Complaints

- Impaired attention/concentration
- Difficulty with learning and memory
- Slowing of information-processing speed
- Manual dexterity difficulties

Psychological and Somatic Complaints

- Depression
- Anxiety
- Irritability
- Personality change
- Loss of interest in work and hobbies
- Decreased libido
- Sleep disturbance (ranging from insomnia to somnambulism)

Differential Diagnosis

Lead poisoning in adults is difficult to diagnose because of the nonspecific nature of the symptoms. Therefore, a history of significant occupational or environment exposure should be present.

Laboratory Findings

1. In adults, a lead blood level higher than 30 µg/dl is considered to be elevated and reflects recent exposure. In children, a blood lead level over 10 µg/dl is considered elevated. Blood level rises rapidly within a few hours after an acute exposure and remains elevated for several weeks.

2. Zinc protoporphyrin (ZPP) or free erythrocyte protoporphyrin level (FEP) begins to rise in adults once the blood lead levels reaches 30 to 40 ug/dl. Once elevated, the FEP remains so for several months even after exposure has ceased and the blood lead level has fallen. The threshold FEP level is 100 µg/dl blood. Both blood lead level and ZPP should be obtained to determine the presence of significant lead exposure.

3. The most widely available method for measuring body burden of lead is diagnostic chelation. Urine lead excretion is measured after infusion of calcium ethylenediaminetetra-acetic acid (EDTA). Urinary excretion of more than 600 g of lead in 72 hours is considered elevated.

4. A new noninvasive method for measuring body burden of lead in bone is x-ray fluorescence (XRF). Because it is rapid and safe, XRF promises to be the new gold standard for measuring lifetime accumulation of lead in bone. It is rapidly becoming an important alternative to chelation testing for monitoring lead burden with chronic exposure.

5. In patients with significant cognitive, psychological, and somatic complaints, neuropsychological testing is worthwhile.

6. Nerve conduction studies are indicated in patients with symptoms of peripheral nervous system damage.

Radiologic Features

Electroencephalogram, computed tomography, and magnetic resonance imaging are not useful in determining lead toxicity, except as they exclude other causes of symptoms.

Treatment

1. Patients with suspected lead toxicity should be removed immediately from the potential source of exposure.

2. Whether chelation therapy should be initiated in addition to removal from exposure depends on the blood lead concentration, the severity of clinical symptoms, biochemical and hematologic abnormalities, and the nature of exposure. The primary indication for treatment in adults is brief, high-level exposure (blood lead above 80 µg/dl) causing acute, severe symptoms. The most commonly used chelating agent is EDTA. Because chelating agents can produce renal toxicity because of increased levels of circulating lead, adequate hydration should be maintained.

Prognosis and Complications

1. Children with lead poisoning may have persistent cognitive and emotional difficulties.

2. In adults, the reversibility of symptoms is unclear because research is lacking in this area.

Prevention

1. Avoid exposure when increased levels of lead are suspected.

2. Use mandatory personal protective equipment in situations with increased risk of lead exposure.

3. Routine medical monitoring should be conducted for individuals at high risk for lead toxicity.

Pregnancy

Lead exposure increases the frequency of miscarriages and stillbirth.

ARSENIC

Epidemiology and Risk Factors

1. Occupational and environmental sources: artificial flowers, bookbinding, brass, bronze, cosmetics, dyes, enamels, gardening, glass, insecticides, paints, rubber, and taxidermy.

2. National Institute for Occupational Safety and Health (NIOSH) estimates that about 900,000 workers have potential daily exposure to arsenic.

Etiology and Pathophysiology

1. The most common routes of absorption of arsenic are dermal and ingestion.

2. Arsenic is stored in the liver, kidney, intestines, spleen, lymph nodes, and bones. It remains in the bones for extended periods of time. The pathways involved in oxidative metabolism are sensitive to arsenic toxicity. Arsenic prevents transformation of thiamine into acetylcholinesterase (acetyl-CoA), causing thiamine deficiency.

Clinical Findings

Like all the heavy metals, symptoms associated with arsenic exposure differ depending on the length and intensity of exposure.

1. Sequelae of acute high-level exposure include rise in temperature, headache, vertigo, abdominal pain, nausea and vomiting, nervousness and apprehension, convulsions, coma, nystagmus, paralysis, positive Kernig's sign with neck stiffness,

hyperreflexia, Mee's lines (white lines in the nails) that usually appear 2 to 3 weeks after acute exposure, and acute peripheral neuropathy.

2. Symptoms of chronic mild to moderate arsenic toxicity include headaches, physical and mental fatigue, cognitive decline, visual changes or optic neuropathy, seizures, painful sensorimotor peripheral neuropathy, vertigo, and restlessness.

Key Clinical Findings: Arsenic Toxicity

- Peripheral neuropathy
- Mee's lines
- Dementia
- Seizures

Differential Diagnosis

A history of occupational or environmental exposure to arsenic should be present.

Laboratory Findings

1. A level of arsenic in urine (24 hour) greater than 50 μg/g creatinine is considered to be elevated. However, a high urinary level may be seen after ingestion of seafood and thus a dietary history should be obtained. A better measurement can be obtained from the inorganic arsenic metabolites, monomethylarsonic acid (MMA) and dimethylarsinic acid (DMA) in the urine. If urinary arsenic comes back elevated and is not fractionated, wait 3 days without seafood intake and repeat.

2. In patients with significant cognitive and mood complaints, neuropsychological testing is worthwhile.

3. Nerve conduction studies are indicated in patients with symptoms of peripheral nervous system damage.

Radiologic Features

Electroencephalogram, computed tomography, and magnetic resonance imaging are not useful in determining arsenic toxicity, except as they exclude other causes of symptoms.

Treatment

1. Patients should be removed from potential sources of exposure.

2. For acute ingestion, treatment involves gastric lavage, and administration of British anti-lewisite (BAL), with electrolyte replacement.

3. Patients with significantly elevated levels of arsenic and moderate to severe symptoms can be treated with chelation therapy using dimercaprol (British anti-lewisite [BAL], d- or dimercaptosuccinic acid [DMSA]).

Prognosis and Complications

In cases of severe poisoning, the prognosis is poor, with a mortality rate of 50% to 75% usually within 48 hours of poisoning.

MERCURY (INORGANIC)

Epidemiology and Risk Factors

1. Occupational and environmental sources: antiseptics, disinfectants, felt manufacturing, alcohol distillation, cosmetics, dentistry, dyes, paints, paperworks, painting, pottery/ceramics, storage batteries, and taxidermy.

2. NIOSH currently estimates that 65,000 workers are potentially exposed to mercury.

Etiology and Pathophysiology

1. The most common routes of absorption are ingestion or inhalation from mercury vapors.

2. Alters cell membranes; causes combination of metabolic disturbance, disturbance of Ca^+ homeostasis, oxidative injury, and aberrant protein phosphorylation.

Clinical Findings

Chronic exposure to inorganic mercury is associated with the following symptoms:

1. Physical: salivary gland swelling, excessive salivation, visual disturbances, intentional tremor, parkinsonism, seizures, painful parasthesias, and peripheral polyneuropathy (sensorimotor axonopathy) affecting the lower limbs more than the upper limbs

2. Cognitive: decreased learning and memory and visuospatial difficulties

3. Psychological and somatic complaints: shyness, fatigue, weakness, personality changes, hyperirritability, insomnia, and depression

Key Clinical Findings: Inorganic Mercury Toxicity

- Intentional tremor
- Sensorimotor neuropathy
- Dementia

Differential Diagnosis

A history of occupational or environmental exposure to mercury should be present, together with elevated mercury levels in blood, urine, or hair. Early differential diagnosis includes Parkinson's disease (PD). The tremor seen with mercurial intoxication in not solely a resting tremor and is usually coarser than that found in PD.

Laboratory Findings

Blood serum concentrations greater than 15 µg/L are considered elevated; however, because of intraindividual and interindividual variability, serum concentrations of mercury are not reliable indications of toxicity. In urine, 35 µg/g creatine is considered elevated. However, this biomarker is also questionable because there is little correlation between symptoms and the amount of mercury excreted in the urine. The measurement of mercury in hair and nails can be problematic unless the potential for external exposures can be excluded.

Radiologic Features

Decreased bilateral attenuation on computed tomography scans in the visual cortex and diffuse atrophy of the cerebellum, especially the vermis, was found years after mercury poisoning in survivors of Minamata disease.

Treatment

Removal from the source of exposure and chelation with oral DMSA or 2,3-dimercapto-1-propane sulfonic acid (DMPS).

ORGANIC SOLVENTS

Common organic solvents include acetone, benzene, carbon tetrachloride, ethylene glycol (antifreeze), formaldehyde, gasoline, methyl-N-butyl ketone (MBK), methyl alcohol (methanol), n-hexane, trichloroethylene (TCE), tetrachlorethane, toluene (methyl benzene), and turpentine. Because most solvents that cause health problems are mixtures of solvents, the neurologic consequences of exposure to organic solvents in general will be discussed.

Epidemiology and Risk Factors

1. Occupational and environmental sources include the plastics and chemical industries.
2. Ten million workers were exposed to solvents in the United States (NIOSH estimate, 1987). The number of workers suffering adverse effects from exposure to organic solvents has decreased with closer adherence by industry to safe airborne concentrations as well as the use of mandatory personal protective equipment by workers. Unfortunately, the abuse of solvents by "huffing" is still a public health concern. Substances such as paint, airplane glue, and gasoline are placed in plastic bags, which are then placed over the face and inhaled to produce a "high."

Etiology and Pathophysiology

1. The most common route of absorption is the respiratory system. Solvents are highly volatile, and volatility corresponds to the amount of solvent that becomes airborne. The amount of uptake is related to workload, respiratory rate, use of respirators, and adequacy of ventilation.
2. Organic solvents are lipophilic and thus concentrate in organs rich in lipids (brain and adrenal glands). Solvents are metabolized and eliminated through the kidneys. The metabolites may be more toxic than the original compounds.
3. At high doses, depending on the specific chemical, solvents may act as anesthetics, convulsants (e.g., fluorothyl), anticonvulsants or anxiolytics (e.g., toluene), antidepressants (e.g., benzene chloride), and narcotics (e.g., TCE).
4. The mechanisms involved in solvent neurotoxicity are generally unknown. Neurotoxicity may be related to effects on neurotransmitters such as dopamine and gamma-aminobutyric acid (GABA).

Clinical Findings

A variety of symptoms are associated with solvent exposure and differ depending on the length and intensity of exposure. Change in mental status, delirium, seizures, and unconsciousness are sequelae of acute high-level exposure.

Key Clinical Findings: Chronic Mild-to-Moderate Solvent Toxicity

Physical Complaints

- Headaches (begin shortly after arriving at work and disappear at night, on weekends, and during vacations)

- Nasal irritation
- Decreased olfaction
- Sleep difficulties
- Alcohol intolerance
- Decreased libido
- Peripheral neuropathy (pain and numbness starting in feet and progressing to the hands)
- Nausea and vomiting (acetone)
- Ataxia, muscle twitching, paralysis, seizures, unconsciousness (benzene)
- Delirium, vertigo, seizures, parkinsonism, optic atrophy, visual difficulties (carbon tetrachloride)
- Absent corneal reflexes (ethylene glycol)
- Somnolence, coma, death (very high level of exposure, as with "huffing")

Cognitive Complaints

- Poor attention/concentration
- Decreased learning and memory
- Poor manual dexterity
- Decreased executive functioning
- Decreased psychomotor/motor functioning
- Alcohol intolerance

Psychological and Somatic Complaints

- Irritability
- Personality change
- Depression
- Confusion

Differential Diagnosis

1. Solvent encephalopathy is confirmed by the presence of positive exposure history, objective findings on neurobehavioral tests, and negative findings on neurologic examination, with the exception of the possible presence of a polyneuropathy. Biomarkers of solvent exposure are unreliable or difficult to obtain. Therefore, the diagnosis is generally one of exclusion. Differential diagnosis includes cerebrovascular disease, tumor, heavy alcohol use, and neuropsychiatric disorders such as affective, anxiety, and somatoform disorders.

2. A classification for solvent encephalopathy includes

   a. Type I: subjective nonspecific symptoms only

   b. Type IIa: sustained personality and mood change. Negative neurobehavioral findings. Unclear if symptoms are reversible.

   c. Type IIb: impairment of intellectual function documented by objective neurobehavioral test results and possible mild neurologic signs. After removal from exposure, symptoms should remain stable or improve, not become worse.

   d. Type III: dementia with neurologic signs, neurobehavioral deficits and possible neuroradiologic findings (e.g., frontal lobe atrophy). Related to repeated severe exposure (i.e., paint huffers). May be irreversible but generally does not progress.

Laboratory Testing

Nerve conduction studies can be useful because solvents affect the peripheral nervous system before the central nervous system. Sensory polyneuropathy is more pronounced in the feet than in the hands.

Treatment

Removal from the source of exposure. Treatment of anxiety and depression secondary to exposure may be necessary. Treatment with psychotropic medications and psychotherapy may be helpful.

Prognosis

Once removed from the source of exposure, symptoms should remain stable or improve over time. Deterioration is common and can be attributed to psychological disorders that develop secondary to the organic solvent exposure.

PESTICIDES

ORGANOPHOSPHATE INSECTICIDES

Epidemiology and Risk Factors

1. Occupational and environmental sources: manufacturing of insecticides, farming, and gardening.
2. Occurrence in the United States of organophosphate poisoning is low; epidemics have been reported in developing countries.

Etiology and Pathophysiology

1. Most common routes of exposure are dermal and respiratory.
2. Organophosphates inhibit acetylcholinesterase and pseudocholinesterase in the brain, spinal cord, myoneural junctions, and pre- and postganglion sympathetic nerve endings. Cholinesterase-

inhibiting insecticides include chlorpyrifos (Dursban), diazinon, Malathion, ethyl and methyl parathion, and trichlorofon. Increases in acetylcholine overstimulates the postsynaptic receptors in the cholinergic system, which inhibits cholinergic synaptic transmission.

Clinical Findings

1. Acute mild symptoms include fatigue, headache, dizziness, increased salivation, nausea and vomiting, diaphoresis, and abdominal cramps (symptoms always develop within 24 hours of exposure).
2. With more moderate poisoning, symptoms may include difficulty speaking or swallowing, shortness of breath, and muscular fasciculation.
3. High exposure can result in diminished levels of consciousness and marked myosis with no pupillary response.
4. After initial recovery from acute poisoning, an organophosphate-induced delayed polyneuropathy (OPIDP) can develop. OPIDP is observed as cramping muscle pain in legs, parasthesias, motor weakness, possible foot drop, and weakness of intrinsic hand muscles, beginning 10 days to 3 weeks after initial exposure.
5. Chronic low level exposure is associated with weakness, malaise, headache, lightheadedness, anxiety, irritability, altered sleep, tremor, numbness and tingling of the extremities, constricted pupils, decreased capacity for information processing, decreased memory and learning abilities, and poor visuoconstructional skills.

Key Clinical Findings: Organophosphate Insecticides

Mild Poisoning

- Fatigue
- Headache
- Dizziness
- Increased salivation
- Nausea and vomiting
- Diaphoresis
- Abdominal cramps

Moderate Poisoning

- Difficulty with speaking or swallowing
- Shortness of breath
- Muscular fasciculation

Severe Poisoning

- Diminished levels of consciousness
- Myosis with no pupillary response

Chronic Low-Level Poisoning

- Many different signs. See above, Clinical Findings, entry 5.

Differential Diagnosis/Laboratory Testing

1. Diagnosis depends on exposure history, clinical symptoms, and low cholinesterase activity in the blood (below 70% of baseline). There is wide interindividual variability in normal cholinesterase activity. A low level is useful diagnostically; however, a low-normal level in an individual with symptoms does not exclude poisoning.
2. A rise in serial cholinesterase levels weeks to months after removal from exposure can confirm the diagnosis.
3. Fasciculations with miosis, while not always present, are diagnostic of organophosphate poisoning.
4. Neurologic evaluation including elctrophysiological studies to assess for neuropathy and neuropsychological evaluations should be done in cases of persistent neurologic and cognitive complaints.

Treatment

1. Induced vomiting at the time of ingestion
2. Primary treatment is the administration of atropine sulfate and pralidoxime (2-PAM).
3. Complications of atropine include flushed, hot and dry skin, fever, and delirium. 2-PAM can cause dangerous increases in blood pressure.

Prognosis

Prolonged high exposure and central and parasympathic nervous system symptoms may be associated with incomplete recovery. After a lower level of exposure, recovery is complete within weeks to months after exposure.

ORGANOCHLORINE INSECTICIDES

Epidemiology and Risk Factors

Chlorinated hydorcarbon insecticides are highly soluble in fat and oils and last a long time in the environment, which contributes to chronic toxicity. Common insecticides in this class include aldrin, chlordane, DDT, endrin, heptachlor, chlordecone (kepone), and lindane. Most of these have been banned in the United States but are still used in developing countries.

Etiology and Pathophysiology

1. Absorption is through respiration, oral, or dermal routes.

2. Neurotoxic mechanisms are not defined well but may involve the excessive and spontaneous release of acetylcholine.

Clinical Findings

1. With acute DDT toxicity, symptoms may include metallic taste, dryness of the mouth, thirst, drowsiness or extreme insomnia, burning eyes, gritty sensation in the eyelid, aching of the limbs, muscular spasms, tremors, stiffness and pain in the jaw, difficulty concentrating, and night blindness.

2. Chronic exposure may be associated with tremor and convulsions, upper limb weakness (with possible wrist drop), mononeuropathy, optic neuropathy, and polyneuropathy.

Key Clinical Findings: Organochlorine Insecticides

DDT Toxicity

• Many signs. (see above under Clinical Findings, entry 1)

Chronic Exposure

• Tremor and convulsions

• Upper limb weakness

• Mononeuropathy

• Optic neuropathy

• Polyneuropathy

Differential Diagnosis

Determined by history. While organochlorines and their metabolites can be found in blood and fat, this test is generally not available.

Treatment

Generally supportive. Anticonvulsants for seizures.

Bibliography

American Conference of Governmental Industrial Hygienists (ACGIH): Threshold Limit Values and Biological Exposure Indices for 1994–1995. Cincinatti: ACGIH, 2001.

Bolla K, Cadet JL: Exogenous acquired metabolic disorders of the nervous system: toxins and illicit drugs. In Goetz CG, Pappert EJ (eds): Textbook of Clinical Neurology. Philadelphia, W.B. Saunders, 1999.

Chang LW, Dyer RS (eds): Handbook of Neurotoxicology. New York, Marcel Dekker, 1995.

Goetz CG: Neurotoxins in Clinical Practice. New York, Spectrum, 1985.

Hartman DE: Neuropsychological Toxicology: Identification and Assessment of Human

Neurotoxic Syndromes (Critical Issues in Neuropsychology), 2nd ed. New York, Plenum, 1995.

Rosenstock L, Cullen MR (eds): Textbook of Clinical Occupational and Environmental Medicine. Philadelphia, W. B. Saunders, 1994, pp. 847–865.

9 Venoms and Bacterial Toxins

Brian W. Smith

This chapter will focus on selected biologic toxins and their effects on the nervous system. Topics covered will include envenomation from snakes, spiders, and scorpions and the toxic effects of diphtheria, tetanus, and botulism.

SNAKE VENOM

Epidemiology

1. There are approximately 120 species of snakes in North America. Thirty of these are dangerous. Most are members of the Crotalid (rattlesnakes, copperheads, and water moccasins) and Elapidae (coral snakes) families.

2. Non-native venomous snakes account for a small percentage of snake bites in the United States, usually illegally imported or found in zoos and pet shops. The most frequently involved species are from the Elapidae family and include cobras, kraits, and mambas.

3. Each year there are approximately 8000 venomous snakebites in the United States associated with 9 to 15 deaths. These numbers are much greater in underdeveloped countries, with thousands of deaths worldwide.

Etiology and Pathophysiology

1. Envenomation usually occurs in subcutaneous tissue. Venom is absorbed via lymphatic and venous drainage.

2. The venom is a complex mixture of enzymes, polypeptides, glycoproteins, and metallic ions. The effects are both localized and systemic, with tissue necrosis at the bite site and systemic effects that include coagulopathy, cardiac toxicity, and neurotoxicity.

3. The neurologic effects are associated with neuromuscular blockade at presynaptic postsynaptic, or terminal portions of motor fibers.

Clinical Features

1. The initial presentation is usually localized and may include swelling, pain, ecchymoses, petechiae, blistering, parasthesias, and tissue necrosis. Mild neurologic symptoms such as parasthesias and fasciculations are common.

2. Systemic manifestations of snakebite may include weakness, malaise, restlessness, confusion, emesis, abdominal pain, diaphoresis, dyspnea, tachycardia, and blurred vision. More severe cases may manifest with coagulopathy, renal failure, acute respiratory distress syndrome, cardiac arrest, and multisystem failure.

3. The full envenomation process and symptom development usually occurs over a few hours with a varying and unpredictable course. Exceptions occur with certain snakes such as the elapids and the Mojave Rattler where there are limited localized symptoms and then a prolonged (up to 12-hour) delay in systemic symptoms. Both of these snake venoms produce severe neurotoxic syndromes that may mimic an acute myasthenic syndrome.

4. Neurologic symptoms include parasthesias, blurred vision, loss of taste, anxiety, and dizziness. Signs may include fasciculations, confusion, dysarthria, diplopia, ptosis, facial diplegia, muscle weakness, areflexia, loss of consciousness, seizures, and respiratory failure.

Key Signs: Snakebite

Initial Signs
- Swelling
- Pain
- Ecchymoses
- Petechiae
- Parasthesias
- Fasciculations

Systemic Signs
- Weakness
- Malaise
- Restlessness
- Confusion
- Emesis
- Abdominal pain

Neurologic Signs

- Paresthesia
- Blurred vision
- Loss of taste
- Anxiety
- Dizziness

Laboratory Tests

1. Laboratory work-up includes a complete blood count, electrolytes, urinalysis, and coagulation panels. Enzyme-linked immunosorbent assay (ELISA) testing to identify the type of snake has been developed but is not commercially available in the United States.

2. Electroencephalographic (EEG) abnormalities in venomous snakebites have been documented. EEG findings and symptoms of cortical dysfunction such as confusion and seizures may be related to hypoxia or other metabolic abnormalities, as it is believed that the toxin does not cross the blood–brain barrier.

Key Tests: Snakebite

Laboratory Work-up

- CBC, electrolytes, urinalysis, and coagulation panels

Other

- ELISA
- EEG

Treatment

1. Treatment for snakebite may include supportive care, antivenin therapy, antibiotics, tetanus immunization, surgical debridement, blood products, and respiratory support.

2. Patients with the delayed neurologic syndrome seen with the elapids and crotalid snakes usually improve with supportive care over a period of 1 week, but full return of muscle strength may require several weeks.

3. There are case reports of the use of neostigmine resulting in temporary though rapid reversal of neurologic symptoms. This treatment should be considered with these snakebites, especially if antivenin treatment will be delayed.

Key Treatment: Snakebite

- Supportive care
- Antivenin
- Antibiotics
- Tetanus immunization
- Surgical débridement
- Blood products
- Respiratory support

SPIDER VENOM

Epidemiology

1. Only a small number of spiders are potentially dangerous to humans.

2. Spiders found in the United States associated with marked systemic and neurologic symptoms include the widow spiders (black, brown, and red), the brown recluse, and the hobo spiders.

Pathophysiology

The spider toxin affects neuromuscular synaptic membranes resulting in extensive release of norepinephrine and acetylcholine with overstimulation of motor end plates.

Clinical Features

1. The manifestations of spider bites may vary from localized pain and skin necrosis to systemic hemolysis and neurologic dysfunction.

2. The most pronounced reaction occurs with the bite of the female widow spiders (*Latrodectus* sp.) and is referred to as latrodectism. The reaction consists of diaphoresis and severe generalized muscle cramping. It is most pronounced in the abdomen and face, resulting in rigidity mimicking a surgical abdomen and facial grimacing and contortions (fascies latrodectismica). Death has been reported secondary to respiratory impairment.

3. Neurologic manifestations of widow spider bites include parasthesias, fasciculations, tremor, ptosis, hallucinations, psychosis, and seizures.

Key Signs: Widow Spider Bites

- Severe muscle cramping
- Fasciculations
- Ptosis
- Hallucinations
- Seizures

Treatment

Treatment consists of supportive care, muscle relaxants, and pain control; latrodectus antivenin is given for severe reactions.

Key Treatment: Widow Spider Bites

- Supportive care
- Muscle relaxants
- Latrodectus antivenin for severe reactions

SCORPION VENOM

Epidemiology

Each year in the United States there are approximately four deaths associated with scorpion envenomation. Most deaths occur in children.

Etiology and Pathophysiology

Scorpion toxin produces prolonged depolarization of nerves of the adrenergic and cholinergic systems, which accounts for the systemic and neurologic symptoms.

Clinical Features

1. The clinical manifestations include pain at the site, restlessness, tachycardia, hypertension, tachypnea, sialorrhea, and respiratory distress that may progress to paralysis and respiratory failure.

2. Neurologic features include; nystagmus, oculogyric movements, roving eye movements, blurred vision, fasciculations, dysarthria, dysphagia, hyperstartle response, ataxia, generalized muscle weakness, involuntary body jerking, and seizures.

Key Signs: Scorpion Bite

- Pain at the site of sting
- Restlessness
- Tachycardia
- Hypertension
- Tachypnea
- Sialorrhea
- Respiratory distress, possibly leading to paralysis and respiratory failure

Neurologic Signs

- Nystagmus
- Oculogyric movements
- Roving eye movements
- Blurred vision
- Fasciculations
- Dysarthria
- Dysphagia
- Ataxia
- Generalized muscle weakness

Treatment

1. Management consists of supportive care and scorpion antivenins.

2. Antihypertensive agents and atropine may be necessary to treat hypertension and the parasympathetic responses.

Key Treatment: Scorpion Bite

- Supportive care
- Scorpion antivenins
- Antihypertensive agents and atropine for hypertension and parasympathetic responses

DIPHTHERIA

Definition

Diphtheria is an acute infectious disease caused by the *Corynebacterium diphtheriae*. There are two major forms of the disease, respiratory and cutaneous.

Epidemiology

1. The disease is now rare in the United States secondary to immunization. However, large numbers of cases have been reported in the former Soviet Union.

2. The cutaneous form of the disease is more common in tropical areas, although there have been recent epidemics in Europe and North America.

Etiology and Pathophysiology

C. diphtheriae is an aerobic, nonsporulating, gram-positive rod. It produces diphtheria toxin, which produces demyelination of the proximal aspect of spinal nerves.

Clinical Features

1. The respiratory form of diphtheria is characterized by a localized inflammatory reaction consisting of a fibrinous pseudomembrane, usually in the upper respiratory mucosa, and by a toxic reaction that primarily involves the heart and peripheral nervous system, producing a myocarditis and polyneuropathy.

2. Bulbar symptoms including dysphagia and nasal voice are the first indicators of neurologic dysfunction and occur during the first 3 weeks after infection. They may be followed by other cranial nerve involvement.

3. Ciliary nerve paralysis causing blurred vision secondary to loss of accommodation takes place around the third to fifth weeks.

4. Diphtheric neuropathy occurs in approximately 20% of patients but in up to 75% of severe cases. It may consist of mild sensory changes or resemble Guillain-Barré syndrome and occurs 3 to 12 weeks after the infective phase.

5. A delayed sensory neuropathy has been reported, occurring several months after infection.

6. Rare neurologic complications include cerebral infarction secondary to cardiac complications and encephalitis.

Key Signs: Diphtheria

- Fibrinous pseudomembrane in the upper respiratory mucosa

- Dysphagia

- Nasal voice

- Blurred vision

- Mild sensory changes

Laboratory Testing

1. Cerebrospinal fluid results are identical to those in Guillain-Barré syndrome.

2. Diagnosis can be made on clinical grounds when the diphtheric membrane is found in the pharynx. However, definitive diagnosis requires demonstration of the organism by gram stain and culture.

Key Tests: Diphtheria

- Cerebrospinal fluid

- Gram stain and culture

Treatment

1. Diphtheria antitoxin will reduce neurologic complications if given within the first few days of infection. Treatment after that time has little effect, as the antitoxin only neutralizes toxin not yet bound to cells.

2. Delay in treatment is associated with increased mortality, so antitoxin should be given if strong clinical suspicion of this disease exists.

3. Antibiotics are given primarily to prevent further transmission of the disease. Treatment otherwise consists of supportive care.

4. Patients usually recover completely from the neuropathy, but with a prolonged recovery period of up to 1 year.

Key Treatment: Diphtheria

- Diphtheria antitoxin

- Antibiotics

- Supportive care

TETANUS

Definition

Tetanus is an acute infectious disease caused by an exotoxin elaborated by *Clostridium tetani*, a gram-positive, anaerobic, sporulating bacillus. The spores may remain viable for years and can be found in the intestinal tract of humans and animals and in soil. It is clinically characterized by skeletal muscle rigidity and spasm.

Epidemiology

1. Approximately 100 cases occur each year in the United States, with a mortality rate of approximately 50%. It occurs almost exclusively in non-immunized individuals.
2. An increased risk of tetanus is seen in older individuals, drug abusers, and infants.

Etiology and Pathophysiology

1. The bacterium is noninvasive and enters the body at sites of trauma or infection, usually through a laceration or puncture wound. *C. tetani* is probably a frequent contaminant of all types of wounds, but spore germination is a rare occurrence because it requires an environment of low oxygen tissue tension.
2. The infection caused by the bacillus is localized, but the elaborated toxin, tetanospasmin, is transported to the central nervous system via retrograde axonal transport in peripheral motor nerves or by blood-borne delivery.
3. The toxin prevents release of neurotransmitter by blocking synaptic vessels from fusing with the cell membrane. Its most pronounced effects are on the inhibitory spinal neurons.

Clinical Features

1. The incubation period is between 2 and 50 days, with most patients becoming symptomatic within the first 2 weeks. The longer the incubation, the less severe the disease.
2. The clinical manifestations may be localized or generalized.
3. The usual initial and most common symptom is jaw stiffness, which leads to trismus (lockjaw). Additional rigidity develops and may involve other areas, including the abdomen, back, and neck. Facial rigidity produces a characteristic expression referred to as *risus sardonicus*.
4. Additional clinical features may include autonomic dysfunction, sphincteric involvement, and dysphagia. Laryngospasm may result in inadequate ventilation, hypoxia, and death.
5. Convulsive spasms may be a prominent and distressing feature.
6. The symptoms usually increase for 3 days and then stabilize. Patients who survive usually recover in 4 weeks.

7. Neonatal tetanus, a severe form of the disease, occurs in infants within the first 10 days of life. The clinical features include rigidity, facial grimacing, opisthotonus, irritability, and excessive crying.
8. The diagnosis of tetanus is clinical and does not depend on bacterial confirmation.

Key Signs: Tetanus

- Jaw stiffness leading to lockjaw
- Rigidity of the abdomen, back, and neck
- Autonomic dysfunction
- Dysphagia
- Convulsive spasms

Differential Diagnosis

The differential diagnosis includes strychnine poisoning, rabies, drug-induced dystonic reactions, hypocalcemia, stiff-person syndrome, and widow spider bite.

Treatment

Treatment consists of early immunization with tetanus antitoxin; management of muscle spasms with benzodiazepines, barbiturates, and phenothiazines; and general supportive care.

Key Treatment: Tetanus

- Tetanus antitoxin
- Benzodiazepines, barbituates, and phenothiazines for muscle spasms
- General supportive care

BOTULISM

Definition

An acute form of poisoning caused by an exotoxin produced by *Clostridium botulinum* and characterized by progressive neuromuscular paralysis. The three major forms of the disease are foodborne, wound, and infantile.

Epidemiology

1. Foodborne botulism most commonly occurs from eating foods contaminated by the exotoxin of *C. botulinum,* usually, improperly canned or home-preserved foods.

2. Wound botulism was previously rare but has increased during the past decade in injectable drug users and has resulted in epidemics in some areas.

3. Honey has been considered the source of botulinum spores in approximately 20% to 30% of cases of infantile botulism. It should not be given to children less than one year of age.

Etiology and Pathophysiology

1. *C. botulinum* is an anaerobic, spore-forming, gram-positive rod that elaborates a potent exotoxin.

2. The disease occurs after absorbtion of the preformed exotoxin from the intestinal tract or wound. It then travels via blood-borne delivery to peripheral presynaptic terminals.

3. The exotoxin blocks presynaptic release of acetylcholine, affecting both motor and autonomic nerves.

4. It is usually caused by toxin types A, B, and E.

Clinical Features

1. The onset of foodborne botulism is abrupt, with symptom presentation 2 to 36 hours after ingestion of the toxin.

2. The initial symptoms may include dry mouth, nausea, vomiting, abdominal cramps, constipation, and diarrhea.

3. The neurologic features are the primary manifestations of the disorder and are usually bilateral and symmetrical. Symptoms include diplopia, blurred vision, dysarthria, dysphagia, and muscle weakness. Signs may include ptosis, ophthalmoplegia, and areflexia. Pupils may be dilated and unreactive. There are no sensory disturbances, and consciousness is usually preserved.

4. Symptoms progress rapidly over several days with a descending flaccid paralysis and respiratory involvement.

5. The infantile form is caused by ingestion of *C. botulism* which colonizes in the intestinal tract with local production of the toxin. The clinical course ranges from asymptomatic carriers to paralysis and sudden infant death. It occurs during the first 6 months of life, is self-limiting lasting 2 to 6 weeks, and may be associated with relapses. Treatment is supportive.

Key Neurologic Signs: Botulism

- Diplopia
- Blurred vision
- Dysarthria
- Dysphagia
- Muscle weakness
- Ptosis
- Ophthalmoplegia
- Areflexia

Differential Diagnosis

1. The initial bulbar findings may be mistaken for myasthenia gravis and the later features for Guillain-Barré syndrome. Additional disorders in the differential diagnosis include tick paralysis, diphtheria, poliomyelitis, and Lambert-Eaton myasthenic syndrome.

2. The pupillary findings, lack of sensory complaints, and severe constipation may be helpful differentiating features. Occurrence of other cases after ingestion of the same food is also helpful.

Differential Diagnosis: Botulism

- Myasthenia gravis
- Guillain-Barré syndrome
- Tick paralysis
- Poliomyelitis
- Diphtheria
- Lambert-Eaton myasthenic syndrome

Laboratory Testing

1. Laboratory confirmation is performed at the Centers for Disease Control and Prevention and some state laboratories. Testing may consist of determination of toxin or *C. botulinum* in serum, stool, or wound.

2. Electromyography (EMG) may be helpful in diagnosis, showing an incremental response to repetitive nerve stimulation or a small evoked muscle action potential in response to a single supramaximal nerve stimulus.

3. Cerebrospinal fluid and routine laboratory tests are normal.

4. Diagnosis is based on clinical, laboratory, and EMG findings.

Treatment

1. Treatment includes botulinum antitoxin and supportive care. Antitoxin reduces mortality if administrated early; thus its use should not be delayed pending microbial confirmation. Recovery is prolonged but usually complete.

2. Guanidine and 4-aminopyridine may result in improvement in ocular and limb muscle strength. Use of plasma exchange or intravenous immunoglobulin is unproven.

3. Prognosis and disease severity are related to the amount of toxin absorbed. Improved and aggressive supportive care have decreased mortality from approximately 50% to 10%.

Key Treatment: Botulism

- Antitoxin

- Supportive care

Bibliography

Blackman JR: Spider bites. J Am Board Fam Pract 8:288–294, 1995.

Cherington M: Clinical spectrum of botulism. Muscle Nerve 21:701–710, 1998.

Hahn I, Levin NA: Arthropods. In Goldrank LR, et al (eds): Goldfrank's Toxicologic Emergencies, 7th ed. New York, McGraw-Hill, 2002, pp. 1573–1588.

Juckett G, Hancox JG: Venomous snakebites in the United States: Management review and update. Am Fam Physician 7;1367–1374, 2002.

Kitchens CS, Van Mierop LHS: Envenomation by the Eastern coral snake. JAMA 12:1615–1618, 1987.

McDonald WI, Kocen RS: Diphtheric neuropathy. In Dyck PJ, Thomas PK, Griffin JW, et al (eds): Peripheral Neuropathy, 3d ed. Philadelphia, W.B. Saunders, 1993, pp. 1412–1417.

Roberts JR, Otten EJ: Snakes and other reptiles. In Goldfrank LR, et al (eds): Goldfrank's Toxicologic Emergencies, 7th ed. New York, McGraw-Hill, 2002, pp. 1552–1567,

10 Illicit Drugs

Russell C. Packard

Definition

1. Illicit drug use or substance abuse is best conceptualized as a biopsychosocial disease resulting from an interplay of physical, psychological, and social factors unique to each patient.
2. Substance abuse is use of an illicit drug in a way that is not medically or socially (legally) sanctioned and/or causes harm to self or others.

Epidemiology and Risk Factors

1. About 35% of the U.S. population will use illicit drugs at some time in their lives, not including abuse of alcohol or prescription drugs.
2. 6% to 8% will meet criteria for dependence (physical adaptation so that rapid removal of the drug will cause a withdrawal syndrome).
3. There are some populations at greater risk for substance abuse.
   a. Adolescents and young adults: Children are experimenting with drugs at an earlier age. Between 40% and 50% of high school seniors admit to some illicit drug use.
   b. Use of alcohol and tobacco are also correlated with illicit drug use.
   c. Use of one substance is often associated with using more than one substance simultaneously.
   d. Disadvantaged populations: Members of racial minorities, people who are homeless, and those who are disabled have a higher incidence of illicit drug use.

Clinical Features

Table 10–1 covers the primary actions of the drugs covered in this chapter.

1. Opioids
   a. The terms "opioids" and "narcotics" are often

TABLE 10–1. KEY SITES OF ACTION FOR ILLICIT DRUGS

Drug	Action
Opiates	Agonist of opioid receptors
Cocaine	Inhibits monoamine uptake
Amphetamine	Stimulates monoamine release
Marijuana (THC)	Agonist at cannabinoid receptors
Hallucinogens	Partial agonist at 5HT2 serotonin receptors
PCP	Antagonist at NMDA glutamate receptors

used interchangeably. The actions of opioids mimic those of morphine.
   b. Examples include heroin, morphine, meperidine, methadone, codeine, pentazocine, butorphanol, hydrocodone, and propoxyphene.
   c. Mild narcotic intoxication includes mood change, sometimes euphoria; drowsiness, nausea, miosis, and pain relief.
   d. Tolerance develops rapidly for euphoria and central nervous system (CNS) depression; less rapidly for analgesia.
   e. Dependence to short-acting drugs (morphine, heroin) develops rapidly; less rapidly to longer-acting drugs (codeine and partial agonist drugs).
   f. Overdose may cause respiratory depression, peripheral vasodilation, pinpoint pupils, pulmonary edema, coma, and death.
   g. Withdrawal symptoms from opioids generally include symptoms and signs of CNS hyperactivity.
      (1) Early symptoms include craving, anxiety, yawning, tearing, rhinorrhea, and perspiration.
      (2) Other symptoms include mydriasis, piloerection ("gooseflesh"), tremors, muscle twitching, hot and cold flashes, and generalized aching.
   h. Complications of opioid abuse are often related to needle sharing and include hepatitis, human immunodeficiency virus (HIV) infection, and endocarditis.

Key Withdrawal Symptoms

- Early symptoms: Craving, anxiety, yawning, tearing, rhinorrhea, perspiration

- Other symptoms: Mydriasis, piloerection ("gooseflesh"), tremors, muscle twitching, hot and cold flashes, generalized aching

1. Cocaine
   a. Cocaine is a stimulant that causes blockade of the uptake of monoamines into the presynaptic terminals. This blockade leads to increased levels of dopamine, norepinephrine, and serotonin. Cocaine hydrochloride is the salt form

and is most commonly used. Free base, a purer and stronger derivative is called "crack."

b. Desired effects are euphoria, increased energy, and appetite control. Tolerance develops rapidly but physical dependence has not been confirmed. No stereotypical withdrawal syndrome occurs when the drug is discontinued. The tendency to continue taking the drug however is quite strong.

c. Most users are episodic recreational users who voluntarily curtail their use. Most cocaine in the United States is snorted intranasally with an onset of action within 2 to 3 minutes. The purity of the cocaine is the major determinant of the "high." Smoking crack cocaine has also become widely publicized.

d. The combined used of cocaine and alcohol produces a more intense and long-lasting effect.

e. Cocaine users may present with unexplained nasal bleeding, headaches, fatigue, insomnia, anxiety, depression, and chronic hoarseness. Transient ischemic attacks, seizures, strokes, and migraine symptoms have also been reported. An acute stroke in a young person should be evaluated with a urine toxicology screen for cocaine within 24 hours of presentation.

f. Overdose may produce tremors, convulsions, and delirium. There may be cardiovascular collapse and/or arrhythmias. Pupils are widely dilated. If hallucinations, paranoia, or aggressive behavior occurs, the person may be dangerous.

Key Overdose Signs

- Tremors
- Convulsions
- Delirium
- Cardiovascular collapse and/or arrhythmias
- Widely dilated pupils

g. Treatment is imprecise and difficult. Usually a structured program is needed. The dopamine agonist bromocriptine, 1.5 mg 3 times a day, may help alleviate the craving.

Key Treatment

- Treatment is imprecise and difficult.
- Bromocriptine (to alleviate craving)

1. Amphetamines
   a. Amphetamines are stimulants. Methedrine ("speed") is commonly used and gives an intense and fairly long-lasting high. Methylphenidate is under prescription control but street availability remains high. Unlike cocaine, amphetamines produce a prolonged rush when taken intravenously.
   b. Acute stimulant intoxication includes sweating, tachycardia, elevated blood pressure, mydriasis, hyperactivity, and an acute brain syndrome with confusion and disorientation.
   c. Tolerance develops quickly and, as the dosage is increased hypervigilance, paranoid ideation, and hallucinations (often of insect infestation) occur. Psychotic symptoms may be indistinguishable from schizophrenia.
   d. Stimulant withdrawal is characterized by depression and hypersomnia.
   e. Several cerebrovascular complications have been reported.
      (1) Amphetamine-induced cerebral vasculitides cause occlusive as well as hemorrhagic strokes.
      (2) Methamphetamine can cause necrotizing angitis or cerebral arteritis if it is used intravenously.
      (3) Severe headaches may precede amphetamine-induced stroke.
      (4) Hypertension may induce some cerebrovascular complications.
   f. Treatment
      (1) Monitor vital signs for hypertension and/or hyperthermia.
      (2) Antipsychotics are used for psychosis or paranoia. Rarely, these may cause a neuroleptic-malignant syndrome.
      (3) Usually a structured treatment program is needed.

Key Treatment

- Antipsychotics
- Structured treatment program

4. MDMA (Ectasy)
   a. MDMA is a derivative of methylenedroxymethamphetamine. It is reported to cause severe damage to the serotonergic neurons in nonhuman primates.
   b. MDMA acts as a stimulant and a hallucinogen. It is abused by individuals to intensify their emotional and sensory experiences.

c. MDMA can also cause increases in blood pressure and heart rate, anxiety, and hyperactivity. Neurologic side effects include pupillary dilatation and tremors.

d. Seizures, strokes, and coma have also been reported with the use of MDMA.

5. Hallucinogens

a. Examples: lysergic acid diethylamide (LSD), MDMA, mescaline (peyote cactus), psilocybin (mushrooms).

b. Many of these compounds have been used by Native Americans in religious ceremonies.

c. The most commonly abused hallucinogen in the United States is LSD. LSD and many other hallucinogens are structurally similar to serotonin. It is the most powerful hallucinogen known.

d. Symptoms consist of euphoria, intense arousal, panic, or even depression. Perceptual distortions are common, as are hallucinations. Patients report visual changes of increased intensity of colors and alteration of shape.

e. Neurologic abnormalities include pupillary dilatation, lacrimation, and hyperreflexia. Some LSD users have recurrent episodic visual disturbances, flashes of color, or geometric pseudohallucinations. Formerly known as "flashbacks," these are now called "the hallucinogen persisting perception disorder."

f. Some heavy users of LSD have been reported to suffer from impaired memory, poor attention span, and confusion.

g. The best treatment is "talking the patient down." Further treatment may be required for anxiety, depression, or suicidal ideation.

Key Treatment: LSD

• "Talking the patient down"

• Treatment for anxiety, depression, or suicidal ideation may be necessary.

6. Phencyclidine (PCP)

a. Initially developed as an anesthetic. However, a large number of patients developed postoperative psychosis after its administration. The drug was discontinued, but during the 1970s PCP reappeared on the street as "angel dust."

b. Because it is simple to produce, it is often used as a deceptive substitute for LSD or mescaline. It can be inhaled, injected, swallowed, or smoked (commonly sprinkled on marijuana).

c. Mild intoxication produces euphoria and a feeling of numbness. Moderate intoxication produces disorientation, a feeling of detachment from surroundings, distortion of body image, combativeness, unusual feats of strength, and loss of ability to integrate sensory input, especially touch and proprioception. High doses can cause a psychotic picture similar to schizophrenia.

d. Neurologic signs of intoxication include miosis, horizontal and vertical nystagmus, and ataxia. Increased muscle tone, hyperreflexia, and tremors have also been reported. Very high doses have caused hypertensive crisis, seizures, and coma.

e. Differential diagnosis involves the whole spectrum of street drugs, because in some ways, PCP mimics sedatives, psychedelics, and marijuana. Blood and urine testing can clarify the diagnosis.

f. Treatment of an intoxicated PCP user involves putting the subject in a very calm environment. Neuroleptic drugs have the potential to precipitate a neuroleptic malignant syndrome. Benzodiazepines can be helpful and are the drug of choice in PCP-induced intoxication.

Key Treatment: PCP Intoxication

• Patient should be kept in a very calm environment

• Benzodiazepines

7. Marijuana

a. *Cannabis sativa*, a hemp plant, is the source of marijuana. The parts of the plant vary in potency. The resinous exudate of the flowering tops of the female plant (hashish) is the most potent. Chemically the substance is a tetrahydrocannabinol (THC).

b. The drug is usually inhaled by smoking. Effects occur in 10 to 20 minutes and last 2 to 3 hours. Conjunctival injection is characteristic. THC causes euphoria, feelings of relaxation, and heightened sexual arousal. There may be altered time perception. Some individuals will have increased hunger, suspiciousness, paranoia, and irritability or aggressiveness. Some withdraw socially.

c. Neurologic signs and symptoms include confusion, disorientation, and an organic delusional syndrome. Some recurrent users develop short-term memory deficits. Nystagmus, ataxia, and tremor have also been reported. Seizures may be precipitated in patients with seizure disorders.

d. Marijuana frequently aggravates preexisting

psychiatric disorders. Panic attacks can begin with marijuana usage or be aggravated. It also adversely affects motor performance and slows the learning process in children.

e. Long-term effects have conclusively shown abnormalities in the pulmonary tree. Laryngitis and rhinitis are often present with prolonged use. Cognitive impairments are probable but studies have not been conclusive.

f. Withdrawal suddenly may cause insomnia, nausea, aching muscles (like "flu"), and irritability.

g. Treatment of a "bad trip" generally just calls for reassurance. Symptoms usually clear within a few hours. Neurologic effects of the drug may take up to 8 hours to clear.

Key Treatment: Marijuana

- Reassuring the patient is usually all that is needed for a "bad trip."

Bibliography

Beers MH, Berkow R (eds): Drug usage and dependence. In the Merck Manual of Diagnosis and Therapy, 17th ed. Totowa: New Jersey, Merck Research Laboratories, 1999, pp. 1578–1595.

Bolla KI, Cadet JL: Exogenous acquired metabolic disorders of the nervous system: Toxins and illicit drugs. In Goetz CG, Pappert EJ (eds): Textbook of Clinical Neurology. Philadelphia, W.B. Saunders, 1999, pp. 791–797.

Eisendrath SJ, Lichtmacher JE: Substance use disorders. In Tierney LM, McPhee SJ, Papadakis MA (eds): Current Medical Diagnosis and Treatment, 39th ed. New York, McGraw-Hill, 2000, pp. 1067–1072.

Gawin FH, Ellinwood EH: Cocaine and other stimulants. Actions, abuse and treatment. N Engl J Med 1988;318: 1173–1182.

Montoya AG, Sorrentino R, Lukas SE, Price BH: Long-term neuropsychiatric consequences of "ecstasy" (MDMA): a review. Harv Rev Psychiatry 10:212–220, 2002.

Nestler EJ, Self DW: Neurobiologic aspects of ethanol and other chemical dependencies. In Yudofsky SC, Hales RE (eds): Textbook of Neuropsychiatry. Washington DC, American Psychiatric Press, 1997, pp. 773–798.

1 Hydrocephalus

Michael E. Seiff

Definition

1. Relative, pathologic accumulation of excess intraventricular cerebrospinal fluid (CSF) in the brain, often leading to elevated intracranial pressure (ICP) with resultant signs and symptoms. There are several classification schemes that overlap.

   a. Congenital versus acquired hydrocephalus

      (1) Congenital hydrocephalus is usually a developmental disorder, most often detected during the perinatal period or early infancy. It is either idiopathic or due to well described mechanisms.

      (2) Acquired hydrocephalus results from injury or illness, whether due to hemorrhagic, infectious, or neoplastic processes; it can also be idiopathic.

   b. Obstructive (noncommunicating) versus nonobstructive (communicating) hydrocephalus

      (1) Obstructive hydrocephalus results from blockage to CSF flow. CSF normally circulates through the ventricular system, out into the subarachnoid space (SAS) at the basal cisterns, and then into the venous system from the SAS overlying the convexity. An obstruction in the pathway therefore causes noncommunication between the intraventricular and extraventricular CSF.

      (2) Nonobstructive hydrocephalus allows communication between ventricular and subarachnoid CSF and is most commonly due to impaired absorption into the venous system overlying the convexity. Rarely, it is caused by CSF overproduction from a choroid plexus tumor or a low-flow state due to increased CSF viscosity.

2. Enlarged ventricles due to increased CSF volume (ventriculomegaly) can exist without elevated ICP.

   a. Normal pressure hydrocephalus (NPH) is an acquired communicating syndromic form with several well defined progressive symptoms. Usually ICP is not elevated despite the presence of ventriculomegaly.

   b. Arrested or compensated hydrocephalus similarly involves normal ICP with enlarged ventricles, often impressively so; but in contrast to NPH, the patients are stable clinically and radiographically. This is usually an incidental finding, and patients can have a high level of function.

3. Some conditions of ventricular enlargement are excluded from the definition of hydrocephalus.

   a. "Hydrocephalus ex vacuo," a term increasingly falling into disfavor, is secondary to the diffuse cerebral atrophy seen with aging or dementing disorders.

   b. Encephalomalacia is secondary to focal destructive lesions, leading to adjacent ventricular expansion toward the weakened, more compliant brain tissue.

Epidemiology

1. The incidence of congenital hydrocephalus is approximately 3 to 4 per 1000 live births.

2. The incidence of acquired hydrocephalus is unknown, although about 100,000 shunts are implanted yearly in developed countries.

3. A bimodal incidence curve shows one peak during infancy and one during adulthood. There may be a slight male predominance in both peaks, perhaps due to a known X-linked pediatric form, as well as a slight male predominance in NPH.

Risk Factors

1. Congenital hydrocephalus can be associated with malformations or syndromes of known genetic basis.

2. There is high risk of hydrocephalus in siblings and first cousins of children born with uncomplicated congenital hydrocephalus, suggesting a genetic tendency.

3. Theoretically, there may be population-based factors predisposing an individual to intracranial hemorrhage, neoplasia, infection, or trauma; there are no other well accepted risk factors.

Pathophysiology

1. Ventricular dilatation causes cytoarchitectural, cytologic, and metabolic changes that affect the periventricular white matter and cerebral cortex.

   a. Acute changes

      (1) Damage to the ependymal lining of the ventricle, which allows permeation of CSF into the surrounding periventricular white matter (transependymal flow)

      (2) White matter edema

   b. Chronic changes

      (1) White matter gliotic scarring

      (2) Abnormal proliferation, migration, and differentiation of neurons in the developing brain

      (3) Alterations in neurotransmitters

2. Elevated ICP, which usually accompanies hydrocephalus, manifests clinically with the same well known signs and symptoms as that of other etiologies that increase the ICP.

Etiology

1. Congenital causes (pediatric)

   a. Stenosis of aqueduct of Sylvius (aqueductal stenosis)

   b. Dandy-Walker syndrome. Posterior fossa malformation includes atresia of outflow foramina of Luschka and Magendie from the fourth ventricle to the basal cistern SAS.

   c. Myelomeningocele, Chiari malformation, or both: often occur together

   d. Vein of Galen aneurysm (rare): compresses posterior third ventricle and/or cerebral aqueduct

   e. Infections: toxoplasmosis, cytomegalovirus (CMV), varicella, rubella, mumps, cysticercosis

   f. Neoplasia: rare

   g. Posthemorrhagic: from intraventricular hemorrhage (IVH) of preterm infant

   h. Idiopathic

2. Acquired causes (pediatric)

   a. Aqueductal stenosis: can follow an infection

   b. Neoplasia: CSF flow obstructed; rarely from overproduction of CSF by choroid plexus tumor

   c. Infection: especially bacterial meningitis

   d. Severe head injury

   e. Venous sinus thrombosis: inhibits absorption of CSF from SAS overlying the convexity

   f. Postoperative: after posterior fossa surgery; due to edema or hemorrhage

   g. Idiopathic

3. Acquired causes (adult)

   a. Infection: usually meningitis, less commonly abscess

   b. Posthemorrhagic: subarachnoid, parenchymal, or IVH

   c. Neoplasia: CSF flow obstructed; rarely due to overproduction of CSF by choroid plexus tumor

   d. Severe head injury

   e. Postoperative

   f. Idiopathic

4. Normal pressure hydrocephalus

   a. Known cause: Any of the above etiologies for hydrocephalus with increased ICP can also lead to ventriculomegaly without elevated ICP in pediatric patients or adults.

   b. Unknown cause: Idiopathic form is the classic presentation, primarily in patients over 60 years of age.

Clinical Features

1. Infants

   a. Symptoms

      (1) Irritability

      (2) Increased sleeping/lethargy

      (3) Emesis

      (4) Poor feeding

   b. Signs

      (1) Increasing head circumference

      (2) Tense or bulging anterior fontanelle

      (3) Dilated scalp veins: reversal of blood flow from intracranial venous sinuses due to increased ICP

      (4) Suture diastasis: palpable separation or visible on radiographs (or both)

      (5) Parinaud's phenomenon ("sun-setting sign"): downward deviation of the eyes with lid retraction due to pressure on the tectal plate of the midbrain

Key Signs and Symptoms: Hydrocephalus in Infants

Symptoms

- Iirritability
- Increased sleeping/lethargy
- Emesis
- Poor feeding

Signs

- Increasing head circumference
- Tense/bulging anterior fontanelle
- Dilated scalp veins
- Suture diastasis
- Parinaud's phenomenon

2. Children and adults

   a. Symptoms

     (1) Headache

     (2) Nausea/vomiting

     (3) Lethargy

     (4) Visual changes

       (a) Diplopia: sixth nerve palsy possibly from increased ICP

       (b) Blurred: from stretch of periventricular optic radiations, or papilledema

     (5) Neck pain: from pressure at foramen magnum due to tonsillar herniation

     (6) Mental status changes: dulled mentation, confusion, or behavioral changes

     (7) Gait difficulty: stretching of periventricular pyramidal tract fibers

     (8) Seizure

     (9) Urinary incontinence: pressure on frontal lobe micturition centers (adults)

   b. Signs

     (1) Papilledema: increased CSF pressure in the optic nerve sheath, impeding venous and axoplasmic outflow and causing swelling of the optic disc

     (2) Sixth nerve palsy: unilateral or bilateral

     (3) Upward gaze palsy: pressure on tectal plate of midbrain

     (4) Spasticity or hyperreflexia: stretching of periventricular pyramidal tract fibers

     (5) Macewen's sign: "cracked pot" sound on cranial percussion (children)

Key Signs and Symptoms: Hydrocephalus in Children and Adults

Symptoms

- Headache
- Nausea/vomiting
- Lethargy
- Visual changes: diplopia and blurred vision
- Neck pain
- Mental status changes: dulled mentation, confusion, behavioral changes
- Gait difficulty
- Seizure
- Urinary incontinence

Signs

- Papilledema
- Sixth nerve palsy
- Upward gaze palsy
- Spasticity, hyperreflexia
- Macewen's sign

3. Normal pressure hydrocephalus

   a. Classic triad

     (1) Gait disturbance: usually precedes other symptoms; short-stepped and broad-based

     (2) Dementia: primarily memory impairment earlier, then slowness of thought (bradyphrenia)

     (3) Urinary incontinence: poor realization of need to void; fecal incontinence rare

   b. CSF pressure less than 18 cm H_2O by definition. Higher readings can accompany classic symptoms, supporting the concept of a clinical spectrum with differing CSF pressures.

Key Signs: Normal Pressure Hydrocephalus

- "Classic triad"
  - —Gait disturbance
  - —Dementia
  - —Urinary incontinence
- CSF pressure < 18 cm H_2O

Laboratory Testing

1. Lumbar puncture (LP)

   a. Most useful as part of NPH work-up. Symptoms may diminish within 1 day after high-volume tap (>20–50 cc) in an adult, allowing favorable prognostication for patient and family.

   b. Brain imaging by computed tomography (CT) or magnetic resonance imaging (MRI) is necessary prior to the tap to rule out an intracranial mass lesion.

   c. Controlled CSF drainage over several days with CSF pressure recordings via lumbar catheter is used in some centers as part of selection criteria for shunt candidates with NPH.

2. CSF analysis

   a. To rule-out or follow infection as an etiology for hydrocephalus

      (1) Samples are traditionally obtained for cell count, chemistry (protein and glucose), and culture.

      (2) Bacterial infection is rare in the absence of low glucose (hypoglycorrhachia), elevated white blood cell count (pleiocytosis), and elevated protein (hyperproteorrhachia).

      (3) Additional studies may include viral and fungal cultures, bacterial antigen assays, and acid-fast bacilli stains.

   b. Protein measurements in posthemorrhagic hydrocephalus should confirm levels of less than 100 mg/dL prior to shunting; otherwise increased viscosity may cause a clog in the catheter, malabsorption of fluid, or ileus.

3. Genetic testing may be indicated with counseling when a family history is suspected for some of the associated syndromic malformations or X-linked hydrocephalus.

4. Of historical interest, the terms communicating and noncommunicating derive from the ability of a dye to be recovered by lumbar puncture shortly after injection into the ventricular system.

Radiologic Features

1. Plain radiographs (of little clinical utility): enlarged cranium relative to facial bones, split sutures, evidence of chronic high ICP such as parasellar erosion, and "beaten copper" appearance to the inner table

2. Ultrasonography through anterior fontanelle: useful for following neonatal IVH and development of hydrocephalus, though imaging is recommended before any invasive treatment

3. CT of the head allows experienced clinicians to recognize most cases of hydrocephalus on sight.

   a. Ventricular dilatation is out of proportion to sulcal enlargement (in proportion suggests atrophy).

   b. Patterns of dilatation proximal to the pathology suggest the etiology.

      (1) Lateral and third ventricular dilatation with a normal fourth ventricle suggests aqueductal stenosis.

      (2) Lateral and third ventricular dilatation with displaced fourth ventricle suggests posterior fossa mass.

   c. Transependymal flow appears as hypodense capping around dilated frontal horns.

   d. Dilated temporal horns of the lateral ventricle in the middle fossa (owing to increased compliance of adjacent parenchyma relative to other periventricular parenchyma) and a slightly rounded third ventricle are often signs of early hydrocephalus.

   e. There may be loss of the convexity sulcal pattern with or without compression of basal cisterns.

4. MRI affords improved imaging for certain findings relative to CT.

   a. Indicated in congenital cases to assess the extent of potential associated anomalies (e.g., agenesis of corpus callosum, Chiari malformation, disorders of neuronal migration)

   b. Upward bowing of corpus callosum on sagittal cuts suggestive of acute process

   c. Improved delineation of brainstem and cerebellar lesions

5. Ventricular cisternography for NPH: Delayed radionuclide washout study after lumbar injection (48–72 hours) is supportive of the diagnosis and a favorable response to shunting.

Radiologic Findings: CT Findings of Hydrocephalus

- Ventricular dilatation out of proportion to sulcal enlargement

- Patterns of dilatation proximal to the pathology

- Transependymal flow

- Dilated temporal horns

- Rounded third ventricle

- Loss of convexity sulci

Key Tests

- Lumbar puncture
- CSF analysis
- Genetic testing
- Ultrasonography
- CT
- MRI
- Ventricular cisternography (NPH)

Treatment

1. Medical therapy
   a. Usually a temporizing measure until surgery can be performed. There is occasional success with transient conditions such as neonatal IVH, infection, or sinus thrombosis.
   b. Acetazolamide (Diamox) and furosemide (Lasix) decrease CSF production by choroid plexus.

2. Lumbar puncture
   a. Can sometimes temporize until surgery is appropriate or help avoid surgery until a transient condition improves, as mentioned above
   b. Safe only with communicating hydrocephalus

3. Shunt placement for CSF diversion is the treatment of choice in most patients with hydrocephalus, allowing drainage of excess fluid to a terminal reabsorption site.
   a. Ventricular shunts
      (1) Ventriculoperitoneal (VP) shunts are used in most cases. The frontal horn of the right lateral ventricle is cannulated through a frontal burr hole (easier placement) or parietooccipital burr hole (more cosmetic). The catheter is tunneled underneath the skin to a separate abdominal incision, and the distal length of tubing is then placed in the peritoneal cavity for drainage.
      (2) Ventriculoatrial (VA) shunts have the distal catheter tip placed in the jugular vein at the neck, through the superior vena cava and into the right atrium of the heart. This technique is used when abdominal abnormalities preclude peritoneal placement (i.e., prior surgical scarring, morbid obesity, malabsorptive lining, recent abdominal sepsis).
      (3) Ventriculopleural shunts can also be used if the peritoneal cavity is not appropriate,

with the tip resting between the visceral and parietal pleural layers, accessed via the second or third intercostal space anteriorly. Absorption may not be as efficient as with VP and VA shunts.
      (4) Other termini for shunt placement
         (a) Gallbladder: still used rarely in extreme cases when all other termini are inappropriate
         (b) Ureter, fallopian tube, stomach: of historical interest only
   b. Lumbar shunts are occasionally used to treat pseudotumor cerebri. The proximal end is placed in the lumbar thecal sac via a small open or percutaneous posterior approach and then tunneled subcutaneously around the flank to a peritoneal terminus (lumboperitoneal shunt).
   c. Shunt design
      (1) Three basic components
         (a) Proximal catheter to access the CSF space
         (b) Valve to regulate the flow
            (i) Usually a pressure differential mechanism functions over a preset range of ICP.
            (ii) Programmable valves allow external adjustment of the pressure range (magnetic).
         (c) Distal catheter to drain into the absorptive cavity (usually the peritoneum)
      (2) Reservoir is usually included proximal to the valve or as part of the valve construct, allowing percutaneous needle aspiration of CSF (or rarely injection of a dye) for analysis.

4. Endoscopic third ventriculostomy
   a. Indicated for obstructive cases only (i.e., aqueductal stenosis), not for communicating hydrocephalus. CSF absorptive mechanisms from the subarachnoid space must be intact.
   b. Endoscope is inserted through a small frontal craniotomy or burr hole, traversing the foramen of Monro and penetrating the floor of the third ventricle. The fenestration allows communication between the intraventricular and subarachnoid spaces.
   c. It eliminates the need for complication-prone mechanical shunting devices.

5. Emergent treatment for acute hydrocephalus
   a. Immediate life-threatening emergency. Most common etiologies are trauma, tumor, and hemorrhage; shunt dysfunction is not usually as dire but can be.

b. Ventriculostomy is attached to an external drainage system. Usually a neurosurgeon drills a right frontal burr hole and passes a catheter to the dilated frontal horn, which is then connected to a drainage bag.

c. In extreme situations without neurosurgical coverage, a spinal needle can be used to decompress the dilated ventricles. Entry point is 9 to 10 cm posterior to the glabella in the right midpupillary line. If no hand drill is available, twist a needle to bore through in a trajectory perpendicular to the skull and advance the needle 5 to 6 cm until CSF issues. It may take about three spinal needles to get through an adult skull owing to dulling of the tip. It must be perpendicular to the scalp.

d. In dire cases of shunt dysfunction, usually percutaneous aspiration of CSF (10–20 cc) from the reservoir with a 23-gauge needle temporizes until a revision can be performed; if a proximal obstruction is suspected, a spinal needle can be passed through the ventricular catheter itself, sacrificing the catheter, which would need to be revised anyway but potentially saving the patient's life.

 Key Treatment

- Acetazolamide (Diamox) and furosemide (Lasix)

- Lumbar puncture

- Shunts for diverting CSF (treatment of choice)

- Endoscopic third ventriculostomy

- Acute hydrocephalus

  —Ventriculostomy attached to external drainage system

  —Spinal needle for decompressing dilated ventricles

  —Percutaneous aspiration of CSF (10–20 cc)

Complications and Prognosis

1. Untreated hydrocephalus can cause permanent neurologic or cognitive deficit due to pathophysiologic mechanisms discussed above. With progressive hydrocephalus and rising ICP, herniation syndromes and death can result.

2. Shunt dysfunction is a well known complication in these patients, the risk of failure being highest during the first few months to 1 year after surgery, and approximating 4% to 5% per year thereafter.

a. Mechanical failure
   (1) Occlusions: account for more than 50% of failures. Can be due to blood, bacteria, debris, choroid plexus ingrowth, or immune reactions. Proximal catheter obstruction is most common, but it can also occur at the valve or the distal catheter.
   (2) Disconnection or fracture
       (a) Can occur at any point in the system, most common at sites of component connection or increased subcutaneous mobility (i.e., at the neck)
       (b) "shunt series": AP/lateral radiographs of head, chest, abdomen/pelvis showing discontinuity
   (3) Valve malfunction can occur without obstruction.
   (4) Migration of distal length of catheter: Multiple sites are reported for almost any cavity or orifice.
   (5) Improper placement of catheter, either proximally or distally, can lead to failure.

b. Infection. Rates vary greatly from surgeon to surgeon and from one institution to another, with a mean incidence of 10% to 15% per patient. It may require temporary externalization (distal catheter externalized through a small thoracic or abdominal incision and attached to a drainage system) until the infection clears, followed by revision. Typical skin flora are the most common agents.

c. Functional
   (1) Overdrainage: can cause subdural hematoma, slit-ventricle syndrome, or craniosynostosis, depending on the age of the patient; may require a valve change to a higher-pressure system
       (a) Slit ventricle syndrome is the rare occurrence of headache, vomiting, and sometimes alteration of consciousness in shunted hydrocephalic children in whom slit-like ventricles are seen on the neuroimaging examination.
       (b) Brain compliance is unusually low and the disorder typically occurs when there has been prior ventriculitis or shunt infection. The symptoms are usually those of high rather than low pressure.
       (c) The syndrome is usually seen in older hydrocephalic children operated on in early infancy, even though it has also been observed occasionally in young children and adults.

(2) Underdrainage: recurrent or persistent symptoms requiring a valve change to a lower-pressure system

3. Work-up of suspected shunt dysfunction

   (a) Shunt series (AP/lateral radiographs of head, chest, abdomen/pelvis) and non-contrast head CT to rule out shunt fracture and ventriculomegaly; can be difficult to interpret CT without prior studies for comparison

   (b) Shunt tap if infection or occlusion suspected

   (1) Shave a small area over a palpable reservoir; obtain radiographs first (or a scout film on CT) to check for reservoir type and location.

   (2) Prepare the area with povidine-iodine solution and drape if possible.

   (3) Access the reservoir with a 25- or 23-gauge needle attached to butterfly tubing and note if CSF flows spontaneously up elevated tubing. If yes, it is not proximally obstructed; can also diagnose elevated ICP if fluid flows very high up the tubing.

   (4) Connect a 10- or 20-cc syringe and slowly aspirate 10 to 20 cc depending on the patient's age and send for analysis. If there is no aspirate, it may be occluded proximally (or slit ventricle syndrome may be present, as suspected on CT).

   (5) Disconnect syringe and assess if fluid runs out of the elevated butterfly tubing into the distal system; if not, there may be a distal occlusion.

4. Prognosis is strongly influenced by the causative factors of hydrocephalus (if known), the duration and degree of disease, and the response to treatment.

   a. Pediatric: strongly depends on co-morbidities

   (1) Isolated idiopathic communicating hydrocephalus patients can achieve normal intelligence quota (IQ) distribution with successful and timely shunting.

   (2) History of a shunt infection has been associated with significant lowering of IQ scores.

   b. Outcome for adult NPH patients is better with a known cause. It can be as high as 80%; patients with idiopathic NPH are at about 50%. Incontinence is the most likely symptom to diminish, followed by gait difficulty and then dementia.

Pregnancy

Transient symptoms of elevated ICP can exist in pregnant women, especially during the third trimester, without significant problems. A relatively large study of gestational shunt-related complications found significant incidences of antepartum and postpartum malfunction, about 9% each. Ventriculopleural shunts have been recommended as perhaps the most appropriate for women of childbearing age.

Bibliography

Black PM: The normal pressure hydrocephalus syndrome. In Scott RM (eds): Hydrocephalus. Baltimore, Williams & Wilkins, 1990, pp. 109–114.

Bradley N, Liakos A, McAllister J, et al: Maternal shunt dependency: implications for obstetric care, neurosurgical management, and pregnancy outcomes and a review of selected literature. Neurosurgery 43:448–461, 1998.

Bruce DA, Weprin B: The slit ventricle syndrome. Neurosurg Clin N Am 12:709–717, 2001.

Drake JM, Sainte-Rose C: Shunt complications. In The Shunt Book. Cambridge, Blackwell Science, 1995, pp. 121–192.

Greenberg MS: Hydrocephalus. In Handbook of Neurosurgery, 3rd ed. Lakeland, FL, Greenberg Graphics, 1994, pp. 224–244.

Rekate HL: Treatment of hydrocephalus. In Cheek WR (ed): Pediatric Neurosurgery, 3rd ed. Philadelphia, W.B. Saunders, 1994, pp. 202–220.

2 Neurofibromatoses

Kevin C. Ess
David H. Gutmann

Definition

1. Neurofibromatosis 1 (NF1) is the most common genetic disorder affecting the nervous system. It is transmitted as an autosomal dominant disorder that manifests with a wide variety of clinical findings. The *NF1* gene product is neurofibromin.
2. Neurofibromatosis 2 (NF2) is a less common autosomal dominant disorder. It has a distinct clinical profile from NF1. The *NF2* gene product is merlin or schwannomin.

Epidemiology

1. Population-based studies estimate NF1 prevalence at 1:3000 worldwide, regardless of gender, ethnicity, or race.
2. NF2 occurs approximately 10 times less frequently than NF1 with a prevalence of 1:40,000 worldwide.

Etiology and Pathophysiology

1. *NF1* is a tumor suppressor gene.
   a. Neurofibromin is believed to function as an inhibitor (negative regulator) of RAS, a key growth-promoting molecule.
   b. Most tumors are benign. Rare cancers (<5% to 10%) can develop including malignant peripheral nerve sheath tumors, myeloid leukemias, and pheochromocytomas.
   c. Loss of heterozygosity (*both* copies of *NF1* mutated or inactivated) occurs in tumors.
   d. Non-tumor phenotypes may result from reduced but not absent expression of neurofibromin.
2. *NF2* is a tumor suppressor gene. Loss of function mutations lead to distinct tumors.
   a. Merlin is believed to function as negative growth regulator that links the actin cytoskeleton to cell surface proteins.
   b. Loss of heterozygosity occurs in NF2-associated tumors.

Clinical Findings

1. NF1
   a. Cutaneous pigmentary lesions are the most common manifestations (café-au-lait macules, axillary or inguinal freckling, Lisch nodules in the iris).
   b. Neurofibromas manifest as either cutaneous or plexiform lesions.
      (1) Cutaneous (dermal) lesions are discrete "fleshy" tumors typically first seen in the pre-adolescent and teenage years. They never become malignant.
      (2) Plexiform lesions are believed to be congenital in origin. They are more diffuse and may involve multiple nerves. Continued growth of these tumors can result in bony abnormalities and disfigurement. These tumors also have the capacity to transform into malignant peripheral nerve sheath tumors (previously termed *neurofibrosarcomas*).
   c. Optic pathway gliomas are World Health Organization grade I neoplasms and are typically seen in children younger than 7 years of age. They may be asymptomatic or lead to visual dysfunction. Precocious puberty may also be a presenting sign of these gliomas as a consequence of hypothalamic involvement.
   d. Bony abnormalities include scoliosis, sphenoid wing, or long bone dysplasias.
   e. Learning disabilities are seen in 40% to 60% of affected individuals.
   f. Macrocephaly is frequently noted but is not correlated with learning disabilities. Hyperintense T_2-bright lesions are often seen on brain magnetic resonance imaging (MRI) scans (unidentified bright objects–UBOs). These are not tumors and have limited clinical significance.
   g. Other associated rare malignancies include juvenile chronic myeloid leukemia and pheochromocytoma.
2. NF2
   a. Bilateral vestibular schwannomas (acoustic neuroma) are the hallmark of this disease.
   b. Other tumor types frequently seen include meningioma (50% of affected individuals), ependymoma, and schwannoma involving other cranial or peripheral nerves.
   c. Ocular involvement is common with juvenile

posterior subcapsular or cortical wedge cataracts, retinal hamartomas, and epiretinal membranes.

NF1 Differential Diagnosis

1. Café-au-lait macules in early childhood suggest the diagnosis of NF1, however rare cases of isolated café-au-lait macules have been reported. As almost all children with greater than six café-au-lait macules will go on to develop additional criteria by age 10, the finding of multiple café-au-lait macules in a child warrants further evaluation and surveillance for NF1.

2. McCune-Albright syndrome includes hyperpigmented macules with irregular borders. In addition, affected individuals may have polyostotic fibrous dysplasia, hyperthyroidism, and precocious puberty.

3. LEOPARD syndrome skin findings include diffuse small hyperpigmented lesions (freckle-like "lentigenes"). This autosomal dominantly transmitted disorder does not include neurofibromas or Lisch nodules.

4. Noonan's syndrome presents with dysmorphic facies, cardiac anomalies (valvular pulmonic stenosis), short stature (Turner syndrome-like features), and mental retardation.

5. Russell-Silver syndrome often manifests with congenital hemihypertrophy, triangular facies, increased head circumference, intrauterine growth retardation, and undescended testis.

6. Watson syndrome is associated with café-au-lait macules, short stature, mental retardation, and pulmonary stenosis.

7. Mosaic NF1. Individuals may present with features of NF1 restricted to one somatic compartment as a result of *NF1* gene inactivation within a localized body region. This clinical presentation raises important issues for genetic counseling.

8. Proteus syndrome is believed to have afflicted Joseph Merrick, "the Elephant Man". The film of the same name gave rise to a widespread misbelief that Mr. Merrick had NF1. Proteus syndrome does not include neurofibromas.

Key Clinical Features and Diagnostic Criteria: NF1*

The diagnosis of NF1 requires the presence of two or more of the following

- Six or more café-au-lait macules measuring 0.5 cm or greater in prepubertal individuals or 1.5 cm or greater in postpubertal individuals

- Two or more cutaneous neurofibromas or one plexiform neurofibroma

- First-degree relative with NF1

- Freckling in axilla or inguinal region

- Optic pathway glioma

- Two or more Lisch nodules (iris hamartomas)

- Dysplasia of sphenoid bone or dyplasia/thinning of cortex of long bone

*Adapted from Gutmann et al.: The diagnostic evaluation and multidisciplinary management of NF1 and NF2. JAMA 278:51–57, 1997.

NF2 Differential Diagnosis

1. Schwannomatosis without vestibular nerve involvement
2. Multiple meningiomas
3. Mosaic NF2 restricted to one segment of the body

Key Clinical Features and Diagnostic Criteria: NF2*

Definite NF2

- Bilateral vestibular schwannomas

or

- First-degree family history of NF2 and
  1. Unilateral vestibular schwannoma younger than 30 years of age *or*
  2. *Two or more of the following: meningioma, glioma, schwannoma, juvenile posterior subscapular cataracts/juvenile cortical cataracts*

Probable NF2

- Unilateral vestibular schwannoma younger than 30 years of age plus one of the following: meningioma, glioma, schwannoma, juvenile posterior subscapular cataracts/juvenile cortical cataracts

or

- Two or more meningiomas plus vestibular schwannoma younger than 30 years of age or one of the following: glioma, schwannoma, juvenile posterior subscapular cataracts/juvenile cortical cataracts

*Adapted from Gutmann et al.: The diagnostic evaluation and multidisciplinary management of NF1 and NF2. JAMA 278:51–57, 1997.

Laboratory Testing

1. NF1 remains a clinical diagnosis.
   a. *NF1* genetic testing can detect approximately 70% of mutations, but its role as a stand-alone screening tool is not established.

b. Yearly ophthalmologic evaluation including slit-lamp and dilated funduscopic examination is essential in the evaluation and management of children with NF1.

2. NF2 is a clinical diagnosis.

a. Genetic testing is available, but current methods are not stand-alone tests.

b. Ophthalmologic evaluation is essential to identify ocular manifestations.

c. Brainstem auditory evoked responses (BAER) and audiology consultation are important in the evaluation of vestibular schwannoma.

Key Laboratory Findings

- NF1 genetic testing can detect 70% of mutations.

- Yearly ophthalmologic evaluation in children with NF1

- NF1 and NF2 remain clinical diagnoses.

Radiologic Features

1. NF1

a. Clinical signs and symptoms should dictate imaging studies; baseline "screening" tests are not necessary.

b. When indicated, MRI of the brain and optic pathway should be employed.

c. Any rapidly enlarging or painful plexiform neurofibroma warrants evaluation to exclude a malignant peripheral nerve sheath tumor.

2. NF2

a. Annual head MRI, audiometry, and BAERs may be indicated for NF2 surveillance.

b. Head MRI should include 3-mm cuts through the internal auditory canal with and without gadolinium enhancement.

c. Newly diagnosed NF2 patients should have MRI of the spine.

Treatment of NF1

1. Overall, most patients with confirmed NF1 have few serious medical problems. NF1 patients require a multidisciplinary, age-based anticipatory management approach.

2. Increasing numbers of café-au-lait macules and the possible emergence of a plexiform neurofibroma are noted in infancy and the toddler stage. Scoliosis and tibial dyplasia should be evaluated.

3. The pre-school years are notable for the emergence of axillary and inguinal freckling. Optic pathway gliomas are more frequent in children younger than 7 years. Once discovered, most optic pathway gliomas do not progress radiographically or clinically. Annual dilated funduscopic examination by an experienced ophthalmologist is mandated in the first decade of life.

4. In late childhood/pre-adolescence, cutaneous neurofibromas become increasingly evident. Those causing impairment of function or cosmetic concern can be surgically removed. Scoliosis may also appear in this age group.

5. Learning disabilities are common and should be screened for to allow early and aggressive intervention.

6. Adult issues include hypertension, headaches, and chronic pain. Malignant peripheral nerve sheath tumors are generally treated with surgery and/or radiation. The role of chemotherapy is not clear.

7. Women with NF1 may note increased neurofibroma growth during pregnancy.

Treatment of NF2

Management of NF2 patients is dictated by clinical symptoms and signs and requires a multidisciplinary team.

Bibliography

Friedman J, Gutmann D, MacCollin M, Riccardi V (eds): Neurofibromatosis, 3rd ed. Baltimore, The Johns Hopkins University Press, 1999.

Gutmann D, Aylsworth A, Carey J, et al.: The diagnostic evaluation and multidisciplinary management of neurofibromatosis 1 and neurofibromatosis 2. JAMA 278:51–57, 1997.

Listernick R, Louis D, Packer R, et al.: Optic pathway gliomas in children with neurofibromatosis 1: consensus statement from the NF1 Optic Pathway Glioma Task Force. Ann Neurol 41:143–149, 1997.

North K, Riccardi V, Samango-Sprouse C, et al.: Cognitive function and academic performance in neurofibromatosis 1: consensus statement from the NF1 Cognitive Disorders Task Force. Neurology 48:1121–1127, 1997.

3

Tuberous Sclerosis Complex and Other Neurocutaneous Disorders

Kevin C. Ess
David H. Gutmann

Definitions

1. Tuberous sclerosis complex (TSC) is an autosomal dominant disorder caused by mutations in the *TSC1* or *TSC2* genes. Multi-organ involvement is almost obligate for diagnosis, commonly affecting the central nervous, dermatologic, renal, and cardiac systems.

2. Ataxia-telangiectasia (AT) is characterized by ataxia, telangiectasias of skin and conjunctivae, immune deficiencies, malignancies, and oculomotor apraxia. It is an autosomal recessive disease.

3. Von Hippel-Lindau disease (VHL) is an autosomal dominant disorder with variable penetrance characterized by retinal angiomata and cerebellar capillary hemangioblastomas.

4. Sturge-Weber syndrome (SWS) is a sporadic condition defined by a "port-wine" facial nevus as well as leptomeningeal blood vessel malformations.

Key Neurocutaneous Syndromes

• Neurofibromatoses (see Part XXII, Chapter 2)

• Tuberous sclerosis complex

• Ataxia telangiectasia

• Von Hippel-Lindau disease

• Sturge-Weber syndrome

Epidemiology

1. TSC incidence is approximately 1:7500.

   a. Only one third of patients inherit mutations in either *TSC1* or *TSC2*. Parents of newly diagnosed children should be closely examined for clinical signs of TSC.

   b. The mutation rates in *TSC1* and *TSC2* are approximately equal.

2. AT incidence is estimated to range from 3 to 11 births per million. It should be considered in any child presenting with progressive ataxia.

3. VHL has an estimated prevalence of 1:36,000 to 1:40,000.

4. SWS occurs in approximately 1 to 2 per 10,000 individuals. While isolated port-wine stains are relatively common, only a few of these individuals have the classic intracranial pathology associated with SWS.

Etiology and Pathophysiology

1. TSC is caused by mutations in *TSC1* or *TSC2*.

   a. *TSC1* on chromosome 9 encodes hamartin. The function of this protein is unclear but it is believed to act as a tumor suppressor.

   b. *TSC2* on chromosome 16 encodes tuberin. This protein likely has a role in intracellular signaling, possibly by regulating RAS-like proteins.

2. Hamartin and tuberin physically interact and may coordinately regulate cell growth. This is consistent with the observation that mutations in either gene lead to the TSC phenotype.

3. TSC2 mutations tend to be associated with more severe symptoms; and this may be partially explained by contiguous deletions that involve the closely linked polycystic kidney disease gene (*PKD1*).

4. Most TSC tumors are benign (hamartomas).

5. AT is caused by a mutation in the *ATM* (ataxia-telangiectasia, mutated) gene.

   a. ATM normally has an important role in signaling cell cycle growth arrest after DNA damage.

   b. Cells lacking ATM function acquire a growth advantage, leading to tumorigenesis.

6. VHL is a tumor suppressor gene that may normally function by (a) regulating transcription through binding to molecules in the elongin complex or (b) promoting the destruction of hypoxic-inducible factor (HIF). Absence of the VHL protein may allow HIF to increase the transcription of growth-promoting genes such as epidermal growth factor and transforming growth factor alpha.

7. SWS may result from a developmental malformation of the vascular plexus supplying early neuroectoderm. A malformed vascular system may lead to secondary hypoxia and ischemia. This mecha-

899

nism may explain the progressive decline seen in SWS patients.

Clinical Findings

1. TSC consensus diagnostic criterion have been formulated (see Key Clinical Features: TSC)
   a. Though not a major diagnostic criterion, infantile spasms, a severe generalized seizure disorder, can be the initial presentation of TSC.
   b. Cardiac rhabdomyomas can be identified in utero with obstetrical ultrasound.

Key Clinical Features: TSC*

Major Features

- Facial angiofibromas (adenoma sebaceum) or forehead plaque
- Periungual fibromas
- Three or more hypopigmented macules
- Shagreen patch
- Multiple retinal nodular hamartoma
- Cortical tuber
- Subependymal nodule
- Subependymal giant cell astrocytoma
- Cardiac rhabdomyoma, single or multiple
- Renal angiomyolipoma or pulmonary lymphangiomyomatosis

Minor Features

- Multiple pits in dental enamel
- Hamartomatous rectal polyps
- Bone cysts
- Cerebral white matter migration lines
- Gingival fibromas
- Nonrenal hamartoma
- Retinal achromic patch
- "Confetti" skin lesions
- Multiple renal cysts

Definite TSC: either two major features **or** one major and two minor features

Probable TSC: one major and one minor feature

Possible TSC: Either one major **or** two or more minor features

*Adapted from Hyman M, Whittemore V: NIH consensus conference: tuberous sclerosis complex. Arch Neurol 57:662–665, 2000.

2. AT often presents with cerebellar signs and cutaneous manifestations.
   a. Neurologic signs include cerebellar dysfunction and nystagmus in infancy. Choreoathetosis, oculomotor apraxia, and cognitive impairment are common.
   b. Telangiectasias involve the conjunctivae, ears, nose, and neck. They are usually first noted after 3 years of age and become more apparent with time due to sunlight exposure.
   c. AT patients commonly experience recurrent infections and a propensity for developing neoplasms (leukemias or lymphomas).
   d. AT sensitivity to radiation has important implications regarding radiotherapy for malignancies.
   e. Atypical diabetes in the second decade of life is characterized by hyperglycemia without glycosuria and insulin resistance.

Key Clinical Features: AT

- Cerebellar dysfunction and nystagmus in infancy
- Telangiectasias involving the conjunctivae, ears, nose, and neck
- Recurrent infections and a propensity for developing hematologic malignancies
- Atypical diabetes characterized by hyperglycemia without glycosuria and insulin resistance

3. VHL patients present with tumors in multiple tissues.
   a. Cerebellar and spinal cord hemangioblastomas are common CNS manifestations.
   b. Retinal angiomas are frequent.
   c. Renal cell carcinomas and pheochromocytomas are also seen.
   d. Cysts of the kidneys, liver, and pancreas are fairly common.

Key Clinical Features: VHL

- Cerebellar and spinal cord hemangioblastomas are common CNS manifestations
- Retinal angiomas
- Renal cell carcinomas and pheochromocytomas
- Cysts of the kidneys, liver, and pancreas

4. SWS is usually first suspected by the presence of a port-wine nevus involving a unilateral cranial

nerve V₁ distribution. Intractable seizures may be encountered, usually beginning in the first year of life. Other manifestations include glaucoma, developmental delay, mental retardation, and cognitive decline.

Key Clinical Features: SWS

- Port-wine nevus involving a unilateral cranial nerve V₁ distribution

- Seizures, usually beginning in the first year of life

- Other manifestations such as glaucoma, developmental delay, mental retardation, and cognitive decline

Differential Diagnosis

1. The combination of clinical findings is quite specific for TSC, though isolated renal angiomyolipoma or pulmonary lymphangiomyomatosis occur.
2. In addition to AT, other important causes of ataxia include neoplasms, drug exposure, acute cerebellar ataxia, Friedreich's ataxia, and abetalipoproteinemia. AT is usually correctly diagnosed when the cutaneous signs become evident.
3. Sturge-Weber syndrome. Other syndromes with similar features to SWS include isolated facial nevus, Klippel-Trenaunay-Weber syndrome, and Dandy-Walker syndrome.

Laboratory Testing

1. TSC is generally diagnosed by the critera listed in Key Clinical Features: TSC.
2. Genetic testing of *TSC1* and *TSC2* can be performed in selected individuals.
3. Direct *ATM* testing is available, with a sensitivity of 70% to 80%. Other cell-based methods assay the sensitivity of lymphocytes to irradiation.
   a. Associated laboratory findings are increased alpha-fetoprotein and carcinoembryonic antigen.
   b. Impaired humoral and cellular immunity can usually be demonstrated.
4. *VHL* mutations are extremely diverse, hampering the development of molecular tests. 15% to 20% of patients harbor large deletions that may be detected by Southern blot. There is no commercially available diagnostic test. VHL remains a clinical diagnosis.
5. No definitive test for SWS exists. Ophthalmologic evaluation is essential for the detection of glaucoma.

Radiologic Features

1. In TSC, brain magnetic resonance imaging (MRI) demonstrates subependymal nodules and giant cell astrocytomas. Calcified tubers are best visualized with head computed tomography (CT).
2. Renal ultrasound or abdominal CT is essential in patients presenting with hypertension or hematuria.
3. Cardiac rhabdomyomas are usually visualized by echocardiogram.
4. AT patients usually have atrophy of the cerebellum evident on MRI.
5. VHL-associated hemangioblastomas are usually visualized on MRI or CT. Magnetic resonance arteriography (MRA) or conventional angiogram may also demonstrate these lesions.
6. SWS
   a. Head CT will reveal the classic "railroad track" calcifications in the majority of patients by the end of the second decade.
   b. MRI is the modality of choice for demonstrating leptomeningeal involvement and cortical atrophy.
   c. MRA may be used to demonstrate vascular anomalies.
   d. Positron emission tomography or single photon emission CT may demonstrate hypometabolism or hypoperfusion.

Treatment

1. No specific treatment exists for TSC. Individual tumors can be resected if symptomatic. This includes cortical tubers if implicated as epileptogenic foci.
2. TSC is a frequent cause of infantile spasms. For this devastating condition, vigabatrin is probably the most effective anti-seizure medication.
3. AT patients should avoid exposure to sunlight and radiologic procedures. Passive immunotherapy with intravenous immunoglobulin may attenuate recurrent infections.
4. VHL patients may undergo surgical resection of hemangioblastomas.
5. SWS treatment.
   a. Seizures usually respond to standard medical therapy. Resectional surgery can be considered in medically refractory patients.
   b. Ophthalmologic surveillance is essential to prevent permanent loss of vision from glaucoma.

c. There is some evidence that aspirin may reduce the incidence of stroke in these patients.

Bibliography

Arzimanoglou A, Andermann F, Aicardi J, et al.: Sturge-Weber syndrome: indications and results of surgery in 20 patients. Neurology 55:1472–1479, 2000.

Crino P, Henske E: New developments in the neurobiology of the tuberous sclerosis complex. Neurology 53:1384–1390, 1999.

Hyman M, and Whittemore V: National Institutes of Health consensus conference: tuberous sclerosis complex. Consensus Development Conference, NIH. Archives of Neurology 57:662–665, 2000.

Kondo K, Kaelin W: The von Hippel-Lindau tumor suppressor gene. Exp Cell Res 264:117–125, 2001.

McClintock WM: Neurologic manifestations of tuberous sclerosis complex. Curr Neurol Neurosci Rep 2:158–163, 2002.

Spacey S, Gatti R, Bebb G: The molecular basis and clinical management of ataxia telangiectasia. Can J Neurol Sci 27:184–191, 2001.

4 Arnold-Chiari Malformation and Syringomyelia

Alireza Minagar
J. Steven Alexander

ARNOLD-CHIARI MALFORMATION

Definition

1. Arnold-Chiari malformation is a congenital or acquired hindbrain deformity characterized by caudal displacement of the posterior fossa structures below the plane of the foramen magnum into the cervical cord.
2. Primary abnormalities of the hindbrain and skeletal structures cause four types of cerebellum and hindbrain malformation relative to the foramen magnum and upper cervical canal.
   a. Type I malformation is the least severe and consists of caudal displacement of medulla into the spinal canal and herniation of the inferior pole of the cerebellar hemispheres through the foramen magnum. Syringomyelia occurs in 50% to 75% of patients and is the anomaly most frequently associated with this malformation.
   b. Type II malformation is most common and is identified by any combination of components of the type I malformation accompanied by noncommunicating hydrocephalus and lumbosacral spina bifida.
   c. Type III malformation can have any of the features of type I or II plus herniation of the entire cerebellum through the foramen magnum with cervical spina bifida cystica. Hydrocephalus is regularly present due to varying degrees of atresia of the fourth ventricle foramina, aqueductal stenosis, or impaction at the foramen magnum.
   d. Type IV malformation comprises extreme cerebellar hypoplasia and is covered with other malformations of the posterior fossa. It has no relation to the other Arnold-Chiari malformations.

PEARLS

- Syringomyelia

—Most common anomaly in patients with type I Arnold-Chiari malformation

—Occurs in 50% to 75% of these patients

- Type II Arnold-Chiari malformation is seen in most patients with myelomeningocele.

Epidemiology and Risk Factors

The exact incidence, prevalence, and risk factors of this malformation are unknown.

Etiology

1. The exact cause of Arnold-Chiari malformation remains to be established.
2. It appears that in most cases Arnold-Chiari malformation is congenital, arising from an embryologic defect during the formation of neural and craniovertebral structures. Stovner (1993), who measured the posterior fossa, found patients frequently to have small posterior cranial fossae.
3. Others have hypothesized that an underdeveloped occipital enchondrium and basilar invagination play a role in worsening overcrowding in the posterior cranial fossa (Nishikawa et al., 1997).
4. In certain patients, altered cerebrospinal fluid (CSF) dynamics may contribute to the formation of an acquired Arnold-Chiari malformation. Arnold-Chiari malformation has also been seen after lumboperitoneal shunting.
5. Genetic factors may play a role in the pathogenesis of Arnold-Chiari malformation. Herman and associates (1990) were the first to report symptomatic Chiari malformation type I in siblings.
6. The presence of other associated syndromes (e.g., neurofibromatosis, holoprosencephaly, epidermal nevus syndrome) and craniofacial and craniovertebral defects (e.g., achondroplasia, Klippel-Feil syndrome, Jarcho-Levin syndrome) in patients with Arnold-Chiari malformation may have a role in its pathogenesis.

Pathophysiology

There are several prevailing hypotheses of the pathogenesis of the Arnold-Chiari malformations.

1. The "traction hypothesis" states that tethering of the spinal cord draws the caudal medulla

903

oblongata and posterior cerebellum through the foramen magnum as the spinal column grows faster than the spinal cord.

2. The "pulsion hypothesis" notes that fetal hydrocephalus generates pressure with caudal displacement of the brainstem and cerebellum during early development.

3. The "crowding hypothesis" suggests that owing to the small size of the posterior fossa, the restricted neural structures within it are forced through the foramen magnum as they grow.

4. According to the "molecular genetic hypothesis" (which is consistent with all aspects of Arnold-Chiari malformations, particularly types II and III) the malformation is the result of ectopic expression of homeobox genes of rhombomere segmentation.

Clinical Features

1. Arnold-Chiari malformation type I is generally asymptomatic during childhood; it usually manifests during adolescence or adult life.

   a. Symptoms are due to direct medullary compression, compression of the vascular supply of the medulla, or hydrocephalus secondary to aqueductal stenosis or obstruction of the fourth ventricle at its outlet foramina or at the foramen magnum. Clinical manifestations of obstruction at the foramen magnum consist of torticollis, opisthotonus, and cervical cord compression.

   b. Other manifestations are headache, vertigo, laryngeal paralysis, and progressive cerebellar signs.

   c. Symptoms include recurrent apneic attacks and pain in the neck and occipital area that are exacerbated by exertion or laughing.

   d. It has been reported that in pediatric patients Arnold-Chiari malformation type I can present with seizures and motor or language developmental delay.

2. Type II manifests with respiratory difficulties and lower cranial nerve palsies. Death may result from aspiration pneumonia or apneic attacks or from other associated malformations such as spina bifida.

3. Type III variant may have any of the features of types I and II.

Key Clinical Signs: Arnold-Chiari Malformation

- Respiratory abnormalities
- Apneic attacks
- Gait ataxia
- Dissociated sensory loss
- Spastic quadriparesis
- Nystagmus
- Lower cranial nerve palsies
- Occipital headaches
- Downbeat or rotatory nystagmus

Differential Diagnosis

1. The differential diagnosis of Arnold-Chiari malformation includes a number of congenital and acquired disorders.

2. Such disorders are brain tumors, hydrocephalus, other disorders of the craniovertebral junction, chronic meningitis, multiple sclerosis, cervical myelopathy, and traumatic syringomyelia.

Laboratory Testing

There are no known laboratory tests to diagnose Arnold-Chiari malformation. The diagnosis is based on clinical and neuroradiologic findings.

Key Laboratory Findings: Arnold-Chiari Malformation

- No specific laboratory tests are available for the diagnosis of Arnold-Chiari malformation.
- Diagnosis is based on clinical and neuroradiologic evidence.

Radiologic Features

1. Plain radiographs of the skull [searching for platybasia, basilar impression, or lacunae (vault defects)], cervical spine [searching for increased canal width or fusion of vertebrae, particularly C2, 3 (Klippel-Feil syndrome)], and lumbosacral spine (seeking any associated spina bifida) are obtained.

2. Brain and spinal cord MRI are the most significant tests in patients with possible Arnold-Chiari malformation.

3. Sagittal views of the brainstem are particularly significant for determining and measuring the degree of cerebellar and brainstem herniation.

4. Brain computed tomography (CT) scanning sometimes indicates that the Chiari malformation is present by revealing such associated anomalies as a beaked tectum and cerebellar tissue around the brainstem on axial views. It cannot adequately identify the degree of herniation, however, and it can miss cases of Chiari malformation (particularly type I).

5. In all patients with Arnold-Chiari malformation, magnetic resonance imaging (MRI) of the cervical cord is mandatory to search for an accompanying syrinx or hydromyelia.

6. It is recommended that individuals with myelomeningocele have their entire neuraxis imaged because of the high likelihood that a tethered cord or hydromyelia is also present. They should also be assessed for uncompensated hydrocephalus.

7. Based on MRI findings it has been found that most patients with spinal symptoms had syringomyelia, and a number of individuals with significant tonsilar herniation were clinically asymptomatic.

8. Deformities of the midbrain can be observed with Arnold-Chiari malformation type I.

9. Based on MRI studies, Arnold-Chiari malformation type 1 appears mainly to be associated with syringomyelia and craniovertebral changes, whereas Arnold-Chiari malformation type II has many associated intracranial findings, such as beaking of the midbrain tectum, caudal displacement of the fourth ventricle, large massa intermedia, kinking of the lower brainstem, craniolacunia, and hypoplasia of the falx with interdigitation of the cerebral gyri.

Key Radiologic Findings: Arnold-Chiari Malformation

- MRI is the test of choice.

- T_1-weighted sagittal and axial scans are used to determine and measure cerebellar ectopia and to affirm the presence or absence of associated syringomyelia.

Treatment

1. Two major issues should be addressed.

   a. Surgical management of the primary disorder

   b. Management of neurologic deficits and disability

2. Surgical management should address the following issues:

   a. Need for and degree of decompression of the posterior fossa

   b. Management of any accompanying syrinx or hydromyelia and determining if any concurrent craniovertebral anomalies exist that require surgical management, such as basilar impression or invagination

   c. In cases of coexisting hydrocephalus, whether shunting or shunt replacement is required

3. Many patients improve with decompression and release of adhesions in the posterior fossa.

4. Patients with an associated syrinx may also require shunting of the cyst with a syringe (subarachnoid) or a shunt, especially if the syrinx is large.

5. Management of pediatric cases may be different. In a survey of the pediatric section of the American Association of Neurological Surgeons, it was determined that there was substantial agreement that surgery should not be performed on asymptomatic patients and that it is indicated for patients with brainstem dysfunction, cranial nerve dysfunction, hydromyelia, or scoliosis associated with these malformations (Haines and Berger, 1991).

Key Treatment: Arnold-Chiari Malformation

- Posterior fossa decompression

- Ventriculoperitoneal or atrial shunting

Prognosis and Complications

1. Some of the clinical manifestations stabilize or improve with time, including myelomeningocele and symptomatic Chiari malformation in some newborns.

2. General neurologic function improves following craniocervical decompression in some patients.

Prevention

There are no known primary preventive methods to decrease the incidence of Arnold-Chiari malformation.

Pregnancy

1. A case report describing a 30-year-old woman with a Chiari malformation who presented with severe pregnancy-induced hypertension suggested the need for caution and close monitoring (Semple and McClure, 1996).

2. Another case report demonstrated the therapeutic effects of acetazolamide for hindbrain hernia headache (Chalaupka, 2000).

SYRINGOMYELIA

Definition

1. The term "syringomyelia" indicates the presence of a fluid-filled cavity in the spinal cord.
2. "Hydromyelia" means dilatation of the central canal of the spinal cord: cavities partially or completely lined by ependymal cells.
3. Syringomyelia indicates cavities located outside the central canal that do not have an ependymal lining but that may have partial connection with the central canal.
4. "Communicating" syringomyelia refers to cavities with a direct communication with the fourth ventricle through the obex. It is usually associated with hindbrain malformations.
5. "Noncommunicating" syringomyelia consists of cavities without communication with the fourth ventricle. It is usually secondary to trauma and tumors of the spinal cord but is also associated with hindbrain malformations.

Epidemiology and Risk Factors

1. A prevalence of 5.6 to 8.6 per 100,000 population has been reported in England.
2. Proportional rates from several series range from 0.4% to 1.0% of cases admitted to neurologic clinics.
3. Males and females are affected equally.

Etiology

1. Syringomyelia associated with Arnold-Chiari I anomaly is possibly of genetic origin.
2. Syringomyelia may complicate basal or spinal arachnoiditis following bacterial meningitis, subarachnoid hemorrhage, tuberculosis, trauma, and reaction to radiopaque material, spinal anesthesia, or detergents.
3. Syringomyelia may be due to intramedullary or extramedullary spinal tumors and infratentorial tumors.
4. Certain tumors, such as ependymomas and hemangioblastomas, have a 50% incidence of associated syringomyelia.
5. The following classification based on etiologic factors has recently been recommended (Moufarrij and Awad, 1997).
   a. Communicating syringomyelia, in which there is a demonstrable communication with the fourth ventricle by neuroimaging studies
   b. Blockage of CSF circulation at (1) the posterior fossa–craniovertebral junction level by an Arnold-Chiari malformation, basal adhesive arachnoiditis, masses, basilar impression, or meningeal carcinomatosis or (2) the spinal level by tumors, arachnoid cysts, adhesive arachnoiditis, or infectious masses
   c. Spinal cord tissue injuries due to trauma, radiation necrosis, infarction, hemorrhage, infection, associated transverse myelitis, demyelinating disease, amyotrophic lateral sclerosis, or compressive myelopathy
6. Syringomyelia may be idiopathic.

Pathophysiology

Pathophysiologic mechanisms of syringomyelia formation include

1. For syringomyelia due to basal arachnoiditis and in a small number of cases associated with Arnold-Chiari malformation type I, the "hydrodynamic theory" may be applicable. CSF may be pushed through the obex into a patent central canal generating communicating syringomyelia. In most such cases, however, there is no identifiable communication at the obex.
2. Anatomic and physiologic blockage of the CSF circulation, which occurs in response to brain expansion during cardiac systole, causes flow from the cranial to the spinal subarachnoid space and forces the cerebellar tonsils into the partially enclosed spinal subarachnoid space (Oldfield et al., 1994). Exaggerated spinal pulse pressures are generated, pushing CSF from the subarachnoid space into the spinal cord through the Virchow-Robin spaces.
3. In patients with posttraumatic syringomyelia, necrosis and cysts resulting from fluid egress from damaged axons may develop at the site of cord injury.
4. With syringomyelia due to spinal arachnoiditis, a vascular mechanism may be causal.
5. In tumor-associated syringomyelia, neoplastic growth may interfere with the blood supply to the spinal cord and cause ischemia, necrosis, and cavity formation.

Clinical Features

1. The onset of syringomyelia is insidious; it manifests between 25 and 40 years of age.
2. Initial manifestations consist of pain, numbness of the hands, stiffness of the legs, scoliosis,

vertigo, oscillopsia, diplopia, dysphonia, dysphagia, laryngeal stridor, sweating abnormalities, torticollis, drop attacks, and neurogenic arthropathy.

3. The dissociated sensory loss is commonly first observed along the ulnar border of the hand and forearm: it then extends to the arm, upper part of the chest, and back in a cape or half-cape distribution, uni- or bilaterally, and to the face following an "onion skin" distribution. All sensory modalities may be impaired or lost in a limb owing to involvement of the root entry zone. In advanced cases, with compression of the spinothalamic tracts or the posterior columns, long tract signs develop in the legs.

4. Wasting and weakness first appear in the hands and progress to the forearms, arms, and trunk.

5. Hypotonia, areflexia, and fasciculations are commonly observed.

6. Involvement of corticospinal tracts in advanced cases gives rise to spastic paraparesis.

7. In patients with lumbar syringomyelia, upper and lower motor neuron signs are present in the lower extremities.

8. Horner's syndrome is common and is frequently the only manifestation of the disease.

9. Trophic changes in the hands consist of hyperkeratosis, scars from old burns, subcutaneous edema, or hematomas.

10. Rotatory or vertical nystagmus is the most common sign of syringobulbia.

11. The onset of posttraumatic syringomyelia ranges from 3 months to 35 years after trauma and consists of an ascending sensory level, pain in the neck or arms, increased muscle weakness, and spasticity.

Key Clinical Signs and Symptoms: Syringomyelia

- Onset usually insidious

- Initial manifestations: pain, numbness of the hands, stiffness of the legs, scoliosis, vertigo, oscillopsia, diplopia, dysphonia, dysphagia, laryngeal stridor, sweating abnormalities, torticollis, drop attacks, neurogenic arthropathy

- Dissociated sensory loss along the ulnar border of the hand and forearm

- Sensory loss—unilateral or bilateral—extending to the arm, upper part of the chest, and back in a cape or half-cape distribution and to the face following an "onion skin" distribution

- Wasting and weakness, first appearing in the hands and progressing to the forearm, arm, and trunk

- Hypotonia, areflexia, and fasciculations

Differential Diagnosis

1. The absence of sensory abnormalities and a normal MRI scan of the spinal cord can exclude motor neuron disease.

2. Multiple sclerosis can be ruled out based on the rarity of trophic changes, neurogenic arthropathies, and dissociated sensory loss in multiple sclerosis (MS) patients. Furthermore, the presence of a high immunoglobulin G (IgG) level and myelin basic protein levels and abnormal visual evoked potentials in MS differentiate these two conditions.

3. Spinal cord syphilis is excluded by the absence of dissociated sensory loss, elevated CSF protein and cell count with a positive VDRL test.

4. Cervical spondylotic myelopathy manifests with lower motor neuron signs in the upper limbs and upper motor neuron signs in the lower limbs. It is common in elderly patients. Bulbar signs, trophic changes, and neurogenic arthropathy are absent.

5. Spinal cord tumors can be differentiated from syringomyelia based on the presence of more severe and progressive pain and an absence of trophic changes or neurogenic arthropathies in patients with tumors. Elevated CSF protein, enlargement of the cord on MRI, and enhancement of the lesion with gadolinium favor the diagnosis of an associated spinal cord tumor.

PEARL

- Analgesia and thermoanesthesia with preservation of other sensory modalities associated with atrophy of the hands may indicate syringomyelia.

Laboratory Testing

There are no known laboratory test to diagnose syringomyelia. The diagnosis is based on clinical and neuroradiologic grounds.

Key Laboratory Findings: Syringomyelia

- No specific laboratory tests are available to diagnose syringomyelia.

Radiologic Features

1. Diagnosis is best made by MRI studies. T_1-weighted images best characterize cord and syrinx morphology, and T_2-weighted sequences best show associated conditions such as myelomalacia, gliosis, or tumor.

2. For patients with type I Arnold-Chiari anomaly, axial and sagittal T_1-weighted images of the cervical spine should be obtained to assess for a cervical syrinx. In patients with caudal extension of the syrinx cavity, a thoracic spine scan should be done to define the full extent of the central syrinx cavity.

3. Intracranial neuroimaging should be done to exclude hydrocephalus. Tonsilar descent is considered abnormal when it is more than 5 mm below the foramen magnum.

4. MR phase contrast imaging shows pulsatile fluid motion in syrinx cavities in synchrony with the adjacent subarachnoid space, mainly in large cavities.

Key Radiologic Findings: Syringomyelia

- MRI is the diagnostic procedure of choice.

- T_1-weighted images best demonstrate cord and syrinx morphology.

- T_2-weighted sequences best reveal associated conditions such as myelomalacia, gliosis, or tumors

Treatment

1. Posterior fossa and upper cervical decompression currently is the recommended procedure for the most common type of syringomyelia in pediatric patients (i.e., syringomyelia associated with Arnold-Chiari malformation type II).

2. In those with decompression failure and in whom a dilated cyst persists, shunting of the CSF from the cystic cavity into the adjacent structures is suggested.

3. Because shunting of the syrinx is associated with a risk of cord damage, it is strongly suggested that surgical treatment of syringomyelia associated with the Chiari malformation be aimed at reestablishing normal CSF pathways (Holly and Batzdorf, 2001; Nishizawa et al., 2001).

Key Treatment: Syringomyelia

- Posterior fossa and upper cervical decompression

Prognosis and Complications

1. Untreated syringomyelia runs a slowly progressive course, and almost one-half of patients stay on a plateau for up to 10 years.

2. Syringobulbia usually complicates syringomyelia possibly through the "slosh" mechanism. When intraspinal pressure is elevated during straining or tightening of the abdominal muscles and the individual cannot equalize intracranial pressure due to ectopia, this pressure is transmitted to the syrinx and the fluid cyst moves upward.

3. Other long-term complications consist of neurogenic arthropathies, cervical spondylosis, central and obstructive sleep apnea, and sudden death.

4. Even patients whose operations were adequate may show subtle deterioration, most likely due to gliosis alongside the walls of the syringomyelic cavities, even though the syrinx is no longer distended.

5. Poor prognostic indicators include symptoms of more than 2 years' duration and the presence of ataxia, nystagmus, bulbar symptoms, muscle atrophy, or dorsal column dysfunction.

6. Complications of foramen magnum decompression consist of cord injury by neck hyperextension or hyperflexion during intubation, spinal cord ischemia due to arterial hypotension, CSF leakage with development of a symptomatic pseudomeningocele, posterior fossa bleeding, infection, hydrocephalus, and cerebellar ptosis.

7. Complications of shunting procedures include shunt malfunction, local hematoma, infection, or a collapsed syrinx.

Prevention

1. Avoidance of traumatic, prolonged labor (including the use of forceps) may prevent the formation of syringomyelia in predisposed newborns.

2. Cautious application of epidural anesthesia, avoiding entry into the subarachnoid space, may prevent the formation of spinal arachnoiditis and syringomyelia.

3. In patients with Arnold-Chiari anomaly and impaired CSF flow across the foramen magnum, avoidance of any maneuver that may induce "craniospinal" dissociation may prevent enlargement of an established syrinx until appropriate decompression has been performed.

Pregnancy

No information is available.

Bibliography

Chalaupka FD: Therapeutic effectiveness of acetazolamide in hindbrain hernia headache. Neurol Sci 21:117–119, 2000.

Haines SJ: Berger M: Current treatment of Chiari malformations types 1 and 2: a survey of the Pediatric Section of the American Association of Neurological Surgeons. Neurosurgery 28:353–357, 1991.

Herman MD, Cheek WR, Storrs BB: Two siblings with the Chiari 1 malformation. Pediatr Neurosurg 16:183–184, 1990.

Holly LT, Batzdorf U: Management of cerebellar ptosis following craniovertebral decompression for Chiari I malformation. J Neurosurg 94:21–26, 2001.

Moufarrij N, Awad IA: Classification of the Chiari malformations and syringomyelia. In Benzel EC, Awad IA (eds): Syringomyelia and the Chiari Malformations. Washington, DC, American Association of Neurological Surgeons 1997, pp. 27–34.

Nishikawa M, Sakamoto H, Hakuba A, et al.: Pathogenesis of Chiari malformation: a morphometric study of the posterior cranial fossa. J Neurosurg 86:40–47, 1997.

Nishizawa S, Yokoyama T, Yokota N, et al.: Incidentally identified syringomyelia associated with Chiari I malformations: is early interventional surgery necessary? Neurosurgery 49:637–640, 2001.

Oldfield EH, Muraszko K, Shawker TH, et al.: Pathophysiology of syringomyelia associated with Chiari I malformation of the cerebellar tonsils: implications for diagnosis and treatment. J Neurosurg 80:3–15, 1994.

Semple DA, McClure JH: Arnold-Chiari malformation in pregnancy. Anaesthesia 51:580–582, 1996.

Stovner LJ: Headache associated with the Chiari type 1 malformation. Headache 33:175–181, 1993.

1 Vasovagal Syncope

Daniel M. Bloomfield

Definition

1. Vasovagal syncope is a transient loss of consciousness caused by an abrupt drop in blood pressure.

2. Patients who present with syncope need an evaluation to determine the cause of syncope.

3. Vasovagal syncope is only one cause of syncope (see Differential Diagnosis).

4. Sir Thomas Lewis coined the phrase vasovagal syncope in 1932 in a paper that described a form of syncope that involved both vasodilation and vagally mediated bradycardia.

   a. Since that time, there have been many terms used to describe this type of syncope, including *neurally mediated syncope, neurocardiogenic syncope, cardioinhibitory syncope, vasovagal syncope,* and *vasodepressor syncope.*

   b. For all practical purposes, these terms are synonymous, although some have distinguished patients according to their heart rate response: *vasovagal syncope* refers to patients with hypotension and bradycardia, and *vasodepressor syncope* refers to patients with hypotension without bradycardia.

   c. Throughout this chapter, I refer to vasovagal syncope in its generic sense without reference to any specific heart rate response.

Epidemiology

1. There are no rigorous estimates of the incidence of vasovagal syncope, although it is clearly the most common cause of syncope.

2. It is thought that between one third and one half of all people will have at least one syncopal episode from vasovagal syncope.

3. There are data indicating that 3% to 6% of all emergency room visits are for syncope and that it results in 1% to 3% of hospital admission. These data include syncope from all causes, although it is likely that a significant number of patients who present to the emergency room or are admitted with syncope have vasovagal syncope.

4. Many patients with vasovagal syncope are either evaluated and treated as outpatients or never seek medical attention for a single apparently benign syncopal episode.

Etiology of Syncope

1. Many patients who present with syncope can have a diagnosis made during the history, physical examination, and the electrocardiogram (ECG), such as

   a. Orthostatic hypotension

   b. Long QT syndrome

   c. Brugada's syndrome

   d. Complete heart block

   e. Sick sinus syndrome with a long pause or marked sinus bradycardia (<30 bpm)

   f. Sustained ventricular tachycardia

   g. Aortic stenosis or hypertrophic obstructive cardiomyopathy

2. The evaluation of the patient with unexplained syncope requires an initial neurologic assessment.

   a. In the absence of symptoms or physical signs suggesting a neurologic etiology, the likelihood of a neurologic cause of syncope is extremely uncommon.

   b. Brain imaging studies rarely make a diagnosis of syncope.

   c. Carotid Doppler ultrasound studies are often done in the evaluation of syncope, although rarely fruitful.

   d. Electroencephalograms (EEG) rarely make a diagnosis of syncope. Indications for an EEG in the evaluation of a patient with unexplained syncope would include patients:

      (1) Who had witnessed convulsions

      (2) Who were confused for a long time following an event, suggesting post-ictal confusion

      (3) Who had lateral tongue biting

      (4) See Part VII, Chapter 2, Epilepsy Syndromes

3. The evaluation of the patient with unexplained syncope also requires an assessment of the risk of ventricular arrhythmia.

   a. This assessment often begins with an evaluation of cardiac structure and function, often with an echocardiogram.

   b. This evaluation must exclude outflow track obstruction either from aortic stenosis or hypertrophic obstructive cardiomyopathy.

c. If there is left ventricular dysfunction or an abnormal electrocardiogram (ECG), then the diagnosis of ventricular tachycardia needs to be entertained and evaluated by a cardiologist or an electrophysiologist.

Pathophysiology

1. Considerable uncertainty remains in our understanding of the mechanism of vasovagal syncope.

2. In most cases, the provocative stimulus is venous pooling in the lower limbs and in the splanchnic vasculature while upright, which requires a compensatory response including an increase in chronotropy, inotropy, and sympathetic vasomotor tone.

   a. The initial stimulus in vasovagal syncope is thought to result from a relative central hypovolemia (reduced ventricular preload) that occurs because of venous pooling.

   b. The afferent end of this reflex is mediated by left ventricular mechanoreceptors that are activated during vigorous contraction around an underfilled chamber.

   c. Information from these mechanoreceptors travels along vagal C fibers to the brainstem, which mediates an abrupt and characteristic efferent response consisting primarily of withdrawal of sympathetic vasomotor tone and often, but not always, a vagally mediated bradycardia.

   d. This characteristic efferent response is often referred to as a "Bezold-Jarisch reflex" and most likely represents a hypersensitive response to an otherwise normal stimulus.

3. The characteristic efferent "vasovagal-like" response that results in hypotension and a paradoxical relative bradycardia can also occur in other settings.

   a. Mechanoreceptor activation can occur from other sources such as the bladder in micturition syncope and the rectum in defecation syncope.

   b. This characteristic efferent response is also observed in carotid sinus hypersensitivity, and during what appears to be vasovagal syncope during phlebotomy.

   c. Vasovagal syncope during blood-injury phobia highlights the possibility of a central nervous system mechanism directly initiating the vasovagal efferent response.

4. This proposed pathophysiology has been called into question by the observation of vasovagal-like syncopal episodes in patients who have undergone cardiac transplantation (and thus have a denervated heart).

   a. These observations either implicate the poten-tial importance of other vascular mechanoreceptors or an alternative afferent mechanism.

   b. In addition, the role of increased sympathetic activity in the pathogenesis of vasovagal syncope has been called into question by a number of studies.

      (1) In one study, clonidine worsened and yohimbine improved orthostatic tolerance in patients with vasovagal syncope.

      (2) Another study found that patients with vasovagal syncope have impaired sympathetically mediated vasoconstriction.

5. It is important to recognize the differences in the pathophysiology of vasovagal syncope and the dysautonomic response to upright posture.

   a. These two disorders can be distinguished based on the cardiovascular and autonomic response to upright posture.

   b. In both disorders, the provocative stimulus is an orthostatic challenge caused by venous pooling in the lower limbs and in the splanchnic vasculature while upright.

   c. In vasovagal syncope, the initial cardiovascular response to upright posture appears to be relatively normal.

      (1) Syncope occurs after an abrupt fall in blood pressure sometimes accompanied by a fall in heart rate (suggesting a "hypersensitive response") after a delayed period of standing or head-up tilt.

      (2) In a few large series of patients undergoing tilt-table testing, the mean time to syncope was ~25 minutes with a standard deviation of 10 minutes.

   d. The dysautonomic response results when the autonomic nervous system appears to be failing.

      (1) These patients are unable to compensate for the drop in venous return that occurs acutely with upright posture.

      (2) When this failure to compensate becomes severe, frank orthostatic hypotension occurs.

      (3) However, in many patients, frank orthostatic hypotension may not develop immediately after the assumption of upright posture.

         (a) Patients with a failing autonomic nervous system may demonstrate a progressive type of orthostatic hypotension after prolonged periods of head-up tilt: as blood continues to pool in the lower limbs with prolonged periods of upright posture, blood pressure continues to fall.

    (b) This has been described as delayed or progressive orthostatic intolerance or a dysautonomic response to upright posture.

6. This distinction between a hypersensitive and a failing autonomic response to upright posture is particularly important in understanding differences in this condition in younger and older patients.

    a. Younger patients almost exclusively suffer from the hypersensitive, classic vasovagal response; a dysautonomic response is extremely rare in otherwise healthy young patients.

    b. In contrast, elderly patients often have an inadequate or failing autonomic response to upright posture which may result in progressive orthostatic hypotension or a Bezold-Jarisch reflex and vasovagal syncope.

    c. This distinction in the mechanism of vasovagal syncope and the dysautonomic response to upright posture has important ramifications in the choice of the treatment of syncope.

Clinical Features

1. The clinical features associated with the classic presentation of vasovagal syncope are listed in Table 1–1. While these clinical features are common, it is important to recognize that vasovagal syncope can have an atypical presentation.

2. Elderly patients can have vasovagal syncope without having any prodromal symptoms.

    a. This is often documented by tilt-table testing.

    b. These patients present with syncope and report waking up on the ground, unsure of what had happened.

TABLE 1–1. KEY CLINICAL FEATURES OF VASOVAGAL SYNCOPE

1. Syncope often occurs
   a. In the upright posture
   b. In warm closed spaces
   c. Following (but not during) exercise
2. Syncope is often preceded by characteristic prodromal symptoms
   a. Lightheadedness
   b. Nausea
   c. Warmth
   d. Diaphoresis
   e. Visual dimming
3. Syncope can often be avoided by sitting or lying down
4. The loss of consciousness is most often brief (usually under 1 minute)
5. After regaining consciousness, patients have a clear sensorium without confusion or disorientation

c. There are two potential explanations for this phenomenon.

    (1) They may develop retrograde amnesia after the syncopal event from profound and sometimes prolonged hypotension.

    (2) When witnessed, witnesses often report that the patient complained of lightheadedness prior to losing consciousness despite the patient's history of having no prodromal symptoms.

3. Elderly patients may not develop symptoms attributable to hypotension during a vasovagal episode.

    a. This is sometimes made clear during tilt-table testing when patients become hypotensive with systolic blood pressures of 70 to 80 mm Hg and report feeling fine and then abruptly lose consciousness as their blood pressure falls further.

4. Vasovagal syncope can occur in the sitting position rather than in the upright position.

5. Vasovagal syncope can occur *following* a bout of exercise, but it is thought to be rare during exercise.

    a. Syncope that occurs while the patient is actively exerting him/herself needs a careful evaluation to exclude the diagnosis of a malignant ventricular arrhythmia triggered in the setting of intense sympathetic excitation.

6. Patients may become incontinent of urine and/or stool during a vasovagal episode, although this is uncommon and suggests either a long asystolic pause or profound hypotension.

7. Patients with vasovagal syncope may develop "convulsive" type movements or posturing during an episode.

    a. These are rarely seizures and are most often a form of myoclonic movements from profound hypotension.

    b. These movements and posturing tend to occur in the setting of a prolonged asystolic pause (often longer than 15–30 seconds).

8. Most patients regain consciousness quickly and have a clear sensorium although they may feel weak, diaphoretic, and nauseated for some time (5–30 minutes) after the event.

    a. There are patients who continue to feel extremely fatigued and generally unwell for a few hours following a vasovagal syncopal episode despite having a normal blood pressure.

    b. Migraine headaches can occur following a vasovagal syncopal episode.

Differential Diagnosis

1. The differential diagnosis of syncope of unclear etiology is long and beyond the scope of this chapter.

2. The most common or most worrisome diagnoses in the differential include

   a. Left ventricular outflow tract obstruction (aortic stenosis or hypertrophic cardiomyopathy)

   b. Ventricular tachyarrhythmias (including those related to Long QT syndrome)

   c. Bradyarrhythmias

   d. Pulmonary embolism

   e. Disorders in blood pressure regulation

3. In most cases, an ECG and an echocardiogram exclude the diagnosis of structural heart disease, suggesting that ventricular tachyarrhythmias are less likely. In these cases, the final differential diagnosis is often between bradyarrhythmias and disorders in blood pressure regulation.

4. Vasovagal syncope is one of a number of disorders of orthostatic control of blood pressure, many of which result in syncope. A classification of these disorders has been proposed.

   a. Reflex syncope (including vasovagal syncope, carotid sinus hypersensitivity, micturition and defecation syncope)

   b. Postural orthostatic tachycardia syndrome

   c. Multisystem atrophy

   d. Pure autonomic failure

5. The focus of this chapter is on vasovagal syncope, a reflex type of syncope. The other three types of disorders of blood pressure regulation are discussed elsewhere in this text.

Laboratory Testing

1. In many cases, the diagnosis of vasovagal syncope can be made based on the clinical history, especially in young patients who present with the characteristic clinical features listed in Table 1–1.

   a. Elderly patients with unexplained syncope, however, often do not present with the typical prodromal symptoms associated with vasovagal syncope.

   b. In patients with unexplained syncope who do not present with the typical presentation of vasovagal syncope, tilt-table testing may be useful.

2. Tilt-table testing is a type of provocative testing used to determine an individual's orthostatic tolerance and susceptibility to vasovagal syncope.

   a. In addition to its utility in establishing the diagnosis in a patient with unexplained syn-

TABLE 1–2. CHARACTERISTIC ABNORMAL FINDINGS DURING TILT-TABLE TESTING

1. A vasovagal response is characterized by an abrupt fall in blood pressure, usually after the patient has been hemodynamically stable for some time. The vasovagal response always includes an abrupt fall in blood pressure but may also include a fall in heart rate, sometimes with an asystolic pause.

2. An orthostatic response is one in which the blood pressure falls immediately (within 1–3 minutes) upon the assumption of upright posture.

3. A dysautonomic response (also called *delayed orthostatic hypotensive response*) is characterized by a gradual and progressive fall in blood pressure, often with little if any compensatory increase in heart rate. This response is indicative of autonomic dysfunction.

4. A Postural Orthostatic Tachycardia Syndrome (POTS) response is characterized by an immediate increase in heart rate (>30 bpm) often to a heart rate > 130 bpm within 3 minutes of assuming upright posture. Patients with POTS often also have a fall in blood pressure and they may also develop vasovagal syncope subsequently during the tilt-table test.

cope, tilt-table testing also provides the physician with the opportunity to observe the pathophysiologic evolution of the patient's syncope.

   b. Observations from tilt-table testing have significantly enhanced our understanding of the pathophysiology of vasovagal syncope and have provided insights into potentially useful treatments.

3. There are a number of different hemodynamic responses to tilt-table testing.

   a. The different hemodynamic patterns of collapse seen during tilt-table testing may provide subtle clues suggesting an initial line of therapy (Table 1–2).

4. There are numerous variations in the methodology used for tilt-table testing, a review of which is beyond the scope of this chapter.

   a. Tilt-table tests are often done in two stages:

      (1) A prolonged period of head-up tilt in the drug-free state.

      (2) This is followed by a shorter period of head-up tilt after the administration of a provocative agent such as isoproterenol or nitroglycerin.

   b. Given that the most valuable information is obtained during drug-free passive tilt, tilt-table testing with a provocative agent should not be done alone and should only follow a negative drug-free tilt.

Treatment

1. Not all patients with vasovagal syncope need treatment.

   a. Given that vasovagal syncope is a benign

disorder that has a good prognosis, the decision to treat a patient with vasovagal syncope or orthostatic intolerance should be based primarily on quality of life.

b. Patients with recurrent syncope have a poor quality of life that is similar to patients with severe rheumatoid arthritis or chronic low back pain.

c. Moreover, the reduction in quality of life is proportional to the frequency of syncopal episodes; those patients with more frequent recurrent syncope have a poorer quality of life.

d. Therefore, patients with frequent episodes are more likely to benefit from treatment.

2. The vast majority of patients with vasovagal syncope do not require specific pharmacologic treatment.

a. Educating the patient about the pathophysiology of vasovagal syncope and ways to avoid it may be extremely effective in preventing recurrent syncope.

b. Several studies that have demonstrated that the probability of having recurrent syncope is significantly diminished after a tilt-table test, presumably because of the counseling and education that occurs after the test is completed.

3. In some patients, medications can be adjusted to reduce the risk of developing syncope.

a. This is especially true with the peripherally active α-antagonists, which are known to cause orthostatic hypotension and syncope and which can be substituted with antihypertensives that are less potent vasodilators and that may be less likely to cause syncope.

b. Nitrates are another class of drug that can cause syncope and can often be safely discontinued.

4. In patients with Parkinson's disease, the disease itself causes autonomic dysfunction and the medications useful in treating Parkinson's disease can further exacerbate the drop in blood pressure with standing and can cause syncope or recurrent lightheadedness.

a. Stopping anti-parkinsonian medications, however, may significantly reduce the quality of life in patients with Parkinson's disease. It may be preferable to support their blood pressure with drugs like fludrocortisone or midodrine to allow the patient to take anti-parkinsonian medications.

5. Salt and fluid intake may be extremely important.

a. Many patients adhere to the American Heart Association guidelines for a healthy diet and maintain a diet that is extremely low in salt.

b. A low-salt diet may make some patients more likely to develop vasovagal syncope, and increasing the amount of salt in their diet may be all that is necessary to prevent recurrent syncope. Increasing salt intake will help expand blood volume and may reduce the hemodynamic impact of venous pooling during upright posture.

c. Normotensive patients with vasovagal syncope should increase their fluid and dietary salt intake. Some will have difficulty increasing their dietary salt intake (because they don't like the taste of salt, or because someone else in their household is hypertensive), in which case salt tablets can be given as a supplement.

6. Drugs that have been used to treat vasovagal syncope are listed in Table 1–3.

a. Relatively few of the drugs have been shown to be effective in randomized placebo-controlled clinical trials.

b. In addition, the few clinical trials that have been done were small, enrolling fewer than 100 subjects, primarily younger patients and enrolling very few elderly subjects.

c. Some of the drugs listed in Table 1–3 have been shown to be ineffective in the treatment of vasovagal syncope in small studies.

7. It is important to determine if the patient has vasovagal syncope in contrast to a dysautonomic response to upright posture.

a. β-Blockers, which often are used to treat vasovagal syncope, would be contraindicated in a patient with a dysautonomia in whom the autonomic response to upright posture is already blunted.

8. The treatment of vasovagal syncope primarily attempts to prevent the afferent triggering of the

TABLE 1–3. DRUGS USED TO TREAT PATIENTS WITH VASOVAGAL SYNCOPE

ACE inhibitors*	Midodrine*
β-Blockers*	Phenylephrine
Clonidine†	Propantheline†
Dextroamphetamine	Pseudoephedrine
Disopyramide†	Salt
Erythropoietin	Scopolamine patches†
Etilefrine†	Serotonin reuptake inhibitors*
Fludrocortisone	Theophylline
Fluids	Verapamil
Methylphenidate	

Abbreviation: ACE: angiotensin converting enzyme inhibitors.
*Benefits shown in randomized placebo-controlled trials.
†Data suggest that these drugs are ineffective in randomized placebo-controlled trials.

Bezold-Jarisch reflex or to modify the central processing of the afferent input.

   a. β-Blockers are thought to blunt the intense inotropic triggering of the Bezold-Jarisch reflex.

   b. Volume expansion with salt and fludrocortisone is thought to limit the impact of venous pooling.

   c. Midodrine may also prevent the afferent triggering of the Bezold-Jarisch reflex by causing venoconstriction, thereby limiting the amount of venous pooling that occurs with upright posture.

   d. β-Blockers or fludrocortisone tend to be used as the first line of treatment because of dosing convenience and physicians' large experience with them.

   e. Selective serotonin reuptake inhibitors (SSRIs) are being used increasingly as first-line therapy. Midodrine, though effective, requires multiple doses and thus is often reserved for patients who have frequent symptoms.

9. Relatively few patients will continue to have recurrent syncope after education, reassurance, and treatment (β-blockers, fludrocortisone, midodrine).

   a. In patients with recurrent syncope despite the optimum use of these treatments, alternative treatments that could be considered include other drugs, tilt training, and permanent pacing.

   b. Generally, pacemakers should be reserved for patients who continue to have recurrent syncope despite the use of multiple medications.

10. The hypertensive patient with vasovagal syncope is challenging because volume expansion with salt and fludrocortisone, and midodrine are contraindicated.

   a. In these patients, β-blockers or SSRIs are often the first line of therapy. Pacemakers may be useful in this population if β-blockers or SSRIs are not effective or well tolerated.

Key Treatment

- Not all cases require treatment
- Pharmacologic treatment not required in many cases
- Increase salt and fluid intake
- β-blockers, fludrocortisone, or SSRIs (often used as first-line therapy)
- Midodrine for patients with frequent symptoms

Prognosis

1. Vasovagal syncope is thought to be a benign disorder with a good prognosis.

2. There are data, however, that allow us to identify patients who have a high likelihood of having recurrent syncope.

   a. Three factors have been shown to be associated with an increased risk of developing recurrent syncope: The absolute number of prior syncopal episodes, the frequency of historical syncope, and recurrent syncope after a tilt-table test.

   b. The probability of having recurrent syncope increases significantly as the number of prior syncopal episodes increases from 1 to 3.

   c. In addition, there is an association between frequent spells over a short period and increased risk of developing syncope (this when compared with a similar number of syncopal episodes that occurred over a long time period)

3. The only patients in whom treatment may affect their prognosis are patients whose syncope puts them at high risk for developing trauma.

   a. These are patients who develop syncope without a warning or prodromal symptoms, and patients who develop syncope while driving without enough warning to safely stop the car.

   b. In addition, there are certain occupational issues that place patients at high risk for injury because of vasovagal syncope such as pilots, truck drivers, roofers etc.

Bibliography

Benditt DG, Ferguson DW, Grubb BP, et al.: Tilt table testing for assessing syncope. American College of Cardiology. J Am Coll Cardiol 28:263–275, 1996.

Bloomfield DM, Sheldon R, Grubb BP, et al.: Putting it together: A new treatment algorithm for vasovagal syncope and related disorders. Am J Cardiol 84:33Q–39Q, 1999.

Grubb BP, Karas B: Clinical disorders of the autonomic nervous system associated with orthostatic intolerance: An overview of classification, clinical evaluation, and management. Pacing Clin Electrophysiol 22:798–810, 1999.

Mosqueda-Garcia R, Furlan R, Tank J, Fernandez-Violante R: The elusive pathophysiology of neurally mediated syncope. Circulation 102:2898–2906, 2000.

Sutton R, Bloomfield DM: Indications, methodology, and classification of results of tilt-table testing. Am J Cardiol 84:10Q–19Q, 1999.

2 Postural Hypotension

Louis H. Weimer

Definition

1. Postural or orthostatic hypotension (OH) is a clinical sign seen in numerous and diverse neurologic and non-neurologic conditions.

2. One consensus agreement defined OH as a fall in systolic blood pressure of 20 mm Hg or 10 mm Hg diastolic within 3 minutes of standing or similar orthostatic challenge, such as upright tilt of at least 60 degrees.

3. OH may be symptomatic or asymptomatic and varies according to underlying conditions or confounding factors. Symptoms develop as a consequence of upright posture or tilt and include diverse complaints including but not limited to dizziness, faintness, and impending loss of consciousness.

4. Confounding variables are numerous when considering the significance of an individual blood pressure measurement. Prominent exacerbating factors include:
   a. Meals (especially a high carbohydrate load)
   b. Early morning
   c. Dehydration or volume contraction
   d. Warm temperature
   e. Recent prolonged recumbency
   f. Postural deconditioning
   g. Medications
   h. Advanced age

Etiology and Pathophysiology

1. Maintaining an adequate blood pressure and cerebral perfusion on standing involves a complex cascade of physiologic events. The effects of gravity and large fluid shifts must be rapidly accommodated. Some understanding of underlying mechanisms is useful in approaching rational therapy.

2. In neurogenic causes of OH, the sympathetic nervous system is not adequately activated. Plasma catecholamine levels fail to sufficiently increase on standing with neurogenic OH, but this assay is not highly sensitive or specific. Some important mechanisms include:
   a. Lack of neurally mediated peripheral vasoconstriction, especially in large skeletal muscle and splanchnic vascular beds

   b. Lack of baroreceptor detection of a blood pressure drop from bilateral receptor injury, deafferentation from neuropathy, or central disruption
   c. Postprandial conditions can lead to splanchnic vasodilation with inadequate peripheral vasoconstriction and resultant hypotension.

3. Non-neurologic conditions can also cause hypotension and must be considered. Mild forms of these processes will exacerbate neurogenic causes. Broad categories include:
   a. Intrinsic cardiac disease, obstruction, or dysrhythmia with low cardiac output
   b. Excessive non-neurologic vasodilation from drugs, alcohol, heat, severe varicosities, or mastocytosis
   c. Low intravascular volume from fluid loss (orthostatic tachycardia), electrolyte imbalance, nephropathy, diabetes insipidus, or endocrinopathy—notably adrenal insufficiency (Addison's disease)
   d. Pheochromocytoma patients demonstrate OH in addition to paroxysmal hypertension.

4. Many chronic causes of OH are relatively asymptomatic due to adaptive mechanisms such as shift of cerebral autoregulatory curves and stimulation of the renin-angiotension-aldosterone system. When these adaptations are overcome, symptoms, including syncope, can rapidly follow.

Clinical Features

1. Dizziness or light-headedness soon after standing is the most common complaint but is far from universal. Other postural symptoms that occur in isolation without light-headedness include:
   a. Pure vertigo with sensation of movement mimicking positional vertigo
   b. "Coat hanger" neck ache or fatigue, likely from muscle ischemia
   c. Confusion or cognitive slowing, especially in the elderly
   d. Syncope without warning

2. Other commonly associated postural symptoms include general weakness and fatigue, blurred vision, tremulousness, anxiety, nausea, pallor, and a clammy sensation.

3. Other symptoms of generalized autonomic failure

may be evident; some are nonspecific in isolation but may be relevant in the OH patient.

a. Dry eyes and mouth; paroxysmal or gustatory tearing

b. Loss or inappropriate sweating especially distally; heat intolerance

c. Urinary incontinence, retention, or frequency

d. Abdominal pain, obstinate constipation, nocturnal or paroxysmal diarrhea

e. Gastric dysmotility, vomiting, early satiety, bloating, anorexia, weight loss

f. Vasomotor complaints, acral discoloration or coldness, Raynaud's sign

g. Sexual dysfunction; erectile or ejaculatory failure

h. Visual blurring, photophobia, or inappropriate glare perception

i. Autonomic neuropathy signs include distal limb trophic or vasomotor changes, excessive skin dryness or reduced resistance (excess smoothness) and loss of hair. Mucosal dryness or pupillary changes may be evident.

4. Bedside blood pressure measurement is a defining screening test. Ideally the patient should rest supine for 5 to 15 minutes then quickly stand. Blood pressure and heart rate are measured for at least 2 minutes but the pressure drop may be delayed 3 to 10 minutes in some cases.

5. Other coincident neurologic findings useful in diagnosis include parkinsonian or cerebellar signs and evidence of large or small-fiber somatic peripheral neuropathy.

Key Symptoms

- Dizziness or light-headedness soon after standing

Postural Symptoms without Light-Headedness

- Vertigo with sensation of movement
- "Coat hanger" neck ache or fatigue
- Confusion or cognitive slowing, especially in the elderly
- Syncope (without warning)

Other Postural Symptoms

- General weakness and fatigue
- Blurred vision
- Tremulousness
- Anxiety

- Nausea
- Pallor
- Clammy sensation

Differential Diagnosis

1. Symptoms of dysautonomia are common in neurologic disease. Diverse disorders such as multiple sclerosis, epilepsy, mass lesions, spinal cord injury, myelopathy, and stroke often affect the numerous autonomic structures and pathways. OH may be a manifestation of numerous conditions, but severe or isolated OH is seen in relatively few conditions.

2. Non-neurologic conditions should also be considered and excluded: cardiac disease, volume depletion, environmental conditions, Addison's disease, and pheochromocytoma.

3. Severe OH may be a manifestation of primary generalized autonomic failure (AF).

   a. In pure autonomic failure (Bradbury-Eggleston syndrome, idiopathic OH), AF is marked, without evidence of other neurologic dysfunction. Diagnosis is not possible for at least 3 years of AF without development of other signs. Patients tend to have severe OH but few cholinergic symptoms such as dry eyes and mouth, incontinence, and hypohidrosis. The condition progresses slowly over years.

   b. Multiple system atrophy (Shy-Drager syndrome) also shows AF but with more pronounced cholinergic signs. Coincident parkinsonism (usually without tremor), ataxia, or both are seen. Other useful markers include poor Dopa response, stridor, sleep disorders, and sphincter denervation. The disease is progressive with a generally poor prognosis and susceptibility to sudden death.

   c. Parkinson's disease (PD) commonly includes minor dysautonomia, but some patients have PD and frank autonomic failure with OH, which is designated "Parkinson's disease with AF." Autonomic signs are similar to PAF but with true Lewy bodies in the brain and in peripheral sympathetic neurons.

   d. Acute or subacute autonomic neuropathy is not rare and may be of immune-mediated or paraneoplastic origin. Many but not all forms manifest OH, which may be severe. 50% of cases are preceded by a viral illness. Strong anecdotal evidence points to benefit from intravenous immunoglobulin therapy. A malignancy screen is usually warranted.

   e. Chronic autonomic neuropathy. Many different causes of peripheral neuropathy cause autonomic dysfunction, although many are limited to distal loss of sweating and vasomotor regulation, usually without OH. Causes that more commonly lead to OH include:

(1) Diabetic autonomic neuropathy

(2) Familial or acquired amyloidosis

(3) Toxic neuropathies, such as from chemotherapy, vacor, podophyllin, heavy metals, hexacarbons, and amiodarone

(4) Hereditary sensory and autonomic neuropathies, Fabry disease, dopamine β-hydroxylase deficiency, hyperbradykininism

(5) Paraneoplastic syndromes

f. Medication effects. Mild or borderline OH can be produced, unmasked, or made symptomatic by medications (see Medications that May Induce Orthostatic Hypotension). Mild supine hypertension may prompt therapy that unmasks OH, especially in the elderly. There are 145 current drug listings in the current *Physician's Desk Reference* with OH as a treatment side effect.

Medications that May Induce Orthostatic Hypotension

- Anticholinergics: tricyclic antidepressants, atropine, oxybutynin

- β-adrenergic blockers: propranalol and others

- α_2-adrenergic agonists: clonidine, prazosin, α-methyldopa, terazosin, doxazosin

- α_1-adrenergic antagonists: phentolamine, phenoxybenzamine, guanabenz

- Ganglionic blockers: guanethidine, hexamethonium, mecamylamine

- Other agents: hydralazine, nitrates, diuretics, acetylcholinesterase inhibitors, antihistamines, combination preparations, antipsychotics, antiparkinsonian agents, narcotics, sidenafil

---

g. Orthostatic intolerance. An increasing number of patients with orthostatic symptoms without OH are known. Symptoms arise from cerebral hypoperfusion despite maintained blood pressure. The hallmark is persistent orthostatic tachycardia despite normovolemia. Criteria are an increase in heart rate ≥30 bpm or an absolute heart rate ≥120 bpm on standing. Half or more of cases have evidence for an attenuated bout of restricted acute autonomic neuropathy.

h. Measurable asymptomatic OH is common over age 70 for multifactorial reasons. New medications or other exacerbating factors can convert the condition to symptomatic OH with hypoperfusion.

Laboratory Testing

1. The clinical situation will dictate work-up, and a regimented algorithm is not practical. The pattern of autonomic testing abnormalities and associated clinical findings can limit possibilities. Items to consider include:

a. Autonomic testing battery

b. Blood counts, electrolytes, VDRL (Venereal Disease Research Laboratory test), human immunodeficiency virus, rheumatologic screen

c. Urine metanephrines, morning and evening cortisol measures, electrocardiogram, and echocardiogram. Additional cardiac workup or Doppler ultrasound studies if warranted.

d. Fasting glucose or Hb A_{1C}; consider a glucose tolerance tests in suspicious neuropathy settings

e. Genetic screen or nerve or fat biopsy for amyloid if suggestive pattern or family history of neuropathy

f. General approach to small-fiber neuropathy work-up if present including serum protein electrophoresis, immunofixation electrophoresis, cryoglobulins, and quantitative immunoglobulins

g. Organ-specific or system-specific tests if appropriate

(1) Pupillography, Schirmer tear test, or Sjögren lip or gland biopsy.

(2) Cystometrics, gastrointestinal manometry or motility studies, sexual function testing

h. Malignancy screen and antibody studies in acute or subacute setting

i. Magnetic resonance imaging

j. For MSA: optional sleep studies, sphincter electromyogram, positron emission tomography scan

Treatment

1. Treatment of symptomatic OH depends on the severity of symptoms. Nonpharmacological measures may be adequate in mild cases, whereas a combination of therapies may be needed in more severe autonomic failure.

2. Autonomic testing and clinical evaluation may reveal underlying mechanisms that can be approached rationally. Also, treating an underlying

disease may improve or arrest the autonomic failure.

3. Nonpharmacological measures include avoiding specific postures and situations.

   a. Beneficial physical maneuvers include moving from lying to standing in slow graded stages, especially early in the morning. Isotonic exercise without strain; swimming, leg crossing, stooping, and squatting can also be used.

   b. Avoid straining, coughing, arm raising, isometric exercise, prolonged recumbency, and hot environments or baths.

   c. Reconsider medications that may worsen or elicit OH. Patients may also be overly sensitive to over-the-counter cold remedies that acutely affect blood pressure.

   d. Raise the head of the bed (reverse Trendelenburg) by 20 degrees at night to reduce nocturnal diuresis, limit supine hypertension, and stimulate baroreceptors. This can be done by placing blocks under the legs at the head of the bed or with a home hospital bed.

   e. Increase salt and fluid intake: Especially critical with signs of volume contraction; salt tablets may be needed

   f. Elastic stockings are of benefit in cases of excess venous pooling, but must be waist high and provide abdominal compression for effect. They are often too cumbersome for elderly or neurologically impaired patients.

   g. Adjust meal size and content. Postprandial hypotension is not uncommon in OH patients. Small frequent meals, avoidance of high carbohydrate loads (pasta), and minimized alcohol should be tried. Advise patient to take extra care on rising after meals.

4. Medications of diverse mechanisms are useful when other measures fail. Goals of treatment are to minimize symptoms and eliminate syncope, not necessarily to restore normotension. Supine hypertension is produced or worsened by many agents but is generally better tolerated than in other patient types.

   a. Fludrocortisone acetate, a long-acting, well-tolerated mineralocorticoid, is the usual first-line agent. The starting dose is 0.1 mg/day, which can be increased, but shows little added benefit over 0.5 mg/day. Potassium supplements may be needed. Side effects including ankle edema, headache, and supine hypertension are seen but are not generally problematic. Heart failure rarely can precipitate.

   b. If fludrocortisone is insufficient, a sympathomimetic agent can be substituted or added. Midodrine (a direct-acting α-adrenergic ago-

nist) is approved for OH treatment. The dosage is titrated between 2.5 and 10 mg three times a day, but not after 6 PM. Side effects include scalp itching and pilomotor (goosebump) reactions that improve with time but can be disconcerting if the patient is not cautioned. Other agents (ephedrine, pseudoephedrine, amphetamines, phenylpropanolamine) are also used but show tachyphylaxis and some limiting central effects.

   c. Erythropoietin increases systolic blood pressure an average of 10 mm Hg and improves orthostatic tolerance. Many chronic autonomic failure patients have anemia. The dose is 25 to 75 μg per kg of body weight 3 times per week until the hematocrit normalizes. Supplementary $FeSO_4$ may be needed as well.

Key Treatment

First-Line Treatment

- Increased salt and fluid intake

- Minimize confounding environmental factors and medications

- Gentle isotonic exercise without straining

- Nocturnal raising of the head of the bed

- Fludrocortisone (Florinef)

- Midodrine (ProAmatine)

- Small, more frequent low-carbohydrate meals

   d. Second- and third-line agents that work sporadically or have less efficacy can supplement in severe cases or if other agents are not tolerated.

   (1) Nonsteroidal antinflammatory agents raise blood pressure a small degree.

   (2) Caffeine 100 to 250 mg 3 times a day through food or tablet

   (3) Octreotide (25–200 μg SQ) may attenuate postprandial OH but is limited by nausea and cramping.

   (4) Dihydroxyphyenylserine (L-DOPS) is a norepinephrine precursor. It is essential in the treatment of the rare genetic disorder dopamine β-hydroxylase deficiency, and it may be helpful in other causes of OH. This agent is not yet available in the United States.

   (5) Vasopressin analogues (e.g., desmopressin acetate) are useful in some cases.

   (6) Third-line agents include dihydroergotamine, β-blockers pindolol and xamoterolol,

clonidine, and yohimbine can be tried in refractory cases.

Key Treatment

Second-Line Treatment

- Nonsteroidal anti-inflammatory agents
- Caffeine
- Octreotide
- Vasopressin analogues

Third-Line Treatment

- Dihydroergotamine, β-blockers pindolol and xamoterolol, clonidine, and yohimbine for refractory cases

Prognosis

Prognosis depends on the underlying disorder, a major reason for proper diagnosis. Of the common severe causes, multiple system atrophy is progressive and carries a poor prognosis, whereas pure autonomic failure is only slowly progressive. Autonomic neuropathy varies with type, but the degree of autonomic neuropathy is an unfavorable prognostic marker, best validated in diabetes mellitus.

Bibliography

The Consensus Committee of the American Autonomic Society and the American Academy of Neurology: Consensus statement on the definition of orthostatic hypotension, pure autonomic failure and multiple system atrophy. Neurology 46:1470, 1996.

Freeman R, Miyawaki E: The treatment of autonomic dysfunction. J Clin Neurophysiol 10:61–82, 1993.

Low PA, Guillermo SA, Benarroch EE: Clinical autonomic disorders: Classification and clinical evaluation. In Low PA (ed): Clinical Autonomic Disorders, 2nd ed. Philadelphia, Lippincott-Raven, 1997, pp. 3–15.

Mathias CJ: Orthostatic hypotension: causes, mechanisms, and influencing factors. Neurology 45(Suppl 5):S6–S11, 1995.

Robertson D, Davis TL: Recent advances in the treatment of orthostatic hypotension. Neurology 45(Suppl 5):S26–S32, 1995.

3 Sexual Dysfunction

George D. Baquis

Definition and Epidemiology

1. Sexual dysfunction is common among men and women and can result from psychological, endocrine, vascular, and neurologic disorders.

2. Male sexual dysfunction manifests as disorders of erectile and ejaculatory function.

3. Females experience abnormalities of clitoral swelling and vaginal lubrication.

4. Men and women can experience alteration of the intensity and quality of orgasm as a consequence of neurologic disease.

5. It has been estimated that 20 million to 30 million men in the United States experience erectile dysfunction, and the prevalence increases with age. However, disorders of sexual function are often not discussed by patients with their physicians.

Facts About Sexual Dysfunction

- Sexual dysfunction in both men and women can result from psychological, endocrine, vascular, and neurologic disorders.

- 20 million to 30 million men in the United States experience erectile dysfunction.

- Prevalence of erectile dysfunction increases with age.

Pathophysiology

1. Penile erectile tissue consists of the corpora cavernosa and spongiosum, which are composed of smooth muscle and fibroelastic sinusoids. Pudendal artery branches supply blood to the penis.

2. Penile erections can result from both psychogenic and reflex stimulation, and are mediated via parasympathic outflow. The sympathetic nervous system also plays a role in the development of psychogenic erections. Relaxation of smooth muscle increases penile blood flow, leading to development of tumescence. Sympathetic efferents close retrograde flow at the bladder neck and induce the emission of semen through rhythmic smooth muscle contraction.

3. Nitric oxide release raises intracellular cyclic guanosine monophosphate resulting in smooth muscle relaxation. It is a principal neurotransmitter mediating penile erection.

4. Parasympathetic outflow regulates reflex erection in men and increased vaginal secretions with lubrication and changes in genital blood flow with clitoral swelling in women. Mechanical stimulation of the anterior vagina may result in sexual arousal. Normal lubrication depends on adequate estrogen levels.

5. Multiple central nervous system (CNS) structures play a role in normal sexual function, including the hypothalamus, limbic system, and frontal lobes. However, CNS integration of sexual function is incompletely understood.

Clinical Features

1. History

   a. Inquiry should be made regarding libido, symptoms of erectile or ejaculatory dysfunction, orgasm, perineal skin sensation, and the situational circumstances of sexual dysfunction.

   b. A full menstrual history should be requested of women.

   c. A psychiatric and social history including drug and alcohol use should be obtained.

   d. All medications should be recorded, with attention to those known to cause sexual dysfunction including antidepressant, antipsychotic and antihypertensive agents.

   e. History should be directed toward medical and neurologic illnesses known to complicate sexual function.

2. Physical examination

   a. In addition to a careful abdominal, pelvic, and general neurologic examination, assessment should be made of the external genitalia, bladder fullness, hernias, peripheral pulses, and anal sphincter function.

   b. Superficial skin sensation should be tested over the abdomen, pelvis, buttocks, inner thighs, and external genitalia.

   c. Several superficial skin reflexes can be evaluated, including the bulbocavernosus reflex, cremasteric reflex, cutaneous anal reflex, and superficial abdominal reflexes.

921

Differential Diagnosis

1. Erectile dysfunction can result from hypogonadism, vascular diseases that reduce penile blood supply or cause venous leakage, and diseases of the central and peripheral nervous system. It is possible that a loss of lubrication in women could result from similar mechanisms

2. Diseases affecting the frontal and temporal lobes (such as stroke and tumors) may result in sexual disinhibition and hypersexuality.

3. Failure of the internal urethral sphincter to close may result in retrograde ejaculation. Anejaculation can result from diseases that impair sympathetic nerve function to the sexual organs and from spinal cord injury. Premature ejaculation is usually a psychiatric problem.

4. Libido may be diminished as a result of psychogenic or neurologic diseases. Depression and medications can contribute. Libido is hormone dependent and alterations can result from disease of the hypothalamic-hypophyseal axis.

5. Anorgasmia can be medication induced, a consequence of neurologic disease including spinal cord injury, or psychogenic.

Diagnostic Testing

1. Tests should be chosen based on clinical diagnostic considerations. General laboratory studies include urinalysis, complete blood count, glucose, blood urea nitrogen, creatinine, serum prolactin, serum total and free testosterone, luteinizing hormone, follicle stimulating hormone, cholesterol, lipid profile, and thyoid function tests.

2. Penile tumescence tests assess the function of the organs supplied by the nerves of concern and are usually performed by urologists and gynecologists. Penile tumescence can be measured by the stamp and snap-gauge tests. These are inexpensive and easily performed studies but are not sensitive or specific measures of erectile dysfunction. Home nocturnal portable monitoring devices can record number and magnitude of erections but may fail to identify patients with mild erectile dysfunction. Results may not correlate with ability to achieve vaginal peretration during sexual intercourse.

3. Vascular tests include Doppler ultrasound after administration of a pharmacological vasodilatory agent, measurement of the penile brachial blood pressure index (lack of standardization), and evaluation of pharmacological penile erection (can support the diagnosis of vascular insufficiency but does not distinguish between arterial and venous disease). Iliac and pudendal arteriography is an invasive study that does not quantify blood flow (there is a lack of consensus regarding what constitutes a positive or negative test).

4. Neurophysiologic tests can directly assess peripheral and central nervous system function. These include the penile dorsal nerve conduction test, pudendal nerve evoked potentials, and the bulbocavernosus reflex test. They directly measure neurologic function, but their sensitivity and specificity for diagnosis of sexual dysfunction is unclear.

Key Tests

General

- Urinalysis
- Complete blood count
- Many others including testing of glucose, blood urea nitrogen, creatinine

Penile Tumescence Tests

- Stamp and snap-gauge tests

Vascular Tests

- Doppler ultrasound (requires administration of a vasodilatory agent)
- Penile brachial blood pressure index

Neurophysiologic Tests

- Penile dorsal nerve conduction test
- Pudendal nerve evoked potentials
- Bulbocavernosus reflex test

Neurologic Disorders

1. Parkinsonism: Erectile dysfunction (ED) is often the first symptom of multiple system atrophy, and this diagnosis should be questioned if erectile function is preserved. ED is less frequent in patients with Parkinson's disease (PD) and usually occurs later in the course of the illness. Increased libido has been described in some PD patients treated with L-dopa.

2. Stroke: Erectile and ejaculatory dysfunction in men and problems with vaginal lubrication and orgasm in women are the most commonly reported difficulties. Frequency and duration of sexual intercourse have been reported to decline, but increased sexual interest has also been described. Direct injury to neural structures important for sexual function may alter sexual activity. Paralysis, sensory loss, spasticity, communication

difficulty, personality change, and depression may interfere with formation and maintenance of interpersonal relationships.

3. Multiple sclerosis (MS): Approximately 70% of men develop erectile failure, which usually occurs several years after initial MS symptoms and is usually accompanied by lower limb pyramidal abnormalities. Loss of ejaculatory function may also complicate MS. Approximately 50% of women have significant sexual problems which include abnormal vaginal lubrication, decreased sensation, loss of libido, and problems achieving orgasm.

4. Spinal cord injury: Male erectile and ejaculatory function are lost during the period of spinal shock. Most men regain erectile function, but ejaculatory function returns in only a minority of patients. Male fertility may be reduced because of poor semen quality. Women may achieve pregnancy, which can be complicated by urinary tract infection, deep venous thrombosis, and autonomic dysreflexia. Abdominal muscle paralysis and absence of perineal sensation can predispose to pelvic floor tears during delivery. A study of 64 premenopausal women compared to 21 able-bodied age matched controls revealed that preservation of T11–L2 dermatomal sensation in women is associated with psychogenically mediated genital vasoconstriction. Less than 50% of spinal cord injured women, and only 17% of those with S2–S5 spinal dysfunction, could achieve orgasm compared to 100% of controls.

5. Cauda equina damage: Men may describe erectile dysfunction, abnormal ejaculation, or decreased penile sensation. Women may experience loss of perineal sensation and inability to appreciate sexual stimuli.

6. Peripheral neuropathy: Erectile dysfunction is a well-described complication of diabetes affecting approximately 50% of men, and retrograde ejaculation can also occur. Decreased libido, slow arousal, inadequate lubrication, anorgasmia, and dyspareunia may affect diabetic women, but studies are limited.

7. Pelvic plexopathy: Injury in women after major pelvic surgery such as radical hysterectomy or abdominoperineal resection can result in diminished lubrication, dyspareunia, and diminished orgasm. A population-based study of radical prostatectomy for clinically localized prostate cancer reported erectile dysfunction in 59.9% of men 18 or more months after surgery.

8. Pudendal neuropathy: Trauma after prolonged bicycle riding, or due to perineal traction on a fracture post in patients undergoing surgery on a fracture table, has been associated with male erectile dysfunction, penile and scrotal numbness, and female perineal numbness.

9. Epilepsy: Partial epileptic seizures can rarely have a sexual sensory aura. Partial complex seizures may include pelvic movements, masturbation, and undressing. Lubrication and orgasm are rare complex seizure components. Epileptic seizures can be provoked by hyperventilation during sexual intercourse, masturbation, orgasm, and specific sexual stimuli.

Neurologic Conditions Associated With Sexual Dysfunction

- Parkinsonism
- Stroke
- Multiple sclerosis
- Traumatic spinal cord injury
- Epilepsy
- Peripheral neuropathy
- Post-surgical plexopathy (prostatectomy, hysterectomy)

Treatment

1. Treatment should be individualized based on the underlying neurologic diagnosis. Modifiable disease-related factors should be identified (see Modifiable Clinical Features).

Modifiable Clinical Features

- Medication (iatrogenic)
- Spasticity
- Depression and other psychological disorders
- Bladder or bowel incontinence
- Pain
- Fatigue

---

2. Because most of the available neurophysiology, vascular, and penile tumescence diagnostic tests lack specificity, and because available medications effectively treat a broad spectrum of disorders with various causes, it is often reasonable to proceed to treatment in the absence of these tests.

3. Oral sildenafil is the medication of choice for treatment of male erectile dysfunction. It is taken 1 hour before sexual activity and can be an effective treatment for erectile dysfunction resulting from a

variety of causes including diabetes mellitus, spinal cord injury, radical prostatectomy, depression, and psychogenic causes. It is absolutely contraindicated in men taking nitrate drugs. Rare serious cardiovascular events, including myocardial infarction and death have occurred, and cardiovascular status should be assessed prior to use. Side effects include headache, flushing, dyspepsia, and transient visual disturbance.

4. Alprostadil is a synthetic form of prostaglandin E_1 that can be administered as a transurethral therapy or as an intracavernosal injection. Advantages include local application and minimal systemic effects. Drawbacks of the transurethral formulation include penile pain, low response rate, and inconsistent effect. Alprostadil can cause priapism and fibrosis. The optimal dose varies between patients.

5. Other intracavernosal medications include papaverine and phentolamine, which may be prescribed in combination. Papaverine can cause priapism and corporal fibrosis, and phentolamine can cause hypotension and reflex tachycardia. Oral yohimbine, an alpha-adrenergic blocker, has been reported to improve erectile function but is only marginally effective for treatment of organic erectile dysfunction.

6. Vacuum devices induce an erection through a canister tube connected to a vacuum pump. Negative pressure draws blood into the penis and tumescence is maintained by a band placed at the penile base. Adverse effects include impaired ejaculation, decreased penile sensation, ecchymosis, and rare penile necrosis.

7. Surgical placement of a prosthesis can restore penile rigidity, but possible complications include infection, erosion, mechanical malfunction, and penile gangrene.

8. Ejaculatory dysfunction after spinal cord injury may respond to mechanical penile vibration or electrical stimulation.

9. Data on neurogenic female sexual dysfunction is lacking, and treatment options remain empirical. These include lubricants for management of vaginal dryness. Sildenafil has been described for treatment of medication-induced sexual dysfunction in both women and men. Further investigation is needed to determine its usefulness for treatment of sexual dysfunction in women with neurologic disease.

Key Treatment

Medications

- Sildenafil
- Alprostadil
- Papaverine*
- Phentolamine*
- Yohimbine

Other

- Vacuum devices
- Surgical placement of a prosthesis
- Mechanical vibration or electrical stimulation
- Lubricants for vaginal dryness

*Can be prescribed together

Bibliography

Baquis GD: Micturition and sexual disorders. In Evans RW (eds): Diagnostic Testing in Neurology. Philadelphia, W.B. Saunders, 1999, pp. 367–389.

Betts CD: Bladder and sexual dysfunction in multiple sclerosis. In Fowler CJ (eds): Neurology of Bladder, Bowel, and Sexual Dysfunction. Boston, Butterworth Heinemann, 1999, pp. 289–308.

Hatzichristou DG: Treatment of sexual dysfunction and infertility in patients with neurologic diseases. In Fowler CJ (eds): Neurology of Bladder, Bowel, and Sexual Dysfunction. Boston, Butterworth Heinemann, 1999, pp. 209–223.

Lechtenberg R, Ohl DA: Normal sexual function. In Sexual Dysfunction. Philadelphia, Lea & Febiger, 1994, pp. 21–43.

Lue TF: Erectile dysfunction. N Engl J Med 342:1802–1813, 2000.

Lundberg PO: Physiology of female sexual function and effect of neurologic disease. In Fowler CJ (eds): Neurology of Bladder, Bowel, and Sexual Dysfunction. Boston, Butterworth Heinemann, 1999, pp. 33–46.

Sipski ML, Alexander CJ, Rosen R: Sexual arousal and orgasm in women: Effects of spinal cord injury. Ann Neurol 49:35–44, 2001.

Stanford JL: Urinary and sexual function after radical prostatectomy for clinically localized prostate cancer. The prostate cancer outcomes study. JAMA 283:354–360, 2000.

4 Sphincter Dysfunction

George D. Baquis

Definition and Epidemiology

1. Disturbances of bladder and bowel sphincter function are common complications of central and peripheral nervous system diseases.
2. Urinary and fecal incontinence are socially disabling. Patients may be embarrassed to tell their physicians, and physicians are often reluctant to inquire about symptoms.
3. Urinary incontinence affects approximately 13 million Americans, with a prevalence of about 15% to 35% of noninstitutionalized people older than 60 years of age and over 50% of nursing home patients.
4. The prevalence of fecal and urinary incontinence differ depending on the neurologic diagnosis and illness severity. For instance, although more than one third of stroke patients have fecal incontinence upon hospital admission, the number decreases to about 10% at 6 months. About 50% of multiple sclerosis patients experience fecal incontinence, and micturition dysfunction occurs in approximately 50% to 80% at some point during their illness. The incidence of urinary incontinence complicating Parkinson's disease ranges from 37% to 71%. Spinal cord injury is a common cause of fecal incontinence, with 11% reporting incontinence weekly and as few as 39% reporting reliable continence.

Facts about Incontinence

Urinary Incontinence

- Approximately 13 million Americans affected
- About 15% to 35% of noninstitutionalized people older than 60 years of age
- Nursing home patients: over 50% affected
- Parkinson's disease patients: 31% to 71% affected

Fecal Incontinence

- Stroke patients: More than one third affected upon hospital admission; decreases to about 10% at 6 months
- Multiple sclerosis patients: approximately 50% affected
- Spinal cord injury patients: 11% report incontinence weekly; only 39% report reliable continence

---

Pathophysiology

1. The lower urinary tract and distal bowel store and periodically eliminate their contents. Normal function requires coordinated integration of multiple voluntary and reflexive neurologic structures and pathways.
2. Anatomic neurologic pathways to the urethral and anal sphincters extend from the frontal lobes through the brainstem, spinal cord, and conus medullaris, to peripheral nerves via sacral 2, 3, 4 nerve roots.
3. The sphincters are composed of external striated muscle and internal smooth muscle components.
4. The striated muscle sphincter innervation derives from pudendal nerve branches originating in anterior spinal cord segments of S1 to S3, the nucleus of Onufrowicz. The puborectalis muscle, a pelvic floor muscle that forms a sling around the anal sphincter, contributes to fecal continence and receives separate innervation from direct sacral pelvic nerve branches.
5. The smooth muscle internal sphincters receive excitatory alpha-adrenergic and inhibitory beta-adrenergic sympathetic innervation from the lower thoracic and upper lumbar spinal cord via the sympathetic chain and hypogastric nerves.
6. Preganglionic efferent parasympathetic neurons in the S2 to S4 spinal cord synapse with cholinergic postganglionic parasympathetic neurons in the pelvic plexus ganglia or visceral ganglia that supply bladder detrusor and distal rectal wall smooth muscle innervation.
7. Pelvic visceral and sympathetic hypogastric nerves convey rectal and bladder sensation. The pudendal nerves convey sensory information from the distal urethra, anal canal, and perineum.

Clinical Features

1. History
   a. Inquiry should be made regarding urinary voiding habits (frequency, urgency, initiation and termination of stream, stream quality, nighttime and daytime patterns), dysuria, hematuria, sensation of bladder or pelvic fullness, episodes of incontinence, relationship to fluid intake, and association with physical activity. A

926 • XXIII Neuromedical and Autonomic Disorders

sexual, psychiatric, and social history should be obtained.

b. An obstetric history should be recorded for all women, which includes birth weight of children, mode of delivery, and use of forceps or episiotomy.

c. Stool consistency, incontinence of flatus, protrusion of rectal material suggestive of prolapse, and leakage of material suggestive of infection should be inquired of patients with fecal incontinence.

d. Severity of fecal and urinary incontinence can be assessed by the need for and number of perineal pads used.

e. All medications should be recorded.

f. Inquiry should be made regarding neurologic, surgical, and medical conditions known to complicate bladder and bowel function.

2. Neurologic examination

a. The "classic" neurologic examination should be supplemented by a careful abdominal examination, assessment for bladder fullness, assessment of external genitalia, palpation of extremity pulses, and hernia evaluation.

b. The prostate of males should be assessed during rectal examination. Women should undergo gynecologic examination with assessment for cystoceles, rectoceles, and to evaluate pelvic floor muscle strength and tone.

c. During rectal examination, undergarment fecal staining, hygiene, inspection of perianal skin for fistulas, scars in women suggestive of prior perineal lacerations or episiotomies, rectal prolapse, anal deformity, and stool consistency can be evaluated.

d. Anal sphincter and puborectalis muscle tone and strength should be observed at rest and during sphincter contraction.

e. Superfical skin sensation can be tested over the external genitalia, abdomen, pelvis, buttocks, and inner thighs.

f. Superficial reflexes include the cutaneous anal, cremasteric, bulbocavernosus, and superficial abdominal reflexes.

Diagnostic Tests

1. Urologic studies

a. Postvoid residual urine: Measurement can be performed by ultrasound or catheterization.

b. Urinalysis

c. Cystometry: Bladder filling and voiding are evaluated after fluid instillation through a catheter. Multichannel instruments measure or calculate pressure, detect involuntary contractions, and measure bladder capacity. Compliance, the relationship of pressure to volume, is recorded. Inquiry is made regarding filling sensation, urgency, and pain. Videourodynamic recording is possible with instillation of radiographic contrast material.

d. Uroflowmetry: Urine volume passage per unit time can be measured with a uroflowmeter. Voided volume, maximum flow rate, time to reach maximum flow, and time to void are determined.

e. Urethral pressure profile: A pressure profile along the length of the urethra is measured with a triple-lumen catheter containing pressure transducers as the catheter is slowly withdrawn.

f. Cystoscopy: Structural urethral and bladder lesions are sought through direct visualization. Excessive bladder trabeculation is associated with spasticity.

2. Anorectal studies

a. Anal manometry: Anal sphincter pressure is measured at rest and during maximal contraction through a catheter pressure transducer.

b. Anal ultrasonography: An intra-anal ultrasound probe can sensitively measure the structural integrity of the internal and external sphincters and detect stretch injury or tears.

c. Cinedefecography: A dynamic radiologic study of rectal emptying is performed after rectal instillation of barium paste. The anal sphincter length, anorectal angle, and perineal descent are measured. Puborectalis function and rectal emptying are qualitatively assessed.

d. Balloon distension: Rectal sensation during rectal balloon distension, anal sphincter relaxation after balloon expulsion, and the rectoanal inhibitory reflex (decrease in anal pressure after rectal distension) can be measured.

3. Electrodiagnostic studies

a. Pudendal nerve terminal motor latency: The motor response of the striated urethral or rectal sphincter muscles is recorded to stimulation of the pudendal nerve at the ischial spine. The St. Mark's electrode, a disposable electrode printed on a flexible circuit board, stimulates and records from the anal sphincter, and the urethral response is recorded from a Foley catheter–mounted intraurethral surface electrode.

b. Penile dorsal nerve conduction: Several techniques have been described that directly measure dorsal nerve conduction.

c. Needle electromyography: Quantitative information can be obtained about neurogenic or myogenic conditions affecting striated sphincter and pelvic floor muscles. The presence of denervation or reinnervation after motor axonal injury can be determined.

d. Bulbocavernosus reflex: A sacral segmental response is recorded from the bulbocavernosus muscle to stimulation of the dorsal penile or clitoral nerves. Other measureable segmental sacral reflexes include the urethroanal, vesicoanal, and cutaneoanal reflexes.

e. Pudendal somatosensory evoked potentials: Conduction values along peripheral and central somatosensory pathways are obtained by recording electrical responses from spine or scalp surface electrodes after stimulation of the dorsal penile or clitoral nerves.

f. Posterior urethral and bladder evoked potentials, sympathetic skin response, and transcranial/spinal magnetic and electrical stimulation are neurophysiologic techniques of unclear clinical usefulness for which limited information exists.

 Key Tests

Bladder Sphincter Dysfunction

- Post-void residual urine

- Urinalysis

- Cystometry

- Pudendal nerve conduction

- Sphincter needle electromyography

Anal Sphincter Dysfunction

- Anal ultrasonography

- Cinedefecography

- Anal manometry

- Pudendal nerve conduction

- Sphincter needle electromyography

Differential Diagnosis

1. Bladder sphincter dysfunction: Neurogenic urinary frequency, urgency, retention, and incontinence can result from detrusor hyperreflexia (involuntary bladder contraction due to neurologic disease), detrusor sphincter dyssynergia (loss of sphincter inhibition preceding detrusor contraction), urethral sphincter deficiency (loss of muscle strength and contractility), or bladder overflow (due to loss of bladder contractility or bladder outlet obstruction).

2. Anal sphincter dysfunction: Constipation and incontinence can occur simultaneously and may be related to stool consistency. Peripheral and central nervous system diseases must be distinguished from non-neurologic medical disorders such as diarrheal illnesses, local neoplasms, direct traumatic injury, infections, and inflammatory bowel disorders.

Neurologic Disorders

1. Parkinsonism: Parkinson's disease (PD), Shy-Drager syndrome, progressive supranuclear palsy, and multiple system atrophy (MSA) are all associated with urinary incontinence. Frequency, urgency, urge incontinence, hesitancy, and retention can occur. Urodynamic testing may demonstrate detrusor hyperreflexia or bladder hypotonia. Needle electromyographic findings of denervation and reinnervation may be more common in patients with MSA and uncommon in PD. Constipation in PD may result from slowed colonic transit time or from outlet type obstruction due to failure of striated anal sphincter and puborectalis muscle relaxation. Reduced resting anal tone could explain episodes of liquid stool fecal incontinence. MSA patients experience a high incidence of postoperative incontinence after transurethral resection of the prostate.

2. Stroke: Disruption of micturition pathways, stroke-related cognitive and language deficits, concurrent neuropathy, and medication effects may cause urinary incontinence. The pattern depends on stroke size, location, acuteness, and the presence of other strokes. Retention may be present initially, followed later by frequency, urgency, and incontinence.

3. Dementia: Disturbances of micturition and defecation have been associated with anteromedial frontal lobe lesions. Urinary incontinence is a common feature of multiple infarction dementia, Alzheimer's disease (AD), and normal pressure hydrocephalus. It is generally felt to develop earlier in the course of Lewy body disease than AD and is predictive of the need for institutionalization of AD patients.

4. Multiple sclerosis: Bladder emptying may be incomplete. Urinary urgency, urge incontinence, frequency, and staccato voiding patterns are common. The latter may result from detrusor sphincter dyssynergia. Cystometrogram abnormalities can be present in the absence of symptoms, and the urodynamic pattern can change over time. Constipation and fecal incontinence

are common, and may be related to abnormal rectal filling sensation, poor anal sphincter contraction, or reduced rectal compliance.

5. Spinal cord injury: Detrusor atonia accompanies spinal shock followed after 6 to 8 weeks by a reflexive hypercontractile bladder with external sphincter dyssynergia. Autonomic dysreflexia can be minimized through careful management. Intractable constipation, fecal impaction, and overflow fecal incontinence can occur.

6. Cauda equina damage: Urinary retention and incontinence, bowel atonia with chronic constipation, and bowel overflow incontinence can occur.

7. Peripheral neuropathy: Bladder hypotonia is a common complication of diabetes mellitus and correlates with the presence of a generalized polyneuropathy. Onset is insidious and may reflect coexistent neurologic disease such as stroke. Bladder dysfunction has been described with other toxic and metabolic polyneuropathies. Fecal incontinence complicating diabetes mellitus is often nocturnal and may be related to altered sphincter tone or impaired perception of rectal fullness.

8. Pelvic plexopathy: Postsurgical urinary incontinence and constipation may occur after abdominoperineal resection or radical hysterectomy. Urinary incontinence can complicate transurethral resection of the prostate for clinically localized prostate cancer. Ogilvie syndrome, functional colonic obstruction, can result from malignant tumor invasion of retroperitoneal sympathetic and parasympathetic nerves.

9. Pudendal neuropathy: Delayed stress urinary incontinence after vaginal childbirth can result from pudendal nerve injury and can be detected by pudendal nerve terminal latency and pelvic floor needle electromyographic testing. Occult lacerations and direct muscle injury to the anal sphincter can accompany pudendal neuropathy and contribute to fecal incontinence.

10. Aging: Detrusor overactivity is an important accompaniment of bladder dysfunction of elderly men and women and could represent an aging effect. The causes and pattern of urodynamic test abnormalities are variable. Reduced sensation of bladder filling and altered cognition may contribute to incontinence.

Treatment

1. Detrusor hyperreflexia may respond to anticholinergic therapy with oxybutynin or tolterodine.

2. Botulinum toxin type A urinary striated sphincter injection has been used for treatment of sphincter dyssynergia in spinal cord–injured patients. Intravesical detrusor injections have been described for treatment of detrusor overactivity.

3. Incomplete bladder emptying can respond to mechanical voiding techniques such as the Crede maneuver. However, intermittent catheterization may be indicated if this is unsuccessful or if bladder sphincter dyssynergia is present.

4. An indwelling urethral or suprapubic catheter is a last option for patients who are incontinent or cannot perform intermittent catheterization.

5. Pelvic floor muscle exercises and biofeedback are used for treatment of stress urinary incontinence, but the role of exercises for management of other neurogenic voiding problems is unclear.

6. Sacral nerve root stimulation after percutaneous electrode implantation is a new technique that has been used for treatment of refractory urgency-frequency syndrome, urge incontinence, and idiopathic urinary retention.

7. Constipation is treated with different types of laxatives and stool softeners.

8. Urge fecal incontinence may respond to a constipating medication such as loperamide.

9. Biofeedback has been described for treatment of fecal incontinence associated with diabetes, spinal cord injury, and multiple sclerosis.

10. Surgical approaches include direct anal sphincter repair, gracioplasty, artificial bowel sphincter, or creation of a stoma.

11. The management of bladder and bowel dysfunction is complex, and cooperation of a team that may include an internist, neurologist, physiatrist, urologist, gynecologist, and psychiatrist ultimately contributes to optimal care.

 Key Treatment: Anal Sphincter Dysfunction

- Stool softeners, laxatives, and bulking agents
- Anticholinergics
- Narcotics (loperamide)
- Biofeedback
- Disposable pads
- Surgical repair
- Percutaneous sacral stimulation (investigational)

Bibliography

Baquis GD: Micturition and sexual disorders. In Evans RW (ed): Diagnostic Testing in Neurology. Philadelphia, W.B. Saunders, 1999, pp. 367–389.

Fowler CJ: Neurological disorders of micturition and their treatment. Brain 122:1213–1231, 1999.

Kamm MA: Diagnostic, pharmacological, surgical, and behavioural developments in benign anorectal disease. Eur J Surg 582(Suppl):119–123, 1998.

Madoff RD, Williams JG, Caushaj PF: Fecal incontinence. N Engl J Med 326:1002–1007, 1992.

Norton C, Henry M: Investigation and treatment of bowel problems. In Fowler CJ (ed): Neurology of Bladder, Bowel, and Sexual Dysfunction. Boston, Butterworth Heinemann, 1999, pp. 185–207.

Rushton DN: Neuro-urological history and examination. In Rushton DN (ed): Handbook of Neuro-urology. New York, Marcel Dekker, 1994, pp. 117–128.

Vaizey DJ, Kamm MA, Roy AJ, Nicholls RJ: Double-blind crossover study of sacral nerve stimulation for fecal incontinence. Dis Colon Rectum 43:298–302, 2000.

Stuart R. Chipkin
Erik A. Cohen
Brian W. Smith

5 Pituitary Tumors

Definition

1. Pituitary adenomas are tumors of the anterior pituitary that are benign but are true neoplasms as shown by clonality studies. They are the most common form of sellar mass from the third decade of life on.

2. Adenomas are classified by size and function. Lesions smaller than 1 cm are classified as *microadenomas* and larger lesions are classified as *macroadenomas*. They can arise from any type of cell of the anterior pituitary and may result in increased secretion of the hormone(s) produced by that cell and/or decreased secretion of other hormones as a result of compression of other cell types.

Epidemiology

The true incidence of pituitary adenomas is difficult to ascertain because they are often asympotomatic; autopsy estimates range from 2.7% to 27%. Pituitary adenomas represent 10% to 15% of all intracranial neoplasms. There is no sexual predilection, but the tumors are most common in adults, with the incidence peaking in the third and fourth decades of life; children and adolescents account of about 10%. These tumors are not hereditary except for rare families with multiple endocrine neoplasia, an autosomal dominant trait manifested by a high incidence of pituitary adenomas and tumors of other endocrine glands.

Etiology and Pathophysiology

1. The functional classification of pituitary adenomas is based on endocrinologic activity, dividing tumors into secreting and non-secreting types.

2. Non-secretory pituitary adenomas are more common. The neoplasm is a space-occupying lesion whose secretory products (if any) do not cause a specific disease state. However, these lesions may produce significant neurologic symptoms through their mass effect.

3. Secretory tumors are less common. Each is associated with a specific pathologic condition.

4. Acromegaly is the disease state characterized by a pituitary adenoma that secretes growth hormone.

5. A prolactinoma secretes prolactin and is associated with hyperprolactinemia.

6. Cushing's disease is a disease state in which there is hypersecretion of adrenocorticotropic hormone (ACTH).

7. Thyrotropin-secreting pituitary adenomas secrete primarily thyroid-stimulating hormone and result in hyperthyroidism.

8. Regardless of their functional status, pituitary tumors have the potential to become invasive. They may invade surrounding structures such as the cavernous sinus, cranial nerves, blood vessels, sphenoid bone, and sinus or brain. Suprasellar extension may compress the foramen of Monro to cause hydrocephalus and symptoms of increased intracranial pressure. Hypothalamic dysfunction may be expressed as diabetes insipidus, although diabetes insipidus is relatively rare with adenomas and, if present, is more suggestive of conditions associated with inflammation or tumor invasion of the pituitary stalk. Extensive subfrontal extension with compression of both frontal lobes may cause personality changes or dementia. There may be seizures or motor and sensory dysfunction.

9. Lateral extension of the tumor with compression or invasion of the cavernous sinus can comprise cranial nerve III, IV, or VI function manifesting as diplopia. The third cranial nerve is most commonly affected. There may be numbness in the V1 or V2 distribution. Overall, however, cranial nerve dysfunction is not a common feature of adenoma and may be more suggestive of other neoplasms of the cavernous sinus.

Clinical Manifestations

1. Sellar masses can present with neurologic symptoms, with abnormalities related to undersecretion or oversecretion of pituitary hormones, or as an incidental discovery on a radiologic examination.

2. Nonfunctional adenomas—neurologic symptoms: Impaired vision is the most common symptom that leads a patient with a macroadenoma to seek medical attention. Visual impairment is caused by suprasellar extension of the adenoma that compresses the crossing fibers in the optic chiasm, first affecting the superior temporal quadrants and then the inferior temporal quadrants. Further expansion compromises the non-crossing fibers and affects the lower nasal quadrants and finally the upper nasal quadrants. Formal visual field testing is important because some tumors affect

only the macular fibers to cause central hemianopic scotomas that may be missed on routine screening. One or both eyes may be affected, and if both, to variable degrees. Diminished visual acuity occurs when the optic chiasm is severely compressed. Other patterns of visual loss may also occur. Thus, an intrasellar lesion should be suspected when there is any unexplained pattern of visual loss. The onset of the deficit is usually so gradual that many patients do not seek ophthalmologic consultation for months or even years. Even at this time, the reason for the deficit may not be recognized unless a visual field examination is performed, further delaying the diagnosis.

3. Other neurologic symptoms that may cause a patient with a macroadenoma to seek medical attention include headaches resulting from stretching of the diaphragm sella and adjacent dural structures that transmit sensation through the first branch of the trigeminal nerve. The quality of the headache is not specific. Diplopia can be induced by oculomotor nerve compression from lateral extension of the adenoma. Cerebrospinal fluid rhinorrhea can be caused by inferior extension of the adenoma. Pituitary apoplexy can be induced by sudden hemorrhage into the adenoma, causing excruciating headache and diplopia. At the time of initial presentation because of a neurologic symptom, many patients with sellar masses, when carefully questioned, admit to symptoms of pituitary hormone deficiencies. However, these symptoms are not usually the reason that the patient seeks medical attention. The most common pituitary hormone deficiency is impaired secretion of luteinizing hormone. The result in men is a subnormal serum testosterone concentration which produces symptoms of decreased energy and libido. The result in premenopausal women is amenorrhea.

4. Secretory adenomas—neurologic symptoms, Prolactinomas: Females: galactorrhea, amenorrhea, oligomenorrhea with anovulation, infertility, estrogen deficiency leading to hirsutism, decreased vaginal lubrication, osteopenia. Males: large tumors more common secondary to delayed diagnosis, possible impotence or decreased libido or hypogonadism; galactorrhea rare because males lack the estrogen-dependent breast growth and differentiation.

5. Growth hormone—secreting pituitary adenoma: Coarse facial features; oily skin; prognathism; carpal tunnel syndrome; osteoarthritis; increased hat, glove, or shoe size; decreased exercise capacity; visual field defects; diabetes mellitus; muscle weakness.

6. Corticotrophin secreting pituitary adenoma: Truncal obesity, round facies, dorsocervical fat accumulation, hirsutism, acne, menstrual disorders, hypertension, wide pigmented, striae, bruising, thin skin, hyperglycemia, proximal muscle weakness (see Part XXI, Chapter 4, Endocrine Disorders).

7. Thyrotropin—secreting pituitary adenoma:thyrotoxicosis, goiter, visual impairment.

Key Clinical Findings

- Headache

- Visual field deficits

- Features related to specific hormonal excess/deficiency

Differential Diagnosis

1. Physiologic enlargement of the pituitary. Two forms are recognized: lactotroph hyperplasia during pregnancy; thyrotroph and gonadotroph hyperplasia due to long-standing primary hypothyroidism and primary hypogonadism, respectively.

2. Other benign tumors: Craniopharyngiomas: These solid or mixed solid-cystic benign tumors arise from remnants or Rathke's pouch along a line from the nasopharynx to the diencephalon. Most are either intrasellar or suprasellar. Although they usually occur during childhood and adolescence, about 50% present clinically after age 20, and some do not present until age 70 or 80. The major symptoms are growth retardation in children and abnormal vision in adults. In addition, pituitary hormonal deficiencies including diabetes insipidus, are common. Meningioma: usually benign tumor arising from the meninges anywhere within the head. Some arise near the sella, causing visual impairment and hormonal deficiencies.

3. Malignant tumors: some arise within or near the sella, and others metastasize to that site.

4. Primary malignancies: those malignancies that arise in the parasellar region including germ cell tumors, sarcomas, and chordomas.

5. Germ cell tumors: also called *ectopic pinealomas,* usually occur through the third decade of life and present with symptoms of hydrocephalus, diabetes insipidus, and anterior pituitary hormonal deficiencies. A mass in the third ventricle is seen by imaging, and human chorionic gonadotropin beta (hCGβ) subunit is found in the serum. Although these lesions are highly malignant and

metastasize readily, they are also highly radiosensitive.

6. Chordomas: usually locally aggressive tumors that can metastasize. They often arise in the clivus and cause headaches, visual impairment, and anterior pituitary hormonal deficiencies. Pituitary carcinomas have been reported but they are rare. Metastases to the hypothalamus and pituitary gland occur most commonly from breast cancer in women and lung cancer in men, but can also be seen with many other cancers. Metastases to the hypothalamus frequently present with diabetes insipidus. Other presentations are hypopituitarism or retro-orbital pain. Survival in 36 patients in one series averaged 6 months.

7. Cysts: Rathke's cleft, arachnoid, and dermoid cysts can produce sellar enlargement, possibly resulting in visual impairment, diabetes insipidus, anterior pituitary hormonal deficiencies, and hydrocephalus.

8. Abscess: Pituitary abscesses are rare; they can occur in a normal or diseased pituitary gland. Those occurring in a previously normal gland may have the appearance of an adenoma but can be distinguished by the absence of central enhancement on contrast-enhanced imaging. Arteriovenous fistula of the cavernous sinus can cause modest enlargement of the pituitary gland. Pituitary size returns toward baseline after the fistula is blocked. Lymphocytic hypophysitis from lymphocytic infiltration of the pituitary gland usually occurs in postpartum women, but can also be seen in women at other times and rarely in men. It is characterized by headaches of an intensity out of proportion to the size of the lesion and hypopituitarism, in which adrenal insufficiency is unusually prominent. With magnetic resonance imaging the enlarged pituitary shows delayed or even absent enhancement in the posterior pituitary area. At least partial recovery of both anterior and posterior pituitary function and regression of the anatomic lesion is possible. Corticosteroid therapy may speed these processes.

9. Secretory adenomas: prolactinoma: pregnancy, primary hypothyroidism, breast disease, breast stimulation. Medications: phenothiazine, antidepressants, haloperidol, opiates, amphetamines, cimetidine. Chronic renal failure, liver disease, polycystic ovarian disease.

10. Acromegaly: ectopic production of growth hormone releasing hormone from a carcinoid or other neuroendocrine tumor.

11. Cushing's disease: diseases that cause ectopic sources of ACTH (small cell carcinoma of the lung, bronchial carcinoid, intestinal carcinoid, pancreatic islet cell tumor, medullary thyroid carcinoma, or pheochromocytoma). Adrenal adenomas, adrenal carcinoma. Nelson's syndrome.

Laboratory Testing

1. Hormonal evaluation: hypothalamic-pituitary hormonal function should be evaluated wherever a sellar mass is encountered. Tests must address both functionality of the tumor and physiologic function of pituitary–end organ axes.

2. Hormonal hypersecretion: hypersecretion, with the exception noted below, is caused only by pituitary adenomas. Consequently, the demonstration of hormonal hypersecretion identifies both the sellar mass as a pituitary adenoma and the kind of adenoma. A serum prolactin concentration greater than 200 mg/ml generally identifies a lactotroph adenoma. Values between 20 and 200 mg/ml could be due to a lactotroph adenoma or to any other sellar mass that may be impinging on the pituitary stalk. Supranormal serum growth hormone levels after an oral glucose load or an elevated IGF-1 concentration indicate a somatotroph adenoma. Elevated 24-hour urine cortisol excretion associated with a high-normal or high ACTH concentration usually indicates a corticotroph adenoma. Gonadotroph adenomas can be identified by characteristic patterns of basal and thyroid releasing hormone–stimulated concentrations of gonadotropins and their subunits. These patterns differ somewhat in men and women.

3. Hormonal hyposecretion: hormonal hyposecretion can be caused by any hypothalamic or pituitary lesion and therefore usually has no value in the differential diagnosis of a sellar mass. One exception is that the spontaneous development of central diabetes insipidus indicates that the lesion affects the hypothalamus or the stalk and is therefore not a pituitary lesion. Although not generally useful diagnostically, the possibility of hormonal hyposecretion should be evaluated in all patients who have a sellar mass in order to identify and replace hormone deficiencies. Hormonal function should focus on demonstrating an intact pituitary–end organ axis. For example, a normal TSH value is inappropriate in the setting of a low free T_4 level.

4. Pituitary incidentaloma: The extent of the evaluation in a patient with an incidentally discovered intrasellar MRI signal abnormality depends on its size. If it is larger than 10 mm it should be evaluated as described above. If it is smaller than 10 mm and the patient has no clinical evidence of

pituitary dysfunction, the most cost-effective approach is to measure the serum prolactin concentration. If the value is normal it is unlikely that other significant hormonal abnormalities are present. Further evaluation is not necessary unless symptoms develop.

Key Laboratory Findings

- Specific hormone excess/deficiency

- Prolactin elevation

Radiologic Features

1. Magnetic resonance imaging (MRI) is the best imaging procedure for most sellar masses and there is usually no need to perform any other imaging study. Certain MRI findings suggest a greater likelihood of some kinds of sellar masses than others, but no finding is pathognomonic of any kind of mass.

2. Unenhanced image: Normal pituitary tissue and most sellar lesions, pituitary adenomas, and other tumors emit a signal that is similar to or slightly greater in intensity than that of central nervous system tissue. Cystic lesions, such as Rathke's cleft cysts, often emit a low-intensity signal on T_1-weighted imaging; however, craniopharyngiomas and even pituitary adenomas may be partially cystic and will also emit low-intensity signals. Furthermore, the signal intensity on T_1-weighted images will be high if the protein or lipid concentration of the cyst fluid is high. On T_2-weighted images, cystic lesions may emit a high-intensity signal. Hemorrhage into the pituitary gland results in a high intensity signal on both T_1- and T_2-weighted images.

3. Gadolinium-enhanced image: Normal pituitary tissue takes up gadolinium to a greater degree than CNS tissue and therefore emits a higher intensity signal than the surrounding CNS. Microadenomas of the pituitary often take up gadolinium to a lesser degree than the normal pituitary. Macroadenomas take up gadolinium to a greater degree than the CNS, but so do other lesions, such as craniopharyngiomas and meningiomas. The post-contrast enhancement of meningiomas is usually homogeneous. If a sellar lesion can be seen as separate from the normal pituitary, whether using unenhanced or (more commonly) enhanced images, the lesion is not a pituitary adenoma.

Key Radiologic Findings

- MRI of pituitary demonstrating adenoma

Treatment

1. Nonpharmacologic—surgery: Selective transsphenoidal resection of the adenoma is the treatment of choice for acromegaly, Cushing's disease, and thyrotropin-secreting pituitary adenomas, which all tend to be microadenomas at the time of onset of symptoms. Macroadenomas, such as the non-secretory pituitary adenoma or prolactinomas, may also be surgically removed, but risk of recurrence is greater and adjunctive therapy such as irradiation may also be necessary. Radiotherapy is reserved for patients who have failed surgical treatment and who still experience the symptoms of their adenoma. Bilateral adrenalectomy has been done in patients with Cushing's disease on failure of other therapies, but complications requiring lifelong hormone replacement or Nelson's syndrome may occur.

2. Radiotherapy: Generally reserved for patients who have failed surgical treatment. Used with varying degrees of success in all of the different pituitary adenomas.

3. Pharmacologic therapy, prolactinoma: bromocriptine, pergolide or carbergoline. Side effects include orthostatic hypotension, nausea, and dizziness.

4. Acromegaly octreotide, a somatostatin analog 100 μg subcutaneously, is the medical therapy of choice, but it is limited by side effects such as biliary sludge and gallstones, nausea, cramps, steatorrhea, and its parenteral administration. Long acting analogs are also available. Bromocriptine is less effective than octreotide, but it has the advantage of oral administration.

5. Cushing's disease: Ketoconazole which inhibits the cytochrome P-450 enzymes involved in steroid biosynthesis, is effective in managing mild to moderate disease in daily oral doses of 600 to 1200 mg. Metyrapone and aminoglutethimide can be used to control hypersecretion of cortisol but are generally used when preparing a patient for surgery or while waiting for a response to radiotherapy.

6. Thyrotropin secreting pituitary adenoma: Ablative therapy with either radioactive iodine or surgery is indicated. Treatment directed to the thyroid alone may accelerate growth of the pituitary adenoma. Octreotide has been shown to be effective in doses similar to those used for acromegaly.

7. Nonsecretory pituitary adenoma: there is no role for medical therapy at this time. Surgery and radiotherapy are indicated.

Key Treatments

- Transphenoidal resection
- Bromocriptine or other dopamine agonist

Prognosis and Complications

Variable prognosis depending on the skill of the surgeon. Complications: Nelson's syndrome. Patients who have undergone irradiation should have close follow-up with back-up medical therapy because response to radiotherapy may be delayed. Incidence of hypopituitarism also increases with time. Pregnancy: Pituitary adenomas may enlarge during pregnancy. Sometimes pregnancy is induced in a woman treated for infertility problems who has an unrecognized pituitary adenoma.

Bibliography

Atchison JA, Lee PA, Albright AL: Reversible suprasellar pituitary mass secondary to hypothyroidism. JAMA 262: 3175–3177, 1989.

Klibanski A, Servas NT: Diagnosis and management of hormone secreting pituitary adenomas. N Engl J Med 342:822–830, 1991.

Melmed S: Acromegaly. N Engl J Med 322:966–977, 1990.

Molitch ME: Pituitary incidentalomas. Endocrinol Metab Clin North Am 26:724–740, 1997.

Molitch ME, Thorner MO, Wilson C: Management of prolactinomas. J Clin Endocrinol Metab 26:996–1000, 1997.

Penar PL: Nathan DJ, Nathan MH, Salsali A: Pituitary tumor diagnosis and treatment. Curr Neurol Neurosci Rep 2:236–245, 2002.

Shimon I, Melmed S: Management of pituitary tumors, Ann Intern Med 129:472, 1998.

Young WF, Scheithauer BW, Kovacs KT, et al.: Gonadotropin adenoma of the pituitary gland: a clinicopathologic analysis of 100 cases. Mayo Clin Proc 71:649–656, 1996.

1 Vascular Surgery

Cathy A. Sila

Overview

1. The most commonly performed vascular surgeries are coronary artery bypass grafting (CABG) and carotid endarterectomy (CE); adverse neurologic events are important contributors to morbidity and mortality.

2. The complications of CABG include: ischemic stroke (2% to 5%), encephalopathy (3% to 12% clinically evident, 35% to 75% with neurocognitive testing batteries), seizures (<5%), coma (0.2%), intracerebral hemorrhage (ICH) (0.03%), peripheral nerve injuries (2% to 13%), and rarely optic neuropathy and pituitary apoplexy.

3. More complex cardiac surgeries, such as valve replacement or repair, ventricular aneurysmectomy, and hypothermic circulatory arrest for reconstruction of the aortic arch are associated with higher rates of stroke at 5% to 15%.

4. Perioperative stroke morbidity and mortality after carotid endarterectomy ranges from 3% to 4% for asymptomatic to 5% to 7% for symptomatic patients in clinical trials although it may be as high as 5% to 10% in clinical practice.

Etiology and Pathophysiology

1. Neurologic complications of cardiac surgery
   a. Stroke
      (1) Ischemic stroke: The presumed mechanisms of ischemic stroke after cardiac surgery with cardiopulmonary bypass (CPB) include embolism from the aortic arch in one third, another one third evenly distributed between cardio-embolism, hypoperfusion, and concomitant cerebrovascular disease, and the remaining one third cryptogenic. Risk factors for stroke after CABG include advanced age, aortic arch atheromatous disease, prior stroke or documented cerebrovascular disease, recent myocardial infarction, left ventricular dysfunction, hypertension, diabetes, chronic renal insufficiency, and postoperative atrial fibrillation. Patients with stroke were more likely to have longer cross-clamp and total CPB times and postoperative low cardiac output.
      (2) Intracranial hemorrhage: Rare, due to hemorrhagic transformation of bland infarcts, coagulopathies in the critically ill, or after cardiac transplantation.

   b. Encephalopathy and cognitive dysfunction: Associated with markers of systemic hypotension, such as postoperative pressor or intraaortic balloon pump support, as well as multifocal microembolization. Risk factors for cognitive decline include advanced age, hypertension, diabetes, excessive alcohol consumption, postoperative atrial fibrillation, a history of peripheral vascular disease or prior CABG, and cerebral atrophy by neuroimaging.

   c. Seizures: Occur typically in the setting of an ischemic stroke.

   d. Peripheral nerve injuries: Typically due to traction or compression, although the phrenic nerve can be injured by iced solution in the mediastinum.

   e. Coma: Results from multifocal cerebral infarction, infarction with herniation, or a diffuse global hypoxic-ischemic insult.

   f. Pituitary apoplexy

2. Neurologic complications of CE
   a. Stroke: The most feared complication of CE; stroke prevention is the primary goal of surgery.
      (1) Ischemic stroke: Complicates 3% to 10% of surgeries. Embolism of plaque or platelet-fibrin debris can produce minor or major cerebral ischemia, but major stroke is more often due to carotid thrombosis.
      (2) Intracerebral hemorrhage: Rare, <1%, attributed to cerebral hyperperfusion from abnormal cerebral autoregulation. Risk factors for hemorrhage include preoperative cerebral infarction, postoperative hypertension, and correction of a severe stenosis.

   b. Seizures: May precede a hemorrhagic stroke or complicate an ischemic stroke.

   c. Peripheral nerve injuries: Frequent complications (3% to 9%) manifest as assymetric grimacing, hoarseness, or dysphagia.

Mechanisms of Cerebral Injury

• Embolization

• Macro and/or microemboli of various composition (e.g., platelet-fibrin thrombus, atherosclerotic plaque, material in the CPB circuit) can be multi-focal

• Hypoperfusion

  • Inadequate collateral flow

  • Low cerebral perfusion pressure

• Impaired cerebral microcirculation from activation of the inflammatory cascade

---

Clinical Features

1. Stroke: Ischemic syndromes are those of embolism or borderzone infarcts while hemorrhages are typically seen in the lobar white matter or basal ganglia.

2. Coma: "Failure to awaken" from surgery without metabolic cause

3. Encephalopathy: Confusional state with inattention or agitated delirium, cognitive impairment, personality change with depression

4. Seizures: Often in association with a stroke and reflect the focal deficits.

5. Peripheral nerve injuries

   a. After cardiac surgery: Lower trunk brachial plexus, phrenic, ulnar, peroneal, and femoral nerves as well as other sites of vein or artery harvesting.

   b. After carotid endarterectomy: Mandibular branch of the facial nerve, greater auricular, superior laryngeal, hypoglossal, and glossopharyngeal nerves

   c. Pituitary apoplexy: Painful ophthalmoplegia and visual loss upon awakening from surgery.

Complications of Cardiac or Carotid Artery Surgery

• Stroke, ischemic or hemorrhagic

• Coma, "failure to awaken" after surgery

• Encephalopathy and cognitive dysfunction

• Seizures

• Peripheral nerve injuries

Laboratory Testing and Radiologic Features

1. Neuroimaging: Computed tomography (CT) scanning is typically performed to exclude hemorrhage or assess for major infarction that could be complicated by life-threatening brain swelling. Magnetic resonance imaging (MRI) is more sensitive for infarction but requires compatible infusion and ventilator equipment and additional patient cooperation.

2. Vascular imaging: Ultrasound techniques, Duplex carotid ultrasound or transcranial Doppler are useful in the acute setting to assess for stenosis or thrombosis; transthoracic or transesophageal echocardiography can evaluate for proximal sources of embolism.

3. Neuropsychological testing: Although more commonly performed in clinical research, test batteries can be helpful in assessing unresolved cognitive complaints.

4. Electrodiagnostic studies: Electroencephalography is used in the diagnosis and monitoring of patients with seizures, and electromyography is useful in the evaluation of peripheral nerve injuries.

5. Miscellaneous: Suspected vocal cord dysfunction can be assessed with fiberoptic laryngeal examination, and visual complaints can be clarified with ophthalmologic evaluation and assessment of visual fields.

 Key Tests

• CT

• MRI

• Duplex carotid ultrasound

• Transcranial Doppler ultrasound

• Transesophageal echocardiography

• Fiberoptic laryngeal examination

• Ophthalmologic evaluation and assessment of visual fields

Treatment

1. Thrombolysis for acute ischemic stroke: Options for treating acute ischemic stroke are complicated by determining the time of onset in an anesthetized patient as well as the postoperative state, which is an exclusion criterion in clinical trials. Preliminary experience with intraarterial thrombolysis within hours of acute ischemic stroke has met with mixed

success in recanalization but few major hemorrhagic complications when performed within several days of cardiac surgery.

2. Endovascular therapies for postoperative acute ischemic stroke: The technology of mechanical clot disruption and extraction methods is under investigation.

3. Neuroprotective strategies: Under investigation; surgery offers a clinical setting in which the nature and exact timing of a potential cerebral injury can be predicted. It affords a unique opportunity to ameliorate neural injury with treatment prior to and during the operation.

Key Treatment

Acute Ischemic Stroke

- Thrombolysis

Postoperative Acute Ischemic Stroke

- Mechanical clot disruption and extraction methods (under investigation)

Prognosis and Complications

1. Stroke: Patients who develop stroke after CABG have a 3–5-fold higher in-hospital mortality rate, as well as greater ICU and hospital length of stay, and discharge to extended-care facilities.

2. Coma: The prognosis of postoperative nonmetabolic coma, with or without nonconvulsive status epilepticus, is extremely poor, with an 85% mortality rate and a <5% chance of useful neurologic recovery.

3. Encephalopathy

   a. Mental status screening exam: Abnormal in 3% to 12% on the fourth postoperative day, although 80% recover by the time of discharge.

   b. Neuropsychological testing: Prospective studies employing extensive neuropsychological test batteries have found that 35% to 75% of patients have impairments in cognitive function after cardiac surgery and 10% to 30% have persistent significant deficits at 3 to 6 months, particularly in attention, concentration, memory, and the speed of mental and motor responses. Those who experience early cognitive decline, particularly older patients and those with lower levels of education, are also more likely to develop late cognitive deterioration.

Prevention

1. Complications of cardiac surgery

   a. Modifications of the CPB circuit: Membrane oxygenators, in-line filtration, and aortic embolic capture devices to reduce macroembolization; heparin-bonded and closed circuits to reduce activation of the inflammatory and coagulation systems

   b. Eliminating CPB: "Off-pump" surgery to avoiding the risks of aortic manipulation.

   c. Prophylactic treatment of concomitant carotid stenosis: Controversial, as prophylactic carotid endarterectomy has not been proven to reduce the risk of stroke with coronary artery bypass surgery; however, carotid stenting is currently being evaluated in several trials targeting high-risk patients with coronary artery disease warranting revascularization.

   d. Aspirin, started within 48 hours after surgery, results in a 62% reduction in stroke and encephalopathy.

2. Complications of carotid surgery: Some surgeons shunt routinely and others use intraoperative monitoring to shunt selectively. Monitoring techniques include electroencephalography, measurement of stump pressure, somatosensory evoked potentials, and transcranial Doppler ultrasound.

Bibliography

Katzan I, Masaryk TJ, Furlan AJ, et al.: Intra-arterial thrombolysis for perioperative stroke after open heart surgery. Neurology 52:1081–1084, 1999.

Lederman RJ, Breuer AC, Hanson MR, et al.: Peripheral nervous system complications of coronary artery bypass graft surgery. Ann Neurol 12:297–301, 1982.

Mangano DT: Aspirin and mortality from coronary bypass surgery. N Engl J Med 347:1309–1317, 2002.

Newman MF, Kircher JL, Phillips-Bute B, et al.: Longitudinal assessment of neurocognitive function after coronary artery bypass surgery. N Engl J Med 344: 451–452, 2001.

Roach GW, Kanchuger M, Mangano CM, et al.: Adverse cerebral outcomes after coronary bypass surgery. N Engl J Med 335:1857–1863, 1996.

Rothwell PM, Slattery J, Warlow CP: A systematic comparison of the risks of stroke and death due to carotid endarterectomy for symptomatic and asymptomatic stenosis. Stroke 27:266–269, 1996.

Wolman RL, Nussmeier NA, Aggarwal A, et al.: Cerebral injury after cardiac surgery: Identification of a group at extraordinary risk. Multicenter Study of Perioperative Ischemia Research Group (McSPI) and the Ischemia Research Education Foundation (IREF) Investigators. Stroke 30:514–522, 1999.

2 Organ Transplantation

Jin-Moo Lee
Evan Allen

Definition

1. Organ transplantation has seen exponential growth over the last 4 decades, owing to the advent of more powerful and precise immunosuppressive agents and improved surgical techniques. With this growth in transplants, neurologic complications have become a large contributor to iatrogenic disorders evaluated and managed by neurologists.

2. Transplantation is reserved for patients suffering imminent or impending organ failure, frequently resulting in signs and symptoms referable to the nervous system. These neurologic disorders of organ failure, which are often evident in patients early after transplantation, are discussed in Part XXI, Chapter 2, Liver and Kidney Failure.

3. Some neurologic complications resulting from major surgical procedures or immunosuppression are common to all organ transplants; however, others are unique to specific transplanted organs.

Neurologic Complications Common to All Transplanted Organs

1. Encephalopathy (and seizures)

    a. Definition: Derangement in consciousness, ranging from confusion, to drowsiness, to stupor, to coma. Seizures are frequently associated with encephalopathy.

    b. Etiologies: Often multifactorial; the time course of symptom onset may help determine the underlying cause.

        (1) Immediate postoperative period (<48 hours)

            (a) Hypoxic-ischemic insults or strokes

            (b) Metabolic abnormalities caused by renal and/or hepatic dysfunction or sepsis

            (c) Sedative or anesthetic agents, especially in the setting of poor excretion or metabolism as a consequence of renal or liver failure

        (2) Two to 14 days after transplant

            (a) Cyclosporine or FK506 toxicity, especially if administered intravenously

            (see Part XXIV, Chapter 6, Effects of Immunosuppressive Therapies)

            (b) Intensive care unit psychosis: May resolve with neuroleptics or environmental reorientation

            (c) Central pontine myelinolysis (CPM) (see below)

        (3) Beyond 2 weeks

            (a) Sepsis

            (b) Central nervous system (CNS) infections, including meningitis or abscess (see below)

            (c) Steroid psychosis

    c. Clinical features

        (1) Hepatic encephalopathy: Associated with asterixis; sometimes seizures

        (2) Uremic encephalopathy: Associated with nausea, vomiting, and uremic myoclonus

        (3) Cyclosporine or FK506 toxicity: May manifest with cortical blindness and visual hallucinations, or ataxia, cerebellar tumor, and seizures (focal or generalized)

        (4) Focal seizures are often associated with structural lesions (e.g., stroke or abscess).

    d. Laboratory testing

        (1) Serum metabolic panel, including blood urea nitrogen, creatinine, liver function tests

        (2) Cyclosporine or FK506 levels

        (3) For acute evaluation, head computed tomography (CT) to evaluate intracerebral hemorrhage

        (4) Magnetic resonance imaging (MRI) can detect focal lesions (e.g., stroke, abscess) or diffuse lesions (e.g., hypoxic-ischemic injury, posterior leukoencephalopathy consistent with cyclosporine or FK506 toxicity, or pontine demyelination consistent with CPM).

        (5) Electroencephalography (EEG) is helpful in diagnosing hepatic encephalopathy (triphasic waves), sedative toxicity (excess fast activity), and helpful in localizing a focus for seizures.

        (6) Lumbar puncture should be performed with any suspicion of infection

Key Tests: When Indicated

- Metabolic panel
- Cyclosporine or FK506 levels
- CT or MRI of the head
- EEG
- Lumbar puncture

e. Treatment
  (1) Encephalopathy
    (a) Rapid diagnosis and treatment of multifactorial etiologies may hasten resolution.
    (b) Often dose reduction, rather than discontinuation, of immunosuppressants is effective.
  (2) Seizures
    (a) Frequently, seizures in the setting of transplantation are transient and merely require correction of the metabolic derangement or adjustment of immunosuppressant dosing.
    (b) In cases of refractory seizures, benzodiazepines are best for short-term management. Gabapentin, which has no enzyme-inducing properties, few systemic side effects, and little interaction with commonly used drugs in transplantation, may also be used.

Neuropathies

1. Incidence ranges from 5% of renal transplants to 13% of patients undergoing cardiac procedures.
2. Causes: Occur during the transplant procedure
   a. Malpositioning of pharmacologically paralyzed patients
   b. Stretching due to prolonged retraction
   c. Local hematoma formation with compression
3. Syndromes
   a. Ulnar nerve
     (1) The most common nerve injured under general anesthesia, usually at the cubital tunnel
     (2) Hypesthesia of the 4th and 5th digits and difficulty with finger flexion
   b. Femoral and lateral femoral cutaneous nerves
     (1) Complications of renal transplants
     (2) Femoral nerve: Loss of leg extension at the knee, and weakness of hip flexion
     (3) Lateral femoral cutaneous nerve: Hypes-

thesia or hyperesthesia of the anterolateral aspect of the thigh
   c. Lower brachial plexus stretch injury
     (1) Complication of heart transplants
     (2) Weakness and numbness in the distal arm, often with diminished triceps reflex
   d. Phrenic nerve
     (1) Complication of heart transplants
     (2) Diaphragmatic paralysis and difficulty weaning from mechanical ventilation or prolonged postoperative hiccups
4. Laboratory testing
   a. EMG and nerve conduction studies may be helpful for localizing and diagnosing compression/stretch neuropathies and may provide prognostic information.
   b. Chest x-ray assessing diaphragmatic positioning may help diagnose phrenic nerve injury.
5. Treatment: Mainly conservative management and physical therapy

Complications from Immunosuppressants
(see Part XXIV, Chapter 6)

1. CNS infections
   a. Epidemiology
     (1) CNS infection complicates 5% to 10% of all transplantations, with a mortality rate of 44% to 77%.
     (2) CNS infections are largely due to long-term immunosuppression.
     (3) The causative organism can frequently be deduced by the time interval between the transplant and infection and clinical features.
   b. Etiology: The timing of the infection may help determine the causative organism.
     (1) During the first month after transplantation: Risk for CNS infection is low, but indwelling catheters, endotracheal intubation, and donor organ infections may contribute to systemic infections. Primary organisms found in donor organs or in recipients prior to transplant include *Mycobacterium tuberculosis* and *Stongyloides stercoralis.*
     (2) Between months 1 and 6: Immunosuppression is maximal, thus the risk for CNS infection is at its highest. Viruses (e.g., cytomegalovirus, Epstein-Barr virus) and opportunistic organisms (e.g., *Listeria monocytogenes, Cryptococcus neoformans,* and *Aspergillus fumigatus,* which

cause up to 80% of CNS infections) predominate.

(3) Beyond the sixth month: The patient is at risk for pathogens that infect the general community and activation of opportunistic organisms.

Organisms Causing CNS Infections

Viruses

• CMV

• EBV

Opportunistic Organisms

• *Listeria monocytogenes*

• *Cryptococcus neoformans*

• *Aspergillus fumigatus*

---

c. Clinical features

(1) Typical signs of CNS infection may be blunted or absent in immunosuppressed patients.

(2) The causative organism is often found outside of the CNS.

(a) *Cryptococcus* skin lesions (ranging from small papules to large cellulitic lesions) occur in 20% of patients in the weeks preceding CNS infection.

(b) CNS *Aspergillus* is often accompanied by pulmonary or paranasal sinus infection.

(3) The causative organism is sometimes suggested by clinical symptoms.

(a) Acute bacterial meningitis is most commonly caused by *Listeria monocytogenes*.

(b) Subacute and chronic meningitis are most commonly caused by *Cryptococcus neoformans*.

(c) CNS abscesses are most commonly caused by *Aspergillus fumigatus, Nocardia asteroides,* and *Toxoplasma gondii*.

d. Laboratory testing (see Part XVIII, Infectious Disorders, for specifics)

(1) A very low threshold for lumbar puncture is essential for early diagnosis to improve patient survival and functional recovery.

(2) MRI is superior to CT in diagnosing CNS abscesses.

(3) A CNS work-up is indicated when *Aspergillus* or *Cryptococcus* infections are found

in the lungs because these organisms frequently spread to the CNS.

Key Tests

• Lumbar puncture

• MRI is superior to CT for diagnosing CNS abscesses.

• CNS work-up is indicated when *Aspergillus* or *Cryptococcus* infections are found in the lungs.

e. Treatment (see Part XVIII, Infectious Disorders, for treatment of specific organisms)

Neurologic Complications Unique to Each Organ System

1. Kidney

a. Epidemiology

(1) Most frequently transplanted organ (>10,000 transplants per year worldwide)

(2) Most accepted therapy for end-stage renal failure from glomerulonephritis, diabetes, hypertensive kidney disease, pyelonephritis, polycystic kidney disease, or systemic lupus erythematosus (SLE)

(3) One-year survival for transplant recipients is 100%, but neurologic complications occur in up to 30%.

b. Perioperative complications

(1) Renal transplantation itself carries little risk aside from the risks of general anesthesia

(2) Compressive neuropathies: Seen in 1.5% to 8.4% of patients

(a) Femoral nerve: Caused by local hematoma formation

(b) Lateral femoral cutaneous nerve: Usually caused by retraction

(3) Spinal cord ischemia

(a) Rare complication

(b) Seen in patients with anomalous blood supply to the distal spinal cord (blood to caudal cord is supplied by branches of the internal iliac artery, rather than intercostal arteries)

(c) When the iliac artery is used to supply blood to the allograft, spinal cord ischemia may result.

c. Long-term complications: Cerebrovascular events

(1) Most common neurologic complication after renal transplant (9.5% of patients)

(2) Most events occur well after transplant (>6 months)

(3) High incidence related to underlying disease for which renal transplants are performed: Diabetes, hypertension, and SLE

(4) Other risk factors found in this population: Elevated cholesterol, triglycerides, and lipoproteins; hematologic abnormalities; and secondary polycythemia vera

2. Liver

a. Epidemiology

(1) Indications for liver transplant include viral hepatitis, alcoholic liver disease, primary biliary cirrhosis, acute liver failure or toxins, and cholangitis.

(2) One-year survival for transplant recipients is 83% and carries a high risk of complications.

(3) Neurologic complications occur in up to 80% of patients.

(a) Most important causes of morbidity and mortality

(b) Due to difficulties of the surgical procedure itself, *and* the precarious state of the patient before surgery (patients usually have some degree of hepatic encephalopathy before surgery, and patients are prone to CNS hemorrhages as a result of coagulopathies associated with liver failure)

b. Neurologic complications

(1) Encephalopathy

(a) Most common neurologic complication

(b) Causes

(i) Metabolic derangements include preexisting hepatic encephalopathy (see Part XXI, Chapter 2, Liver and Kidney Failure)

(ii) Hypoxic-ischemic injury: Significant blood loss during the transplant procedure, often requires massive replacement of blood and electrolytes, predisposing patients to hypoxic-ischemic injury

(iii) Drug toxicity, especially due to cyclosporine or FK506

(iv) Sepsis

(2) Central pontine myelinolysis

(a) Unusual neurologic disorder that occurs at increased frequency in liver transplant patients (7% to 19% in autopsy series)

(b) Symmetric noninflammatory demyelination of the basis pontis with relative sparing of neurons and axons (can be diagnosed by MRI)

(c) Cause is unknown, but it is thought to be the result of rapid correction of hyponatremia (during the transplant procedure, wide fluctuations in serum sodium concentrations occur as a result of the rapid replacement of intraoperative blood loss with intravenous fluids and blood products that contain high concentrations of sodium)

(d) Clinical manifestations include altered mental status or coma, pseudobulbar palsy, and quadriplegia.

(3) Lower brachial plexopathy

(a) Most common peripheral nerve injury (6% of transplant patients)

(b) Injury occurs during the axillary dissection required for access to the axillary vein for venovenous bypass.

3. Heart

a. Epidemiology

(1) Indications for heart transplant include cardiomyopathies, atherosclerotic cardiovascular disease, valvular heart disease, and congenital heart defects.

(2) Although graft rejection and infection are major complications, neurologic complications may occur in up to 60% of patients.

b. Neurologic complications

(1) Complications of cardiopulmonary bypass

(a) Embolic stroke: Causes

(i) Cannulation of a diseased aorta can dislodge atheromatous material.

(ii) Risk of air emboli introduced after release of aortic cross-clamp

(iii) During extracorporeal circulation, exposure of blood to nonendothelial surfaces increases the risk of embolus formation from platelet aggregation or disruption of fibrin.

(b) Intracerebral hemorrhage: Causes

(i) Consumption of platelets and coagulation factors during extracorporeal circulation

(ii) Use of anticoagulants during cardiopulmonary bypass

(c) Hypoxic-ischemic events: Causes
  (i) Prolonged bypass times
  (ii) Hypotension

(2) Encephalopathy and seizures: Time of symptom onset may suggest etiology

  (a) Immediate postoperative period: Suggests hypoxic-ischemic injury (for encephalopathy) or focal stroke (sometimes leading to focal seizures)

  (b) Late postoperative period: Suggests metabolic disturbances, drugs, multiple organ failure, or sepsis

(3) Peripheral nervous system injuries

  (a) Lower brachial plexus injury caused by stretching during chest wall retraction or compression by hematoma

  (b) Recurrent laryngeal nerve injury (due to traction) may result in vocal cord paralysis.

  (c) Phrenic nerve injury, a cold-induced injury from packing the heart in ice at the time of transplantation, may lead to diaphragmatic paralysis and difficulty weaning from mechanical ventilation or prolonged postoperative hiccups.

(4) After transplantation, patients remain at risk for cerebrovascular events from cardiac emboli, underlying atherosclerosis, and postoperative arrhythmias

4. Lung
  a. Epidemiology
    (1) Relatively new procedure (first successful transplant in 1983) with little data available regarding neurologic complications
    (2) Indications for lung transplant include emphysema (including α_1-antitrypsin deficiency), cystic fibrosis, pulmonary hypertension, idiopathic pulmonary fibrosis, and obliterative bronchiolitis.

    (3) One-year survival: 90% for single-lung transplant; 80% for bilateral lung transplant
  b. Neurologic complications are similar to heart transplant patients and include encephalopathy, cerebrovascular events (ischemic stroke, watershed infarcts, and hemorrhages), seizures, and neuropathy (including phrenic nerve injury).

5. Pancreas
  a. Epidemiology
    (1) Relatively rare procedure
    (2) Transplants are performed in type 1 diabetes patients with extensive end-organ damage (frequently in combination with renal transplants).

  b. Neurologic complications are mostly related to the underlying diabetes and resultant end-organ damage, including nephropathy, neuropathy, retinopathy, accelerated atherosclerosis with resultant stroke, myocardial infarction, and peripheral vascular disease.

Bibliography

Adams H, Dawson G, Coffman T, et al.: Stroke in renal transplant patients. Arch Neurol 43:113, 1986.

Andrefsky JC, Frank JI: Complications of organ transplantation. In Biller J (ed): Iatrogenic Neurology. Boston, Butterworth-Heinemann, 1998, p. 89.

Beresford TP: Neuropsychiatric complications of liver and other solid organ transplantation. Liver Transpl 7(Suppl 1) S36–S45, 2001.

Lee J-M, Raps EC: Neurological complications of transplantation. In Evans RW (ed): Neurologic Clinics of North America: Iatrogenic Disorders, vol. 16. Philadelphia, W. B. Saunders, 1998, p. 21.

Patchell RA: Neurological complications of organ transplantation. Ann Neurol 36:688, 1994.

Sila C: Spectrum of neurologic events following cardiac transplantation. Stroke 20:1586, 1989.

Stein D, Lederman R, Vogt D, et al.: Neurological complications following liver transplantation. Ann Neurol 31:644, 1992.

3 Drug-Induced Movement Disorders

Alireza Minagar
Lisa M. Shulman
William J. Weiner

Definition

1. Movement disorders can be categorized as primary idiopathic conditions and those that are precipitated secondarily owing to a specific cause or insult. Drugs, especially those used for treatment of psychiatric diseases (also known as neuroleptics) (Table 3–1) are the most single cause of secondary movement disorders. Movement disorders can also be an adverse reaction to nonneuroleptic drugs. The clinical spectrum of drug-induced movement disorders includes both hyperkinetic movements (excessive motor activity such as dyskinesia) and hypokinetic movements (decreased spontaneous movements such as bradykinesia).

2. Drug-induced movement disorders (DIMDs) include (Sethi, 2001; Wirshing, 2001)
   a. Acute dystonia
   b. Akathisia
   c. Neuroleptic malignant syndrome
   d. Tardive dyskinesia
   e. Neuroleptic-induced parkinsonism (see Part V, Chapter 1, Parkinson's Disease)
   f. Asterixis (Table 3–2)
   g. Chorea (Table 3–3)

Epidemiology and Risk Factors

1. The incidence of DIMDs is unknown and difficult to define. Many drugs administered for various

TABLE 3–1. NEUROLEPTIC DRUGS AND RELATED AGENTS

Phenothiazines	**Thioxanthenes**
Prochlorperazine	Thiothixene
Perphenazine and amitriptyline	Chlorprothixene
Thioridazine	
Promethazine	**Benzamide**
Fluphenazine	Metoclopramide
Mesoridazine	
Trifluoperazine	**Dihydroindolone**
Chlorpromazine	Molindone
Thiethylperazine	
Perphenazine	**Dibenzoxazepine**
	Loxapine
Butyrophenones	
Haloperidol	**Dibenzodiazepine**
Droperidol	Clozapine

TABLE 3–2. DRUGS ASSOCIATED WITH ASTERIXIS

Antiepileptics: phenobarbitone, valproic acid, primidone, carbamazepine
Ceftazidime
Methyldopa
Metrizamide used for myelography

reasons are potentially insulting. Such estimation is further confounded by the diversity of the clinical manifestations and their varied severity. It is likely that DIMDs are common and frequently unrecognized. Patients with acquired immunodeficiency syndrome (AIDS) and degenerative neurologic disorders such as Parkinson's disease are highly susceptible to DIMD.

2. Approximately 2% to 5% of patients develop dystonia within days (occasionally) or hours of beginning therapy with neuroleptics. Acute dystonia is more common in men and young patients in general, with the peak incidence under age 15 years. It decreases with age and becomes uncommon after age 40.

3. Akathisia has no age or gender predilection; however, both dystonia and akathisia are more common with high-potency neuroleptics, high doses of drugs, and depot injections.

4. Neuroleptic malignant syndrome (NMS) is rare, occurring in fewer than 1% of neuroleptic-treated patients. Preexisting physical exhaustion, dehydration, thyroid disorders, and metabolic disorders are risk factors for NMS.

5. It is estimated that almost 15% of patients treated chronically with neuroleptics have tardive dyskinesia (TD). It occurs relatively late in the course of drug therapy. The first manifestations of TD usually appear after many months or years of neuroleptic therapy; occasionally, the movements present only when the insulting drug is discontinued or the dose is decreased. TD appears to be dependent on age, with a dramatic rise in occurrence in individuals over 40 years of age. Women are affected more often than men, and neuroleptic-treated patients with affective disorders (in contrast to schizophrenia) may be more susceptible to TD.

TABLE 3–3.   DRUGS ASSOCIATED WITH CHOREA

Neuroleptics
Aminophylline
Theophylline
Amphetamines
Amoxapine
Anabolic steroids
Anticholinergics: benzhexol
Antiepileptics
   Carbamazepine
   Ethosuximide
   Phenobarbital
   Phenytoin
   Valproic acid
   Gabapentin (Neurontin)
Cimetidine
Cocaine
Cyclosporin
Levodopa
Lithium
Oral contraceptives
Tricyclic antidepressants

Etiology and Pathophysiology

1. All theoretical explanations are based on the clinical observation that dopaminergic receptor blockade induces acute dystonia and akathisia. Two major hypotheses on mechanism of acute dystonia are based on a hypo- or hyperdopaminergic state associated with dopamine (DA) receptor blockade in the caudate, putamen, or globus pallidus.

2. It is also known that neuroleptics induced an increase in striatal acetylcholine and cholinergic agents induced dystonia in neuroleptic-primed monkeys, both of which were reversed by anticholinergic agents.

3. The role of γ-aminobutyric acid (GABA) and serotonin in acute dystonia is much less well studied. GABA agonists such as picrotoxin exacerbate dystonia.

Clinical Features

1. Acute dystonia consists of involuntary sustained muscular contractions, causing an abnormal posture that usually persists 20 to 30 minutes at a time and is painful. It may take the form of overextension or overflexion of the head, torsion of the spine with arching and twisting the back, or forceful closure of the eyes and a fixed grimace (Table 3–2).

2. Akathisia is the inability to rest and stay still because of a sense of inner restlessness. It manifests with wiggling legs, pacing, or rocking from foot to foot.

3. NMS manifests with hyperthermia, severe muscle rigidity, altered sensorium (confusion, disorientation, mutism, stupor, coma), and autonomic dysfunction (tachycardia, tachypnea, fluctuations of blood pressure, excessive sweating, incontinence). Occasionally, hyperkinetic features such as tremor and dystonia are observed. Seizures and coma may ensue. NMS is a potentially life-threatening idiosyncratic reaction that demands immediate attention and treatment. Patients who have recovered from NMS are at higher risk of developing NMS once again with future antipsychotic use.

4. Tardive dyskinesia is an abnormal involuntary movement disorder resulting from the chronic (<3 months) use of neuroleptics. TD is a choreic disorder. The choreic movements are usually nonpatterned, but in the context of TD they may be patterned. The most frequent clinical manifestation is orofacial dyskinesias, but it may affect the truck and extremity muscles too. Variants of TD include tardive dystonia, tardive akathisia, tardive Tourette-like syndrome, tardive myoclonus, and withdrawal dyskinesia.

5. Asterixis consists of arrhythmic lapses of sustained posture in which the sudden interruptions of muscular contraction allow gravity or the inherent elasticity of muscles to generate a movement, which the patient then corrects, sometimes with overshoot. Asterixis was originally observed in patients with hepatic encephalopathy. It is also observed in patients with drug-induced hepatic encephalopathy.

6. Chorea consists of involuntary, sudden, abrupt nonrhythmic, unpatterned muscular jerks with variable and unpredictable timing and anatomic distribution.

Key Signs

- Acute dystonia

  —Overextension or overflexion of the head

  —Torsion of the spine, with arching and twisting the back

  —Forceful closure of the eyes and a fixed grimace

- Akathisia

  —Wriggling legs

  —Pacing

  —Rocking from foot to foot

- Neuroleptic malignant syndrome

  —Hyperthermia

  —Severe muscle rigidity

  —Altered sensorium (confusion, disorientation, mutism, stupor, coma)

  —Autonomic dysfunction (tachycardia, tachypnea, fluctuations of blood pressure, excessive sweating, incontinence)

- Tardive dyskinesia

  —Orofacial dyskinesias; truck and extremity muscles may also be affected

- Asterixis

  —Arrhythmic lapses of sustained posture

- Chorea

  —Involuntary, sudden, abrupt nonrhythmic, unpatterned muscular jerks

  —Jerks of variable and unpredictable timing

Differential Diagnosis

1. Acute reactions to drugs are easily recognized. Naturally occurring dystonic reactions (e.g., torticollis, blepharospasm, writer's cramp) are of gradual onset, present in nonpsychiatric patients, involve no precipitating drugs, and do not resolve.

2. Other differential diagnoses of acute dystonic reaction include tonic focal seizures, hypocalcemia with carpopedal spasm, and muscle spasm due to bony injury or subluxation.

3. Akathisia may be mistaken as mania, intoxication with psychostimulant agents, drug withdrawal, an agitated emotional state, or restless leg syndrome.

Laboratory Testing

Usually no laboratory work-up is necessary for dystonia or akathisia. The diagnosis of NMS is supported by finding an elevated serum creatine kinase level, but this finding is highly nonspecific.

Key Tests

- No laboratory tests are necessary for dystonia or akathisia.

Treatment

1. Dystonia is treated by reducing the neuroleptic dosage or total withdrawal of the drug. Acute dystonia is treated with intramuscular or intravenous administration of benztropine, diphenhydramine, or diazepam; or it resolves spontaneously regardless of whether the insulting drug is discontinued. Prophylaxis with anticholinergic agents or diphenhydramine decreases the risk.

2. Akathisia can be treated.

   a. Beta-blockers: propranolol at doses as low as 10 to 20 mg three times daily

   b. Benzodiazepines such as diazepam and lorazepam

   c. In summary, the best approach to akathisia depends on the clinical picture and if the psychosis is diminishing. Akathisia should be treated with anticholinergics if parkinsonism is present. If parkinsonism is absent, propranolol should be administered. If psychosis persists with akathisia present, a neuroleptic of a different class and with lower potency is recommended.

3. The significant steps for treating patients with NMS are discontinuing the neuroleptic and basic supportive care, including correction of fluid and electrolyte imbalance, cooling the patient, and management of renal, pulmonary, and cardiac complications. Drugs that have been used in the management of NMS are dantrolene, bromocriptine, lisuride, benzodiazepines, and N-methyl-D-aspartate (NMDA) receptor blockers (amantadine, memantine).

4. There are various treatment approaches for the treatment of drug-induced TD.

   a. Lowering the neuroleptic dose or, if not possible, switching to a lower-potency neuroleptic

   b. Propranolol, a β_1 and β_2 lipophilic antagonist, 40 to 240 mg/day

   c. Clonidine 0.1 to 0.3 mg/day

   d. GABA agonists: clonazepam 0.5 to 3.0 mg/day, diazepam 2 to 20 mg/day, valproate 250 to 1500 mg/day, baclofen 10 to 60 mg/day

   e. Anticholinergics: trihexylphenidyl 2 to 20 mg/day

   f. Dopamine-depleting agents: tetrabenazine 50 to 200 mg/day

Key Treatment

- Dystonia
  - Reduction or discontinuance of neuroleptic
- Acute dystonia
  - Benztropine
  - Diphenhydramine or diazepam
  - Condition may resolve spontaneously
- Akathisia
  - Propranolol
  - Diazepam
  - Lorazepam
- Neuroleptic malignant syndrome
  - Discontinuation of neuroleptic
  - Supportive care (i.e., correction of fluid and electrolyte imbalance, cooling the patient, and management of renal, pulmonary, and cardiac complications)
  - Various drugs (e.g., dantrolene, bromocriptine, lisuride, benzodiazepines)

- Tardive dyskinesia
  - Reducing the dose or switching to a lower-potency neuroleptic
  - Propranolol
  - Clonidine
  - GABA agonists: clonazepam, diazepam, valproate, baclofen
  - Trihexylphenidyl
  - Tetrabenazine

Bibliography

Caroff SN, Mann SC, Campbell EC, Sullivan KA: Movement disorders associated with atypical antipsychotic drugs. J Clin Psychiatry 4(Suppl):12–19, 2002.

Rodnitzky RL: Drug-induced movement disorders. Clin Neuropharmacol 25:142–152, 2002.

Sethi KD: Movement disorders induced by dopamine blocking agents. Semin Neurol 21:59–68, 2001.

Susman VL: Clinical management of neuroleptic malignant syndrome. Psychiatr Q 72:325–336, 2001.

Wirshing WC: Movement disorders associated with neuroleptic treatment. J Clin Psychiatry 62(Suppl 21):15–18, 2001.

4 Cognitive Side Effects of Medications

Brian W. Smith

Definition

This chapter will focus on the primary or direct effect of drugs on cognitive function. Drugs producing secondary effects (i.e., by drug-induced disturbances of other organs or systems, e.g., drug-induced hepatic or hypoglycemic encephalopathy) will be only briefly covered. Cognitive effects will include delirium and dementia, with occasional mention of other neurologic effects if directly related or part of a syndrome.

Epidemiology and Risk Factors

1. Numerous factors influence the response to medications. The following items address the risk factors related to patients and to drugs. Direct mechanisms of neurotoxicity are discussed later, under Etiology and Pathophysiology.

2. Advanced age is a risk factor for increased side effects to medication and may be related to various factors, including decreases in albumin with increased levels of free drug; decrease in blood flow and metabolism in liver and kidneys; brain changes including loss of neurons, synaptic connections, neurotransmitters; and increased use of medications.

3. Neurologic disorders with compromised brain function such as strokes, degenerative diseases (Alzheimer's, multiple sclerosis, AIDS), tumors, seizures, and head injuries may result in an increase in adverse responses.

4. Systemic diseases, especially those with involvement of the liver and kidneys, may result in decreased threshold to medication effects.

5. Drug-related factors that increase adverse response include dose, route of administration, rate of delivery, and drug interactions.

6. Polypharmacy markedly increases the risk of side effects, with possible mechanisms including changes in plasma concentration, receptor activities, and idiosyncratic interactions.

7. Alcohol, drug addiction, and recent surgery may predispose patients to cognitive side effects.

Key Risk Factors

- Age
- Dosing schedule
- Polypharmacy
- Underlying systemic or neurologic disease

Etiology and Pathophysiology

1. Several factors may both influence drug effects on the central nervous system (CNS) and produce neurotoxicity.

2. These factors may include the ability to penetrate the blood–brain barrier, disturbance of brain energy metabolism via changes in adenosine triphosphate function, oxygen delivery effects, and impact on enzyme activity.

2. Additional disturbances may include calcium influx, free radical formation, and effects on neurotransmitters.

3. Direct effects on neurotransmitters include inhibitory effects on the cholinergic system (e.g., anticholinergic medications); agonist effects on GABA receptors (e.g., benzodiazepines); and inhibition of noradrenergic receptors (e.g., antihypertensive agents).

Clinical Features

1. The two changes in cognitive function that will be primarily considered include delirium and dementia.

2. *Delirium* refers to an acute organic reaction consisiting of alteration in consciousness and attention. Disturbances may include hallucinations, emotional lability, memory impairment, sleep cycle disturbance, incoherent speech, and psychomotor agitation.

3. *Dementia* refers to a loss of intellectual function, which may include disturbances of memory, abstract thinking, or personality change that affects social function. In this context, the term refers to a drug reaction, and not to the development of a degenerative form of dementia.

947

4. Additional neurologic or clinical symptoms may be mentioned if associated with the cognitive changes (e.g., depression or leukoencephalopathy) or if part of a syndrome.

Key Signs

Delirium

- Hallucinations
- Emotional lability
- Memory impairment
- Sleep cycle disturbance
- Incoherent speech
- Psychomotor agitation

Dementia

- Memory disturbances
- Impaired abstract thinking
- Personality change that affects social function

Medications Causing Direct Cognitive Effects

Psychotropic Medications

1. Antidepressants
   a. Primarily seen with the tricyclic agents (amitriptyline, nortriptyline, amoxapine) secondary to anticholinergic effects. Confusional states, delirium, and memory impairment occur primarily in the elderly.
   b. Medication side effects may be difficult to differentiate from cognitive impairment caused by depression.
   c. The serotonin-specific reuptake inhibitors (SSRIs) such as fluoxetine, sertraline, and paroxetine, do not significantly produce the effects presented under Key Signs.
   d. Serotonin syndrome
      (1) Rare disorder resulting from central serotonergic hyperstimulation, usually from the simultaneous use of two or more serotonergic drugs.
      (2) Drugs associated include SSRIs, monoamine oxidase inhibitors (including selegiline), tricyclic antidepressants, St. John wort, L-tryptophan, lysergic acid diethylamide (LSD), lithium, L-dopa, buspirone, sumatriptan, 3,4-methylenedioxyethamphetamine (MDMA/Ectasy), dextromethorphan, meperidine, pentazocine, trazodone, cocaine, fenfluramine, and carbamazepine.
      (3) Diverse symptoms and signs with an onset from within minutes after receiving the second drug to weeks after being on a stable dose.
         (a) Neuromuscular: Myoclonus, hyperreflexia, Babinksi's sign, muscle rigidity, tremor, ataxia, shivering/chills, nystagmus, opisthotonos, trismus, oculogyric crisis, and rhabdomyolysis
         (b) Autonomic: Hyperthermia, diaphoresis, sinus tachycardia, hypertension, hypotension, tachypnea, dilated pupils, unreactive pupils, flushed skin, diarrhea, abdominal cramps, and salivation
         (c) Neuropsychiatric: Confusion, coma, dizziness, agitation, anxiety, hypomania, lethargy, seizures, insomnia, and hallucinations
         (d) Myoclonus and hyperreflexia present in over 50% of cases and shivering in up to 25%.
      (4) Diagnosis of exclusion
         (a) Neuromuscular malignant syndrome has some overlapping features including fever, rigidity, and altered consciousness.
         (b) Need to exclude infection, metabolic disorders, and drug withdrawal.
      (5) Treatment
         (a) Discontinuing medications that enhance serotonin transmission and supportive care
         (b) Benzodiazepines first choice for neuromuscular disorders and seizures
         (c) Many of the symptoms may respond to cyproheptadine.
         (d) With treatment, patients usually improve within 12 to 24 hours.
2. Neuroleptics
   a. Cognitive changes are not a common side effect and occur more prominently with neuroleptics that have anticholinergic effects (e.g., chlorpromazine and thioridazine) and with use in nonpsychotic individuals.
   b. Neuroleptic malignant syndrome should be considered when confusion is associated with hyperthermia and rigidity.
3. Lithium
   a. Cases of encephalopathy and memory loss occur more frequently with toxicity but can

also be seen with serum levels in the normal range.

b. Drug accumulation and intoxication may occur with renal failure.

c. Case reports include a Wernicke's encephalopathy and a reversible Creutzfeldt-Jakob–type syndrome.

Antiparkinson Medications

1. Includes both the dopaminergic (levodopa, bromocriptine, pergolide, pramipexole, and ropinirole) and anticholinergic (trihexyphenidyl, benztropine) agents.

2. Anticholinergics produce the more significant confusional states.

3. Hallucinations are the most common side effect of dopaminergic agents, but confusional events and delusions are reported, especially with higher doses.

Benzodiazepines

1. Confusional episodes occur from direct effects but more commonly from withdrawal, especially in the elderly.

2. Marked memory impairment and anterograde amnesia are well-documented side effects.

Cardiac Drugs

1. Anti-hypertensives

   a. The reports are somewhat sporadic and these side effects are generally felt to be uncommon except for the centrally acting agents. Chronic hypertension may also have an effect on cognitive function and may be difficult to differentiate from drug effects.

2. Beta-blockers

   a. Memory difficulties and depression are the most common negative cognitive effects.

   b. Psychoses, hypnagogic hallucinations and vivid nightmares usually occur with higher dosing.

3. Centrally acting agents

   a. Include the drugs methyldopa, clonidine, and reserpine.

   b. Clonidine has produced delirium, psychosis, and a reversible dementia.

   c. Methyldopa is associated with memory difficulties and confusion.

   d. Reserpine produces a dose-related depression.

4. Calcium channel blockers: This class of drugs may produce confusion and depression.

5. Angiotensin-converting enzyme inhibitors: Do not produce any significant cognitive side effects.

6. Digitalis

   a. Well documented to produce delirium, dementia, psychosis, and depression, which may result from drug-associated alterations in cardiac function.

   b. Cognitive side effects may occur in up to 15% of patients and correlate with plasma levels.

   c. Events suggestive of transient global amnesia have occurred and may represent intermittent cerebral hypoperfusion.

7. Antiarrhythmic drugs

   a. Lidocaine is associated with psychosis, agitation, and disinhibition, possibly secondary to diffuse neuronal excitation.

   b. Bretylium tosylate has been linked to reports of confusion, paranoid psychosis, and mood disturbance.

   c. Amiodorone produces a syndrome consisting of encephalopathy, ataxia, neuropathy, tremor, and dizziness.

   d. Disopyramide, flecainide, tocainide, and quinidine may produce a delirium.

Anticholinergics

1. Include several classes of drugs discussed in other sections, including the antidepressants and neuroleptics, in addition to the antihistamines such as meclizine and scopolamine.

2. This class commonly produces memory dysfunction, hallucinations, and delusions, especially in the elderly.

3. Additional features of toxicity may include fever, gait disturbance, and dilated pupils.

H2 Antagonists

1. Side effects are reported with cimetidine and less frequently with ranitidine and other newer agents.

2. Cognitive side effects may include delirium, psychosis, and depression.

Analgesics

1. Narcotics produce the most significant effects on cognition, resulting in delirium and impairment in memory.

2. Nonsteroid anti-inflammatory drugs rarely produce delirium and cognitive dysfunction.

Antimicrobials

1. Intravenous penicillin G, amoxicillin, erythromycin, and the cephalosporins have been associated with encphalopathy.

2. Sulfonamides may rarely produce an encephalopathy, most commonly occurring in patients with AIDS.

3. Isoniazid is associated with psychosis, probably secondary to deleting vitamin B_6, producing a pellagra-like syndrome.

4. Cycloserine is associated with delirium and worsening of psychosis in predisposed patients.

5. Chloramphenicol has been linked to encephalopathy and delirium.

6. Clioquinol may produce a global amnesia and encephalopathy.

7. Quinolones are associated with psychosis, delirium, and agitation.

Antineoplastic Agents

1. Cisplatin may produce encephalopathy.

2. Cytosine arabinoside may cause confusion and somnolence or an encephalopathy with marked cerebellar features.

3. Fludarabine has a rare effect consisting of an encephalopathy with cortical blindness and seizures.

4. 5-fluorouracil is associated with memory impairment and encephalopathy in addition to cerebellar dysfunction and leukoencephalopathy.

5. Levamisole may produce confusion in addition to tremor, myalgias, and leukoencephalopathy.

6. Methotrexate-induced encephalopathy and leukoencephalopathy are more common with cumulative dosing and intrathecal format.

7. Ifosfamide encephalopathy consists of confusion and mutism, possibly reversed or prevented by methelene blue.

8. Vincristine side effects are rare, but both encephalopathy and cortical blindness have been reported.

Anticonvulsants

1. Cognitive function changes in patients with epilepsy may be related to several factors including underlying structural lesions, postictal states, brain damage from seizures, and anticonvulsant medications.

2. The older agents produce more prominent cognitive effects and depression. Phenobarbital in particular has been shown in several studies to have especially significant effects, but such changes are also common with dilantin, carbamazepine, and valproic acid.

3. Drugs with a favorable cognitive profile include lamotrigine, gabapentin, tiagabine, oxcarbazepine, and levitiracetam.

4. Gabapentin produces limited cognitive differences when compared to placebo.

5. Levitiracetam studies have shown a tendency of improvement in cognition. There are several

reported cases of psychosis, irritability, and hostile behavior.

6. Topiramate may produce significant cognitive side effects. Psychosis and depression have also been reported.

7. Oxcarbazepine is associated with side effects similar to phenytoin but less prominent than carbamazepine. It may rarely produce a hyponatremic encephalopathy.

8. Tiagabine studies have not shown any significant cognitive, behavioral, or EEG changes.

9. Zonisamide has produced impaired cognition in small studies. Psychosis has been reported.

10. Lamictal may produce positive effects on cognition.

Steroids

1. Corticostertoids can produce severe disturbances including psychosis, memory loss, and depression with chronic use.

2. Anabolic steroids have been associated with psychotic reactions, cognitive impairment, mood disturbance and rage reactions. Symptoms can occur both with use and with withdrawal.

Antimalarials

1. Psychoses have been related to the use of chloroquinine and mefloquine. Mefloquine is relatively contraindicated in patients with a history of psychiatric illness.

Interferons

1. Interferon alpha and gamma can produce an "interferon syndrome" consisting of confusion, memory problems, and leukoencephalopathy.

2. Interferon alpha may also produce significant depressive symptoms requiring treatment with antidepressants.

Interleukins

1. Interleukin–2 (IL-2) is associated with neuropsychiatric symptoms in up to one third of patients.

2. Features of IL-2 toxicity may include confusion, agitation, hallucinations, monocular blindness, coma, and leukoencephalopathy.

Other Agents

1. Acyclovir has been reported to produce an encephalopathy. It differs from viral encephalitis by a more acute onset, normal cerebrospinal fluid, and the absence of focal neurologic findings, fever, and headache. It is more common with renal failure and high serum concentrations.

2. Baclofen has been linked to an acute encephalopathy in addition to chronic effects including psychosis and depression.

3. Bromides can produce delirium, confusion, excessive sedation, ataxia, and tremor with chronic ingestion. Two features distinguish bismuth toxicity from other diagnoses: cachexia and skin lesions consisting of acne, folliculitis, or pemphigoid.

4. Bismuth toxicity may manifest with encephalopathy with dementia, encephalopathy with myoclonus, or a Creutzfeldt-Jakob like syndrome. Diagnosis may be assisted by blood levels, radiopaque findings on abdominal films, or increased cerbral cortex density on CT.

5. Theophylline encephalopathy may be associated with seizures and cortical edema on CT.

6. Cyclosporine side effects may include encephalopathy, ataxia, and a reversible leukoencephalopathy. Occurrence may be as frequent as 25%.

Common Secondary Cognitive Syndromes

1. Hepatic encephalopathy may be secondary to elevated ammonia levels and/or effects on neurotransmitters. Drugs associated with this effect include valproic acid, propranolol, and propylthiouracil.

2. Hyponatremic encephalopathy occurs with several classes of medications including diuretics, antidepressants, oral hypoglycemic agents, and antineoplastic agents. There are also reported cases with the anticonvulsant agent oxcarbazepine.

3. Hypertensive encephalopathy may be secondary to elevation in blood pressure from erythropoietin, cyclosporine, corticosteroids, amphetamines, phenylpropanolamine, ephedrine, nonsteroidal anti-inflammatory drugs, and beta-agonists.

4. Hypoglycemic encephalopathy is most common in diabetics using insulin, captopril, beta blockers, or lithium. It also occurs in patients with renal failure treated with disopyramide and sulfamethoxazole.

Laboratory Tests

1. Electroencephalogram (EEG)
   a. Diffuse theta and delta slowing is seen with metabolic, toxic, infectious, and less commonly with vascular or traumatic etiologies.
   b. Triphasic waves are most commonly seen with hepatic and uremic encephalopathy but are also associated with other metabolic etiologies including medications. They have been reported with baclofen, lithium, and levodopa toxicity.

   c. Periodic sharp waves, depending on the location and pattern, may represent disorders including herpes encephalitis, Creutzfeldt-Jakob disease, subacute sclerosing panencephalitis, seizure activity, and stroke.

2. CT or MRI of brain should be performed to rule out lesions described in the differential diagnosis (see below).

3. Laboratory tests may include complete blood count, electrolytes, divalents, liver function tests, ammonia, thyroid stimulating hormone, vitamin B_{12}, rapid plasma reagin, human immunodeficiency virus (HIV), Lyme titer, urinalysis, and toxicology screen.

4. Lumbar puncture should be performed if there is any suspicion of infection.

Key Tests

- EEG
- CT/MRI
- Lumbar puncture
- Blood work

Differential Diagnosis

1. Infections
   a. HIV
   b. Syphilis
   c. Viral encephalitis
   d. Bacterial or fungal meningitis
   e. Lyme disease
   f. Progressive multifocal leukoencephalopathy
2. Inflammatory conditions
   a. CNS vasculitis
      (1) Isolated angiitis of the CNS
      (2) SLE
      (3) Temporal arteritis
      (4) Wegener's granulomatosis
      (5) Polyarteritis nodosa
3. Paraneoplastic: Limbic encephalitis
4. Intracranial lesions
   a. Tumor
   b. Stroke
   c. Intracerebral hemmorhage
   d. Leukoencephalopathy
5. Degenerative disorders
   a. Alzheimer's disease
   b. Creuztfeldt-Jacob disease

6. Psychiatric disorders
   a. Depression
   b. Psychosis
7. Seizures
   a. Partial seizures
   b. Post-ictal state
   c. Nonconvulsive status epilepticus
8. Migraine: Basilar migraine
9. Withdrawal syndrome: Alcohol or drug
10. Trauma: Concussion or postconcussion syndrome
11. Metabolic
    a. Hepatic or renal dysfunction producing encephalopathy
    b. Wernicke's encephalopathy
    c. Heavy metal intoxication
    d. Hypoxic-ischemic encephalopathy
    e. Vitamin deficiencies (B_{12}, niacin)

Prevention

1. Attempt to avoid polypharmacy.
2. Be aware of medication history including prescription drugs, over-the-counter medications, and substances of abuse.

Bibliography

Brunbech L, Sabers A: Effect of antiepileptic drugs on individuals with epilepsy: A comparative review of newer versus older agents. Drugs 62:593–604, 2002.

Jain KK: Drug-Induced Neurologic Disorders. Seattle, Hogrefe & Huber, 1996, pp. 5–86.

Meador KJ: Cognitive side effects of medications. Neurol Clin 16:141–55, 1998.

Meador KJ: Cognitive effects of epilepsy and of antiepileptic medications. In Wyllie E (ed): The Treatment of Epilepsy: Principles and Practice, Baltimore, Williams & Wilkins, 1996, pp. 1121–1127.

Meador KJ, Loring DW, Ray PG, et al.: Differential cognitive and behavioral effects of carbamazepine and lamotrigine. Neurology 56:1177–1182, 2001.

5 Iatrogenic Seizures

Steven C. Schachter

General Considerations

1. Iatrogenic seizures are defined as seizures that result from physician-directed interventions.

Categories of Iatrogenic Seizures

- Administration of medications
- Surgery
- Medical procedures
- Diagnostic tests

---

2. The incidence of iatrogenic seizures is unknown.

3. Estimates of the relatively common causes of iatrogenic seizures among patients in intensive care units are as follows: drug withdrawal, 33% (for example morphine, propoxyphene, midazolam, meperidine); postoperative iatrogenic fluid loading, 15%; drug toxicity, 15%.

4. The treatment of iatrogenic seizures involves removal of the offending agent and symptomatic treatment.

5. Physicians should exercise caution in administering medications associated with iatrogenic seizures to patients with a previous history of seizures, underlying brain diseases, neurologic or neuropsychiatric disorders, or positive family history of epilepsy.

6. The evaluation of new-onset seizures should include a search for possible iatrogenic causes.

Iatrogenic Seizures from Administration of Medications

Prescription medications are the most common cause of iatrogenic seizures.

1. Respiratory agents
   a. Theophylline
      (1) Most patients have no prior history of seizures.
      (2) The most common seizure types are generalized (33%) and partial with secondary generalization (30%).
      (3) Nearly half of the patients have at least three seizures; status epilepticus may also occur.
      (4) Peak serum theophylline concentrations are over 21 mg/L in two thirds of the cases.
      (5) Mechanism probably involves adenosine receptors.
   b. Terbutaline

2. Psychotropic medications
   a. Phenothiazines
      (1) Overall incidence in nonepileptic patients is approximately 1.2%, ranging from 0.5% for patients taking low doses to 10% for patients receiving large doses.
      (2) Pretreatment epileptiform electroencephalogram pattern may increase risk.
   b. Antidepressants
      (1) Risk factors
         (a) Previous or family history of epilepsy
         (b) Barbiturate withdrawal
         (c) Previous electroconvulsive therapy
         (d) Cerebrovascular disease
      (2) Tricyclic antidepressants: Imipramine, amitriptyline
      (3) Clozapine: Up to 3% of treated patients have generalized tonic-clonic seizures during treatment.

Features of Clozapine-Induced Seizures

- Overall risk of seizures is approximately 3%.
- High dosages (>600 mg/day) are more likely than low dosages (<300 mg/day) to be associated with seizures (4.4% vs 1.0%).
- Rapid dosage titration increases the risk of seizures.

---

      (4) Lithium
         (a) Symptoms and signs range from mild lethargy and nausea to seizures and coma.
         (b) EEG may show multifocal spike and waves.
      (5) Miscellaneous: maprotiline, bupropion, amoxapine

3. Analgesics: pentazocine, meperidine

4. Anesthetic agents: lidocaine, enflurane, isoflurane

953

5. Anti-infectives and immunosuppressnats
   a. Isoniazid, nalidixic acid, chlorambucil, metronidazole
   b. Cyclosporine: Mechanisms may involve hypertension, hypomagnesemia, and nephrotoxicity.
   c. Anti-epileptic drugs (AEDs)
      (1) Typical signs of AED toxicity include ataxia, diplopia, nystagmus, and altered mental status.
      (2) Seizures may also occur, particularly with phenytoin at supertherapeutic serum concentrations, although the cause and effect relationship remains controversial.
      (3) Carbamazepine may exacerbate generalized atypical absence seizures.
6. Withdrawal seizures: May occur after sudden cessation of therapy with sedatives or tranquilizers; described also for chlordiazepoxide and baclofen.

Iatrogenic Seizures from Surgical and Medical Procedures

1. Surgery
   a. Brain surgery
      (1) Relative risk is high for patients with brain malignancies, implicating the underlying disease process, rather than the surgical procedure, as responsible for postoperative seizures in some patients.
      (2) Risk is also increased after craniotomies (compared to burr holes), and in patients with a preoperative history of epilepsy.
      (3) Particular procedures associated with postoperative seizures are glioma biopsies, ventricular shunt insertions (especially when complicated by infection or when revision was necessary), craniotomies for tumor excisions and aneurysmal repairs (particularly middle cerebral artery aneurysm repair followed by postoperative neurologic deficits).

   b. Organ transplantation: Seizures after organ transplantation may be due to immunosuppressive therapy, the neurologic complications of end-stage organ failure, or the transplantation procedure.
   c. Nonspecific surgery-related seizures: Generalized seizures may result from the severe hyponatremia associated with inappropriate secretion of antidiuretic hormone that rarely complicates the early recovery period after elective surgery, particularly in otherwise healthy women.
2. Medical procedures
   a. Myelography
      (1) Associated with ionic contrast medium
      (2) Treatment consists of removal of contrast material from the spinal canal as the head and trunk are elevated, as well as supportive management of seizures, rhabdomyolysis, and metabolic abnormalities.
   b. Electroconvulsive therapy
      (1) Rarely associated with the induction of spontaneous seizures independent of electroconvulsive treatments, especially if oxygenation during the procedure is inadequate.

Bibliography

Devinsky O, Duchowny MS: Seizures after convulsive therapy: A retrospective case survey. Neurology 33:921–925, 1983.

Devinsky O, Honigfeld G, Patin J: Clozapine-related seizures. Neurology 41:369–371, 1991.

Foy PM, Copeland GP, Shaw MDM: The natural history of postoperative seizures. Acta Neurochir 57:15–22, 1981.

Jabbari B, Bryan GE, Marsh EE, et al.: Incidence of seizures with tricyclic and tetracyclic antidepressants. Arch Neurol 42:480–481, 1985.

Lerman P: Seizures induced or aggravated by anticonvulsants. Epilepsia 27:706–710, 1986.

Schachter SC: Iatrogenic seizures. Neurol Clin 16:157–170, 1998.

Wijdicks EFM, Sharbrough FW: New-onset seizures in critically ill patients. Neurology 43:1042–1044, 1993.

6 Side Effects of Immunosuppressive Therapies

Hazem Machkhas

As the list of neurologic disorders with presumed or proven autoimmune etiology continues to grow, neurologists have found themselves increasingly ordering, supervising, and monitoring immunosuppressive and immunomodulatory therapies. Although most conditions respond to familiar first-line treatments, refractory cases require that we delve into an armamentarium previously reserved for oncologists. Successful planning and supervision of immunomodulatory therapy requires, in addition to familiarity with the indications and dosages of these agents, an intimate knowledge of their common and uncommon (but serious) side effects.

1. General guidelines

   a. Goals of therapy: slow the progression of the disease process and improve clinical deficits while keeping side effects to a minimum.

   b. Adequately establish diagnosis before initiation of therapy. Only in rare and select cases should empiric treatment trials be employed.

   c. Establish baseline variables that will be monitored on follow-up visits to gauge the response to therapy (e.g., muscle strength, vital capacity, timed walking, timed swallow).

   d. Be aware of coexisting medical conditions that may be contraindications to immunosuppression in general (e.g., active infections) or to specific agents (uncontrolled diabetes with steroids, congestive heart failure with intravenous immunoglobulin). Check PPD on all patients.

   e. Patient compliance is of paramount importance for ensuring a proper response to therapy and keeping side effects to a minimum. Often patient noncompliance is the only absolute contraindication to therapy. Establish a contract with your patients: Repeated violations of its terms result in stoppage of treatment.

   f. Always use optimal doses of each agent and give it time to act. Often agents that have been labeled "treatment failures" were given in suboptimal doses or for too short periods of time.

2. Prednisone

   a. Side effects. The list of potential side effects of oral prednisone therapy is extensive. The treating physician must be aware of the most important side effects and share that information with the patient from the onset of therapy.

      (1) Osteoporosis is one of the most concerning side effects of prednisone use and occurs mainly during the first 6 months of treatment. At highest risk are postmenopausal women.

      (2) Avascular necrosis is infrequent but devastating when it occurs. It has a predilection for the hips but may be seen in any joint. Magnetic resonance imaging (MRI) is the most sensitive tool for detecting the earliest changes.

      (3) Abnormalities of glucose metabolism range from glucose intolerance to overt diabetes. In diabetics it causes loss of glycemic control.

      (4) Obesity is secondary to increased appetite and abnormal distribution of fat. Cushingoid appearance develops in most patients.

      (5) Suppression of the hypothalamic-pituitary-adrenal axis lasts in some patients for 9 to 12 months beyond discontinuation of treatment. Exogenous steroid supplementation is necessary in potentially stressful situations such as surgery.

      (6) Neurologic complications (most commonly neuropsychiatric disturbances) range from mild mood swings to euphoria, depression, and rarely frank psychosis. A steroid-induced muscle weakness secondary to selective type II muscle atrophy may also be seen.

      (7) Other complications include hypertension, hyperlipidemia, menstrual irregularities, delayed wound healing, and increased susceptibility to infections. A high index of suspicion is required: Any new symptom that arises during prednisone therapy requires consideration of an appropriate dose reduction or switch to another immunomodulatory therapy.

955

Key Side Effects: Prednisone

- Osteoporosis

- Avascular necrosis

- Glucose intolerance

- Hypertension

- Neuropsychiatric disturbances

b. Prevention and monitoring

(1) Patient education at the onset of therapy is paramount for minimizing some of the side effects. The reassurance that some of them are transient ensures maintained compliance as some of the side effects appear.

(2) Dietary modification to a low-calorie, low-salt, low-carbohydrate, high-protein diet helps reduce the risk of developing glucose intolerance, weight gain, hypertension, and cushingoid features. If necessary, a dietary consultation should be obtained.

(3) Antacids should be started concomitantly to minimize gastrointestinal (GI) discomfort.

(4) Calcium and vitamin D supplementation reduces the risk of osteoporosis. Axial exercises (walking, swimming) are also good preventive measures. Postmenopausal women should be on hormonal replacement therapy.

(5) Promptly switching to an alternate-day regimen has been shown to reduce most side effects while maintaining an adequate clinical response.

(6) Baseline studies include a complete blood count (CBC), liver function tests, lipid profile, and routine chemistry panel (including fasting blood glucose). Careful history and physical examination help identify patients at risk for developing certain side effects. The value of baseline bone densitometry is unclear, but it is advisable to obtain one on all elderly patients and postmenopausal women. The baseline studies must be repeated monthly at least twice, and every 3 to 6 months subsequently. Bone densitometry is recommended at 6 months.

3. Intravenous methylprednisolone

a. Intravenous methylprednisolone therapy is usually given in regular pulses at monthly intervals. It has long been observed that intravenous methylprednisolone has a more benign side effect profile than oral prednisone. The reason is suspected to be the intermittent nature of the treatment as well as the delivery route.

b. The main complications are transient and resolve a few days after each pulse. They include mood changes (mainly euphoria but also depression), sleep disturbances, increased appetite, facial flushing, epigastric discomfort, and palpitations.

c. Prevention of these complications is not possible. It is important to have prepared the patient about their potential occurrence and offer reassurance about their transient, benign nature.

d. Routine monitoring guidelines have not been set. It is recommended that a CBC and detailed chemistry panel be obtained periodically.

4. Intravenous immunoglobulin (IVIG)

a. Side effects: the perception of IVIG as a safe modality is not accurate. More than half of patients receiving IVIG develop some side effect. In up to 10% the side effect is serious enough to warrant discontinuation. Major and most common side effects include

(1) Renal failure. Although rare, at obvious increased risk are patients with preexisting renal disease and those at increased risk for nephropathy (diabetics). Typically, discontinuation of therapy restores normal renal function.

(2) Headaches. These are a common, benign complication of IVIG therapy.

(3) Aseptic meningitis. In a small number of patients a syndrome of headache, stiff neck, photophobia, fever, and vomiting develops, associated with cerebrospinal fluid (CSF) findings consistent with aseptic meningitis.

(4) Thromboembolic events. An IVIG-induced increase in serum viscosity is believed to be the underlying cause of the observed increased risk of cerebrovascular accidents, pulmonary emboli, and deep venous thrombosis. This is particularly observed in the elderly.

(5) Others. There are also anaphylactoid reactions [mainly in patients with immunoglobulin A (IgA) deficiency], rash (rarely eczema), myalgias, and congestive heart failure. The potential for propagation of transmissible infections exists but so far has been limited to early reports of hepatitis C transmission, all linked to the same commercial preparation.

Key Side Effects: IVIG

- Renal failure
- Headaches
- Aseptic meningitis
- Thromboembolic events

b. Prevention and monitoring

(1) Careful patient selection reduces the potential for adverse events. IVIG should be used with extreme caution in patients with compromised renal function, at risk for nephrotoxicity (e.g., diabetics), or at risk for (or with a history of) thromboembolic events.

(2) Before each infusion it is important to ensure that the patient is not volume-depleted.

(3) In patients with preexisting renal dysfunction or those at risk for nephrotoxicity, it is recommended that the lowest concentration of IVIG be used and that it be infused very slowly. It is also recommended that IVIG preparations containing sucrose as a stabilizer be avoided.

(4) Screening for IgA deficiency is not recommended.

(5) Baseline studies should include a CBC and a basic chemistry panel. Routine monitoring guidelines are not well established. Periodically checking renal function [blood urea nitrogen (BUN) and creatinine] is recommended for all patients. Close monitoring is required in patients at risk of nephrotoxicity (prior to each infusion). All patients should be instructed to report any reductions in their urine output.

5. Azathioprine
   a. Side effects
      (1) Hematologic complications. Myelosuppression is the most common and potentially most serious complication of azathioprine therapy. It usually develops early in the treatment course and may be abrupt. Leukopenia and thrombocytopenia are the usual manifestations. Therapy must be stopped if the leukocyte count decreases below 2500 cells/μL or if the absolute neutrophil count decreases below 1000 cells/μL. When counts normalize, therapy may be restarted at a lower dose.

      (2) Hepatic complications. Hepatotoxicity can develop 2 weeks to 33 months after initiation of therapy. Typically, there is a mild increase in liver transaminases that responds to dose reduction.

      (3) GI complications. These include epigastric discomfort, nausea, anorexia, and diarrhea. They are typically mild and respond to dividing the dose or reducing it.

      (4) Drug interactions. They are seen mainly with allopurinol, which causes elevated levels of azathioprine and consequently increases the potential for side effects. When used with allopurinol, the azathioprine dose should be reduced by 75%.

      (5) Others. A hypersensitivity reaction can produce a flu-like syndrome of malaise, fever, and myalgias. As with most immunosuppressive agents, an increased susceptibility to opportunistic infections is observed. An increased risk of neoplasia has been well documented only after organ transplantation.

Key Side Effects: Azathioprine

- Leukopenia
- Hepatotoxicity
- Drug interaction with allopurinol

b. Prevention and monitoring

(1) There are no specific preventive measures to reduce the risk of any of the side effects. GI complications may be reduced by taking the drug with food.

(2) Routine monitoring laboratory investigations include CBC with differential and platelet count, as well as liver function tests. These tests should be obtained at the onset of treatment, at the time of each scheduled dose increment, monthly for about 3 months, and subsequently at regular intervals not to exceed 3 months once a stable nontoxic dose has been reached.

6. Methotrexate
   a. Side effects
      (1) Hepatotoxicity ranges from a transient mild increase in liver transaminases (in up to 30% of patients during the first 3 weeks of therapy) to full-blown hepatic cirrhosis and fibrosis (seen in approximately 3% of patients).

      (2) Hematologic complications include megaloblastic anemia, leukopenia, thrombocytopenia, and pancytopenia. Cytopenias occur in 5% to 25% of patients and respond

to dose reduction or discontinuation of therapy. Megaloblastic anemia responds to folate supplementation. Pancytopenia is rare but requires cessation of therapy and intravenous leukovorin (10–20 mg q6h) until counts normalize.

(3) Pulmonary complications appear, the most common of which is an acute or subacute interstitial pneumonitis, manifesting as dyspnea, dry cough, and flu-like symptoms. It requires discontinuation of treatment and supportive therapy as needed.

(4) Neurologic complications include seizures, as methotrexate is known to lower the seizure threshold. More serious complications occur with intrathecal or high-dose intravenous treatment, routes never used for common neurologic therapy. They include transverse myelitis, transient stroke-like syndromes with encephalopathy, and a severe protracted leukoencephalopathy.

(5) Others include GI complaints, increased risk of abortion, and opportunistic infection.

Key Side Effects: Methotrexate

- Hepatotoxicity
- Interstitial pneumonitis
- Leukopenia
- Megaloblastic anemia

b. Prevention and monitoring

(1) Pretreatment liver biopsy is recommended as a screening tool in patients with a history of excessive alcohol use, persistent transaminase elevations, and chronic hepatitis B or C infection.

(2) Routine folate supplementation may have a beneficial effect in reducing the risk of developing megaloblastic anemia and may reduce other side effects, including GI discomfort, diarrhea, and liver function test abnormalities.

(3) Baseline studies include liver function tests, serology for hepatitis B and C, CBC, and routine chemistry panel.

(4) It is recommended that liver function tests, CBC, and a routine chemistry panel be performed with every dose escalation. Once a stable dose has been reached, these monitoring studies should be done every 3 to 4 months.

(5) Carefully remind patients that their medication is dosed *weekly*, not daily.

7. Cyclosporine

a. Side effects

(1) Hypertension. This is the most common complication, with an incidence ranging from 20% to 30% in nontransplant patients. It is reversible with discontinuation of treatment but is not an indication for such a drastic measure so long as it can be controlled with medications. The drug of choice is nifedipine.

(2) Renal dysfunction. This is seen in 5% of cases when using routine doses.

(3) Neoplastic complications. There is a 3.0- to 4.9-fold increased risk of developing a malignancy with high-dose cyclosporine therapy (e.g., as is used in transplant cases). The risk is unknown with more conventional doses.

(4) Neurologic complications. These include seizures, ataxia, tremor, leukoencephalopathy, peripheral neuropathy, and myalgias. They are more common with high-dose therapy.

(5) Drug interactions. Drugs that interfere with cytochrome P-450 cause elevated or reduced blood concentrations of cyclosporine.

Key Side Effects: Cyclosporine

- Hypertension
- Renal dysfunction
- Increased risk of malignancy

b. Prevention and monitoring

(1) Careful review of patient's medications is needed prior to onset of therapy.

(2) Identify patients at risk of developing side effects (mostly patients with hypertension, compromised renal function).

(3) Baseline studies include CBC with differential, routine chemistry panel, liver function tests, and urinalysis.

(4) Follow-up studies include monthly BUN and creatinine. The rest of the baseline studies should be monitored every 3 months.

(5) Periodic blood pressure measurements.

8. Cyclophosphamide
   a. Side effects
      (1) Hemorrhagic cystitis has been observed in 10% to 50% of patients. It can be severe, causing a drop in hematocrit that necessitates transfusion.
      (2) Bladder cancer may occur. The risk is dependent on the cumulative dose, with a 14.5-fold increased risk with cumulative doses of more than 50 g.
      (3) Other complications include myelosuppression, nausea, vomiting, alopecia, and infertility.

Key Side Effects: Cyclophosphamide

• Hemorrhagic cystitis

• Bladder cancer (cumulative dose)

• Myelosuppression

   b. Prevention and monitoring
      (1) Baseline studies include a routine chemistry panel, liver function tests, CBC with differential, and urinalysis.
      (2) With oral therapy, monthly CBC and urinalysis are performed.
      (3) With IV therapy, the same monitoring profile should be obtained before each round of treatment.
      (4) Prevention of hemorrhagic cystitis is through vigorous intravenous hydration and infusion of mesna.
      (5) Prevention of nausea is achieved with concomitant administration of ondansetron.
9. Others
   a. Mycophenolate mofetil
      (1) Mycophenolate mofetil (CellCept; Roche, Nutley, NJ) is a potent immunosuppressant with proven efficacy in preventing acute rejection after organ transplantation. It has also shown a potential role in other immune-mediated disorders, including Crohn's disease, rheumatoid arthritis, and systemic lupus erythematosus. Open-label trials have suggested that it may be an efficacious and well tolerated agent for refractory myasthenia gravis.
      (2) Available experience to date suggests that mycophenolate has a favorable profile of side effects when compared with other immunosuppressants. Common side effects include diarrhea, abdominal pain, nausea and vomiting, peripheral edema, leukopenia, and increased risk of infection and sepsis.
   b. Tacrolimus
      (1) Tacrolimus is a potent immunosuppressant with a mode of action similar to that of cyclosporine. It is predominantly used for transplantation. There is limited experience in its use for autoimmune neurologic diseases, including polymyositis, dermatomyositis, and experimental autoimmune myasthenia gravis.
      (2) Side effect profile is similar to that of cyclosporine.

Bibliography

Machkhas H, Harati Y: Side effects of immunosuppressant therapies used in neurology. Neurol Clin 16:171–188, 1998.

Machkhas H, Harati Y, Rolak LA: Clinical pharmacology of immunosuppressants: guidelines for neuroimmunotherapy. In Rolak LA, Harati Y (eds): Neuroimmunology for the Clinician. Boston, Butterworth-Heinemann, 1997, pp. 77–104.

Wiles CM, Brown P, Chapel H, et al.: Intravenous immunoglobulin in neurological disease: a specialist review. J Neurol Neurosurg Psychiatry 72:440–448, 2002.

1   Mood Disorders

Jeffrey P. Staab
Christos Ballas

Definitions

1. *The Diagnostic and Statistical Manual of Mental Disorders, 4th Edition* (DSM-IV) defines nine major categories of mood disorders and scores of possible subcategories.

   a. This level of precision is better suited to research than clinical purposes.

   b. A simple, clinically effective, diagnostic scheme has emerged from investigations of mood disorders in primary care settings and a convergence of treatment outcome data.

      (1) Primary care

         (a) Major and minor depression

         (b) Bipolar type I and other bipolar disorders

      (2) Treatment outcome data: A few subtypes of mood disorders require particular pharmacologic considerations.

2. See Table 1–1 and Table 1–2, respectively, for the main clinical features and main medication treatments for mood disorders

Major Depression

1. Definition. A disturbance of mood, neurovegetative functions, and cognition that may be accompanied by suicidality, homicidality, or psychosis

   a. Mood: disturbance may be dysphoria or anhedonia (or both)

      (1) Dysphoria: low, sad, blue, or depressed mood

      (2) Anhedonia: loss of interest in, or pleasure from, activities

   b. Neurovegetative functions

      (1) Sleep: increased or decreased

         (a) Early morning awakening (e.g., 3:00–4:00 a.m.) is the classic sleep disturbance in depression.

         (b) Difficulty falling asleep also is common, especially when anxiety accompanies depression.

      (2) Appetite: increased or decreased

         (a) The diagnostic criterion specifies a 10% change in weight.

TABLE 1–1.   MAIN CLINICAL FEATURES OF MOOD DISORDERS

Mood Disorder	Mood Changes	Neurovegetative Changes	Duration	Psychosis	Suicide Risk
Major depression (typical)	Depressed Irritable Labile (moody) Withdrawn	Decreased sleep Weight loss Decreased energy Impaired concentration	> 2 Weeks	May occur in severe cases	Moderate to high
Major depression (atypical)	Depressed Labile Highly reactive to situations	Increased sleep Weight gain	> 2 Weeks	May occur in severe cases	Moderate to high
Minor depression	Depressed Irritable Disinterested	Mild to moderate insomnia, appetite and energy changes	Days to years	No	Low to moderate
Bipolar disorder— manic	Grandiose or irritable	Decreased sleep Decrease appetite Increased energy Hyperkinetic	1 Week	Common in severe cases	Moderate
Bipolar disorder— hypomanic	Same as manic Not as severe	Same as manic Not as severe	> 4 Days	No	Low
Bipolar disorder— depressed	Same as major depression	Same as major depression	Same as major depression	Same as major depression	Same as major depression

TABLE 1–2. MAIN MEDICATION TREATMENT CHOICES FOR MOOD DISORDERS*

Mood Disorder	First Line	First-Line Alternatives	Second Line	Adjunctive Medications
Major depression	SSRIs	Venlafaxine Buproprion Mirtazapine Nefazodone	Tricyclic antidepressants MAOIs	Benzodiazepines Neuroleptics
Minor depression	SSRIs	Venlafaxine Buproprion Mirtazapine Nefazodone	Tricyclic antidepressants MAOIs	Hypnotics
Bipolar—mania	Lithium	Divalproex	Carbamazepine Oxcarbazepine Lamotrigine Topiramate Gabapentin	Benzodiazepines Neuroleptics
Bipolar—depressed	Lithium	Divalproex	Lamotrigine Carbamazepine Oxcarbazepine Topiramate Gabapentin	SSRIs Other first-line antidepressants MAOIs Benzodiazepines Neuroleptics

Abbreviations: SSRIs, Selective serotonin reuptake inhibitors; MAOIs, monoamine oxidase inhibitors.
*Effective psychotherapies exist for all of these disorders. Psychotherapy may be used with or without medications for major and minor depression. Medications have superior efficacy in patients with severe major depression. Patients with bipolar disorder (especially type I) should not be treated with psychotherapy alone. Electroconvulsive therapy is effective for all these disorders.

(b) Many patients report a subjective change in appetite without an alteration in weight (e.g., "I have no appetite, but I'm forcing myself to eat.")

(3) Energy: usually low, though some patients complain of an uncomfortable edginess or inability to relax

(4) Motor activity: restless or sluggish

c. Cognition

(1) Memory and concentration: short-term memory loss, absent-mindedness, difficulty sustaining attention, easy distractibility, poor concentration

(a) May give the appearance of mild dementia (previously called "pseudodementia")

(2) Self-concept: decreased self-esteem, worthlessness, unwarranted guilt about past mistakes or present circumstances, excessive pessimism, hopelessness

d. Suicidality

(1) Ideation

(a) Passive: thoughts of dying or wishes to be dead (e.g., "I want go to sleep and never wake up.")

(b) Active: thoughts of taking one's own life

(2) Intent: suicidal ideation or behaviors in which the patient hopes for one of the following outcome

(a) Death: a definite wish to be dead

(b) Attention: a hope that others will notice one's pain, suffering, or distress (e.g., "Nobody would pay attention to me any other way")

(c) Revenge: a wish to get back at others (e.g., "If I kill myself, my parents will have to live with it the rest of their lives")

(d) Ambivalence/uncertainty: Many patients (perhaps most) have mixed feelings about dying or are not clear about the factors driving their suicidal ideation or behaviors.

(3) Plan: thoughts about the method(s) and timing of potential suicidal behaviors

(a) Premeditated: time, place, and method considered in advance, often in the face of chronic stressors or long-standing psychopathology

(b) Impulsive: spur of the moment response to an acute stressor

(4) Behaviors: acts in furtherance of suicidal ideation or plans

(a) Preparations: writing notes, putting affairs in order, acquiring the means to carry out a suicide plan

(b) Attempts: physically harming oneself

(i) Some clinicians make a distinction between "true suicide attempts" and "suicide gestures" based on their interpretation of psychological factors underlying the patient's behavior. This distinction may be speculative, particularly if the clinician does not know the patient well, and may not correlate with potential lethality. A more productive initial approach is to define the ideation, intent, and plan as outlined above.

e. Homicidality or assaultiveness

(1) The definitions of homicidal or assaultive ideation, intent, plans, and behaviors parallel those just described for suicidality, except that the potential victim is someone else.

(2) Intended victim

(a) Specific: a clearly specified target

(b) General: not directed at a specific person (e.g., "I'm going to kill the next person who bothers me")

f. Psychosis: In severe cases, psychotic symptoms may accompany major depression.

(1) Hallucinations

(a) Auditory hallucinations are the most common to occur with major depression (see Part IX, Chapter 11).

(i) Auditory hallucinations usually are negative, pessimistic, or deprecating.

(ii) Command auditory hallucinations may occur, including directives about harmful behaviors.

(b) Other hallucinations usually have negative content as well (e.g., "I see the shadow of death in my room").

(2) Delusions

(a) The delusions of major depression are rigidly held beliefs that tend to be persecutory or self-deprecating in nature. They often are highly exaggerated reflections of actual circumstances in the patient's life, but they may have a bizarre content that has no basis in reality.

(b) Nihilistic delusions: unshakeable, overwhelming preoccupation with thoughts of hopelessness and worthlessness (e.g., "I have nothing to live for" "Nobody needs me" "I don't amount to anything anymore"). Most commonly encountered in older patients

(3) Behavioral disturbances

(a) Response to internal stimuli: observable behavioral responses to hallucinations and delusions (e.g., fearful startle,

grimacing, or talking as if an external stimulus is present)

(b) Acting on command hallucinations

Caveats

- Early morning awakening (e.g., 3:00–4:00 a.m.) is the classic sleep disturbance in major depression.

- In severe cases, psychotic symptoms may accompany major depression.

---

2. Epidemiology. The incidence and prevalence of major depression vary with age, gender, and medical morbidity but not with ethnicity, education, marital status, or socioeconomic status.

a. Incidence

(1) New cases of major depression are most common from the late teenage years through the late twenties, with a peak during the mid-twenties.

(2) When the first onset of major depression occurs after 40 years of age it is more likely to have a medical etiology.

b. The point prevalence and lifetime risk of major depression vary with gender.

(1) Point prevalence

(a) Women 5% to 9%

(b) Men 2% to 3%

(2) Lifetime risk

(a) Women 10% to 25%

(b) Men 5% to 12%

(3) Many biologic variables (e.g., hormonal effects) and psychosocial variables (e.g., women's role in society) have been postulated to account for these differences, but the actual cause is unknown and is likely to be multifactorial.

c. General medical health also affects the prevalence of major depression.

(1) Some medical conditions cause depression because of their adverse effects on the brain [e.g., stroke, central nervous system (CNS) lupus].

(2) For many other medical conditions, the specific causal factors are not known. Potential etiologies include

(a) Psychosocial burdens of illness and disability

(b) Unknown biologic factors (e.g., cytokine activation, autonomic nervous system dysregulation)

(3) Effect of medical morbidity is most striking

among adults older than age 65, the demographic group that bears the greatest burden of medical illness. The prevalence of major depression is

    (a) Community dwelling elderly 5%

    (b) General medical outpatients 8% to 10%

    (c) Nursing home residents 25% to 40%

    (d) Patients in acute care medical/surgical settings 30% or more

d. Impact on society

  (1) Financial

    (a) The financial impact of depression in terms of direct costs of care, lost wages, and poor work productivity is more than $40 billion annually in the United States.

    (b) The economic impact of depression is equivalent to that of heart disease and diabetes.

  (2) Medical utilization

    (a) Patients with major depression use significantly more inpatient and outpatient general medical services than their nondepressed counterparts, even after controlling for medical morbidity.

    (b) Strongly consider a diagnosis of depression (or anxiety) in patients with persistent, nonspecific medical or neurologic complaints.

Caveat

• Strongly consider a diagnosis of depression in patients with persistent, nonspecific medical or neurologic complaints.

---

3. Pathophysiology

  a. Biologic agents

  (1) Monoamines. The role of monoamines was inferred initially from the efficacy of drugs that affect monoamine neurotransmission and from the results of dietary depletion studies.

    (a) Norepinephrine

      (i) During the 1960s tricyclic antidepressants were found to inhibit reuptake of norepinephrine.

      (ii) Animal models: Manipulations of norepinephrine systems altered "depressive" behaviors.

      (iii) Thus was born the "chemical imbalance" theory of mood disorders.

    (b) Serotonin

      (i) Tertiary tricyclic antidepressants (e.g., imipramine, amitriptyline) and monoamine oxidase inhibitors enhance serotonin and norepinephrine neurotransmission.

      (ii) Newer antidepressants specifically target serotonin.

      (iii) Humans fed diets deficient in the serotonin precursor tyramine lost the benefits of antidepressant medication treatment.

    (c) Dopamine

      (i) It does not appear to play a central role in the development of depression.

      (ii) It may have a modulating influence. Dopaminergic agonists (bromocriptine, methylphenidate) can augment antidepressant treatment.

  (2) Cortisol

    (a) A significant effort has been expended to understand alterations in the hypothalamic-pituitary-adrenal axis during depression.

    (b) Two reasonably consistent findings have emerged from investigations of the dexamethasone suppression test (DST), neither of which is used clinically.

      (i) In psychotic depression, cortisol levels are elevated and are not suppressed by administration of dexamethasone.

      (ii) Among depressed patients with abnormal DSTs, those whose DST does not normalize with antidepressant treatment are highly prone to relapses.

  (3) Cytokines

    (a) Induction of cytokine pathways (e.g., by interferon) produces "sickness behaviors" akin to depression in animals and humans.

    (b) This can be blocked by administering antidepressant medications.

  (4) Biologic rhythms

    (a) Several lines of evidence suggest that circadian and other biologic rhythms may be altered in patients with mood disorders.

    (i) Phase advances in cortisol secretion

    (ii) Shortened rapid eye movement (REM) sleep latency

    (iii) Seasonal susceptibility to depressive episodes

  (b) This suggests that midbrain structures play an important but incompletely understood role in the pathophysiology of mood disorders.

b. Psychosocial agents

  (1) Many psychological theories of mood disorders have been advanced over the years.

  (2) Several are supported by rigorous clinical investigations.

    (a) They give an explanation for certain clinically observable symptoms.

    (b) They provide effective methods for psychological treatment of mood disorders.

  (3) Cognitive theory

    (a) Negative mindsets dominate the patient's daily life, biasing his or her perception of events in a negative manner (e.g., "Why study, I'll just fail this test anyway" "Nobody will care if I'm not there").

    (b) It develops into a pattern of self-reinforcing, sometimes self-fulfilling thoughts and behavior that sustain depressive emotional responses.

  (4) Interpersonal theory

    (a) Conflicted or unsatisfying aspects of interpersonal interactions move to the forefront, negatively affecting the patient's sense of self-worth and feelings of competence in important roles (e.g., parent, spouse, occupation).

    (b) This also can create a self-fulfilling, vicious circle in which the patient appears negativistic to others, and they react in kind.

4. Clinical features

  a. Alterations in mood or interests (or both) for at least 2 weeks

    (1) "Bad," not just "sad," moods. Mood may be down, labile, irritable, numb, detached, or a combination.

    (2) Loss of interest or pleasure in activities may predominate (anhedonia).

      (a) This is more common in geriatric patients.

      (b) They may deny depressed mood but are not participating in usual activities.

  b. Neurovegetative changes for at least 2 weeks

    (1) Alteration in sleep and appetite are most diagnostic.

      (a) Most often insomnia (early morning awakening)

      (b) "Atypical depression"—*increased* sleep and appetite

  c. Suicidality. Clinicians must always evaluate the possibility of suicidal or homicidal ideation, intent, and plans.

  d. Psychosis. May be present in those with severe depression

  e. Somatization

    (1) Many depressed patients present with physical complaints.

    (2) For patients with medically unexplained physical symptoms, the odds ratio for an active depressive episode is 15 (compared with the general population).

  f. Typical lifetime course of depression

    (1) There is an 80% likelihood of recurrent major depressive episodes.

    (2) There is a similar likelihood of periods of lesser depressive symptoms.

    (3) Both of these conditions suggest a need for long-term follow-up and treatment.

Key Signs: Major Depression

- Alterations in mood or interests for at least 2 weeks
- Neurovegetative changes for at least 2 weeks; alteration in sleep and appetite most diagnostic
- Suicidality
- Apathy
- Irritability
- Somatic preoccupation

5. Differential diagnosis

  a. Psychiatric diagnoses

    (1) Other mood disorders

      (a) Bipolar affective disorder (BAD)

        (i) Clinicians must screen depressed patients for evidence of bipolar disorder (e.g., past episodes of mania or hypomania).

  (ii) Treating depression alone in patients with BAD may have undesirable short- and long-term consequences.

- Inducing a manic episode
- Increasing the frequency and severity of BAD cycles

(c) Minor depressive disorders. The diagnosis of minor versus major depression may affect choice, dose, and duration of antidepressant treatment

(2) Anxiety disorders. Commonly coexist with depression

(3) Substance-related disorders. Misuse of any CNS-active substance (not just CNS depressants) may cause depression.

(4) Psychotic disorders

(a) Specific diagnosis may be difficult when both depressive and psychotic symptoms are present.

(b) Diagnostic precision is essential for planning maintenance treatment.

(c) Collect data on the lifetime course of the patient's psychiatric symptoms.

(5) Somatoform disorders. Depression is common in patients with somatoform disorders.

(a) Evaluate extent and persistence of physical versus depressive symptoms.

(b) Treat depression.

(c) If physical complaints persist, develop a treatment plan for somatoform disorders (see Part XXV, Chapter 5).

b. Neurologic diagnoses

(1) Stroke

(a) Some data indicate that frontal lobe infarctions (particularly on the left side) are most likely to cause depressive episodes.

(b) Magnetic resonance imaging (MRI) studies in geriatric patients suggest that the extent of white matter disease (small vessel infarctions) correlates with susceptibility to depression.

(2) Head trauma

(a) Mood lability and irritability are common after head trauma, including mild traumatic brain injury (e.g., postconcussive syndrome).

(b) Fully developed depressive episodes also occur frequently.

(3) CNS tumors, particularly tumors in the frontal lobes

(a) Meningiomas

(b) Astrocytomas

(4) CNS infections

(a) Human immunodeficiency virus (HIV)

(i) Data are conflicting on whether HIV infection itself is a risk factor for depression.

(ii) "HIV dementia" is somewhat of a misnomer.

- Clinical symptoms are a combination of affective and cognitive changes.
- They respond to aggressive antiretroviral and psychiatric treatment.

(b) Herpes simplex virus (HSV)

(i) Herpes encephalitis

(ii) Affective (depressive, manic, mixed) and psychotic symptoms are common during the acute illness.

(iii) Depression may persist or occur for the first time during the post-encephalitic period.

(5) Autoimmune disease affecting the CNS

(a) Systemic lupus erythematosus (SLE) is the major autoimmune cause of depression. CNS lupus may produce severe depression or mania (or both) accompanied by psychosis.

(b) Other autoimmune illnesses may be associated with depression. The mechanism is more likely the psychological burden of chronic illness than a direct CNS effect.

(6) Demyelinating diseases (multiple sclerosis)

(a) Direct effect: demyelination of neural circuits linking frontal with midbrain and limbic structures

(b) Indirect effect: psychological burden of illness and disability

c. Medical diagnoses

(1) Endocrine and metabolic

(a) Hypothyroidism

(b) Occasionally hyperthyroidism

(c) Hypercalcemia, particularly chronically elevated serum calcium

(d) Hypercortisolemia

(2) Malignancy

    (a) High rates of depression in pancreatic carcinoma

(3) Cardiac disease

    (a) Heart failure may present with fatigue and sleep disturbances, leading to a reduction in social activities and anhedonia.

    (b) Coronary artery disease

        (i) The period after a myocardial infarction is a high risk time for depression.

        (ii) Depression is a risk factor for adverse cardiac events. It has multiplicative interaction with other cardiac risk factors.

(4) Pulmonary disease

    (a) Chronic obstructive pulmonary disease (COPD): fatigue, reduced social activities, anhedonia, sleep disturbance

    (b) Sleep apnea: sleep disturbance, daytime fatigue, mental sluggishness

(5) Infectious disease

    (a) Tertiary syphilis: does not usually cause depression alone

---

Caveats

Psychiatric Caveats

• Screen depressed patients for evidence of bipolar affective disorder (BAD) because treating depression alone may induce a manic episode or increase the frequency and severity of BAD cycles.

• It may be difficult to arrive at specific diagnosis when both depressive and psychotic symptoms are present.

Neurologic Caveats

• Some data indicate that frontal lobe infarctions (particularly on the left side) are most likely to cause depressive episodes.

• Mood lability and irritability are common after head trauma.

• SLE is the major autoimmune cause of depression. CNS lupus may produce severe depression or mania accompanied by psychosis.

Medical Caveats

• Hypothyroidism may be the most commonly overlooked medical cause of depression.

• High rates of depression are found with pancreatic carcinoma.

• The period after a myocardial infarction is a high risk time for depression.

---

6. Laboratory testing

  a. The extent of medical evaluations for patients with depression should be based on their medical histories and findings on physical examination.

  b. For a patient with a benign medical history and unremarkable physical examination, screen for

    (1) Thyroid-stimulating hormone

    (2) Drugs in the urine

  c. Additional testing

    (1) Look for any evidence of illnesses described under the Differential Diagnosis.

    (2) For treatment-resistant cases, evaluate for a broader range of medical illnesses.

    (3) A more extensive medical evaluation is indicated for patients over age 40 with a first-ever episode of depression.

Key Tests: Major Depression

• Thyroid-stimulating hormone

• Urine drug screening

• Testing for evidence of illness

• Broader medical evaluation for patients over 40 years of age with a first episode of depression

---

7. Treatment

  a. Medications

    (1) There are no cures for depressive disorders, but symptoms can be substantially reduced in more than 90% of patients, with a full remission in 30% to 40%.

    (2) Duration of treatment

        (a) High rates of depressive recurrence suggest longer, rather than shorter, treatment duration.

            (i) First lifetime episode: 6 to 12 months of treatment

            (ii) Second lifetime episode: 12 months of treatment

            (iii) Subsequent episodes: maintenance treatment

        (b) Maintenance treatment

            (i) Goal is prophylaxis; treatment is indefinite.

              • Evidence suggests that 80% reduction in recurrence risk is achievable.

              • Medications are superior to psychotherapy, though a combination of medications and therapy is best for some patients.

(ii) Continue the acute treatment regimen (no dose reductions from acute to maintenance treatment period).

(3) First-line agents include the selective serotonin reuptake inhibitors (SSRIs).

　(a) Fluoxetine (Prozac, Sarafem)

　(b) Sertraline (Zoloft)

　(c) Paroxetine (Paxil)

　(d) Fluvoxamine (Luvox)

　(e) Citalopram (Celexa)

　(f) Escitalopram (Lexapro)

　(g) None of these medications is clearly superior to the others.

　(h) They are effective for atypical depression.

　(i) Typical side effects include

　　(i) Mild gastrointestinal (GI) symptoms

　　(ii) Increased sleep (citalopram, paroxetine, fluvoxamine) or decreased sleep (fluoxetine)

　　(iii) Sexual dysfunction
　　　• More often anorgasmia than impotence
　　　• Loss of libido

　　(iv) Sweating, especially at night

　　(v) Headache, usually transient at initiation of therapy

　　(vi) Restlessness or jitteriness

　(j) Withdrawal symptoms sometimes occur in patients who stop an SSRI suddenly or forget to take a dose.

　　(i) Headache, dizziness

　　(ii) Arthralgias

　　(iii) Confusion

　　(iv) "Out of body" or "unreal" feelings
　　　• Most often seen with paroxetine because of its relatively short half-life
　　　• Rarely seen with fluoxetine

(4) Growing body of evidence suggests that "dual-action" antidepressants may be superior to the SSRIs.

(5) "Dual-action" agents affect serotonin and norepinephrine systems in the brain.

　(a) Venlafaxine (Effexor), a direct serotonin and norepinephrine reuptake inhibitor (SNRI)

　　(i) Typically affects serotonin at low doses (<75 mg/day) and norepinephrine at high doses (>225 mg/day)

　　(ii) Side effects include GI upset, increased blood pressure, sexual dysfunction.

　(b) Mirtazapine (Remeron)

　　(i) Stimulates serotonin (5-hydroxytryptamine, 5HT) and norepinephrine secretion.

　　(ii) Blocks 5HT2 and 5HT3 receptors.

　　(iii) Side effects include sedation and mild weight gain.
　　　• It is useful for depression with anxiety and insomnia.
　　　• 5HT3 blockade helps manage nausea.

(6) Other antidepressants

　(a) Bupropion (Wellbutrin)

　　(i) Enhances norepinephrine and possibly dopaminergic function

　　(ii) Side effects
　　　• Insomnia
　　　• Increases anxiety or restlessness in some patients
　　　• Greater seizure risk (0.4%) than other antidepressants (most likely at total daily doses above 450 mg)
　　　• No sexual side effects

　　(iii) Good alternative to SSRIs
　　　• Different mechanism of action
　　　• Different side effect profile

　(b) Nefazodone (Serzone)

　　(i) SNRI and postsynaptic 5HT2 blocker

　　(ii) Reduces the metabolism of benzodiazepines

　　(iii) Rare instances of hepatic necrosis (routine monitoring of transaminases not recommended)

　　(iv) Sedating, likely due to α_1-adrenergic antagonism

　　(v) No sexual side effects

(7) Tricyclic antidepressants

　(a) Clomipramine (Anafranil)

　(b) Amitriptyline

　(c) Imipramine

　(d) Nortriptyline

　(e) Desipramine

　(f) Protriptyline

　(g) Efficacy similar to SSRIs but with more side effects

　　(i) Anticholinergic side effects: dry

mouth, constipation, urinary retention

(ii) Sedation (due to antihistamine activity)

(iii) Cardiac effects

- Increased heart rate

- High doses may predispose to arrhythmias (prolonged QTc interval, torsades de pointes)

(iv) Orthostasis (due to α_1-adrenergic effects)

(8) Monoamine oxidase inhibitors (MAOIs)

(a) Phenelzine (Nardil)

(b) Tranylcypromine (Parnate)

(c) Extremely effective but more difficult to use than other medications

(i) Effective for atypical depression

(d) Dietary and medication restrictions

(i) Dietary restrictions (reduced tyramine)

- Main limitations are naturally aged meats and cheeses, broad beans, and foods with a high yeast content.

- These limitations are not as severe as in the past owing to a larger variety of acceptable foods in the marketplace.

(ii) Medication interactions

- Includes over-the-counter medications, such as decongestants and diet aids

- Serious adverse interaction with meperidine (Demerol)—may be fatal

(e) Side effects

(i) Orthostasis: almost universal when initiating treatment

(ii) Sleep changes: sedation (phenelzine), insomnia (tranylcypromine)

(iii) Hypertensive crisis: if dietary and medication restrictions are not followed

(f) Reversible MAOIs have shown inconsistent results for treating major depression, so they are not recommended as a principal therapy.

b. Psychotherapy

(1) Several types of psychotherapy have proven to be effective in clinical trials.

(a) Equal to medications for mild to moderate depressive episodes

(b) Less effective as a sole treatment for severe episodes or depression with psychosis or for maintenance antidepressant treatment

(2) Cognitive behavioral therapy

(a) Focuses on automatic thought patterns that sustain depression.

(b) Extensive research data support this treatment.

(3) Interpersonal psychotherapy

(a) Focuses on conflicted and unsatisfying interpersonal relationships.

(b) Considerable research data support this treatment.

(4) Psychodynamic psychotherapy

(a) Focuses on unresolved developmental conflicts

(b) It has a long tradition but limited rigorous research support.

(c) Investigations have found that time-limited, psychodynamic therapy that specifically targets the patient's current symptoms can be helpful.

c. Electroconvulsive therapy (ECT)

(1) It is still the most effective treatment for depression: more than 80% versus 60% success for medications or psychotherapy.

(2) Typically 6 to 12 treatments (given 3 per week) are required for major depression.

(a) May be used as maintenance treatment

(b) One treatment every 2 to 4 weeks

(3) Common side effects

(a) Myalgias

(b) Headache

(c) Disorientation and amnesia around the time of treatment (includes limited anterograde and retrograde amnesia, as is found with naturally occurring seizures). No convincing evidence for long-term memory impairment

Key Treatment: Major Depression

Medications

- First-line agents include the SSRIs.

- A growing body of evidence suggests that dual-action (affecting the serotonin and norepinephrine systems) antidepressants may be superior to the SSRIs.

- TCAs and MAOIs are second-line treatment options.

ECT

- Electroconvulsive therapy is still the most effective treatment for major depression.

Psychotherapy

- Cognitive behavioral therapy

- Interpersonal therapy

- Time-limited psychodynamic therapy

Caveat

- When given to a patient on MAOIs, meperidine (Demerol) can have serious adverse interactions that may be fatal.

MINOR DEPRESSION

1. Definition. Minor depression is disturbance of mood, neurovegetative function, and cognition, occasionally accompanied by suicidal or homicidal ideation.

   a. Minor depression has fewer or less severe symptoms than major depression.

   b. Duration of illness may be short (days to weeks) or long (many years).

   c. Dysthmic disorder is the prototype of minor depression in the DSM-IV.

      (1) Depressive mood most days for 2 years

      (2) Accompanied by mild to moderate, but nagging changes in sleep, appetite, energy, concentration

2. Epidemiology

   a. It is much the same as for major depression.

   b. Elderly are at significantly higher risk for minor depression.

   c. It may be more common than major depression.

      (1) Recent longitudinal research shows that depressive illness is a chronic, waxing and waning condition with periods of euthymia interspersed with episodes of major and minor depression of varying lengths.

         (a) This suggests that major and minor depression are not separate illnesses but different manifestations of the same pathophysiologic process(es).

         (b) This is the strongest evidence to date for the lifetime nature of depressive illness.

Caveat

- The elderly are at significantly higher risk for minor depression.

---

3. Pathophysiology: not known but is likely to be the same as for major depression

4. Clinical features

   a. Symptoms the same as for major depression but fewer or less severe

   b. Generally fewer vegetative symptoms

      (1) Somnolence and fatigue

      (2) Appetite disturbance

   c. More subjective symptoms

      (1) Guilt

      (2) Worry

      (3) Pessimism

   d. Patients are at higher risk for major depression.

   e. Overall level of lost productivity is higher for minor depression than major depression, as the population experiences more total days of minor depression.

Key Symptoms: Minor Depression

- Symptoms are the same as for major depression but are fewer or less severe.

5. Differential diagnosis

   a. It is the same as for major depression.

   b. Most likely source of confusion is between minor and major depression.

6. Laboratory testing

   a. There are no specific laboratory tests for minor depression.

   b. Same guidelines as for major depression can be used.

Key Tests

- There are no specific laboratory tests for minor depression.

- The same guidelines as for major depression can be used.

7. Treatment

   a. It is substantially the same as for major depression.

   b. Pharmacology is the same.

      (1) No evidence that smaller doses of antide-

pressants are needed should medications be warranted.

(2) Some evidence indicates that higher doses and more prolonged treatment may be necessary for an adequate response.

c. Formal studies of specific psychotherapies and medication-psychotherapy combinations are underway.

(1) At present, similar psychotherapies are used for major and minor depressive episodes.

 Key Treatment: Minor Depression

• Pharmacology for minor depression is the same as that for major depression.

BIPOLAR AFFECTIVE DISORDERS

1. Definition

   a. Disturbance of mood, neurovegetative function, and cognition, which may be accompanied by suicidal or homicidal ideation and psychosis

   b. Not always two completely opposite poles, despite the name of the illness

      (1) Manic symptoms may or may not be the opposite of those encountered in patients with depression.

      (2) Manic and depressive periods typically occur separately or sequentially, but patients may demonstrate mixed manic-depressed states.

2. Epidemiology

   a. BAD affects approximately 1% of the population.

   b. There is an equal preponderance of males and females.

   c. Onset usually occurs at around 20 years of age.

      (1) Onset before 12 years of age or after 60 is uncommon. When the first episode occurs in an elderly person, it suggests a medical etiology.

      (2) Onset is usually marked by a manic episode.

   d. There is strong heritability, with twins having up to 50% concordance and first-degree relatives approximately 10% to 20%.

Caveats

• Onset is usually marked by a manic episode.

• A first episode of BAD in an elderly person suggests a medical etiology.

3. Pathophysiology

   a. Pathophysiology is unknown.

      (1) Many of the same factors involved in depression are likely relevant in BAD.

      (2) Abnormal circadian and ultradian rhythms are being actively investigated.

   b. Genetic factors are likely, and putative genetic loci on chromosomes 18 and 22 are being investigated.

4. Clinical features

   a. Diagnosis of BAD type I requires the patient to have experienced at least one episode of mania.

      (1) Periods of sleeplessness (days)

      (2) Racing thoughts

      (3) Impulsivity

      (4) Grandiosity ("feeling like you can do anything and everything")

      (5) Spending money excessively

   b. Less severe symptoms and those of shorter duration are diagnosed as hypomania. Patients with exclusively hypomanic episodes have BAD type II or cyclothymia.

   c. There may or may not be a history of recurrent depressive episodes.

   d. In some cases, psychotic features are present.

      (1) Hallucinations

      (2) Paranoia

      (3) Delusions

         (a) Grandeur

         (b) Reference: belief that things somehow refer back to the patient (e.g., the color of a passing car indicates that the patient is to do something special)

   e. Mania and major depressive episodes: BAD, type I

   f. Hypomania and major depressive episodes: BAD, type II

   g. Hypomania and minor depressive episodes: cyclothymic disorder

5. Differential diagnosis

   a. Differential diagnosis of bipolar disorder includes all the illness listed in the differential diagnosis for depression and psychotic illnesses.

   b. Type I versus type II versus cyclothymia

c. Additionally, there may be

    (1) Stimulant abuse

        (a) Caffeine

        (b) Amphetamines

        (c) Cocaine

    (2) Sedative withdrawal

        (a) Alcohol

        (b) Barbiturates

        (c) Benzodiazepines

    (3) Medical illness

        (a) Hyperthyroidism, including overadministration of thyroid medication

        (b) Hypocalcemia/hypomagnesemia

        (c) Poststroke period

    (4) Sleep deprivation

6. Laboratory testing. There is no formal laboratory testing for bipolar disorder. Routine investigation is the same as for depression.

    a. Thyroid-stimulating hormone (TSH)

    b. Urine drug screen (UDS)

    c. Levels of mood stabilizers, when prescribed

        (1) Lithium

        (2) Valproic acid

        (3) Carbamazepine

    d. Other laboratory tests, guided by historical or physical examination evidence of conditions in the differential diagnosis

Key Tests: Minor Depression

- There is no formal laboratory testing for bipolar disorder.

- The same guidelines as for major depression can be used.

7. Treatment

    a. Treatment can be divided into acute and chronic management of symptoms.

    b. Even with good compliance to the treatment, relapse rates are fairly high (30%).

    c. Chronic management

        (1) Mood stabilizers

            (a) Lithium

                (i) Levels should be checked 3–5 days after starting or changing dose.

                (ii) Effective dose is usually 900 to 1200 mg.

                (iii) Side effects.

                    • Hypothyroidism: 20% of those taking lithium for 5 years develop minor hypothyroidism.

Check thyroid status before and periodically during lithium treatment.

- Peripheral edema
- Peripheral neuropathy
- Weight gain
- Polyuria/polydipsia: urine output more than 3 L/day
- Tremor: It may be a sign of toxicity, though some patients on long-term lithium maintenance develop a persistent tremor.
- Renal dysfunction: Change in creatinine clearance with normal aging probably outweighs that induced by lithium for patients who have not had bouts of lithium toxicity.
- Toxicity: nausea, tremors, ataxia, seizures. Level above 2.5 mg/dL or above 2.0 mg/dL with symptoms of toxicity is an indication for immediate dialysis.

    d. Teratogenicity: rare cause (<1%) of Ebstein's anomaly if used during first trimester of pregnancy

        (b) Valproic acid

            (i) Average dose is 1500 to 2000 mg.

            (ii) Levels necessary for bipolar disorder may be higher than for seizure disorder.

            (iii) Side effects

                • Weight gain

                • Sedation

                • Uncommon cause of thrombocytopenia

                • Teratogenicity (neural tube defects during first trimester)

                • Controversial cause of polycystic ovary syndrome

        (c) Other antiepileptic medications: overall efficacy of these medicines still being investigated

            (i) Carbamazepine/oxcarbazepine

            (ii) Gabapentin

            (iii) Lamotrigine

            (iv) Topiramate

        (d) Antipsychotics. There is considerable evidence that these medications are useful for acute mania and some evidence that they are useful for preventing mania (see Part XXV, Chapter 4 for dosing and side effects).

(i) Olanzapine

(ii) Risperidone

(iii) Clozapine

(iv) Typical antipsychotics may be useful for extremely short periods during acute mania, though there is some evidence that patients with mood disorders are more vulnerable to tardive dyskinesia than patients with schizophrenia.

(2) Psychotherapy

(a) Several psychotherapies have been developed or adapted specifically for bipolar disorder, particularly cognitive-behavioral therapy.

(b) It is useful as an adjunct to maintenance medication but not as an alternative.

d. Acute management

(1) Patients should be started on a first-line mood stabilizer. If they are already on one, its serum level should be checked.

(2) Benzodiazepines or antipsychotics are used to manage the acute symptoms.

(a) They should be discontinued once the acute episode has resolved.

(b) Mood stabilizers should be maintained.

(3) Patients with mania and decreased sleep may improve markedly simply by promoting significant increases in sleep.

(4) ECT is highly effective for both manic and depressed episodes of bipolar disorder.

Key Treatment: Bipolar Disorder Type I

- Chronic management

  —Mood stabilizers

  —Psychotherapy

- Acute management:

  —First-line mood stabilizer; if patient is taking one, check serum level

  —Benzodiazepines or antipsychotics

  —Promote sleep

  —Electroconvulsive therapy

Bibliography

Doris A, Ebmeier K, Shajahan P: Depressive illness. Lancet 16:1369–1375, 1999.

Hilty DM, Brady KT, Hales RE: A review of bipolar disorder among adults. Psychiatr Serv 50:201–213, 1999.

Moore JD, Bona JR: Depression and dysthymia. Med Clin North Am 85:631–644, 2001.

Muller-Oerlinghausen B, Berghofer A, Bauer M: Bipolar disorder. Lancet 359:241–247, 2002.

Mulrow CD, Williams JW Jr, Trivedi M, et al: Treatment of depression: newer pharmacotherapies. Psychopharmacol Bull 34:409–795, 1998.

Thase ME: Long-term nature of depression. J Clin Psychiatry 60(Suppl 14):3–9, 1999.

2 Hyperventilation Syndrome
Randolph W. Evans

Definition

Hyperventilation syndrome (HVS) is a syndrome characterized by a variety of somatic symptoms induced by physiologically inappropriate hyperventilation and usually reproduced in whole or in part by voluntary hyperventilation.

Epidemiology and Risk Factors

1. Acute hyperventilation with obvious tachypnea accounts for about 1% of all cases.
2. The other 99% are due to chronic hyperventilation where there may be a modest increase in respiratory rate or tidal volume, which may not even be apparent to the patient or a medical observer.
3. Occurs in about 6% to 11% of the general patient population and is one of the most common causes of dizziness.
4. Acute HVS occurs 2 to 7 times more commonly in females than in males with most patients ranging in age from 15 to 55 years; it is especially common in females in their late teens.
5. Chronic HVS is more prevalent in middle-aged women.
6. Greatly underrecognized and misdiagnosed by physicians. Misdiagnoses include epilepsy, migraine, multiple sclerosis, cerebrovascular disease, angina, malingering and functional illness, vasovagal attacks, brain tumor, and hypoglycemia.

Etiology and Pathophysiology

1. Frequently associated with anxiety or stress, although some patients have no detectable psychiatric disorder and develop a habit of inappropriately increased ventilatory rate or depth.
2. Common triggers of acute HVS include anxiety, nausea and vomiting, and fever due to the common cold.
3. Less than 5% of cases of HVS have a solely organic cause, 60% have a psychogenic (emotional and habitual) basis, and the remainder have varying combinations.
4. Acute HVS reduces arterial pCO_2, resulting in alkalosis.
   a. Respiratory alkalosis produces the Bohr effect, a left shift of the oxygen dissociation curve with increased binding of oxygen to hemoglobin and reduced oxygen delivery to the tissues.
   b. The alkalosis also causes a reduction in plasma Ca^{2+} concentration.
   c. Hypophosphatemia may be due to intracellular shifts of phosphorus caused by altered glucose metabolism.
5. In chronic HVS, bicarbonate and potassium levels may be decreased because of increased renal excretion.
6. Stress can produce a hyperadrenergic state that may trigger hyperventilation through beta-adrenergic stimulation.
7. Central and peripheral mechanisms have been postulated for production of neurologic symptoms during hyperventilation.
   a. Voluntary hyperventilation can reduce cerebral blood flow by 30% to 40%. Headache, visual disturbance, dizziness, tinnitus, ataxia, syncope, and psychological symptoms may be produced by diminished cerebral perfusion.
   b. The precise cause of generalized slowing of brain waves on an electroencephalogram during hyperventilation is not certain.
      (1) The response is most common and pronounced in children and teenagers, diminished in adults, and is rare in old age.
      (2) Hypoglycemia can accentuate the slowing.
      (3) A brainstem-mediated response to hypocarbia may be responsible.
   c. Muscle spasms and tetany may be due to respiratory alkalosis and hypocalcemia.
   d. Hypophosphatemia can result in tiredness, dizziness, poor concentration, disorientation, and paresthesias.
   e. A hyperadrenergic state may result in tremor, tachycardia, anxiety, and sweating.
   f. Hypokalemia can cause muscle weakness and lethargy.
   g. The cause of bilateral and unilateral paresthesias is not certain.
      (1) A reduction in the concentration of extracellular Ca^{2+} may increase peripheral nerve axonal excitability, resulting in spontaneous bursting activity of cutaneous axons, perceived as paresthesias.
      (2) Lateralization of symptoms might be ex-

973

plained by anatomic differences in the peripheral nerves and their nutrient vessels.

(3) Alternatively, symmetrically decreased cerebral perfusion could account for bilateral paresthesias; asymmetrically decreased perfusion, for unilateral paresthesias.

(4) It is not known why unilateral paresthesias occur more often on the left side of the face and body.

    (a) One hypothesis is that psychosomatic symptoms are associated with right hemisphere psychic processes. During stress and arousal, the right hemisphere is activated more than the left. Symptoms of conversion or hyperventilation are more likely to occur on the left side of the face and body.

    (b) However, this hypothesis does not account for the increased frequency of left-sided paresthesias in normal subjects who are asked to hyperventilate.

Clinical Findings

1. There are numerous manifestations of HVS (see Key Symptoms and Signs). Patients may have one or multiple symptoms and signs which can occur in symptom clusters.

2. Patients with different symptoms may see different specialists. Cardiologists may see those complaining of chest pain, palpitations, and shortness of breath while neurologists frequently see those with dizziness and paresthesias.

3. Paresthesias

    a. HVS is the most common cause of distal symmetrical paresthesias.

    b. May be bilateral or unilateral.

       (1) In normal volunteers asked to hyperventilate, predominantly unilateral paresthesias reported by 16% involving the left side in over 60%. Also predominantly left-sided in symptomatic patients.

       (2) Patterns of numbness may be perioral and just the 4th and 5th fingers. Unusual patterns such as one side of the abdomen or forehead can occur.

4. A patient's anxiety about the unexplained symptoms of HVS may result in feelings of impending death, fear, or panic.

5. Complaints such as déjà vu, auditory, and visual hallucinations are rare.

Key Symptoms and Signs

General

- Fatigability, exhaustion, weakness, sleep disturbance, nausea, sweating

Cardiovascular

- Chest pain, palpitations, tachycardia, Raynaud's phenomenon

Gastrointestinal

- Aerophagia, dry mouth, pressure in throat, dysphagia, globus hystericus, epigastric fullness or pain, belching, flatulence

Neurologic

- Headache, pressure in the head, fullness in the head, head warmth

- Blurred vision, tunnel vision, momentary flashing lights, diplopia

- Dizziness, faintness, vertigo, giddiness, unsteadiness

- Tinnitus

- Numbness, tingling, coldness of face, limbs, trunk

- Muscle spasms, muscle stiffness, carpopedal spasm, generalized tetany, tremor

- Ataxia, weakness

- Syncope, seizures

Psychological

- Impairment of concentration and memory

- Feelings of unreality, disorientation, confused or dream-like feeling, déjà vu

- Hallucinations

- Anxiety, apprehension, nervousness, tension, fits of crying, agoraphobia

- Neuroses, phobias, panic attacks

Respiratory

- Shortness of breath, suffocating feeling, smothering spell, inability to get a good breath or to breathe deeply enough, frequent sighing, yawning

Differential Diagnosis

1. Numerous organic disorders can cause hyperventilation.

    a. Drugs including salicylate and caffeine

    b. Cirrhosis and hepatic coma

    c. Acute pain

d. Splenic flexure syndrome, cholecystitis, fever, and sepsis

e. Dissecting aortic aneurysm, respiratory dyskinesia, pulmonary embolism, pneumothorax, interstitial lung disease, asthma, and heat and altitude acclimatization

2. Neurologic disorders

a. Rett, Joubert, and Reye syndromes

b. Pyruvate dehydrogenase deficiency and biotic-dependent multiple carboxylase deficiency

c. Malignant hyperthermia, brainstem tumor, thalamic hemorrhage, syringobulbia, and neurogenic pulmonary edema due to intracranial hypertension.

3. Cardiac disease should certainly be considered in patients with chest pain.

a. Hyperventilation can mimic cardiac disease by producing electrocardiogram changes including T wave inversions, systolic time-segment depression, and systolic time-segment elevation in patients without coronary artery disease.

b. Some patients with angina pectoris may hyperventilate in response to their pain and anxiety

c. The symptoms of hyperventilation and mitral valve prolapse may overlap and, in some cases, the symptoms may be due to HVS rather than prolapse.

4. Symptoms of panic attacks (see Part XXV, Chapter 1, Mood Disorders) greatly overlap with HVS, and the differential diagnosis is quite similar.

5. Tonic spasms (paroxysmal dystonia) of multiple sclerosis (see Part VI, Chapter 1, Multiple Sclerosis) can be somewhat similar to the muscle spasms, tetany, and paresthesias of HVS.

Testing

1. The acute form is easily recognized, but the chronic form may be overlooked because the respiratory rate is not reported as rapid or does not appear rapid, and because the symptoms may appear to be atypical.

a. For example, a respiration rate of 18 per minute may lead to overbreathing that is not easily detectable.

b. Because the chronic disorder is intermittent, spot arterial or end-tidal volume pCO_2 results can be normal.

2. The hyerventilation provocation test

a. Can be performed with either an increased ventilation rate of up to 60 per minute or simply deep breathing for 3 minutes.

b. Dizziness, unsteadiness, and blurred vision commonly develop within 20 to 30 seconds, especially with the patient in the standing position. Paresthesias have a later onset.

c. Chest pain is reported by 50% of patients after 3 minutes of hyperventilating.

d. For clinical purposes, measurement of end-tidal volume pCO_2 is not necessary. In addition, there is no clear correlation between $Paco_2$ and neurologic symptoms.

e. The diagnosis is often made by reproducing some or all of the symptoms with the provocation test and excluding other possible causes by either clinical reasoning or laboratory testing when indicated. Patients frequently report only one or two symptoms but, on performing the provocation test, report other symptoms that appear during typical episodes but that they had forgotten.

f. For some patients with HVS, symptoms cannot be reliably reproduced during the provocation test or on consecutive tests.

(1) In some cases, the provocation test lacks test-retest reliability.

(2) For some patients, antecedent anxiety and stress, not present during the test, may predispose to symptom formation because of a hyperadrenergic state.

(3) Differerent patterns of hyperventilation with different respiratory rates, tidal volumes, and durations may induce different symptoms.

g. Contraindications to the provocation test include patients with ischemic heart or cerebrovascular disease, pulmonary insufficiency, hyperviscosity states, significant anemia, sickle cell disease, or uncontrolled hypertension.

Treatment

1. In many cases, reassurance and education of the patient is all that is required.

2. Some patients may be able to terminate an attack by decreasing their respiratory rate or breathing into a paper bag for 1 to 2 minutes.

3. Others may respond to other approaches such as breathing exercises, diaphragmatic retraining, biofeedback, progressive relaxation, hypnosis, psychological and psychiatric treatment.

4. Medications such as beta blockers, benzodiazepines, and antidepressants may also be of benefit for some patients.

Key Treatments

- Reassurance and education
- Decreasing respiratory rate
- Breathing into a paper bag
- Other approaches: breathing exercises, diaphragmatic retraining, biofeedback, progressive relaxation, hypnosis, psychological and psychiatric treatment
- Medications

Prognosis

1. Fifty percent of patients with acute HVS recover without treatment.
2. In 10% of those with chronic HVS, symptoms may persist for more than 3 years.
3. With proper management, 70% to 90% of adults become symptom free.
4. Forty percent of children and adolescents with HVS may still have episodes as adults with many suffering from chronic anxiety.

Bibliography

Beumer HM, Bruyn GW: Hyperventilation syndrome. In Goetz CG, Tanner CM, Aminoff MJ (eds): Handbook of Clinical Neurology, vol. 19. Amsterdam, Elsevier, 1993, pp. 429–448.

Evans RW: Neurologic aspects of hyperventilation syndrome. Semin Neurol 15:115–125, 1995.

Evans RW: Hyperventilation syndrome. In Gilman S (ed): Medlink Neurology. San Diego, Medlink, 2003.

Folgering H: The pathophysiology of hyperventilation syndrome. Monaldi Arch Chest Dis. 54:365–372, 1999.

Lum LC: Hyperventilation syndromes in medicine and psychiatry: a review. J R Soc Med 80:229–231, 1987.

3 Anxiety Disorders

Jeffrey P. Staab
Christos Ballas

Definition

Anxiety disorders are syndromes characterized by excessive or chronic worry. There are several subtypes of anxiety disorders, including panic disorder, obsessive-compulsive disorder, posttraumatic stress disorder, social phobia, and generalized anxiety disorder. Each comes with its own set of symptoms.

Epidemiology

1. The lifetime prevalence of anxiety disorders is approximately 15%.
2. Social phobia is the most common anxiety disorder and the third most common psychiatric diagnosis. It has a lifetime prevalence of 10% to 15%, with onset usually during the teenage years.
3. Panic disorder has a lifetime prevalence of 3%, with onset during the twenties.
4. Posttraumatic stress disorder is experienced by 3% of Americans per year, although the exact epidemiology is difficult to assess given the nature of the disorder.
5. Obsessive-compulsive disorder is found in 3% of the population; and most of these patients (75%) manifest symptoms by age 30.

Pathophysiology

1. The pathophysiology of the anxiety disorders is not completely understood, but there are two neuroanatomic regions that appear to be involved. This is supported by the efficacy of medications that act on them.
   a. Overactivation of noradrenergic systems (locus ceruleus)
      (1) Medical conditions that activate the noradrenergic systems cause anxiety (i.e., pheochromocytoma, cocaine or amphetamine intoxication)
   b. Underactivity of or diminished inhibitory control by serotonergic systems (medial and dorsal raphe nuclei)
      (1) Medicines that increase serotonin modulate anxiety.
         (a) Selective serotonin reuptake inhibitors (SSRIs)
         (b) Buspirone

Symptoms

See Table 3–1.
1. Panic disorder
   a. Panic disorder is characterized by discrete episodes of terror and autonomic arousal.
      (1) Panic attacks are often spontaneous with no known precipitant.
      (2) Panic attacks also may be triggered by one or more identifiable stimuli, which leads to avoidance of known precipitants.
      (3) Intense autonomic symptoms of panic attacks include
         (a) Chest pain
         (b) Tachycardia, palpitations
         (c) Shortness of breath
         (d) Choking, dysphagia
         (e) Dizziness, lightheadedness
         (f) Sweating
         (g) Flushing
         (h) Numbness, paresthesias
      (4) Medical causes of these symptoms must be ruled out, including myocardial infarction, dysrhythmias, asthma, chronic obstructive

TABLE 3–1. MAIN SYMPTOMS AND PROVOCATIVE STIMULI OF ANXIETY DISORDERS

Anxiety Disorder	Major Symptom(s)	Provocative Stimuli
Panic disorder	Panic attacks	Spontaneous and/or multiple provocative places and situations
Agoraphobia	Avoidance	Multiple "unsafe" or fear-provoking situations (usually unfamiliar settings or when alone)
Generalized anxiety	Chronic worry	Multiple daily life events
Social phobia	Episodic anxiety Avoidance	Social situations (particularly unfamiliar settings or people)
Obsessive-compulsive disorder	Obsessions Compulsions	Dirt or contamination Things perceived as undone Perceived untidiness
Posttraumatic stress disorder	Reexperiencing Avoidance Hyperarousal	Reminders of traumatic event (people, places, things, conversations)

pulmonary disease (COPD), and vestibular disorders.

(5) Panic disorder may occur with or without agoraphobia.

    (a) Agoraphobia was originally described as "fear of the marketplace" or "fear of open spaces," but it now refers to a widespread fear and avoidance of situations perceived to be unsafe or that provoke panic symptoms.

    (b) The patient remains at home or in other safe, familiar environments as a means of avoiding stimuli that induce panic attacks.

Caveat

• For intense symptoms of panic attack (e.g., chest pain, tachycardia, shortness of breath, choking, dizziness, sweating, flushing, numbness), medical causes must be ruled out, including heart attack, asthma, COPD, vestibular disease, hyperthyroidism, and mitral valve prolapse.

---

2. Obsessive-compulsive disorder (OCD)

  a. Obsessions: recurrent, intrusive thoughts

    (1) Often these are repeated words, phrases, or ideas. Patients may recognize the unusual nature of the thoughts but may not be able to stop or resist them.

    (2) Common obsessive themes

      (a) Dirt, contamination, infection

      (b) Things not done or improperly done

        (i) Doors unlocked

        (ii) Lights, stove left on

        (iii) Mistakes on job-related tasks

      (c) Order, tidiness: closets, rooms, clothes, and so on, are out of order.

      (d) Repulsive, violent images or impulses: Patients fear they may have or will harm another.

    (3) Some of these themes are similar to the intrusive thoughts of Tourette's syndrome, although with OCD the thoughts may not have to be expressed verbally.

  b. Compulsions: rituals or rigid routines

    (1) Compulsions are performed most often in response to obsessions to reduce the anxiety associated with the obsessions. Inability to complete the ritual increases the anxiety.

    (2) Compulsions often include magical think-

ing (i.e., the compulsive act will "prevent" horrible events, such as a family member's death).

    (3) Common behavioral compulsions

      (a) Checking

        (i) Doors, locks

        (ii) Oven, gas

        (iii) Toilets

      (b) Washing, showering, cleaning

      (c) Precise ordering or arranging of objects

      (d) Hoarding

    (4) Compulsions may be mental rather then physical activities.

      (a) Counting. Some patients need to organize objects around a certain number (e.g., having seven of everything).

      (b) Mental repetition of songs, prayers, or slogans

  c. Up to 20% of patients with OCD manifest motor tics.

  d. There is a higher than expected co-morbidity with Tourette's syndrome

---

Caveats

• Compulsions are performed in response to obsessions to reduce the anxiety associated with the obsessions.

• Compulsions may be mental rather than physical activities.

---

3. Generalized anxiety disorder

  a. This disorder is characterized by excessive or chronic worry.

    (1) Some avoidance of stressors is common.

    (2) Occasionally "anxiety attacks" occur, but these attacks are more often described by patients as a gradually increasing spiral of worry rather than the sudden onset of autonomic arousal that occurs with panic disorder.

  b. Insomnia and fatigue are the most common somatic symptoms.

    (1) Patients may describe difficulty falling asleep because of excessive thoughts.

    (2) They may awaken in the middle of the night with an "anxiety attack."

      (a) Tachycardia, sweating, autonomic arousal

      (b) Fear

    (3) Little sleep or poor quality sleep may lead to daytime fatigue.

c. Other somatic symptoms are common.
  (1) Paresthesias or muscle tension
  (2) Dizziness, headaches
4. Social phobia
  a. It is characterized by an intense fear of social situations or unfamiliar people or performances. The fear is understood as unreasonable, but it still causes the patient distress and promotes avoiding social situations. Typically, this disorder first manifests during the teen years.
    (1) Patient avoids making a call to a repairman out of fear that he will think ill of her.
    (2) Patient is uncomfortable in the supermarket line because he feels everyone is looking at him.
    (3) Patient has difficulty interacting with the boss, even on a social level, for fear of saying the wrong thing or "making a fool of myself."

Caveat

• Social phobia is the most common anxiety disorder and the third most common psychiatric diagnosis.

---

5. Posttraumatic stress disorder (PTSD)
  a. PTSD is triggered by exposure to a traumatic stressor (i.e., a life-threatening event), not just a stressful occurrence such as a divorce or job loss.
  b. There are three clusters of PTSD symptoms.
    (1) Reexperiencing: Patients may relive the experience in several ways.
      (a) Recurrent or intrusive memories of the event
      (b) Flashbacks: intense sensations as if the event were recurring
        (i) The patient behaves as if he or she is back at the time and place of the traumatic event.
        (ii) It often occurs at times of high stress or when his "guard is down" (e.g., riding a bus, walking on the street).
      (c) Physical or psychological reactions as if one is reliving the experience
        (i) This may include panic attacks or other autonomic hyperarousal.
        (ii) It may last only seconds, but the patient experiences it as if it were much longer.
        (iii) It differs from a flashback in that

the patient does not have the sensation of returning to the time and place of the trauma.
      (d) Nightmares
    (2) Avoidance
      (i) Trauma-specific avoidance
        (i) Avoidance of cues and reminders of the event
        (ii) This would include avoiding conversations about the trauma and may lead to more severe pathologic reactions, such as repression or denial.
      (b) Generalized avoidance
        (i) Estrangement from others
        (ii) Social isolation
    (3) Hyperarousal
      (a) Irritability
      (b) Insomnia
      (c) Tension
      (d) Easy startle

Caveats

• PTSD is triggered by exposure to a traumatic stressor (a life-threatening event), not just a stressful occurrence such as a divorce or job loss.

• Reexperiencing, avoidance, and hyperarousal are the three clusters of PTSD symptoms.

Differential Diagnosis

1. Psychiatric differential diagnosis includes mood disorders and substance use.
  a. Depression
  b. Substance-related
    (1) Stimulant use, abuse
      (a) Amphetamines
      (b) Cocaine
      (c) Caffeine
        (i) 1 cup brewed coffee: 110 mg
        (ii) 12 oz of soda: 45 mg
        (iii) 1 cup tea: 45 mg
        (iv) 1 oz dark chocolate: 20 mg
    (2) Lithium toxicity
      (a) Generally presents first with tremor, then ataxia and confusion
    (3) Beta-agonists and other sympathomimetic medications, including anticholinergics
    (4) Steroids

(5) Neuroleptics—akathisia (restlessness) may mimic anxiety

c. Substance withdrawal

(1) Alcohol

(2) Barbiturates

(3) Benzodiazepines

2. Medical differential diagnosis

a. Cardiac disease

(1) Dysrhythmias

(a) Superventricular tachycardias

(b) Atrial fibrillation

(c) Ventricular tachycardia

(2) Mitral valve prolapse

(3) Coronary artery disease: particularly for patients over 40 years of age

b. Respiratory causes

(1) Asthma

(2) COPD

(3) Hypoxia

(4) Pulmonary embolus

c. Endocrine disorders and metabolic abnormalities

(1) Hyperthyroidism: includes symptoms from increases in thyroid replacement hormone

(2) Hypoglycemia

(3) Hypocalcemia

(4) Hypomagnesemia: particularly important in alcoholics

(5) Pheochromocytoma: extremely rare

d. Neurologic diseases: seizures

e. Otologic conditions: peripheral and central vestibular deficits

Laboratory Studies

1. There are no specific studies for anxiety disorders. Diagnostic investigations are geared toward ruling out medical causes.

2. When the psychiatric symptoms are clear and the medical history is benign, only a few studies are needed.

a. Drug screening

b. Thyroid-stimulating hormone

3. For persistent or unremitting anxiety and for clinically ambiguous situations, a greater range of studies may be needed.

a. Electrocardiography

b. Pulse oximetry

c. Calcium, magnesium, glucose assays

4. In some cases, extensive diagnostic evaluations are needed, but they tend to be undertaken much more often than is clinically necessary, particularly in young patients with unremarkable medical histories and examinations.

a. 24-Hour Holter monitoring

b. Exercise stress test

c. Pulmonary function tests

d. Vestibular and balance function tests

e. 24-Hour urinary catecholamines

f. Brain imaging

g. Electroencephalography

Key Tests: Anxiety Disorders

• There are no specific studies for anxiety disorders.

• Diagnostic investigations are geared toward ruling out medical causes.

• Extensive diagnostic evaluations may be needed but tend to be undertaken more often than clinically necessary, particularly in young patients.

Treatment

See Table 3–2.

1. There are no cures for anxiety disorders, but a substantial reduction of symptoms is expected and full remission can be achieved in 30% to 40% of cases.

2. The newer antidepressants have superseded ben-

TABLE 3–2. MAIN MEDICATION TREATMENT CHOICES FOR ANXIETY DISORDERS*

ANXIETY DISORDER	FIRST LINE	FIRST LINE ALTERNATIVES	OTHER CHOICES
Panic disorder	SSRIs	Venlafaxine Mirtazapine Nefazodone	Benzodiazepines Tricyclic antidepressants MAOIs
Generalized anxiety disorder	SSRIs	Venlafaxine Mirtazapine Nefazodone	Benzodiazepines Tricyclic antidepressants MAOIs
Social phobia	SSRIs	Venlafaxine Mirtazapine Nefazodone	Benzodiazepines Beta blockers Tricyclic antidepressants MAOIs
Obsessive-compulsive disorder	SSRIs	Clomipramine	Venlafaxine
Posttraumatic stress disorder	SSRIs	Nefazodone	Sedating tricyclic antidepressants

*Abbreviations: SSRIs, selective serotonin reuptake inhibitors; MAOIs, monoamine oxidase inhibitors.
Effective psychotherapies exist for all of these disorders and may be used with medications or as an alternative to pharmacotherapy.

zodiazepines as the treatment of choice for anxiety disorders for several reasons.

  a. High co-morbidity of depression with anxiety, for which benzodiazepines are ineffective

  b. High likelihood of symptom relapse after stopping benzodiazepines, when they are used as the sole treatment

  c. Abuse liability of benzodiazepines

3. Most antidepressants are effective for most anxiety disorders.

  a. Initial doses used to treat anxiety disorders are lower than those used for depression.

   (1) Most newer antidepressants can exacerbate anxiety if started at too high a dose.

   (2) Begin with half the dose recommended for depression.

  b. Full therapeutic dose ranges are the same for anxiety and depressive disorders. Titrate the medication to full clinical effect.

  c. Strongly noradrenergic antidepressants do not relieve anxiety.

   (1) Bupropion (Wellbutrin, Zyban)

   (2) Activating tricyclic antidepressants (e.g., desipramine, protriptyline)

  d. Obsessive-compulsive disease must be treated with a serotonergic agent (e.g., an SSRI or clomipramine).

4. First-line agents are the SSRIs.

  a. Fluoxetine (Prozac, Sarafem)

  b. Sertraline (Zoloft)

  c. Paroxetine (Paxil)

  d. Fluvoxamine (Luvox)

  e. Citalopram (Celexa)

  f. Escitalopram (Lexapro)

  g. None of these medications is clearly superior to the others.

  h. Typical side effects include

   (1) Mild gastrointestinal (GI) symptoms

   (2) Increased sleep (citalopram, paroxetine, fluvoxamine) or decreased sleep (fluoxetine)

   (3) Sexual dysfunction

    (a) More often anorgasmia than impotence

    (b) Loss of libido

   (4) Sweating, especially at night

   (5) Headache, usually transient at initiation of therapy

   (6) Restlessness or jitteriness

  i. Withdrawal symptoms sometimes occur in patients who stop an SSRI suddenly or forget to take a dose.

   (1) Headache, dizziness

   (2) Arthralgias

   (3) Confusion

   (4) "Out of body" or "unreal" feelings

    (a) Most often seen with paroxetine, because of its relatively short half-life

    (b) Rarely seen with fluoxetine

5. Effective alternatives to SSRIs as first-line agents

  a. Venlafaxine (Effexor): serotonin and norepinephrine reuptake inhibitor (SNRI)

   (1) Typically affects serotonin at the lower dosages (<75 mg/day) and norepinephrine at the higher dosages (>225 mg/day)

   (2) Side effects of GI upset, increased blood pressure at higher doses (>150 mg/day), sexual dysfunction

  b. Mirtazapine (Remeron)

   (1) Stimulates serotonin (5-hydroxytryptamine, 5HT) and norepinephrine secretion

   (2) Blocks 5HT2 and 5HT3 receptors

   (3) Side effects include sedation and mild weight gain

    (a) Useful for anxiety with insomnia

    (b) 5HT3 blockade helps manage nausea

6. Less commonly used antidepressants

  a. Tricyclic antidepressants

   (1) Clomipramine (Anafranil)

   (2) Amitriptyline

   (3) Imipramine

   (4) Nortriptyline

   (5) Efficacy similar to SSRIs, but with more side effects

    (a) Anticholinergic side effects

     (i) Dry mouth

     (ii) Constipation

     (iii) Urinary retention

    (b) Sedation

    (c) Cardiac effects

     (i) Increased heart rate

     (ii) High doses may predispose to arrhythmias (prolonged QTc, torsades de pointes)

  b. Nefazodone (Serzone): SNRI and postsynaptic 5HT2 blocker

   (1) Reduces the metabolism of benzodiazepines

   (2) Rare instance of hepatic necrosis

   (3) Sedating, likely due to α_1 antagonism

c. Monoamine oxidase inhibitors
  (1) Phenelzine (Nardil) is used more frequently than tranylcypromine (Parnate) for anxiety disorders.
  (2) Extremely effective, but they are more difficult to use than other medications.

7. Benzodiazepines
  a. Although effective, especially in the short term, tolerance and abuse potential limits their use.
  b. Anxiety relapse likely after discontinuing benzodiazepines when they are used alone.
  c. In patients with bona fide anxiety disorders, tolerance to good control of anxiety symptoms is *not* common (i.e., consistent dosing is the rule). Reevaluate the use of benzodiazepines in patients who request frequent dose increases.
  d. Generally, benzodiazepines are not used chronically.
    (1) Used for acute episodes of panic attack
    (2) For situational anxiety
      (a) Performance anxiety
      (b) Specific phobias
  e. Choice of benzodiazepines is based on half-life and onset of action.
    (1) Clonazepam (Klonopin)
      (a) Longer acting (half-life 8–12 hours)
      (b) Moderate onset of action
    (2) Alprazolam (Xanax)
      (a) Short acting (half-life 4 hours)
      (b) Extremely fast onset of action
    (3) High-potency benzodiazepines (clonazepam, alprazolam, lorazepam) are most effective for panic disorder.

8. Beta-blockers
  a. Limited utility except in specific situations
    (1) Effective for performance anxiety but not for other anxiety subtypes
    (2) Effective for essential tremor
  b. Nonspecific beta-blockers such as propanolol (Inderal) are most commonly used.

9. Antihistamines
  a. Most often used in place of benzodiazepines for patients with addiction potential
  b. Have a nonspecific sedative effect

10. Buspirone (Buspar): serotonin agonist at 5HT1a receptors
  a. Generally given in two- or three-times-a-day dosing
  b. Effective for mild to moderate GAD
  c. Not effective for panic disorder
  d. May be useful as an adjunct in OCD and PTSD

Caveats

- Most antidepressants are effective for most anxiety disorders.

- Many antidepressants can exacerbate anxiety if started at too high a dose; begin with half the dose recommended for depression, then titrate up for clinical effect.

- Consistent dosing of benzodiazepines is the rule because tolerance to good symptom control is uncommon.

- OCD should be treated with a serotonergic agent.

Bibliography

Gorman JM, Kent JM, Sullivan GM, Coplan JD: Neuroanatomical hypothesis of panic disorder, revised. Am J Psychiatry 157:493–505, 2000.

Hidalgo RB, Davidson JR: Posttraumatic stress disorder: epidemiology and health-related considerations. J Clin Psychiatry 61(Suppl 7):5–13, 2000.

Jenike MA: An update on obsessive-compulsive disorder. Bull Menninger Clin 65:4–25, 2001.

Lang AJ, Stein MB: Anxiety disorders. how to recognize and treat the medical symptoms of emotional illness. Geriatrics 56:24–27, 2001.

Lang AJ, Stein MB: Social phobia: prevalence and diagnostic threshold. J Clin Psychiatry 62(Suppl 1):5–10, 2001.

Lydiard RB: An overview of generalized anxiety disorder: disease state—appropriate therapy. Clin Ther 22(Suppl A):A3–19, 2000.

4 Psychotic Disorders

Christos Ballas
Jeffrey P. Staab

Definition

1. A psychotic disorder is one in which there is a defect in thinking or in reality testing. This would include the presence of
   a. Positive symptoms
      (1) Hallucinations
      (2) Delusions
         (a) Ideas of reference (i.e., that things relate back to the patient)
         (b) Paranoid delusions
         (c) Somatic delusions
      (3) Disorganization in thoughts or behavior
   b. Negative symptoms
      (1) Decreased motivation
      (2) Decreased interest in things

Epidemiology

Worldwide epidemiologic studies have found a prevalence of schizophrenia of 1% across races, cultures, and the developmental levels of countries.

Pathophysiology

1. Although not completely understood, several factors appear to be relevant in the development of psychotic disorders.
   a. Genetic factors
      (1) Lifetime risk to a patient of a first-degree relative with schizophrenia is 10% (i.e., 10 times higher than the normal population).
         (a) Apparently there is no increased risk of psychotic illness in children adopted by schizophrenic parents.
         (b) This suggests that schizophrenia cannot be induced in individuals who have no predisposing factors.
      (2) Concordance rate is 50% in monozygotic twins. This is evidence for a strong genetic predisposition but indicates that prenatal and childhood developmental factors play a role as well.
      (3) Lifetime risk of a psychotic disorder is 40% to 50% in children of two parents with schizophrenia.

   b. Infectious: Viruses seem most likely candidates.
      (1) Herpes simplex virus 2 infection in a pregnant mother significantly increases the risk.
      (2) Other viruses may be implicated.
      (3) Second trimester appears to be the vulnerable period.

2. Neuroanatomic and biochemical correlates
   a. Dopamine
      (1) D2 receptors appear most relevant.
         (a) D2 receptor saturation of 55% to 65% by antipsychotic medications is associated with reduced psychotic symptoms.
         (b) Receptor occupation above this proportion is associated with motoric side effects.
      (2) Dopamine agonists such as amphetamines can induce a psychotic syndrome, especially paranoia.
   b. Glutamate
      (1) N-Methyl-D-aspartate (NMDA) receptor blockade by phencyclidine (PCP)-induces psychosis
      (2) More schizophrenic-like than psychotic syndromes induced by dopamine agonists (e.g., amphetamines)
         (a) Hallucinations
         (b) Negative symptoms
         (c) Thought disorder

Symptoms

1. Psychotic illnesses vary in symptomatology, but the most common symptoms are
   a. Hallucinations
      (1) Auditory hallucinations predominate.
      (2) Prominent visual hallucinations are more symptomatic of organic disorders (i.e., delirium, medical and neurologic illness). Cross-modal hallucinations are often the result of toxic states or drugs.
      (3) See Part IX, Chapter 11, Auditory Hallucinations, for more details.
   b. Delusions
      (1) Self-referential delusions
      (2) Paranoia

983

c. Problems with thinking (i.e., thought process abnormalities)
   (1) Thoughts being implanted by others
   (2) Thoughts being removed by others
   (3) Extrasensory perception
   (4) Depersonalization
d. Problems with motivation
   (1) Lack of initiation
   (2) Negativism
   (3) Reduced spontaneity of speech, alogia
e. Problems with affect
   (1) Emotional blunting
   (2) Feeling perplexed
   (3) Inappropriate affect
f. Social isolation

Key Symptoms: Schizophrenia

Positive Symptoms

• Hallucinations

• Delusions

• Thought disorder

• Disorganized behavior

Negative Symptoms

• Restricted affect

• Decreased motivation

• Decreased interest

Course

• First 5 years: waxing, waning, deteriorating

• Middle years: chronic symptoms with acute exacerbations

• Later years: increasing cognitive impairment

Differential Diagnosis

1. Includes psychiatric, medical, and substance-related diagnoses
   a. Psychiatric disorders
      (1) Schizophrenia
      (2) Schizoaffective disorder
      (3) Bipolar disorder with psychotic features: generally associated with severe mood symptoms (i.e., severe mania)
      (4) Psychotic depression
         (a) Generally, psychotic symptoms are mood congruent (i.e., depressive themes).
         (b) Voices are derogatory or disparaging.

(5) Shared psychotic disorder
   (a) Develops because of a close relationship with another who already has the delusion
   (b) Folie à deux: mental disorder affecting two persons who share the same delusions
(6) Somatoform disorders. Although not typically psychotic disorders, patients with extreme somatoform disorders may develop a fixed delusion concerning symptoms.
   (a) Belief that one is infested (i.e., delusional parasitosis)
   (b) Belief that one has an extremely rare disease
(7) Postpartum psychosis
(8) Dissociative disorders: Patient may relate the experience of being "out of their body" or "missing time."
(9) Personality disorders
   (a) Patients with severe borderline personality disorder may be prone to brief periods of psychosis, especially when stressed.
   (b) Schizotypal personality disorder is characterized by odd, magical thinking that does not reach the level of psychosis but may be mistaken for such. These ideas typically do not interfere with daily functioning.
      (i) Example: Belief the FBI is watching them
      (ii) Example: belief that aliens are among us
   (c) Paranoid personality disorder: generally limited to an overarching sense of mistrust, suspiciousness of others, and paranoia, without other psychotic symptoms

b. Medical disorders
   (1) Infectious
      (a) Tertiary syphilis
      (b) Acute encephalitis or postencephalitic sequelae
   (2) Central nervous system tumor
   (3) Delirium: all causes
   (4) Advanced dementia complicated by psychosis
   (5) Vitamin deficiencies
      (a) Dementia and subsequent psychosis due to vitamin B_{12} or folate deficiency

(b) Vitamin B$_1$ (thiamine) deficiency: Korsakoff's psychosis

(c) Pellagra (niacin deficiency)

(i) Skin, mucosal sores

(ii) Diarrhea: seen in patients with malabsorption syndromes, alcoholics, and those who eat primarily corn

(6) Addison's disease

(a) Most common symptoms are memory problems and irritability.

(b) Delirium and psychosis are seen in rare, severe cases.

(c) Vitamin B$_{12}$ deficiency is found in about 25%.

(7) Cushing's disease

(8) Thyroid conditions

(a) Thyrotoxicosis

(b) Myxedema

(9) Hepatic encephalopathy

(10) Seizures: Temporal lobe seizures may produce psychotic symptoms.

(a) Visual hallucinations, auras

(b) Religious experiences

c. Substance-related

(1) Alcohol

(a) It does not produce hallucinations by itself.

(b) Chronic use may cause alcoholic hallucinosis.

(i) Commonly seen with some motor dysfunction

(ii) Atrophy of cerebellar vermis

(c) Withdrawal

(i) Agitation in early stages

(ii) Full psychotic symptomatology indicative of delirium tremens (DTs). DTs are found in those with

• History of seizures

• Preceding high blood alcohol level

• Infection, especially pulmonary

• Fever

(2) Marijuana

(a) Hallucinations are not common.

(b) Misperceptions and illusions are more common.

(3) Cocaine

(a) Generally agitation

(b) Hallucinations possibly cross-modal

(4) Amphetamines: most commonly paranoia

(5) Hallucinogens

(a) LSD: cross-modal: auditory to visual (e.g., "seeing" sounds as colors)

(b) Ketamine: dissociation

(6) Steroids

(a) Problems are found in 20% of patients whose dosages of prednisone are above 80 mg/day, most commonly during the first 10 days of steroid use.

(b) Agitation, confusion, and mood changes are more common than delusions and hallucinations.

(7) Anticholinergic drugs

(a) Scopolamine

(b) Atropine

(c) Procainamide

(i) Overt hallucinations are uncommon.

(ii) Disorientation and delusions are more common.

Laboratory Studies

1. There are no specific tests for psychotic disorders; studies are used to rule out medical or other causes.

2. Typical studies include

a. Rapid plasmin reagin

b. Thyroid-stimulating hormone

c. Drug screening

d. Other tests as indicated by the medical history and examination

Key Tests: Psychotic Disorders

• There are no specific tests for psychotic disorders; tests are used to rule out medical or other causes (e.g., rapid plasmin reagin, thyroid-stimulating hormone, drug screening).

Treatment

Treatment may be divided into acute psychosis and chronic psychosis.

1. Acute psychosis (particularly due to non-psychiatric conditions)

a. Managed with neuroleptics as needed

(1) Typical neuroleptics are favored because of their faster action.

(a) Haloperidol

(b) Chlorpromazine

(2) Intravenous and intramuscular administra-

tion produces more rapid results than oral dosing.

    (a) It is associated, however, with more extrapyramidal symptoms (EPSs).

    (b) Prolonged QTc and hypotension are potential side effects.

(3) In some instances, short-term standing doses are helpful.

    (a) Psychosis due to dementia

    (b) Sundowning: For these cases, atypical neuroleptics are favored (see choices below).

    (c) Delirium: High potency typical neuroleptics (e.g., haloperidol, fluphenazine) are cost-effective treatments for short-term use, but atypical antipsychotic medications are gaining favor.

2. Chronic psychosis

For schizophrenia and other psychoses that are persistent and not due to the effects of medical illness or substances, chronic treatment with neuroleptics is indicated.

  a. Typical neuroleptics

    (1) EPSs more likely at high doses

    (2) Risk of tardive dyskinesia

      (a) Incidence is 5% per year of treatment during first 4 to 5 years.

      (b) Prevalence is 20% to 25% for those on long-term therapy.

    (3) For chronically noncompliant patients, depot preparations of fluphenazine and haloperidol can be given every 2 weeks and every month, respectively.

  b. Atypical antipsychotic medications

    (1) These are favored owing to much lower risk of EPSs or tardive dyskinesia.

    (2) Each comes with its own side effect profile.

      (a) Risperidone (Risperdal)

        (i) Increased prolactin

        (ii) EPSs at higher doses

      (b) Olanzapine (Zyprexa)

        (i) Increased appetite

        (ii) Sedation

        (iii) Possible risk of diabetes

      (c) Quetiapine (Seroquel)

        (i) Sedation

      (d) Ziprasidone (Geodon)

        (i) QTc prolongation (average increase 20 ms)

      (e) Clozapine (Clozaril)

        (i) Agranulocytosis: requires weekly or biweekly monitoring of complete blood cell count

        (ii) Sedation

        (iii) Weight gain

        (iv) Not a first-line agent but most effective for treating resistant cases

(3) Studies do not clearly favor one atypical antipsychotic medication over the others.

    (a) Exception is that clozapine may be the best choice for treatment-resistant psychotic illnesses.

    (b) Medication choice is based on the side effect profile and patient response.

(4) Atypical antipsychotic medications are preferred for patients with Parkinson's disease and psychosis.

    (a) These agents are much less likely to worsen motor symptoms than are typical agents.

    (b) Clozapine is particularly useful for this purpose.

Key Treatment: Psychotic Disorders

- Acute psychosis is managed with neuroleptics.

  —Haloperidol and chlorpromazine are chosen because of their fast action.

  —Intravenous and intramuscular administration produces results more quickly than does oral dosing.

  —Short-term standing doses are helpful for psychosis due to dementia, sundowning, or delirium.

- Chronic psychosis (e.g., schizophrenia) is managed with neuroleptics.

  —First-line: atypical neuroleptics

  —Alternative: typical neuroleptics

  —Others: depot neuroleptic to enhance compliance; mood stabilizer for lability or aggression despite adequate antipsychotic therapy

Bibliography

American Psychiatric Association: Practice guidelines for the treatment of patients with schizophrenia. Am J Psychiatry 154(Suppl):1, 1997.

Knoll JL IV, Garver DL, Ramberg JE, et al: Heterogeneity of the psychoses: is there a neurodegenerative psychosis? Schizophr Bull 24:365–379, 1998.

Menezes NM, Milovan E: First-episode psychosis: a comparative review of diagnostic evolution and predictive variables in adolescents versus adults. Can J Psychiatry 45:710–716, 2000.

5 Somatoform Disorders

Christos Ballas
Jeffrey P. Staab

Definition

1. Emotional stresses and worries experienced as physical symptoms. There may or may not be conscious awareness of this shift.

2. Subtypes of somatoform disorders

   a. Somatization disorder

   b. Conversion disorder

   c. Pain disorder

   d. Hypochondriasis

Epidemiology

See Table 5–1.

1. More than 50% have a concomitant mood or anxiety disorder.

2. More than 50% have a personality disorder.

3. Somatization and conversion disorders

   a. Female predominance (>90%) is strong for somatization disorder but less so for conversion disorder.

   b. Onset is before 30 to 35 years of age; when onset occurs over the age of 35 years, the likelihood of medical illness is increased.

   c. As many as 30% of patients diagnosed with conversion disorders are later determined to have actual neurologic dysfunction.

   d. Patients with somatoform disorders may develop medical complications from their psychiatric disorder (e.g., disuse atrophy and contractures in a limb "paralyzed" by a chronic conversion disorder).

      (1) The potential for medical etiologies and complications indicate the need for continued medical surveillance for patients with these somatoform conditions.

   e. There is a possible relation to sexual abuse.

4. Hypochondriasis

   a. Onset at 20 to 40 years of age

Caveats

- More than 90% of patients with somatization disorder are female; the incidence is lower for conversion disorder.

- Up to 30% of patients diagnosed with conversion disorders are later determined to have actual neurologic dysfunction.

Symptoms

1. Somatoform disorder (Briquet's syndrome)

   a. Medically unexplained physical symptoms

   b. Complaints of pain or dysfunction involving multiple organ systems

   c. Highly resistant to precise diagnosis and management

      (1) Neurologic: headache, paresis, paresthesias, loss of coordination, "seizures"

      (2) Cardiorespiratory: chest pain, palpitations, dyspnea, choking

      (3) Gastrointestinal: nonspecific abdominal pain, cramping, bloating, diarrhea, constipation

      (4) Genitourinary: dysuria, dyspareunia

      (5) Constitutional: chronic fatigue

2. Conversion disorders

   a. Medically unexplained physical symptoms

      (1) Usually one or a small number of related symptoms

      (2) Resists diagnosis and management

   b. Most common neurologic symptoms

      (1) Pseudoseizures

      (2) Ocular (blindness, diplopia)

         (a) "Hysterical blindness" with normal papillary reaction

      (3) Cognitive (memory loss, loss of single discrete ability)

      (4) Visceral

         (a) Psychogenic vomiting

         (b) Urinary retention

         (c) Pseudocyesis (false pregnancy)

TABLE 5–1. MAIN FEATURES OF SOMATOFORM DISORDERS

Diagnosis	Physical Symptoms	Pain/Dysfunction	Psychological Aspects
Somatoform disorder	Multiple symptoms related to various organ systems	Complaints of pain and dysfunction	Focus on symptoms
Conversion disorder	Single or small number of related symptoms	Dysfunction of a voluntary muscle group	"La belle indifference"
Pain disorder	Chronic pain	Pain	Impairment from pain
Hypochondriasis	Few to many	Relatively minor	Belief in serious illness

(5) Sensory dysfunction

  (a) Notably paresthesias or pain in specific region or system

  (b) Often across dermatomes

(6) Motor dysfunction

  (a) Characteristically a *voluntary* motor dysfunction

3. Pain disorder

  a. Pain is perceived to be so great or chronic that it interferes with normal life.

  b. Indicators of somatoform pain

    (1) There is a delay between injury and beginning of pain.

    (2) Pain is of a specific quality that distinguishes it from other pain.

      (a) "It feels like needles."

      (b) "First it starts to throb, then it travels here, where it is sharp."

    (3) Some level of analgesic dependence is evident.

    (4) Multiple visits to clinician are common.

  c. Most common neurologic symptoms

    (1) Headache or "migraine"

    (2) Major physical groups that preclude normal functioning (e.g., hip or back, not finger or ear)

    (3) Seizures

4. Hypochondriasis

  a. Primarily a preoccupation with illness, rather than symptoms ("I have a brain tumor"—not "I am dizzy")

  b. There may or may not be any physical symptoms or complaints.

  c. It is the fear of illness that is incapacitating.

  d. Illness in question is usually life-threatening (e.g., myocardial infection, cancer).

  e. Symptoms and other perceived evidence of illness are described in exceptional detail.

  f. Doctor visits are frequent.

  g. Patient already suspects diagnosis and is unsatisfied without full medical and neurologic work-up.

Differential Diagnosis

1. Includes all *plausible* medical and psychiatric illnesses. Somatoform disorders should be considered as a part of the medical differential diagnosis, not conditions to be diagnosed after excluding all conceivable medical illnesses in an exhaustive work-up.

2. Psychiatric differential diagnoses

  a. Catatonia

  b. Personality disorder

  c. Factitious disorder or malingering

    (1) Patients purposefully produce their medical signs and symptoms (e.g., they may inject themselves with foreign substances such as insulin or infectious materials, or they may contaminate laboratory samples).

  d. Anxiety disorder

  e. Mood disorder

3. Medical disorders to be excluded

  a. Cancer

  b. Chronic infection: Lyme disease, syphilis, human immunodeficiency virus (HIV)

  c. Chronic or remitting neurologic illnesses

    (1) Multiple sclerosis

    (2) Myasthenia gravis

  d. Metabolic disorders

    (1) Acute intermittent porphyria

    (2) Thyroid and adrenal diseases (hyperactive or hypoactive)

  e. Rheumatologic illnesses

    (1) Systemic lupus erythematosis

    (2) Other arthritides

  f. Trauma: physical injury

Treatment

1. After excluding plausible medical illness, treatment of these disorders is focused on management of symptoms, not cure.

2. A single medical provider must be designated to act as the main medical contact and manage all

issues. Multiple visits to specialists should be discouraged.

3. Schedule frequent, regular, short visits; 15 minutes per month is usual.

4. Therapeutic alliance

    a. It is acceptable to differ on the *cause* of the symptoms, but the savvy clinician agrees with the patient about the *existence* of symptoms.

    b. Recruit patient into active participation in care by setting health goals.

        (1) Emphasize daily functioning rather than symptoms.

        (2) Concentrate on routine health maintenance.

        (3) Maintain vigilance for new or changing symptoms that suggest a medical condition, particularly one that can run an indolent course.

5. Medications

    a. Antidepressants can be helpful for managing co-morbid depression or anxiety and may provide some pain benefit as well (notably amitriptyline and gabapentin).

    b. Analgesic prescriptions should be proportional to the identifiable organic pathology.

        (1) Somatoform pain symptoms respond erratically and often temporarily to analgesics (likely a placebo effect).

        (2) Chronic use of analgesics is best avoided.

Key Treatment

- Management of symptoms, not cure
- One medical provider
- Frequent, regular, short visits
- Therapeutic alliance
- Antidepressants

Caveats

- For these disorders, one medical provider must act as the main medical contact, manage all issues, and discourage multiple visits to specialists.

Bibliography

Bass C, Peveler R, House A: Somatoform disorders: severe psychiatric illnesses neglected by psychiatrists. Br J Psychiatry 179:11–14, 2001.

Escobar JI: Overview of somatization: diagnosis, epidemiology, and management. Psychopharmacol Bull 32:589–596, 1996.

Fritz GK, Fritsch S, Hagino O: Somatoform disorders in children and adolescents: a review of the past 10 years. J Am Acad Child Adolesc Psychiatry 36:1329–1338, 1997.

Smith GR: Somatization Disorder in the Medical Setting, Washington, DC, American Psychiatric Press, 1991.

Walker EA: Dealing with patients who have medically unexplained symptoms. Semin Clin Neuropsychiatry 7:187–195, 2002.

6 Personality Disorders

Christos Ballas
Jeffrey P. Staab

Definition

1. A personality disorder is a repetitive pattern of thinking or behavior that usually impairs functioning, though this may not be apparent to the patient.
2. The DSM-IV classifies personality disorders into three general subtypes.
   a. Cluster A: odd, eccentric
   b. Cluster B: dramatic
   c. Cluster C: anxious, inhibited

Epidemiology

1. Approximately 10% to 20% of the population meets the criteria for at least one personality disorder, and at least half of them meet criteria for two or more personality disorders.
   a. Cluster A: 6% of the population; more common in men
   b. Cluster B: 10% of the population; more common in women, except for antisocial personality disorder, which is more common in men
   c. Cluster C: 5% of the population, more common in women
   d. Gender differences may be the result of diagnostic biases.

Symptoms

See Table 6–1.
1. Cluster A: "odd" personalities
   a. General characteristics
      (1) Introverted and self-absorbed
      (2) Prone to daydreaming and fantasy
      (3) Insecure about themselves (believe they are right and others wrong, and thus beneath them)
      (4) Project their feelings and hostilities onto others
      (5) Lack of trust, inhibiting interpersonal relationships (hence difficult to establish an effective doctor-patient relationship)
   b. Specific characteristics
      (1) Schizotypal personality disorder
         (a) Eccentric beliefs, odd perceptions of reality (not delusions)

TABLE 6–1. MAIN FEATURES OF PERSONALITY DISORDERS

DISORDER	PRIMARY FEATURE(S)
A—odd cluster	
Paranoid	Suspicious, distrustful
Schizoid	Loner
Schizotypal	Eccentric
B—dramatic cluster	
Antisocial	Disregard for rules, laws, mores
Borderline	Labile, highly reactive to others
Histrionic	Dramatic, but shallow
Narcissistic	Egotistical
C—anxious cluster	
Avoidant	Intense social anxiety
Dependent	Needy, meek
Obsessive-compulsive	Rigid, "by the book," restricted affect

       (b) May be preoccupied with the occult, paranormal theories, and so on
     (2) Schizoid personality disorder
       (a) Stereotypical loner does not desire relationships with others
     (3) Paranoid personality disorder
       (a) "Conspiracy theorist"
       (b) Suspicious; believes others always have selfish or malevolent intentions

---

Caveat

• It is difficult to establish an effective doctor-patient relationship with these patients.

---

2. Cluster B: dramatic personalities
   a. General characteristics
      (1) Immature, upset when their needs are not met
      (2) Self-centered with distorted understanding of others' emotions and perceptions
      (3) Impulsive
      (4) Overtly or covertly manipulative
      (5) Unstable interpersonal relationships
      (6) May overstep the bounds of the doctor-patient relationship
         (a) "Emergency" phone calls
         (b) Special requests
         (c) Seductiveness, manipulative
      (7) May be associated with childhood deprivation or abuse

b. Specific characteristics

(1) Antisocial personality disorder

(a) Disregard for laws, rules, societal mores, social obligations

(b) May or may not engage in criminal activity

(c) Quick to take advantage of others

(2) Borderline personality disorder

(a) Emotionally labile, moody

(b) Overly responsive (positively and negatively) to interactions with others (interpersonal relationships are chronically unstable)

(c) May engage in self-mutilating behaviors (e.g., cutting, biting, burning)

(d) May have recurrent thoughts of death or suicide

(3) Histrionic personality disorder

(a) Showy in presentation

(b) Rapidly shifting, shallow emotional expressions

(4) Narcissistic personality disorder

(a) Intensely self-centered, egotistical

(b) Constant need for attention, admiration

Caveat

• These patients may overstep the bounds of the doctor-patient relationship by making special requests or so-called emergency phone calls, or by being seductive or manipulative.

3. Cluster C: anxious/inhibited personalities

a. General characteristics

(1) Socially inhibited, shy, awkward

(2) Hypersensitive to actual or perceived criticism

(3) Fretful, ruminative

(4) Avoidance of conflict or reliance on others to manage conflict

(5) May compensate by being overly controlling, lack of flexibility

(6) In the doctor-patient relationship, they may

(a) Need repeated explanations and reassurances

(b) Be overly compliant (e.g., fail to report side effects to avoid being perceived as a difficult patient)

(c) Be quietly noncompliant (e.g., delay evaluations and treatment)

b. Specific characteristics

(1) Avoidant personality disorder

(a) Strong desire for interpersonal relationships but intensely anxious in new social settings ("wallflower")

(2) Dependent personality disorder

(a) Tremendous need for close interpersonal relationships

(i) Often appear clingy, needy

(ii) Alternatively, may adopt an excessive caretaker role (pseudoindependence) to maintain contact with others

(b) Avoids conflict or engages in passive-aggressive, rather than overtly hostile, responses to others

(3) Obsessive-compulsive personality disorder

(a) Rigid, inflexible, "plays by the rules"

(b) Excessive attention to detail that impairs productivity

(c) Emotionally isolated

Caveat

• In the doctor-patient relationship, these patients may need repeated reassurance and explanations; they also may be overly compliant (e.g., not to be seen as difficult, they fail to report side effects) or quietly noncompliant (e.g., they delay treatment).

Differential Diagnosis

1. The psychiatric differential diagnosis includes disorders that often coexist with personality disorders.

a. Cluster A

(1) Schizophrenia or schizophreniform disorder

(2) Mood disorders with psychotic features

b. Cluster B

(1) Bipolar disorder, especially bipolar II disorder

(2) Depressive disorders

(3) Anxiety disorders

(4) Substance abuse

(5) Dissociative disorders

c. Cluster C

(1) Anxiety disorders

(2) Depressive disorders

2. Medical differential diagnoses can be investigated if there are symptoms or signs to suggest a medical illness or if there has been a noticeable change in personality.

   a. Central nervous system disturbances

     (1) Head injury

     (2) Cerebrovascular accident

     (3) Tumor

     (4) Infection

       (a) Syphilis

       (b) Encephalitis

       (c) Meningitis (unusual)

     (5) Seizures, especially postictal states

     (6) Dementia (normal pressure hydrocephalus)

     (7) Toxins

       (a) Toxic metals: mercury, thallium, lead, arsenic

       (b) Pesticides, organophosphates

       (c) Solvents

     (8) Metabolic

       (a) Wilson's disease

       (b) Porphyria

         (i) Presence of bizarre behavior

         (ii) Abdominal pain secondary to alcohol

       (c) Renal or hepatic insufficiency

         (i) May manifest as emotional lability or belligerence

     (9) Endocrine

       (a) Hypothyroid: may appear slow, socially isolated, unmotivated

       (b) Hyperthyroid: may appear irritable, restless, "high strung"

       (c) Hypoglycemia or hyperglycemia

       (d) Hypoparathyroidism or hyperparathyroidism

       (e) Menstrual or menopausal hormone changes

Laboratory Investigations

1. There are no specific laboratory tests for personality disorders.

2. Tests are used to rule out medical illness.

   a. Drug screening

   b. Thyroid function tests (when mood or anxiety symptoms are prominent)

   c. Others as indicated by medical history and physical examination. More extensive diagnostic investigations are indicated for a change in personality rather than personality characteristics present over a lifetime.

Key Tests

- Tests to rule out medical illnesses

- Drug screening

- Thyroid function tests when mood and anxiety symptoms are prominent

Treatment

1. Treatment is an ongoing therapeutic process.

2. For the primary clinician and nonpsychiatric specialist, management of the patient's personality traits is necessary to prevent interference with medical care.

   a. Set reasonable, firm limits (e.g., appointment times, emergency access procedures).

   b. Be consistent in availability, demeanor, and treatment.

   c. Expect patients to project their feelings onto the clinician.

     (1) Do not take it personally or overreact when it occurs.

     (2) Reinforce setting limits and being consistent in availability, demeanor, and treatment.

3. Treat co-morbid mood and anxiety or thought disorders.

4. Refer to a psychiatrist or psychotherapist.

   a. Several types of psychotherapy (e.g., cognitive-behavioral therapy) have demonstrated utility for the treatment of personality disorders.

   b. Select medications may minimize extreme symptoms, such as mood lability, social anxiety, or minor psychotic symptoms under stress.

Key Treatment

- Therapeutic process is ongoing.

- Manage of personality traits that may interfere with medical care.

- Psychotherapy is useful in the treatment of personality disorders.

- Select medications may minimize symptoms.

- Refer to a psychiatrist or psychologist.

Bibliography

Akhtar S, Thomson JA Jr: Overview: narcissistic personality disorder. Am J Psychiatry 139:12–20, 1982.

American Psychiatric Association: Practice guideline for the treatment of patients with borderline personality disorder. http://www.psych.org/clinres/borderline.index.cfm, 2001.

Sadock BJ, Sadock VA: Kaplan and Sadock's Comprehensive Textbook of Psychiatry, 7th ed. Philadelphia, Lippincott Williams & Wilkins, 1999.

Siever LJ, Davis KL: A psychobiological perspective on the personality disorders. Am J Psychiatry 148:1647, 1991.

7 Substance-Related Disorders

Jeffrey P. Staab
Christos Ballas

Definition

1. There are various definitions of substance related disorders. The most prominent are the *Diagnostic and Statistical Manual of Mental Disorders, 4th Edition* (DSM-IV) categories of abuse and dependence and the National Institutes of Alcohol Abuse and Alcoholism (NIAAA) definition of problem drinking.
2. DSM-IV
   a. Definitions are based on biologic, psychological, and social consequences of central nervous system (CNS)-active substance use.
   b. DSM-IV has no measurement of quantity of substances consumed.
   c. Abuse is the continued use of alcohol or other CNS active substances despite adverse legal, occupational, or personal consequences.
   d. Dependence is the continued use of alcohol or other CNS-active substances despite symptoms in the following areas.
      (1) Biologic
         (a) Tolerance
         (b) Withdrawal
      (2) Psychological
         (a) Failed attempts to reduce substance use
         (b) Loss of control (i.e., substance often used in larger quantities than intended)
      (3) Social
         (a) Failure to meet personal and occupational obligations
         (b) Legal problems
         (c) Considerable time spent using or recovering from substances
   e. Categories of common substances of abuse
      (1) Alcohol
      (2) Amphetamines and other stimulants
      (3) Cannabis
      (4) Cocaine
      (5) Hallucinogens
      (6) Inhalants
      (7) Opioids
      (8) Phencyclidine (PCP)
      (9) Sedatives/hypnotics/anxiolytics
      (10) Caffeine and nicotine
3. NIAAA
   a. Definition based on population norms of weekly alcohol consumption in the United States
      (1) Problem drinking is more than the 90th percentile on this measure.
      (2) There is no assessment of the sequelae of alcohol use, though this level of drinking is associated with increased health risks.
   b. Problem drinking, by weekly consumption
      (1) Men
         (a) More than 14 drinks total per week
         (b) More than 4 drinks total per occasion on more than one occasion per week
      (2) Women
         (a) More than 7 drinks total per week
         (b) More than 3 drinks per occasion on more than one occasion per week
      (3) Seniors (age 65 and older)
         (a) More than 7 drinks total per week
         (b) More than 2 drinks per occasion on more than one occasion per week
   c. There are no similar criteria for drug abuse.

Epidemiology

1. Prevalence estimates of substance related disorders vary, depending on the definitions and screening methods employed in epidemiologic studies.
2. In the population with which physicians have the most contact—general medical outpatients—alcohol and drug abuse are present in 16% to 20% of individuals.
   a. It is likely underdetected.
   b. In one survey, less than half of primary care physicians routinely screened their patients for substance related problems.
      (1) 41% for alcohol
      (2) 20% for drug of abuse

Pathophysiology

1. Development of substance related disorders is likely a nature–nurture interaction.
   a. There may be genetic vulnerability to addiction.
      (1) Familial aggregation of substance dependence

(2) Genetic variability in response to intoxication

(3) Research example

   (a) Intravenous infusion of alcohol equivalent to three drinks

   (b) Children of alcoholics, nonaddicted themselves, experienced a mild euphoria.

   (c) Comparison group with a negative family history reported mostly a sedative effect.

b. Environmental influences likely provide models of problematic substance use, which stimulates early experimentation and misuse.

c. Stressful events also may trigger overuse.

2. Substances with multiple CNS effects (e.g., sedatives, stimulants, hallucinogens) can be addicting. Common biologic vulnerability may be abnormal reinforcement generated in the dopaminergic reward pathways of the brain.

Clinical Features

1. Lifetime patterns of substance-related problems

a. Experimentation and misuse that remits spontaneously: adolescence and early adulthood

b. Abuse and dependence

(1) Early onset—early adolescence: most common in individuals with genetic predispositions, exposure to heavy-use environments, or both

(2) Late onset—adulthood, even senior years: new or increased use during a time of stress

(3) Early- and late-onset substance-related problems follow a common clinical course once initiated.

   (a) Social problems first

      (i) More time devoted to substance use

      (ii) Neglect of personal, occupational obligations

   (b) Psychological changes next

      (i) Loss of control

      (ii) Failed attempts to quit or cut down

   (c) Biologic sequelae

      (i) Increased risk of withdrawal (alcohol and sedatives)

      (ii) Medical problems

   (d) Hallucinogen or inhalant abuse often follows a more erratic course.

      (i) Episodic use

      (ii) Potential for early CNS injury due to direct toxicity of the substances

2. Intoxication

a. Clinical presentation depends on the pharmacology of the substance(s) used.

3. Withdrawal

a. Alcohol and sedative withdrawal can be life-threatening.

(1) Mortality as high as 15% for severe, untreated withdrawal

b. Opiate withdrawal is highly uncomfortable but not life threatening.

c. Other substances do not produce a biologic withdrawal, although fatigue, somnolence, and dysphoria may occur after ceasing stimulant use (e.g., cocaine crash).

d. Alcohol withdrawal

(1) Autonomic instability (temperature, heart rate, blood pressure): best (objective) marker of severity of withdrawal state

(2) Motor excitability (tremor, increased reflexes)

(3) Agitation, restlessness, insomnia

(4) Delirium

(5) Begins several hours after last drink; peaks at 24 to 72 hours; may persist for 7 to 10 days depending on severity

e. Sedative withdrawal (benzodiazepines, barbiturates)

(1) It is similar to alcohol withdrawal.

(2) Time course depends on half-life of sedative used.

   (a) Short half-life: similar to alcohol withdrawal

   (b) Long half-life: may produce motor excitability, agitation, insomnia, even delirium, with less autonomic instability

f. Opiate withdrawal

(1) Subjective symptoms: precede overt clinical signs

   (a) Abdominal cramping, malaise, myalgias

   (b) "Drug seeking" behavior

(2) Objective signs

   (a) Dilated pupils, lacrimation, rhinorrhea, piloerection

   (b) Motor excitability

   (c) Agitation, restlessness, insomnia

(3) Time course depends on half-life of opiate used.

Stimulant Withdrawal

• Fatigue, somnolence, dysphoria

Alcohol Withdrawal

• Autonomic instability

• Motor excitability (tremor, increased reflexes)

• Agitation, restlessness, insomnia

• Delirium

• Signs begin several hours after last drink, peak at 24 to 72 hours, may persist for 7 to 10 days depending on severity.

Sedative Withdrawal

• Time course depends on half-life of sedative.

—Short half-life: similar to alcohol withdrawal

—Long-half-life: motor excitability, agitation, insomnia, even delirium, with less autonomic instability

Opiate Withdrawal

• Subjective symptoms (precede overt clinical signs)

—Abdominal cramping, malaise, myalgias

—"Drug seeking" activity

• Objective signs

—Dilated pupils, lacrimation, rhinorrhea, piloerection

—Motor excitability

—Agitation, restlessness, insomnia

Differential Diagnosis

1. Psychiatric disorders
   a. Substance use without abuse or dependence
      (1) Occasional overuse of legal substances
      (2) "Recreational" use of illegal substances
      (3) No pattern of use resulting in repeated adverse consequences
   b. Mood disorders
      (1) Poor judgment or erratic behaviors during mania and hypomania
      (2) Social isolation, neglect of obligations during depression
   c. Psychotic disorders: hallucinations, delusions
   d. Anxiety disorders
   e. Attention deficit hyperactivity disorder

   f. Antisocial personality
      (1) Illegal behaviors
      (2) Disregard for personal responsibilities
2. Medical and neurologic conditions
   a. Episodic or waxing and waning illnesses may give the appearance of intoxication, impaired judgment, or irresponsibility.
   b. Poorly controlled endocrine/metabolic diseases may be present.
      (1) Diabetes
      (2) Thyroid disease, particularly with erratic use of replacement hormone
      (3) Adrenal insufficiency or excess (including exogenous steroids)
      (4) Hypoxia: chronic pulmonary disease
   c. Brain injury (traumatic and other causes)
   d. Transient ischemic attacks
   e. Neurotologic conditions
   f. Side effects of prescribed medications
3. Coexisting disorders
   a. Substance use disorders are commonly associated with other psychiatric conditions.
   b. Diagnosis and treatment of all disorders is necessary for a good outcome.

Laboratory Testing

1. Drug detection
   a. The most sensitive and specific test for substance related disorders is the clinical history, not any laboratory test.
      (1) Use of a clinical screening tool can enhance detection rates.
      (2) Example: CAGE-AID (the *CAGE* screen *A*dapted to *I*nclude *D*rugs) (Table 7–1)
         (a) Have you tried to *C*ut down on your use of drugs or alcohol?
         (b) Do you feel *A*nnoyed when others criticize your drinking or drug use?
         (c) Do you feel *G*uilty about your drinking or drug use?
         (d) Do you ever have an *E*ye-opener or use alcohol or drugs to "get going," steady your nerves, or get rid of a hangover?
   b. Clinical laboratory tests
      (1) Urine
         (a) Most urine assays screen for six to eight classes of substances.
         (b) Cocaine, amphetamines, opiates, benzodiazepines, barbiturates, PCP, alcohol, marijuana

TABLE 7–1. DIAGNOSIS AND TREATMENT STRATEGIES

PARAMETER	COMMENT
Diagnosis	Made by history—use a clinical screening tool such as the CAGE-AID
Abuse	Persistent use despite personal or professional consequences
Dependence	Persistent use despite biologic, psychological, and social symptoms
Treatment	
Detoxification	For patients at high risk of complicated withdrawal from alcohol, benzodiazepines, barbiturates, or opiates
Rehabilitation	Inpatient, outpatient, day, and residential programs—should provide services for social, occupational, financial, legal problems
Medications	Alcohol dependence—naltrexone, disulfuram
	Opiate addiction—methadone, naltrexone

(2) Serum

    (a) Blood alcohol concentration is measured.

    (b) Availability of assays for other substances vary widely among clinical laboratories.

(3) Hair: most commonly used in forensic settings

(4) Breath: alcohol

(5) Clinical laboratories cannot detect several drugs of abuse.

    (a) Inhalants

    (b) "Designer" or "club" drugs

2. Screening for medical sequelae of substance use. Consider the following tests, if clinically indicated, to detect medical problems arising from alcohol and drug use. These should not be used as "screening tests" for substance use because their sensitivities for that purpose are quite low (<40%).

a. Alcohol dependence

    (1) Complete blood count

    (2) Transaminases, γ-glutamyl transferase (GGT)

        (a) GGT is quite specific for alcohol related problems (>90%)

        (b) Suspect alcohol abuse or dependence when it is elevated.

        (c) However, sensitivity is low (~ 40%), so it is a poor screening test.

    (3) Head imaging for patients with evidence of dementia

b. Intravenous drug use

    (1) Hepatitis B and C serologies

    (2) Human immunodeficiency virus (HIV)

    (3) Complete blood count (CBC) and blood cultures (if evidence of endocarditis)

    (4) Chest radiograph and ventilation perfusion scan to detect pulmonary emboli from injection of insoluble "fillers" (for respiratory distress)

Treatment

1. Detoxification (Table 7–1)

a. Patients at high risk for complicated withdrawal should undergo medically monitored detoxification, usually as hospital inpatients. Some individuals are at high risk.

    (1) Patients with a history of complicated withdrawal in the past

    (2) Patients with a history of seizures

    (3) Patients in active withdrawal at the time of examination

2. Rehabilitation (Table 7–1)

a. General principles

    (1) It is common practice to match the level of rehabilitation placement (i.e., inpatient, outpatient, day program) to the apparent severity of addiction.

    (2) Evidence suggests that the level of treatment may not be the most important factor for outcomes.

        (a) Program retention, regardless of level of care, is more important.

        (b) Providing for psychosocial needs, not just drug counseling, is essential.

            (i) Family interventions

            (ii) Vocational assessment and training

            (iii) Housing and financial counseling

            (iv) Legal services

b. Clinician-led programs

    (1) Inpatient, outpatient, and day treatment programs with services provided by physicians, psychologists, nurses, social workers, drug and alcohol counselors

c. Self-help programs

    (1) Abstinence programs: Emphasize the need to refrain totally from substance use to achieve recovery: Alcoholics Anonymous, Narcotics Anonymous.

    (2) Nonabstinence programs: goal is responsible substance use.

d. Medications

    (1) Alcohol dependence

        (a) Adversive agent: disulfiram produces nausea, malaise when used with alcohol

(b) Therapeutic agent: naltrexone reduces alcohol craving and positive reinforcing effects

(2) Opiate addiction

  (a) Substitution: provide controlled, safe opiate to reduce illicit use

    (i) Methadone

    (ii) By law, may be administered only in Drug Enforcement Agency (DEA)-registered clinics.

  (b) Therapeutic agents: reduce craving, blunt opiate effects

    (i) Naltrexone

    (b) Buprenorphine

Bibliography

Anton RF, Litten RZ, Allen JP: Biological assessment of alcohol consumption. In Allen JP, Columbus M (eds): Assessing Alcohol Problems: A Guide for Clinicians and Researchers, National Institutes of Health Publication 95-3745, Bethesda, U.S. Department of Health and Human Services, Public Health Service, 1995, p. 31.

Brown R, Rounds LC: Conjoint screening questionnaires for alcohol and other drug abuse: criterion validity in a primary care practice. Wis Med J 94:135, 1995.

Ewing J: Detecting alcoholism: the CAGE questionnaire. JAMA 252:1905, 1984.

Kreek MJ, Laforge KS, Butelman E: Pharmacotherapy of addictions. Natl Rev Drug Discov 1:710–726, 2002.

Staab JP, Datto, CJ, Weinrieb RM, et al: Detection and diagnosis of psychiatric disorders in primary medical care settings. Med Clin North Am 85:579–596, 2001.

8 Attention Deficit Hyperactivity Disorders

Christos Ballas
Jeffrey P. Staab

Definition

1. Attention deficit hyperactivity disorder (ADHD) is a syndrome of inattention and hyperactivity/impulsivity that significantly impairs normal functioning. There are three subtypes (Table 8–1).

   a. Hyperactive/impulsive: predominantly excessive motor activity (fidgeting, squirming, pacing, running, talking), difficulty engaging in sedate activities, and a tendency to act spontaneously or without considering consequences (disrupting activities or conversations of others, blurting out answers in class, cutting in lines)

   b. Inattentive: predominant features are inability to sustain focus on a task, difficulty organizing and completing tasks, forgetfulness, difficulty following instructions, easy distractibility)

   c. Combined: features of hyperactivity/impulsivity and inattention

Epidemiology

1. ADHD is a condition that begins during childhood, almost always before the age of 7 years.

   a. It may persist into adolescence and adulthood but does *not* begin during adulthood.

2. The prevalence of ADHD is not precisely known.

   a. Most studies suggest a prevalence of 3% to 5% in school age children, though other studies have found it to be higher.

   b. Prevalance during adolescence and adulthood is unclear.

TABLE 8–1. KEY CLINICAL FEATURES OF ADHD

Inattentive
Distractible
Forgetful
Difficulty sustaining effort on tasks

Hyperactive/Impulsive
Excessive motor activity
Fidgety, squirmy
Disruptive of others' tasks and conversations

Combined
Elements of both

3. Girls are more likely to have only the inattentive form.

4. The disorder tends to run in families.

5. ADHD is highly associated with other psychiatric illnesses, complicating epidemiologic studies and diagnosis.

   a. Conduct disorder

   b. Oppositional-defiant disorder

   c. Depressive disorders

   d. Childhood-onset bipolar disorder

   e. Mental retardation, autism, other developmental disorders

   f. Neurologic disorders

   g. Substance-related disorders in adolescents and adults

Pathophysiology

1. Pathophysiology is unknown.

2. Genetic factors are likely because of the familial aggregation of this disorder.

3. It is unclear whether ADHD is a distinct pathophysiologic entity or the extreme of a continuum of behaviors involving attention deficits and hyperactivity (much as hypertension is on a continuum of blood pressures).

Clinical Features

1. The symptoms of ADHD fall into two categories (Table 8–1), as defined above.

   a. Inattention

      (1) Distractibility

      (2) Forgetfulness

      (3) Difficulty sustaining even enjoyable tasks

   b. Hyperactivity/impulsivity

      (1) Fidgetiness

      (2) Restlessness

      (3) Inability to "wait one's turn"

      (4) Aggressivity

2. Many, perhaps most, patients have features of both subtypes.

Differential Diagnosis

1. The differential diagnosis of ADHD includes both medical/psychiatric disorders and social factors.
   a. Psychiatric disorders
      (1) Mood/anxiety disorders
         (a) Depression
         (b) Childhood-onset bipolar disorder
            (i) Hypomanic states
         (c) Anxiety disorders
            (i) Generalized anxiety
            (ii) Situational anxiety
               • Social and other phobias
               • Separation anxiety
      (2) Mental retardation
      (3) Developmental disorders
         (a) Pervasive developmental disorder
         (b) Autism
      (4) Substance abuse
      (5) Physical/sexual abuse or neglect
         (a) Posttraumatic stress disorder
      (6) Understimulating or overstimulating environment
         (a) Poor socialization
      (7) Psychotic disorders
   b. Neurologic disorders
      (1) Sequelae of central nervous system (CNS) insults
         (a) Traumatic brain injury
         (b) Anoxic brain injury
         (c) Infection: meningoencephalitis
      (2) Tic disorders
   c. Medical disorders
      (1) Not a common cause of the entire syndrome of ADHD.
      (2) They may cause some symptoms suggestive of ADHD.
      (3) Consider endocrine/metabolic diseases.
         (a) Thyroid disease
         (b) Poor diabetic control

Laboratory Testing

1. There is no formal laboratory testing for ADHD. Routine investigation is the same as for most other psychiatric illnesses.
   a. Thyroid-stimulating hormone (TSH): most useful in adolescents and adults in whom thyroid diseases are more common.
   b. Urine drug screen, especially for adolescents and adults

c. Other laboratory tests, guided by the history or physical examination evidence of conditions in the differential diagnosis

 Key Tests

• There is no formal laboratory testing for ADHD.

Treatment

1. Medications
   a. Stimulants are the most widely used treatments for ADHD, although there are few long-term studies (almost none beyond 2 years).
   b. There is no difference in efficacy among stimulants.
   c. Although alleviation of symptoms is common, there is no evidence that medications improve school performance.
      (1) Stimulants
         (a) Methylphenidate (Ritalin)
            (i) Best studied
            (ii) Twice-daily or thrice-daily dosing
            (iii) Long acting forms available.
            (iv) Single stereoisomer, dexmethylphenidate (Focalin) available.
         (b) Dextroamphetamine (Dexedrine)
            (i) Twice-daily or thrice-daily dosing
         (c) Mixed amphetamine salts (Adderall): short- and long-acting forms available.
         (d) Pemoline (Cylert)
            (i) Not a first-line choice
            (ii) Requires monitoring for hepatotoxicity
      (2) Antidepressants. Few data overall but some evidence to support their usage
         (a) Bupropion most widely used antidepressant for this purpose
            (i) Nonamphetamine, dopamine reuptake inhibitor
            (ii) Requires some caution in those with a history of seizures
         (b) Tricyclic antidepressants
            (i) Most widely studied
            (ii) Better than placebo but less efficacious than stimulants
      (3) Clonidine (α_2-agonist)
         (a) Controversial; some evidence that it works in ADHD with tic disorder
         (b) Used for oppositional behavior
         (c) Sedating; benefits may be transient

(4) Neuroleptics

  (a) Occasionally effective, especially for hyperactivity/impulsivity

  (b) Useful with co-morbid tic disorders

(5) Modafinil, a novel stimulant, may be effective in children and adults.

2. Behavioral and social interventions (contingency management)

a. "Time out" for problematic behaviors

b. Reward or token system for acceptable behaviors

c. Teachers, parents, and other involved parties must be trained to use consistent contingency management strategies.

Key Treatment

First Line

- Stimulants: methylphenidate, dextroamphetamine, mixed amphetamine salts

- Behavioral management

Second Line

- Antidepressants: bupropipon, tricyclic antidepressants

- Clonidine

- Neuroleptics

Bibliography

American Academy of Pediatrics: Clinical practice guideline: diagnosis and evaluation of the child with attention-deficit/hyperactivity disorder. Pediatrics 105:1158–1170, 2000.

Gallagher R, Blader J: The diagnosis and neuropsychological assessment of adult attention deficit/hyperactivity disorder: scientific study and practical guidelines. Ann NY Acad Sci 931:148–171, 2001.

Kirby K, Rutman LE, Bernstein H: Attention-deficit/hyperactivity disorder: a therapeutic update. Curr Opin Pediatr 14:236–246, 2002.

Mental Health Report: A Report of the Surgeon General, http://www.surgeongeneral.gov/library/mentalhealth/chapter3/sec4.html#treatment.

Pary R, Lewis S, Matuschka PR, et al.: Attention deficit disorder in adults. Ann Clin Psychiatry 14:105–111, 2002.

Medical-Legal Issues and Neurology *Michael I. Weintraub*

Malpractice awards against neurologists are the highest of all specialties. Critical analysis reveals failure to diagnose, lack of informed consent, and poor chart documentation as major factors.

I. Records

    A. Documentation: Physicians are obligated by state laws to maintain records. Penalties and sanctions can be imposed on the physician who does not maintain and keep medical records for a prescribed period. Documentation of history, exam, conclusions, testing, treatment, and informed consent are often the key to success or failure in a lawsuit that reaches trial several years later. Remember, *the medical record is the malpractice witness that never dies.*

    B. Spoliation of records: Do not tamper with or erase records after receiving notice of a lawsuit. Ink analysis and handwriting pattern analysis are so scientifically sophisticated and accurate that if there is evidence of "doctoring" the record, the physician will not only lose the lawsuit but may face punitive damages and even loss of licensure.

    C. Record correction: Put a clean line through any erroneous statement, followed by your initials, the date and the time, preferably witnessed. Write "retrospective" or "correct" on the next available line, again with signature, date, time, and witness.

    D. Handwriting: Clear and legible are acceptable. If illegible, may lead to errors in prescriptions, rejection by Medicare, and at trial poor defense (i.e., sloppy records, sloppy care).

    E. Consultation and management: Document allergy and medication history. If two or more disorders are considered in differential diagnosis, i.e., migraine vs epilepsy, should state why one is favored, etc. Courts accept the notion of what a "reasonable" physician would do.

    F. Laboratory/radiology tests: Results of pertinent tests, i.e., CT scan, MRI scan, prothrombin time must be known *prior to discharge.*

    G. Family members: These are usually the individuals who initiate lawsuits. Maintain good contact and document every conversation, even if there are no legal concerns. Indicate which family member or members were present.

    H. Drug interactions: Physicians should acknowledge the potential interaction of an anti-epileptic drug with contraceptives, coumadin, Theophylline, etc. and demonstrate that vigilance will be maintained.

    I. Compliance: Document if patient is medication and treatment compliant, that the patient keeps appointments, etc.

II. Informed Consent

    A. Patients and families need to know "material" information regarding risks and rewards of diagnostic procedures and treatments so that they can make an informed decision. Failure to provide such information in obtaining consent exposes the physician not only to lawsuits but also to criminal charges of assault and battery, etc.

    B. Document the specific risks of a particular medicine on a prescription form or consultation note; list family members at any session present. Anti-epileptic medication and corticosteroids are two common and frequent classes of drugs used by neurologists that have serious side-effects.

    C. Pregnancy: Discuss possible teratogenic effect of any drug on fetus; and make sure that the patient understands the issues.

    D. Telephone calls: Document when a call was originated, by whom, for what reason, and your response. Often drug side-effects lead to symptoms that need to be discussed. A *strong* doctor–patient relationship must be maintained.

    E. Testamentary capacity: If a patient is demented, obtain permission to treat or perform research from the proper legal guardian. Both federal and state laws protect the rights of vulnerable individuals.

III. Subpoena

Neurologists usually learn that they are named in a lawsuit or that their testimony is needed via a subpoena. A subpoena is a legal document/summons given in person or through registered mail showing that a person will be part of a pending action or that certain records are required by the court. Legal advice should be obtained from the malpractice insurance carrier and personal attorney to determine exactly what is being requested.

IV. Confidentiality

Despite a subpoena for records, certain sensitive and confidential information is protected by statute, i.e., HIV status, sexual abuse, substance abuse, domestic violence, sexually transmitted diseases, and psychiatric history. Persons who mistakenly violate an individual's right of privacy under these statutes have been punished. Obtain legal advice before sending out records if they contain sensitive information.

V. Expert Testimony

Trials are adversarial in the United States, and physicians are often asked for their legal opinion either by the plaintiff, the defense, or the Court.

A. Expert (FRE 702): Any licensed physician can testify based on knowledge, skill, expertise, training, or education. Physicians must be familiar with the specific issues of a given case, however, and their opinions can be reviewed by other physicians for deviations, perjury, etc. The American Medical Association (AMA) passed Resolutions 121 and 216, declaring that expert witness testimony should be considered the practice of medicine and subject to peer review. False testimony is intolerable and the AMA suggests disciplining physicians by reporting them to state licensing authorities.

VI. Epilepsy

Epilepsy is a common condition confronting the neurologist and has dimensions that generate a variety of lawsuits from patients, third parties, and the public.

A. Should people be treated after a first seizure?

B. When and how does withdrawal of anticonvulsant medication occur?

C. Can the patient drive?

D. What constitutes informed consent regarding medication?

E. What is a rational monitoring schedule?

Case 1

A thirteen-year-old boy with persistent headache, abnormal EEG with paroxysmal sharp waves. Differential diagnosis was childhood migraine vs partial complex seizures (PCS). Tegretol was started, and 2 weeks later the boy developed Stevens-Johnson syndrome (SJS).

Action: Plaintiff experts stated that the correct diagnosis was migraine and that the patient should have received ergotamine.

Defense expert claimed diagnosis PCS was a "reasonable exercise of medical judgment" and that the more serious disease should be treated first.

Verdict: $1.5 million.

Case 2

A 28-year-old epileptic treated with valproic acid (VA). One week prior to admission the patient experienced abdominal pain which led to emergency admission for suspected pancreatitis. The dosage of VA was reduced but *not* discontinued. The patient became comatose and died.

Action: Plaintiff expert claimed VA caused pancreatitis, coma, and death and that if the medication had been discontinued at the time of hospitalization, the patient would have had an excellent chance of recovery.

Defendant expert testified that tapering the dosage was appropriate because abrupt withdrawal could cause status epilepticus or uncontrolled seizures, a life-threatening condition.

Verdict: $500,000.

Comment: Need to monitor liver enzymes and amylase and if elevated, adjust or discontinue accordingly. Proper documentation, informed consent, and possible need for second opinion would be helpful in reducing potential risks of death and subsequent litigation.

Pregnancy and epilepsy represents a high-risk condition not only for the fetus but also for the mother.

A. Increased risk of seizures during pregnancy, labor, and delivery.

B. Increased incidence of stillbirths and neonatal and perinatal deaths.

C. Increased risk of congenital malformations in mothers with diagnosis of epilepsy (4% to 6%).

D. Specific drugs produce defects, i.e., tegretol/valproic acid produces neural tube defects; dilantin produces fetal hydantoin syndrome (FHS).

Case 3

Mrs. Harbeson developed epilepsy while pregnant with her first child and was prescribed dilantin (DPH). The child was born healthy. Desiring to become pregnant again, she asked physicians about side effects of DPH and was informed *only* about temporary hirsutism and cleft palate. She subsequently bore two children with "Fetal Hydantoin Syndrome" with characteristics of wide-set eyes, ptosis, hypoplasia of the fingers, small nails, broad nasal bridge, growth deficiency, etc.

Action: Harbeson sued Parke-Davis, the physicians, and the federal government (was treated at a military hospital) under the Tort Claims Act for Medical Malpractice, lack of informed consent, "wrongful birth" and "wrongful life."

Verdict: Physicians and government were guilty. Parke-Davis exonerated.

Washington Supreme Court and subsequent Appellate review sustained a verdict for lifetime damages.

Message: Must provide informed consent and proper documentation that FHS can occur with various anti-epileptic drugs in pregnant women.

VII. The Epileptic Driver

Six states (California, Delaware, Pennsylvania, Nevada, New Jersey, and Oregon) compel physicians to report individuals with epilepsy to the Department of Motor Vehicles. Failure to comply with these mandatory rules exposes physicians both legally and financially. Know your responsibility based on state statute.

Case 1

A 15-year-old epileptic applied for a driver's license, and the neurologist completed the mandated form of California Health and Safety Code Section 410. Three years later, the patient was hospitalized for focal seizures and advised not to drive, but was *not* reported to the DMV. Six months later, after good control, the neurologist advised the patient to resume driving. Two months later, while driving with a friend, she had a presumed seizure; the car veered into oncoming traffic, killing a man and leaving the passenger paraplegic.

Action: Passenger sued neurologist for not reporting patient hospitalization to DMV.

Verdict: Jury awarded $3.1 million. The AAN, EFA and Epilepsy Society of San Diego County filed an Amicus Brief with the Court of Appeals leading to subsequent reversal.

Case 2

A patient suffered "spells" of epigastric aura followed by aphasia for two and a half years. Neurologists found focal EEG slowing and normal carotid imaging, and concluded that the spells were secondary to cerebral ischemia. The patient was driving and suffered a major convulsion, lost consciousness, and crashed into a home, killing its occupant.

Action: The neurologist *claimed* to have told the patient not to drive, but this was not documented, and no MRI studies were performed.

Verdict: $900,000.

Comment: Poor documentation led to a poor defense.

Case 3

A 73-year-old patient was in rehabilitation after a stroke. She decided to leave the rehabilitation facility and drive; she had a seizure and injured a pedestrian. The pedestrian sued the physician and nursing facility claiming negligence for failing to prohibit the patient from driving based on her neurologic status.

Verdict: The New York Appellate Division dismissed the suit and the Court of Appeals affirmed the summary judgment.

Case 4

A non-insulin-dependent diabetic patient struck four pedestrians while driving.

Action: The pedestrian filed suit against the driver and a secondary action against the physician, asserting that the patient's diabetes caused a temporary lapse of consciousness at the wheel, which caused the accident.

Verdict: Trial court dismissed the suit indicating that diabetes was *not* a reportable disease to the DMV.

Settlement: None.

Comment: The last two cases demonstrate a creative form of litigation whereby the physician is held libel to third party actions because their patients injure others. This is becoming more common in patients who have the diagnosis of Alzheimer's disease and sleep disorders which usually leads to increased incidents of accidents.

Thus, more of this type of litigation is anticipated. Document in chart if patient is driving and if you believe restrictions should be placed. Speak with family.

VIII. Conclusions

It is well known that the patient's recall of informed consent varies dramatically over time to the point where it is not reliable. Thus, the *physician's best defense is appropriate documentation* in the chart or in a letter to referring doctor. Because trials usually occur several years after the fact, the only accurate and true recording of events will be in the chart. Juries and the Court firmly believe that *"if it is not written, it didn't happen."*

Bibliography

Beresford HR: Neurology and the law. Private Litigation and Public Policy. New York, Oxford, 1998.

Holloway RG, Panzer RJ: Lawyers, litigation and liability: can they make patients safer?

Saper JR: Medicolegal issues: headache. Neurol Clin 17:197–214, 1999.

Weintraub MI: Expert witness testimony: An update. Neurol Clin 17:363–369, 1999.

Weintraub MI: Documentation and informed consent. Neurol Clin 17:371–381, 1999.

Weintraub MI: Medicolegal aspects of iatrogenic injuries. Neurol Clin 16:217–227, 1998.

Index

Note: Page numbers followed by the letter f refer to figures and those followed by t refer to tables.

E

ISBN 0–7216–9761–5

9 780712 697613

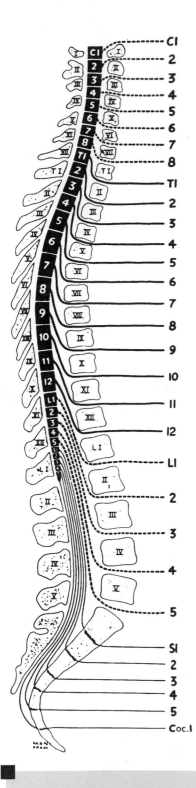

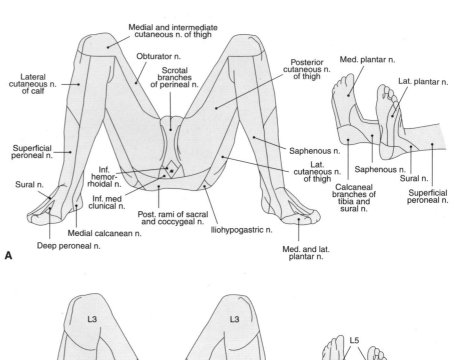

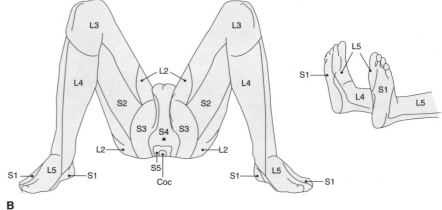

A

A, Cutaneous fields of the peripheral nerves of the perineum and limbs. Labels include: Medial and intermediate cutaneous n. of thigh, Obturator n., Scrotal branches of perineal n., Posterior cutaneous n. of thigh, Med. plantar n., Lat. plantar n., Lateral cutaneous n. of calf, Superficial peroneal n., Saphenous n., Lat. cutaneous n. of thigh, Saphenous n., Sural n., Superficial peroneal n., Sural n., Inf. hemorrhoidal n., Inf. med clunical n., Calcaneal branches of tibia and sural n., Deep peroneal n., Medial calcanean n., Post. rami of sacral and coccygeal n., Iliohypogastric n., Med. and lat. plantar n.

B

Perineum and limbs. A, Cutaneous fields of the peripheral nerves of the perineum and limbs. B, Segmental (dermatomal) innervation of the skin of the perineum and limbs. (Modified from Haymaker W, Woodhall B: Peripheral Nerve Injuries. Philadelphia, W.B. Saunders, 1953.)

The relationship of spinal segments and nerve roots to the vertebral bodies and spinous processes in the adult. The cervical roots (except C8) exit through foramina above their respective vertebral bodies, and the other roots issue below these bodies. The spinal cord is much shorter than the spinal column, ending between vertebral bodies L1 and L2. The lumbar and sacral roots form the cauda equina and descend caudally, beside and below the spinal cord, to exit at the intervertebral foramina. (From Haymaker W, Woodhall B: Peripheral Nerve Injuries [2d ed]. Philadelphia: Saunders, 1953.)